THE NURSE'S ALMANAC

Edited by Howard S. Rowland

Director of Research
Beatrice L. Rowland

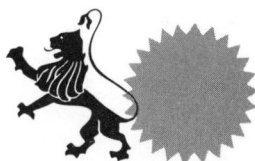

AN ASPEN PUBLICATION

Library of Congress Cataloging in Publication Data

Rowland, Howard S.
The nurse's almanac.

Includes index.
1. Nursing. 2. Nursing—United States.
I. Rowland, Beatrice L. II. Title.
RT41.R78   610.73   78-311
ISBN 0-89443-031-9

Library of Congress Catalog Card Number: 78-311
ISBN: 0-89443-031-9

Printed in the United States of America
1 2 3 4 5

Dedicated to the American Nurse—
The World's Finest

BOARD OF ADVISORS

TABLE OF CONTENTS

TABLE OF CONTENTS

X

ACKNOWLEDGMENTS

Collection of the comprehensive background information and detailed data necessary for a publication such as this, would not have been possible without the dedication and energy of our research staff, the cooperation of countless federal officials in a vast range of U.S. government agencies and the resource assistance of national professional associations, private health organizations, major health care publications and special library centers.

Our special thanks go to Beatrice Rowland, the project's research director. Without her creative approach to this massive search for information and her ability to plan and organize an immensely successful research apparatus this book would never have been produced. She was ably assisted by staff members Mark Goldberg, Phyllis Sokol, Peter Rush, Amy Anders, and Fred Shuttleworth.

Among our primary sources of information were the Congressional hearings and reports on health care matters. These included House of Representatives hearings by the Committee on Interstate and Foreign Commerce, the Subcommittee on Health and Environment, and the Subcommittee on Oversight and Investigation, and the Ways and Means Committee; and Senate hearings by the Committee on Labor and Public Welfare, the Subcommittee on Health, the Subcommittee on Children and Youth, the Subcommittee on Alcoholism and Narcotics, the Committee on Nutrition/Human Need, the Senate Finance Committee and the Senate Ways and Means Committee.

No less important were the contacts and communications with a host of federal officials who enabled us to locate and identify the thousands of statistical studies, research reports, annual surveys, critical reviews, policy summaries, projection analyses and handbooks which were reviewed in the course of preparing this book. Among the administrators and agency staff members who were particularly helpful were: Evelyn S. Mathis, Chief, Health Facilities Statistics Branch, National Center for Health Statistics; Bill Shell, Bureau of Quality Assurance, Health Services Administration; Mary Ann Hatcher, Bob Taylor and Mr. Elkin of Community Health Service, Health Service Administration; Anne Jacobs, Institute of Alcoholism; Joan Dunlavey, Institute of Drug Abuse; Earle Edminton, Publications Officer, Social and Rehabilitation Services; Geneva Woodson, Bureau of Health Resources Development, Health Resources Administration; Grace Henry, National Center for Social Statistics, Social and Rehabilitation Services; Gale Chipman, Office of Consumer Affairs; Phil Edsel, U.S. Civil Service Commission; Emily Boile, Emergency Medical Services; Patricia Kuntze, Bureau of Medical Devices, Food and Drug Administration; Ms. Stafford, Publications Director, Equal Employment Opportunity Commission; Joe Duncan and Dennis Johnston, Office of Management and Budget; T. Bell, Office of Human Development, HEW; George Bradshaw, Public Affairs Office, Commissioned Personnel Operations Division; Robert Robinson, Alfred Skolnik and Ophelia Baxter, Social Security Administration; Lorraine Desbordes, Director, National Injury Information Clearinghouse, Consumer Product Safety Commission; Maxine Cullin and Betsy Dericott, National Institute for Occupatioṇ. Safety and Health; Doreen Mead, National Institute of Child Health and Human Development; Ann Urban, Clinical Center, National Institutes of Health; Jay Roland, President's Committee for the Employment of the Handicapped; Ruth Shenker, Food and Nutrition Service, Department of Agriculture; N. Karlin, Bureau of Labor Statistics, Department of Labor; Dr. Sals, Heart and Lung Institute, National Institutes of Health; Shirley Wilner, Biometry Branch, National Institute of Mental Health; Economic Research Service, Department of Agriculture; Janet Anderson, Office of Assistant Secretary (PHS); Helen Davis and Ella Green, Women's Bureau, Department of Labor; Frank Sis, Office of Communications, Bureau of Health Manpower, Health Resources Administration; Janet Blanken, Office of Nursing Home Affairs, Office of Assistant Secretary (PHS); from the Center for Disease Control—Anthony Lowell, James R. Allen, M.D., Charles H. Hoke, Jr., M.D., Donald L. Eddins, Joseph H. Blount and others; Gloria Kapantis, Division of Manpower and Facilities Statistics, National Center for Health Statistics; Margaret Stevens, Publications Officer, Health Resources Administration; International Education Branch, Fogarty Center; Barbara Weimer and Wayne Richie, Division of Long Term Care Facilities; George Armstrong, National Clearinghouse for Poison Control Centers; Julia Rosenberg, Office of Public Affairs, Food and Drug Administration; Beulah Land, Bureau of Census, Department of Com-

ACKNOWLEDGMENTS

xvi

merce; Grace Madison, Division of Associated Health Professions, Health Resources Administration; Betty Spence, Office of Communications, Health Resources Administration; Renee Gallop, Bureau of Domestic Commerce, Department of Commerce; from the Bureau of Health Manpower Education—Dr. Marie Bourgeois, Mr. Bellin, Jean Rader and Dr. Levine; Evaleen Leon, Bureau of Standards, Department of Commerce; Sandy Suber, National Center for Health Statistics; Howard Stambler, Chief, Manpower Analysis Branch, Health Resources Administration.

Among those health professional associations who have so generously made available background material, information and data from their literature and publications, we would like to single out: the American Nurses' Association, the National League for Nursing, the National Federation of Licensed Practical Nurses, the National Association for Practical Nurse Education, a number of specialized nurse and state nurse associations, the American Hospital Association, the American Medical Association, the American Dietetic Association, the American Public Health Association, the Joint Commission for Accreditation of Hospitals, and the American Society of Allied Health Professionals.

A number of private health organizations which contributed time and/or material deserve special mention: American Association of Blood Banks, Association for Voluntary Sterilization, American Cancer Society, National Council on Aging, Metropolitan Life Insurance Company, National Health Council, Blue Cross Association, Health Insurance Institute, Public Citizens Inc. (Health Research Group), The National Foundation: March of Dimes, American Diabetes Association, Association for the Study of Abortion, National Genetics Foundation, Family Service Association of America, American Foundation for the Blind, Arthritis Foundation, American Heart Association, Allergy Foundation, Nutrition Foundation, American Geriatrics Society, Mental Health Materials Center, National Association for the Prevention of Blindness, Planned Parenthood Federation of America, Medic Alert, American Lung Association, National Hemophilia Foundation, National Multiple Sclerosis Society, National Kidney Foundation, United Cerebral Palsy Association, Allen Guttmacher Foundation, N.Y./N.J. Transplant Center, Leukemia Society of America, Muscular Dystrophy Association, and the American National Red Cross.

In addition to Federal depository and government resource centers, several specialized libraries have provided assistance through use of their facilities: the AJN library (with particular thanks to Cosey Brown and Fred Patterson), Pace University (Nursing Division), the Institute of Life Insurance and the American Academy of Medicine.

As lengthy as the acknowledgments for this book may seem, there may still be a number of remarkably helpful people and associations that have not been included in this listing. Such was not our intention but merely an oversight in the last harried minutes of meeting a publication deadline.

1

INTRODUCTION

Calendars

Calendar of Health-Related Events and Major Holidays

JANUARY

1–31	Birth Defects Prevention Month
1st	March of Dimes
9th	National Smoking Education Week

Holiday

1st	New Years Day

FEBRUARY

1–28	American Heart Month
6th	Children's Dental Health Week

Holidays

12th	Lincoln's Birthday
14th	Valentine's Day
3rd Mon.	Washington's Birthday

MARCH

1–31	Red Cross Month
6th	Save Your Vision Week
20th	Poison Prevention Week

APRIL

1–30	Cancer Control Month
4th	Rural Health Week
7th	World Health Day
23rd	National Baby Week
24th	National Volunteer Week

MAY

1–31	Mental Health Month
8th	World Red Cross Day
8th	National Hospital Week
8th	National Nursing Home Week

Holidays

2nd Sun.	Mother's Day
4th Mon.	Memorial Day

JUNE

1st	Muscular Dystrophy March
20th	Suicide Prevention Congress

Holidays

14th	Flag Day
3rd Sun.	Father's Day

JULY

Holiday

4th	Independence Day

AUGUST

1–31	Good Nutrition Month
1st	National Smile Week

SEPTEMBER

17th	Expectant Father's Day

Holiday

1st Mon.	Labor Day

OCTOBER

2nd	Employ the Physically Handicapped
3rd	Child Health Day
10th	National Pet Health Week

Holiday

2nd Mon.	Columbus Day

NOVEMBER

1–30	Diabetes Month
1–30	Retarded Citizens Month

Holidays

11th (Tr.)	Veterans Day
1st Tues.	Election Day
4th Thurs.	Thanksgiving

DECEMBER

2nd	Pan-American Health Day

Holiday

25th	Christmas Day

3-Year Calendar

1978

January	1978
S M T W T F S
1 2 3 4 5 6 7
8 9 10 11 12 13 14
15 16 17 18 19 20 21
22 23 24 25 26 27 28
29 30 31

February 1978
S M T W T F S
1 2 3 4
5 6 7 8 9 10 11
12 13 14 15 16 17 18
19 20 21 22 23 24 25
26 27 28

March 1978
S M T W T F S
1 2 3 4
5 6 7 8 9 10 11
12 13 14 15 16 17 18
19 20 21 22 23 24 25
26 27 28 29 30 31

April 1978
S M T W T F S
1
2 3 4 5 6 7 8
9 10 11 12 13 14 15
16 17 18 19 20 21 22
23 24 25 26 27 28 29
30

May 1978
S M T W T F S
1 2 3 4 5 6
7 8 9 10 11 12 13
14 15 16 17 18 19 20
21 22 23 24 25 26 27
28 29 30 31

June 1978
S M T W T F S
1 2 3
4 5 6 7 8 9 10
11 12 13 14 15 16 17
18 19 20 21 22 23 24
25 26 27 28 29 30

July 1978
S M T W T F S
1
2 3 4 5 6 7 8
9 10 11 12 13 14 15
16 17 18 19 20 21 22
23 24 25 26 27 28 29
30 31

August 1978
S M T W T F S
1 2 3 4 5
6 7 8 9 10 11 12
13 14 15 16 17 18 19
20 21 22 23 24 25 26
27 28 29 30 31

September 1978
S M T W T F S
1 2
3 4 5 6 7 8 9
10 11 12 13 14 15 16
17 18 19 20 21 22 23
24 25 26 27 28 29 30

October 1978
S M T W T F S
1 2 3 4 5 6 7
8 9 10 11 12 13 14
15 16 17 18 19 20 21
22 23 24 25 26 27 28
29 30 31

November 1978
S M T W T F S
1 2 3 4
5 6 7 8 9 10 11
12 13 14 15 16 17 18
19 20 21 22 23 24 25
26 27 28 29 30

December 1978
S M T W T F S
1 2
3 4 5 6 7 8 9
10 11 12 13 14 15 16
17 18 19 20 21 22 23
24 25 26 27 28 29 30
31

1979

January 1979
S M T W T F S
1 2 3 4 5 6
7 8 9 10 11 12 13
14 15 16 17 18 19 20
21 22 23 24 25 26 27
28 29 30 31

February 1979
S M T W T F S
1 2 3
4 5 6 7 8 9 10
11 12 13 14 15 16 17
18 19 20 21 22 23 24
25 26 27 28

March 1979
S M T W T F S
1 2 3
4 5 6 7 8 9 10
11 12 13 14 15 16 17
18 19 20 21 22 23 24
25 26 27 28 29 30 31

April 1979
S M T W T F S
1 2 3 4 5 6 7
8 9 10 11 12 13 14
15 16 17 18 19 20 21
22 23 24 25 26 27 28
29 30

May 1979
S M T W T F S
1 2 3 4 5
6 7 8 9 10 11 12
13 14 15 16 17 18 19
20 21 22 23 24 25 26
27 28 29 30 31

June 1979
S M T W T F S
1 2
3 4 5 6 7 8 9
10 11 12 13 14 15 16
17 18 19 20 21 22 23
24 25 26 27 28 29 30

July 1979
S M T W T F S
1 2 3 4 5 6 7
8 9 10 11 12 13 14
15 16 17 18 19 20 21
22 23 24 25 26 27 28
29 30 31

August 1979
S M T W T F S
1 2 3 4
5 6 7 8 9 10 11
12 13 14 15 16 17 18
19 20 21 22 23 24 25
26 27 28 29 30 31

September 1979
S M T W T F S
1
2 3 4 5 6 7 8
9 10 11 12 13 14 15
16 17 18 19 20 21 22
23 24 25 26 27 28 29
30

October 1979
S M T W T F S
1 2 3 4 5 6
7 8 9 10 11 12 13
14 15 16 17 18 19 20
21 22 23 24 25 26 27
28 29 30 31

November 1979
S M T W T F S
1 2 3
4 5 6 7 8 9 10
11 12 13 14 15 16 17
18 19 20 21 22 23 24
25 26 27 28 29 30

December 1979
S M T W T F S
1
2 3 4 5 6 7 8
9 10 11 12 13 14 15
16 17 18 19 20 21 22
23 24 25 26 27 28 29
30 31

1980

January 1980
S M T W T F S
1 2 3 4 5
6 7 8 9 10 11 12
13 14 15 16 17 18 19
20 21 22 23 24 25 26
27 28 29 30 31

February 1980
S M T W T F S
1 2
3 4 5 6 7 8 9
10 11 12 13 14 15 16
17 18 19 20 21 22 23
24 25 26 27 28 29

March 1980
S M T W T F S
1
2 3 4 5 6 7 8
9 10 11 12 13 14 15
16 17 18 19 20 21 22
23 24 25 26 27 28 29
30 31

April 1980
S M T W T F S
1 2 3 4 5
6 7 8 9 10 11 12
13 14 15 16 17 18 19
20 21 22 23 24 25 26
27 28 29 30

May 1980
S M T W T F S
1 2 3
4 5 6 7 8 9 10
11 12 13 14 15 16 17
18 19 20 21 22 23 24
25 26 27 28 29 30 31

June 1980
S M T W T F S
1 2 3 4 5 6 7
8 9 10 11 12 13 14
15 16 17 18 19 20 21
22 23 24 25 26 27 28
29 30

July 1980
S M T W T F S
1 2 3 4 5
6 7 8 9 10 11 12
13 14 15 16 17 18 19
20 21 22 23 24 25 26
27 28 29 30 31

August 1980
S M T W T F S
1 2
3 4 5 6 7 8 9
10 11 12 13 14 15 16
17 18 19 20 21 22 23
24 25 26 27 28 29 30
31

September 1980
S M T W T F S
1 2 3 4 5 6
7 8 9 10 11 12 13
14 15 16 17 18 19 20
21 22 23 24 25 26 27
28 29 30

October 1980
S M T W T F S
1 2 3 4
5 6 7 8 9 10 11
12 13 14 15 16 17 18
19 20 21 22 23 24 25
26 27 28 29 30 31

November 1980
S M T W T F S
1
2 3 4 5 6 7 8
9 10 11 12 13 14 15
16 17 18 19 20 21 22
23 24 25 26 27 28 29
30

December 1980
S M T W T F S
1 2 3 4 5 6
7 8 9 10 11 12 13
14 15 16 17 18 19 20
21 22 23 24 25 26 27
28 29 30 31

2

Nursing Conventions

American Association of Colleges of Nursing—1978 Feb. 6–8, Oct. 9–11; Washington, D.C.

American Association of Critical-Care Nurses—1978 May 9–12, St. Louis

American Association of Industrial Nurses—1978 April 9–14, New Orleans

American Association of Neurosurgical Nurses—1977 April 24–28, Toronto

American Association of Nurse Anesthetists—1977 August 21–25, Hollywood, Fla.

American College of Nurse-Midwives—

American Indian Nurses Association—1977 April 17–20, Albuquerque

American Nurses Association—1978 June 11–16, Honolulu

American Society of Hospital Nursing Service Administrators—1977

Assembly of Hospital Schools of Nursing—1977, Chicago

Association of Operating Room Nurses—1978 March 12–17, New Orleans

Association of State and Territorial Directors of Nursing—1977 May 16–18, Washington, D.C.

E/WAHA Council of Nurse Healers—1977 June 10–12, San Francisco

Emergency Department Nurses Association—1977 November 8–10, San Francisco

National Association for Practical Nurse Education and Service—1978 May 8–11, Phoenix

National Federation of Licensed Practical Nurses—1978 October, Louisville, Ky.

National League for Nursing—1979 April 29–May 1, Atlanta; 1981 May 12–15, Las Vegas

National Student Nurses Association—1978 April 27–30, St. Louis

Nurses Association of American College of Obstetricians and Gynecologists—1978 Autumn, District Workshops; 1979 National Convention

Oncology Nursing Society—1977 May 14–15, Denver

Health and Professional Conventions—1977

American Association of Medical Assistants—October, San Francisco

American Health Care Association—October, San Diego

American Hospital Association—August, Atlanta

American Public Health Association—October, Washington, D.C.

American School Health Association—October, Chicago

American Society of Allied Health Professions—November, Dallas

Association for Practitioners in Infection Control—April, Hollywood, Fla.

National Council for International Health—March, Arlington

Who's Who in Nursing

Nursing Award Winners

National League for Nursing

Mary Adelaide Nutting Award: For outstanding leadership and achievement in nursing.

1944	Mary Adelaide Nutting
1947	International Council of Nurses
	Isabel Maitland Stewart
1949	Annie Warburton Goodrich
	Mary M. Roberts
1951	Frances Payne Bolton
	Maternity Center Association of New York
1955	Stella Goostray
1957	Nell V. Beeby
1959	Effie J. Taylor
1961	Mary Breckenridge
1963	R. Louise MacManus
1965	Lulu Wolf Hassenplug
1967	Helen Nahm
	Ruth B. Freeman
1969	Helen Bunge
	Milfred E. Newton
1971	Jessie M. Scott
	The W. K. Kellogg Foundation
1973	Lucille Petry Leone
	Esther Lucille Brown
1975	Jo Eleanor Elliott
	Mary Kelly Mullane
1977	Virginia Henderson

The Lucille Petry Leone Award: For contributions to nursing education by an outstanding teacher.

1967	Martha Clyde Davis
1969	Kathryn E. Barnard
1971	Ada Sue Hinshaw
1973	Rhoda B. Epstein

4

| 1975 | Lillian G. Stokes |
| 1977 | Gail Stuart |

The Linda Richards Award: For meritorious contribution of a unique, pioneering nature.

1963	Mildred L. Montag
1967	Signe S. Cooper
1969	Billie B. Larch
1973	Hildegard Peplau
	Mabel Keaton Staupers
1975	Rosemary Wood
1977	M. Lucille Kinlein

The NLN Distinguished Service Award: For outstanding leadership and service in the implementation of NLN goals.

1967	Mildred Gaynor
	Marion Sheahan
1969	Alma B. Gault
	Frances Reiter
1971	Mary C. Rockefeller
	Alabama League For Nursing
1973	Ruth Sleeper
1975	Anna Fillmore
1977	Lulu W. Hassenplug

The Anna M. Fillmore Award: For leadership in community health services.

| 1977 | Eva M. Reese |

American Nurses' Association

Honorary Recognition Award: For distinguished service, contributions and/or accomplishments which are of national or international significance to nursing.

1954	Katherine DeWitt
1962–64	Clara Hardin*
1964–66	Lucille Petry Leone
1966–68	Senator Lister Hill*
	Barbara Schutt
1968–70	Pearl Parvin Coulter
	Rozella Schlotfeldt
1970–72	Mary Kelly Mullane
	Jessie Scott
1972–74	Adele Herwitz
	Virginia Stone
1974–76	Helen E. Browne
	Signe S. Cooper

*Not a nurse

Honorary Membership Award: For outstanding leadership and for contributions which furthered the purposes of the American Nurses' Association

| 1958–60 | Ella Best |
| | Agnes Ohlson |

1960–62	Katharine D. Dreves
	Mina Kenworthy
1962–64	Margaret B. Dolan
	Pearl McIver
	Elizabeth Porter
	Mathilda Scheuer
1964–66	Jo Eleanor Elliott
	Frances L. A. Powell
	Fannie Warncke
1966–68	Frances Reiter
	Helen Salmon
	Anne Zimmerman
1968–70	Eleanor Lambertsen
1970–72	Dorothy Cornelius
1972–74	Hildegard E. Peplau
1974–76	Mary E. Macdonald

Mary Mahoney Award: For an individual or group of nurses who have opened or advanced equal opportunities in nursing for members of minority groups and who have also made a significant contribution to nursing.

1936	Adah B. Thoms
1937	Nancy L. Kemp
1938	Carrie E. Bullock
1939	Petra Pinn
1940	Lulu G. Warlick
1941	Ellen Woods Carter
1942	Ruth Logan Roberts
1943	Ludie Andrews
1944	Mabel Northcross
1945	Capt. Susan Freeman (ANC)
1946	Estelle M. Riddle Osborne
1947	Mabel K. Staupers
1949	Mary E. Merritt
1951	Eliza M. Pillars
1952	Marguerette C. Jackson
1952–54	May Maloney
1954–56	Mildred Ann Vogel
1956–58	Fay O. Wilson
1958–60	Marie C. Mink
1960–62	Mildred P. Adams
1962–64	Alice M. Sundburg
	M. Elizabeth Pickens
1964–66	Katharine Ellen Faville
1966–68	Helen S. Miller
1968–70	Vernice D. Ferguson
1970–72	Mary Lee Mills
1972–74	Fostine Glenn Riddick
1974–76	Carolyn McGraw Carter

Pearl McIver Public Health Nurse Award: For an ANA member who has contributed to the field of public health on a national level and who has shown professional expertise and leadership in public health nursing.

1954–56	Pearl McIver
1956–58	Ruth B. Freeman
1958–60	Emilie Sargent
1960–62	Pearl Parvin Coulter
1962–64	Judith E. Wallin
1964–66	Olive M. Klump
1966–68	Margaret B. Dolan
1968–70	Marion I. Murphy
1970–72	Kathryn A. Robeson
1972–74	Doris L. Wagner
1974–76	Virginia M. Ohlson

Honorary Nurse Practitioner Award: For a registered nurse for outstanding nurse practice devoted to direct patient care.

1972–74	Ruth Murphy
1974–76	Deanna Sebestyn

Shirley Titus Award: For recognition of individual contributions made to the Economic and General Welfare Program of the ANA.

1974–76	Edna Behrens
	Elizabeth K. Porter

Arnold and Marie Schwartz Awards: For a significant contribution to nursing research which has influenced nursing care.

1974–76	Jeanne Q. Benoliel
	Carol A. Lindeman

American Association of Nurse Anesthetists

Agatha Hodgkins Award: For dedication to excellence and furthering the art and science of nurse anesthesia.

1975	Ruth P. Satterfield
1976	Helen Lamb Frost

American Association of Colleges of Nursing

Honored in 1976: For key roles in founding and guiding AACN since its inception in 1969.

Dr. Dorothy Mereness
Dr. Mary K. Mullane
Dr. Martha Rogers
Dr. Ada Fort
Dr. Madeline Leininger
Dr. June Rothberg
Dr. Emily Holmquist
Dr. Rozella Schlotfeldt
Dr. Marguerite Schaefer
Dr. Mildred Quinn
Dr. Margaret Shetland

Current Outstanding Nurses

*Abdellah, Faye G.—Assistant Surgeon General and chief nurse officer of U.S. Public Health Service. Background as a nurse researcher; served on faculty of Yale University School of Nursing and Columbias Teachers College; functioned as chief of the Nursing Education Bureau, 1949–59, and senior consultant in nursing research. Recipient of many awards, including Federal Nursing Service award. Holds the commission of admiral in USPHS, one of two first women to hold the title. Author of several books including *New Directions in Nursing Service,* 1973 and *New Directions in Patient-Centered Care,* 1973.

*Aguilera, Donna C.—nurse educator; associate professor, Department of Nursing, California State University. Author: *Crisis Intervention: Theory and Methodology,* 1970.

*Aydelotte, Myrtle K.—nurse educator, on faculty of University of Iowa School of Nursing. Served as captain in U.S. Army Nurse Corps, 1942–46, president of NLN, 1962–66, on editorial board of *Nursing Research.*

*Bahr, Sister Rose Therese—associate professor at University of Kansas School of Nursing. Served on Comprehensive Health Planning Council, 1969–70, on Kansas Master Planning Commission for Nursing and Nursing Education, as president of Kansas League for Nursing, 1973–75.

Burgess, Ann—appointed by HEW as head of the new Rape Prevention and Control Advisory Committee; cofounded one of the first rape victim counseling programs, at Boston City Hospital; coauthor of *Rape: Victims of Crisis.*

Coulter, Pearl P.—former dean of University of Arizona College of Nursing. Served as member and president of Arizona State Board of Nursing, president of Colorado League for Nursing and Colorado State Nurse's Association; as board member of American Journal of Nursing Company and NLN. Recipient of Public Health Nurse award, 1962. Author, works include *The Nurse in the Public Health Program,* 1954.

*Carnegie, Mary E.—editor, *Nursing Research.*

---

* Members of the American Academy of Nursing.

6

*Chow, Rita K.—Deputy chief officer of U.S. Public Health Service and deputy director of the federal Office of Nursing Home Affairs.

*Dyer, Elaine D.—Director of nursing research at College of Nursing, Brigham Young University. Served on Task Force Measuring Quality of Nursing Care for VA, 1968–71; president of Utah Nurses Association. Functioned as USPHS fellow in 1967 and NIH grantee in 1971–74. Inventor, pressure breathing therapy. Coauthor of *Improved Patient Care Through Problem Oriented Nursing,* 1974.

Elliott, Jo E.—nurse educator. Served as director of nursing programs for the Wester Interstate Commission for Higher Education. Recipient of Mary A. Nutting award, 1975.

*Fagin, Claire M.—Dean at University of Pennsylvania School of Nursing. Served on WHO's 1974 Expert Panel on nursing as NIMH fellow, Author of several books, including *Nursing in Child Psychiatry,* 1972.

Freeman, Ruth B.—nurse educator and consultant. Served as national administrator of National Red Cross nursing services, as consultant to National Security Resources Board, as member of WHO's Expert Panel on Nursing and the White House Conference on Children and Youth. Recipient of many awards.

*Harkins, Sister Elizabeth C.—Dean, University of Southern Mississippi School of Nursing. Served with Mississippi Health Planning Advisory Council, as president of Mississippi State Board of Nursing and as president of Mississippi Nurses' Association.

*Harty, Margaret B.—Vice president, Institute of Health Sciences, Texas Woman's University. Served as chairman of the editorial advisory committee of International Nursing Index, president of California League of Nurses, as consultant and lecturer.

Hassenplug, Lulu W.—nurse educator and consultant. Dean emiritus of the School of Nursing, University of California, Los Angeles. Served on Surgeon General's Consultant Group on Nursing (preliminary

basis for Nurse Training Act of 1964) and recently on California's Advisory Committee on Physician's Assistant Programs. Recipient of many awards including two honorary doctor of science degrees.

Haynes, Inez—Held the post of Chief of the Army Nurse Corps with rank of colonel. Served as general director of NLN; with executive committees of National Health Council and National Assembly for Social Policy and Development; as vice president of WHO's Citizen Committee.

Herwitz, Adele—executive director of the newly established Commission on Graduates of Foreign Nursing Schools. Served as executive director of International Council of Nurses since 1970; as associate director at ANA.

*Kelly, Lucy S.—professor of nursing, School of Public Health, Columbia University. Serves as consultant on city and state level. Author: *Dimensions of Professional Nursing,* 1975.

*Leininger, Madeline—Dean, College of Nursing, University of Utah. Served as president of American Association of Colleges of Nursing; as editor of *Health Care Dimensions.* Author: *Two Worlds to Blend: Anthropology and Nursing,* 1970; *Contemporary Issues in Mental Health Nursing,* 1973.

Leone, Petry L.—first woman in United States to hold rank of brigadier general. Served as chief nurse officer and assistant surgeon general, 1949; as director of nursing education for USPHS, as technical expert on nursing for WHO; as administrator of the Cadet Nurse Corps program. An award was established in her name by NLN in 1966 for her contribution to nursing education.

McManus, R. Louise—designer of the first national testing service for the nursing profession. Helped establish the Institute of Research and Service in Nursing education and a national project in two year academic nursing programs. Served as consultant to Navy's Bureau of Medicine and Surgery and the National Advisory Health Council. Coauthor: *The Hospital Head Nurse.*

Montag, Mildred L.—nurse educator. Served as professor of nursing education at Teachers College, Columbia for 20 years; as director of major research project in

---

*Members of the American Academy of Nursing.

junior and community college education for nursing, 1952–57. Recipient of many awards, including two honorary doctoral degrees. Author: works include *Fundamentals in Nursing Care*.

Mullane, Mary K.—professor of nursing administration, College of Nursing, University of Illinois. Served as chairman of Illinois Study Commission on Nursing, 1965–70; as special consultant on nurse training to HEW; as dean of several nursing colleges. Recipient of NLN's Nutting Award in 1975 for leadership in management of nursing services.

* Murillo-Rohde, Ildaura—professor and associate dean of University of Washington's School of Nursing. Served as psychiatric consultant to Guatemala (WHO, 1963–64); as director of various mental health/psychiatric nursing educational programs.

Nahm, Helen—created a national accrediting service for schools of nursing and was first director of the National Nursing Accrediting Service, founded by NLN in 1952. Served as director of NLN's Division of Nursing Education, as dean of the School of Nursing, University of California at San Francisco.

* Rogers, Martha E.—professor, Division of Nursing, New York University. Served as president of the New York State League for Nursing. Recipient of many awards. Author: many articles and books, including *Educational Revolution in Nursing*.

* Rothberg, June S.—Dean, School of Nursing, Adelphi University. Served as president of American Association of Colleges of Nursing, on board of directors of Nurses for Political Action.

Scott, Jessie M.—served as assistant surgeon general and director of the Division of Nursing, National Institutes of Health; one of the first two women to receive the commission rank of admiral from USPHS.

Wood, Rosemary—Chief of Nursing Branch, U.S. Indian Health Service, first American Indian to hold that position. Served as executive director of the American Indian Nurses Association; as research consultant for IHS. Recipient of NLN's Linda Richards Nursing Award, 1975.

Famous American Nurses of the Past

Barton, Clara (1821–1912)—Founder of American Red Cross in 1862. Never actually a nurse, Barton was active in the distribution of supplies for wounded soldiers and in aid to war victims.

Beard, Mary (1876–1946)—Contributor to field of public health nursing; as director of the International Health Division for the Rockefeller Foundation financially assisted nursing education and community health systems abroad. Served as director of American Red Cross during WWII.

Beck, Sister M. Berenice (1893–1960)—Nurse educator who promoted collegiate programs for nurses. Chaired ANA's Ethical Standard Committee and was instrumental in formulating the Code for Professional Nurses.

Breckinridge, Mary (1881–1965)—Founder of the Frontier Nursing Service in 1925 to offer maternal-child care in isolated communities of Kentucky. In 1919 originated France's first Child Hygiene and Visiting Nurse Service, now a permanent agency.

Burgess, May Ayres (1883–1953)—Leader in evaluation and upgrading of nursing schools in the 1930s. Author of *Nursing Schools Today and Tomorrow*, 1934.

Crandall, Ella P. (1871–1938)—Leader in public health nursing. As first executive secretary of NOPHN, organized public health nurses around the country. As educator, developed courses in district nursing at Columbia Teachers College.

Davis, Mary E. (1858–1924)—First business manager of the *American Journal of Nursing*, assisting Sophia Palmer in the organization and financing of the publication, insisting it be "owned, edited and controlled by nurses."

Delano, Jane A. (1862–1919)—Military nurse organizer. Served as Superintendent of the Nurse Corps, U.S. Army in 1909; as nursing director for ARC during WWI, supervising the recruitment, selection and assignment of all military nursing units. Early president of the ANA.

** Dix, Dorothea (1802–1887)—Civil War superintendent of army nurses. Instru-

---

* Members of the American Academy of Nursing.

mental in reforming care and treatment of the mentally ill.

*Dock, Lavinia (1858–1956)—Author of *Textbook of Materia Medica for Nurses,* 1889, first of its kind, and coauthor of *History of Nursing.* First secretary of the International Council of Nurses and leading activist in women's rights.

*Goodrich, Annie W. (1866–1954)—Supporter of higher educational standards for nurses: served as state inspector of nursing schools, dean of the Army School of Nurses during WWI and dean of the first nursing program at Yale University. Director of Visiting Nurse Service at Henry Street Settlement, 1916–1923.

*Franklin, Martha—Organizer and first president of the National Association of Colored Graduate Nurses in 1908.

Gardner, Mary S. (1871–1961)—Leader in public health nursing. Instrumental in establishing the NOPHN journal *Public Health Nurse* and developing public health services in ARC. Author of *Public Health Nursing,* 1916.

Goodnow, Minnie (c.1883–1952)—Pioneer in textbooks for nurses, writing the first nursing text on chemistry in 1911.

Gretter, Lystra E. (1858–1951)—Nurse innovator: as director of nursing, employed graduate nurses to supervise student nurses, established the first eight hour day for student nurses in 1891. Inspired the writing of the "Nightingale Pledge" in 1893.

*Maass, Clara (1876–1901)—Dedicated army nurse who served during the Spanish-American War and lost her life as a volunteer in the experiments which revealed a type of mosquito as the carrier of yellow fever. A 1976 U.S. postage stamp honored her memory.

*Mahoney, Mary E. (1845–1926)—First professionally trained black nurse, graduated in 1879. Helped organize NACGN. ANA award named in her honor.

Maxwell, Anna C. (1851–1929)—Nurse educator, established and headed nurse training school at Presbyterian Hospital for 30 years. Instituted standardization of nursing techniques and procedures.

---

*Honored in American Nurses' Association's Hall of Fame.

Noyes, Clara (1869–1936)—Leading organizer; served in the early years as president of NLN, and of ANA (helped establish national headquarters); director of nursing service in ARC after WWI.

*Nutting, Mary A. (1858–1947)—First professor of nursing in the world, at Columbia Teachers College, 1907–25. Coauthor with Lavinia Dock of the four-volume *History of Nursing.* Influential in the formation of ICN and in progressive reform at Johns Hopkins as director of nursing.

*Palmer, Sophia (1853–1920)—First editor of *American Journal of Nursing,* from 1900–1920. Instrumental in promoting state registration and licensure; first president of NYS Board of Examiners.

Powell, Marie (1871–1943)—Formulator of a model for collegiate nursing education as first superintendent (1910–24) at University of Minnesota's School of Nursing, the first collegiate nursing program.

*Richards, Linda (1841–1930)—First graduate nurse in the United States. Director of nursing and training program at Massachusetts General Hospital. Established first nursing school in Japan. Pioneer in industrial and psychiatric nursing.

*Robb, Isabel A. (1860–1910)—Organizer and first president of Nurses Associated Alumnae (1896) which became the ANA. Served as first principal of Johns Hopkins School of Nursing. Instrumental in establishing university affiliation for nursing education courses. Author of *Nursing Ethics,* 1890s.

*Stewart, Isabel M. (1878–1963)—Important nurse educator: on faculty of Columbia's Teachers College since 1909, advanced to become director of nursing department from 1925–43. Author of numerous curriculum guides. Chairman of ICN committee on education for 22 years; chairman of Committee on Nursing Education Personnel, War Manpower Commission, WWII.

*Thoms, Adah B. (1863–1943)—Instrumental in gaining acceptance of black nurses into the Army Nurse Corps and Red Cross. First treasurer and later president of NACGN. Assistant director at Lincoln School of Nursing.

*Wald, Lillian (1867–1940)—Leader in public health nursing with emphasis on the social aspects. Founder of the precursor to the Henry Street Settlement and Visiting Nurse Service of New York. First president of the National Organization for Public Health Nursing. Originator of the concept of Federal Children's Bureau. Championed many social causes, including national health insurance.

History of Nursing

Nursing in the Ancient World

Early practices of nursing and medicine are so closely interwoven that it is often impossible to distinguish one from the other. Nursing in primitive societies was evident as early as 4000 B.C. A nurse was identified as a mother-nurse working with a priest. She, in a sense, was a magician, a medicine man, a dispenser of witchcraft, of black magic. Nursing was inextricably bound up with all these practices and was associated especially with the feeding and care of infants, attending of invalid and aged relatives, and the administration of practical household remedies such as herbs, fomentations, poultices and baths.

Real nursing, as medicine, seems to have begun with the Egyptians. Workers on some jobs were excused from work to nurse their fellow workers, and perhaps some people were specialized in this task. There were also wet nurses, at least for the nobility. Nursing techniques, such as feeling the strength of the pulse, using bandages, and midwifery, were also practiced. Egyptian temples served as the first hospitals, and a public hospital system had emerged by the 11th century, but there is no evidence that they made use of nurses.

There is a record of nursing in 2000 B.C. in Babylonia, Assyria and Chaldea, where nurses are referred to as "wet nurses" and "children's nurses." They were also mentioned in the Code of Hammurabi, King of Babylonia. There are references to nursing duties such as giving baths to patients, massaging patients' bodies with butter, and dressing and bandaging his wounds.

The Hebrews made much of nursing care of the sick by the family. However, they are better known for their comprehensive sanitary and dietary laws, which are health-related. Nurses and wet nurses are frequently referred to in the Old Testament.

In India, 800–600 B.C., the health religions had a strong influence on the development of nursing, medicine, surgery, hygiene and sanitation, which for that period were well developed. The annals of India give details of nursing principles and practices. Nurses were young men, since women remained restricted to the home. Young male nurses belonged to the Brahmin caste. India introduced a pattern for lay brothers to work in hospitals during the Christian era. By the third century B.C., an edict establishing hospitals throughout the kingdom was issued. Much Hindu medical knowledge was acquired from Egypt.

By 770 B.C. Greece came to be identified as a seat of medical excellence. There are records of hospital wards, baths and gymnasiums which were used extensively.

The women of the family typified the skill of nursing and health conservation. Hippocrates, 460–370 B.C. and his school were responsible for turning medicine into a science instead of a branch of magic. Strict cleanliness for doctors and sterilization of bandages in boiled water or wine were practiced. Hippocrates also recorded detailed notes about nursing. However, nursing was only taught to his medical students, who carried out what we now define as nursing services.

Rome added little to medicine or nursing. Its eminence was in sanitation and hygiene—public sauna baths, well-ventilated and heated houses, improved water supply, sewers and drains. The first hospitals were built for Caesar's frontier armies, but later Rome established even free clinics for the poor. There is no record of nursing during this time apart from the work of military orderlies in the army. In Rome, slaves performed nursing for the rich.

Concurrently, pre-Christian nursing in Ireland was remarkably developed. Laws were established providing very basic instruction and codes for the construction of hospitals and kinds of nursing services to be provided; provision was made for a hospital in every camp and for women to be trained for the care of the sick and wounded.

Nursing in the Christian Era to 1850

In the early Christian Church, deaconesses performed visiting nurse services, caring for orphans, the poor, travelers and the ailing. Phoebe, a friend of St. Paul, organized nursing for the poor. Nursing was one of the many forms of service undertaken by the various religious orders before and as part of the monastic movement. In 390 A.D., a Roman Christian matron, Fabiola founded the first public hospital under Christian auspices in the West and worked as a nurse. In the Eastern Empire, Constantine founded one in 330 A.D.; a huge hospital in Athens was built a little later. Under the immediate auspices of the Roman Catholic Church, the Hotel Dieu was established at Lyons in 542, and still exists, being the hospital with the longest record of continuous service. The Hotel Dieu in Paris was founded about 650 and became the prototype of the medieval hospital. However, there is no record of nursing services provided there. Nursing was relegated largely to monks and to the lady of the castle who nursed the sick in her family as well as tenants and serfs.

The medicine and hospital system of the Greeks and Romans was kept alive and passed on in Constantinople, where the works of Galen (130–201 A.D.), the greatest Roman physician, were employed. In the tenth century, Arabia became the center of world medicine because of its remarkable hospitals and the writings of the great scholar Avicenna (980–1037). Baghdad had 60 medical institutions by 1160. Nursing is not reported, but nursing activities must have been performed on a large scale during this period.

In the West, nursing and hospital care was provided mainly by specialized nursing orders such as the Augustinian Sisters in Paris, the Third Order of St. Francis in Italy, and the Beguines of Belgium. By the 13th century, the influence of the Crusades brought back to Europe Islamic medical knowledge and hospital practices. The Pope built a large hospital in Rome on the Arabian model and ordered it copied throughout Europe. Thousands were built under the Order of the Holy Ghost. As medicine received new emphasis and doctors reappeared, these hospitals, with their nursing services rendered by the orders, resembled the modern hospital system. The Knights Hospitalers of Jerusalem, the Teutonic Knights and others were male nursing orders.

However, from the 15th century to the 19th century, these hospitals suffered a progressive decline and collapse of quality. The religious wars brought on by the Reformation made a shambles of care for the poor and sick, and in the Protestant areas, no hospital system was established to replace those of the Catholic orders. Even the quality of persons entering the orders deteriorated drastically, while overcrowding, disregard of cleanliness and hygiene, and crowding as many as six into a bed made infection endemic in hospitals, turning them into pesthouses for the poor, mere places to die. The wealthy sought medical treatment at home. This deterioration of hospitals and correspondingly of nursing occurred, ironically, at a time when medicine, now definitively separated from nursing, was developing at a rapid rate.

A new, modern chapter for nursing started in 1826. The Kaiserswerth deaconesses came into prominence and were prepared for many kinds of services: nursing, teaching, management of children and convalescents. And it was at Kaiserswerth that Florence Nightingale, the founder of modern nursing, received a brief period of training that strongly influenced her. Nightingale rose to prominence as a result of her service during the Crimean War, where, even without knowledge of microbes, she successfully utilized the weapons of soap, hot water, sunshine, fresh air and reduced crowding to reduce the death rate in the military hospital where she worked from 40% to 2%. These reforms restored the practices of the ancients and set the stage for the development of modern nursing. Nightingale began this era with the founding in 1860 of the first nurses' training school and home, connected to St. Thomas's Hospital in London. She not only applied her nursing practices here, but also established patterns of nursing service, laundries, diet kitchens, and even developed a system for the collection of hospital statistics. Her school became the model and training ground for nurses and hospital-nurse training schools from all over the world.

American Nursing: 1850–1900

Nursing as it is now known in the United States hardly existed before 1850. The first enduring hospital founded in America was the Pennsylvania Hospital, founded by the Quakers in 1751. Others followed, especially after the Revolutionary War. Massachusetts General was founded in 1813. Nursing, such as it was, was performed by members of religious orders and poorly trained attendants. A few women served as nurses in Washington's army, including the famous "Molly Pitcher" (Mary Mc-

Cauley), but most nursing was done by untrained men.

Before the Civil War, hospitals were considered places to avoid because their mortality rates were notoriously high. In lay hospitals, the nursing was particularly inept. However, several Catholic sisterhoods, most famous, the Sisters of Charity, set up dozens of hospitals staffed with well-trained, disciplined nurses. On a smaller scale, Protestant churches also trained nurses.

The Civil War created a sudden demand for large numbers of nurses. Three thousand women formed a volunteer group in the North; Dr. Elizabeth Blackwell, the first woman U.S. physician, set up nurse training courses at New York's Bellevue; Dorothea Dix, a teacher, was appointed superintendent of U.S. Army nurses; other nurses also came forward, including Clara Barton, later first president of the American National Red Cross.

In the 35 years after the Civil War, nursing schools proliferated, the numbers and competence of nurses increased tremendously and nursing became a major profession, producing many famous nurses.

Chronology of Nursing History, 1850–1900:

1872: First training school for nurses in the United States opened at New England Hospital for Women and Children, Boston; director, Susan Dimock.

1872: Similar school opened at Women's Hospital of Philadelphia.

1873: First three nursing schools operated on Nightingale principles opened: Bellevue Training School for Nurses, N.Y., superintendent, Helen Bowdin; Connecticut Training School for Nurses, New Haven, run by Miss Bayard; Boston Training School for Nurses at Massachusetts General Hospital, superintendent, Linda Richards. None of these schools was founded or run by the hospitals, but by nurses.

1879: Mary Eliza Mahoney graduates from New England Hospital for Women and Children as first professional black nurse in America.

1880s: Nursing schools attached to hospitals proliferated.

1885: Clara Weeks Shaw wrote first textbook for nurses.

1885: Buffalo, N.Y., District Nursing Association established, first in U.S.

1888: *The Trained Nurse,* first nursing journal in U.S., appeared, edited by a trained nurse.

1889: Johns Hopkins Hospital opened in Baltimore, first on a modern model, to have strong impact on nursing as well; Isabel Hampton Robb is first director, and Mary Adelaide Nutting and Lavinia L. Dock attend first class of Training School, 1890.

1890: Lavinia Dock wrote *Textbook on Materia Medica for Nurses,* the first of its kind.

1890: Number of nursing schools reaches 35 with 1,552 students.

1893: A congress of nurses is convened at Chicago World's Fair under chairmanship of Isabel Hampton Robb; "American Society of Superintendents of Training Schools for Nurses" founded, first U.S. nurses association (becomes National League of Nursing Education in 1912 and NLN in 1952).

1893: Lillian D. Wald and Mary Brewster rent tenement to serve the poor, later becomes Henry Street Settlement, beginning social and community-oriented nursing in the country.

1896: Isabel H. Robb founded Associated Alumnae of the United States and Canada, first association to bring together all nurses; became American Nurses Association, 1911.

1898: Nurses volunteered to help in Spanish-American War; in great demand to treat epidemics of typhoid fever, malaria and yellow fever.

1899: First program for nurses under auspices of a university begun at New York Teachers College, in hospital economics.

1900: *American Journal of Nursing* founded; first editor Sophia F. Palmer.

1900: Number of nurse training schools soars to 432 schools with 11,164 students.

American Nursing: 1900–1950

In the first half of the 20th century, nursing grew to be one of the largest single professions in the United States and remained one of the most important occupations for women. Early

12

in this period, nursing schools attached to hospitals became the prime source of cheap labor for the hospitals through the use of student nurses.

In 1880, there were only 15 nursing schools—by 1910 there were more than 1,000. Since the hospitals were staffed primarily by students, most graduates had to find jobs as private duty nurses or working with doctors where they competed with untrained workers and correspondence school graduates.

Later this trend was reversed, and hospitals employed many more graduates. Also during this period various studies appeared on the inadequacies of nurse training; as a result nursing education was vastly improved.

The federal government also became involved with nursing during this period, hiring its first public health nurse in 1935 and, during World War II, financing nurse training.

Finally, in the late 1940s, the trend toward collegiate training of nurses, away from hospital schools, began. Then the junior college "associate" degree was initiated.

Chronology of Nursing History, 1900–1950

1901: Nurses accompanied U.S. Army team of doctors led by Walter Reed to Cuba to investigate cause of yellow fever, and Clara Maass, 25-year old nurse, dies testing out effect of mosquito bite.

1901: Permanent Army Nurse Corps formed based on splendid record of nurses in Spanish-American War.

1902: First state nursing association formed in North Carolina; purpose of early state associations was to pressure for state nurses registration laws.

1903: North Carolina became the first state to pass a nurse registration law, inaugurating "registered nurse" profession; New York, New Jersey and Virginia followed the same year.

1905: Mary Adelaide Nutting became first nurse in the world to become a professor in a university when she headed the new Department of Household and Institutional Administration at Columbia Teachers College.

1908: National Association for Colored Graduate Nurses organized.

1909: University of Minnesota School of Nursing opened as first basic program for nursing education run on sound educational basis.

1910: Columbia Teachers College offered first program of special preparation in public health nursing.

1910: Number of hospital nursing schools reached 1,630.

1912: National Organization for Public Health Nursing founded.

1912: Book, *Educational Status of Nursing*, published, influences nursing education, written by Mary Adelaide Nutting; calls for moving nursing school out from under hospital control.

1916: *Public Health Nursing*, publication of NOPHN, began appearing.

1917 –18: Nurses serve in World War I; Major Julia C. Stimson a noted leader.

1923: *Nursing and Nursing Education in the United States*, result of four years of investigation funded by Rockefeller Foundation, published, known as Goldmark Report; provided comprehensive survey of hospitals, pointed out inadequacies in nurse training.

1925: Mary Breckinridge founded Frontier Nursing Service of Kentucky, servicing 10,000 people in isolated Appalachian communities.

1926: Number of schools of nursing reached 2,155, the high point before the Depression again reduced the number.

1929: Great Depression confronted nursing with problem of overproduction of nurses, many inadequately trained; hundreds of smaller schools closed, concern for quality training enhanced.

1931: American Association of Nurse Anesthetists organized.

1933: Federal Emergency Relief Act provides for reimbursement for nursing services to those unable to pay.

1934: United States Public Health Service employed first public health nurse.

1934: Nursing Information Bureau of ANA set up, published first issue of *Facts about Nursing*, 1935.

1937: *RN* began publication.

1941 –45: Nurses played vital role in World War II, stimulated federal concern for training nurses.

1942: American Association of Industrial Nurses founded.

1943: Nurse Lucille Petry headed the U.S. Cadet Nurse Corps, an organization of student nurses created that year, to provide specially trained nurses for the war effort.

1948: *Nursing for the Future,* by Esther L. Brown (the Brown Report), published; very influential in moving nursing from hospital-apprenticeship type training to university educational settings.

1950: 195 collegiate programs for nurse training were in existence.

American Nursing: 1950 to the Present

From 1950 to the present, nursing has been undergoing a further revolution toward increasing professionalization, and partially back toward medicine, from which field it had separated in the Middle Ages. During the 1950s and 1960s, the federal government played an increasing role in funding nurse training, while federal legislation in all areas of health care led to sizable investment in health, affecting nursing as well. By the 1970s, specializations such as nurse practitioner and clinical nurse specialist created a new role for the nurse as a primary health care dispenser, able to replace some of the less sophisticated functions of the physician. At the same time, nurses were taking on increasing responsibility for public and community health care. These trends seem likely to dominate nursing through the rest of this century.

Other Significant Events—Chronologies

U.S. Health Care and Health Professions

1665: Earliest law to regulate practice of medicine in the colonies; passed in Massachusetts.

1699: Legislation for the control of communicable disease enacted in Massachusetts.

1752: Pennsylvania Hospital opened, first to do free outpatient work for indigent outpatients.

1767: College of Physicians and Surgeons (Columbia University) opened in New York.

1768: First state insane hospital incorporated in Williamsburg, Virginia, later known as Eastern State Hospital.

1786: Philadelphia Dispensary established, first dispensary to supply free medicine to the needy.

1797: *Medical Repository* appears, first original medical journal.

1799: First general Quarantine Act passed by Congress.

1802: First vaccine institute, organized in Baltimore; U.S. Vaccine Agency established in 1813.

1817: Work on "Therapeutics and Materia Medica," the first in the U.S.

1821: Philadelphia College of Pharmacy opened.

1846: Organization of American Medical Association, first national medical society of permanence.

1848: First woman's medical school, Boston Female Medical School, established; absorbed in 1874 by Boston University School of Medicine which then became the first coeducational medical school in the world.

1853: New York Infirmary for Women and Children incorporated, first such infirmary staffed by women physicians, including Dr. Elizabeth Blackwell, the first academically trained female physician.

1855: Woman's Hospital established in New York, the first hospital in the world founded for the exclusive use of women.

1861: First school for nurses to award a diploma was chartered: the School of Nursing, Woman's Hospital of Philadelphia.

1862: Establishment of the first U.S. Army field hospital, in a tent, at the battle of Shiloh, Tennessee.

1872: American Public Health Association founded.

1874: Introduction of the first hospital record system, by head nurse Linda Richards, at Bellevue Training School for Nurses.

1876: First woman physician elected to the AMA, Dr. Sarah H. Stevenson, a delegate of the Illinois State Medical Society.

1878: Pathological laboratory for the study of bacteriology opened at Columbia's College of Physicians and Surgeons.

1882: Establishment of the American Red Cross, through the efforts of Clara Barton, its first president.

1886: First nurses' magazine, *The Nightingale,* a monthly publication.

1887: Establishment of a bacteriological research laboratory at Marine Hospital, Staten Island; retitled the Hygienic Laboratory in 1892, the research arm of the projected USPHS and eventually the nucleus of National Institutes of Health.

1891: First interracial hospital, the Provident Hospital, incorporated in Chicago.

1893: Founding of the first national organization in nursing, the American Society of Superintendents of Training Schools for nurses, renamed the National League for Nursing Education in 1912.

1896: Establishment of Nurses Associated Alumnae, renamed American Nurses' Association in 1911.

1901: Legislation to establish the Army Nurses' Corps; Dita M. Kenney, the first superintendent.

1902: United States Public Health Service established.

1903: First state law establishing requirements for state examination and registration of nurses, by North Carolina.

1906: Passage of Pure Food and Drug Act, first legislation of its kind.

1908: First university school of nursing, instituted as part of the University of Minnesota.

1909: Passage, in Chicago, of a compulsory milk pasteurization law, the first in the United States.

1910: Publications of Dr. Abraham Flexner's "Medical Education in the United States," a report which condemned poor teaching and substandard conditions in existing medical schools and led to sweeping reforms.

1918: First national standardization program, initiated by the American College of Surgeons, established in 1913.

1934: First graduate degree program in hospital administration at university level, instituted at University of Chicago.

1935: Social Security Act includes health provisions for maternal and child health, welfare and community public health services.

1946: Passage of Hill-Burton Act provides funds for new hospital facilities; in 1954, amended to include construction of nursing homes, rehabilitation facilities and health centers.

1948: World Health Organization established.

1952: Joint Commission on Accreditation of Hospitals established.

1964: "Smoking and Health" report issued by the Surgeon–General's Advisory Committee cites cigarette smoking as a major cause of lung cancer.

1965: Passage of Medicare and Medicaid legislation.

1972: Professional Standards Review Organization program adopted by Congress.

1975 –78: Congressional debate on enactment of a national health insurance program (National Health Planning and Resources Development Act)

Medicine

1628: Discovery of blood circulation by William Harvey.

1667: First transfusion of blood performed (on man) by Edmund King.

1674: Tourniquet invented by Morel.

1675: Observation under microscope of "little animals" in droplets of water, by Van Leeuwenhock.

1690: The pulse was first counted by watch.

1717: Introduction of innoculation by the Asiatic method, for preventing smallpox.

1736: First successful appendectomy by Claudius Amyand.

1796: First successful antitoxin by Edward Jenner, to prevent smallpox.

1809: First removal of an ovarian tumor, by Ephraim McDowell.

1816: Invention of the stethoscope, by René Laennec.

1836: Observation and description of the process of digestion, by William Beaumont.

1836: Modern germ theory first suggested by discovery of the yeast plant.

1842: Administration of ether as an anesthetic during surgery, by Crawford W. Long.

1865: Introduction of antiseptic surgery, by Joseph Lister.

1866: Invention of the clinical thermometer, by Thomas C. Allbut.

1870: Bacteriological researches commence, revealing discoveries relating to rabies by Pasteur, tuberculosis by Koch, typhoid fever by Eberth, diphtheria by von Behring.

1883: Discovery of the diphtheria-causing bacillus, by Edwin Klebs.

1889: Discovery of antitoxins to treat diphtheria and tetanus, by Emil von Behring. Introduction of tuberculin to treat tuberculosis, by Robert Koch.

1890: Discovery of the bacillus of bubonic plague, by Alexandre Yersin.

1895: Discovery of the x-ray, by Wilhelm Roentgen.

1901: Identification of the mosquito-spreading etiology of yellow fever, by Walter Reed and others.

1905: Discovery of the spirillum which causes syphilis, by Schaudinn.

1921: Isolation of hormone insulin for effective treatment of diabetes, by Frederick Banting and Charles Best.

1924: Invention of the electrocardiograph, by William Einthoven.

1926: Isolation of liver extract to treat pernicious anemia.

1928: Discovery of penicillin, by Alexander Fleming.

1929: Identification of growth-producing vitamins, by Hopkins; of antineuritic vitamin group, by Eijkman.

1933: Description of the hereditary function of chromosomes, by Thomas H. Morgan.

1940: Invention of the bronchoscope, by Chevalier Jackson.

1941: Development of the "Pap smear" test, by George Papanicolaou.

1943: Use of newly discovered streptomycin in treating tuberculosis, by Selman Waksman.

1944: Use of corrective heart surgery for "blue-baby" survival, by Alfred Blalock and Helen Taussig.

1949: Introduction of cortisone, by Philip Hench and others.

1954: Establishment of hypodermic poliomyelitis vaccine, by Jonas E. Salk; oral vaccine by Albert Sabin in 1957.

1954: Introduction of open-heart surgery, C. W. Lillehei.

1963: Innovative use of artificial heart during heart surgery, by Michael deBakey.

1963: Demonstration of successful measles vaccine, based on work of John F. Enders.

1967: First surgical transplant of a human heart, by Christian Barnard.

1969: Analysis of gamma globulin, one of the body's chief defenses against disease, by Gerald Edelman and others.

1969: Perfection of rubeola vaccine.

2
NEWS HIGHLIGHTS

Health and Health Services

Facts and Trends

Following are some of the current highlights and trends in health conditions, costs and services.

- The nation's state of health is "generally good," with improvements made over the last ten to twenty years, comments the Department of Health, Education and Welfare in the first overall U.S. health report issued.
- The cost of health care escalated 300% in the last decade and is growing 50% faster than the rate of general inflation, reports the U.S. Public Health Service.
- Hospital admissions decreased for the first time in 15 years, reported the American Hospital Association in its annual summation of 1975 data. To save costs, a National Medical Institute panel (National Academy of Science) recommended a 10% reduction of hospital beds over the next five years.
- In an economy move, Blue Cross announced a campaign to have laboratory tests made prior to hospital admission, a procedure which could reduce the length of patient stays by as much as two days.
- The national birth rate continues to decline, recorded at 14.8 live births per 1,000 population for 1975, latest annual figures available.
- The national death rate hit lowest level in U.S. history, 9.2 per 1,000 population, according to 1974 data. Evaluations by the National Center for Health Statistics indicate that the 4.8% decrease of heart disease and stroke deaths balanced out the increased rates of cancer, suicide and homicide deaths.
- The suicide rate among young people has been in a rapid upward trend over the last decade (1965–74), reports the NCHS in a survey on mental health. For those in their 20s, the current rate is about 15.5 suicides per 1,000, with a major 70% increase for those in the 20–24 year old group.
- Heroin deaths in Detroit outnumber the combined toll of such fatalities in five large cities, including New York and Philadelphia. The rate of heroin usage in Detroit is 1 in 41, up 900% since 1971.
- An estimated $735 million is spent on cold remedy products, with little effect on the prevention or cure of colds, reports the Food and Drug Administration.
- Live-virus oral vaccine caused more than half the U.S. polio cases in 1973–75, reports the Center for Disease Control.
- The nationwide swine flu vaccine campaign ended in a fiasco with the linkage of the vaccine to deaths and a rare nervous disease.
- The shortage of doctors in the U.S. appears to have been curtailed, announced the Carnegie Council on Policy Studies in Higher Education; but the unequal distribution of physicians still leaves the problem of insufficient medical services within low-income urban and rural areas.
- Nearly all medical school scholarship aid was "tied" to future enlistment in the National Health Service Corps in the $2.1 billion health manpower bill signed at the end of 1976.

Issues and Controversy

- The delivery of medical services was at the center of much controversy recently as investigations exposed Medicaid fraud, physician malpractice and nursing home scandals. Other issues centered on the rights and protection of persons in medical situations: euthanasia and the right to die, experimentation on humans, and consumer health protection.
- "Abysmal administration" and "rampant abuse" by both health services and Medicaid recipients uncovered in the Medicare/Medicaid investigation report by the Senate Subcommittee on Long-Term Care. Senator Frank Moss claimed that $45 million of Medicare/Medicaid payments to clinical laboratories goes for kickbacks and waste.
- Physicians, laboratories and pharmacists who received more than $100,000 in Medicaid reimbursements were made publicly known in a release from the Department of Health, Education and Welfare.
- Criticism of numerous existing "Medicaid mills" was made by New York City Coordinator of Nurses, Shirley Sanderson, who commented that wretched service was provided to the Medicaid patients, and then inflated bills were submitted to Medicaid for reimbursement.

18

- Fraud against Medicare/Medicaid within nursing home operations was highlighted by the case of operator Bernard Bergman who committed an alleged $1.2 million fraud against the government.
- Incompetent doctors number 16,000 (5% of the physician population) *The New York Times* reported in an investigative series on doctors. Evidence included excessive surgery and faulty prescriptions resulting in deaths. The *Times* also noted the reluctance of doctors to criticize their peers.
- Testing laboratories were on the firing line as the Center for Disease Control identified, out of a representative sample of 22 laboratories, 16 that made frequent errors in analyzing samples.
- The issue of medical malpractice was openly aired as more suits with large settlements were brought against physicians and hospitals by a more informed public. Malpractice insurance rates have risen accompanied by open protests from medical personnel. Physicians complain that the upsurge in medical costs is in part due to the higher overhead of malpractice insurance costs. A growing number of hospitals have "gone bare," underwriting their own risk against suits, in an effort to avoid high premiums. At the same time, most hospitals are looking into procedures which lower their susceptibility to malpractice suits.
- The right-to-die became a legal controversy in the case of young Karen Quinlan who had been sustained for months on life-supporting equipment. The final court decision permitted disconnection of the respirator lifeline if the medical advisors indicated there was no reasonable chance of recovery. Across the country, California recognized the social issue and signed a right-to-die bill.
- The use of federal prisoners in medical research experiments was stopped by the Bureau of Prisons when the issue was made public. Director Carlson indicated the stoppage was necessary as truly voluntary consent was impossible in the situation. Shortly afterwards, the rights of human subjects in research experiments were provided protection by a watchdog commission established by the Senate.
- A major controversy took place over genetic research involving recombinant DNA; whether the hazards would justify suspen-

sion or at least control of further research. The National Institutes of Health issued guidelines to govern the research.
- The rapid accumulation of sophisticated health obstructions—the bans on cyclamates, red dyes #2 and #4, the problems of drug interaction, the questionable use of breast x-rays for standard, repeated examinations—required an alert consumer. To supply information on drugs, surgery and other health matters which would serve the public interest, a new Consumer Center for Health Information was formed.

Labor Disputes and Health Personnel

- In various parts of the country, physicians, nurses and nonmedical hospital personnel were included in unprecedented protests over a variety of conditions.
- The United Physicians of California sponsored a 35-day slowdown strike in the southern portion of the state in protest over a 35–45% increase in malpractice insurance premiums. The protestors were satisfied when Governor Jerry Brown proposed a bill which would establish a state-run malpractice insurance pool.
- Nurses picketed all but one of Honolulu's seven major hospitals in a 19-day strike over wage demands and won an acceptable two-year contract.
- For over two months, 1,800 registered nurses, members of the Washington State Nurses' Association, set up picket lines at 15 Seattle hospitals in a demand for higher wages, better staffing and an end to 16-hour work shifts. The nurses' strike was the first in the state's history. A separate strike was conducted by nurses from Seattle Group Health Hospital and ten clinics.
- Two major Chicago hospitals were confronted by 1,000 nurses on strike over the hospitals' attempt to reduce benefits, including elimination of pay for the first two sick days allowed.
- An all-out strike of nurses in Israel resulted in 15,000 nurses out for ten days, seeking higher wages and better working conditions.
- A unified group of 200 LPNs and laboratory technicians at United Hospital of Newark (New Jersey) walked out in a dispute over layoffs and stalled talks.

A massive 11-day walkout of around 30,000 nonmedical personnel hit 33 voluntary hospitals, 10 municipal hospitals and 14 nursing homes in New York City. Members of the organized District 1199 of the National Union of Hospital and Health Care Employees, the strikers consisted of technicians, nursing aides, orderlies, dietary and housekeeping staff and clerks. Demands were for a cost-of-living wage increase while the hospitals' representative, the League of Voluntary Hospitals and Homes, indicated a financial bind because of frozen Medicaid and Blue Cross payments. The matter went into arbitration with federal mediators; the hospitals increased what had been a reduced patient load and phased back the striking workers.

Another strike hit 16 more New York City municipal hospitals, a month after the city's largest hospital strike; this time the 18,000 nonmedical hospital workers were organized by District 37 of AFSCME and were out for three days.

Advances in Medical Technology

Further refinements of devices that "see" into the body have been developed: a special x-ray scanner that can scan a cross-section of the brain, producing a picture which can even be computer-coded to show up in color; a special scintillation camera that is able to trace a tiny amount of radioactive substance as it travels, and so determine the location of blockage; and ultrasound beams which can be used for examination of internal body structures, for example fetuses, without harm.

An operation to bypass blocked coronary arteries by inserting sections of veins from the patient's leg, thereby correcting coronary heart disorders likely to lead to heart attacks, has now reached the stage of success where it is being done in many community hospitals.

An easy-to-read disposable oral thermometer that gives an accurate reading in 30 seconds promises to save nursing time and avoid crosscontamination among patients.

Radio waves have been used to apply heat locally to malignant cancer tumors and melt them down. The method has shown positive results experimentally with small numbers of patients, but several problems remain to be solved before it can be applied generally.

A researcher at the University of California at Berkeley has developed a new technique that will allow biologists to process up to 100 million cultures of live cells at once, vastly increasing the scope of experiments on cellular growth and abnormality, and allowing computer-programmed research to be carried out.

A new artery technique, based on x-ray technology, allows measurement of fatty deposit build-ups in the arteries of heart attack victims.

Medical Drug and Vaccine Advances

Work has been in progress on controlled delivery drugs, drugs that release measured amounts continuously for days or longer, for such diseases as glaucoma, malaria, motion sickness and even tooth decay.

Progress has been made in manufacturing interferon, the body's main substance for killing viruses, and in new combination drugs effective against all known disease-carrying bacteria, including strains resistant to antibiotics now in use.

A new drug against schistosomiasis, an illness which debilitates millions in the Third World, has been developed and found to be effective against one common form of the causative parasite.

A safer, more reliable and faster test for syphilis is now available.

A researcher has found a human virus linked with diabetes in mice, which raises the possibility of a vaccine against the disease.

A four-drug combination used to treat Hodgkin's Disease (cancer of the lymph system) has proved completely effective in 81% of cases treated recently; a three-drug combination has shown itself largely effective in reducing the recurrence of breast cancer in women who had surgery *after* the cancer had reached the lymph nodes, which often leads to relapse.

Vaccines effective against drug-resistant strains of bacterial pneumonia, which kills 70,000 people a year, have been used with

20

success in Africa; they are being prepared for use here, and may save 20,000 lives a year. Vaccines against two strains of meningitis have worked well in adults—none effective for young children has been found. Meningitis is the fifth leading type of infectious disease.

- Drugs are being tested that can dissolve gallstones and kidney stones, problems which together afflict over one million people a year.
- A new rabies vaccine requiring two-thirds fewer injections has been found effective.
- The first laboratory culturing of a malaria parasite was achieved, a factor which enhances the possibility of producing a malaria vaccine.
- A new asthma drug that can be swallowed in syrup form is expected to be useful for juvenile patients.
- Experimenters report success in manufacture, by bacteria, of human hormones for medical use.
- A major step was taken toward the understanding of heredity with the first construction of bacterial genes, complete with regulatory mechanisms.

Public Attitudes Toward Health*

Only 42% of the public, pointing to increased medical knowledge, better facilities and drugs, and more nutritious foods, feel that today's generation is healthier than their parents. A smaller but still significant 27%, pointing to diet problems and increased stress, feel people today are actually less healthy than their parents. Twenty-eight percent feel that there is not much difference between the health of the two generations.

When asked to describe their own health, 34% said "excellent," 46% said "pretty good," 15% said "only fair" and 5% said "poor."

Sixty-seven percent of the general public said they had been to a doctor or a clinic for a physical check-up within the last 12 months.

When individuals rated the seriousness of various diseases for someone of their age, cancer was rated highest, followed by stroke, heart condition, diabetes and high blood pressure.

---

*Source: National Institutes of Health, 1975.

3

RELIGION, UNUSUAL PRACTICES
AND QUACKS

Religion and Patient Care*

Following are brief descriptions—drawn from 16 major religions—of the practices and beliefs that affect patient health care.

Adventist

Seventh Day Adventist
Church of God
Advent Christian Church

Birth: Opposed to infant baptism. Adults baptized by total immersion.

Death: The dead are asleep until the return of Jesus Christ, at which time final rewards and punishment will be given.

Health crisis: Believe in man's choice and God's sovereignty. Taking of Communion or undergoing baptism may be desired. Some believe in divine healing and practice anointing with oil and use of prayer.

Diet: No alcohol, coffee or tea. The taking of all narcotics and stimulants is prohibited because the body is the temple of the Holy Spirit and should be protected. Many groups prohibit meat.

Beliefs: Some sects regard Saturday as Sabbath. They accept the Bible literally, and keeping the commandments is the evidence of salvation. They believe their duty is to warn mankind to prepare for the second coming of Christ. Some oppose use of hypnotism in therapy.

Baptist Bodies

(27 bodies)

Birth: Opposed to infant baptism. Only believers should be baptized, and it must be done by immersion.

Death: Clergy seeks to minister by counsel and prayer with patient and family.

Health crisis: Some Baptists believe and practice healing by the "laying on of hands."

Diet: Some groups condemn coffee and tea.

Beliefs: Supreme authority of Bible in all matters of faith and practice. Many Baptists condemn what the American Baptist Association terms "... so-called modern

science." Although the practical expression of this view is largely confined to opposition to "Darwinism," resistance to medical therapy may be encountered. Most, however, believe that God works through the physician. Some who believe in predestination respond passively to care.

Black Muslim

Birth: No baptism.

Death: Carefully prescribed procedure for washing and shrouding the dead, and performing funeral rites.

Diet: Prohibits alcoholic beverages, pork and meat of dead animals; also corn bread, collard greens, or other foods traditional among American blacks.

Beliefs: General adherence to Moslem tenets is overlaid in many instances by antagonism to Caucasians, especially Christians and Jews. They do not indulge in activities such as sleeping more than is necessary to health and always maintain personal habits of cleanliness.

Church of Christ, Scientist
(Christian Scientist)

Health crisis: They deny the existence of health crises; sickness, sin, and death are errors of the human mind and can be destroyed by altering thoughts, not by drugs or medicines. They do not allow hypnotism or any form of psychotherapy which alters the "Divine Mind." A Christian Science Practitioner can be called to administer spiritual support; the *Christian Science Journal* contains a directory of Christian Science nurses available to help bandage wounds, set bones, etc.

Diet: Alcohol, coffee, tobacco are seen as drugs, so not used.

Beliefs: Disease is a human mental concept that can be dispelled by "spiritual truth." Many Christian Scientists adhere to this belief to the extent that they refuse all medical treatment, but each individual may decide whether he wishes to rely completely on Christian Science. Many adherents desire the services of a Practitioner or Reader. The Church operates several nursing homes that rely solely on such "spiritual" means of health maintenance. They do not use drugs or blood transfusions, accept vaccines only when required by law, and do not seek biopsies or physical examinations.

---

*Reprinted with permission from the July 1976 issue of *Nursing Update,* Intermed Communications, Inc., 132 Welsh Rd., Horsham, Pa. 19044. Further reproduction in whole or in part expressly prohibited by law.

22

Church of Jesus Christ of Latter Day Saints (Mormon)

Birth: Baptism by immersion at 8 years or older.

Death: Believe it proper to bury in ground; cremation is discouraged. Baptism of the dead is held essential, though a living person may serve as proxy. Preaching the Gospel to the dead is also practiced.

Health crisis: Devout adherents believe in divine healing through the "laying on of hands," though many do not prohibit medical therapy. The Church maintains an extensive and well-funded welfare system, including financial support for the sick.

Diet: Prohibits alcoholic beverages, tobacco, hot drinks (tea, coffee), or any other substance which may be injurious to the body. Encourages sparing use of meats but prohibits none outright.

Beliefs: There is a strong tradition of revelation through visions. A special undergarment is often worn. Patients may desire to have a Church Priesthood holder administer the sacrament to them while in the hospital. This would be on Sunday.

Eastern Orthodox Churches

(Turkey, Egypt, Syria, Romania, Bulgaria, Cyprus, Albania, Poland, Czechoslovakia)

Birth: Generally, these denominations believe in infant baptism by total immersion, followed immediately by confirmation.

Death: Last rites obligatory if death is impending.

Health crisis: Anointing of the sick is a form of healing by prayer.

Diet: Restrictions dependent on particular sect.

Episcopalian

Birth: Infant baptism is mandatory and especially urgent if prognosis is grave, although aborted fetuses and stillborns are not baptized.

Death: "Last Rites" ("Rite for the Anointing of the Sick") is not mandatory for all members.

Health crisis: Some believe in spiritual healing.

Diet: Some abstain from meat on Fridays and some fast before receiving Holy Communion, which may be daily.

Beliefs: Many practice confession of sins and absolution.

Friends (Quakers)

Birth: Do not baptize—at birth, an infant's name is recorded in official books.

Death: Do not believe in life after this life.

Beliefs: Are pacifists and conscientious objectors in wartime. Believe in plain speech and dress and refusal of tithes, oaths. Believe God is in every man and can be approached directly—religion inward, personal.

Greek Orthodox Church

Birth: Baptism is significant. Prefer to baptize the child at least 40 days from birth. If it is not possible to baptize by sprinkling or immersion, the church allows the child to be baptized "in the air" by moving the child in the form of the sign of the cross as appropriate words are said.

Death: Last rites are the administration of the Sacrament of Holy Communion. The priest should be called early enough so that the patient is still conscious.

Health crisis: In most cases, these health crises situations must be handled by an ordained priest, though a Deacon of the Church may also serve in some cases. Usually a priest administers Holy Communion in the hospital room in a procedure that takes only a few minutes. Some patients may also want the Sacrament of Holy Unction which the Priest can conduct in the hospital room in a brief time in an abbreviated service.

Diet: The Church usually prescribes a fast period which means avoidance of meat and, in many cases, dairy products. These rules need not be enforced in cases of illness, especially when they may be of some harm to the health of the patient. Sometimes Orthodox patients will insist upon fasting even when in the hospital. If decision and desire to fast in the hospital do not interfere with medical procedures, there would be no reason for this to be refused. However, if this would adversely influence the medical condition of the patient, a priest should be called to convince the patient to forego fasting until his health is restored. The usual fasting days are Wednesday, Friday, and Lent.

Jehovah's Witnesses

Birth: No infant baptism.

Death: No last rites.

Health crisis: Adherents are generally absolutely opposed to blood transfusion, though individuals can sometimes be persuaded in emergencies. When parents refuse consent for a child's transfusion, it is often possible to obtain a court order appointing some key hospital official temporary guardian of the child. The official may then legally consent to the transfusion.

Beliefs: The sect opposes the "false teachings" of other sects; opposition often extends to modern science, including medicine. Some are pacifists and conscientious objectors in wartime; conversion of others is important. They don't participate in nationalistic ceremonies or celebrate holidays by gift giving.

Judaism

Birth: Ritual circumcision is mandatory among Orthodox and Conservative adherents on the 8th day. Reform Jews favor ritual circumcision, but not as a religious imperative. A fetus is to be buried, not discarded.

Death: Human remains are ritually washed following death by members of the Ritual Burial Society, and the burial should take place as soon as possible. Cremation is not in keeping with Jewish law. All Orthodox Jews and some Conservatives are opposed to autopsy.

Diet: Orthodox and Conservative Jews observe strict kosher dietary laws, which mainly prohibit pork, shellfish, and the eating of meat with any milk products. There are complex proscriptions and prescriptions regarding food preparation. Reform Jews do not usually observe kosher dietary laws.

Beliefs: Orthodox and Conservative adherents observe the Sabbath from sundown Friday to sundown Saturday. They may resist surgical procedures during this period unless a rabbi counsels that such procedures are medically necessary and are therefore permitted by Talmudic law. Amputated limbs or organs or surgically removed body tissues should be available to the family for burial. Parts of the body are not donated or removed, even during autopsy.

Lutheran

Birth: Baptize (only living) persons at 6–8 weeks following birth by pouring, sprinkling, or immersing.

Death: "Last Rites" are optional.

Health crisis: If the prognosis is grave, the patient may request the anointing and blessing of the sick.

Beliefs: Accept developments of science and technology but would raise objections if such techniques are administered unjustly or are clearly contrary to Christian theology.

Methodist

Birth: Baptism for children or adults.

Death: Believe in divine judgment after death. Good will be rewarded and evil punished.

Health crisis: Communion may be requested prior to surgery or similar crisis.

Beliefs: Ministers counsel but do not hear confession. Donation of one's body or part of body at death is encouraged.

Pentecostal (Assembly of God, Foursquare Church)

Birth: Water baptism by complete single immersion after age of accountability.

Death: No last rites.

Health crisis: No inhibitions against blood transfusions or medical care. Believe in possibility of divine healing through prayer. Anointing with oil may be practiced with laying on of hands.

Diet: Abstain from alcohol, tobacco, eating blood and strangled animals. Individual may resist pork.

Beliefs: Some insist illness is divine punishment but most consider illness an intrusion of Satan. Deliverance from sin and sickness are provided for in atonement. Pray for divine intervention in health matters and seek to reach God in prayer for themselves and others when ill.

Orthodox Presbyterian

Birth: Sprinkling most common in infant baptism.

Death: Last rites not a sacramental procedure; they read Scripture and pray.

Health crisis: Communion administered when appropriate and convenient; blood transfusion acceptable when advisable; no formal laying on of hands ceremony; prayer appropriate; local pastor or elder should be called.

Belief: True science to be utilized for relief of suffering and recognized as a gift of the Creator. Full forgiveness through genuine repentance for any illness connected with a sin. Think of heaven and hell in material terms.

Roman Catholic

Birth: Infant baptism is mandatory and especially urgent if prognosis is grave. Baptism is demanded if an aborted fetus may not be clinically dead. For baptismal purposes, "death" is a certainty only if there is obvious evidence of tissue necrosis.

Death: The Rite for the Anointing of the Sick is mandatory. If the prognosis is grave, the patient or the family may request it.

Health crisis: The patient or family may desire that a major amputated limb be buried in consecrated ground. There is no blanket mandate for this but it may be required within a given diocese.

Diet: Most hospital patients are exempt from fasting or abstaining from meat on Ash Wednesday and Good Friday. Some older Catholics may still adhere to the former rule of abstaining from meat on all Fridays.

Unusual Practices

Biorhythms*

The time for administering medications, taking vital signs, serving meals, executing treatments and procedures, regulating rest and activity, and analyzing blood and urine studies may one day be based on the concepts of biorhythmology.

This new branch of biology known as biorhythmology or chronobiology has emerged as a result of research findings that support the concept of biological clocks or living rhythms in plants, animals, and man.

A biological rhythm (biorhythm) is a self-sustaining oscillation apparently controlled from within the body. Biorhythms are synchronized to environmental cycles such as light and darkness, gravity, cosmic stimuli, and electromagnet fields. Dysynchronization of the biorhythms takes place when changes occur in the environmental cycles such as transatlantic flight where the cycle of light and darkness is altered or when eastern standard time is changed to daylight savings time and vice versa. In these instances, the biorhythms shift in phase to adjust to the new environmental cycles and it takes the body, in most instances, a few days to adjust to the new environmental cycle.

Types of Human Rhythmic Cycles

Human beings demonstrate behavioral, biochemical, and physiological rhythmic cycles over definite time periods. There are various types of cycles including circadian, ultradian,

and infradian. The most common of these is the "circadian" which comes from the Latin, *circa dies,* meaning "about a day." Physiological rhythms, such as body temperature, heart rate, blood pressure, respirations, brain function, and muscle function, demonstrate this rhythmicity. Rhythmicity is also demonstrated in biochemical analyses of urine, blood enzymes, and plasma serum. That is, they present a pattern of rhythmicity which persists for about 24 hours with a peak and trough time. The peaks occur as a rule in the early evening, and troughs, in the early morning hours. It is a well-known fact that each day the body temperature has a low value in the morning and highest value toward evening.

"Ultradian" rhythmicity has a higher frequency than circadian and usually persists for minutes or hours. It is seen in the rapid eye movement (REM) cycle of the rest-activity cycle of sleep. It has been demonstrated that babies' rest activity cycle in sleep ranges from 55 to 60 minutes as compared to 90 to 100 minutes for adults.

The menstrual cycle is an example of "infradian" rhythmicity, meaning it persists for a period of weeks or a month. Consisting of an internal cyclical process which proceeds from a point of origin, through hormonal stages, back to the original point, it usually operates on a 28-day cycle.

Faith Healing**

"Therapeutic touch," is the ancient art of voluntary transfer of some undefined energy from a well person to one who is ill. This art has been called the laying-on of hands in the western world, and records of its continued use go back to the cradle of western culture in the hieroglyphics of early Egypt and the cuneiform writings of ancient Assyria. This practice is characterized by the touching of another person, coupled with a strong intent to help or to heal that person.

[Although] our society supports a no-touch culture, nurses are a notable exception to these bans. Literature from the East, particularly from India and Tibet, states that the life energies in man, which we in the West call vitality, are an expression of an energy system called *prana.*

---

*Source: Margaret L. O'Dell, "Human Biorhythms," *Nursing* Forum, Vol. XIV, No. 1, 1975.

**Source: Dolores Krieger, Ph.D., RN, "Therapeutic Touch," *Journal, NYSNA,* August, 1975.

The healer [was] an individual whose health gave him access to an over-abundance of *prana,* and whose strong sense of commitment and intention to help ill people gave him a certain control over the projection of this vital energy. The act of healing then would entail the channeling of this energy flow by the healer for the wellbeing of the individual.

[Only a few scientists have] successfully studied healing by a laying-on of hands with the rigor demanded by scientific methodologies. In the early 1960s Grad, of McGill University in Montreal, conducted two studies using the services of Oskar Estebany. In the first study he divided 300 standardized mice whose backs had been artificially wounded in a specific manner into three equal groups. In the first group no attempt was made to interfere with any natural healing process. Estebany held the second group in the manner he used when doing the laying-on of hands. The third group were held by medical students who "did not profess to heal." After fourteen days it was found that the group held by Estebany had accelerated their rate of wound healing beyond the other two groups at a probability which was determined to occur less than once in a thousand times by chance alone.

The second study was conducted on barley seeds which were first soaked in saline solution to simulate a "sick" condition. The methodology was similar to the study with mice. In this case it was found that the seeds watered from flasks held by Estebany sprouted earlier, the plants grew taller, and they had more chlorophyll in the leaves.

Integrating this literature from the East and the studies noted above from the West, I selected hemoglobin (one of the body's most sensitive indicators of oxygen uptake) as a dependent variable in a study designed to elicit clues to the bio-energetic change that might underlie the effects of therapeutic touch. I designated a group of sick people who would have treatment by Estebany as the experimental group and a second group who would have no treatment, as the control group. I took pre-test hemoglobin samples on all subjects in both groups to determine whether there was any significant difference in their mean hemoglobin values, and upon analysis found none. I also controlled for differences in age, sex, diet, medications and some biorhythms. My hypothesis was that there would be a sig-

nificant change in the hemoglobin values of the experimental group after treatment by the laying-on of hands, while there would be no significant difference between the control group's pre-test and post-test hemoglobin values.

I conducted another study in 1974 in which nurses learned how to utilize therapeutic touch. The design again included an experimental and a control group, the nurses in the former group engaged in therapeutic touch on their patients, while the nurses in the control group only performed the kinds of touch necessary to daily nursing procedures without any attempt to heal.

It was found that the hemoglobin values of the experimental group, the group that had had therapeutic touch, had changed at a probability that exceeded .001. The control group's hemoglobin values simultaneously showed no significant difference between their pre-test and post-test values.

Folk Medicine, Superstition and Herbal Remedies

Folk Medicine and Old-Time "Cures"

In ancient and primitive cultures, magic, incantation and conjuration were used to heal diseases and "cast out" death, thought to be caused by malignant spirits. The concept of incantation, recited or worn as an amulet, was regarded as effective well into the European Middle Ages. There were exceptions. The ancient *Egyptian Book of Surgery,* dating from 2500 B.C., makes only a single reference to a method of magic in its discussions of 48 separate surgical operations.

One of the most influential concepts of medical practice was the *doctrine of signatures,* originating in either Egypt or Babylonia and holding sway until the 17th century. The doctrine held that all natural objects (plants, herb, animals, animal parts) were marked by a sign which revealed their medicinal benefit for specific ailments. Basically these plants or animal parts were used because of some resemblance to the disease to be cured or to the diseased part of the body. Thus, the poppy was used for brain disorders because its fruit was shaped like a head; red roses were considered beneficial for blood problems, gummy plants for pus-exuding sores, many-seeded plants for barrenness, trefoiled plants for heart trouble and so on.

With time for increased observation of the effectiveness—or ineffectiveness—of medicinal plants, folk medicine did grow more sophisticated. After all, some traditional remedies are related to modern cure: the drug digitalis is derived from the foxglove plant; quinine, to treat malaria, is refined from Peruvian bark; and ephedrine, used in the treatment of allergies, comes from the herb, ma huang, used by the Chinese for generations. Even today, the Chinese are reviving their very ancient and systematic knowledge of herbal medicine to combine it with Western medical methods for treatment of disease. Since 1949 they have collected and identified more than 2,000 medicinal herbs and clinically isolated many useful chemical compounds from them.

However, many of the traditional remedies were linked to superstitions and persisted not as a result of scientific scrutiny but because coincidence or the self-limiting character of many milder diseases helped establish their reputation.

Superstitious Remedies for Illnesses:

Aches: a poultice of cow manure; ground worms simmered in lard.

Asthma: poultices of black pepper and lard.

Bronchitis: an onion cut in half and applied to the soles of the feet; for a simple croup, a teaspoon of kerosene "sweetened" by a few drops of sugar; for relief from coughing, lemon extract blended with butter and sugar.

Burns: mashed potatoes; fresh cow dung; for soothing, lard; to reduce the feel of heat, scraped flesh of raw potatoes.

Colds: bear grease as protection and to alleviate muscle aches; other greases used included camphorated oil, goose grease.

Communicable diseases: wear camphor around the neck.

Cramps: apply an eel's skin on bare leg, for leg cramps; lay shoes on stomach, for stomach cramp; tie a cormorant skin to the stomach.

Cuts and wounds: human urine; a piece of salt pork to draw out the infection and prevent lockjaw.

Diarrhea: eat green apples (modern therapy now includes apple pectin).

Earache: blow smoke or spit tobacco juice into ear; warmed oil; application of a hot baked potato held against the ear.

Frostbite: poultice of cow manure and milk; to restore circulation, rub area with snow.

Headache: tie around the neck the head of a buzzard; mustard poultice.

Jaundice: treat with warmed turkey dung bitters.

Lung congestion: poultice of sliced raw onions; turpentine heated with lard and applied to the chest.

Nosebleeds: stopped by cobwebs; for prevention, a nutmeg worn on a string around the neck.

Rheumatism: carry in pocket the bone of a racoon's penis; or a new potato until it is hard and black; buckshot in the hip pocket.

Sciatica: a plaster of onions, rum and neat's foot oil.

Skin diseases: sulfur and rum for boils; gunpowder boiled in water for ringworm.

Sore throat: wear gold or amber bead necklaces; salt pork worn around the neck; for relief, powdered sulfur or a hot fomentation of vinegar; for treatment, vinegar with soda, salt or pepper.

Herbal Remedies:

Aromatic Weeds: Such as spearmint, used to treat nausea.

Asafetida: Pieces of this ill-smelling gum, tied in small cloth bags, and suspended about the neck, were worn by schoolchildren to ward off "catching" diseases. The word was pronounced: "assafidetty."

Bitters: A tonic and blood purifier brewed from yellow-root, burdock root, and bark of prickly ash.

Blackberry: A tea made at home from its leaves and roots, and a purchased cordial, were used to control diarrhea.

Boneset: An herb, more properly called thoroughwort, used in a severe form of influenza.

Buckeye: The large, shiny, brown seeds were carried on the person to forestall or alleviate rheumatism.

Camomile: An almost universal remedy, for relief from colds to rheumatic pains.

Castor-oil: This replaced the calomel of the pioneers as a cathartic. Much disliked by children, it called, more than any other medicine, for the rude treatment of "holding the nose" to force swallowing.

Catnip: Tea made from the leaves was given to young babies before a mother's milk was available.

Chestnuts: For the treatment of croup.

Clover (red): Reputed especially effective for whooping cough; in syrup form, used for general cough medicine.

Goldthread: In infusion form, used by the Indians to treat "canker," sores in the mouth or throat.

Herbal tea: Teas made with herbs, such as sage, catnip or yarrow were used to bring down fever.

Jimson-weed: Leaves cooked in lard to make a salve for the treatment of old unhealed wounds.

Lobelia: Commonly known as "pukeweed," used to encourage vomiting and reduce stomach cramps.

Mint: Infusion of leaves for upset stomach.

Mullen: Leaves cooked in vinegar made poultices for the relief of rheumatism. Dried and pulverized, they were smoked in clay pipes in the treatment of asthma and lung congestion.

Pennyroyal: Made into tea for allaying fever. Taken in infusion, it was regarded as a regulator of menses.

Poke: The berries were crushed and strained through a colander; the juicy pulp was heated and then combined with sweet anise dissolved in grain alcohol. This was a specific for rheumatism.

Sassafras: Roots were dug in spring and a tea made by boiling them was taken to "thin the blood." This drink was pungent and bitter as opposed to the delicious tea that can be made by mild infusion of the bark of the roots.

Sumac: Cure for stomach disturbances. When boiled in beer it will break up colds, its gum will help a tooth-ache, its seeds will cure hemorrhoids and its powder and honey will stop bleeding.

Tansy: Tea made from the leaves was taken to relieve cramps accompanying menstruation.

Tree bark: The barks of certain trees were believed to have a laxative effect when stripped downward, but would cause vomiting when stripped off in an upward movement.

Yellow dock: Boiled in vinegar, for use on athlete's foot rashes.

Walnut: Bruised leaves were used as a poultice.

Watermelon: Tea made from the seeds was administered to stimulate kidney action.

Quackery*

What is a Quack?

A quack is one who professes skill or knowledge in any matter in which he knows little or nothing. Quackery can take several forms:

- *worthless drugs* which could include so-called baldness cures, face creams to "wipe away the years," and pills, salves and tablets to "cure" diabetes and cancer.
- *food fads*—many so-called health foods are a misnomer, implying they actually give health or a cure when the most they have are nutritive qualities generally found in wholesome foods.
- *"medical" devices*—these could range from worthless vibrating devices to complicated machines that look impressive but don't do a thing to cure or help disease. Many manufacturers or promoters have been convicted of fraud for the sale of such "medical" devices.

Spotting a Quack

The AMA Department of Investigation lists six simple indicators for spotting a quack:

1. He uses a special or "secret" machine or formula he claims can cure disease.
2. He guarantees a quick cure.
3. He advertises or uses case histories and testimonials to promote his cure.
4. He clamors constantly for medical investigation and recognition.
5. He claims medical men are persecuting him or are afraid of his competition.
6. He tells you that surgery or x-rays or drugs will cause more harm than good.

He may also have an unusual degree such as N.D. (doctor of naturopathy); Ph.N. (philosopher of naturopathy) or Ms.D. (doctor of metaphysics)?

Target Areas for Quackery

Cancer Cures

Cancer is a prime target of quacks, and it is estimated that cancer victims spend ten million

*Source: *FDA Consumer*, DHEW Pub. No. (FDA) 76-4001, 1976.

dollars a year on worthless cancer cures. According to the American Medical Association: "In one report of 64 cancer patients referred to a reputable hospital after treatment by quacks, 27 patients died who might have been saved if they had received proper treatment earlier. Ten patients were mutilated for life. Only 27 patients were fortunate enough to have quit using unproven remedies in time to receive proper medical care, and live."

Through the years, the following have been touted as cancer cures: expensive bottled seawater, tea made from red clover to bathe external cancer, salves and plasters (escharotics) to "draw out" the cancer, worthless diets to correct the so-called "imbalance" that produces cancer, a drink of vegetable juice and calf liver juice (combined with a treatment of coffee enemas), anti-carcergen Z-50, prepared from pooled cancer tissue and the patient's blood or urine, a zinc-lined pine box in which a patient sat to absorb "orgone energy," and other bizarre devices, machines and cures. All were worthless.

A device promoted to diagnose and treat diseases, including cancer, for example, was the "Film-O-Sonic." The innocent person who had (or only thought he had) cancer was "treated" at fees as high as $500. In actuality, the fake machine was a tape play-back device without a speaker. The patient would apply two pads, wired to the machine, over the region of his body presumably affected by his cancer. Then, switched on, the device played either "Smoke Gets in Your Eyes" or "The Lord's Prayer"—backwards.

Arthritis Cures

Arthritis also has a huge following of quacks. Among the 1,200 worthless "cures" for arthritic sufferers have been: "immune milk" (cost: $1.75 a quart) which allegedly got its immunity from antibodies produced in the udders of cows injected with special vaccines, vibrating devices, copper bracelets, copper and zinc discs in the shoes, drugs with alfalfa seeds, and herbs and vitamins. There was also the silly "uranium tunnel" cure (one had to sit in a uranium tunnel!) and colonic irrigation (pressurized flushing of the bowel).

Other "remedies" include salts from the Dead Sea and oil of wintergreen. Some people even go to an abandoned uranium mine in Utah, hoping that radiation from the mine will relieve their pain.

The Arthritis Foundation in New York estimates that arthritis victims spend $400 million a year on quack remedies.

The Chiropractor

A recent investigation by the American Medical Association revealed that almost anybody can get into chiropractic school from age 18 on—without a high school education, or with grade averages so low as to be at the failing level.

A study made in California of two schools of chiropractic showed that of 29 faculty members only 10 claimed to have bachelor's degrees (in four of these cases the college named by the faculty member denied that such a degree had been granted).

The Bioelectrometer Electrophysical Resistance Instrument," used by many chiropractors, was recently condemned after seizure under the food and drug laws. This marvel was supposed to find disjointed parts of the spine. It also was supposed to discover—and treat—all kinds of sickness, including bursitis, piles, kidney, heart, and stomach ailments, dizziness, and migraine headaches!

Breast Enlargement*

Silicone injections became something of a craze in the 1960s with the advent of "topless" dancers.

Plastic surgeons in Las Vegas estimate that 12,000 women there had silicone injections during the height of the fad. Now, each year about 120 of these women seek surgical help for problems that developed within one to 14 years after injection.

Serious injury, and at least four known deaths, have been attributed to the use of silicone injections. Reported reactions include severe pain, swelling, lumpiness, discoloration, and infection. Surgical removal of the breasts has been necessary in some cases to prevent gangrene or potentially fatal migration of silicone particles from the breasts to the brain, lungs or heart.

Another practice involves the use of liquid silicone in a pliable silicone bag placed between the breast tissue and the chest muscles. When used in this manner, silicone is classified as an implanted device and none of the problems connected with liquid silicone injections has been reported for this procedure.

---

*Source: U.S. Food and Drug Administration, 1976.

In spite of the injuries and disfiguration that have occurred, some doctors are continuing the practice of breast injections, using an industrial grade silicone, which is available to anyone. Also, breast injections of silicone are available in Mexico, and medical grade silicone from Mexico can be purchased by unethical U.S. practitioners.

Medical Devices*

After Benjamin Franklin's discovery of the electrical force present in lightning, numerous individuals sought to use electrical energy to treat human ailments. At the time of the American Revolution, a gadget known as the Perkins Tractor became quite popular. This device was claimed to be capable of drawing disease out of the body by its electrical current.

A quack device which was the subject of FDA action in the late 1940s was the Spectochrome, of one Dinshah P. Ghadiali, which consisted of a 1,000-watt lamp, in a cabinet supplied with colored glass slides to fit an aperture through which the light bathed the patient. By becoming a member of Ghadiali's "Institute" for a fee of $90 a person could obtain the lamp plus voluminous literature which sought to cloak the scheme in oriental mysticism and sanctity. Claims were made for its value in treating such diseases as diabetes, cancer, tuberculosis and syphilis, and several thousand lamps were distributed.

The "Zerret Applicator," popularly called the "Plastic Dumbbell," which consisted of two plastic water tumblers filled partially with water, sealed with paraffin, joined at their mouths by scotch tape, and set into paraffin in the handle of plastic baby rattles. It was claimed to introduce in the human body the energy given off by "expanded hydrogen atoms" or "Z rays" alleged to be present in the liquid sealed in the tumblers. The user was to hold the article in his hands keeping the feet flatly on the floor without crossing the legs, or while reclining. This, it was claimed, caused the atoms of the body to expand and bring health through the hands. This article, costing $50, was offered to correct obesity and abnormal thinness due to glandular malfunctioning, correct diarrhea and constipation, reverse the aging process, rejuvenate the user, and cure "any disease known to mankind."

*Source: "Medical Devices Amendments of 1975," Senate Report, 1975.

The "Vrilium Tube" was a small pencil-shaped tube containing a glass vial of a white granular substance (barium chloride) worth one two-thousandths of a cent, but this tiny gadget, also called the "Magic Spike," was sold for $300 to gullible sick people. They were told that it had radioactive powers that would cure disease when it was worn on the body, and these trusting purchasers were using it for cancer, diabetes, leukemia, ulcers and other serious diseases.

One popular area for quack devices has been diagnostic products. During the 1950s, the biggest source of such devices was the Electronic Medical Foundation of San Francisco. On March 16, 1954, an injunction barred shipment in interstate commerce of "Blood Specimen Carriers" for use in the Foundation's diagnostic machine, the "Radioscope." There were estimated to be about 5,000 of the devices throughout the country. The diagnostic service was based upon the theory that any ailment can be diagnosed by measuring enanations from a dried blood spot on sterile paper. Practitioners who mailed in the blood spots taken from their patients received, for a fee, a diagnosis blank filled in with the diseases which the patient was supposed to have, their location in the body, and the recommended "dial settings" for treatment with the Foundation's devices. The blood-spotted paper was put into a slot of the electrical device called the "Radioscope" while the operator stroked with a wand the abdomen of a person holding metal plates connected to the device. If a wand "stuck" to a particular location, that was supposed to be a manifestatiion of an "electronic reaction," and the operator determined from this the identity, kind, location, and significance of any disease present. Investigation disclosed that this diagnostic service was incapable of distinguishing the blood of animals or birds from that of man, or that of the living from the dead. Even a spot of coal-tar dye was reported as indicating systematic toxemia. The Foundation's literature listed hundreds of disease conditions which could be treated by their machines once the diagnoses had been made by means of the "Radioscope." Other devices for which diagnostic as well as therapeutic claims were made were the "Drown Radio Therapeutic Instrument," the "Magnetic Affinitizer," and the "Neuromicrometer." These devices involved their own bizarre intricacies of operation.

30

A considerable number of devices for applying electricity to the body were subject to regulatory action. They included: (1) devices which produced galvanic (direct) current of low voltage by means of dry cells or batteries ("Electreat," "Acme Electric Machine"), (2) devices which used alternating current with a transformer to reduce the voltage ("Sinuothermic," "Elector-Way"), (3) devices in which alternating current was added to galvanic in order to obtain a rippled or pulsating galvanic current ("Facial and Body Genie," "Vitalitone," "Elector-Pulse"). Other devices sought to use radioactivity, ultrasonic energy or infrared or ultraviolet light to diagnose or treat disease.

Some fraudulent devices have been sold to practitioners rather than consumers. One such device as the Micro-Dynameter, a string galvanometer for measuring minute electrical currents which was claimed to be capable of allowing diagnosis of particular diseases based on each disease's electrical potential. Nearly 1,200 units of the product were destroyed during one 12-month period after FDA obtained an injunction against continued shipment of the device in 1963.

Hundreds of consumers bought a device called Relaxicisor during the 1950s and 1960s. This device was represented as an aid in reducing weight and operated by sending shocks through the muscles. Testing revealed the device could aggravate muscular, gastrointestinal, and other disorders. It took FDA five years to complete court proceedings necessary to eliminate Relaxicisors from the market. FDA expended some half-million dollars in this effort.

4
COST OF HEALTH CARE

National Health Expenditures

Figure 4-1   National health expenditures: percent of gross national product, selected fiscal years 1950–75

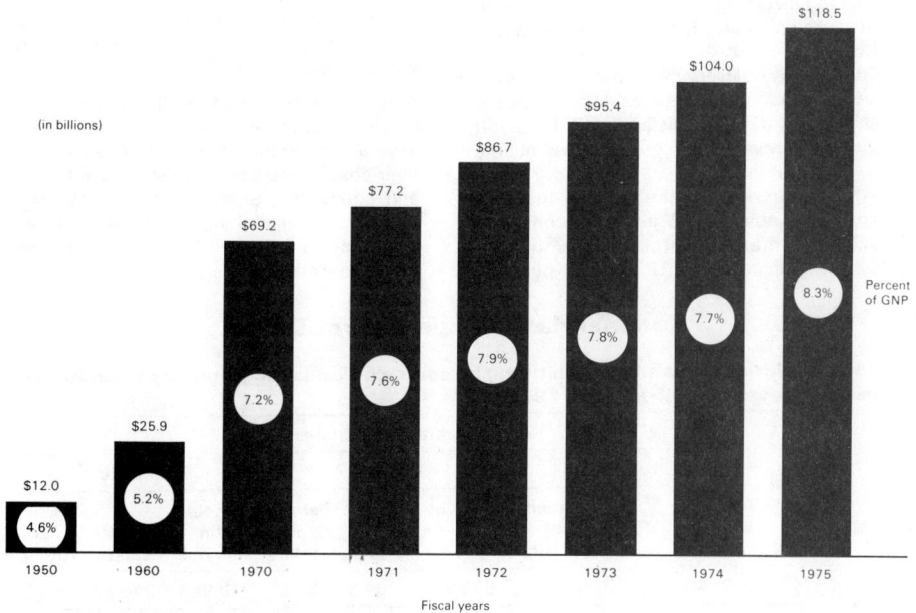

(in billions)

Year	Amount	Percent of GNP
1950	$12.0	4.6%
1960	$25.9	5.2%
1970	$69.2	7.2%
1971	$77.2	7.6%
1972	$86.7	7.9%
1973	$95.4	7.8%
1974	$104.0	7.7%
1975	$118.5	8.3%

Percent of GNP

Fiscal years

Source: U.S. Social Security Administration, 1976.

Factors Affecting Rising Costs of Medical Services*

The following is a summary of research findings concerning escalation of cost of medical services:

*Source: House Appropriations Committee Hearings, 1977.

1. Increased demand for hospital care has led to the offering of a more technologically sophisticated, and more expensive, hospital product. Hospital wages have also evidenced a dramatic catchup in the recent past. Contributing factors have been exist-

32

4

ing biases in existing health insurance and the increasing emphasis on defensive medicine (M. Feldstein).

2. Changes in treatment of selected illnesses (for example, appendicitis, maternity care, myocardial infarction) have tended to be cost-raising; that is, costs have risen more than they would have if prices only had changed (Scitovsky).

3. An increase in collection ratios and/or decrease in free care to the elderly by physicians has been associated with Medicare supplemental insurance benefits (Sloan).

4. Existing insurance is heavily biased in favor of surgical and in-hospital procedures (Sloan).

5. The quantity of services provided per physician appears to decline as prices increase suggesting that physicians will trade off increased revenue for greater leisure time (M. Feldstein).

6. A comparison of the usual–customary–reasonable (UCR) and traditional fee schedule methods of reimbursing physicians indicates that UCR, used by most

private health insurance plans, results in both higher fee levels and faster rates of fee inflation (Sloan).

7. Extended care facilities are complements rather than substitutes for short-term hospitals, and their coverage increases per episode costs (M. Feldstein).

8. While hospital costs increased faster than the Consumer Price Index during 1964–73, inflation did slow appreciably during the period of Cost of Living Council (COLC) regulations. The extent to which this can be ascribed to COLC is not entirely clear, however, since the decline in the hospital inflation rate started in 1970 before COLC was established (Lave).

9. Although certificate-of-need laws have successfully curbed bed expansion, such laws have also prompted hospitals to accelerate their costly investment in services, facilities and equipment. Such programs may tend to increase hospital inpatient costs per day while days and admissions per capita have been reduced (Salkever).

National Health Expenditures Data*

Table 4-1   National health expenditures, by source of funds: aggregate, per capita and percent of gross national product, 1975

| | Gross national product (in billions) | Health expenditures | | | | | | | | | |
| | | Total | | | Private | | | Public | | |
Fiscal year		Amount (in millions)	Per capita	Percent of GNP	Amount (in millions)	Per capita	Percent of total	Amount (in millions)	Per capita	Percent of total
1975	1,424.3	118,500	547.03	8.3	68,552	316.46	57.8	49,948	230.57	42.2

Table 4-2   National health expenditures by type of expenditure and source of funds, 1975 (In millions)

| | | Source of funds | | | | | |
| | | Private | | | Public | | |
Type of expenditure	Total	Total	Consumers	Other	Total	Federal	State and local
Total	$118,500	$68,552	$63,784	$4,768	$49,948	$33,828	$16,119
Health services and supplies	111,250	65,665	63,784	1,881	45,585	30,776	14,808
Hospital care	46,600	20,957	20,413	544	25,643	18,264	7,380
Physicians' services	22,100	16,245	16,230	15	5,855	4,262	1,593
Dentists' services	7,500	7,085	7,085	—	415	255	160

*Source: U.S. Office of Management and Budget, 1976.

Table 4-2 (continued)

Type of expenditure	Total	Private			Public		
		Total	**Consumers**	**Other**	**Total**	**Federal**	**State and local**
Other professional services	2,100	1,591	1,551	40	509	342	167
Drugs and drug sundries	10,600	9,695	9,695	—	905	478	427
Eyeglasses and appliances	2,300	2,198	2,198	—	102	57	45
Nursing-home care	9,000	3,799	3,767	32	5,201	2,982	2,220
Expenses for prepayment and administration	4,593	3,389	2,845	544	1,204	997	207
Government public health activities	3,457	—	—	—	3,457	1,201	2,256
Other health services	3,000	706	—	706	2,294	1,939	355
Research and medical-facilities construction	7,250	2,887	—	2,887	4,363	3,052	1,311
Research	2,750	235	—	235	2,515	2,418	97
Construction	4,500	2,652	—	2,652	1,848	634	1,214
Publicly owned facilities	1,266	—	—	—	1,266	68	1,198
Privately owned facilities	3,234	2,652	—	2,652	582	566	16

Figure 4-2   National health expenditure: health services and source of funds

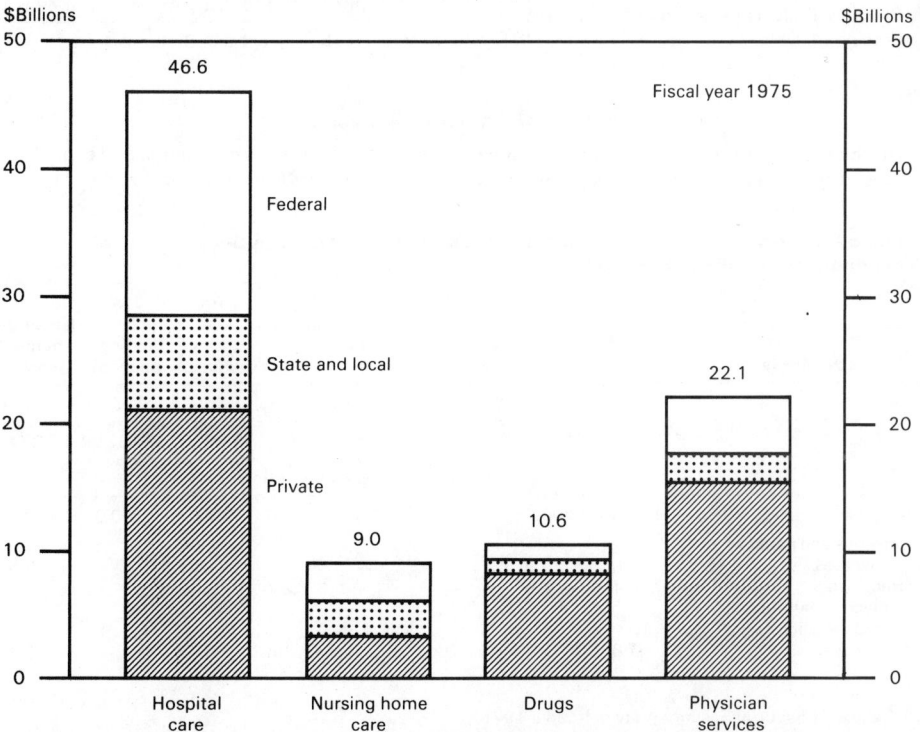

Health Care Cost Index

Table 4-3   Consumer health care cost index—May 1976 (1967 = 100)

Medical care	182.8
Drugs and prescriptions	125.5
Physicians' fees	186.8
Dentists' fees	170.6
Hospital daily services	146.7
Hospital, semiprivate rooms	263.2

Source: U.S. Bureau of Labor Statistics.

Table 4-4   Consumer health care cost index—selected cities or SMSA's (1967 = 100. Annual averages)

City/SMSA	Medical care
City average	168.6
Atlanta, Ga.	183.7
Baltimore, Md.	180.4
Boston, Mass.	166.4
Buffalo, N.Y.	155.3
Chicago, Ill.-Northwestern Ind.	169.1
Cincinnati, Ohio-Ky.	176.7

Table 4-4   (continued)

City/SMSA	Medical care
Cleveland, Ohio	183.0
Dallas, Tex.	162.8
Detroit, Mich.	187.4
Honolulu, Hawaii	164.8
Houston, Tex.	173.7
Kansas City, Mo.-Kans.	160.5
Los Angeles-Long Beach, Calif.	165.7
Milwaukee, Wis.	163.6
Minneapolis-St. Paul, Minn.	159.6
New York, N.Y.-Northeast N.J.	181.0
Philadelphia, Pa.-N.J.	184.3
Pittsburgh, Pa.	162.9
Portland, Oreg.	166.0
St. Louis, Mo.-Ill.	155.9
San Diego, Calif.	161.5
San Francisco-Oakland, Calif.	164.9
Scranton, Pa.	171.2
Seattle, Wash.	158.5
Washington, D.C.-Md.-Va.	179.5

Source: U.S. Bureau of Labor Statistics.

Costs of Specific Illnesses*

The direct cost of illness represents expenditures for prevention, detection, treatment, rehabilitation, research, training, and capital investment in medical facilities.

Table 4-5   Direct costs, selected categories: estimated distribution, by type of expenditure and diagnosis, 1972

Diagnosis	Total	Hospital care	Physi-cians' services	Dentists' services	Other profes-sional services	Drugs and drug sundries	Eye-glasses and ap-pliances	Nursing-home care
				Amount (in millions)				
Total	$75,231	$34,219	$16,916	$5,581	$1,717	$8,628	$1,896	$6,274
				Percentage distribution				
Total	100.0	100.0	100.0	100.0	100.0	100.0	100.0	100.0
Infective and parasitic diseases	1.9	1.9	2.0	—	.3	2.2	—	3.5
Neoplasms	5.1	8.6	3.1	—	2.7	2.2	—	2.5
Endocrine, nutritional, and metabolic diseases	4.6	2.7	7.6	—	1.5	10.0	—	5.2

*Source: U.S. Social Security Administration, 1976.

Table 4-5   (continued)

Diagnosis	Total	Hospital care	Physi- cians' services	Dentists' services	Other profes- sional services	Drugs and drug sundries	Eye- glasses and ap- pliances	Nursing- home care
Diseases of the blood and blood-forming organs	.7	.7	.9	—	.2	.9	—	.5
Mental disorders	9.3	15.4	4.0	—	.5	5.0	—	9.5
Diseases of the nervous system and sense organs	7.9	3.0	7.6	—	38.1	6.9	100.0	7.6
Diseases of the circula- tory system	14.5	15.4	9.9	—	5.0	15.1	—	41.1
Diseases of the respira- tory system	7.9	7.2	10.9	—	1.7	16.9	—	1.9
Diseases of the diges- tive system	14.8	11.7	5.2	100.0	2.5	5.1	—	2.5
Diseases of the geni- tourinary system	5.9	7.9	6.4	—	2.0	6.6	—	1.2
Complications of pregnancy, childbirth, and the puerperium	3.5	6.8	.9	—	2.3	1.0	—	—
Diseases of the skin and subcutaneous tissue	2.0	1.4	3.9	—	.3	4.1	—	.3
Diseases of the mus- culoskeletal system and connective tissue	4.8	4.9	4.6	—	21.4	4.9	—	6.7
Congenital anomalies	.5	.9	.3	—	.2	.1	—	.2
Accidents, poisonings, and violence	6.8	9.2	7.2	—	2.2	4.1	—	9.1
Other	9.8	2.3	25.4	—	18.9	14.7	—	8.3

The indirect costs or loss in output due to disability (morbidity) and premature death (mortality) are the costs to society rather than to the sick individuals or their families. These are not estimated here.

Personal Health Care Expenditures

Table 4-6   Expenditures for personal health care by direct payment and third parties

Fiscal year	Total	Direct pay- ments	Third-party payments			
			Total	Private health insurance	Govern- ment	Philan- thropy and industry
			All ages			
Total amount (in millions)	103,200	33,600	69,600	27,340	40,924	1,337
Per capita amount	476.40	155.11	321.30	126.21	188.92	6.17
Percentage distribution	100.0	32.6	67.4	26.5	39.7	1.3

Table 4-6 (continued)

| Fiscal year | Total | Direct payments | Third-party payments | | | |
			Total	Private health insurance	Government	Philanthropy and industry
			Under age 65			
Total amount (in millions)	72,817	24,890	47,926	25,699	21,007	1,220
Per capita amount	374.79	128.11	246.68	132.28	108.12	6.28
Percentage distribution	100.0	34.2	65.8	35.3	28.8	1.7
			Aged 65 and over			
Total amount (in millions)	30,383	8,709	21,674	1,640	19,917	116
Per capita amount	1,360.16	389.88	970.28	73.44	891.63	5.22
Percentage distribution	100.0	28.7	71.3	5.4	65.6	.4

Source: U.S. Social Security Administration, 1975.

Figure 4-3 Distribution of per capita personal health care expenditures by type of expenditure and source of funds, fiscal year 1975

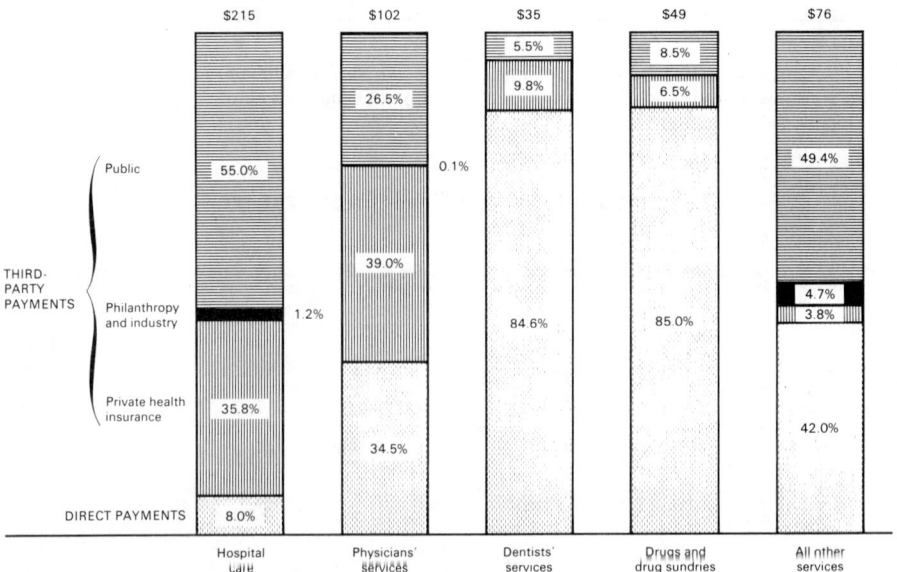

Source: U.S. Social Security Administration, 1976.

Table 4-7 Estimated personal health care expenditures by type of expenditure, source of funds and age group, 1975 (In millions)

	All ages			Under 19			19–64			65 and over		
	Total	Private	Public	Total	Private	Public	Total	Private	Public	Total	Private	Public
Total	$103,200	$62,276	$40,924	$15,406	$11,657	$3,749	$57,411	$40,153	$17,258	$30,383	$10,466	$19,917
Hospital care	46,600	20,957	25,643	5,173	3,063	2,110	27,960	16,515	11,445	13,467	1,379	12,088
Physicians' services	22,100	16,245	5,855	5,083	4,431	652	12,155	9,826	2,329	4,862	1,987	2,875
Dentists' services	7,500	7,085	415	1,545	1,387	158	5,415	5,196	219	540	502	38
Other professional services	2,100	1,591	509	462	378	84	1,197	993	204	441	220	221
Drugs and drug sundries	10,600	9,695	905	2,014	1,893	121	5,957	5,517	440	2,629	2,285	344
Eyeglasses and appliances	2,300	2,198	102	379	365	15	1,415	1,335	80	506	498	8
Nursing-home care	9,000	3,799	5,201	225	139	86	1,125	88	1,037	7,650	3,571	4,079
Other health services	3,000	707	2,293	525	1	524	2,187	682	1,505	288	24	264

Source: U.S. Social Security Administration, 1976.

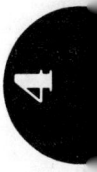

Table 4-8 Estimated per capita personal health care expenditures by type of expenditure, source of funds and age group, 1975

Type of expenditure	All ages			Under 19			19–64			65 and over			65 and over percentage distribution		Public	
	Total	Private	Public	Total	Private	Public	Total	Private	Public	Total	Private	Public	Total	Pri-vate	Medi-care	Other
Total	$476.40	$287.48	$188.92	$212.14	$160.52	$51.62	$471.88	$330.03	$141.85	$1,360.16	$468.53	$891.63	100.0	34.4	42.0	23.5
Hospital care	215.12	96.74	118.38	71.23	42.17	29.05	229.82	135.74	94.07	602.89	61.75	541.14	100.0	10.2	72.2	17.6
Physicians' services	102.02	74.99	27.03	69.99	61.02	8.98	99.91	80.77	19.14	217.66	88.96	128.69	100.0	40.9	54.1	5.1
Dentists' services	34.62	32.71	1.92	21.27	19.10	2.17	44.51	42.71	1.80	24.17	22.45	1.72	100.0	92.9	.0	7.1
Other professional services	9.69	7.35	2.35	6.36	5.21	1.15	9.84	8.17	1.67	19.74	9.83	9.91	100.0	49.8	38.0	12.2
Drugs and drug sundries	48.93	44.76	4.18	27.73	26.07	1.66	48.96	45.35	3.62	117.68	102.30	15.38	100.0	86.9	.0	13.1
Eyeglasses and appliances	10.62	10.15	.47	5.23	5.03	.20	11.63	10.97	.65	22.65	22.29	.36	100.0	98.4	.0	1.6
Nursing-home care	41.55	17.54	24.01	3.10	1.91	1.19	9.25	.73	8.52	342.47	159.88	182.58	100.0	46.7	3.1	50.3
Other health services	13.85	3.26	10.59	7.23	.01	7.22	17.98	5.61	12.37	12.89	1.05	11.84	100.0	3.2	.0	91.8

Source: U.S. Social Security Administration, 1976.

4

Health Insurance

Third Party Payments

Third party payments are those made by private health insurance, government, philanthropy, and industry. The contribution of third parties to personal health care financing—expenditures for health services and supplies—though climbing rapidly in recent years, particularly in government spending, still leaves the consumer with direct out-of-pocket expense for a third of his health care bills. Although third parties accounted for 92 cents of every hospital care dollar spent, the consumer paid directly more than a third of his charges for physicians' services, 85% of his dentist's bills and 85% of his prescription drug costs. Looked at another way, for each insurance claim dollar, 61 cents goes for hospital bills, 31 cents for physicians' services, 3 cents for the dentist, 3 cents for drugs and drug sundries, and the remaining 2 cents for private-duty nursing, vision care, nursing-home care, visiting-nurse service, and other types of care.

Table 4-9   Distribution of personal health care expenditures met by third parties by type of expenditure, 1975

| Type of expenditure | Total | Direct pay-ments | Third-party payments | | | |
			Total	Private health insur-ance	Govern-ment	Philan-thropy and in-dustry
			Aggregate amount (in millions)			
Total $	$103,200	$33,599	$69,601	$27,340	$40,924	$1,337
Total %		32	67	26	40	1
			Per capita amount			
Total	$476.40	$155.10	$321.30	$126.21	$188.92	$6.17
Hospital care	215.12	17.25	197.87	76.99	118.38	2.51
Physicians' services	102.02	35.17	66.85	39.76	27.03	.07
Dentists' services	34.62	29.30	5.32	3.41	1.92	—
Drugs and drug sundries	48.93	41.60	7.34	3.16	4.18	—
All other services[1]	75.71	31.79	43.91	2.90	37.42	3.59

[1]Includes other professional services, eyeglasses and appliances, nursing-home care, and other services not elsewhere classified.

Source: U.S. Social Security Administration, 1976.

Private Health Insurance*

Table 4-10   Private health insurance: percent of population covered, by age and type of care, as of January 1975

Type of service	Percent of civilian population (All ages)	Percent of civilian population (Under age 65)	Percent of civilian population (Aged 65 and over)
Hospital care	77.6	79.9	57.9
Physicians' services:			
Surgical services	75.7	78.3	54.0
In-hospital visits	73.6	77.6	40.3

*U.S. Social Security Administration, 1976.

Table 4-10   (continued)

Type of service	Percent of civilian population (All ages)	Percent of civilian population (Under age 65)	Percent of civilian population (Aged 65 and over)
X-ray and laboratory examinations	72.7	77.5	31.7
Office and home visits	59.4	62.3	35.5
Dental care	15.8	17.4	1.9
Prescribed drugs (out-of-hospital)	67.3	73.2	16.9
Private-duty nursing	67.0	72.9	16.8
Visiting-nurse service	64.9	70.1	21.0
Nursing-home care	33.2	35.2	15.8
HIAA estimates:			
Hospital care	81.6	85.2	51.0
Surgical services	77.2	81.4	41.7

Group Practice Prepayment

Table 4-11   Private health insurance: enrollment under independent group-practice prepayment plans, by type of care, 1974 (In thousands)

	Physicians' services				
Hospital care	Surgical services	In-hospital visits	Office, clinic, or health center	Dental care	Drugs
4,976	5,779	5,424	6,174	997	1,821

Blue Cross/Blue Shield

Background

The first Blue Cross Plan was formed by a group of school teachers in Dallas, Texas, in 1929, ending that year with 1,500 members. Blue Cross nationally now serves more than 80 million persons. In addition, using much of the same systems, people, and facilities, the Blue Cross Association is an intermediary, under contract with government, for Part A of Medicare in all parts of the country as well as for Medicaid, CHAMPUS, and other public programs in a number of states.

Group enrollment covers 72 million Plan members in an estimated 650,000 groups. Another 13 million are enrolled for individual (nongroup) coverage which is available to all persons. Within those totals, 7,860,000 aged persons look to the Plans for Medicare complementary coverage—to pay costs not covered by the federal program.

In addition to their primary role in the private market, Blue Cross and Blue Shield Plans perform intermediary roles for state and federal health programs such as Medicare (for the aged), Medicaid (for the poor or near-poor) and CHAMPUS (for retired members and dependents of active and retired members of the uniformed services).

In these programs, the Plans provide service, in behalf of government, for more than 30 million persons. (Blue Shield Plans provide their intermediary services for 6 million under Medicare; 4,600,000 under Medicaid; and 1,500,000 under CHAMPUS. Blue Cross Plans provide other services to 21,800,000 under Medicare; 6,900,000 under Medicaid; and 4,200,000 under CHAMPUS. The figures cannot be added to a grand total because of overlap in some cases.)

All together, more than 115 million Americans look to Blue Cross and Blue Shield Plans for services and/or benefits of one kind or another.

Manpower

The Blue Cross and Blue Shield organizations are composed of 110 Plans. (There are 74 U.S. Blue Cross Plans and 71 Blue Shield Plans, but in many cases they operate as a single corporation.) In addition to the home office of

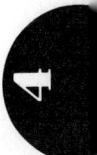

each Plan, there are 400 district and field offices.

Plans are operated by a staff of 73,000 employees, including management, administrative and technical specialties in such areas as electronic data processing, claims administration, actuarial science, subscriber relations, provider relations, marketing, communications, benefit design, statistical analysis, cost containment, research and training.

The Plans paid $11,608,000,000 in claims expense on their private programs in 1974, and another $15,192,000,000 as intermediaries for state and federal programs. Operating expense was $905,900,000, which represented only 7.2% of total income.

Survey of 1975 New Group Health Insurance Plans and Their Coverage

Source: Adapted from *New Group Health Insurance,* Health Insurance Institute, 1975.

Employees w/Health Insurance Coverage

Paid entirely by employer	38%
Employer shared cost	59
Employee paid in full	3

Basic Hospital Expenses

Forty-one percent of the employees were covered for basic hospital expenses. For those covered:

● Daily room and board benefits of $50 or more	34%
● Full coverage for semi-private accommodations	41
● Full coverage for miscellaneous hospital expenses of $500 or more	90

Maximum Number of Days Covered

31 days	29%
70 days	29
120 days	26
180 days and over	10

Basic Surgical Expenses

Forty-six percent of the employees were covered for basic surgical expenses. For those covered:

● Schedules with maximum benefits of $500 or more	84%
● Coverage for reasonable and customary charges	10%

Maximum Surgical Benefit	Percentage of Employees 1975
Less than $300	.4
$300–$399	5.4
$400–$499	10.0
$500–$599	5.8
$600–$999	13.6
$1,000 or more	54.5
Reasonable and customary	10.3

In-Hospital Private Physician Fees

Thirty-seven percent of the employees had medical benefits to help pay in-hospital private physicians' fees, the most common maximum was $5 per visit.

Basic Diagnostic X-ray Coverage (out-of-hospital)

Thirty-two percent had basic diagnostic x-ray coverage. For those covered 98% had benefits of $50 or more. Seventy percent had benefits of $100 or more.

Supplementary Major Medical Expense Coverage

Fifty-one percent of the employees were covered by supplementary major medical expense plans (90% had a $100 single deductible). Seventy percent had full plan benefits for treatment of nervous and mental disorders.

Comprehensive Major Medical Expense Coverage

Thirty-one percent of the employees were covered by comprehensive major medical expense plans:

● an initial deduction of $100	25%
● maximum benefits:	
$25,000 or more	90
$50,000 or more	80
$100,000 or more	70
● Nearly all had some type of daily room and board benefit limit; however, 59% had this limit on private room accommodations only.	
● Benefits for treatment of nervous and mental disorders (includes 80% with full plan benefits)	90%
● Additional room and board benefits for intensive care accommodation	60

Maximum Major Medical Benefit	Percentage of Employees
$20,000	8%
$25,000	5
$25,000–$49,999	1
$50,000	9
$50,001–$99,999	1
$100,000	4
More than $100,000	71

Nursing Home Coverage

Fifty percent of the employees had nursing home or extended care facility coverage. Of those with this coverage:

- Daily room and board benefits of $30 or more (including 4 in 10 with full payment for semiprivate rooms) — 80%
- Over 60 days of nursing home or extended care facility confinement coverage — 50

Dental Coverage

Fifteen percent of the employees had dental coverage. Of this group:

- Dental care integrated with a major medical plan — 30%
- Comprehensive dental plans (of these 1 in 4 had a maximum annual benefit of $1,000 or more or no limit) — 40

Short-Term Disability Income Coverage

Thirty-one percent of those in plans had short term disability coverage. Seventy-five percent of these enjoyed benefits from the first day of total disability due to accident and from the eighth day because of sickness.

- 13-week benefit plans — 30%
- 26-week plans — 60
- 52-week plans or more — 10

Long-Term Disability Income Coverage

Twelve percent of those in plans had long term disability coverage. Of these, benefits are paid:

- after 3 months disability — 60%
- after 6 months disability — 30
- benefits extended to age 65 for both accident and sickness (for group plans of 25–499 employees: 89%) — 60
- average monthly benefit of $400 or more — 60
- average monthly benefits of $600 or more — 30
- maximum available monthly income benefit of $1,000 or more — 94

Intensive Care Benefits

Thirty-four percent of those in group plans had it (usually double the room and board benefit).

Maternity Benefits (Employee & Spouse) — 60%

Continuation or Conversion of Coverage at Retirement — 90%

Medicaid and Medicare

Differences Between Medicaid and Medicare

Medicaid

A. Designed for certain kinds of needy and low income people:
   The aged (65 and over).
   The blind.
   The disabled.
   Members of families with disabled children.
   Some other children.
   Some states also include (at state expense) other needy and low income people.
   Some people can have both Medicaid and Medicare.

Medicare

A. For almost everyone 65 or older whether rich or poor. It also protects disabled people who have received Social Security disability payments for at least two years.

Differences Between Medicaid and Medicare (continued)

Medicaid	*Medicare*
B. Is an assistance program with funds derived from federal, state, and local taxes for eligible people.	B. Is an insurance program with money derived from federal trust funds for insured people.
C. A federal-state partnership which varies from state to state.	C. A federal program which is the same throughout the United States.
D. Medicaid pays for at least these services: Inpatient hospital care. Outpatient hospital services. Other laboratory and x-ray service. Skilled nursing facility service. Physician services. Screening, diagnosis, and treatment of children. Home health care services. Family planning services.	D. Medicare provides basic protection against costs of: Inpatient hospital care. Posthospital extended care. Posthospital home health care.
E. In many states, Medicaid pays for such additional services as dental care, prescribed drugs, eyeglasses, clinic services, intermediate care facility services and other diagnostic, screening, preventive and rehabilitation services.	E. Medicare provides supplemental protection against costs of physician services, medical services and supplies, home health care services, outpatient hospital services and therapy and other services.
F. Is financed by federal and state governments.	F. Medicare hospital insurance is financed by a separate payroll contribution; and the medical insurance is financed by monthly premiums paid by the federal government and the insured person.
G. Is run by state governments within federal guidelines.	G. Is run by the federal government.

Medicaid

Medicaid in 1976 was expected to cost $13 billion. The federal share average—55%. Roughly 25 million Americans received such services and met their state's eligibility rules related to income and resources. All states and territories operate a Medicaid program except for Arizona. Most recipients of Aid to Families with Dependent Children (AFDC) and Supplementary Security Income (SSI) are automatically considered eligible for Medicaid.

Services Covered Under Medicaid

Required

Hospital services (inpatient and outpatient).
Physician services.
Labs and x-ray services.
Skilled nursing facility services for persons over 21.
Screening, diagnosis, and treatment of children (includes outreach and referral services).
Family planning.
Medically related home health care services.
Transportation to necessary medical care.

Optional

Private nursing services.
Clinic services.
Dental services.
Physical therapy.
Drugs.
Intermediate care facility services.
Mental hospital services for persons over 65.
Prosthetic devices, eyeglasses, and hearing aids.
Inpatient psychiatric hospital services for persons under 21.
Other diagnostic, screening, preventive, and rehabilitative services.
Skilled nursing facility services for persons under 21.
Services of other practitioners licensed under state law.

Proportional Expenditures

Figure 4-4   Medicaid services and funds

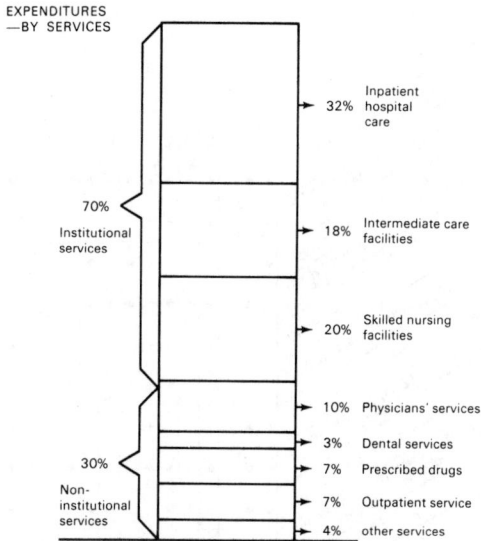

EXPENDITURES
—BY SERVICES

32% Inpatient hospital care

70%

Institutional services

18% Intermediate care facilities

20% Skilled nursing facilities

10% Physicians' services

3% Dental services

30%

7% Prescribed drugs

Non-institutional services

7% Outpatient service

4% other services

Source: DHEW, Nov. 1975.

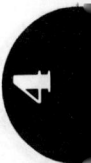

Figure 4-5   Medicaid patients and dollars

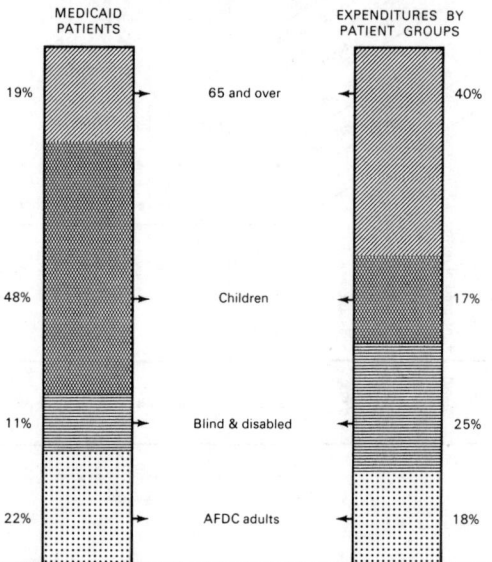

MEDICAID PATIENTS		EXPENDITURES BY PATIENT GROUPS
19%	65 and over	40%
48%	Children	17%
11%	Blind & disabled	25%
22%	AFDC adults	18%

Source: DHEW, Nov. 1975.

Analysis of States' Medicaid Services

Table 4-12 Medicaid Services State by State, June 1, 1976[1]

Services provided only under the Medicare buy-in or the screening and treatment program for individuals under 21 are not shown on this chart.

Definitions and limitations on eligibility and services vary from state to state. Details are available from local welfare offices and state Medicaid agencies.

Legend

- ● offered for people receiving federally supported financial assistance
- + offered also for people in public assistance[2] and SSI[3] categories who are financially eligible for medical but not for financial assistance

Basic* Required Medicaid Services See following page

Additional services for which federal financial participation is available to states under Medicaid.

State	FMAP[4]	Basic Required	Clinic services	Prescribed drugs	Dental services	Prosthetic devices	Eyeglasses	Private duty nursing	Physical therapy and related services	Other diagnostic, screening, preventive and rehabilitative services	Emergency hospital services	Skilled nursing facility services for patients under 21	Optometrists' services	Podiatrists' services	Chiropractors' services	Care for patients 65 or older in institutions for mental diseases	Care for patients 65 or older in institutions for tuberculosis	Care for patients in psychiatric hospitals under 21 / institutional services	Intermediate care facilities
Alabama	74	●	●			●	●			●	●	●				●			● 5
Alaska	50	●				●	●			●	●	●				●			● 5
Arizona	60	+																	
Arkansas	75	+	+	+	+	+		+	+	+	+	+	+	+	+	+	+	+	● 5
California	50	+	+	+	+	+	+	+	+	●	+	+	+	+	+	+	+	+	+ 5
Colorado	55	+	●		●	●		●	+	●	+	+	+	+	+	+	+	+	+ 5
Connecticut	50	+	●	+	●	●	+	●	+	●	+	+	+	+	+	+	+	+	+ 5
Delaware	50	●	+		●	+	●		+	●	+	+	+	+		+			+ 5
D.C.	50	+	+		●	●	●	+	+	+	+	+							● 5
Florida	57	●	●	+	●		●	+	●	●	●				●				● 5
Georgia	66	●	●	●					+	●	+	+			●				● 5
Guam	50	+	+				+		+	+	+	+	+			+	+		
Hawaii	50	+	+	+	+	+	+	+	+	+	+	+	+	+	+	+	+		+
Idaho	68	●	+		●		●	+	+	+	+	+	●	●					● 5
Illinois	50	+	+	+	●	+	●	+	+	●	+	+	+	●	+		+	●	+ 5
Indiana	57	●	●		●		●		●	●	+	+	+	+	●				+ 5
Iowa	57	+	●		●	+	●	+	●	●	+	+	+	●	+	+	+		● 5
Kansas	54	+	+		+	+	+	+	+	●				+	+	+	+	+	+ 5
Kentucky	71	+	+		+		●	+	●	●	+	+	+	●	+				+ 5
Louisiana	72	●	●		●		●		+	●	+	+			●				● 5
Maine	71	+	+		+	+	+	+	+	+	+	+	+		+				● 5
Maryland	50	+	+	+	+	+		+	+	+	+	+	+	+	+	+			+ 5
Massachusetts	50	+	+	+	+			+	+	+	+		+	+	+	+	+	+	+ 5
Michigan	50	+	+	+	+	+	+	+	+	+	+	+	+	+	+	+	+	+	● 5
Minnesota	57	+	+	+	+		+	+	+	+	+	+	+	+	+	+	+		+ 5
Mississippi	78	●	●	●					+	+	+				●				● 5

State FMAP percentages (leftmost data column):

State	FMAP
Missouri	59
Montana	63
Nebraska	56
Nevada	50
New Hampshire	60
New Jersey	50
New Mexico	73
New York	50
North Carolina	68
North Dakota	58
Ohio	54
Oklahoma	67
Oregon	59
Pennsylvania	55
Puerto Rico	50
Rhode Island	57
South Carolina	74
South Dakota	67
Tennessee	70
Texas	64
Utah	70
Vermont	70
Virgin Islands	50
Virginia	58
Washington	54
West Virginia	72
Wisconsin	60
Wyoming	61
Total (●)	21
Total (+)	32
Total	53

*BASIC REQUIRED MEDICAID SERVICES: Every Medicaid program must cover at least these services for at least everyone receiving federally supported financial assistance: inpatient hospital care; outpatient hospital services; other laboratory and x-ray services; skilled nursing facility services and home health services for individuals 21 and older; early and periodic screening, diagnosis, and treatment for individuals under 21; family planning; and physician services. Federal financial participation is also available to states electing to expand their Medicaid programs by covering additional services and/or by including people eligible for medical but not for financial assistance. For the latter group states may offer the services required for financial assistance recipients or may substitute a combination of seven services.

Intermediate Care Facilities (ICF): P.L. 92-223 transferred the ICF program to Medicaid (Title XIX) as an optional service, effective 1-1-72. States may at their option include in-stitutions for the mentally retarded, both public and private. See footnote five.

1 Data from Regional Office reports of characteristics to state programs and state plan amendments.
2 People qualifying as members of families with dependent children (usually families with at least one parent absent or incapacitated).
3 People qualifying as aged, blind, or disabled under the Supplemental Security Income program.
4 FMAP.—Federal Medical Assistance Percentage: Rate of federal financial participation in a state's medical vendor payment expenditures on behalf of individuals and families eligible under Title XIX of the Social Security Act. Percentages, effective from July 1, 1975, through June 30, 1977, are rounded.
5 Including ICF services in institutions for the mentally retarded.

Source: U.S. Social and Rehabilit. Service.

46

Medicare

Program Types and Enrollment

The Medicare program was enacted on July 30, 1965, as Title XVIII—Health Insurance for the Aged—of the Social Security Act.

The program makes available two separate but coordinated insurance programs: hospital insurance, covering nearly all persons reaching age 65 as well as disabled persons under 65 years entitled to disability benefits for at least 24 consecutive months, and covered workers and their dependents with chronic renal disease who require renal dialysis or kidney transplant; and supplementary medical insurance, covering those persons eligible for hospital insurance who voluntarily pay the premiums for medical insurance.

The hospital insurance (HI) program pays for part of the costs of inpatient hospital care and related health care services provided by skilled nursing facilities (formerly termed extended care facilities) and home health agencies following a period of hospitalization. For the services to be covered, they must be provided by institutions and organizations which have been certified as qualified providers of services and which have signed an agreement to participate in the program. An exception exists for hospitals certified under special provisions to provide only emergency services.

Supplementary medical insurance (SMI) pays for physician and other outpatient services.

Table 4-13   Insurance coverage under Medicare: Enrollment by type and age

Type of coverage	Enrollment (in thousands)		
	Total	65 years and over	Under 65 years
Hospital insurance and/or supplementary medical insurance	23,545	21,815	1,731
Hospital insurance	23,301	21,571	1,731
Supplementary medical insurance	22,491	20,921	1,570

Source: Social Security Administration, 1976.

Source of Funds

To be eligible for coverage under SMI, each older person must sign up for the program and pay $6.70 per month ($80.40 per year). In addition, each beneficiary must pay a deductible of the first $60 in doctor bills and outpatient services as well as 20% of all eligible services incurred after the deductible payment is satisfied. (See Table 4-14)

Table 4-14   Medical charges soar: 1965–1975

	1966	1975	Percent Increase
Hospital Insurance (HI)			
Deductible	$40	$92	130%
Co-Insurance			
Hospital			
1st–60th day	None	None	—
61st–90th day	$10 Daily	$23 Daily	130%
Lifetime reserve days	$20	$46	130%
Nursing home/extended care			
1st–20th day	None	None	—
21st–100th day	$5 Daily	$11.50 Daily	130%
Medical Insurance (SMI)			
Premium	$3.00	$6.70	123⅓%
Deductible	$50.00	$60.00	20%
Co-insurance	20%	20%	—

Source: Social Security Administration.

Strong cost control regulations restrict what Medicare will pay the physician to a "reasonable" fee in light of prevailing charges in the area. Any charge in excess of this rate must be absorbed by the older person.*

Medicare is the largest publicly financed health care program. HI is financed largely through Social Security taxes on earnings, while SMI is financed by premiums from enrollees and contributions from general tax revenues. Both insurance components are administered primarily through private insurance companies under contract with the Social Security Administration.

Medicare has increased rapidly in cost in recent years—rising 123% from 1972 to 1977. Estimated outlays of $19.6 billion in 1977 will provide average benefits of nearly $2,200 for the 5.9 million persons receiving HI benefits, and over $400 for the 14.2 million persons receiving SMI benefits.

Coverage

As of January 1975, the number of disabled persons eligible for Medicare hospital insurance had increased to 1.9 million, including 10,000 with renal diseases; 1.7 million of the disabled were also eligible for supplementary medical insurance.

Table 4-15   Medicare coverage, benefits, and administration (dollars in millions)

	1975 actual	1976 estimate	1977 estimate
Hospital insurance (HI):			
Persons with protection (millions)	23.7	24.3	24.9
Beneficiaries receiving services (millions)	5.5	5.7	5.9
Benefit payments	$10,353	$11,869	$12,960
Administrative expenses	$259	$327	$321
Claims received (millions)	10.3	11.9	12.7
Supplementary medical insurance (SMI):			
Persons with protection (millions)	23.3	23.9	24.6
Beneficiaries receiving services (millions)	12.6	13.2	14.2
Benefit payments	$3,765	$4,687	$5,804
Administrative expenses	$405	$550	$561
Claims received (millions)	97.5	107.8	121.1

Utilization and Reimbursement

Table 4-16   Medicare utilization and reimbursement, by geographic region

	North-east	North Central	South	West
Hospital insurance (HI):				
Hospital beds per 1,000 population[1]	4.4	4.8	4.3	3.9
Hospital admissions per 1,000 enrollees[1]	290	350	360	330
Average length of hospital stay (days)[1]	13.9	11.9	10.7	9.2
HI reimbursement per enrollee	$400	$350	$290	$360
Supplementary medical insurance (SMI):				
Physicians per 100,000 population	161	112	109	148
SMI reimbursement per enrollee	$150	$110	$120	$170

[1]Excludes specialty hospitals.   Source: U.S. Office of Management and Budget, 1976.

*Source: *Senate Special Committee on Aging Report,* June 1975.

Although Medicare offers identical benefits to all enrollees, its reimbursements differ substantially in various regions of the country. These differences reflect variations in resource availability, utilization practices, and service costs.

National Health Insurance

Position Paper of
American Association of Colleges
of Nursing

The AACN incorporates the beliefs of the American Nurses' Association regarding National Health Insurance which state:

1. Health care is a basic right of all people.

2. Government has responsibility for assuring through appropriate legislation the accomplishment of this goal just as government has responsibility for assuring that other requirements for physical, mental, and social well-being of people are met such as adequate income, housing, food and education.

3. There should be partnership between government and the private sector to finance the health care system with government providing a stable source of funding for the purchase of comprehensive health insurance coverage for those segments of the population unable to provide for themselves.

4. The federal government should establish national standards governing health insurance coverage so that each citizen is assured equal benefits.

5. There should be integrated health care systems to deliver comprehensive health care services which are available, acceptable and accessible to all people.

6. Integrated systems for delivery of comprehensive health care services for specified population groups should be developed from community health planning mechanisms in which consumers (prosumers) are involved.

7. As a system evolves there should be continuing opportunity for consumers to evaluate its effectiveness in meeting their needs.

8. Comprehensive health care consists of preventive health maintenance, diagnostic and treatment, restorative and protective services.

9. The general educational system of the nation should prepare health manpower for all types in sufficient numbers to provide an acceptable standard of comprehensive health care services.

10. There should be joint planning by all health professions for recruitment, preparation, utilization and compensation for health manpower.

11. There should be professional, intellectual, social and financial incentive to bring about deployment of health manpower to those areas where there is scarce supply.

12. There should continue to be a system of state licensure for the practice of nursing which facilitates interstate movement of qualified nurses and which permits optimum utilization of the professional nursing function in the health care system.

13. There should be provisions within a health care system for the nursing profession to fulfill its function according to established nursing standards and to collaborate with other disciplines in evaluating health care practices.

Anticipated Changes under National Health Insurance*

For a comprehensive program, estimates of increases in the demand for outpatient medical services range up to 25%. Corresponding estimates for manpower requirements range from 2% for allied health workers to 12% for physicians.

Demand for hospital services is not expected to increase significantly and may, in fact, decrease slightly under many of these proposals. Thus, the nation's aggregate supply of short-term hospital beds should be adequate to meet anticipated demand. The supply of dentists, pharmacists, and nurses should be adequate if current growth rates are maintained and if currently inactive professionals are attracted back into the market.

Foreign Countries Having National Health Insurance

Services for segments of population (e.g. workers, aged) or partial services generally available

Afghanistan	Jordan
Algeria	Kenya
Argentina	South Korea
Barbados	Lebanon
Bolivia	Libya
Brazil	Malta
Burma	Mexico
Taiwan (China)	Morocco
Colombia	Nicaragua
Costa Rica	Nigeria
Dominican Republic	Pakistan
Ecuador	Panama
Egypt	Paraguay
El Salvador	Peru
Ghana	Philippines
Greece	Portugal
Guatemala	Senegal
Guinea	Singapore
Guyana	Spain

Haiti	Sri Lanka
Honduras	Tanzania
India	Trinidad & Tobago
Indonesia	Tunisia
Iran	Turkey
Iraq	Upper Volta
Italy	Uruguay
Ivory Coast	Venezuela

Services essentially complete for whole population

Australia	France
Austria	German Democratic
Belgium	Republic*
Canada	Iceland
Chile	Ireland
China (PRC)*	Israel
Cuba	Jamaica*
Cyprus	Japan
East European bloc:*	Kuwait*
Albania	Luxembourg
Bulgaria	Malaysia*
Czechoslovakia	Netherlands
Hungary	New Zealand
Poland	Norway
Romania	Sweden
Yugoslavia	Switzerland
Federal Republic of	USSR*
Germany	United Kingdom
Finland	

* Services provided by national government.

Source: U.S. Social Security Administration, 1974.

Five Comprehensive National Health Insurance Plans*

Before the Carter administration presented its proposals, a number of comprehensive solutions to the nation's health care crisis had been entertained. The five major proposals under discussion at that time are displayed here, with an eye toward simplifying their main points, and the approaches they have adopted.

---

* Source: National Institutes of Health.

* Source: The Health Insurance Institute.

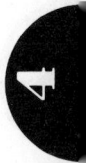

Table 4-17   A descriptive display of five comprehensive

	The benefit	Patient pays
Healthcare (Burleson-McIntyre Proposal) (Developed by Health Insurance Association of America)	Progressively expanding comprehensive coverage including hospital stays; extended care; nursing home treatment; surgery; diagnostic services; general and special physician services; preventive checkups; maternity care; well baby care; prescription drugs; rehabilitation services; dental and visual care; and psychiatric care in and out of hospital.	Patient pays nominal co-payments for hospital, nursing home, home care, physician and surgeon services, drugs, in-hospital psychiatric services. Co-payments for other services range from none for preventive checkups, to 50% for out-of-hospital psychiatric care. For poor and near poor, total co-payments are eliminated or limited by income.
National Health Insurance Standards Program Family Health Insurance Plan (Developed by the Nixon Administration)	Comprehensive coverage including hospital; surgical; extended care; diagnostic workups, general and special physician services; maternity and well-child care; health maintenance services, low income family counselling; vision care for children; acute hospital psychiatric services.	Patient pays first $100 of expenses and cost of first two days of hospital care, plus 25% co-payment on first $5,000 of expense. The $100 deductible is eliminated for well baby care and child vision care. Deductibles as well as co-payments are eliminated for the poor and scaled down for near poor. Part B Medicare monthly premium costs are eliminated.
National Health Security Plan (Kennedy-Griffiths Proposal) (Developed by Committee for National Health Insurance and AFL-CIO)	Immediate comprehensive coverage, including hospital stays; extended care; surgical; general and special physician services; diagnostic workups; preventive care; maternity and well baby care; prescription drugs; rehabilitation services; vision care; dental care for young; psychological and psychiatric services; health and nutrition counselling; prosthetic devices.	Patient pays nothing.
National Health Insurance and Health Services Improvement Program (Developed by Sen. Jacob K. Javits)	Comprehensive medical coverage, including hospital stays; extended care; surgical; diagnostic workups; general and special physician services; annual physical exams; maternity; long term prescription drugs for chronic conditions; dental care for young children; psychiatric care in and out of hospital; medical appliances.	Patient pays first $52 of hospital stay and some co-payments for long term hospitalization and convalescent care. For other services patient pays first $50 plus 20% of the bill. Drug co-payments are limited to $1 per prescription.
Medicredit (Fulton-Hansen Proposal) (Developed by American Medical Association)	Limited comprehensive coverage, including hospital stays; extended care; surgery, radiation therapy, physician services; diagnostic services; preventive checkups; maternity; child well care; psychiatric services in and out of hospital; hospital rehabilitation; catastrophic illness coverage.	Patient pays first $50 per hospital stay, plus nominal co-payments for other services. Patient also pays up to 20% of adjusted gross income before catastrophic illness coverage takes over.

*Several other plans have also been proposed. They include: Minimum Health Benefits and Health Services Distribu- Association; National Health Insurance Plan, sponsored by Rep. Dingle; A catastrophic illness insurance measure de- Insurance Program, introduced by Rep. Hogan.

national health insurance proposals*

Financed by	Underwritten by	The approach
For most, employers and employees will share premium costs. For the poor and near poor, states and federal government will subsidize premium costs up to 100%.	Private carriers regulated by state insurance commissions, except for Medicare benefits.	Establish upgraded benefit standards and provide access to health care financing for all. Phase in benefits to prevent overloading the health care delivery system. Phase poor and near poor into the benefit program faster. Use co-payment system to hold down premium costs and prevent over-utilization. Use grants, loans and other incentives to expand health manpower, to distribute manpower and facilities properly and to create system of comprehensive ambulatory care centers. Absorb Medicaid and supplement Medicare benefits for over 65 population.
Employers and employees will share premium costs with employers eventually paying 75%. Group-rate pools will be set up for state and local government employees, self-employed, small employers and people outside of labor force. For the poor the plan would pay all costs. A sliding scale of subsidies would apply to costs for families with incomes of $3,000 to $5,000. Social Security and Railroad Retirement recipients will be financed through Social Security taxes and Railroad Retirement contributions.	For employed persons, private carriers working under federal regulations. For poor with dependent children—a federal program. For all other poor—the present federal-state Medicaid programs.	Mandate health insurance coverage through the employer-employee mechanism and establish civil court procedures for non-compliance. Establish risk pools for groups not covered by other means. Encourage with grants and loans the development of health maintenance organizations and permit families to elect this type of service. Increase output of health manpower with per-capita grant program to medical-dental training centers. Encourage proper distribution of health personnel under existing incentive legislation. Continue Medicare for aged.
One half with general federal revenues; one half with employer-employee wage taxes, self-employed tax, and tax on unearned income.	Department of Health, Education and Welfare through a federal health security board and state health agencies.	Scrap private health insurance plans and finance costs publicly through new and existing federal taxes. Scrap co-payment system. Absorb Medicare and Medicaid into the new system, to complete federal administration of all health care financing. Encourage group practice and preventive medicine through an incentive system. Establish funds to increase health manpower. Empower HEW secretary to promote proper distribution of health manpower and facilities. No phasing.
General revenues and new Social Security taxes, shared in three equal parts by employers, employees and the federal government. Individuals and employer-employee groups can establish alternative private plans, with benefits equal or superior to the government plan and the financing by employers and employees on a 75%–25% basis.	The Department of Health, Education and Welfare with private carriers as intermediaries. Alternative private plans would be underwritten by private carriers working under HEW guidelines.	Liberalize and extend to the general population provisions of the Medicare Program, retaining the use of private carriers to administer claims. Provide for alternative, or superior plans in the private sector. Encourage organization or comprehensive health care center through incentives. Phase poor, disabled and unemployed into system first, then extend plan to rest of population. Control costs by establishing interplay between private and public systems.
Sliding scale of tax credits based upon income. Poor and near poor would receive assistance through premium payment vouchers.	Private carriers under a national health insurance advisory board, chaired by secretary of Health, Education, and Welfare, and including commissioner of Internal Revenue Service, working through state insurance departments.	Support voluntarily purchased private health insurance premiums for the poor and near poor with payment vouchers. Subsidize these costs for others with a sliding scale of tax credits based upon income. Set minimum federal standards for health insurance plans. Retain present Medicare program for people over 65.

tion and Education Program, sponsored by Sen. Pell and Sen. Mondale; Ameriplan, developed by the American Hospital veloped by Sen. Long; A catastrophic illness insurance measure introduced by Rep. Hall; National Catastrophic Illness

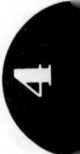

Other Sources of Financial Support

Federal Health Programs

Figure 4-6 Flow of federal health services dollars

($9.2 Billion in Budget Authority in 1976)*

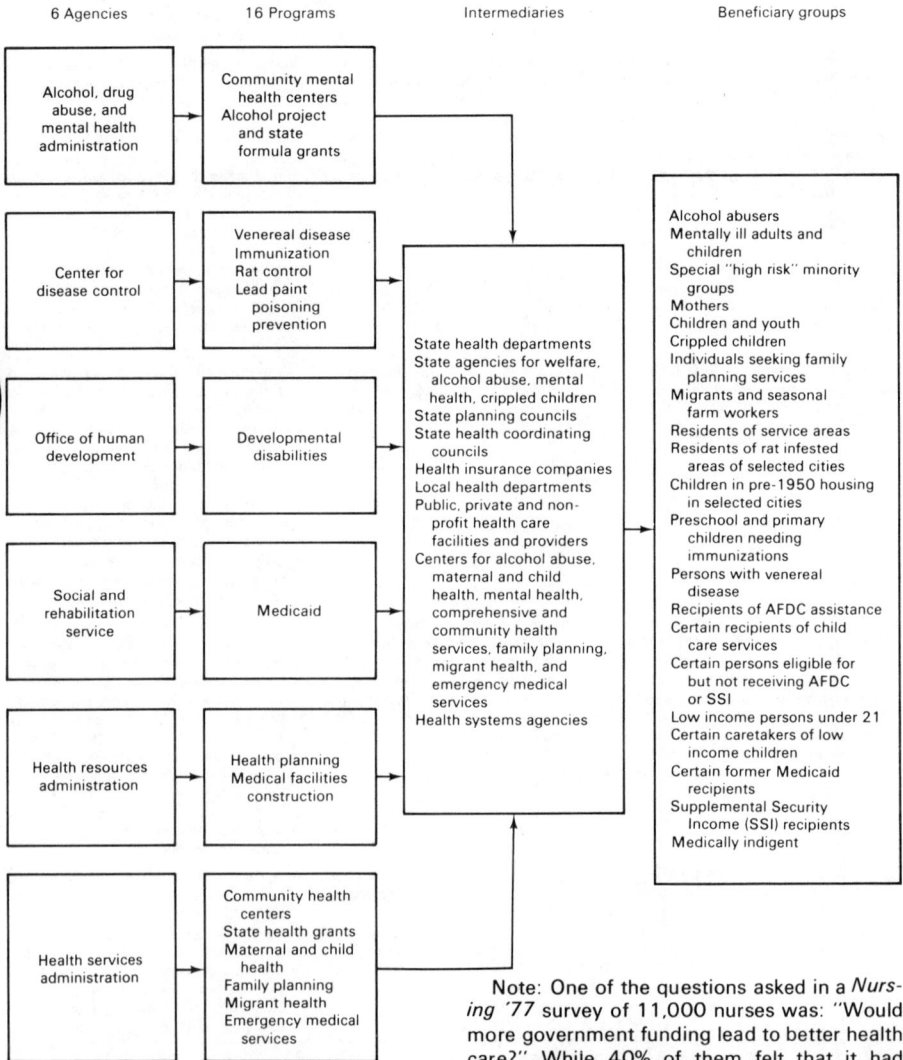

| 6 Agencies | 16 Programs | Intermediaries | Beneficiary groups |

| Alcohol, drug abuse, and mental health administration | Community mental health centers
Alcohol project and state formula grants |

| Center for disease control | Venereal disease
Immunization
Rat control
Lead paint poisoning prevention |

| Office of human development | Developmental disabilities |

| Social and rehabilitation service | Medicaid |

| Health resources administration | Health planning
Medical facilities construction |

| Health services administration | Community health centers
State health grants
Maternal and child health
Family planning
Migrant health
Emergency medical services |

Intermediaries:

State health departments
State agencies for welfare, alcohol abuse, mental health, crippled children
State planning councils
State health coordinating councils
Health insurance companies
Local health departments
Public, private and non-profit health care facilities and providers
Centers for alcohol abuse, maternal and child health, mental health, comprehensive and community health services, family planning, migrant health, and emergency medical services
Health systems agencies

Beneficiary groups:

Alcohol abusers
Mentally ill adults and children
Special "high risk" minority groups
Mothers
Children and youth
Crippled children
Individuals seeking family planning services
Migrants and seasonal farm workers
Residents of service areas
Residents of rat infested areas of selected cities
Children in pre-1950 housing in selected cities
Preschool and primary children needing immunizations
Persons with venereal disease
Recipients of AFDC assistance
Certain recipients of child care services
Certain persons eligible for but not receiving AFDC or SSI
Low income persons under 21
Certain caretakers of low income children
Certain former Medicaid recipients
Supplemental Security Income (SSI) recipients
Medically indigent

*does not include NIH programs.
Source: U.S. Department of Health, Education and Welfare.

Note: One of the questions asked in a *Nursing '77* survey of 11,000 nurses was: "Would more government funding lead to better health care?" While 40% of them felt that it had improved the quality of health care, 33% thought it had lowered the quality of care, and 27% felt that it hadn't made any difference.

Table 4-18   Federal outlays for medical and health-related activities by agency, 1977 (in millions of dollars)

	Health research	Training and education	Construc- tion	Health planning activities	Direct Federal hospital and medical services	Indirect Federal hospital and medical services	Preven- tion and control of health problems	Total
Department of Health, Education, and Welfare (total)	$2,187	$656	$360	$213	$204	$29,634	$531	$33,792
Health Services Administration	2	23	56	10	143	608	104	946
Health Resources Administration	26	388	241	151	—	4	8	819
Alcohol, Drug Abuse, and Mental Health Administration	128	62	27	—	55	343	72	687
Center for Disease Control	38	1	—	—	—	—	88	127
National Institutes of Health	1,955	151	38	—	—	—	44	2,188
Food and Drug Administration	29	—	4	—	—	—	194	227
Assistant Secretary for Health	8	1	1	46	5	8,980	20	9,062
Social Security Administration	—	—	—	—	—	19,646	—	19,646
Social and Rehabilitation Service	1	—	—	1	1	34	—	37
Other HEW	—	30	1	5	—	18	—	53
Department of Defense	125	246	325	—	2,512	585	47	3,841
Veterans Administration	97	271	308	23	3,532	301	—	4,521
Department of Housing and Urban Development	60	—	265	—	—	33	11	308
Department of Agriculture	80	—	5	—	—	—	307	371
Environmental Protection Agency	72	—	—	—	—	—	4	76
National Aeronautics and Space Administration	253	1	19	—	—	—	142	415
Energy Research and Development Administration	6	20	—	17	—	1	99	125
Department of Labor	—	8	—	—	—	—	34	59
Department of State	—	—	—	—	—	1	—	49
National Science Foundation	49	—	—	—	—	—	—	49
Department of the Interior	40	2	2	—	—	9	2	53
Department of Transportation	48	—	1	9	21	—	20	101
Department of Justice	2	14	2	148	26	4	3	37
Other agencies	29	—	15	—	—	37	70	312
Agency contributions to employee health funds	—	—	—	—	—	—	—	1,793
Total outlays for health, 1977	$3,048	$1,217	$1,309	$409	$6,285	$32,396	$1,270	$45,935

Source: U.S. Federal Budget, Fiscal Year 1977.

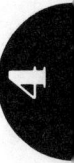

54

Philanthropy & Foundations

In 1975 private philanthropy contributed $730 million for hospital construction; $1260 million for personal health care; $835 million for health agencies; $780 million for endowment; $220 million for medical research.

Foundations contributed $162 million to health related projects, representing 24% of all foundation expenditures.

Table 4-19   Private philanthropy funds: total and health-related—1960 to 1975 (in billions of dollars)

Item	1960	1965	1970	1971	1972	1973	1974	1975
Total	$8.9	$12.2	$19.2	$21.1	$22.7	$23.4	$25.3	$26.9
Health	1.1	2.1	3.1	3.5	3.7	3.8	3.9	4.0

Source: *Statistical Abstracts, USA 1976.*

Table 4-20   Foundations health grants reported, 1972–75 (covers foundations making grants of $10,000 or more in 1972; $5,000 or more thereafter)

Field	Amount (mil. dol.)				Percent			
	1972	1973	1974	1975	1972	1973	1974	1975
Total	$784	$716	$701	$677	$100	$100	$100	$100
Health	131	172	138	162	17	24	20	24

Source: *Statistical Abstracts, USA 1976.*

The Voluntary Health Agency

It has been estimated that over 100,000 voluntary health organizations exist in the United States today.

The voluntary health agency is one that is supported by public donations raised in fund drives rather than by tax moneys. This kind of health organization is unique to the United States and not found in other countries. Its focus is usually delimited to a specific health problem, as exemplified by the American Cancer Society, the American Heart Association, or the United Cerebral Palsy Association.

These agencies often serve to supplement the efforts of the official health agencies of the community. Because they have greater flexibility with regard to their use of funds, they can pioneer in demonstration programs and try new approaches to old problems.

Table 4-21   The National Information Bureau's rough "campaign" tabulation, February 1974

Campaign dates	Organization	Estimates in fiscal year 1973 "campaign income" only
April	American Cancer Society	$ 63,007,000
February	American Heart Association	40,379,000
Nov. 13–Dec. 31	American Lung Association	38,005,000
May	The Arthritis Foundation	8,250,000
Oct.–Dec.	Muscular Dystrophy Associations of America	17,508,000
May	National Association for Mental Health	12,419,000

Table 4-21   (continued)

Campaign dates	Organization	Estimates in fiscal year 1973 "campaign income" only
Nov.	National Association for Retarded Citizens	5,806,000
March 1–Apr. 14	Natl. Easter Seal Soc. for Crippled Child. & Adults	26,000,000
January	The National Foundation (March of Dimes)	40,783,000
May 12–June 16	National Multiple Sclerosis Society	10,130,000
	Planned Parenthood Federation of America	18,400,000
January	United Cerebral Palsy Associations	18,000,000
	Total of 12 National Health Agencies Above	$298,687,000
Fall & March	American National Red Cross	$141,850,000
Fall	Local United Way campaigns in U.S.	$918,000,000

5
MANPOWER AND JOBS FOR NURSES

Overview

The number of active professional nurses (R.N.s) has risen by 50% over the past decade, much more rapidly than population growth. However, more and more nurses are working only part time, thereby dampening somewhat the actual increase in nursing services implied by these large numerical gains. Figure 5-1 gives a graphic display of the decade's changes in the supply of physicians, dentists and nurses.

Figure 5-1   Changes in number of active health personnel

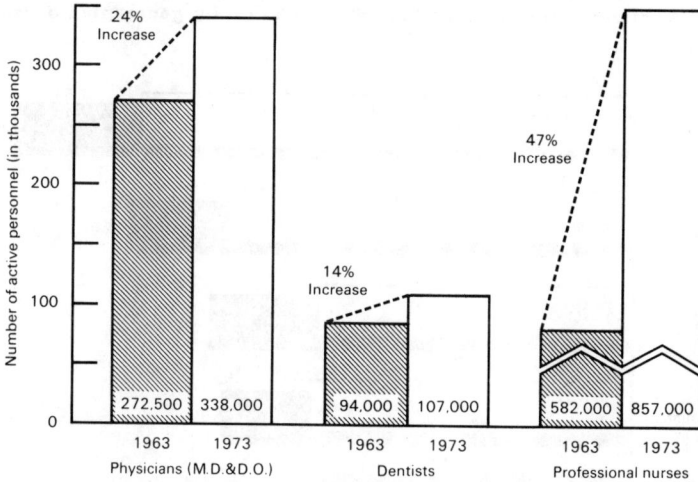

Source: DHEW, Nov. 1975.

Figure 5-2   Active nursing personnel by educational preparation, January 1974

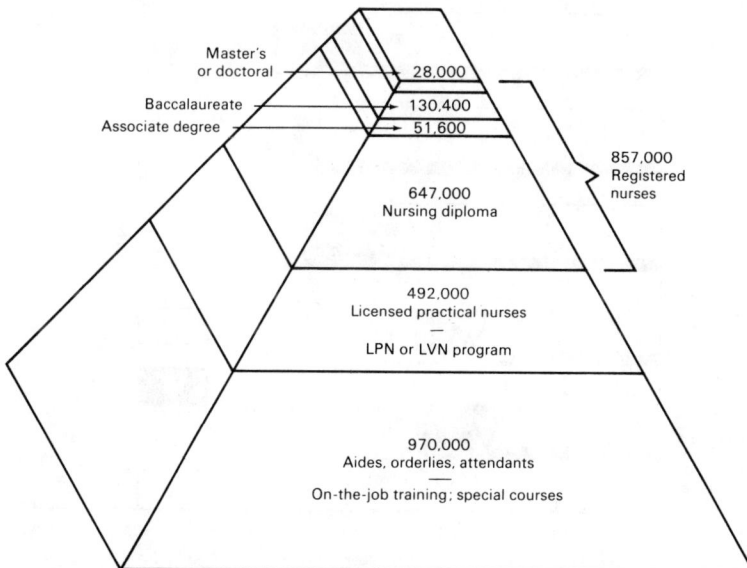

Source: DHEW, 1975.

Nursing salary levels rose sharply in the latter part of the 1960s, making the nursing profession more attractive economically. The employment of registered nurses on a part-time basis also has had a marked influence on the upward trend in nurse supply. In 1960, about 18% of the total were working part time. In 1974 part-time R.N.s represent 29% of the total supply. These nurses have become an integral part of staffing in most fields of nursing employment, particularly in hospitals.

Figure 5-3   Registered nurses per 100,000 population by geographic division: 1962 and 1972

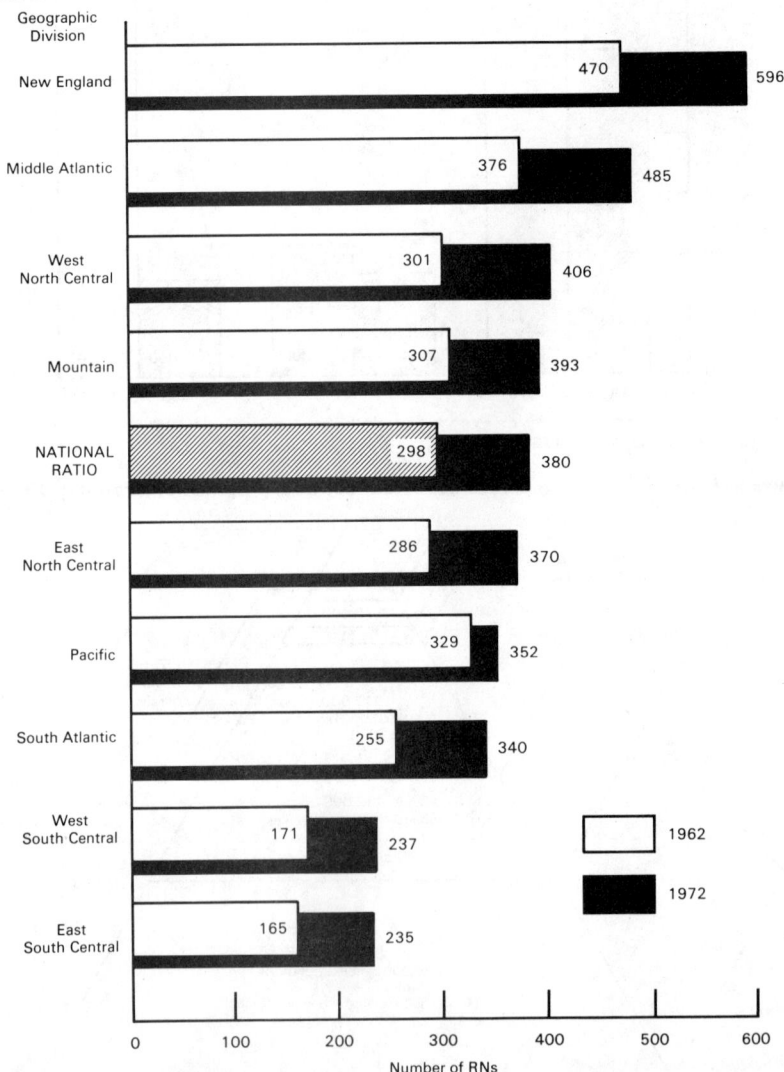

Geographic Division

Geographic Division	1962	1972
New England	470	596
Middle Atlantic	376	485
West North Central	301	406
Mountain	307	393
NATIONAL RATIO	298	380
East North Central	286	370
Pacific	329	352
South Atlantic	255	340
West South Central	171	237
East South Central	165	235

Number of RNs

Source: DHEW, 1975.

The unequal distribution of active registered nurses and licensed practical nurses among the states continues, as shown in Figure 5-3 by the ratios of nurses per 100,000 population.

Even greater variations in nurse–population ratios are evident among counties within states, and among the standard metropolitan statistical areas throughout the nation.

Figure 5-4   Hospitals and nursing homes employ three-fourths of the total RN and LPN supply

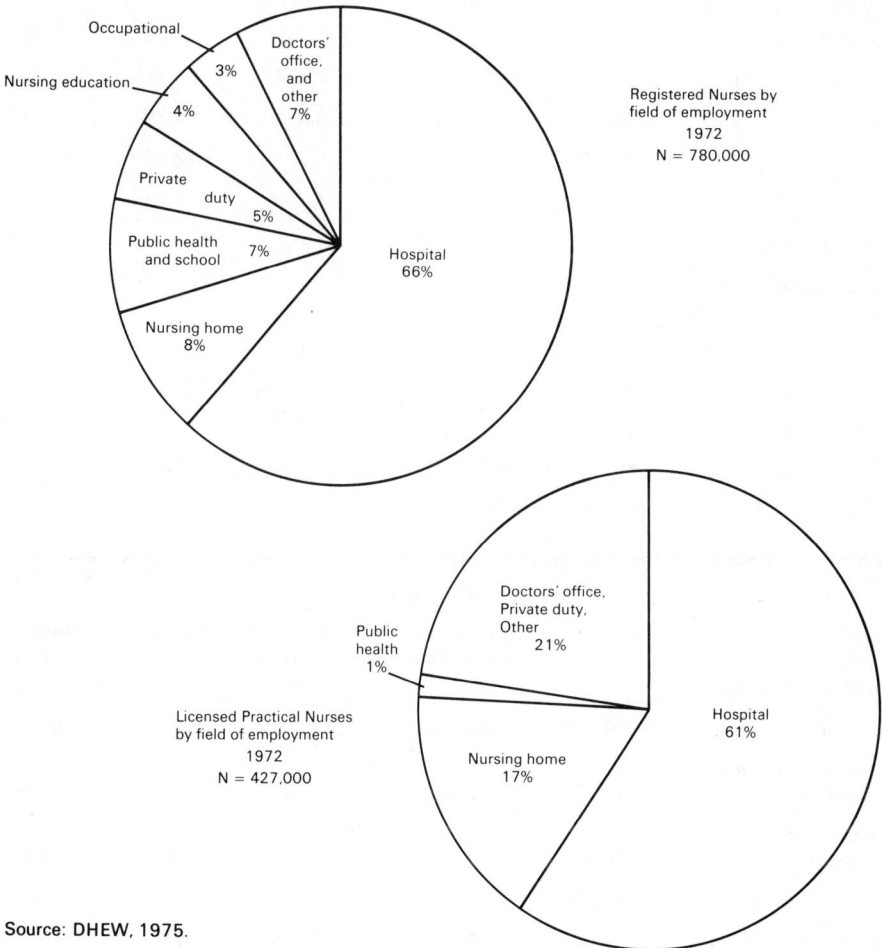

Occupational
3%

Nursing education
4%

Doctors' office, and other
7%

Private duty
5%

Public health and school
7%

Nursing home
8%

Hospital
66%

Registered Nurses by field of employment
1972
N = 780,000

Licensed Practical Nurses by field of employment
1972
N = 427,000

Public health
1%

Doctors' office, Private duty, Other
21%

Nursing home
17%

Hospital
61%

Source: DHEW, 1975.

Hospitals, nursing homes, and related institutions employ nearly three-fourths of all active registered nurses, 78% of licensed practical nurses, and 98% of the nursing aides, orderlies and attendants.

Table 5-1   Active registered nurses by field of practice, by region and state: 1972

	United States	Northeast	North Central	South	West
Total	778,470	248,779	215,198	184,973	129,520
Hospital	499,594	151,285	142,485	120,644	85,180
Nursing home	53,988	20,553	16,161	8,844	8,430
Public health	68,945	24,950	15,137	17,338	11,520
Occupational health	19,403	6,075	6,439	4,652	2,237
Nursing education	28,820	9,522	8,322	7,126	3,850
Private duty	38,923	18,958	5,810	10,263	3,892
Office	52,390	12,357	15,784	12,265	11,984
Other field	4,086	1,031	1,303	1,144	608
Field not reported	12,321	4,048	3,757	2,697	1,819

Source: DHEW, 1974.

Table 5-2   Estimated needs for nursing personnel in 1980 by field of employment

Field of employment	Total	Registered nurses		Licensed practical nurses	Aides, orderlies, attendants
		Baccalaureate and hiCher degree	Diploma and associate degree		
Total	2,800,000	440,000	660,000	700,000	1,000,000
Hospitals and nursing homes	2,240,000	275,000	485,000	530,000	950,000
Public health and school	175,000	70,000	50,000	5,000	50,000
Occupational health	33,000	33,000	—	—	—
Private duty and office	292,000	2,000	125,000	165,000	—
Nursing education	50,000	50,000	—	—	—
Other fields	10,000	10,000	—	—	—

Source: DHEW, 1974.

Table 5-3   Employment status of registered nurses, 1972

Type employment	Number	Percent
Full time	505,201	44.8
Regular part time	159,609	14.1
Irregular part time	78,591	7.0
Full time or part time not known but employed in nursing	35,069	3.1
Not employed in nursing	316,611	28.1
Employment status not known	32,576	2.9
Total	1,127,657	100.0

Source: DHEW, 1975.

Table 5-4   Registered nurses employed part time

Year	Part-time nurses, percent	Year	Part-time nurses, percent
1973	29.1	1967	26.0
1972	29.7	1966	25.0
1971	28.8	1964	22.7
1970	28.7	1962	21.3
1969	27.5	1960	17.9
1968	26.7	1958	16.5

Source: DHEW, 1975.

Table 5-5   U.S. licensure of foreign trained nurses

Year	Estimated first time U.S. licensure of foreign trained nurses[1]	Total first time licenses	Per-centage foreign
1959	2,106	—	—
1960	2,127	—	—
1961	2,111	—	—
1962	2,618	35,312	7.4
1963	2,718	32,080	8.5
1964	3,172	36,088	8.8
1965	3,271	36,432	9.0
1966	3,803	37,466	10.2
1967	5,006	42,499	11.8
1968	5,772	46,456	12.4
1969	4,043	45,708	8.8
1970	4,144	47,010	8.8
1971	4,749	50,171	9.5
1972	6,608	54,682	12.1
1973	6,335	—	—

[1]Values are the sum of first time U.S. licensures of foreign trained nurses by endorsements and the number of foreign trained nurses receiving their license by examination. Some foreign trained nurses obtain their first license by endorsement and are required in another state to take the examination. This results in some double counting and hence, the reported number may be high.

Source: DHEW, 1975.

Table 5-6   Distribution of employed registered nurses by marital status and by sex

	Year	
Classification	1962	1972
Marital status:	Percent	Percent
Married	61.0	68.7
Single	25.6	18.4
Widowed, divorced or separated	11.0	12.0
Not reported	2.4	0.9
Sex:		
Female	98.9	98.5
Male	0.9	1.4
Not reported	0.1	0.1

Source: DHEW, 1975.

Table 5-7   Analysis of all employed registered nurses aged 16 years and over: By selected characteristics and state, 1970

Area	All employed registered nurses, 16 years and over			Place of residence						Negro		Spanish heritage[1]	
				Urban		Rural							
						Farm		Nonfarm					
	Both sexes	Male	Female	Male	Female	Male	Female	Male	Female	Male	Female	Male	Female
United States	829,691	22,332	807,359	18,169	653,210	409	19,274	3,754	134,875	3,318	59,007	1,093	16,275
Alabama	10,588	298	10,290	228	7,677	13	285	57	2,328	49	1,601	—	33
Alaska	940	11	929	5	538	—	—	6	391	—	31	—	21
Arizona	7,419	154	7,265	140	6,472	—	26	14	767	20	135	15	540
Arkansas	5,683	228	5,455	161	3,778	11	275	56	1,402	18	343	—	24
California	86,934	2,986	83,948	2,724	78,864	4	516	258	4,568	379	5,635	401	6,192
Colorado	10,643	172	10,471	161	9,235	—	178	11	1,058	5	247	11	562
Connecticut	17,222	291	16,931	222	13,152	—	87	69	3,692	13	599	—	93
Delaware	2,690	48	2,642	36	2,077	—	33	12	532	4	187	—	14
District of Columbia	3,246	186	3,060	186	3,060	—	—	—	—	161	1,839	—	50
Florida	25,501	769	24,732	661	21,564	15	200	93	2,968	65	1,519	122	751
Georgia	14,673	365	14,308	259	10,164	10	421	96	3,723	83	2,074	19	117
Hawaii	2,915	100	2,815	91	2,529	—	23	9	263	—	17	—	35
Idaho	2,481	65	2,416	43	1,417	7	295	15	704	—	15	—	26
Illinois	43,799	926	42,873	804	37,238	6	1,283	116	4,352	107	3,364	53	623
Indiana	18,387	285	18,102	213	13,049	10	944	62	4,109	27	756	—	98
Iowa	12,009	279	11,730	201	8,341	23	1,424	55	1,965	8	68	—	56
Kansas	9,205	237	8,968	199	6,571	17	649	21	1,748	14	310	30	101
Kentucky	8,843	193	8,650	123	6,263	10	380	60	2,007	6	345	—	48
Louisiana	10,947	281	10,666	226	8,237	7	186	48	2,243	50	1,292	7	194
Maine	5,082	98	4,984	47	3,002	11	120	40	1,862	—	11	—	7
Maryland	16,840	439	16,401	355	13,448	2	182	82	2,771	121	1,921	7	213
Massachusetts	37,000	1,118	35,882	943	30,201	—	105	175	5,576	72	780	16	97
Michigan	32,116	1,180	30,936	798	24,304	27	681	355	5,951	158	2,377	6	241
Minnesota	19,349	415	18,934	313	15,139	29	1,089	73	2,706	8	95	6	81
Mississippi	6,660	137	6,523	94	4,078	—	337	43	2,108	35	778	—	22
Missouri	17,439	511	16,928	417	14,124	17	725	77	2,079	76	1,934	—	129
Montana	2,877	52	2,825	19	1,919	6	114	27	792	—	4	—	20
Nebraska	6,454	179	6,275	138	4,776	13	555	28	944	—	91	—	57
Nevada	1,748	28	1,720	20	1,396	—	23	8	301	—	17	—	43
New Hampshire	4,500	84	4,416	51	2,586	—	60	33	1,770	—	16	—	28
New Jersey	30,997	704	30,293	642	27,263	—	73	62	2,957	172	2,669	—	94
New Mexico	3,320	68	3,252	54	2,651	—	66	14	535	—	36	34	543
New York	85,024	3,163	81,861	2,728	70,017	23	675	412	11,169	861	12,948	115	927
North Carolina	17,565	509	17,056	270	9,990	14	771	225	6,295	115	1,771	5	83
North Dakota	2,624	50	2,574	44	1,699	—	305	6	570	—	14	—	—
Ohio	40,987	629	40,358	488	32,940	28	927	113	6,491	81	2,319	13	245
Oklahoma	8,458	203	8,255	139	6,354	15	387	49	1,514	5	291	7	124
Oregon	8,317	195	8,122	137	6,292	18	283	40	1,547	6	50	6	105
Pennsylvania	55,973	1,228	54,745	970	41,793	—	607	258	12,345	143	2,474	—	26
Rhode Island	4,485	104	4,381	95	3,777	—	5	9	599	—	34	—	34
South Carolina	8,314	123	8,191	108	5,091	—	232	15	2,868	46	895	3	42
South Dakota	2,525	40	2,485	26	1,596	8	317	6	572	—	16	—	23
Tennessee	13,647	443	13,204	323	9,803	23	563	97	2,838	107	1,531	—	90
Texas	39,183	1,308	37,875	1,160	31,787	28	1,071	120	5,017	201	3,419	195	2,888
Utah	3,608	86	3,522	86	3,096	—	33	—	393	—	16	10	61
Vermont	2,711	29	2,682	5	1,184	—	83	24	1,415	—	5	—	23
Virginia	17,948	372	17,576	275	13,173	—	470	97	3,933	74	1,667	5	212
Washington	15,057	333	14,724	294	11,716	—	314	39	2,694	12	251	7	115
West Virginia	5,814	132	5,682	69	3,446	6	92	57	2,144	6	77	—	25
Wisconsin	17,567	457	17,110	351	13,323	—	714	106	3,073	10	139	—	99
Wyoming	1,377	41	1,336	27	1,020	8	90	6	226	—	—	—	23

[1]In 42 states and the District of Columbia, this population is identified as "persons of Spanish language"; in five southwestern states, as "persons of Spanish language or Spanish surname"; and in the three middle Atlantic states, as "persons of Puerto Rican birth or parentage."

Source: U.S. Census Bureau, September 1975.

Jobs Open to Nurses

Note: Other descriptions of nursing jobs can be found in Chapter 6: "Administration" and Chapter 15: "Expanded Role for Nurses."

A registered nurse can work in hospitals, public health, private duty or a variety of other situations. Preparation for licensure may be obtained in a hospital diploma program (two-and-one-half to three years), an associate degree program generally located in junior or community colleges (two years), or a college baccalaureate degree program (four years).

Where Nurses Work

Private Agencies or Institutions
Hospitals, proprietary and nonprofit, general or special
Nursing Homes
Dispensaries, infirmaries, convalescent homes, and foundations
Nonofficial public health nursing organizations
International, national, state and local nurses associations
Religious and missionary associations
Insurance companies
Industrial organizations
   (1) in an employee health service, or
   (2) to promote the use of a product, for example, hospital equipment
Foundations
Specialized clinics
Regional medical planning organizations
Business organizations, such as management consultant firms
Transportation agencies
Nursing Service of the American National Red Cross

Public Agencies or Institutions
International Organizations, such as the World Health Organization
Federal and allied government nursing services
   U.S. Army Nurse Corps
   U.S. Navy Nurse Corps
   U.S. Air Force Nurse Corps
   Public Health Service of the U.S. Department of Health, Education, and Welfare in various divisions and offices
   Veterans Administration Nursing Service
   Children's Bureau, U.S. Department of Health, Education, and Welfare
   U.S. Office of Civil and Defense Mobilization
   U.S. Civil Service Commission, Medical Division

Manpower programs
OEO Health project agencies
Missile Bases
State, county, township and municipal departments and private agencies which are responsible for health or educational work in nursing
Boards of health
Psychiatric and other types of special hospitals
Infirmaries of state institutions for the deaf and the blind
Boards of education
Any health organization or service supported by the state, county, township, or village funds, such as narcotic farms and sanatoria for tuberculosis patients
Combination of official and nonofficial agencies, organizations or institutions
Professional and other health or related organizations

Educational Institutions
Colleges and universities
Associated field centers, such as hospitals and related institutions, public health and other community agencies

Private Service
Private patients cared for at home, in hospitals or in other institutions, and nurse employed through professional nurses registries, or by physician or patient
HMOs

Miscellaneous Positions in Which Nurses Are Sometimes Employed
Airline hostess
Anatomic artist
Assistant to mortician
Author of nursing textbook or other publication
Camp counselor
Dean of women or adviser of girls
Demonstrator of appliances, instruments or food
Editor of a periodical
Executive secretary or field secretary of a health or a social organization, such as
   Heart Association
   Cancer Society
   Red Cross Chapter
   Tuberculosis Association
   Community Chest
   Family Welfare Association
   Council of Social Agencies
   Medicare Agencies

64

Feature writer on nursing subjects
Ghost writer
Health education instructor
Kindergarten worker
Lecturer
Lobbyist
Manager of nurses' clubhouse or hotel
Missionary nurse
Oral hygienist
Personnel or guidance worker
Physical education instructor
Police matron
Probation officer
Promotional educational worker
Publicity specialist
Transport nurse: airline, ship or train
Traveler's-aid counselor
Vocational guidance counselor
Worker with juvenile delinquents
Writer for magazine

For more information on nursing careers write to:

ANA-NLN Nursing Careers Program
American Nurses Association
10 Columbus Circle
New York, N.Y. 10019

Hospital Nursing

Most nurses are employed in hospitals or other related institutions—nursing homes and homes for children, the aged and the chronically or mentally ill.

The hospital nurse normally begins as a general duty nurse, working with all types of patients. From this starting point, the nurse can advance, with further education and experience, to such supervisory positions as head nurse, supervisor, assistant director and director of nursing service. This also is true in clinical practice.

Nursing, like medicine, enables an individual to specialize in an area of particular interest. A pediatric nurse specializes in caring for children ... a psychiatric nurse in caring for the mentally ill or disturbed ... an obstetrical nurse in caring for mothers and their babies. Those entering one of the clinical nursing specialties prepare themselves by obtaining advanced academic training at the master's level in a university.

Some nurses also specialize in caring for patients having specific diseases—cancer, poliomyelitis and tuberculosis, for instance.

General Duty (or Staff) Nurses

Staff nurses constitute the largest single group of nurses. Most provide skilled bedside nursing care and carry out medical treatment plans prescribed by physicians. They may also supervise practical nurses, aides and orderlies. Staff nurses usually work with groups of patients that require similar nursing care. For instance, some nurses work with post-surgery patients; others care for children, the elderly, or the mentally ill.

The general duty nurse utilizes special skill, knowledge, and judgment in observing and reporting the symptoms and condition of the patient; administers highly specialized therapy with complicated equipment; gives medication and notes reactions; maintains records on patient's condition, medication and treatment; assists the physician with treatment; may set up equipment, prepare the patient, etc; may supervise professional and other nursing personnel who are working as members of a nursing team in caring for a group of patients; may spend part-time instructing, supervising or assigning duties to student nurses, practical nurses and nursing aides; may instruct patients and family; may assume some or all the functions of the head nurse in her absence; may bathe and feed acutely ill patients; may take and record temperatures, respiration and pulse.

Operating Room Nurse

Registered nurses who specialize in operating room nursing provide direct care to surgical patients. They work as colleagues in collaboration with other health professionals and assume responsibility for nursing care. The minimal preparation for an operating room nurse is a license to practice as a registered nurse.

Operating room nurse clinicians plan, implement and evaluate patient care and coordinate patient care with other disciplines and other nursing units. They also teach individuals, families or groups in a variety of settings. Nurse clinicians have demonstrated expertise in OR nursing practice. Generally, minimal preparation is the baccalaureate degree in nursing.

Operating room clinical nurse specialists are advanced clinicians with a greater depth of theoretical knowledge, technical skill, and competence in operating room and surgical nursing or a subspecialty of operating room nursing (e.g., orthopedics, neurosurgery).

They work directly with surgical patients and their families, especially in complex situations. Clinical nurse specialists provide care indirectly to the public through guidance and planning of care with patients, nurses, and other health care professionals serving on the surgical team. An operating room clinical nurse specialist holds a master's degree in clinical nursing, preferably with an emphasis in surgical nursing.

Clinical Nurse Specialists

Clinical nurse specialists have a high degree of knowledge, skill, and competence in a specialized area of nursing.

Qualifications for a clinical specialist usually include a master's degree with a major in nursing and considerable experience in clinical care of patients. Working with specific groups of patients she must systematically assess the patient, establish a nursing diagnosis, consider the findings and therapeutic plans of the physician and of others in the health team and delineate the short-term and long-range goals of nursing care. The clinical specialist functions as a consultant to members of nursing teams and to other health workers. She is expected to be informed of scientific progress in her field and in the other health professions and to find appropriate means for incorporating these new findings into her practice.

The National Commission for the Study of Nursing and Nursing Education (*An Abstract for Action,* McGraw-Hill 1970) recommended that personnel policies in all health-care facilities be so designed that they:

1. Differentiate levels of responsibility in accord with the concepts of staff nurse, clinical nurse and master clinician with appropriate intermediate grades. These levels should be designed according to the content of the position and the clinical proficiency required for competent performance.
2. Provide for promotion granted on the basis of acquisition of the knowledge and demonstrated competence to perform in a given position.
3. Develop schedules of substantially increasing salary levels for experienced nurses functioning in clinical capacities.

Team Leaders

A team leader is usually a registered professional nurse who works under the supervision of a head nurse. Other members of the nursing team may include registered nurses, practical nurses, nurse's aides and orderlies. The nursing team is responsible for working with an assigned group of patients and their families in planning for and evaluating the quality and quantity of direct nursing care. The team leader has varying responsibilities, which include direct participation in providing care to selected patients. She supervises other nursing team personnel and assists in planning for and cooperates in the teaching and evaluation of nursing personnel.

Liaison Nurses

The liaison nurse is a relatively new role in nursing service. This position is usually occupied by a registered nurse with a background of education and experience in community health nursing. The liaison nurse assists the nursing staff in identifying nursing needs of patients that will continue following their discharge from the hospital. She also plans and conducts follow-up surveillance after the patient is discharged. She facilitates the coordination of care through referral systems to appropriate community agencies and institutions and cooperates with other hospital-based health professionals.

Other Nursing Jobs

The Nurse Anesthetist

As a key member of the operating team, the nurse anesthetist combines two professions into one, blending professional nursing skill with the science of anesthesia. She administers intravenous, spinal and other anesthetics to render persons insensible to pain during surgical operations, deliveries or other medical and dental procedures: positions patients and administers prescribed anesthetics in accordance with standardized procedures, regulating flow of gases or injecting fluids intravenously or rectally; observes patient's reaction during anesthesia, periodically counting pulse and respiration, taking blood pressure and noting skin color and dilation of pupils; administers oxygen or initiates other emergency measures to prevent surgical shock, asphyxiation or other adverse conditions; informs the physician of patient's condition during anesthesia; records patient's preoperative, operative and postoperative condition, anesthetic and medications administered and related data; may give patient postoperative care as directed.

Overall, 67% of nurse anesthetists are hospital employed, 25% practice in groups, and the remainder (8%) are in a freelance practice.

Of the hospital employed nurse anesthetists, 77% are employed as staff anesthetists; of those that practice in groups, 88% practice in groups composed of both nurse anesthetists and an M.D. anesthetist.

There are three levels of R.N.s providing anesthesia services. The certified registered nurse anesthetist must first engage in the necessary education to become an R.N. and pass the state board examination to be so recognized and then pursue a special course of anesthesia education which now generally requires 2 years of study. Following graduation certification is granted by the American Association of Nurse Anesthetists upon successful completion of a national examination.

The second group is composed of individuals who have taken the necessary education and the state board examination so as to become R.N.s. These R.N.s have pursued the special course in anesthesia education, but have not become certified by the AANA because they either have not taken the examination or passed the examination.

The third group providing anesthesia services is composed of those who have taken the necessary education and passed the state board examination to become an R.N., but have had no special training in anesthesia.

Table 5-8   Who Administers Anesthetics (In percent)

Personnel category	Hospital beds			
	0 to 49	50 to 99	100 to 249	Over 250
C.R.N.A.	67.0	65.0	50.4	42.5
Anesthesiologist	11.0	16.6	35.0	47.5
Medical doctor	16.0	14.0	11.0	7.3
Registered nurse	5.0	4.0	3.0	2.0
Others	.57	.5	.6	.7

Anesthesiologists (M.D.s) are more often located in urban areas, in larger hospitals, and in university settings. C.R.N.A.s function in all types of settings with or without the supervision of anesthesiologists. They provide proportionately more of the anesthesia in smaller hospitals and in rural areas.

In 40% of the hospitals in the United States there are no anesthesiologists. Most Certified Registered Nurse Anesthetists (C.R.N.A.s) are employed by hospitals; and their national average income, based on a 40-hour work week, was $15,338 in 1974. In the same year, the median net income of anesthesiologists was $69,000.

Currently, there are more than 14,000 professionally qualified nurse anesthetists (and an estimated 11,800 anesthesiologists (M.D.s)). Anesthetists work in more than 6,000 community, military service, Public Health Service and Veterans Administration hospitals in the United States.

For more information on nurse anesthetists write to:

American Association of Nurse Anesthetists
Suite 3010, Prudential Plaza
Chicago, Illinois 60601

Camp Nurse

If you plan to take a position in a children's summer camp you should be prepared to deal with the following typical camp illnesses and accidents:*

abrasion	fever
allergies	fractures
asthma	headache
athletes foot	head injury
bites and stings	heat disorders
blisters	home sickness
bruises	impetigo
burns	indigestion
colds	menstrual problems
constipation	nosebleed
corns	pediculous (lice)
diabetes (Mellitus)	pinworms
diarrhea	poison (plants/food)
drowning	pregnancy
drug dependence	prickly heat
earache	ringworm
emotional disturbance	sore throat
enuresis	splinters
epilepsy	sprains
eye injuries	sunburn
fainting	toothache
fatigue	wounds

*For more information, see Mary Hamessey, *Handbook for Camp Nurses* (N.Y.: Tiresias Press, 1976).

Nurse Educator

Since more than 150,000 students enroll each year in schools of professional and practical nursing, many highly qualified nurses are required to prepare them to become expert nurses. These nurse educators teach students the principles of nursing and the skills of nursing through classroom instruction and learning experiences in the clinical area. Some also conduct refresher and in-service courses for nurses. Many of the better-prepared nurse educators are teaching in university graduate programs—both master's and doctorate. The most critical need confronting the nursing profession, in the opinion of most nursing leaders, is for more nurse educators.

A nurse educator is a registered professional nurse who instructs student, professional, or practical nurses in theory and practical aspects of nursing art and science. She assists in planning and preparing curriculum and outline for courses. She lectures to students and demonstrates accepted methods of nursing service, such as carrying out medical and surgical treatments, observing and recording symptoms and applying principles of asepsis and antisepsis. She collaborates with nursing supervisors to supplement classroom training with practical experience in various departments. She renders individual training assistance wherever needed and observes performance of students in actual nursing situations. She may prepare, administer and grade examinations to determine student progress and achievement. A nursing instructor may make recommendations relative to improved teaching and nursing techniques and assist in carrying out hospital in-service training programs by initiating new procedures and practices and training graduate nurses in their application. She may conduct refresher training courses for graduate nurses in theory and practice of general nursing care of clinical specialties. She may train auxiliary workers in administration of nonprofessional aspects of nursing care and teach practical nursing techniques to classes of lay persons.

Gerontological Nurse

This newly emerging field of nursing is concerned not only with the sick geriatrics but with skilled nursing care of those who are well but aged.

There are still few well-qualified nurses who teach or practice gerontologic nursing. A number of geriatric nurse-practitioner programs have been started, but even these are usually taught by faculty qualified in medical/surgical nursing rather than gerontology.

For those who have become specialists in the care of the aged there are a number of career opportunities: serving as high level patient-care managers in nursing homes; assessing patient physical, mental and functional abilities and problems as a supplement to the medical assessment; providing primary-care in senior centers, such as health assessments, treatments, offering health counseling and teaching the elderly self-assessment; acting as independent practitioners; and conducting research in the field of aging.

Nurse-Midwife

The certified nurse-midwife is a registered nurse who has completed additional education in the theory and practice of normal obstetrics, routine gynecology, including family planning and infant care.

The nurse-midwife is qualified to provide prenatal, intrapartum, postpartum and family planning care for the expectant mother. A nurse-midwife works as part of the obstetrical team, consulting the obstetrician whenever there is any deviation from normal.

In 1973, there were an estimated 1,300 nurse-midwives in the United States, most of whom practiced in the eastern part of the country.

Responsibilities—During prenatal care, the nurse-midwife performs the total physical examination of the mother, including breast examination, abdominal palpation, complete pelvic examination and evaluation, and takes the Papanicolaou smear. She provides warmth and support to the woman in labor, encouraging her to participate in the birth process according to her wishes and limits. As long as the course of labor is normal, the nurse-midwife will manage the labor and perform the delivery. The obstetrician to whom she is responsible is consulted whenever there is any deviation from the normal. Any treatments, infusions, and medications such as sedatives and analgesia are prescribed by the nurse-midwife, in accordance with the hospital's approved orders for nurse-midwifery service.

At the time of delivery, if indicated, the nurse-midwife performs a pudendal block or gives a local anesthesia prior to performing an episiotomy. She manages the second and third stages of labor and repairs the episiotomy. She

68

provides immediate care of the newborn, and if necessary performs simple resuscitation. She also gives the official Apgar score and signs the birth certificate. She offers support and reassurance to the delivered mother at times of infant feeding, emphasizing an early positive mother–newborn relationship. She performs the postpartum examinations, and counsels, instructs and administers methods of birth control to mothers seeking help with family planning.

Education and certification—Nurse-midwifery education is offered on the post-R.N. level and the master's degree level. The former program lasts about eight months and leads to a certificate. The latter program is 12 to 24 months long and leads to a certificate in conjunction with a master's degree. Under both programs the preventive components of health care are emphasized.

The American College of Nurse-Midwives administers the certification examination. Upon passing the examination, graduates are entitled to use the official C.N.M. (Certified Nurse-Midwife) after their names.

Currently 18 midwifery educational programs exist in the United States. All are approved by the American College of Nurse-Midwives. Approximately 125 new nurse-midwifery graduates pass the ACNM national certification examination each year.

Scholarships are available to eligible applicants in almost all nurse-midwifery programs. For further information, write to:

American College of Nurse-Midwives
50 East 92nd Street
New York, New York 10028

The license to practice nurse-midwifery is determined by the jurisdiction or state in which the nurse-midwife is employed. Nurse-midwives are now practicing in the following states—Alaska, California, Connecticut, Florida, Georgia, Illinois, Kentucky, Maryland, Mississippi, Missouri, New Mexico, New York, Ohio, Oregon, Pennsylvania, Tennessee, Utah, Vermont and West Virginia, and in Puerto Rico. Legislation is now underway in many other states to encourage the practice of nurse-midwifery.

Types of jobs—You could be employed as a nurse-midwife by a private physician, by a hospital, by a public health agency, or by a health maintenance organization or similar agency. Or you might enter into a partnership with a physician or an incorporated group and be paid on a profit-sharing basis. Most nurse-midwives are salaried professional staff. Salaries vary greatly, but beginning salaries generally range from $13,000 to $16,000. They increase beyond this, of course, with experience.

Many nurse-midwives have used their preparation in nurse-midwifery as background for employment in positions as maternal and child health consultants in federal, state, and local health departments; as supervisors and administrators of maternity care services; in parent education relating to childbirth; as professors and instructors of maternity nursing on all levels of nursing education; and as teachers of nurse-midwifery.

Effectiveness—An example of effectiveness of the nurse-midwife was recently cited in Congressional testimony:

Certified nurse-midwives have improved the health care to mothers and babies in impoverished areas of Mississippi and have reduced both the neonatal and infant mortality rate. Before the initiation of the nurse-midwifery program in 1968, the neonatal mortality rate—death in the first 28 days of life—in Holmes County, Mississippi, was 28.0 deaths per 1,000 live births, whereas in the United States as a whole it was 17.1 per 1,000 live births.

By 1970 this Holmes County rate had fallen to 19.8. The figures from January to November 1971 showed an astonishing 7.0 per 1,000 live births. The infant mortality rate in Holmes County dropped from 39.2 deaths per 1,000 live births prior to initiation of the nurse-midwifery program to 18.8 after 3 years of nurse-midwifery services.

Occupational Health Nurse

To assure that their employees have ready access to basic health protection, many industries and businesses employ occupational health nurses. Sometimes they work alone, or with a physician on call. Often they are public health nurses. In larger organizations they may be part of a health service staff.

Following the instructions of a physician, occupational health nurses treat minor injuries and illnesses, arrange for medical care and offer health counseling to employees. They may assist in health examinations and in giving inoculations. They also keep health records of employees and develop programs designed to prevent or control diseases and accidents among workers.

The occupational health nurse must be willing to accept the concept that the prevention of disease and maintenance of health is as important as the treatment of illness. This necessitates sufficient experience to evaluate an illness or accident, the immediate needs of the employee, as well as possible consequences.

Nursing '76 found that starting salaries for industrial nurses range from $9,175 to $15,977 per year. Salaries and fringe benefits are especially lucrative in large industries such as oil, steel, and automotive.

Education and certification—Continuing education and training geared to the industrial nurse are available through various sources. Perhaps the most valuable is the American Association of Industrial Nurses (79 Madison Ave., New York, N.Y. 10016). State and local chapters of this organization sponsor institutes, workshops, symposia, and conferences on industrial nursing.

Many occupational health nurses seek special training in audiometry, industrial noise monitoring, industrial hygiene, the use of personal protective equipment, toxicology, first aid instruction and organic chemistry.

To obtain certification as an industrial nurse, you must pass an examination administered by the American Board for Occupational Health Nurses (ABOHN). You must have at least five years of experience in industrial nursing and have completed 60 course contact hours in occupational health or related subjects within the past five years to qualify for the exam. ABOHN provides suggested guidelines for self-study to prepare for the examination.

The exam covers the areas of administration, nursing care, illness and injury, physical examination, disease prevention and control and health and safety legislation.

Office Nurse

Many physicians and some dentists require the services of professional nurses in their office practices. The office nurse helps with physical examinations, in giving immunizations and treatment, in caring for and sterilizing instruments and sometimes does secretarial-receptionist and routine laboratory work.

Some doctors have the office nurse take the patient's basic history. Other duties may include: administering injections, dressing wounds and incisions, interpreting physician's instructions to patients, assisting with emergency and minor surgery, keeping records of vital statistics and other pertinent data of the patient, cleaning and sterilizing instruments and equipment and maintaining stocks of supplies.

Profile of office nurse—

● Four of five currently married

● Two of three have children living at home

● One of three work part-time (92 percent of these are married)

● Three of five were employed in hospitals immediately prior to accepting their current positions

Education: 87% diplomas; 7% A.D.s; 6% B.S.s.

Reasons for becoming office nurse— Office nursing is the third largest field for R.N.s with a total of 56,000 working office nurses in 1975.

Convenience of working hours and location were reasons most often given for accepting the office nurse position. Seventy-eight percent were attracted by the working hours and 42% by the location. Eighty-three percent of all those with children at home were attracted by the convenience of the working hours. Ninety percent of the part-time nurses with children at home found this an important reason for accepting the position. The convenience of the location was also somewhat more often given as a reason by all those with children at home when their responses were compared with all the nurses.

Table 5-9   Office nurse annual salary (1973)

	Percent
Total	100.0
Under $5,000	3.5
$5,000–5,999	8.0
$6,000–6,999	19.5
$7,000–7,999	24.0
$8,000–8,999	17.4
$9,000–9,999	7.1
$10,000 and over	7.8
Not determined	12.7

Source: DHEW, March 1975.

Orthopedic Nurse *

If you were an orthopedic nurse, your responsibilities would be divided between the office and the hospital. Your duties would involve administration, recordkeeping, housekeeping (and, most important, patient care).

Patient care duties might include escorting patients from the waiting room to the examining room and making sure they're appropriately attired for the physician's examination. You'd take temperatures, pulses, respirations, and blood pressures as well as patient histories. You'd also administer medications, change dressings, remove sutures, order x-rays, remove bivalve casts, and do any other plaster work needed. You'd assist the physician with application of casts and splints, injections and aspirations, physicals, and other procedures. Since patient teaching opportunities occur with nearly every patient visit, you'd make the most of them. Also, if no physical therapist were available, you'd adjust crutches, instruct patients in gait, and teach them exercises.

In the hospital, your duties on the unit would include making patient rounds (either with the doctor or alone); changing dressings and bivalve casts; removing stitches; and assisting the doctor in keeping patient charts up to date by seeing that orders are signed, progress notes written, operative notes dictated, and so forth. You'd also act as a liaison between the doctor and the hospital unit personnel.

As an orthopedic surgeon's assistant in the OR, you'd assist in all surgery where your assistance is required, see that special equipment is on hand (e.g., camera, special instruments, metal) as needed, see that the patient's x-rays are available from either the office or the hospital x-ray department and provide the hospital with procedure case cards for all operations.

Immediately before surgery, you would check the instruments needed for the case, place the x-rays on the view box, see that the operative area has been scrubbed with pHisoHex, assist the circulating nurse in checking equipment and special supplies and assist in positioning the patient. After the surgery, you'd write the postop orders, note the operation on the progress notes, assist with application of dressings and cast and help transfer the patient to the recovery room bed.

---

*Source: *Nursing '76*, January.

Private Duty Nurse

Representing the second largest employment area of professional nursing is private duty nursing. Engaged at the request of a family or physician, the private duty nurse contracts independently to provide expert bedside nursing care to home patients requiring around-the-clock attention or to hospitalized patients. At a hospital, a private duty nurse may attend several patients needing nursing care, but not requiring constant care. (As more and more hospitals open intensive care units, however, requests for private duty nurses may diminish.)

The private duty nurse: administers medications, treatments, dressings and other nursing services, according to physicians' instructions and the condition of the patient; observes, evaluates and records symptoms; administers independent emergency measures to counteract adverse developments and notifies the physician of the patient's condition; instructs the patient in good health habits; maintains equipment and supplies; may supervise diet when employed in a private home; and may specialize in one field of nursing such as obstetrics, psychiatry or tuberculosis.

Psychiatric Nurse

Psychiatric nurses work with psychologists, social workers, and therapists as part of a team to provide therapy and offer understanding care, usually under the supervision of a psychiatrist or psychiatric nurse clinician.

A psychiatric nurse provides clinical nursing care, is part of the therapeutic milieu, counsels and provides assistance in the planning of treatment, and carries out the administrative and technical aspects associated with nursing.

Psychiatric nurses play an important role in the treatment of mental patients; often they see the patients in more different settings and situations than do the therapists and, hence, may offer emotional support in addition to regular therapy.

For those who desire to go beyond the normal requirements and pursue a master's degree or above in clinical psychiatric nursing, the duties are greatly expanded. For clinical nursing specialists, functions may include individual and group psychotherapy, family therapy, sociotherapy, clinical supervision, administration and direction of staff training programs, or research.

The term psychiatric nurse usually applies to one who has completed advanced training, usually a master's degree in psychiatric-mental health nursing, after completion of a bachelor's degree in nursing. The advanced training requires one or two years.

Beginning nurses in psychiatric settings generally earn from $7,000 to $10,000. Those who have extensive training and experience and occupy administrative, teaching or supervisory positions may earn $15,000 to $20,000.

The Public Health Nurse (Community Health Nurse)

The public (community) health nurse is concerned with preventing illness as well as caring for the ill.

She provides nursing care and counsel to individuals and families, in clinics, in homes, in schools and at work. She also assists in community health education programs involving other nurses, allied health personnel and community groups.

She is employed primarily in local health departments, schools and voluntary agencies such as visiting nurse associations. But she also works in free clinics, health maintenance organizations, health planning agencies, neighborhood health centers and, increasingly, in private practice.

Areas of particular concern in public health nursing include maternal and child health, communicable disease control, chronic illness and rehabilitation, psychiatric care, and nutritional education.

The public health nurse: visits homes to render nursing service and instruct families in care of patients and maintenance of healthful environment; gives specialized treatment, following the physician's instructions, to patients afflicted with mental disorders, physical deformities and communicable diseases; assists persons with social and emotional problems to secure aid through community resources; teaches home nursing, maternal and child care and other subjects related to individual and community welfare; participates in programs to safeguard health of children; assists in preparation of special studies and in research programs; cooperates with families, community agencies and medical personnel to arrange for convalescent care of sick or injured persons and to carry out immunization programs; and may specialize in particular phases of public health nursing such as pediatrics or tuberculosis.

Recently community nurses have been caring for their patients during hospitalization as well as before and after. Community nurses also bring a special perspective into hospital posts as liaison nurses or discharge planners.

Among other developments involving community health nurses, Ruth Spalding in *Professional Nursing* notes:

> Clinical specialties previously bound to institutions are moving more and more into other settings—not only health agencies for ambulatory services but also into non-health settings. Family planning services and abortion counselling have drawn maternity nursing into the community scene. Senior citizen centers provide the setting for a whole new specialty, geriatric nursing. Ambulatory clinics often use specialists in cardiopulmonary nursing to help clients adapt hospital procedures to the home care situation. Psychiatric nurses have moved out of mental hospitals into the burgeoning community mental health field.

School Nurse

The school nurse-teacher is a registered professional nurse, certified to teach health-related subjects, who practices her profession in the school, rather than a clinical setting, one with children who are well rather than ill. The prime focus of her professional practice is on health teaching, health counseling, health consultation, and identifying children with actual or potential health needs (casefinding). Her major responsibilities are (1) helping students and their families to understand and accept the significance of these health needs and to plan and assume responsibility for obtaining the necessary health care; (2) interpretation of the pupil's health needs to the school staff and assisting school personnel to plan and implement all necessary modifications of the educational program for each child. This is accomplished by counseling, conferences and other educational means. Thus, she serves as both a nurse and an educator.

School nurses: assess and evaluate health and developmental status of pupil and interpret their observations for parents, school personnel, and for pupil; interpret results of medical findings concerning pupil for parents, school personnel and for pupil; instruct classes in subjects, such as child care, first aid and home nursing and establish nursing policies to meet emergencies; cooperate with school personnel in identifying and meeting social, emotional and physical needs of school children; administer immunizations and maintain health records of students; recommend modifications in the educational program to administrator when health or developmental status of pupil indicates need for such action; serve as health consultant and resource person in health instruction curriculum planning by providing current scientific information from related fields; use direct health services as vehicle for health counseling; serve as liaison between parent, school, and community in health matters; and serve as a member of placement committee for special educational programs.

Federal Jobs

U.S. Health Service

Within the U.S. Health Services Administration R.N.s work in a broad variety of assignments—general and specialized clinical nursing, public health nursing, occupational health nursing, nursing education, nursing consultation, and nursing administration.

Most of the 2,000 nurses provide direct patient care. Installations vary in size from the extensive facilities of such large hospitals as the U.S. Public Health Service Hospital on Staten Island to small health centers devoted to the care of American Indians and Alaskan natives in remote areas.

Nurses are employed under two systems: the Federal Civil Service and the Commissioned Corps of the U.S. Public Health Service, a uniformed service of the federal government. Most are employed under the Federal Civil Service system. A baccalaureate degree is required for appointment to the Commissioned Corps. Pay and allowances for the corps are the same as for the military services, but you are *not* committed to a specific contract as to the length of your tour of duty.

Health benefits—A choice of various health insurance plans is available, with the government sharing the cost for Civil Service employees. Commissioned officers are entitled to full medical and dental care and hospitalization by the Service. Their eligible dependents qualify for medical benefits.

Education—HSA actively sponsors upward mobility programs for all employees. These opportunities include fully paid long-term support in university courses within degree programs, as well as individual advanced specialty courses.

Travel—Transportation and moving expenses are normally paid to your first and subsequent assignment—AND you may transfer from one location to another without losing health benefits, vacation time or seniority.

Civil Service

Pay scales in most localities are adjusted above the minimum to make them comparable with local salaries. Fringe benefits approximate another third of salary. Appointment grade and salary are based upon education and experience qualifications and upon the level of the position for which you qualify and to which you are assigned. Periodic within-grade salary increases and promotions to higher grades are considered at regular intervals.

Minimum requirements for appointment—

1. United States citizenship;
2. Graduation from an approved school;
3. Physical eligibility.

Salary and allowances—In the Federal Civil Service system, with geographic location; to be competitive with nonfederal hospitals in the area. Periodic increments, Sunday and holiday pay, shift differential, uniform allowances are provided.

Entrance salaries—Depending on qualifications, $7,976–$13,482 per year.

Holiday, vacation and sick leave—Annual leave—Civil Service employees earn from 13 to 26 work days of leave per year, depending on length of service. Civil Service employees are provided 13 work days' sick leave annually.

Benefits—Benefits in the Civil Service System include:

- Premium pay for work on Sundays, holidays and overtime;
- Merit pay increases;
- Low cost health insurance, with premium payments shared by the federal government;
- Low cost group life insurance;
- Retirement plan, with payments shared by the federal government;
- Annual leave of 13–26 work days;
- Sick leave of 13 work days per year;
- Emergency medical care when injured or taken sick in line of duty;

- Transportation expenses to first assignment and for subsequent transfers requested by the service paid by the federal government;
- Employee health service preventive health program at no cost; and
- Cash awards through the employee suggestion program.

Commissioned Corps

A uniformed service—similar to the Army, Navy and Air Force—the Commissioned Corps is comprised largely of professionals in medical and health related fields. Uniquely, an "all officer" corps, it serves as a mobile force to combat disease and hazards to human health.

Qualifications—To qualify, a candidate must:

- Be a U.S. citizen;
- Meet physical standards;
- Have been granted an appropriate academic or professional degree from an approved educational institution;
- Meet educational and other requirements for positions available in the Commissioned Corps.

Selective service—For draft eligibles who qualify for the Commissioned Corps, two years of active duty fulfills obligations under Selective Service.

Career advancement—Through planned Career Development Programs, the service offers opportunity for professional development . . . as well as advancement in the ranks of the Commissioned Corps.

Salaries—Determined by rank and length of service—is similar to that of the Armed Forces. In addition to basic pay, all officers receive tax-free rental and subsistence allowances.

Entrance salary—$12,178 per year without dependents. Commissioned Corps nurses are allowed 30 calendar days of leave annually. Commissioned Corps are granted sick leave as needed.

Benefits—A career in the Commissioned Corps offers unusual professional and personal rewards. It provides a climate of scientific inquiry, application, and achievement, with contemporaries from a variety of other health related disciplines. Pay and allowances are comparable to those of officers of the Armed Forces. In addition, the P.H.S. provides medical care for officers and dependents; tax-free quarters and subsistence allowance; com-missary, post exchange, and officers' club privileges; 30 days annual leave; and other liberal benefits.

U.S. Public Health Service: Agencies and Programs

HEALTH SERVICES
Indian Health Service
Federal Health Programs Service
National Center for Family Planning Services
Maternal and Child Health Service
Community Health Service
National Health Service Corps
Health Maintenance Organization
Quality Assurance
HEALTH RESOURCES
National Center for Health Statistics
National Center for Health Services Research and Development
Regional Medical Programs Service
Health Manpower Education
Comprehensive Health Planning
Health Care Facilities
FOOD AND DRUG
Biologics
Drugs
Foods
Radiological Health
Veterinary Medicine
Regional Operations
National Center for Toxicological Research
CENTER FOR DISEASE CONTROL
National Institute for Occupational Safety and Health
Epidemiology
Laboratories
State Services
Smallpox Eradication Program
Training Program
Tropical Disease Program
National Clearinghouse for Smoking and Health
NATIONAL INSTITUTES OF HEALTH
National Cancer Institute
National Eye Institute
National Heart and Lung Institute
National Institute of Allergy and Infectious Diseases
National Institute of Arthritis and Metabolic Diseases
National Institute of Child Health and Human Development
National Institute of Dental Research
National Institute of Environmental Health Sciences

National Institute of General Medical Sciences

National Institute of Neurological Diseases and Stroke

Research Grants

Research Services

Research Resources

Computer Research and Technology

John E. Fogarty International Center for Advanced Study in the Health Sciences

Clinical Center

National Library of Medicine

ALCOHOL, DRUG ABUSE AND MENTAL HEALTH ADMINISTRATION

Employment Opportunities

VA Hospitals

VA nurses can choose from a variety of work settings. The 171 VA hospitals range in size from 150 to 2,000 beds and are located throughout the country in rural, urban and suburban areas. In addition, the VA offers a competitive salary structure with premium pay for evening, overtime, on call and Sunday duty.

VA nurses earn regular increases and receive periodic consideration for promotion. They generally work a 40-hour week; however, part-time employment is available at many hospitals.

Fringe benefits: VA nurses enjoy a variety of federal benefits including 26 work days of vacation per year, liberal sick leave which may accumulate, life insurance, health insurance, retirement, financial protection and medical treatment for job-related illnesses and injuries, and annual physical examination.

The VA emphasizes a wide variety of learning approaches, technological innovations, and communication systems. These, combined with extensive clinical learning resources, enable each nurse to continue professional growth.

Relocation is possible without any loss in salary, benefits, or career status.

Extensive affiliations: Many VA hospitals are affiliated with the nation's medical and dental schools for internships and residencies, and with schools of nursing for clinical practice. VA nurses practice their professions in a wide variety of settings. Treatment modalities such as intensive care, coronary care, hemodialysis, respiratory care, alcohol and drug treatment, day treatment, epidemiology, extended care, gerontology, spinal cord injury,

nurse administered units, and ambulatory care offer many clinical choices. There are also opportunities for clinical specialists and nurse practitioners, in addition to nurse researchers, educators, and administrators. Opportunities are also available in the fields of nursing administration, education and research.

Requirements: A minimum of a master's degree and three years of responsible nursing practice, and an interest in administration, education or research. For further information, direct inquiries to the Veterans Administration Central Office (111B), Washington, D.C. 20420.

National Health Service Corps

The National Health Service Corps was established in 1971 to improve the delivery of health services to persons living in communities and areas of the United States where health personnel and services are inadequate to meet their health needs. To alleviate the critical health manpower shortage, the corps recruits and places health teams consisting of physicians, dentists, nurses and allied health professionals in shortage areas. The corps seeks to improve health services in communities not only by providing temporary help but principally by helping these areas plan and build their own systems of health care.

Data on every approved community are available through the National Health Service Corps data bank. Each candidate is matched with at least four sites in two regions which most closely resemble preferences expressed by the applicant.

After telephone assessment of all four sites, the applicant has the option of selecting and visiting one of the sites. Based on both applicant and community needs and preferences, the most acceptable match is made.

- In 1975, 551 physicians, dentists, nurses, and other health professionals were placed in 268 communities in 45 states.
- Approximately 85% of the practices are in rural areas with the remainder in urban inner city areas.
- Of the approved sites, 49 are located in rural Appalachia, 31 are migrant health projects, 62 have black populations of at least 25%, 19 have Indian populations of at least 15%, 35 have Spanish-speaking populations of at least 10% and 234 have elderly populations of at least 10%.

Nurse Practitioners

The corps is particularly interested in demonstrating to communities how nurse practitioners may be utilized. Where possible, the corps recruits nurse practitioners locally and gives preference to local nurses for training in the field.

Nurse practitioners must meet the basic nursing education and registration requirements of the states chosen for practice. They may be employed either through the Commissioned Corps or the Civil Service.

Salary rates vary with location, but range from $11,046 to $17,523.

The number of physician extenders has increased steadily since 1972. In 1974, there were 33 nurse practitioners and 11 physician's assistants. By the end of 1975, the corps expects to have nearly 100 in service.

Others

The Regional Medical Programs Service is responsible for assisting local Regional Medical Programs (RMP) to improve health care services to all the residents of their regions. Each of the 56 RMPs constitutes a cooperative arrangement among representatives of the health establishment of each region and includes both providers and recipients of health care.

Authorized by Congress in 1965, Regional Medical Programs are involved with regionalizing resources for the diagnosis and treatment of heart disease, cancer, stroke, kidney disease and related diseases, as well as improving the overall health delivery system.

The Indian Health Service operates 51 hospitals and 77 health centers, located mostly west of the Mississippi and in Alaska. The hospitals range in size from 6 to 307 beds, and 8 have more than 100 beds. About 3,000 beds are provided in the total hospital system. Each hospital has a large outpatient department. Over 2,000,000 visits are made each year to Indian health hospitals and satellite clinics.

The Public Health Service provides medical, psychiatric, surgical, dental, and related services for 21,000 federal prisoners. This health program operates 22 hospitals and 5 dispensaries located in institutions dispersed over the country. These include a 1,000-bed Medical Center for Federal Prisoners, which is located at Springfield, Missouri.

U.S. Armed Forces

All services offer:

- periodic raises in pay;
- comfortable free living quarters or allowance;
- recreational facilities wherever you are stationed;
- sports facilities;
- 30 days paid vacation each year;
- free medical and dental care;
- free hospitalization;
- low cost life insurance;
- travel opportunities;
- $300 initial uniform allowance;
- hospital duty uniforms and free laundering;
- fully paid moving costs when you are transferred, plus travel expenses; and
- shopping at commissaries and post exchanges.

Army Nurse Corps

Army health facilities range in scope from well-baby clinics to out-in-the-community public health care settings to the highly sophisticated wards of intensive care and the newborn nursery. There are more than 100 Army health care facilities throughout the continental United States, Alaska and Hawaii. You may also have the chance to travel and practice clinically in Japan, Germany, Italy, and other countries around the world.

Some nurses further their clinical specialties in areas such as: operating room nursing, intensive care nursing, Army health nursing (public or community health nursing is the civilian equivalent), anesthesia, psychiatric-mental health, midwifery, pediatrics, obstetrics and gynecology, and medical-surgical nursing.

Others participate in in-service programs given at Army hospitals to prepare themselves for administrative positions; nursing methods analyst; even chief of nursing services.

If you are interested in teaching, there is a broad range of opportunities from teaching very basic courses to the most advanced.

Some nurses are selected to pursue an advanced nursing degree, full time, at a civilian university.

New programs: The role of nurse-clinician was created to further the role of the nurse to provide an expanded scope of health care for the patient. The nurse-clinician provides diagnostic, therapeutic, health maintenance and educational services to the community.

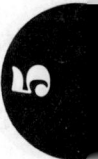

Clinicians may specialize in the following areas: ambulatory care, pediatrics, obstetrics and gynecology, nurse midwifery, psychiatric-mental health, Army health nursing, anesthesia, and infection control.

Rank—advancement—salary: The same salary privileges and opportunities are enjoyed by women and men commissioned in the same rank. Advancement is based on individual performance alone. Performance records are reviewed on a regular basis. If you are a recent graduate of a collegiate program, appointment will be to lieutenant. Nurses with bachelor's or master's degree and additional experience in teaching, supervision or administration may qualify for appointment as a captain or major.

Navy Nurse Corps

There are about 2,500 Navy Nurse Corps officers. They serve in 123 hospitals, dispensaries, schools and other Navy facilities within the United States and at 29 bases in other countries. Navy nurses provide professional nursing care for the men and women of the Navy and Marine Corps and their dependents. In addition, they provide for the teaching, training and supervision of Hospital Corps personnel. Assignments can vary from a five-bed dispensary to a 2,000-bed hospital. In addition, qualified nurses are assigned to research, teaching and administration.

Educational opportunities: Navy Nurse Corps offers comprehensive educational programs. (1) Full-time duty under instruction at civilian colleges and universities to earn baccalaureate degrees, as well as advanced degrees in areas of nursing service administration, nursing education, nursing research and the clinical specialties. (2) Specialty courses in operating room techniques, anesthesia and extended roles in nursing. (3) Nurses are encouraged to attend courses on their off duty time under the Navy's Tuition-Aid Program.

Benefits: Automatic pay increases based on your grade and time in service, liberal policies on paid vacations (30 days a year), housing allowances and retirement. Naval officers are offered medical and dental care, legal assistance, commissary and exchange privileges and the opportunity to travel on military aircraft when space is available or on civilian airlines at reduced fares.

Air Force Nurse Corps

Air Force hospital facilities range from a small outpatient clinic to a 1,100-bed teaching hospital, complete with closed-circuit color television for use in research and training programs.

Assuming that you have graduated from nursing school, you would enter the Air Force as a second lieutenant. Your initial base pay, plus allowances for food and housing, if you live off base, would amount to over $839 a month.

Specialties open to R.N.'s include: coronary care, intensive care, OB-gyn, pediatrics, midwifery, mental health, operating room, anesthesia, medical surgical, aerospace nursing, flight nursing, nurse practitioners.

Benefits: The benefits generally include 30 days of paid vacation each year; full medical and dental care with full pay for the entire time you are unable to work; initial clothing allowance of $300; the more education and experience, the higher your grade when commissioned; and automatic pay increase every two years.

Educational programs: Each year a selected group of career nurse officers are sent to civilian colleges and universities to earn baccalaureate degrees or advanced degrees in clinical nursing administration. In addition, a range of specialty courses is available to career nurse officers. These include: anesthesia, nurse administration, aerospace medicine and nurse midwifery. The flight nurse course, unique to the Air Force, and nurse practitioner courses are also open to those who qualify.

6
NURSING ADMINISTRATION

The Nurses' Views on Administration

Nursing '77 in a survey of 10,000 nurses found that nurses were not exactly enthralled with their administrators and distant supervisors. "Excellent" or "good" ratings were given to the leadership abilities of their *immediate* supervisors by 59% of the nurses, but only 47% rated their nursing service administration that well. Their *overall* administrations were rated positively by 50%.

The nurses had many ideas on improving administration. Among them were:

- Nurses need to be given more responsibility in planning, staffing and determining policies that affect health care.
- Internal audits are too often a whitewash; they should be conducted by a disinterested third party, as financial audits are handled in the banking industry.
- Provide adequate staffing in hospitals so that the few competent nurses there are can assure quality physical and psychological care.
- Hospitals should have some kind of check system to find out if their nurses are competent; if they are incompetent, they should be fired, not shuffled to another floor.
- Revise records, charts and all kinds of forms in cooperation with the medical, nursing, legal, admissions and other related departments to minimize the time spent on unnecessary and repetitive charging.
- The idea of working with a "skeleton staff" on weekends and holidays is ridiculous and should be banned; patient care is an ongoing process—it doesn't suddenly ease off on the weekend.
- Stricter hospital policies for all procedures.
- More staff evaluations of peers and the right to evaluate supervisors.
- More effective use of the health professionals we do have.
- Nurses should be included on most hospital committees.
- Every hospital should have one or more R.N.s in the position of "patient advocate" or ombudsman, to assure that patients receive humane treatment at all times.
- Hiring clerks to cut nurse paperwork, thereby allowing them to spend more time with patients.
- More realistic nurse/patient ratios.*

---

* Source: "Quality of Care," *Nursing '77,* Jan. 1977.

Nursing Administrators—Job Descriptions

Director of Nursing

The director of nursing is a registered professional nurse who directs and supervises all nursing services concerned with care of patients in the hospital. She plans the nursing services needed to achieve the objective of the hospital and is responsible for maintaining such nursing service in accordance with accepted standards. She analyzes and evaluates nursing and related sevices to improve quality of patient care and to plan better utilization of staff time and abilities. She plans and directs the orientation and inservice educational program for nursing personnel. She interprets hospital personnel policies. She administers the budget for the nursing department and may assist in its preparation. The director of nursing may also participate in community health education programs or be responsible for the administration of a school of nursing if such a school is operated by the hospital. She may also delegate any of these responsibilities to an assistant or assume the functions of a supervisor in a small hospital. She often selects and recommends appointment of nursing personnel.

The director of nursing's primary responsibility is not administration of the hospital, nor is she an assistant director who has been delegated responsibility for either nursing service or the school of nursing.

Profile of the Director of Nursing

The most recent comprehensive study of nurse administrators is the 1968 National League for Nursing survey on organizational patterns of nursing service in hospitals. Among the findings were: The ages of the directors ranged from 21 to 77 years, with the median age 48. Eighty-eight percent graduated from diploma schools, 9% were basic baccalaureate graduates. While most had sought education beyond their basic program, slightly less than one-third had earned no academic credential beyond the diploma. Of the 1,172 directors surveyed, 2 had doctorates, 467 (39.8%) had master's, and 310 (26.5%) had bachelor's degrees. About 38% of the directors with master's degrees had majored in nursing service administration; about 34% in nursing education; and about 29% in other fields.

78

Director of Nursing's Functions*

1. **Provide and evaluate nursing service**: to provide and evaluate nursing service for patients and their families in support of medical care as directed by the medical staff and pursuant to the objectives and policies of the hospital.

   Provide nursing service
   Determine patients' basic requirements;
   Determine level of nursing skill required;
   Establish qualifications for personnel;
   Ensure supervision of nursing care.

   Support medical care plans
   Familiarize nursing staff with medical staff organization;
   Participate on committees;
   Work on the patient care committee;
   Foster nurse-physician relationship.

   Evaluate nursing service
   Formulate standards for measuring performance;
   Establish review procedures;
   Design review and report forms.

2. **Define philosophy, objectives, policies and standards**: to define and implement the philosophy, objectives, policies, and standards for nursing care of patients and related nursing services.

   Define the philosophy
   Provide leadership;
   Involve staff;
   Compose a statement of philosophy;
   Obtain acceptance of the philosophy.

   Define objectives
   Establish overall objectives;
   Establish objectives for clinical services;
   Use objectives as an administrative tool.

   Define policies
   Determine the need;
   Set up a policy manual.

   Define standards
   Differentiate between care and service;
   Write nursing care procedures.

   Implement philosophy, objectives, policies, and standards
   Lead;
   Find and develop leaders;
   Inform staff—communicate;
   Involve staff in decision making.

   *Source: Practical Approaches to Effective Functioning of the Department of Nursing Service, 1972. Reprinted by permission of the American Hospital Association.

3. **Provide plan of administrative authority**: to provide and implement a departmental plan of administrative authority that clearly delineates responsibilities and duties of each category of nursing personnel.

   Design a plan of organization
   Pattern control;
   Chart planning and policy structure;
   Plan for interdepartmental communication.

   Differentiate between line and staff responsibility
   Function as staff;
   Advise and counsel medical staff;
   Relate with other departments as staff.

   Delegate authority
   Listen and guide;
   Assign functions.

   Develop job descriptions and classifications
   Use job descriptions to determine function; prepare nursing personnel job descriptions.

4. **Coordinate functions**: to coordinate the functions of the department of nursing service with the functions of all other departments and services of the hospital.

   Know other departments' functions
   Coordinate mutual functions
   Participate in management
   Establish staff-to-staff communication channels
   Inform staff and interpret policies

5. **Estimate department of nursing service requirements**: to estimate the requirements for the department of nursing service and to recommend and implement policies and procedures to maintain an adequate and competent nursing staff.

   Estimate personnel requirements
   Calculate number needed;
   Classify patients;
   Determine time and skill required for patients;
   Analyze and evaluate procedures and assignments.

   Maintain an adequate and competent staff
   Develop a recruitment program;
   Select and assign staff;
   Institute techniques to keep staff;
   Enhance practice of nursing.

6. **Interpret hospital and nursing service objectives:** to provide the means and methods by which the nursing personnel can work with other groups in interpreting the objectives of the hospital and nursing service to the patient and the community.

Maintain standards of service

Share information with patient care agencies
Make agreements with other agencies;
Reassure patients to be transferred;
Exchange information.

Inform nursing personnel about hospital activities

Support volunteer services
Organize the volunteers;
Establish functions;
Instruct the volunteers.

Work with news media

7. **Formulate personnel policies:** to participate in the formulation of personnel policies, to implement established policies and evaluate their effectiveness.

Establish employment policies

Establish administrative procedures

Develop staff trained in personnel techniques

Maintain records

8. **Develop nursing records:** to develop and maintain an effective system of clinical and administrative nursing records and reports.

Develop and maintain nursing care plans and clinical records
Establish nursing care plans;
Document clinical data on patient records.

Maintain administrative records

Maintain nursing department records

9. **Estimate needs for facilities, supplies and equipment:** to estimate needs for facilities, supplies and equipment, and implement a system for evaluation and control.

Estimate needs
Analyze program and service needs;
Record usage.

Implement a system of evaluation and control
Establish a system for selection, procurement and control;
Appraise use of disposable supplies.

10. **Participate in financial planning:** to participate in and adhere to the financial plan of operation for the hospital.

Determine departmental needs

Prepare departmental budget

Control the budget

11. **Participate in studies and research projects:** to initiate, utilize, and participate in studies and research projects designed for the improvement of patient care and the improvement of other administrative and hospital services.

Participate in clinical research
Determine degree of involvement;
Safeguard the patient.

Participate in administrative studies
Assess the problem;
Inform the staff.

Initiate studies

12. **Provide continuing education:** to provide and implement a program of continuing education for all nursing personnel.

Provide an orientation program
Plan orientation to the hospital;
Plan orientation to the nursing department;
Plan induction into the specific job.

Provide a continuing education program

13. **Participate in educational programs:** to participate in and facilitate all educational programs that include student experience in the department of nursing service.

Establish and maintain relationships

Provide clinical facilities for a collaborative program

Provide essentials

Support the programs

Peer Evaluation Factors for a Director of Nursing Service *

General Standards—

1. The standard setting for nursing service, not interrelated service, is 100% under control of the Nursing Department.
2. The results of the problem-identification and decision-making processes utilized in nursing go to the highest level of the hos-

---

* Source: *Quality Assessment and Patient Care,* NLN Division of Community Planning, 1975 (Pub. No. 52–572).

pital administrative echelon for action upon recommendations.
3. Staffing standards indicate patient acuity need related to staff level assignment.

Performance Factors—
What evidence is there that the Director of Nursing Service is functioning well?

1. Staff development—In-Service Education in the facility is actively planned, implemented and outcomes measured and documented.
   - Orientation for new staff to new type of job
   - A reward system exists for staff in regard to participation: recognition given, encouraged and supported involvement in continuing education seminars: director values staff and sends staff, not just self, to pertinent programs.
2. Position in organization in top management
   - Makes decision for patient care by direct input to administrative policy making body (group)
   - Responsibility/Authority/Accountability in position evidenced by documented participation in decision-making policy setting
3. A nursing audit is in effect
   - Patient comfort a concern
   - Patients speak well of care
   - Professional outcomes monitored
4. Interpersonal relations with nursing staff
   - Planned meetings with staff
   - Staff know Director of Nursing, i.e., can identify him/her
   - Expectations for staff performance included in the evaluation process
5. Forecasting trends of patient population to plan to deal with actual problems or potential problems
   - Studies population served and makes attempts to learn client's culture, value system and expectations of health care delivery services
   - Profiles nurses available, their cultures and values and tries to match both
6. Fiscally responsible
   - Quantitative measurement system existent
   - Establishes norms of productivity
   - Regular budget review—annual, other hospital annual

   - Equal management input regarding budget planning
7. Active support and staff support of educational programs
   - Nursing students
   - Community teaching programs for health according to client population
8. Evidence of patient discharge planning and referral
9. Has established a system of support and rescue to facilitate risk taking by staff
10. Has established a climate for growth, risk taking
11. Active in self continuing education
    - Knowledge of systems
    - How system works?
    - How it interdigitates?
    - Using power constructively?
    - How does power structure work?
    - Politically astute
    - Communication system?
      How measure effect?
      What parameters to set?
    - Clinical knowledge
      What kind?
      How current in regard to depth?
      Other factors?

Example of Development of Indicators for a Factor (Criterion)—
Director is educationally oriented

- Has system for orientation, staff development
- Community health training program
- Match staff to jobs
- Publicize what is being presented
- Patient education program
- Who goes to in-service programs?

Nurse Supervisor

Functions

The supervisor of nursing service is usually a professional registered nurse who is responsible for nursing care in a hospital area that involves one or more patient units, each of which has a head nurse. Nursing supervisors are also assigned to such areas as the operating room, the outpatient department, the recovery room, and special or intensive care units. Supervisors generally participate with the director of nursing in the development and implementation of the philosophy and objectives for nursing service. They are usually involved in the development and control of budgets, the selection of supplies and equipment, and the arrangement and design of physical facilities within their assigned area of work. Nursing supervisors assist in planning with other departments within a health agency and are involved in the coordination of activities and services that contribute to the physical environment and to patient care. A nursing supervisor is usually responsible for planning the kind and amount of patient care; that is, staffing, analyzing, evaluating, and revising nursing services as needed. Supervisors are often involved in the evaluation of nursing employee performance and usually take active part in staff development and in-service education programs.

Qualifications *

The beginning supervisor should:

- Have at least five years experience as a head nurse;
- Be intelligent, capable of learning readily and of retaining the knowledge;
- Be able to convey knowledge to others in an understanding and interesting way;
- Be tolerant and understanding;
- Be objective;
- Be able, when necessary, to show authority without being too demanding and without losing the respect of subordinates;
- Have self confidence and be able to gain the confidence of others;
- Have good physical and mental health;
- Be able to promote good public relations;
- Keep up with new trends in nursing and be able to convey this information to others;
- Be able to do new procedures and to use new equipment (as well as older methods) and to instruct others with clarity.

Responsibilities *

- Maintain interest in good nursing care;
- Know administrative regulations of the general hospital and how they apply to you and your coworkers;
- Be a good listener and a sounding board;
- Be able to make sound judgments with confidence in your choices. When you are sure you are right, proceed;
- Give support where needed and a helping hand at times. Let your personnel know you

---

*Source: Betty J. Robinson, "Supervision As I See It," *Supervisor Nurse*, Oct. 1974.

are interested in their work and are willing to help when necessary;
- Be objective. Have an open mind to suggestions given by others. Try the good ones. Give explanations when suggestions cannot be accepted;
- A pleasant and understanding nature is valuable in gaining the confidence of your subordinates;
- Cooperation between coworkers and shifts is most important if you want a smooth running institution. It is your job to set the climate;
- Know your help, whom you can rely on, who needs prodding;
- Know the case load and the type of patients on each unit. Be ready to place extra help where needed;
- Keep your personnel occupied and there will be less strain on all concerned.

Head Nurse

Responsibilities

A head nurse is a registered professional nurse who is usually responsible for the direct and indirect nursing care of patients within an organized unit of a clinical area, such as surgery, medicine, or pediatrics, or a specialized unit, such as the nursery, tumor clinic in the outpatient department, coronary care unit, or the emergency room.

The head nurse assigns patient care duties to (professional and nonprofessional) nursing personnel and supervises and evaluates work performance. She periodically visits patients to insure optimal care and to ascertain need for additional or modified services. She supervises the execution of doctors' orders and related treatments and the maintenance of nursing records. She assists in the orientation of new personnel to the unit, and insures the availability of supplies and equipment. She identifies nursing service problems and assists in their solution. The head nurse may also give direct nursing care in selected situations (i.e., performs duties of general duty nurse), and assist in the in-service education and guidance of nursing personnel. She may spend part of her time supervising or instructing student nurses. She may also be responsible for ward 24 hours a day in the sense that evening and night nurses report to her and she is responsible for assigning duties on other shifts.

Time and Activities

Figure 6-1   Head Nurse: percent of time spent in various functions in typical hospital*

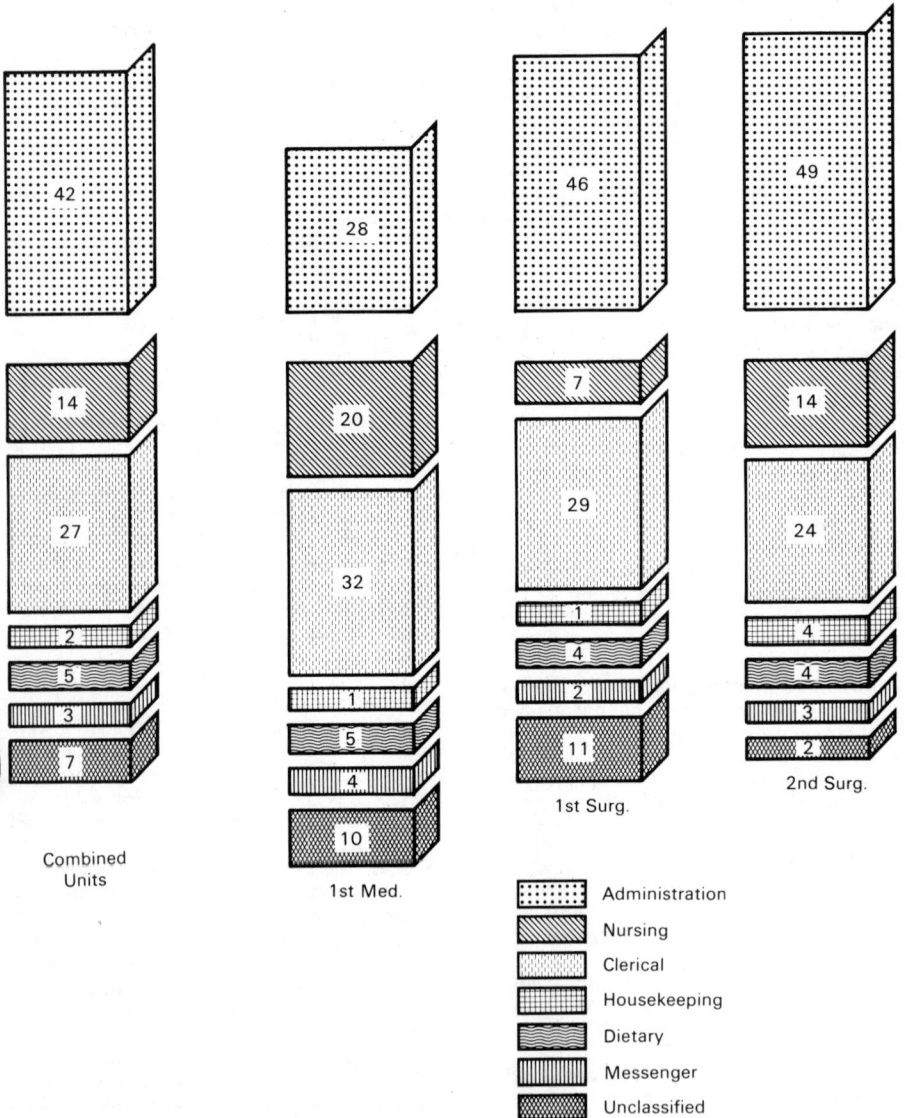

Combined
Units

1st Med.

1st Surg.

2nd Surg.

Administration

Nursing

Clerical

Housekeeping

Dietary

Messenger

Unclassified

*Source: DHEW, 1964.

Unit Manager

Concept of Responsibilities

To various extents in different institutions, unit managers have assumed responsibility for clerical tasks, equipment and supplies, budgeting, coordination with other departments, and sometimes staffing and other administrative responsibilities.

When the unit manager concept first came into vogue, most of the unit managers were trained inside hospitals. More recently, however, associate degree programs have been developed to provide formal two-year hospital unit-management education. As in schools of nursing, students take courses in liberal arts and their particular specialty and receive on-the-job training.

The unit manager provides the administrative direction of the patient unit, while forming a working partnership with the nurse who supervises the nursing practice. He can be responsible either to the administration or the nursing department.

The nonnursing functions for which the unit manager may have responsibility fall into five major categories:*

1. Coordination of related services and departments, for example, requests of housekeeping or of the dietary division
2. Maintenance of satisfactory physical environment of the patient division
3. Maintenance of equipment and supplies, including evaluation and ordering of new equipment
4. Personnel services, which may include scheduling of all staff
5. Direct supervision of and responsibility for nonprofessional nursing staff

History

The unit manager system can be traced back to 1948, when a New York hospital developed it for the purpose of relieving the professional nurse of nonnursing functions and for the provision of hospital management at the unit level. The concept of the unit manager system in the United States has been spreading rapidly: 1960, 3 hospitals; 1965, 20 hospitals; 1970, 170 hospitals.

Patient-Care Benefits

The National Commission for the Study of Nursing and Nursing Education found that staff

---

*Source: From Sloane, Robert M., and Sloane, Beverly LeBov: *A Guide to Health Facilities,* ed. 2, St. Louis, 1977, The C. V. Mosby Co.

nurses devote an average of 40% of their time to patient care, head nurses devote an average of only 15% and supervisors only 7%.

Other utilization studies indicate that at least 25% of nursing activities could be classified as nonnursing. With a unit management system, then, proportionally more time should be available to the nurse for patient care activities.

Another purpose of unit management is the provision of hospital management at the unit level.

A survey of hospitals in 16 states revealed that where unit management systems were in operation, few unit managers were responsible to the nursing division—most were responsible to hospital administration.

Eileen Helger, in *JONA* (January–February 1972) warned, however, that the research thus far had indicated that nurses have not consistently demonstrated a significant increase in direct patient care activities following implementation of unit management.

Nursing Administrators' Salaries

Overview—Administrative Nurses' Salaries (1972)**

Nonfederal Hospitals
In August 1972, the following average salaries for registered nurses in nonfederal hospitals in 21 large metropolitan areas were found:

	Range of Averages in 21 Areas
Director of Nursing:	$12,870—$19,214
Supervisor:	$10,556—$13,884
Head Nurse:	$ 9,386—$12,792
General Duty:	$ 8,502—$11,128

Nurses Employed in Public Health Agencies
As of April 1, 1973, the following median salaries for nurses in local health agencies were found:

	Official	Nonofficial
Nurse Directors:	$15,400	$15,030
Supervisors:	$12,850	$11,469
Staff Nurses:	$10,249	$ 9,062

Nonfederal Hospitals in Miami, August 1972

Director of Nursing:	$16,588
Supervisor:	$11,908
Head Nurse:	$10,686
General Duty:	$ 9,360

**Source: DHEW, Oct. 1975.

Weekly earnings[1]	Atlanta	Balti-more	Boston	Buffalo	Chicago	Dallas	Denver	Detroit	Houston
									All
Under $170	4	—	—	2	8	1	—	—	—
$170 and under $180	9	—	2	6	12	9	—	—	10
$180 and under $190	28	2	—	5	10	8	6	—	29
$190 and under $200	26	20	10	13	31	22	11	—	41
$200 and under $210	20	22	28	29	38	17	18	8	53
$210 and under $220	24	40	42	19	53	16	30	11	26
$220 and under $230	26	34	78	26	72	2	12	15	11
$230 and under $240	6	42	52	19	77	7	24	84	7
$240 and under $250	5	72	68	—	87	6	11	117	6
$250 and under $260	—	47	34	9	77	—	2	79	—
$260 and under $270	—	54	64	31	94	8	5	45	1
$270 and under $280	1	5	22	17	102	1	3	26	4
$280 and under $290	—	11	19	4	19	—	—	15	3
$290 and under $300	—	1	15	—	3	—	—	8	2
$300 and over	2	14	2	—	14	—	3	2	—
Number of employees	151	364	436	180	697	97	125	410	193
Average weekly earnings[1]	$206.00	$241.50	$242.00	$232.50	$243.00	$210.00	$223.50	$248.50	$206.00
									Nongovernment
Under $170	4	—	—	2	8	—	—	—	—
$170 and under $180	9	—	2	6	12	6	—	—	10
$180 and under $190	25	2	—	5	10	5	6	—	28
$190 and under $200	20	20	10	13	30	21	11	—	41
$200 and under $210	8	21	22	25	36	17	18	4	41
$210 and under $220	11	36	39	19	52	10	23	10	26
$220 and under $230	7	31	65	25	70	1	10	10	5
$230 and under $240	2	42	30	14	68	1	23	80	7
$240 and under $250	2	64	57	—	71	—	9	100	4
$250 and under $260	—	29	19	3	53	—	1	28	—
$260 and under $270	—	24	46	1	65	—	—	30	1
$270 and under $280	1	5	17	1	30	—	1	14	—
$280 and under $290	—	3	19	—	11	—	—	15	—
$290 and under $300	—	—	15	—	1	—	—	6	—
$300 and over	2	2	2	—	10	—	—	2	—
Number of employees	91	279	343	114	527	61	102	299	163
Average weekly earnings[1]	$199.50	$234.00	$241.50	$214.00	$236.00	$199.00	$218.00	$247.00	$201.00
									Government (non
Under $190	3	—	—	—	—	7	—	—	1
$190 and under $200	6	—	—	—	1	1	—	—	—
$200 and under $210	12	1	6	4	2	—	—	4	12
$210 and under $220	13	4	3	—	1	6	7	1	—
$220 and under $230	19	3	13	1	2	1	2	5	6
$230 and under $240	4	—	22	5	9	6	1	4	—
$240 and under $250	3	8	11	—	16	6	2	17	2
$250 and under $260	—	18	15	6	24	—	1	51	—
$260 and under $270	—	30	18	30	29	8	5	15	—
$270 and under $280	—	—	5	16	72	1	2	12	4
$280 and under $290	—	8	—	4	8	—	—	—	3
$290 and under $300	—	1	—	—	2	—	—	2	2
$300 and under $310	—	2	—	—	—	—	3	—	—
$310 and under $320	—	6	—	—	4	—	—	—	—
$320 and over	—	4	—	—	—	—	—	—	—
Number of employees	60	85	93	66	170	36	23	111	30
Average weekly earnings[1]	$216.00	$267.00	$243.50	$263.50	$265.00	$228.50	$249.50	$252.00	$234.00

[1] Earnings relate to standard salaries that are paid for standard work schedules and exclude extra pay for work on late shifts, as well as the value of room, board, and other perquisites, if any, provided in addition to cash salaries. Average weekly earnings are rounded to the nearest half dollar.

[2] Workers were distributed as follows: 5 at $300 to $310; 2 at $310 to $320; 3 at $320 to $330; 4 at $330 to $340; and 8 at $340 and over.

6

time supervisors of nurses in nongovernment and government (non-earnings, 21 selected areas, August 1972)

Los Angeles–Long Beach and Anaheim–Santa Ana–Garden Grove	Memphis	Miami	Milwaukee	Minneapolis–St. Paul	New York SMSA	Philadelphia	Portland	St. Louis	San Francisco–Oakland	Seattle–Everett	Washington
hospitals											
—	2	—	—	1	—	24	—	12	—	—	—
—	3	3	—	—	—	33	2	—	—	—	—
3	33	—	7	1	—	22	—	7	—	2	2
15	19	10	—	3	—	35	18	23	—	11	—
—	17	8	10	15	11	44	24	23	—	25	10
40	16	23	18	34	90	139	24	36	3	21	10
22	17	27	15	46	134	99	19	23	6	19	31
112	4	18	25	43	391	23	15	17	15	4	8
94	5	21	24	18	265	53	1	16	32	18	22
69	—	14	24	4	264	19	—	12	52	2	21
35	—	2	12	6	415	12	—	—	30	1	2
50	—	—	3	—	220	7	—	4	35	3	6
43	—	3	4	6	98	18	—	3	24	—	—
58	—	1	2	1	36	3	—	1	33	—	2
53	—	1	—	—	148	21	—	3	19	—	([1])
594	116	131	144	178	2,072	552	103	180	249	106	127
$258.00	$203.00	$229.00	$238.00	$228.50	$257.50	$223.00	$214.00	$220.00	$267.00	$221.50	$256.00
hospitals											
—	—	—	—	—	—	22	—	12	—	—	—
—	—	—	—	—	—	33	2	—	—	—	—
3	28	—	7	—	—	20	—	7	—	2	2
15	17	10	—	3	—	35	18	21	—	11	—
—	10	5	10	7	11	44	19	20	—	21	10
40	7	23	16	31	90	137	22	30	3	18	—
22	4	26	14	45	80	96	16	19	6	14	31
111	2	15	20	28	174	15	4	6	10	2	7
94	4	20	14	8	112	33	1	8	25	3	21
69	—	2	10	1	83	14	—	6	45	—	19
35	—	2	7	—	142	10	—	—	28	1	1
48	—	—	3	—	100	7	—	3	31	3	5
40	—	3	4	—	38	9	—	3	2	—	—
30	—	1	2	—	27	2	—	1	5	—	2
20	—	1	—	—	142	21	—	3	2	—	10
527	72	108	107	123	999	498	82	139	157	75	108
$252.00	$200.50	$228.00	$234.00	$223.50	$258.00	$220.50	$211.00	$215.50	$257.00	$216.50	$245.00
federal hospitals											
—	[4]10	—	—	2	—	4	—	—	—	—	—
—	2	—	—	—	—	—	—	2	—	—	—
—	7	—	—	8	—	—	—	3	—	4	—
—	9	—	2	3	—	2	—	6	—	3	1
—	13	—	1	1	54	3	—	4	—	5	—
1	2	—	5	15	217	8	—	11	5	2	1
—	1	—	10	10	153	20	—	8	7	15	1
—	—	—	14	3	181	5	—	6	7	2	2
—	—	—	5	6	273	2	—	—	2	—	1
2	—	—	—	—	120	—	—	1	4	—	1
3	—	—	—	6	60	9	—	—	22	—	—
28	—	—	—	1	9	1	—	—	28	—	—
13	—	—	—	—	—	—	—	—	9	—	2
[5]20	—	—	—	—	6	—	—	—	8	—	1
67	44	([6])	37	55	1,073	54	([6])	41	92	31	19
$305.00	$207.50	([6])	$249.50	$240.00	$257.00	$246.50	([6])	$235.00	$283.50	$233.50	$319.00

[3]Workers were distributed as follows: 1 at $160 to $170; 3 at $170 to $180; and 3 at $180 to $190.
[4]Workers were distributed as follows: 2 at $160 to $170; 3 at $170 to $180; and 5 at $180 to $190.
[5]Workers were distributed as follows: 9 at $320 to $330; and 11 at $330 to $340.
[6]No data reported or data that do not meet publication criteria.

Source: U.S. Bureau of Labor Statistics, 1974.

Table 6-2   Earnings: Head nurses (Distribution of full-time head straight-time weekly earnings[1],

Weekly earnings[1]	Atlanta	Balti-more	Boston	Buffalo	Chicago	Dallas	Denver	Detroit	Houston
									All
Under $160	14	—	—	12	—	12	18	—	30
$160 and under $170	36	—	—	18	—	58	105	—	104
$170 and under $180	49	4	12	64	22	58	143	—	181
$180 and under $190	57	34	65	89	119	76	62	—	142
$190 and under $200	41	86	109	88	90	49	72	20	60
$200 and under $210	35	80	198	115	185	46	86	93	43
$210 and under $220	34	83	174	46	178	26	48	133	10
$220 and under $230	15	97	116	145	218	9	22	208	5
$230 and under $240	3	45	176	12	200	—	20	220	1
$240 and under $250	2	30	61	—	144	—	—	46	5
$250 and under $260	—	17	35	—	88	—	—	47	—
$260 and under $270	1	16	17	—	32	—	—	3	—
$270 and under $280	—	5	35	—	4	—	—	7	—
$280 and under $290	—	11	4	—	2	—	—	2	—
$290 and over	—	—	—	—	—	—	—	—	—
Number of employees	287	508	1,002	589	1,282	334	576	779	581
Average weekly earnings[1]	$190.00	$217.50	$219.00	$201.00	$221.00	$186.50	$188.00	$226.50	$181.00
									Nongovernment
Under $160	9	—	—	12	—	12	18	—	26
$160 and under $170	28	—	—	18	—	43	105	—	92
$170 and under $180	29	3	12	61	22	58	141	—	168
$180 and under $190	21	33	39	61	107	70	52	—	129
$190 and under $200	23	77	81	39	78	47	49	18	51
$200 and under $210	16	74	160	77	153	24	73	85	25
$210 and under $220	15	69	126	19	139	18	39	118	6
$220 and under $230	6	85	90	1	166	2	3	166	—
$230 and under $240	2	34	56	—	131	—	1	157	—
$240 and under $250	2	12	54	—	87	—	—	42	1
$250 and under $260	—	13	35	—	35	—	—	19	—
$260 and under $270	1	1	17	—	15	—	—	3	—
$270 and under $280	—	—	23	—	4	—	—	7	—
$280 and over	—	—	4	—	2	—	—	2	—
Number of employees	152	401	697	288	939	274	481	617	498
Average weekly earnings[1]	$188.00	$212.00	$218.50	$189.00	$217.00	$184.00	$183.50	$224.50	$179.00
									Government (non
Under $160	5	—	—	—	—	—	—	—	4
$160 and under $170	8	—	—	—	—	15	—	—	12
$170 and under $180	20	1	—	3	—	—	2	—	13
$180 and under $190	36	1	26	28	12	6	10	—	13
$190 and under $200	18	9	28	49	12	2	23	2	9
$200 and under $210	19	6	38	38	32	22	13	8	18
$210 and under $220	19	14	48	27	39	8	9	15	4
$220 and under $230	9	12	26	144	52	7	19	42	5
$230 and under $240	1	11	120	12	69	—	19	63	1
$240 and under $250	—	18	7	—	57	—	—	4	4
$250 and under $260	—	4	—	—	53	—	—	28	—
$260 and under $270	—	15	—	—	17	—	—	—	—
$270 and under $280	—	5	12	—	—	—	—	—	—
$280 and under $290	—	11	—	—	—	—	—	—	—
$290 and under $300	—	—	—	—	—	—	—	—	—
$300 and over	—	—	—	—	—	—	—	—	—
Number of employees	135	107	305	301	343	60	95	162	83
Average weekly earnings[1]	$192.50	$239.50	$221.50	$212.50	$231.50	$197.00	$210.50	$232.50	$191.00

[1] Earnings relate to standard salaries that are paid for standard work schedules and exclude extra pay for work on late shifts, as well as the value of room, board, and other perquisites, if any, provided in addition to cash salaries. Average weekly earnings are rounded to the nearest half dollar.

nurses in nongovernment and government (nonfederal) hospitals by 21 selected areas, August 1972)

Los Angeles–Long Beach and Anaheim–Santa Ana–Garden Grove	Memphis	Miami	Milwaukee	Minneapolis–St. Paul	New York SMSA	Philadelphia	Portland	St. Louis	San Francisco–Oakland	Seattle–Everett	Washington
hospitals											
—	1	—	—	—	3	39	—	16	—	—	—
—	8	2	—	—	1	29	12	12	—	3	—
—	42	42	3	—	—	132	9	77	—	3	4
12	40	17	20	11	28	199	42	81	—	20	6
58	54	96	29	55	329	257	155	70	15	60	32
112	9	67	52	91	366	177	71	96	29	117	87
267	1	41	58	165	1,523	165	—	62	26	25	84
169	1	27	92	32	780	114	—	38	76	2	61
202	—	12	13	8	668	86	—	32	91	1	22
218	—	33	5	7	520	22	—	15	91	—	2
87	—	—	3	—	182	14	—	4	149	—	3
120	—	—	—	—	85	11	—	4	34	—	3
21	—	—	1	—	86	8	—	—	53	—	14
21	—	1	—	—	65	2	—	—	13	—	62
49	—	—	—	—	41	37	—	—	33	—	13
1,336	156	338	276	369	4,677	1,292	289	507	610	231	393
$234.00	$186.00	$205.50	$213.50	$209.50	$225.50	$205.00	$193.00	$200.50	$246.00	$200.50	$229.50
hospitals											
—	—	—	—	—	—	39	—	—	—	—	—
—	2	2	—	—	—	29	12	12	—	3	—
—	38	34	3	—	—	129	2	75	—	1	4
12	32	17	20	3	24	199	23	80	—	17	6
58	47	96	28	39	133	229	115	54	15	33	31
112	6	64	35	68	233	153	71	85	28	98	78
266	—	33	42	147	531	101	—	20	22	15	81
168	—	22	45	24	365	99	—	32	43	2	56
200	—	7	12	—	308	73	—	16	63	—	22
187	—	7	5	—	355	17	—	14	32	—	2
80	—	—	3	—	168	5	—	4	113	—	3
21	—	—	—	—	73	11	—	3	3	—	3
1	—	—	1	—	74	4	—	—	—	—	12
—	—	1	—	—	90	36	—	—	3	—	17
1,105	125	283	194	281	2,354	1,124	223	395	322	169	315
$226.00	$186.00	$201.50	$212.00	$209.50	$230.50	$203.50	$194.50	$198.00	$236.50	$201.00	$219.50
federal) hospitals											
—	1	—	—	—	3	—	—	16	—	—	—
—	6	—	—	—	1	—	—	—	—	—	—
—	4	—	—	—	—	3	—	2	—	2	—
—	8	—	—	8	4	—	—	1	—	3	—
—	7	—	1	16	196	28	—	16	—	27	1
—	3	—	17	23	133	24	—	11	1	19	9
1	1	—	16	18	992	64	—	42	4	10	3
1	1	—	47	8	415	15	—	6	33	—	5
2	—	—	1	8	360	13	—	16	28	1	—
31	—	—	—	7	165	5	—	1	59	—	—
7	—	—	—	—	14	9	—	—	36	—	—
99	—	—	—	—	12	—	—	1	31	—	—
20	—	—	—	—	12	4	—	—	53	—	2
21	—	—	—	—	16	2	—	—	10	—	47
49	—	—	—	—	—	1	—	—	—	—	6
—	—	—	—	—	—	—	—	—	33	—	5
231	31	(²)	82	88	2,323	168	(²)	112	288	62	78
$269.00	$184.50	(²)	$218.00	$210.50	$220.50	$218.00	(²)	$208.50	$257.00	$200.50	$270.50

²No data reported or data that do not meet publication criteria.

Source: U.S. Bureau of Labor Statistics, 1974.

Administrative Practices

Staffing

Staffing Trends

The following trends in staffing were noted in a *Supervisor Nurse* report ("Staffing," E. M. Price, July 1975).

1. There is a movement toward establishing one central staffing office in the nursing department. This increases fairness in scheduling to all employees and reduces the redundancy of effort when each head nurse makes out her own schedules.
2. This central office is being staffed primarily by nonnurses. Of the attendees at the Spring, 1975, workshops 25% are nonnurse staffing coordinators.
3. Personnel policies are being revised to include a Sunday starting day for the pay period.
4. Increasing numbers of hospitals are providing every other weekend off for all personnel in nursing.
5. Benefits of vacation and sick time are being prorated for part-time personnel.
6. There is a movement toward longer vacations.
7. More employees are under contract each year.
8. Nurse administrators are assuming greater responsibility for preparation and control of their budgets and are increasingly able to defend their needs for staffing.
9. Workload data are identified on a shift basis in relation to the usual needs of the patients. The workload data are translated into:

- Average hours of care per patient per day;
- Desired combination of full and part-time personnel by category;
- Percentages of staff by category;
- Numbers of personnel required by category to provide the desired weekend off benefit;
- Ratios of full to part-time personnel; and
- The personnel budget specifying FTEs (full-time equivalents) and fringe benefit replacement needs by each unit.

A Method of Estimating Staffing Needs*

On the average the minimal care patients on nights received five minutes of care. The ratios of categories to each other and between shifts all can be expressed as multiples of the amount of care a minimal care patient receives on the night shift.

On the day shift average patients received twice as much, above average care patients six times as much, and intensive care patients 12 times as much direct nursing care as minimal care patients. The ratio among the categories on the day shift became identified as 1:2:6:12. Subsequently, the ratio of the average direct nursing care times on evening shift was found to be 1:2:7:14, and on the night shift, 1:2:7:25.

Further analysis revealed that, on the average, patients received four times more direct nursing care on the day shift than on the night shift and twice as much care on the evening shift as on the night shift. Thus the ratio of the amount of nursing care received on day, evening, and night shifts was 4:2:1.

These ratios may be used as weighting factors for the corresponding categories on each shift to arrive at an *index of patient load* on the nursing unit for any shift.

Table 6-3 Ratios of direct nursing care time, per shift and patient category

Shift	Category			
	Minimal	Average	Above Average	Intense
Days	4	8	24	48
Evenings	2	4	14	28
Nights	1	2	7	25

Table 6-3 shows the patient load index for all three shifts during one month on one surgical nursing unit. It can be seen that the census ranged from a low of 28 patients on the 21st day to a high of 38 patients on the 28th day. However, the day load index on the 21st day was quite high at 492, but on the 28th, with 10 more patients, the index was much lower at 396. Similarly, on the 5th and the 12th of the month the census was equal at 35

---

*Source: DHEW, May 1972.

patients, but the day load index was 512 and 272, respectively, for the two days.

The number of hours of direct nursing care required could be obtained by multiplying the calculated load index for any shift by 5/60. The activity studies also show that on the average the nursing staff spent 42% of their eight-hour day (3.36 hours) giving direct care to patients.

Scheduling

Nursing '75 in a survey of hospital working conditions found that:

- only 5% of full-time nurses work other than an eight-hour day.
- only 58% reported they are required to rotate shifts.
- 42% said they are often pulled from one unit to another and 54% said sometimes. Only 3% said never.

Ten-Hour Day

A nationwide survey of hospitals funded by the Manpower Administration of the Department of Labor found that 83% of those using a modified scheduling used the ten-hour day, four-day week with predetermined calendar patterns. The ten-hour schedule is particularly favored by the larger hospitals.

Block Scheduling

The block system sets a pattern which provides advance notice of work hours and minimizes long concentrated periods without a day off. In a repeated two-week pattern, each staff member receives every other weekend off plus one weekday off during the beginning or end of the week. The net effect is that no one works more than four consecutive days. Each member is assigned an individual two-week pattern to repeat continuously. There is a present trend toward utilizing block scheduling in hospitals.

Premium Day and Block Scheduling

The premium day off is an innovative approach to avert the issue of overstaffing during the week or of using part-time personnel, both practices which are inherent to block staff scheduling. As used in Rochester Methodist Hospital, the nurse is given an extra day off if she volunteers to work one additional weekend within a four-week scheduling block. From an administrative point of view, the premium day system is a trade-off of three days of weekday coverage for two days of weekend coverage, a flexible system that does not add directly to hospital costs. Nurses can designate their preference and use the premium day to lengthen off-weekend periods or break up patterns of consecutive workdays.

Three-Week Schedule

This three-week schedule of nursing service averages 37-1/3 hours per week per person. Longest work span is four days. Schedule provides for seven days off, including one weekend, and an extra day.

Figure 6-2   Three-Week Schedule for Nursing Unit Staff

NURSE	S	M	T	W	T	F	S	S	M	T	W	T	F	S	S	M	T	W	T	F	S
A	x	o	x	x	x	x	o	o	x	x	x	o	o	x	x	x	o	o	x	x	x
B	o	x	x	x	o	o	x	x	x	o	o	x	x	x	x	o	x	x	x	x	o
C	x	x	o	o	x	x	x	x	o	x	x	x	x	o	o	x	x	x	o	o	x

Source: *Practical Approaches to Effective Functioning of the Department of Nursing Service,* 1972. Reprinted by permission of the American Hospital Association.

Figure 6-3 Seven-Week Schedule

WEEK	1							2							3							4							5							6							7						
NURSE	S	M	T	W	T	F	S	S	M	T	W	T	F	S	S	M	T	W	T	F	S	S	M	T	W	T	F	S	S	M	T	W	T	F	S	S	M	T	W	T	F	S	S	M	T	W	T	F	S
1 Straight days	d	d	d	d	d	o	o	d	d	d	d	d	o	o	d	d	d	d	d	o	o	d	d	d	d	d	o	o	d	d	d	d	d	o	o	d	d	d	d	d	o	o	d	d	d	d	d	o	o
2 Straight evenings	o	e	e	e	e	e	e	o	e	e	e	e	e	e	o	e	e	e	e	e	e	o	e	e	e	e	e	e	o	e	e	e	e	e	e	o	e	e	e	e	e	e	o	e	e	e	e	e	o
3 Straight nights	n	o	o	n	n	n	n	n	o	o	n	n	n	n	n	o	o	n	n	n	n	n	o	o	n	n	n	n	n	o	o	n	n	n	n	n	o	o	n	n	n	n	n	o	o	n	n	n	n
4 Rotating d-e-n	o	d	d	e	e	e	d	d	d	e	e	n	o	o	d	d	o	o	d	d	d	o	n	n	o	o	d	d	d	d	o	o	e	e	d	o	o	d	d	d	o	o	d	d	o	o	d	d	o
5 Rotating d-e-n	d	d	d	o	o	n	n	d	d	d	o	o	d	d	d	d	o	o	d	d	d	o	o	d	d	d	e	e	d	d	o	o	d	d	d	d	d	n	n	o	o	d	d	o	o	d	d	d	d
6 Rotating d-e	e	o	o	d	d	d	d	o	o	d	d	e	e	d	o	o	e	e	d	o	o	e	e	d	o	o	e	e	d	o	o	e	e	d	o	o	d	d	o	o	d	d	o	o	e	e	d	d	e
7 Rotating d-n	d	n	n	o	o	d	d	d	d	d	o	o	d	d	d	d	o	o	d	d	d	o	o	d	d	d	d	d	d	d	o	o	d	d	d	d	d	d	d	o	o	d	d	d	o	o	d	d	d

Staffing standard for this unit calls for three nurses on day tour, one on evening tour, and one on night tour. On basis of 40-hour week, seven nurses are required. Nurse man-hours per week total 280: days, 3 × 56 hours (8 hours × 7 days) = 168; evenings, 1 × 56 hours = 56; nights, 1 × 56 hours = 56. Key: d = day, e = evening, n = night, o = off.

Source: *Practical Approaches to Effective Functioning of the Department of Nursing Service,* 1972. Reprinted by permission of the American Hospital Association.

12-hour Shift Schedule

One of the most innovative scheduling systems is the 12-hour shift. Full daily coverage is split into two shifts of 12 hours each (from 7 a.m. to 7 p.m., and from 7 p.m. to 7 a.m.) with each staff member working seven days in straight succession, followed by seven days off. Instead of head nurse and assistant head nurse being assigned to evening shifts and no night shifts, it is possible to have the busy part of evening shift covered by supervisory personnel and the slow part relegated to limited coverage—a savings for the hospital of at least half of supervisory salaries used formerly for the evening shift.

There are notable benefits and disadvantages to this system. In a survey of "the good and bad aspects" of the 12-hour shift, *RN* (September 1975) reported that: *

> In terms of efficiency, the total number of sick days taken over the surveyed two month period amounted to the number previously taken in an average week. Communication and interaction improved notably at team turnover time. More time was available for preparing patient records; nurses spent more time with patients, parents and doctors.
>
> Nurses felt an intense involvement in patient care. They had the opportunity to prepare children for surgery and still be there when they returned post-op. Another benefit was an emotional continuum with patients and parents. Parents, for example, showed less anxiety when the same nurse was present to receive their child after surgery.
>
> In spite of these benefits, however, the majority of the nurses found that the 12-hour shifts were too exhausting to continue. "By the end of the last day of a four- or five-day stretch, fatigue was close to unbearable," one nurse reported. Cumulative fatigue was the worst aspect of the experiment. During a comparable period the previous year, three minor accidents occurred on the floor, and no medication problems were reported. Dur-

ing the experiment, 10 minor accidents and five medication mix-ups were recorded. The nurses felt the increased incidence was due to extreme fatigue.

The majority felt a 12-hour shift simply doesn't fit the life-style of the average person.

Tips on Evaluating Staff**

A number of hospitals are designing evaluation forms that measure observable and definable behaviors. Ideally, these forms rate each nurse on nearly all of her duties, as defined by the procedure manual or a job description.

An objective form *does* accomplish a lot:

- It does tell the employee what her employer expects of her. (For example, to report to work on time, to attend one in-service class each month, and so on.)
- It does show her what she is doing right and wrong and—if the behaviors are specific enough—it shows clearly what she must do differently in order to improve her evaluation score.
- It does ensure that all nurses throughout the hospital are rated for the same qualities and behaviors—an important feature since promotions and transfers are likely to be competitive throughout the hospital.

Many nurses err on the side of generosity, rating all their employees as excellent.

Others start each new nurse off with a fair rating, then systematically increase her rating at each evaluation. Of course, after a few ratings, the nurses all achieve excellent ratings.

Some tips that will improve any system:

- Never base an appraisal on a single observation. In fact, you should informally observe and evaluate your staff members at least once a month, keeping notes on your opinions. Of course, any deficiencies should be mentioned to the employee at the time so she can improve. Don't save all your ammunition and surprise her with it twice a year.
- If your observations aren't self-explanatory, be sure to include anecdotes to support your conclusions. "This is really important," says a former head nurse. "And staff nurses

should demand it if it isn't done. I have a bad habit of cutting through red tape if something needs to be done, and I once had a supervisor who got very upset about it. Anyway, one time she handed me my evaluation to sign, and I noticed she had put a poor rating next to the category, 'Obeys hospital rules and regulations'—Can you imagine how that would have looked next time I was considered for promotion!

"I asked her to explain, and it turned out my crime was to scribble myself a note and leave it on a spindle by the Kardex every day. (The note was just to remind me of questions I wanted to ask at the next day's report.) The supervisor was mad because I refused to make such notes part of the permanent records."

- Be sure you include complimentary anecdotes, too. Good performances, like flies, thrive on honey. Such anecdotes will soften your criticisms and serve a basic human need to know "How am I doing?"
- Don't ignore your feelings. If your objective evaluation form looks like a computer printout, and you feel that some unmeasurable quality of a nurse's performance ought to be mentioned, mention it. Use the bottom or a separate sheet. Of course, if your subjective evaluation is completely different from the objective evaluation, try a little self-analysis: Is your impression a fair description of the person, or does it arise from one of your own prejudices? (Are you *sure* she is lazy, or did you expect it the minute she came on the floor because all Irish or black or white, etc., nurses are lazy?) Does she really deserve another chance in spite of her bad record or do you just want to give her another chance because you were in training together?
- Try to phrase criticisms in a constructive way. For example, it's less offensive and more helpful to say, "She should clean her shoes and pay more attention to personal grooming," rather than "looks sloppy."
- Give your staff advance notice that evaluation is coming up. You might say, "I'll be giving you your evaluation next week, so you probably want to think over any questions or comments you'd like to make. I'd particularly like to know about any changes you'd like to make in your job, or about any way in which you'd like me to help you over the next year."

- During the evaluation, ask each employee, "What are your most important jobs, as you see them?" If her answers differ greatly from yours, her performance will never meet your standards. The nurse who thinks her job is "to do what the doctors tell me" is never going to raise her score on the "displays initiative" section.
- Ask, "What changes would you like to make in your job?" One nurse told us that this question turned out to be the most important part of an evaluation she did with a new grad.

"I had an uneasy feeling about her patient care, but I couldn't really find anything to criticize. Then, when I asked, she told me she'd like to work on another unit. It turned out her mother and grandmother both had cancer, so that working on our unit—which is mostly cancer patients—was putting her through hell eight hours a day. She's on another unit now, and turning into a terrific nurse."

- Ask, "What's the hardest part of your job?" Many nurses won't tell you they don't know how to do something, but they won't mind ranking their jobs from easiest to hardest. And just think, if you keep a list of all the hard jobs, you may have all your in-service topics for the next six months.
- Ask, "How can I help you more?" Depending on how secure you feel, you may want to follow this question with others that show how your staff evaluate *you.*
- Ask, "Do you have any particular goals you'd like to work toward?" Again, the question gives your staff a chance to admit weaknesses in a supportive atmosphere. *But* studies have shown that goal-setting is not beneficial to employees without continuing support from the supervisor. Don't ask this question unless you're interested in following through with the answer.

Finally, *supervise* and *support* your staff throughout the year. It has been proven beyond question that employee satisfaction and productivity require both these behaviors on your part. If *you* are being evaluated, don't sit there passively. Something very important is happening to you, and you can affect the outcome.

- If your evaluation does not provide enough information or if you think the ratings are unfair, discuss the additions or changes you think the head nurse should make. But discuss them with an open mind and admit it if she convinces you that her evaluation is, in fact, correct. If you still disagree, ask her to make a note of your disagreement. Better yet, make a note yourself, and attach it to the evaluation.

- Ask the head nurse to provide examples of any behavior in which you didn't score well. If she is right, ask her how you can improve. If you can't believe you ever did what she says you did, ask her to point out such behavior to you the next time she sees it.

- If you think you have done something exceptionally well, ask her to put it on the evaluation. Your evaluation is a permanent record of your performance—and that's no place for modesty.

- Start working immediately to improve your performance. Ask your head nurse, "How should I go about improving my performance?" Pin her down to specific things you should do and ask her to help you if your head nurse gives you a poor ER and *can't* tell you how to improve, something is wrong somewhere.)

- If you think your head nurse is unfair, ask her approval for you to meet with the nursing supervisor or director of nursing to discuss your evaluation with them. Don't make matters worse by going over her head without her knowledge.

List of Nursing Tasks and Average Time to Perform Each Task*

Code	Activity	Level of competence	Standard (minutes)
1	Admission of newborn	L.P.N., R.N.	30
2	Admission to postpartum	L.P.N., R.N.	10
3	Admit new patient	L.P.N., R.N.	20
4	Admit new patient, assessment by team leader	R.N.	35
5	Ambulate patients	Att., L.P.N., R.N.	30
6	Analyze oxygen concentration in nursery	L.P.N., R.N.	5
7	Answer call lights	Att., L.P.N., R.N.	5
8	Aqua K-pad	L.P.N., R.N.	20
9	Assist patient to sit up, back to bed, or up in chair	Att., L.P.N., R.N.	10
10	Assist with bedpan, urinal, or commode	Att., L.P.N., R.N.	10
11	Assist with circumcision	L.P.N., R.N.	15
12	Attend seminars and demonstrations	Att., L.P.N., R.N.	50
13	Backrub	Att., L.P.N., R.N.	8
14	Blanket technique in nursery	Att., L.P.N., R.N.	3
15	Bone marrow aspiration	L.P.N., R.N.	30
16	Bottle feeding of infant in nursery	Att., L.P.N., R.N.	20
17	Breast-feeding for infant	Att., L.P.N., R.N.	10
18	Cardiac arrest	R.N.	60
19	Catheter irrigation	L.P.N., R.N.	10
20	Catheterization	L.P.N., R.N.	20
21	Change catheter bags	Att., L.P.N., R.N.	10
22	Change dressings or reinforce	L.P.N., R.N.	10
23	Changing diaper	Att., L.P.N., R.N.	3
24	Charting	L.P.N., R.N.	2
25	Check medicine cards with Kardex	L.P.N., R.N.	15

(continued)

*Source: Mildred Hilliard, *Orientation and Evaluation of Professional Nursing,* The C. V. Mosby Co. (St. Louis, 1974).

List of Nursing Tasks and Average Time to Perform Each Task* (continued)

Code	Activity	Level of competence	Standard (minutes)
26	Clarification report	R.N.	2
27	Clean catch specimen	Att., L.P.N., R.N.	10
28	Clean bassinet	Att., L.P.N., R.N.	15
29	Cleansing enema, prepackaged	Att., L.P.N., R.N.	30
30	Cleansing enema, soapsuds	Att., L.P.N., R.N.	30
31	Clinitest-Acetest	L.P.N., R.N.	10
32	Close charts	L.P.N., R.N.	2
33	Collect intake and output records	Att., L.P.N., R.N.	5
34	Collect soiled linen from nursery	Att., L.P.N., R.N.	4
35	Collect specimen requested	Att., L.P.N., R.N.	5
36	Collect urine specimen from infant	Att., L.P.N., R.N.	10
37	Colostomy care	L.P.N., R.N.	30
38	Colostomy irrigation	L.P.N., R.N.	30
39	Complete bed bath	Att., L.P.N., R.N.	45
40	Complete checklist on pre-ops and chart	L.P.N., R.N.	10
41	Conduct change-of-shift report	L.P.N., R.N.	1-2 per patient
42	Count narcotics	L.P.N., R.N.	2
43	Death procedure, physical care	L.P.N., R.N.	30
44	Decubitus care	L.P.N., R.N.	20
45	Discharge of infant	Att., L.P.N., R.N.	30
46	Discharge of patient	L.P.N., R.N.	10
47	Douche	L.P.N., R.N.	20
48	Eye instillation	L.P.N., R.N.	5
49	Feed patient	Att., L.P.N., R.N.	28
50	Feed patient, assisting	Att., L.P.N., R.N.	30
51	Fill ice bags	Att., L.P.N., R.N.	10
52	Gastric tube irrigations	L.P.N., R.N.	10
53	Give information to visitors	Att., L.P.N., R.N.	5
54	Hand-scrubbing technique	Att., L.P.N., R.N.	5
55	Heat applications	L.P.N., R.N.	10
56	Indirect patient care (assisting with proctoscopic examination)	Att., L.P.N., R.N.	30
57	Infant gavage	L.P.N., R.N.	20
58	Infant lavage	L.P.N., R.N.	30
59	Infant suctioning	L.P.N., R.N.	3
60	Initiation of cardiac monitoring	R.N.	20
61	IV (add to)	R.N.	5
62	IV (discontinue)	L.P.N., R.N.	5
63	IV (set up)	R.N.	10
64	Kardex rounds with unit resident	R.N.	4 per patient
65	Lumbar puncture	L.P.N., R.N.	30
66	Make bed, patient in bed	Att., L.P.N., R.N.	10
67	Make bed, patient not in bed	Att., L.P.N., R.N.	5
68	Make out assignments	R.N.	6 per patient
69	Making of linen pack	Att., L.P.N., R.N.	5
70	Midnight census	L.P.N., R.N.	2
71	Moist heat application	L.P.N., R.N.	15
72	Morning bath in nursery	Att., L.P.N., R.N.	30
73	OB observational rounds	L.P.N., R.N.	3
74	Oral or nasal suction	L.P.N., R.N.	15

List of Nursing Tasks and Average Time to Perform Each Task* (continued)

Code	Activity	Level of competence	Standard (minutes)
75	Patient bed bath	Att., L.P.N., R.N.	20
76	Pass medications, injections	L.P.N., R.N.	3 per patient
77	Pass water	Att., L.P.N., R.N.	3
78	Passive exercises	L.P.N., R.N.	10
79	Patient P.M. care	Att., L.P.N., R.N.	10
80	Patient rounds	R.N.	2
81	Pelvic exam, Pap smear	L.P.N., R.N.	20
82	Perineal care	L.P.N., R.N.	10
83	PKU	L.P.N., R.N.	3
84	Posey restraint on bed patient	L.P.N., R.N.	20
85	Prepare patient for surgery or diagnostic procedure	L.P.N., R.N.	15
86	p.r.n. mealtime assistance	Att., L.P.N., R.N.	5
87	p.r.n. medications, charting, narcotics, barbiturates, sedatives	L.P.N., R.N.	5
88	p.r.n. oxygen therapy, nasal cannula and mask	L.P.N., R.N.	10
89	Proper attire for isolation	L.P.N., R.N.	15
90	Receive report	Att., L.P.N., R.N.	1-2 per patient
91	Receiving newborn	Att., L.P.N., R.N.	15
92	Record verbal or phone orders	R.N.	2
93	Removal of Foley catheter	L.P.N., R.N.	10
94	Removal of Levin or gastric tube	L.P.N., R.N.	10
95	Remove bedpan, urinal, or commode	Att., L.P.N., R.N.	5
96	Remove specimen container from isolation	Att., L.P.N., R.N.	15
97	Reposition patient	Att., L.P.N., R.N.	5
98	Restrain patient in chair	L.P.N., R.N.	20
99	Rounds with doctors	R.N.	2
100	Set up medications and chart	L.P.N., R.N.	2 per patient
101	Setting up room for isolation of patient	Att., L.P.N., R.N.	30
102	Shaving patient	Att., L.P.N., R.N.	30
103	Showing of babies	Att., L.P.N., R.N.	5
104	Sitz bath	Att., L.P.N., R.N.	30
105	Stryker frame	L.P.N., R.N.	20
106	Suppositories	L.P.N., R.N.	5
107	Taking fetal heart tone	L.P.N., R.N.	5
108	Taking infant to mother for the first time	L.P.N., R.N.	10
109	Team conference	R.N.	2
110	To remove infant from blanket in nursery	Att., L.P.N., R.N.	3
111	T.P.R. (oral or rectal)	Att., L.P.N., R.N.	2
112	Tracheostomy care	L.P.N., R.N.	15
113	Tracheostomy suctioning	L.P.N., R.N.	10
114	Transfer of patient	L.P.N., R.N.	2
115	Tube feedings, drip method	L.P.N., R.N.	20
116	Unsolicited visits to patient	Att., L.P.N., R.N.	2
117	Venous pressure	R.N.	10
118	Vital signs	Att., L.P.N., R.N.	3
119	Weigh patient, bed patient	Att., L.P.N., R.N.	10
120	Weigh patient, up patient	Att., L.P.N., R.N.	5
121	Weighing an infant	Att., L.P.N., R.N.	5

Orientation of Nurses

On the first day of orientation, all R.N.s and L.P.N.s are given the same check list. (See Figure 6-4.)

The orientees are expected to complete the check list during the first 90 days of employment (the probationary period). They ask a staff member to observe the performance of each activity. The staff member initials the item in question to indicate that performance was satisfactory. Orientees with previous experience are requested to complete most of the items on the check list during their two week orientation.

Review initially takes place at 30, 60 and 90 days. If deficiencies in the check list are present, the supervisor and the new employee plan experiences to correct them.

Figure 6-4   R.N. & L.P.N. Orientation check list

This procedure should be completed when possible during the 90 day probation, and the new person is responsible for getting it done. When completed, it should be given to the unit supervisor to keep and then turned in to Personnel when the person resigns. This orientation check list allows better evaluation of the new employee.

Responsibility	Discussed and/or demonstrated	Performance satisfactory	Not applicable
1. Intravenous Therapy Technique And Care Of			
a. Butterfly			
b. Angiocath			
c. Blood Transfusion			
d. Addition of fluids to present intravenous			
e. Clysis			
f. Use of IVAC Controller			
2. Tracheostomy			
a. General Hygienic Care			
b. Suctioning			
3. Foley Catheterization			
a. Daily Catheter Care			
b. Irrigation			
c. Foley Kit			
4. Administration of Medications			
a. Oral			
b. Intramuscular and Subcutaneous			
c. Intravenous			
(1) Admixtures			
(2) Direct Push			
d. Rectal			
e. Vaginal			
f. Clerical Responsibility			
(1) Doctor's Order			
(2) Medication Cards and Kardex			
(3) Narcotics, Hypnotic, Sedatives			
(4) Charting of Medications			
(5) Floor Stock			
(6) Obtaining reorders of chargeable drugs from Pharmacy			
(7) Obtaining drugs after hours			
(8) Errors—How to report what constitutes an error			

Figure 6-4   (continued)

Responsibility

5. Naso-gastric Tubes
   a. Levine
   b. Miller Abbott
   c. Blakemore
      (1) insertion
      (2) General Hygienic Care
      (3) Irrigation
      (4) Gomco & Airshield Suction Machines
      (5) Removal

6. Team Nursing For All 3 Shifts
   a. Team Member
   b. Team Leader
      (1) Making Assignment
      (2) Nursing History
      (3) Writing Care Plans and keeping up-to-date
      (4) Leading a Team Conference
      (5) Patient Teaching
         (a) Preop
         (b) Discharge Planning
   c. Doctors' Rounds
   d. Floor Routine—Duties of
      (1) 7–3
      (2) 3–11
      (3) 11–7
      (4) Reports of 3 shifts

7. Equipment—Where obtained, Care of, Use of and Charging
   a. O₂—Mask; Catheter, Tent
   b. Suction Apparatus—Wall Unit
   c. Emerson Chest Suction
   d. Orthopedic Equipment

8. Special Procedures of Unit
   a. Use of Wall O₂ and Suction
   b. Use of Electric Beds
   c. Use of Laundry and Trash Chutes
   d. Use of Dumbwaiter
   e. Use of Bed Status Board
   f. Use of Addressograph and Requisition Chute
   g. Use of IVAC Thermometers
   h. Housekeeping Responsibilities and Care of Linen

9. Special Treatment Trays
   a. Dressing Cart
   b. Lumbar Puncture
   c. Cut-down Trays
   d. Crash Carts
   e. Isolation Carts

Responsibility

10. Safety Devices
    a. Bed Rails—Policies for use of
    b. Restraints—Policies for use of
    c. Fire Regulations
       (1) Reporting a Fire
       (2) Floor Exits
       (3) Fire Extinguishers
       (4) Evacuation Plan
    d. Transportation of Patients
       (1) Stretcher
       (2) Wheelchair
       (3) Patient Bed

11. Ward Administration—Procedure and Policies
    a. Admission of patients
    b. Placement of patients on floor
    c. Transfer of patients (room to room, floor to floor)
    d. Discharge of patients
    e. Care of patients, clothing and valuables
    f. Seriously ill or critical patients
    g. Death of patient
    h. Visiting hours
    i. Private duty nurses and sitters
    j. Accident and Incident Reports

12. Food Service for Patients
    a. Requisitioning—Permissible Floor Stock
    b. Diet Orders and Changes
    c. Serving of the Trays
    d. Requesting Diet Instruction by Dietician
    e. Isolation Trays

13. Nursing Care Procedures
    a. Basic Nursing Procedures (List any you need help with)
       1.
       2.
       3.
    b. Recording Intake and Output
    c. Compresses
       1. Cold
       2. Hot
       3. Sterile
    d. Skin Care
       1. Prevention of decubitis
       2. Care of decubitis
       3. Use of sheep skin

(continued)

Figure 6-4 **(continued)**

Responsibility

e. Collection, Labeling and Delivery of Specimens for:
   1. Clean Catch Urine
   2. Urine Cultures
   3. Diabetic Urines
   4. 24 Hour Urine
   5. Sputum—AFB & Pap
   6. Stool
f. Assisting with:
   1. Physical Examination
   2. Pelvic Examination
   3. Spinal Tap
   4. Thoracentesis, Paracentesis
g. Postmortem Care
h. Preoperative Care
i. Postoperative Care
j. Isolation Technique
   (1) Policies
   (2) Orientation Review
k. Gavage
   (1) Infant
   (2) Adult
l. Sitz Bath
m. Clean Catch Urines for Culture
n. Diabetic Urine
   (1) Ketodiastix
   (2) Clinitest
   (3) Testape
o. Apical Pulse
p. Colostomy
   (1) Care of (dressings)
   (2) Irrigation
q. Ileostomy Care
r. Surgical Dressings
s. Other:

14. Charting
    a. Nurses Notes
    b. Graphic Charts
    c. Noting Doctors' Orders
    d. Nursing Kardex

15. Cardio-Pulmonary Resuscitation
    a. Procedure for Calling Team
    b. A-B-Cs of Resuscitation
    c. Duties and Responsibilities of Unit and Team

16. Miscellaneous
    a. Paging System—General and Unit
    b. Doctors' Call System

Responsibility

c. Disaster Call Schedule
d. Chaplain Service
e. Nursing Administration Call System
f. Sources of Information
   (1) Procedure Books
   (2) Diet Manual
   (3) Reference Material

17. Other (List)
_____
_____
_____
_____
_____
_____
_____
_____

Special Procedures ICU-CCU
1. Routine CCU Orders and Policies

2. Application of Chest Leads

3. Use of Monitors
   a. In Patient Room
   b. At Nurses' Station

4. Recognition of Basic Arrhythmias
   a. PVCs
   b. PACs
   c. PNCs
   d. Atrial Fibrillation
   e. Atrial Flutter
   f. Ventricular Tachycardia
   g. Ventricular Fibrillation
   h. 1°, 2°, 3° Heart Block
   i. Cardiac Standstill

5. Defibrillation

Special Procedures Postpartum-GYN
1. Routine Postpartum Orders

2. Routine Postop Orders

3. Home Going Instructions

4. Clipping Perineal Sutures

5. Sitz Baths

6. Monitoring Fetal Heart Tones With Fetoscope

NAME _____

UNIT _____

Source: Betsy Frank and Betsy Powell, "A Skills Checklist," *Supervisor Nurse*, May 1975. (Developed at Wayne County Memorial Hospital, Goldsboro, N.C.)

Personnel Problems

Communication

The Nurse's View

Experts say we only hear one-quarter of what people say to us.

One researcher [*Nursing '76*] who studied 100 American industries discovered that the president of the average company got only 90% of the information the board of directors wanted him to give company employees. The department heads (listen well, nursing supervisors) got only 50% of the information. The foremen (are you listening, head nurses?) got 30%. And the nonmanagement employees—for whom the information was intended—got only 20% of the information.

A *Nursing '76* survey of 10,000 nurses asked:

"How would you rate communication between..."

	Great	Moderate	Slight	Poor
Nurses & hospital administration	6%	35%	33%	24%
Nurses & doctors	21%	60%	11%	7%

"Do you feel your voice is heard and that your opinions count..."

All nurses responding:

	Frequently	Occasionally	Never
With hospital administration	12%	51%	31%
With nursing administration	23%	60%	15%

Source: Loy Wiley, "Communications," *Nursing '76,* April.

The Communications Gap Between Supervisor and Nurse

In a survey of what nurses and supervisors expected from each other, *Supervisor Nurse* magazine reported that many of the things that nurse supervisors said they needed from their staffs were startlingly similar to what the staff nurses assumed the supervisors would want. However, there remained many supervisory wants and needs of which nurses are unaware as reflected by the shaded items in Figure 6-5. Note also that many of the things supervisors assume that nurses need or want from them are not in fact deemed terribly significant to the nurses.

Figure 6-5   Supervisor-nurse communication

A	A1
WHAT SUPERVISORS SAID THEY NEED OR WANT FROM A NURSE:	WHAT NURSES SAID THEY ASSUMED THEIR SUPERVISORS NEED OR WANT FROM THEM:
1. Dependability in attendance: promptness.	1. Dependability.
2. Competence in technical skills.	2. (a) Basic knowledge of nursing techniques. (b) Ability to handle most situations.
3. Ability to communicate with supervisor, staff, patients and families.	3. Ability to work harmoniously with other members of staff and with patients.
4. Ability to benefit from constructive criticism.	4. Ability to accept constructive criticism.
5. Honesty.	5. Honesty.
6. Willingness to learn new procedures.	6. Willingness to learn and try new things.
7. (a) Willingness to function in any capacity when need arises. (b) Flexibility—can go above and beyond the call of duty.	7. Willingness to do whatever duties or as many duties as are necessary in a day's work.

GENERAL / AGREEMENT

Figure 6-5   (continued)

A	A1
WHAT SUPERVISORS SAID THEY NEED OR WANT FROM A NURSE:	**WHAT NURSES SAID THEY ASSUMED THEIR SUPERVISORS NEED OR WANT FROM THEM:**

GENERAL AGREEMENT

8. (a) Be patient-oriented with the ability to speak with patients of all ages and with any problems.
(b) Alleviate fears and anxieties of patients and families.
(c) Sensitivity to human needs with respect for individual differences.

8. Inventiveness in behalf of patients' comfort within the guidelines of physicians' orders and hospital rules.

9. Loyalty.

9. Conscientious carrying out of duties.

10. Good grooming.

10. To be neat and clean.

LACK OF COMMUNICATION

11. Take responsibility for own actions.

11. Knowledge of routines and policies of hospital.

12. To be calm in stressful situations.

13. To notice and mention the good in people; to comment on a job well done.

14. To be able to take orders as well as give them.

15. To work toward excellent public relations.

16. Good rapport.

17. Enthusiasm for job; a feeling that work can be joy and not "just a job."

B	B1
WHAT NURSES SAID THEY NEED OR WANT FROM A SUPERVISOR:	**WHAT SUPERVISORS SAID THEY ASSUME A NURSE NEEDS OR WANTS FROM THEM:**

GENERAL AGREEMENT

1. To serve as a liaison between staff and administration.

1. Act as a buffer between staff and physicians and other departments including administration.

2. Sharing responsibilities in any problem areas; backing us up.

2. (a) Support for coworkers.
(b) Available to use authority with physicians when conflicts arise.

3. Ability, knowledge and willingness to teach new techniques.

3. Keep up to date on new equipment and procedures and pass this on to me.

Figure 6-5 (continued)

B	B1
WHAT NURSES SAID THEY NEED OR WANT FROM A SUPERVISOR:	WHAT SUPERVISORS SAID THEY ASSUME A NURSE NEEDS OR WANTS FROM THEM:

L
A
C
K

O
F

C
O
M
M
U
N
I
C
A
T
I
O
N

4. Experience.

5. Knowledge of varied ways to deal with unusual situations and willingness to advise.
6. Thorough knowledge of hospital procedures.
7. Willingness to teach routine procedures which may not be familiar to some of the staff.

4. Open door policy to discuss any problem that I feel pertinent.

5. Provide a happy atmosphere to work in.

6. Enthusiasm.

7. Honesty.

8. (a) Keep me posted on how I'm doing and communicate with me as problems arise.
   (b) Need guidance and direction when indicated.
9. Let me know when I've done a good job; recognition.
10. Respect my feelings; keep confidences.
11. Want to feel secure in position assigned.
12. Aware of unit activity and staffing needs.
13. Operates as a "change-agent" in planning, exercising and evaluating.
14. Will perform direct patient care when necessary.
15. Try to alleviate internal conflicts to maintain good morale.

Source: Arthur Giancutti et al., "Creating Harmony Between Supervisor and Nurse," *Supervisor Nurse*, August 1975.

Job Satisfaction

A *Nursing '76* national survey (June 1976) on dissatisfaction among nurses found:

	Nurses	Average U.S. worker[1]
Dissatisfied with their jobs	44%	11%
Satisfied with their jobs	46	77
No answer	10	12

An earlier survey on working conditions had sought to identify the aspects of nurses' jobs that caused their dissatisfaction.[*] (See Figure 6-6 on following page.)

---

[1] 1973 Gallup Poll of U.S. workers
[*] Source: Marjorie Godfrey, "Working Conditions," *Nursing '75,* May.

Figure 6-6   What aspects of your job do you find most dissatisfying?

	Ranked number 1 complaint	Ranked number 2 or number 3	Ranked as major problem (1, 2, or 3)	Typical comments
Inadequate staffing	36%	25%	61%	"I thoroughly enjoy my work and my coworkers. If we were adequately staffed, I could tolerate everything else." "It's hard to give complete and thorough care without enough staff and with inadequately trained staff." "There is no shortage of nurses in the area, just a shortage in the hospital."
Salary	14	28	42	"I'm not dissatisfied with my job. Just the money." "It's a sad society where street cleaners make $13,500 a year and nurses start at $8,200."
Working hours/shifts	13	17	30	"After 15 years of working nights, weekends, and holidays I've had it. You make plans; then something comes up, and there goes your day off."
Physical working conditions	9	20	29	"I'm satisfied with everything except the cramped space we work in."
Opportunities for advancement	8	18	26	"Very little opportunity in the area for continuing education, and little stimulation to advance in the area, especially for the evening and night shifts."
Fringe benefits	4	19	23	"I work part time and get no fringe benefits." "Our hospital has inadequate maternity leave and no leaves of absence. If I stay out over 90 days with the baby, I'll have to resign."
Job authority/ responsibility	5	15	20	"I have the responsibility, yes, but not the authority to do the job."
Job satisfaction	4	12	16	"Team nursing approach takes nurses further from the patients. Now most of my work is supervisory."

Absenteeism*

Table 6-4   Rates of absenteeism among nursing service employees

% of absenteeism		
RN	LPN	Aide
2.7%	3.7%	4.7%

*Source: Mohan Kirtane, "Analyzing Absenteeism," Excerpted with permission from *Hospital Progress,* May 1975. Copyright 1975 by The Catholic Hospital Association.

Table 6-5   Amount of absenteeism in a sample hospital (6-month period)

Days absent	Employees	Days absent	Employees
0	594	10	5
1	127	11	10
2	99	12	8
3	95	13	4
4	52	14	1
5	47	15	2
6	33	16	1
7	26	17	—
8	16	18 or more	4
9	11		

Average absence per employee = 1.5 days
Standard deviation = 2.93 days

Table 6-6   Probability of absenteeism based on sample (6-month period)

Days absent[1]	Probability	Employees
9 or more	10% or less	46
10 or more	7.5% or less	35
11 or more	6% or less	30
12 or more	5% or less	20

[1]Nine or more days of absence in a period of six months could be defined as excessive.
Note: The data for this study was collected in a 300-bed, private hospital in a metropolitan area during a period of 12 months on 11 nursing units.

Turnover

In the metropolitan areas, where job change is easier due to proximity and number of choices, the turnover rate sometimes reaches 150 to 200 percent. It would seem that many nurses change jobs, hoping to find a difference, but generally find the new position quite like the previous one—and quite as frustrating.

- The National Commission on Nursing and Nursing Education (1970) estimated that the staff R.N. turnover rate was 70% per year.
- An HEW study ("The Geographic Distribution of Nurses," 1973) found that the mean number of workdays a new, inexperienced R.N. spent on the job before assuming full responsibilities was 39.1, or about eight workweeks.

Therefore, if the actual turnover rate is 70%, the average position is filled each 68 weeks, and the new inexperienced employee is not fully productive 12% of the average tenure.

Why Nurses Quit Their Jobs *

A three-part questionnaire (returned by 94 staff nurses in two cities who had resigned their positions in the previous four months) revealed that psychological rewards were more important than safety or social rewards in keeping nurses on the job. Younger nurses and new graduates had the highest turnover. Single nurses stayed no longer than married nurses; amount of spouses' salaries did not affect turnover; there was no difference between diploma and baccalaureate nurses; higher pay did not keep a nurse, nor was she influenced by a specialty area. Most nurses wanted opportunities to attend educational programs, continue course work for credit, career advancement other than to the head nurse position, and recognition of work from peers and supervisors.

Table 6-7   Reasons given for leaving a job

Rank	Reason for leaving job
1	Moving
12	Retirement
13	Illness
4	Distance of hospital
14	Leaving nursing
6	Pregnancy
7	To travel
8	To go to school
2	Dissatisfaction
5	Personal and family reasons
3	To increase fringe benefits
10	To try other areas of nursing
11	To get a promotion
15	Poor transportation
9	Other

Salary was not rated as important as many psychological rewards to nurses. Poor salary has been traditionally blamed for the high nursing turnover and nursing shortage. However, in this study a salary raise of $150 per month was rated only fourth in importance while salary raises of $100 and $50 per month

* Source: Joanne McCloskey, "Influence and Incentives on Staff Nurse Turnover," *Nursing Research*, May–June 1973. Copyright © American Journal of Nursing Company.

ranked 17th and 24th. These findings indicated that today's nurses are not very interested in retirement and maternity leave incentives. On the other hand, the findings showed that they were interested in "more opportunity to work part-time, where you can name your own days of the week and areas you want to work in," "more choice to choose a straight day shift" and "better child-care facilities."

Nurse Shortages

There is much more nurse resistance to employment in central cities of metropolitan areas than to rural employment. For this reason, nurse supply problems in central cities merit particularly serious policy consideration. Black nurses are relatively more willing to work in central cities than are whites; on the other hand, whites are more favorably disposed to rural areas.

Table 6-8   Safety, social, and psychological reward items

Number/Reward	Over-all rank	Number/Reward	Over-all rank
Safety		19. Maternity leave of an additional six months	22
1. Salary raise of $50 per month	24	20. Better child-care facilities	17
2. Salary raise of $100 per month	17	21. Different supervisor	12
3. Salary raise of $150 per month	4	22. Different head nurse	18
4. One week more paid vacation each year	20	23. More social contact with your co-workers	25
5. Two weeks more paid vacation each year but the hospital tells you when you have to take off these two weeks	19	24. More social contact with nursing superiors	27
6. Two weeks more paid vacation each year	14	25. More social contact with doctors	28
7. Three weeks more paid vacation each year	6	26. More opportunities to share your opinions and feelings with other registered nurses	15
8. Seven more days sick leave per year	20	27. More opportunities to share your opinions and feelings with doctors	13
9. Fourteen more days sick leave per year	21		
10. One more weekend a month off	19	*Psychological*	
11. Two more weekends a month off	11	28. More opportunities to attend educational programs	1
12. More opportunity to work part-time, even if the hospital names the days you must work and the areas where you must go	26	29. More responsibility on the job	8
		30. More recognition for your work from your peers and supervisors	3
13. More opportunity to work part-time, where you can name your own days of the week and the area you want to work in	10	31. More help to gain job skills from your peers and supervisors	9
		32. More opportunity for career advancement other than an assistant head nurse or head nurse position	2
14. More choice to choose a straight day shift	7	33. More opportunity to continue course work that would earn credits for your next degree	2
15. More opportunity to work shorter hours per day	16	34. More recognition for the good work that your unit did	9
16. A better insurance policy than you had	23	35. More encouragement to write and publish	21
17. A better retirement program than you had	22	36. More encouragement and help to initiate and take part in nursing research on your floor	5
Social			
18. A maternity leave of an additional three months	24		

Table 6-9 Reasons for refusing employment in rural and poor sections of central cities: marital status, training, and ethnicity*

Reasons	Marital status			Type of education			Ethnicity	
	Single	Married	Other	AA	BA	Dip.	White	Black
Small community:								
Inadequate transportation	7.7	3.5	4.6	3.1	5.0	4.7	3.9	7.8
Transportation time	11.9	8.2	7.3	9.3	8.1	9.1	8.3	13.2
Personal danger	4.8	2.1	2.4	2.6	2.2	2.8	2.3	3.9
Types of patients	7.8	2.6	2.8	3.9	6.4	3.2	3.6	6.2
Spouse would oppose it	—	17.2	—	8.9	9.6	13.2	11.9	11.6
Poor schools	2.6	4.1	3.6	3.8	3.5	3.7	3.5	4.7
Poor sections:								
Inadequate transportation	9.3	6.9	6.9	6.9	7.9	7.5	7.5	4.7
Transportation time	15.4	13.6	12.5	14.8	12.4	14.1	14.2	9.3
Personal danger	28.8	18.2	16.1	18.9	21.2	20.4	20.8	15.5
Types of patients	12.3	6.7	6.7	8.9	9.2	7.4	18.0	6.2
Spouse would oppose it	—	30.3	—	18.7	20.0	22.8	22.4	12.4
Poor schools	9.0	14.7	13.3	13.7	12.3	13.6	13.6	13.2

Source: DHEW, May 1975 (1973 data)

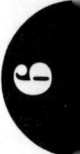

Table 6-10 Reasons for refusing employment in rural and poor sections of central cities: income and dependents[1]*

Reasons	$0–5,000		$5,001–10,000		$10,001–15,000		$15,001–25,000		Over $25,000	
	No dep.	Dep.	No dep.	Dep.	No dep.	Dep.	No dep.	Dep.	No dep.	Dep.
Small community:										
Inadequate transportation	1.7	3.1	3.2	4.7	3.9	3.3	0.0	3.4	12.5	0.0
Transportation time	4.5	6.6	9.7	7.3	11.2	10.0	7.7	10.3	12.5	2.2
Personal danger	1.7	1.3	2.3	1.9	0.7	2.3	2.6	3.4	12.5	0.0
Types of patients	2.8	4.0	3.5	1.8	6.6	1.7	2.6	2.4	0.0	0.0
Spouse would oppose it	12.9	11.9	15.2	17.6	10.5	22.0	10.3	20.0	37.5	13.0
Poor schools	2.2	4.0	2.9	5.3	2.0	4.0	2.6	4.1	12.5	8.7
Poor sections:										
Inadequate transportation	6.7	5.7	8.5	8.3	4.6	7.2	7.7	6.2	12.5	0.0
Transportation time	8.4	12.8	15.2	14.2	15.1	15.7	17.9	15.2	12.5	0.0
Personal danger	19.7	18.9	21.1	17.7	27.6	16.4	25.6	18.3	12.5	6.5
Types of patients	7.9	10.6	9.4	6.6	11.2	4.2	7.7	4.8	12.5	4.3
Spouse would oppose it	29.8	21.1	32.6	34.4	28.9	32.9	25.6	30.0	37.5	23.9
Poor schools	9.0	16.3	15.5	17.7	11.8	15.2	7.7	13.8	12.5	10.9

[1]Includes married nurses only.

Source: DHEW, May 1975 (1973 data)

7

PROFESSIONAL STANDARDS REVIEW ORGANIZATION (PSRO)

Background

Professional Standards Review Organization (PSRO) is a program organized, administered and controlled by local physicians to evaluate the necessity and quality of medical care delivered in their area under Medicare, Medicaid, and Maternal and Child Health programs.

PSRO is an effort to make these federally funded programs more effective through greater participation by the physicians themselves.

Local physicians set the standards and criteria of care, monitor to see that they are applied, and take corrective action when they are not.

PSROs review the medical necessity of services, the quality of care delivered, and the appropriateness of the care in terms of the level, duration, and methods of treatment. In reviewing medical necessity and quality, PSROs determine whether health care services provided are necessary on the basis of professionally developed standards and norms of care, diagnosis, and treatment. In reviewing appropriateness, PSROs must determine whether health care services are provided at the most efficient and effective level. This peer review system is intended to assure that payment is made from federal and state funds for only medically necessary, appropriate, and quality care.

PSROs only review care delivered in institutions and do not cover care delivered in a physician's office, a clinic, or any other ambulatory setting unless the physicians in a PSRO request that it do so. A PSRO does concern itself with the fees for services charged by physicians or institutions.

Types of PSROs

In 1974 the country was divided into 203 PSRO areas designated by HEW. Late in 1974, 102 areas were funded with 11 conditional PSROs and 91 planning PSROs. Of the 203 areas, over 75% had less than 2,000 physicians; about 65% of the areas had populations of 1 million or less; and only about 10% had over 2 million.

By June 1975—there were PSROs in all but four states. One hundred twenty-one separate PSROs and 13 Statewide Support Centers were being funded by the federal government. It was estimated that 90,000 physicians were already members of these existing PSROs.

PSROs involve substantial administrative cost which is financed totally by the federal government. These costs were expected to be reasonable in comparison with the total cost of the health care programs which are subject to PSRO review. Federal funds are also being provided for planning and for establishing conditional PSROs.

Planning PSROs

Planning contracts for potential PSROs are awarded to organizations to help them meet the requirements for conditional designation as a PSRO and to help finance activities, such as recruiting of physician members, designing their review plan, and selecting staff.

Conditional PSROs

Organizations that are ready to conduct PSRO review of medical care can be awarded funds as conditional PSROs. (By the end of 1975, about 30–40 of the existing 91 planning PSROs converted to conditional PSRO status.) These organizations must meet the statutory organizational requirements, such as open and voluntary membership including a substantial proportion of physicians in the PSRO area— which has been set at about 25%. They must have open election of officers and rotate reviewers. As conditional PSROs, they must develop an appropriate review plan approved by HEW.

The hospital peer review system in short term hospitals must include: concurrent review, medical care evaluation studies and profile analysis. Concurrent review includes admission certification and continued stay review. The review is based on the use of explicitly stated norms, criteria, and standards, established by the physicians in each PSRO area. This review essentially replaces existing third party payment review.

In order to conduct review in these hospitals, the conditional PSROs: (1) are developing memoranda of understanding with the Medicare intermediaries and Medicaid agencies; (2) are developing memoranda of understanding with each hospital in which review is initiated; (3) have and continue to establish norms and adopt or adapt criteria and standards; (4) are evaluating and determining capability of each hospital to carry out its own review; (5) are delegating and monitoring review to capable and willing hospitals and conducting review in other hospitals; (6) are continuing to recruit physician members; (7) are working with nonphysician practitioners and (8) are developing internal operating procedures and accounting systems and training reviewers and other personnel.

Organization and Impact

Establishing a PSRO

A proposal is solicited from a physician-sponsored organization to apply for planning funds and subsequently for designation as a PSRO. The requirements are that such an organization must have at least 25% of the practicing licensed physicians in that federally designated PSRO area as members of the organization.

PSROs range from around 300 physicians, the smallest type of PSRO, to about 2,500 to 3,000 for some of the statewides. The metropolitan areas have considerably more than that, but have been retained as single PSRO areas to better coordinate with their peers.

Membership

PSRO membership is open on a voluntary basis to licensed, practicing doctors of medicine or osteopathy in the PSRO area. Members usually include physicians of all medical specialties, representatives from hospital medical staffs, private practitioners, academic physicians, administrative physicians, interns and residents. It has been noted that as PSROs become more mature, as they enter their second and third years of operation, their physician membership acceptance grows remarkably. It takes only 25% membership to qualify. But by the second year most of the PSROs have well over 50 to 90% of all the physicians in the area joining them.

By 1977 a third of the physicians in the country belonged to PSROs, and in areas where PSROs had been established about one-half of the eligible physicians were members.

A PSRO at Work

The Wyoming PSRO is performing admission certification and continued stay review on 100% of the elective and emergency admissions covered under Titles XVIII, XIX, and V in all 37 hospitals in the state. Between September 20, 1974, and January 11, 1975, the PSRO reviewed 5,413 PSRO admissions. During this period, they were phasing-in review activity on a hospital-by-hospital basis. Current review activity is approximately 3,000 admissions per month. The PSRO has signed a Memorandum of Understanding with the Medicaid agency and an interim document with the Medicare intermediary. The PSRO has 320 members out of an eligible 360 physicians. Physician committees have developed critical criteria for 104 diagnoses, and have two Medical Care Evaluation Studies in progress.

Impact of PSRO Review

Conditionally designated PSROs have found evidence that where PSRO review is implemented, hospital lengths of stay are shorter than under previous conditions.

For example, length of stay data available from four newly designated conditional PSROs (South Carolina, Idaho, Hartford County, and Greater Oregon), showed an average decrease of length of stay of 22.75%. For Medicaid patients, length of stay declined from 7.94 days to 5.68 days. At an average cost of about $100 a day the resultant rough estimate of the savings in basic hospitalization costs was approximately $223 per episode of hospitalization. For Medicare patients, length of stay declined from 11.21 to 9.3 days. At a cost of $100 per day, the resultant saving in basic hospitalization costs can be estimated to be approximately $189 per episode of hospitalization.

Standards and Sanctions*

Standards

Each PSRO must establish standards and criteria of care that reflect acceptable patterns of practice in the PSRO's area and that will lend themselves to local review.

---

*Source: DHEW, June 1974

It is expected that the standards and criteria used by a PSRO will be modified as experience is gained and developments in medicine warrant their modification. Norms, standards and criteria must take into account the professional personnel, facilities and equipment available. The National Professional Standards Review Council must approve norms used by a PSRO that are significantly different from professionally developed regional norms.

The national specialty societies are preparing model criteria which will be made available to the PSROs and which they can adopt or adapt to meet local circumstances. The norms, standards and criteria are checkpoints which identify instances of care that fall outside what would normally be expected to occur. These checkpoints will be established for classes of patients with a particular diagnosis or problem. When applied, they screen out cases requiring more in-depth review. It is at this point that peer review really comes into play. All factors related to the particular case in question should be considered before any decision affecting payment is made. For example, consideration of the patient's psychological and social situation and the availability of alternative facilities of course must be considered as must the distinction between the case in question and the criteria themselves.

The PSRO staff is responsible for rotating the peer review responsibilities among the physicians in the area who are members of the PSRO.

Sanctions

If a physician's pattern of practice indicates that he is delivering excessive or insufficient health care or otherwise improperly treating his patients, his peers in the PSRO are supposed to advise the physician and recommend appropriate remedies, such as professional consultation and education. Only in rare cases would sanctions provided by law be imposed, such as suspension or termination of Medicare and Medicaid payments. Appeal mechanisms from any sanctions recommended by the PSRO are also provided by law.

If a physician's peers in the PSRO disapprove a proposed procedure or service or an extension of a length of stay, the immediate effect would be that the government would not pay for those services. The physician is still free to provide the care and services he chooses, and he can appeal the determination of his local PSRO to the statewide Professional Standards Review Council and to HEW.

The PSRO legislation contains strong penalties for breech of confidentiality.

PSROs and the Hospital*

The current PSRO guidelines require that PSROs initially establish a review system for inpatient care in short-stay general hospitals. A PSRO is required to utilize the services of and accept the findings of hospitals in carrying out its responsibilities provided such hospitals demonstrate capability and continue to provide evidence that effective and timely review is being conducted.

The new "Utilization Review" regulations are designed to facilitate the development of effective in-house review capability and thereby expedite the establishment of the PSRO program.

The PSRO may organize itself in many ways to accomplish its responsibilities. In the area of criteria development, for example, it may ask the medical staff of a particular hospital to develop criteria on a particular subject, while, on another topic, it may use a committee representing the medical staffs of several hospitals, or a local specialty society.

Major Characteristics of the PSRO Review System

Concurrent Review

Concurrent review certifies the necessity, appropriateness, and quality of services during the hospital episode and assures that Medicare and Medicaid payments will be made as long as the patient is eligible and the services provided are covered benefits of the program.

Concurrent Admission Certification (CAC)

Concurrent admission certification is a form of review which is meant to assure that a patient's admission to a hospital level of care is medically necessary.

Concurrent Continued Stay Review (CSR)

Concurrent continued stay review is a form of health care review which occurs during a

_____
*Source: "The PSRO Hospital Review," supplement to *Medical Care*, April 1975.

patient's hospitalization and is designed to allow (1) a review of the need for continued stay in the hospital and (2) a review, in selected cases, of some aspects of the quality of the care being provided including the review of ancillary services (concurrent quality assurance). Continued stay review is performed on all patients who are still in the hospital at the time of the initial checkpoint.

Medical Care Evaluation Studies (MCE Studies)

Medical care evaluation studies are a form of health care review in which an indepth assessment is made of the quality and administration of health care services. They are designed to assure that (1) health care services are appropriate to the patient's needs and are of appropriate quality and (2) health care organization and administration support the timely provision of quality care.

Medical care evaluation studies focus on assuring quality much as concurrent review focuses on improving utilization practices. While all components of the PSRO hospital review system are designed to assure the quality of health care services, MCE studies emphasize quality improvement through continuing medical education targeted specifically to correct identified problems.

There is some confusion as to the nature of MCE studies. They are, in fact, medical audits. The reason they are difficult to describe is that their subject matter varies greatly and can include review of the patient care process, patient outcomes, the use of a given procedure, or the operating characteristics of an institution.

Profile Analysis

Profile analysis is a form of retrospective review in which aggregated patient care data are subject to pattern analysis. A "profile" is defined as the presentation of aggregated data in formats which display patterns of health care services over a defined period of time.

The analysis of profiles related to hospital care may be used to focus concurrent review efforts (AC and CSR) or MCE studies, to develop local norms of hospital utilization, and to monitor the effectiveness of hospital review activities.

The process of analysis should include: comparisons of the patterns of care by similar providers (institutions or practitioners), comparisons of current patterns with those from a previous time period, and the identification of exceptional patterns. Some of the comparisons may be performed by computer with the unusual patterns identified in the reports. The additional analysis is done in the hospital or by the PSRO.

Impact of PSRO on the Nurse

There are areas within the PSRO guidelines that pertain specifically to the involvement of nurses in a peer review program. The guidelines from the PSRO Manual indicate that "PSROs must show evidence over time" that nonphysician health care practitioners have become involved in the following activities:

1. Development and ongoing modifications of norms, criteria and standards for their areas of practice.
2. Development of review mechanisms to be used for peer assessment of the performance of nonphysician health care practitioners.
3. Conduct of health care review of nonphysician health care practitioners by their peers.
4. Where care is provided jointly by physicians and nonphysician health care practitioners, there should be joint development of criteria and joint assessment of care by peer physicians and nonphysician practitioners.
5. Where appropriate, participation of both physicians and nonphysician health care practitioners in review committee activities.
6. Working with established continuing education programs to assure utilization of results of review in educational efforts.

Once a program of assessment of nursing services within the frame of PSRO has been established, there are further implications for the nursing service administrators.

The results of review may be used at the PSRO level to prepare composite reports of review findings from all nursing services of similar nature, e.g., from general hospitals, skilled nursing facilities, rehabilitation facilities, etc.

The results of review could also assist the director of nursing service in gaining agency administrative support for corrective actions needed. Such actions may include: (1) changes in staffing, (2) changes in policy, (3) purchase of new equipment and/or supplies to improve

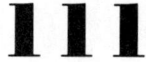

patient care, (4) intensification of inservice educational efforts and (5) even backing to take appropriate action when an individual's performance reflects inability to meet criteria in a sufficient number of patient reviews.

Early Resistance by Doctors

A *Medical World News* national survey of M.D.s and D.O.s in 1974 found that:

- One-fifth of the nation's practicing GPs say they will refuse to treat Medicare and Medicaid patients rather than have a PSRO monitor their performance.
- One-fourth of all practitioners fear PSROs will cut their incomes.
- One-third of all practitioners fear PSROs will trigger more malpractice suits.
- Slightly more than half of all doctors are opposed to PSROs.
- Most doctors who are either hospital-based, under 45 years of age, or live in the northeast favor PSROs.

In the over-all tabulation, 53.1% of all doctors are against the PSRO program.

Related Agencies

National Professional Standards Review Council

The National Council is composed of eleven "physicians of recognized standing and distinc-

tion in the appraisal of medical practice." The majority of members were recommended by organizations representing practicing physicians and the remainder by consumer groups and other health care interests. The major role of the National Professional Standards Review Council concerns the development and use of norms, standards, and criteria in PSRO review and evaluation.

PSRO Support Centers

Since many state level physician organizations had some experience in peer review, it was felt that in the larger states with multiple PSRO areas, they could serve a useful purpose as Statewide Support Centers to PSROs. Thirteen of such organizations have become PSRO Support Centers in states with four or more PSRO areas.

The Support Center contracts were divided into two parts. Part I was to develop a program to *educate physicians about PSROs and provide initial assistance* to physician groups in their desire to organize as planning PSROs or begin to advance toward conditional PSRO status. Part II of the scope of work called for the provision of *additional assistance*. This included the provision of *technical assistance* to planning PSROs in developing the capability to apply for conditional designation. It also included assistance in the actual development of proposals to become both planning and conditional PSROs.

8
UNIONS

The Scene Today

Rates and Success

The tempo of unionization within the health care industry is picking up speed. By 1971, nearly 1,400 hospitals out of the 7,000 questioned by the American Hospital Association had acknowledged at least one union. During fiscal year 1975, representation petitions to the National Labor Relations Board (NLRB) from the health industry numbered 1,659. Unions won 125 of the 200 elections that occurred in hospitals that year. Within the total number of elections, 140 were contested cases in which elections had been ordered by the NLRB. (The majority of these hospitals were not-for-profit hospitals possessing fewer than 300 beds; three-quarters of them registered no union representation among employees.)

The success of unions in all hospital elections held that year was 62%, outdistancing the current union win rate for all industry in the country (50%). However, where the hospital union elections were contested, the union win rate was only 49%, a bit less than the comparable national rate. In a refinement of these figures, *Hospitals, JAHA* (December 16, 1975) reported that where management was aggressive in their campaign, only 35% of the elections went union; where management displayed little effort, 65% of the elections went to the union faction. It was noted that many hospitals believe the rate of unionization can be slowed down through the use of outside consultants to direct management's campaign during union organization efforts. One-third of the hospitals followed such a practice; and in those instances, unions won only 33% of the elections.

Union Organizers

The competition among union organizers within given hospital elections has been relatively low, though there are several unions that cover the varied employees in the hospital industry sector. Recently, the most active union has been the Service Employees International Union (SEIU), with, for example, participation in hospital elections in a 13-state area in 1975. The once predominant Local 1199 of the Retail, Wholesale and Department Store Union was active in eight states. The Teamsters Union has concentrated its efforts in California and the Retail Clerks Union has spread its involvement to six states.

Among nurses, there has been a substantial increase of union activity. During 1975, organizing efforts were undertaken by nearly a third of the state nurses' associations, with particularly aggressive activity in Pennsylvania, New York, Ohio and California. Early in that year, around 571 different contracts were negotiated by state associations, according to the American Nurses' Association. Approximately 84,000 nurses were represented in the collective bargaining process during the year. Estimates of membership among other unions provide approximate tallies of 10–15,000 R.N.s in SEIU and 25,000 nurses in AFL/CIO affiliates.

Survey of Union Sentiment Among Nurses*

Only 4% of the nurses participating in the *Nursing '76* survey said they were union members, and for most, this meant being represented by their state nurses' association.

	Staff Nurses	Directors
Very much in favor of nurses' unions	28%	9%
Someone should represent nurses but not unions	56	50
Unions are acceptable for nonprofessionals but not for nurses	7	6
Very much opposed to nurses' unions	9	35

Pro-union

Those in favor of unions listed these benefits:

- power to make management listen, participation in decision making;
- improved wages and fringe benefits for everyone, including part-time nurses;
- influence over working conditions, including improved staffing;
- a grievance procedure;
- job security and a seniority system;
- more control over their own profession and

---

*Source: Marjorie Godfrey "Someone Should Represent Nurses" *Nursing '76*, June 1976.

a way to strengthen nursing service;

- a way to change outdated procedures and policies.

Anti-union

Negative feelings expressed were that unions:

- are divisive—they pit one employee group against another and pit labor against management;
- are nonprofessional and not capable of dealing with the unique problems of health care institutions;
- are insatiable with ever-increasing demands;
- turn hospitals into assembly lines;
- promote the self-interests of the nurse at the expense of the patient, up to and including strikes;
- make it impossible to reward excellence;
- infringe on personal freedom by forcing some to belong against their will and make it hard to get out once you're in. Contracts are binding on employees as well as management.

Expectations from Union

Nursing '76 asked: "What would you expect the union to achieve for you?"

Expect salary increases with cost-of-living adjustments	89%
Increase in continuing education courses	78
Improved patient care	70
Better health insurance coverage	65
Job security	61
New staffing systems	53

Nursing Committees

An earlier survey (*Nursing '75*, May) queried nurses about nursing committees. Thirty-nine percent of U.S. nurses reported having such committees to represent their concerns to the hospital administration. Some 43% do not, and 16% didn't know if they did or not.

Only 40% of those represented by a committee considered it a suitable substitute for a nurses' union.

Collective Bargaining

By the end of 1975 over 20% of all hospital employees were represented by some type of labor organization. R.N. collective bargaining agreements were in effect in 11.4% in the most recent survey of hospitals. These hospitals were more likely to be large and have medical school affiliations.

Table 8-1 Collective Bargaining Agreements—Hospital R.N.s

	All hospitals	Size (beds)					Census area				Ownership		
		Under 50	50 to 99	100 to 199	200 to 399	400 and over	North-east	North Central	South	West	Non-profit	Govern-ment	Proprie-tary
% R.N. collective bargaining agreements	11.5	9.0	5.9	11.9	16.2	22.5	12.1	10.7	5.0	22.1	9.8	14.6	8.8

Source: DHEW, 1975.

Table 8-2 Collective Bargaining—Hospitals in Cities. Workers in nongovernment and state and local government hospitals having collective bargaining agreements covering a majority of their workers (in percent)

Area	Registered professional nurses		Other professional and technical employees		Office clerical employees		Other non-professional employees	
	Non-government	State and local	Non-government	State and local	Non-government	State and local	Non-government	State and local
Atlanta	—	—	—	—	—	—	—	—
Baltimore	(¹)	10–14	—	35–39	5–9	35–39	50–54	30–34
Boston	20–24	90–94	10–14	25–29	—	70–74	—	85–89
Buffalo	5–9	55–59	—	70–74	—	50–54	40–44	60–64

Table 8-2   (continued)

Area	Registered professional nurses Non-government	Registered professional nurses State and local	Other professional and technical employees Non-government	Other professional and technical employees State and local	Office clerical employees Non-government	Office clerical employees State and local	Other non-professional employees Non-government	Other non-professional employees State and local
Chicago	(1)	60–64	—	(1)	(1)	50–54	20–24	75–79
Dallas	—	—	—	—	—	—	—	—
Denver	—	—	—	—	—	—	—	—
Detroit	(1)	65–69	—	45–49	5–9	70–74	30–34	70–74
Houston	—	—	—	—	—	—	—	—
Los Angeles	(1)	95+	(1)	95+	5–9	95+	10–14	90–94
Memphis	—	—	—	—	—	80–84	—	85–89
Miami	—	—	—	—	—	95+	—	90–94
Milwaukee	—	95+	—	5–9	—	—	15–19	—
Minneapolis–St. Paul	85–89	—	—	5–9	—	(1)	80–84	10–14
New York	15–19	95+	20–24	90–94	15–19	95+	45–49	95+
New York City	15–19	95+	25–29	85–89	20–24	95+	55–59	95+
Philadelphia	—	95+	(1)	75–79	—	95+	10–14	95+
Portland	50–54	95+	—	—	(1)	5–9	55–59	95+
St. Louis	5–9	30–34	—	5–9	5–9	45–49	5–9	85–89
San Francisco	75–79	30–34	50–54	35–39	20–24	45–49	90–94	55–59
Seattle	90–94	95+	—	—	5–9	15–19	5–9	55–59
Washington	—	—	—	—	—	—	5–9	25–29

[1] Estimates of less than 5%.

Note: Dashes indicate no data reported.

Source: U.S. Bureau of Labor Statistics (1972 data), 1974.

Background

Unions and the ANA

1946:   The House of Delegates of the ANA officially initiated the Economic Security Program (a highly stylized approach to collective action) with the policy stating:

The American Nurses' Association believes that the several state and district nurses' associations are qualified to act and should act as the exclusive agents of their respective memberships in the important fields of economic security and collective bargaining. The Association . . . urges all state and district nurses' associations to push such a program vigorously and expeditiously.

1950:   ANA adopted a no-strike policy.
1952:   29 state associations adopted it.
1961:   Mass resignations became a popular technique for pressing demands.
1968:   ANA revoked the no-strike policy and initiated a more militant approach. From there on, ANA's posture was not unlike a trade union's.

Strikes and Mediation

A labor organization is prohibited from striking without giving ten days notice of the intention to strike management. This advance notice is to provide management with an opportunity to make arrangements for continued patient care, even if on a limited basis. Unions and health care facilities are also required by law to notify each other no less than ninety days before a contract modification or termination.

A labor dispute in a health care institution is automatically subject to mediation by the Federal Mediation and Conciliation Service (FMCS). The FMCS may set up fact-finding boards to make recommendations for settlement. Such a board would be established 30 days before the contract expires and would report 15 days before expiration.

Supervisors and Unions

If the NLRB rules that nurses who are supervisors are also part of health care management, and therefore not allowed to participate in organizing efforts, then the ANA and its state nursing associations could be depleted of their main leadership all across the U.S. The

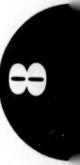

economic and general welfare movement would have to depend more and more on developing collective bargaining support at the staff nurse level.

The ANA has complained that hospital managers are rewriting job descriptions to bring as many nurses as possible under the management umbrella. In other instances, ANA says, directors of nursing and top supervisors are being forced to make a choice: either stay on as management and part of hospital administration or resign from state and national nursing groups.

A Grievance Procedure*

A formal grievance procedure should include:

1. A simple written account of the grievance procedure.
2. Varying steps of appeal (usually three is sufficient) through which the employee can seek regress for his/her perceived unfair treatment.
3. Alternate routes of appeal which can be taken by an employee should he/she feel the need to bypass an immediate super-visor. Ordinarily the personnel department is the alternate route. Figure 8-1 presents an example of a grievance system that might exist in a hospital for the nursing department.
4. A time limit must be set for each step, so management is prohibited from delaying the processing of a complaint. This requires the grievance system to have total support of all management, to avoid the possibility of it becoming just a formality for approving management actions. The grievance (large or small) must be acted on in all cases. This is necessary for the system to build integrity.
5. An appeal mechanism for both management and employees. If an employee is turned down on the initial appeal or if management feels that the decision was truly unfair, each should have the right to continue on to the next appeal.
6. A final review board for arbitration, containing employees as well as management personnel. True representation must be provided. If employee representation is not provided, then employees usually view the

---

*Source: Chaney and Beech, *The Union Epidemic* (Aspen Systems, 1976).

Figure 8-1   Example of a grievance system

EMPLOYEE

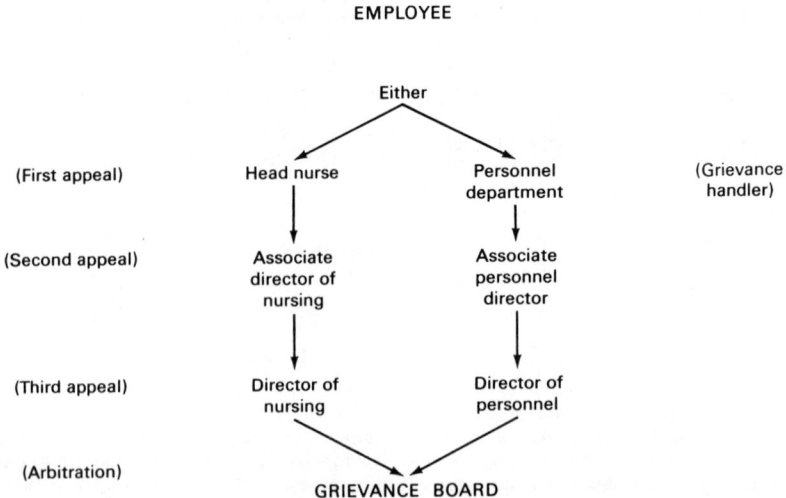

whole grievance process as a mere rubber stamp for the supervisor.

Terminology in Collective Bargaining and Strikes

Collective bargaining refers to the process of negotiation between a union and employer to effect a written labor contract stipulating the terms and working conditions of employees. The strike represents a dramatic "cease-work" form of economic pressure to win acceptance of contract demands, but several methods of arbitration are gaining approval as an attractive alternative for settling demands.

Alternative Methods of Arbitration:

Arbitration is a method in which the two factions of union and employer mutually agree to submit their dispute to a third party for a binding resolution. There are variations on the process:

- *Conciliation* is a fairly traditional step, rather than an alternative, to achieve a voluntary settlement through the efforts of a third party. The decision is nonbinding on the two opposing viewpoints.

- *Compulsory arbitration* is used when strikes are legally forbidden and the disputing parties are required to present their cases before an impartial arbitrator.

- *Mediation–arbitration* involves a three-step phase where an experienced arbitrator sits in on the negotiations; shifts to the position of a mediator when an impasse is reached, and attempts to effect a voluntary agreement; and, at last resort, assumes the position of arbitrator who hands down a binding settlement.

- *Last-offer arbitration* involves the presentation of minimum acceptable demands by both sides before an arbitrator who choses one proposal as a final settlement.

- *Fact-finding* is a review of evidence and arguments from both sides which results in a series of nonbinding recommendations from the individual or panel of impartial experts selected to hear the issues.

Strikes and Related Terms:

- *Cease and desist order* requires an employer or union to refrain from an unfair labor practice. It is issued by the National Labor Relations Board and is enforced through the U.S. Court of Appeals.

- *Cooling-off period* is a legally required ten-day notice period unions give to hospitals; an opportunity for settlement.

- *Economic strike* is motivated by the employer's rejection of union demands for economic considerations—wages, fringe benefits—rather than unfair labor practices.

- *Emergency dispute* involves a strike which endangers national health, thereby involving special procedures under the NLRA.

- *Grievance* refers to a complaint that a provision of the collective bargaining contract has been violated.

- *Picketing* provides the public with evidence of a labor dispute through signs carried at the strike site by members of the union.

- *Recognitional picketing* is an attempt by a labor organization to win recognition as the bargaining agent for all employees by publicizing their presence via the picket line.

- *Sit-down strike* occurs when the striking employees remain on the job site but temporarily stop work.

- *Slowdown* is an attempt to enforce employee demands through a unified reduction of work pace.

- *Unauthorized strikes* occur when employees strike without the consent of their union and contrary to the union's advice. If such a strike is in violation of the labor contract, it is dubbed a "wildcat" strike.

- *Whipsawing* is a practice where a union strikes against a single employer in an area, wins a favorable contract and then presents it to other employers in the area.

The Unionization Process

Union Organizing*

Steps in Organizing

Union organizing attempts primarily incorporate one or more of three steps.

STEP 1: The Hospital Survey—Background information is a necessary part of any campaign. Unless the organizer has a thorough understanding of the hospital, its policies, its key people, its problems, etc., a formalized strategy cannot be developed. Consequently, the first step is to do a "target" survey.

Initially, the organizer spends several hours simply observing the facility, talking to cafeteria employees, workers in housekeeping, nurses, and so on. From such conversations the organizer attempts to determine the number of employees per shift; employee breakdown by sex, age, race, etc.; what eating and drinking facilities are nearby; available transportation facilities for the employees; and special problems the facility might face.

The second part of a survey involves establishing contact with the existing labor movement in the community. Here the organizer determines the labor position of the mass media; the labor history of the organization; names of employees who are active in community work such as churches, civic groups, and politics (these persons often make good initial contacts); names of former employees who belonged to a union; a general idea of wages, conditions, and problems; community relations with the target facility; community reaction to organized labor; and meeting dates and places for local union groups.

STEP 2: Selecting the Employee Leaders—Having completed his initial survey of the facility, the organizer is now ready to make his first contact with the employees of the health care facility. Most union organizers are primarily interested in finding the employee who is respected by his/her fellow workers and who has informal influence within the health care facility. These are the workers that the organizer will depend on for "internal leadership" and information about the specific problems and complaints of the employees.

The labor organizers court potential internal leaders. The benefits of the union are explained, and an attempt is made to build up the trust of the leaders. The organizers try to get leaders for every faction within the organization; for the women, the men, the minority groups, etc. They create committees and encourage mass participation.

STEP 3: Showing the Union Presence—In Step 3 the union will begin actively to distribute handbills and/or begin seeking authorization card signatures for the purpose of forcing an election. The purpose of this first handout distribution is little more than to show union presence. Such leaflets tend to be general in nature and are usually prepared by the union's international or national office.

Once the "internal leaders" begin bringing the organizer the signed union authorization cards, the organizer dramatically steps up the campaign by seeking the trouble spots, evaluating internal leadership, determining the area in which to build additional support and determining the best areas for the key supporters within the health care facility.

Demand for Recognition

Early in a campaign the union usually will send a telegram, letter, or even the organizer in person demanding recognition as the official bargaining unit for the health care employees. This demand for recognition usually asserts that:

1. the union has been officially designated as the exclusive bargaining agent by the majority of employees in the bargaining unit,
2. the union is prepared to begin immediate bargaining with management,
3. the union is prepared to present its authorization cards to management or to a third party to validate its claim of majority representation, and
4. the employer should beware of violating its "employees" statutory rights guaranteed under the National Labor Relations Act.

The purpose in sending this demand is to seek voluntary recognition without an election. Failing that, the demand is reflected in the official petition for an election filed to initiate the National Labor Relations Board's election procedures. Usually, the hospital's labor counsel will send a standard letter to the union stating that the hospital doubts that the union represents an uncoerced majority of employees; the hospital believes that the best

---

*Source: Chaney and Beech, *The Union Epidemic* (Aspen Systems, 1976).

method for determining the true wishes of the employees is through the secret ballot; the hospital has no knowledge of the method by which the union solicited authorization cards and, thus, cannot accept their validity; and the hospital recommends that the union file an election petition with the NLRB, which has jurisdiction over such activities.

Union Authorization Card

The typical union authorization card simply authorizes the union to act as an employee's agent for purposes of collective bargaining with the hospital.

In addition, the card serves four other important purposes. The first one is to satisfy the NLRB's 30% showing of interest requirement. In other words, the union must obtain a 30% show of interest by signed authorization cards or employees' signatures on a petition to file with the NLRB to hold a secret ballot election (conducted by the NLRB).

Second, the authorization cards are usually a reliable barometer of the employee sentiment within the hospital. Third, authorization cards are useful as a check on an overzealous union organizer who might forge or persuade employees to sign cards without regard to the employees' real interest in the union.

Fourth, a hospital can be ordered by the NLRB to bargain with the union, even if the union lost the election. This can happen if 50% or more of the employees have signed authorization cards *and* the employer/hospital commits serious unfair labor practices, which tend to preclude the possibility of conducting a second election.

The Election

Having failed to get management to agree voluntarily to collective bargaining, it now becomes necessary to carry the campaign toward an election. The majority of effort is spent on encouraging those that signed the cards to actually vote for the union. Inside the health care facility the prounion employees try to persuade the other employees to support the effort. Participation is the key word in a union organizing attempt. The organizers create all types of committees:

1. membership (accumulate potential members, names, groups);
2. publicity (to discuss union information within the facility);

3. distribution (mimeographing, handing out pamphlets, maintaining mailing lists, etc.);
4. strategy (works with organizer in developing tactics and strategies for the campaign effort); and
5. community (to explain the need for the union to the community and to try to get its support).

Another primary purpose for getting as many inside workers as possible on committees is to prevent management from claiming that the union activity is the result of "outside agitation," or to protect from the attack that it is the work of "a minority of disgruntled employees."

Collective Bargaining Representation

See Figure 8-2 on the following page for an outline of collective bargaining representation procedures.

Unfair Labor Practices*

Unfair Labor Practices and the NLRB

The NLRB has two basic purposes. First, it defines and eliminates certain practices on the part of labor and employer that are deemed illegal under the act, called unfair labor practices. Second, it supervises and conducts secret ballot elections among employees to determine whether they want to be represented by a labor organization for purposes of collective bargaining. To accomplish these primary directives, the NLRB and the Office of the General Counsel act through 42 regional and field offices located in major cities throughout the United States. If an employer or a labor union is charged with committing an unfair labor practice, the hearing and taking of evidence will be conducted at one of the regional offices located within the area where the union and employer are doing business, or where the unfair labor practice in question took place. Such a hearing is conducted before an administrative law judge from either Washington, D.C., or San Francisco, California, the home bases. However, a hearing officer, usually an employee of the board's regional office, presides as the judge in both preelection and postelection representation hearings.

---

*Source: Chaney and Beech, *The Union Epidemic,* (Aspen Systems, 1976).

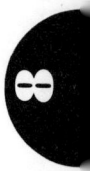

Figure 8-2   Outline of collective bargaining representation procedures

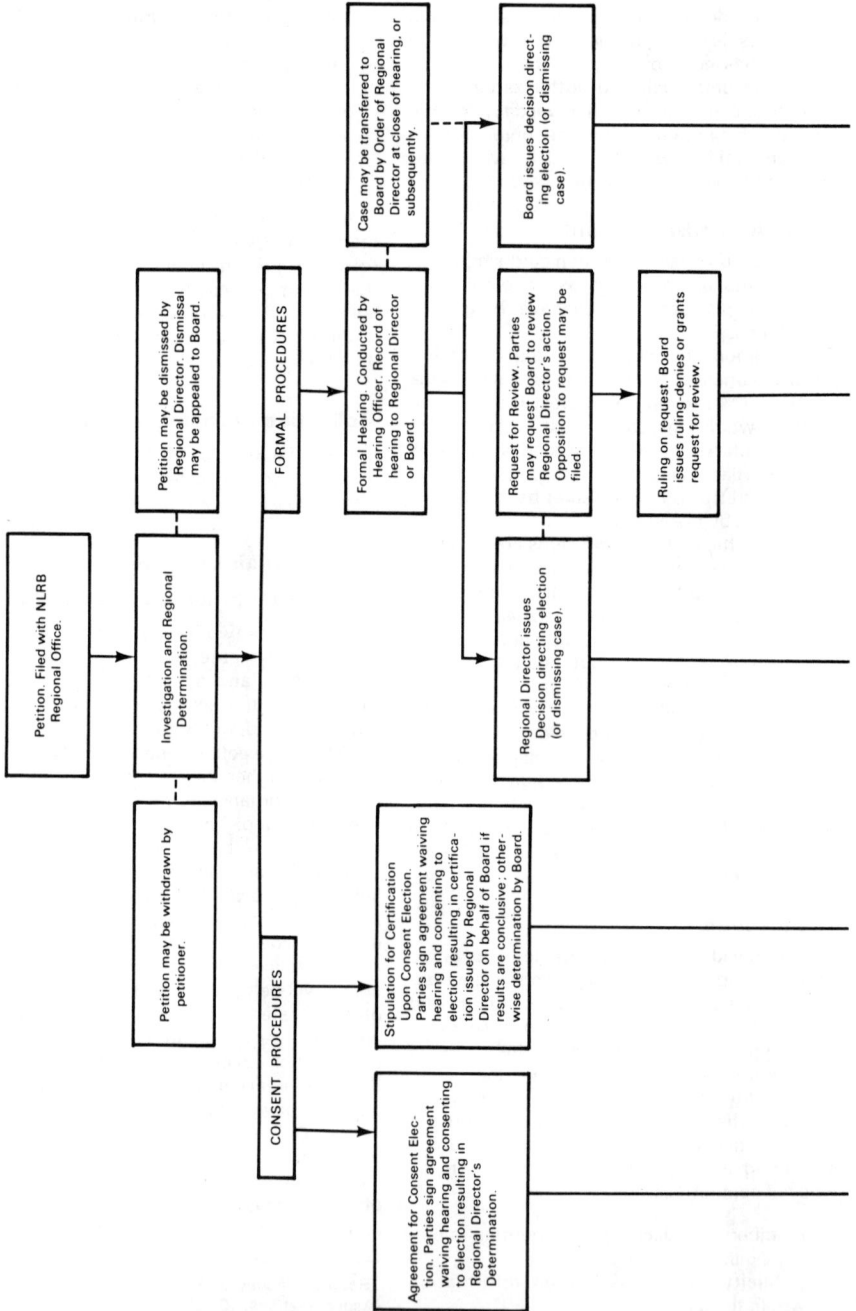

Petition. Filed with NLRB Regional Office.

Petition may be withdrawn by petitioner.

Investigation and Regional Determination.

Petition may be dismissed by Regional Director. Dismissal may be appealed to Board.

CONSENT PROCEDURES

FORMAL PROCEDURES

Agreement for Consent Election. Parties sign agreement waiving hearing and consenting to election resulting in Regional Director's Determination.

Stipulation for Certification Upon Consent Election. Parties sign agreement waiving hearing and consenting to election resulting in certification issued by Regional Director on behalf of Board if results are conclusive ; otherwise determination by Board.

Formal Hearing Conducted by Hearing Officer. Record of hearing to Regional Director or Board.

Case may be transferred to Board by Order of Regional Director at close of hearing, or subsequently.

Regional Director issues Decision directing election (or dismissing case).

Request for Review. Parties may request Board to review Regional Director's action. Opposition to request may be filed.

Board issues decision directing election (or dismissing case).

Ruling on request. Board issues ruling-denies or grants request for review.

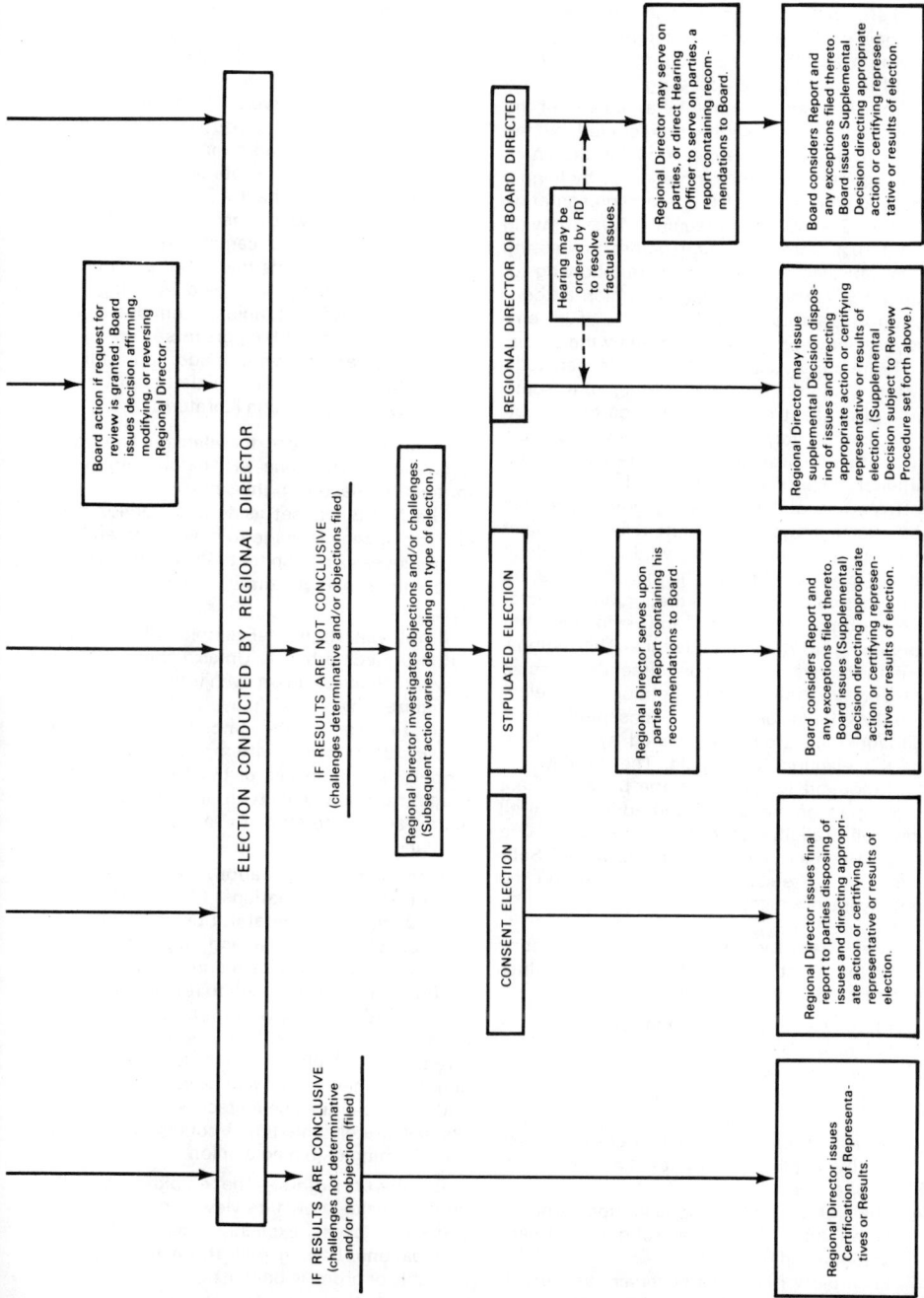

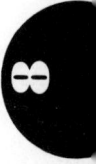

There are two basic ways in which a union can gain exclusive bargaining rights for a group of employees. The union can make formal demand to the employer for recognition based on authorization cards signed by a majority of the employees sought to be represented by the union. The second manner in which the union can become the bargaining agent is by filing a petition with the NLRB for a representation election. The board will require a 30% showing of interest from the union before processing such an election petition. The showing of interest is normally supplied by union authorization cards totaling at least 30% of all employees sought to be represented by the union.

The regional staff will attempt to persuade both the union and employer to agree to some form of consent election. If the parties refuse to enter into a form of consent election, a hearing is then held before a hearing officer of the regional office of the labor board. At this time both parties and the hearing officer can call and examine witnesses without being subject to the procedural rules followed in the federal district courts. After the hearing, the hearing officer submits a report to the regional director summarizing the issues and evidence, but containing no recommendations. The regional director then issues a report, either directing an election or dismissing the petition. If an election has been ordered or consented to by management, a date is selected by the board for the election to be held. The employer is then required to furnish to the board at least two copies of the names and addresses of all employees eligible to vote in the election, one of such copies being sent to the union. Subsequently, an election is held, usually on the employer's premises.

Guidelines for Election—In an election under the direction of the NLRB regional office several guidelines are followed.

1. More than one union may appear on the ballot.
2. Eligibility to vote is determined by a previous payroll roster of the employees.
3. The election is usually held on the employee's premises in an area easily accessible by employees and at a time opportune for the employees.
4. The NLRB supplies the ballot upon which is listed all options, i.e., choice between union(s) and no union.
5. Each party may have observers at the polling place and challenge any employee's right to vote.
6. Ballots are tabulated by the NLRB at the conclusion of the voting period, in the presence of observers. A majority of the votes cast are required for union representation. If more than one union was on the ballot and the vote was split, a runoff election would be held.
7. Within five days of the announcement of results, both parties can challenge the election on the grounds that: (a) the manner in which the election was held was illegal; (b) the employer or union intimidated employees; (c) false promises or misrepresentations were made; and (d) reproductions of the official ballot were misused as campaign literature.

Should the union lose the election, the union must wait at least one year before petitioning for another election in the same unit.

The NLRB will set aside any election if an election speech is made to massed assemblies of employees on hospital time within 24 hours before the scheduled time for starting the election.

Employee Rights—Examples of employee rights protected by the Unfair Labor Practices Law: (1) to join a union even if the union is not recognized by the employer; (2) to assist a union to organize the employees of an employer; (3) to form or attempt to form a union among the employees of the company; (4) to refrain from any activity in or on behalf of the union; and (5) to strike to secure better working conditions.

Employer Unfair Labor Practice—Examples of employer violations: (1) threatening to close down the hospital if a union should win the election; (2) questioning employees about their union activities or memberships in such circumstances as will tend to restrain or coerce the employee; (3) spying on union gatherings or meetings or pretending to spy on them; (4) threatening employees with loss of jobs or benefits if they should join or vote for a union; and (5) granting wage increases or other benefits deliberately timed to discourage employees from forming or joining a union.

Employer Rights—The employer has the right to make known its views on unionization to its employees, explicitly including all communications, barring only those that threaten reprisals or promise benefits.

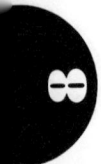

Figure 8-3   Basic procedures in cases involving charges of unfair labor practices

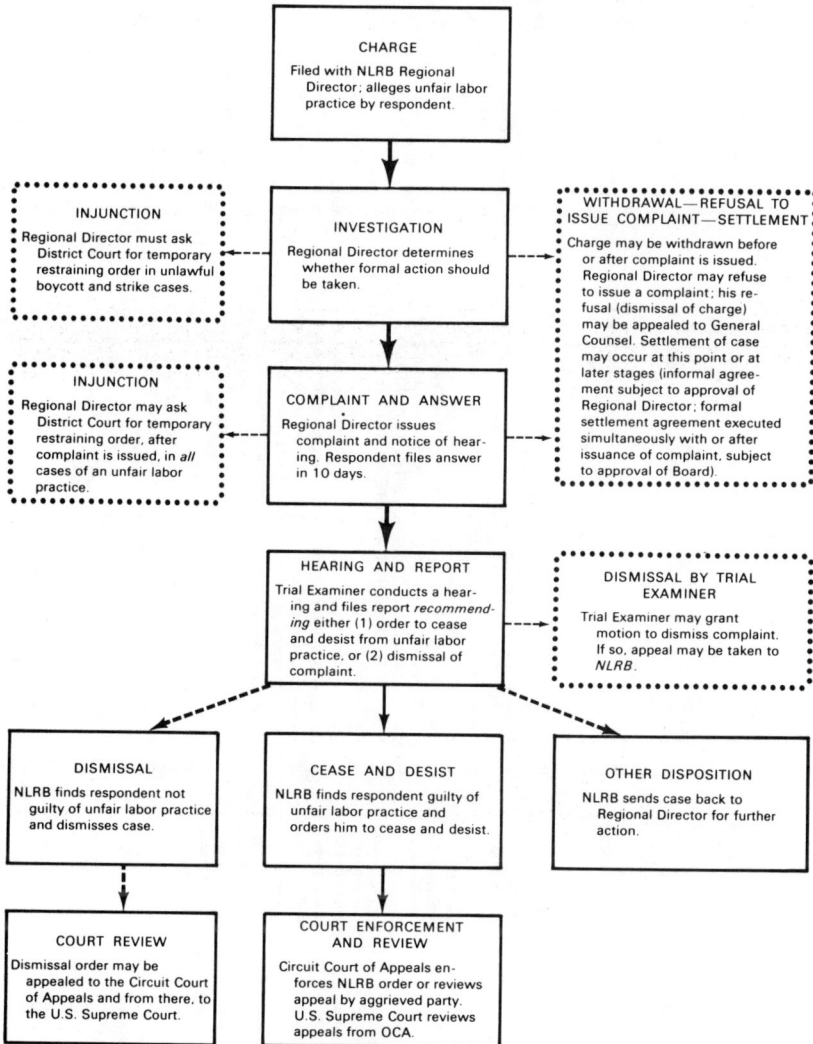

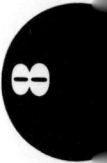

CHARGE

Filed with NLRB Regional Director; alleges unfair labor practice by respondent.

INJUNCTION

Regional Director must ask District Court for temporary restraining order in unlawful boycott and strike cases.

INVESTIGATION

Regional Director determines whether formal action should be taken.

WITHDRAWAL—REFUSAL TO ISSUE COMPLAINT—SETTLEMENT

Charge may be withdrawn before or after complaint is issued. Regional Director may refuse to issue a complaint; his refusal (dismissal of charge) may be appealed to General Counsel. Settlement of case may occur at this point or at later stages (informal agreement subject to approval of Regional Director; formal settlement agreement executed simultaneously with or after issuance of complaint, subject to approval of Board).

INJUNCTION

Regional Director may ask District Court for temporary restraining order, after complaint is issued, in *all* cases of an unfair labor practice.

COMPLAINT AND ANSWER

Regional Director issues complaint and notice of hearing. Respondent files answer in 10 days.

HEARING AND REPORT

Trial Examiner conducts a hearing and files report *recommending* either (1) order to cease and desist from unfair labor practice, or (2) dismissal of complaint.

DISMISSAL BY TRIAL EXAMINER

Trial Examiner may grant motion to dismiss complaint. If so, appeal may be taken to *NLRB*.

DISMISSAL

NLRB finds respondent not guilty of unfair labor practice and dismisses case.

CEASE AND DESIST

NLRB finds respondent guilty of unfair labor practice and orders him to cease and desist.

OTHER DISPOSITION

NLRB sends case back to Regional Director for further action.

COURT REVIEW

Dismissal order may be appealed to the Circuit Court of Appeals and from there, to the U.S. Supreme Court.

COURT ENFORCEMENT AND REVIEW

Circuit Court of Appeals enforces NLRB order or reviews appeal by aggrieved party. U.S. Supreme Court reviews appeals from OCA.

8

Figure 8-4 Unfair labor practices—types of cases

Charge against employer	Charge against labor organization				Charge against Labor organization and employer
Section of the Act *CA*	**Section of the Act** *CB*	**Section of the Act** *CC*	**Section of the Act** *CD*	**Section of the Act** *CP*	**Section of the Act** *CE*
8(a)(1) Interfere with, restrain, or coerce employees in exercise of their rights under Section 7 (to join or assist a labor organization or to refrain).	**8(b)(1)(A)** Restrain or coerce employees in exercise of their rights under Section 7 (to join or assist a labor organization or to refrain).	**8(b)(4)** (i) TO ENGAGE IN, OR INDUCE OR ENCOURAGE ANY INDIVIDUAL EMPLOYED BY ANY PERSON ENGAGED IN COMMERCE OR IN AN INDUSTRY AFFECTING COMMERCE TO ENGAGE IN, A STRIKE OR A REFUSAL IN THE COURSE OF HIS EMPLOYMENT TO USE, MANUFACTURE, PROCESS, TRANSPORT, OR OTHERWISE HANDLE OR WORK ON ANY GOODS OR TO PERFORM ANY SERVICES; OR (ii) TO THREATEN, COERCE OR RESTRAIN ANY PERSON ENGAGED IN COMMERCE OR IN ANY INDUSTRY AFFECTING COMMERCE, WHERE IN EITHER CASE AN OBJECT THEREOF IS:	**8(b)(4)** First Stage - 10(k)* Second Stage - Complaint**	**8(b)(7)** To picket, cause, or threaten the picketing of any employer where an object is to force or require an employer to recognize or bargain with a labor organization as the representative of his employees, or to force or require the employees of an employer to select such labor organization as their collective bargaining representative, unless such labor organization is currently certified as the representative of such employees:	**8(e)** To enter into any contract or agreement (any labor organization and any employer) whereby such employer ceases or refrains or agrees to cease or refrain from handling or dealing in any product of any other employer, or to cease doing business with any other person.
8(a)(2) Dominate or interfere with the formation or administration of a labor organization or contribute financial or other support to it.	**8(b)(1)(B)** Restrain or coerce an employer in the selection of his representatives for collective bargaining or adjustment of grievances.	(A) To force or require any employer or self-employed person to join any labor or employer organization or to enter into any agreement prohibited by Sec. 8(e).	(D) To force or require any employer to assign particular work to employees in a particular labor organization or in a particular trade, craft, or class rather than to employees in another trade, craft, or class, unless such employer is failing to conform to an appropriate Board order or certification.		
8(a)(3) Encourage or discourage membership in a labor organization (discrimination in regard to hire or tenure).	**8(b)(2)** Cause or attempt to cause an employer to discriminate against an employee.		* First Stage—Proceeding under Section 10(k) of the Act		
8(a)(4) Discharge or otherwise discriminate against an employee because he has given testimony under the Act.					
8(a)(5) Refuse to bargain collectively with representatives of his employees.					

AC

Requesting amendment of certification.

UC

(A) where the employer has lawfully recognized any other labor organization and a question concerning representation may not appropriately be raised under Section 9(c).

(B) where within the preceding 12 months a valid election under 9(c) has been conducted, or

(C) where picketing has been conducted without a petition under 9(c) being filed within a reasonable period of time not to exceed 30 days from the commencement of such picketing.

Requesting clarification of bargaining unit.

UD

Whenever it is charged that any person has engaged in an Unfair Labor Practice within the meaning of paragraph (4)(d) of Section 8(b), the Board is empowered and directed to hear and determine the dispute out of which such Unfair Labor Practice shall have arisen. . . .

**Second Stage—Complaint

Complaint under Section 8(b)(4)(D) is issued where there has been no voluntary adjustment of the dispute, and no compliance with the Board's Decision and Determination of Dispute.

9(e)(1) Employees wish to rescind a union security clause.

RD

(B) To force or require any person to cease using, selling, handling, transporting, or otherwise dealing in the products of any other producer, processor, or manufacturer, or cease to doing business with any other person, or force or require any other employer to recognize or bargain with a labor organization as the representative of his employees unless such labor organization has been so certified.

(C) To force or require any employer to recognize or bargain with a particular labor organization as the representative of his employees if another labor organization has been certified as the representative.

9(c)(1)(A)(ii) Asserting that the certified or recognized bargaining agent is no longer the representative.[1]

RM

8(b)(3) Refuse to bargain collectively with employer.

8(b)(5) Require of employees the payment of excessive or discriminatory fees for membership.

8(b)(6) Cause or attempt to cause an employer to pay or agree to pay money or other thing of value for services which are not performed or not to be performed.

9(c)(1)(B) Alleging that one or more claims for recognition as exclusive bargaining agent have been received by employer.[1]

RC

9(c)(1)(A)(i) Requesting the designation of filing party as bargaining agent.[1]

2. Petitions

[1]This statement is not applicable if an 8(b)(7) charge is on file involving the same employer; however, the "R" designation applies.

Source: House Appropriations Committee Hearings. February 1976.

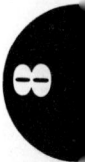

8

Labor Law History*

The first federal labor law was passed in 1935, more commonly referred to as the Wagner Act. This legislation created many new procedures in the field of labor relations. Primarily, the law:

1. delineates those employees and organizations considered to be under the act;
2. specifies the duties of the National Labor Relations Board (NLRB), charged with the administration of the act;
3. describes the rights of employees;
4. delineates management's unfair labor practices;
5. specifies procedures for selecting representatives, designating bargaining units, and conducting elections;
6. empowers the NLRB with authority to determine what are unfair labor practices and provide methods to seek redress and conduct investigations;
7. creates the Federal Mediation and Conciliation Service (FMCS) and specifies its duties;
8. denotes procedures that should be taken in national emergency disputes; and
9. describes how and under what conditions suits can be brought by and against labor unions and employers.

Voluntary nonprofit hospitals were within the jurisdiction of the Wagner Act.

The Taft-Hartley Act of 1947 made it clear that nonprofit hospitals had no legal obligation to recognize or bargain with their employees.

(In the 1960s demonstrations, mass sick calls, picketing, sit-ins, work slowdowns and a variety of other innovative actions for gaining public attention were initiated by nurses. Ultimately the nurses turned to mass resignations (threats and walkouts) and a few landmark strikes in such states as California and New York. These actions resulted in speedy and diligent responses by employers in negotiating grievances with nurses.)

In 1974, Public Law 93-360 was enacted. It amended the federal labor laws to extend guaranteed uniform coverage to all nonpublic health care facilities. Simply put, it states that employees of health care facilities (except federal facilities) have every right to organize, collectively gather, and petition for more bene-

fits, higher pay or better working conditions. For the first time, all nongovernmental hospitals, nursing homes, clinics, health maintenance organizations, homes for the aged and other institutions devoted to the care of infirm or aged persons are brought under the nation's labor laws.

Unions & Nursing Homes

In 1967, the NLRB asserted jurisdiction over proprietary hospitals and nursing homes. At the time of their decision, there were approximately 20,000 nursing homes in the United States, and 18,000 of these were proprietary. The agency ruled that any home with a gross business volume of at least $100,000 would come under its jurisdiction. This figure was discretionary so as to exclude small homes which did not sufficiently affect interstate commerce. The 1967 decision meant that employees of proprietary homes could now petition the NLRB and have it conduct the secret ballot election.

Unionization Process**

Indicators of Union Activity

Six common indicators of union activity should be recognized by every administrator:

1. Buzzing of the home's "grapevine" with frequent small huddles and furtive glances.
2. Unexplained slowdown of work or sagging of the quality of performance.
3. Sudden increase of gripes and complaints with no apparent justification.
4. Noticeable coolness of normally friendly employees.
5. Reports to management by loyal employees that something is brewing.
6. Appearance of union propaganda leaflets.

As a part of the organizing campaign, the union must persuade the employees that a victory will mean a significant wage increase, better fringe benefits, correction of personnel policy inequities, improvement of working conditions and security of jobs.

---

*Source: Chaney and Beech, *The Union Epidemic* (Aspen Systems, 1976).

**Source: Arthur J. Sampson, "Labor Unions and the Nursing Home," *Journal of Long Term Care Administration,* Summer 1974.

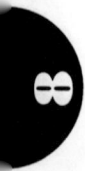

Process of Unionization

Propaganda leaflets are distributed and posted everywhere; i.e., on bulletin boards, walls, car windshields, etc; union buttons are worn which usually say "vote yes;" employees are solicited on-the-job, at home, and outside the nursing home; and a campaign to reach the public is launched to gain their sympathy.

The first active step taken by the union is to pass out union cards which require the employee's signature to the statement that he wants a union to represent him in collective bargaining. After the union has collected a significant number of signed cards (usually 30% of the employees), it petitions the administration for certification. At this point, the employer has two alternatives; he can concede to the union or he can ask for an election. The latter alternative is usually chosen because (1) the administrator does not believe that a majority of his employees wants union representation, and (2) even if 50 or more percent have signed the cards, there is a good possibility that a secret ballot election will "turn the tables" and the union will be defeated.

The election is supervised by the impartial NLRB, and every effort is made to see that every employee votes and that his ballot is, of course, secret. If a majority of the workers vote against the union, the union must wait one year before soliciting the same home again. A union victory means the collective bargaining process has arrived for the institution.

Action to Block Unions

If management tries to regain control of the home, good communication rules must be followed. Five ground rules for communication are:

1. They (management) can talk with employees individually or in groups at any time in any public place or open working area where they would normally talk with employees, but not in any private management office.

2. They can tell the employees that they (the supervisors) disapprove of unions and union policies and explain any bad experience they have had with unions.

3. They can talk about what harm they believe unions have done in the nation and in specific plants.

4. They can state what they believe to be an answer to any union propaganda, argument or claim.

5. They can say that they think employees should vote "no" in a union election.

On the other hand:

1. They cannot ask if an employee has signed a union card or belongs to a union or whether he knows if other employees belong.

2. They cannot ask how an employee has voted or will vote in a union election.

3. They cannot promise benefits or bribes to employees, or threaten, coerce or discipline them in order to influence them to refrain from belonging to a union.

Although money is important, there are other reasons why nursing home employees turn to the union.

Some of the most important are:

1. Working conditions. Long hours, obnoxious odors or fumes, dirty rest rooms and locker rooms and no coffee break time contribute to employee discontent.

2. Employees receive only a minimum of information about the status of the employer's financial health, goals, sales and production achievements. Consequently, they feel insecure in their jobs. They are ignored—not part of the team—and they have not been sold on the employer.

3. Work rules are inconsistently enforced at different times or in different departments or on different shifts.

4. The employer introduces changes in policy or work rules without advanced notice or subsequent explanation to the work force, or the employer is subcontracting work with subsequent layoffs. The union tells the remaining employees that a union contract would have protected their jobs by forbidding subcontracting.

5. The employer uses pressure tactics rather than leadership to obtain high production and productivity.

6. Employees feel stymied as far as future opportunities are concerned.

7. Employees see their supervisors playing favorites while they are losing out, or supervisors are bullying or needling employees.

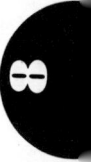

8. Their complaints and grievances are shrugged off or ignored by management instead of being discussed and cleared up promptly.

9. Employees are requested to pay increased contributions for group insurance or pensions.

Handling Grievances

The following procedure was suggested for handling grievances.

1. Develop clear, concise personnel policies.
2. Post your rules and give each employee a copy.
3. Review the rules with your supervisors.
4. Impress your supervisors with the importance of listening to a complaint.
5. Circulate.
6. Listen, but don't comment.
7. Develop a grievance review committee.
8. Do something about problems.

Racial discrimination and exploitation is also an invitation to unionism. In September, 1969, a massive demonstration of soul power and union power was combined at Baltimore's Johns Hopkins Hospital and the result was an overwhelming victory for Local 1199 Hospital and Nursing Home Employees Union (AFL-CIO).

Collective Bargaining

Collective Bargaining—Nursing Homes in Cities*

Establishments having collective bargaining contracts covering at least a majority of their full-time R.N.s were found in only six areas, whereas such unionization for full-time service and maintenance workers was reported in 17 areas.

New York had the largest proportion of union workers among service and maintenance employees and by far the largest number among R.N.s. Most homes in the survey had either a majority or none of the specified employee groups unionized; few homes had only a minority of either group unionized.

Table 8-3   Percent of employees in nursing homes and related facilities with collective bargaining agreements, May 1973

Area	Registered professional nurses	Service and mainte-nance employees
Atlanta	—	—
Baltimore	—	50–54
Boston	(^{1})	5–9
Buffalo	5–9	30–34
Chicago	—	40–44
Cincinnati	—	5–9
Cleveland	—	35–39
Dallas	—	—
Denver	—	—
Detroit	(^{1})	55–59
Los Angeles– Long Beach and Anaheim– Santa Ana– Garden Grove	—	5–9
Miami	—	45–49
Minneapolis– St. Paul	—	10–14
New York	50–54	75–79
Philadelphia	(^{1})	20–24
Portland	—	(^{1})
St. Louis	—	25–29
San Francisco– Oakland	5–9	60–64
Seattle–Everett	—	(^{1})
Washington	—	5–9

^{1} Less than 5%.

Note: Dashes indicate none of the establishments visited had a majority of the workers covered by collective bargaining contracts.

Doctors, Strikes and Unions**

Medical Opinion's 1975 survey of physicians' attitudes found:

- More than two-thirds of practitioners say they would strike, although most would leave emergency services functioning.
- Three out of four physicians believe that the physicians who went on strike recently in

---

*Source: U.S. Bureau of Labor Statistics, 1975.

**Source: Byron T. Scott, "Would You Go on Strike," *Medical Opinion,* December 1975.

Florida, Ohio, California, New York and elsewhere were largely justified in doing so.

- Just as many physicians would strike out of empathy as would leave work to protest issues directly affecting them.

- Despite this, however, only half would join a doctor's guild or a union—a percentage no

greater than existed three years ago when *Medical Opinion* conducted a similar survey.

What issues in particular will cause physicians to close ranks? For many, it's the sky-rocketing premiums of malpractice insurance. Most would like their medical societies and the AMA to be far more active in their behalf.

In 1975 a clear majority of physicians favored strikes or "withholding services."

If a physician strike were called in your area to protest, how would you react? (In percents)

	1975	1973	1972
Would strike, provided emergencies covered	51	33	38
Would strike, under other conditions	14	11	11
Would strike, even if meant total shutdown	4	3	4
Would not strike	23	31	28
Don't really know	8	22	19

How do you feel about joining a physicians' guild or union? (In percents)

	1975	1973	1972
Would join either one	28	31	35
Would join a guild, not a union	22	17	23
Would join a union, not a guild	7	3	3
Wouldn't join either one	31	23	19
Don't really know	12	26	20

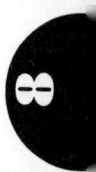

9

THE NURSE'S PERSONAL LIFE

Images and Attitudes

The conventional view of the ideal nurse is suggested by the Department of HEW description of desired personal qualifications for a nurse:

Ideally, the nurse must possess many desirable qualities, but one—a strong motivation to help others—is of uppermost importance. Service is the very heart of nursing and it must be performed for patients of all types and ages, whenever and wherever needed.

Since the nurse-patient relationship is an intimate one, the nurse must exercise sympathy, tact and understanding. This requires tolerance for human frailties, a sense of perspective and a healthy outlook on life, which is particularly needed during life's darker moments. Common sense, integrity, a sense of responsibility and self-discipline are equally important. The nurse must like people well enough to work smoothly with other members of the health team—physicians, nurses, and other professional personnel, and auxiliary workers.

To be suited for a career in nursing, one also must have an alert mind to master the knowledge and techniques required in all sorts of nursing situations. Good health is absolutely essential."

The actual qualities of the nurse are neither that simple nor that ideal.

Dedication*

In spite of their *own* commitment, 61% of nurses (in a survey of 10,000 nurses) felt that the professional dedication of nurses has declined in recent years. Nurses with more education and/or higher positions rated themselves as being more dedicated and as being more strongly of the opinion that professional dedication of nurses has declined.

---

*Source: "Quality of Care," *Nursing '77,* January.

To what extent is nursing central to your life?

	Female	Male
Nursing is my primary, life-long professional career	42%	66%
Nursing is an interesting career as long as it fits into other aspects of my life	52	27
Nursing is an interim thing until I get married, but it is reassuring to know that I can come back	2	0
I would leave if given an opportunity to do so	4	7

Male nurses, not surprisingly, are more career-minded than females.**

Self-Confidence

How sure of yourself do you feel?

Very	27%
Moderately	69.5%
Not very	3%
Not at all	0.5%

How confident do you feel about your nursing abilities?

Very	32%
Mostly	58%
Somewhat	9%
Not very	1%
Not at all	0.1%

Source: "Ethical Problems Survey," *Nursing '74,* September.

Career Goals†

Relatively large proportions of nurses cited leadership opportunities and the availability of jobs as reasons for their career choice. Other common reasons were being able to work with people, having the opportunity to be helpful to others, the chance for steady progress and making a contribution to society.

**Source: "Nursing Ethics," *Nursing '74,* October.
† Source: Health Resources Administration, DHEW, November 1974.

Most nurses expected to work in a hospital or clinic providing services to others. Other major job goals were teaching, administrative duties and counseling.

The average nurse was very modest in her self-ratings, particularly on mathematical and mechanical ability, academic ability, intellectual self-confidence, originality, popularity and drive to achieve. Nonetheless, nurses were more likely than were aspirants in other college groups to rate themselves high on cheerfulness, and over three in four gave themselves superior ratings on understanding of others.

The goal of having administrative responsibility for the work of others was highly valued by most nurses, whereas the goals of making a theoretical contribution to science and becoming a community leader were given low priority.

Attitudes Toward Work

Nurses in their 30s, 40s and 50s plan to remain with their current employer longer than those under 30 or over 60. Hospitals able to attract recent nursing school graduates must expect a higher nurse turnover rate.

Nurses with children aged two to six are likely to intend to stay longer than nurses with no children or children in other age groups. Possibly, the nurse who desires to work even though she has small children is particularly career-oriented.

As earnings of the nurse's spouse increase, nurse work hours decrease. Family income from nonemployment sources also has a negative impact on nurse hours of work. These results are consistent with past research on female labor supply by economists.

Personal Morality and Patient Care*

Nurses tend to respond in a similar way to patients who have performed various "immoral" or criminal acts. Nurses who admit having trouble giving optimal care to drug addicts, also tend to have trouble with alcoholics, attempted suicides and criminals. Difficulties in giving optimal care to homosexuals is

moderately correlated with difficulty in caring for criminals. Nurses who admit difficulty in giving optimal care to very old persons also admit difficulty with patients from minority groups.

Have you found it difficult to give optimal care to any of the following?

	Female nurses Yes	Male nurses Yes
Drug addicts	41%	40%
Alcoholics	34%	29%
Homosexuals	29%	21%
Criminals	25%	16%
Attempted suicides	21%	16%
Very old persons	16%	21%
Welfare patients	7%	11%
Minority group members	3%	7%

Sex and the Nurse**

Doctor and Nurse

What is your opinion about sexual involvement between a nurse and the doctor who work together?

Nothing wrong with it	16%
It's all right if they share affection	16%
It's all right, but it may hamper their work	40%
It's wrong because it's unprofessional behavior	14%
It's morally wrong	14%

Nearly 70% did not condemn involvement between a doctor and nurse who work together, but more than half of those cautioned that it may interfere with their work.

The older a nurse, the more likely she is to condemn sexual involvement between nurse and doctor. The converse is true. Nurses between ages 23 and 28 are most likely to condone it. Nurses in the Northeast and West are more apt to condone liaisons with doctors, whereas those in the South tend to condemn it.

---

*Source: "Ethical Problems," *Nursing '74*, September (Survey of 11,000 nurses).

**Source: "Ethical Problems" *Nursing '75*, September.

Patient and Nurse

Do you know of any nurses who had engaged in sexual intercourse with their patients?

	Female nurses	Male nurses
Yes, many	1%	1%
Yes, several	2%	5%
Yes, one or two	10%	20%
No	87%	75%

How often have you had patients make seductive or sexual advances to you?

Frequently	2%
Occasionally	30%
Only once or twice	43%
Never	25%

Have you ever responded to sexual advances made by someone while he or she was a patient?

	Female nurses	Male nurses
No, because advances never made	22%	29%
Never responded	66%	44%
No, but secretly tempted	9%	21%
Sometimes, but with no sex play	2%	2%
Sometimes, but short of intercourse	0.3%	2%
Yes, including intercourse	0.3%	2%

If we are to believe these self-reports, sexual intercourse between nurse and patient is extremely rare.

Nurses and Pornographic Films*

During the past few years, drive-in circuits and lower-grade movie houses have been showing

---

*Source: Dr. Alan Wheelock, "The Tarnished Image," *Nursing Outlook* August 1976. ©American Journal of Nursing Company.

any number of "X" and "R"-rated films with stories loosely based on a nursing or hospital situation. *Nurses Report, Student Nurses, Night Nurse,* and *Part-Time Nurse* are only some of the titles advertised in local papers these days. And, in what is considered to be the most explicit and controversial pornographic film ever made in this country for commercial distribution—*Deep Throat*—the now famous (or infamous) Linda Lovelace portrays a visiting nurse. Like teachers and stewardesses, nurses are members of a hierarchy that tends to maintain men at the very top.

Women subject to the mandates of male authority provide excellent opportunities for sexual fantasizing, and when the professional services to be rendered are dispensed almost exclusively by women, the fantasy gains considerable strength.

Stanley Kramer's *Not As A Stranger* depicts the struggles of a poor but brilliant medical student who marries a nurse he does not love because she has a steady, well-paying job. The nurse is a first-generation American of Scandinavian extraction. Her accent is pretty thick, and so is she. Incapable of understanding any of her husband's clever jokes or *bons mots,* she can't even repeat them for the benefit of dinner guests. The husband soon runs off with a provocative, highly articulate society woman, succeeds in making himself and his wife a local spectale, and then, in the end, returns to his wife. He is badly compromised, but still an acceptable husband—for a dumb nurse.

In Robert Altman's *M.A.S.H.,* nurses—many of them married—sleep with their superior officers in order to keep morale high during the Korean War. Those who don't—or won't—are subjected to merciless "peeping tomism"; their most intimate conversations are broadcast over the outfit's PA system, and whenever they attempt to shower, the facility collapses suddenly, leaving the poor naked women to face a dozen jeering, cheering doctors.

These films play on the same two themes: obedience to higher authority and assumption of fundamental dull wittedness. The dull but compliant nurse thus emerges as an ideal figure for erotic fantasy. As the films depict her, she does what a man wishes and poses no threat. The vacuity that actresses transmit as they engage in pornographic activities on screen helps to communicate that ideal image of a brainless, compliant, ever so obliging female.

Total Care?

Sexual fantasy films also tend to portray the nurse as a master of many sophisticated sexual techniques—mainly . . . because of her professional dedication to the concept of "total care." Since her knowledge of and exposure to the human body are so extensive, the thinking goes, it would follow that her ability to comfort must have a well-developed sexual dimension.

Marriage and a Nursing Career

Employment Patterns—
Married Nurses

In a recent study on the employment status of 2,000 married nurses in Michigan, some startling information was discovered on the utilization that professional nurses made of their training.

Of the total sample of nurses, 36% were inactive in 1972, while 43% worked part time, and 19% worked full time in nursing positions. The remaining two percent were either employed in the health field but not as a nurse or employed but not as a nurse. Of the 1,998 nurses in the sample, 17% were inactive throughout the five-year period from 1968 through 1972, 14% worked part time, and 7% worked full time. The fact that only 7% (139) of a sample of almost 2,000 married nurses had worked each year for five years is itself an indicant of the seriousness of the problem of labor force participation in nursing. . . .

A majority (80%) obtained their basic nursing education in diploma programs, 6% graduated from associate degree programs, and 14% graduated from baccalaureate programs.*

This employment inactivity, while admittedly of a small select sample (married R.N.s) suggested to the researchers another factor in the high cost of nursing education.

The cost of nurse preparation, which in earlier years was borne principally by the student through her contribution to the health services of a hospital, is now derived from public and private sources which support, in great part, the educational institution wherein the nursing program is located. Twenty-five years ago the majority of students had "paid" for their education by the time they graduated. Society had already received its service. Today the young graduate who becomes inactive denies society a service which has been obligated in part.

Second, large numbers of the academically best-prepared nurses are utilized in educating students who become and remain inactive. The preparation of nurses who possess long-term career commitments would greatly reduce the actual number needed. Preparation of fewer nurses would necessitate fewer schools which would, in turn, free many nurse faculty members for employment in health institutions that provide direct patient services.

Third, shortened and carefully planned periods of employment inactivity and judicious use of part-time employment would reduce the number of nurses who decide never to return to employment because of having been away from a field of practice too long. It would also reduce the cost of reeducating returning nurses for contemporary practice.*

Marital and Age Status

According to the ANA 1972 Inventory, out of a total of 1,127,657 R.N.s, the largest number fall into the 25–29-year-old category (164,-925) and the 30–34-year-old category (143,-914). Their representation in the following two categories is particularly high: those who are single (95.1% and 93.2%, respectively) and those divorced (94.6% and 91.6%, respectively). The highest percentage of employment is maintained by single R.N.s under 25 years of age (97.1%). The lowest, not surprisingly, is evidenced by married R.N.s age 65 and over.

Table 9-1   Registered nurses by marital and employment status, 1972

Marital status and employment status	Total Number	Total Percent
Total	1,127,657	—
Single	163,264	100.0
Employed	143,448	87.9
Not Employed	19,079	11.7
Not Reported	737	0.4
Married	810,348	100.0
Employed	535,028	66.0
Not Employed	268,291	33.1
Not Reported	7,029	0.9
Widowed	63,158	100.0
Employed	43,612	69.1
Not Employed	18,522	29.3
Not Reported	1,024	1.6
Divorced or separated	56,039	100.0
Employed	49,405	88.1
Not Employed	6,311	11.3
Not Reported	323	0.6
Marital status not reported	34,848	100.0
Employed	6,977	20.0
Not Employed	4,408	12.7
Not Reported	23,463	67.3

Source: "The Nation's Nurses, 1972 Inventory" ANA.

Diploma graduates tend to have a greater proportion of nurses who are single than any other group (54%). Following close behind are nurses who graduate from baccalaureate programs.

Marital Status of Nursing Seniors and Newly Licensed Nurses

Table 9-2   Marital status and plans of nursing seniors

Marital status	No.	%
Presently married	2,187	20.6
Plan to marry within a year	3,018	28.5
Not married and no marriage plans	5,115	48.2
Not married; plans not reported	287	2.7
Total	10,607	100.0

Source: Career Goals of Hospital School of Nursing Seniors, 1975. Reprinted by permission of the American Hospital Association.

Table 9-3   Newly licensed nurses by marital status and type of program

Marital status	Number	Type of Program Total	Bacc	AD	Dipl	PN
Single	2,608	42%	52%	30%	54%	32%
Married	3,153	51	41	59	44	53
Separated/divorced	392	6	1	9	2	13
Widowed	61	1	—	2	—	2
Total		100%	100%	100%	100%	100%
N	6,214	(6,214)	(1,150)	(1,650)	(1,956)	(1,458)

Source: DHEW, May 1975.

Parental Status—Newly Licensed Nurses

Both associate degree nurses and practical nurses are more likely to have the responsibility of caring for children under the age of 6 years.

Table 9-4   Newly licensed nurses by children and type of program

Children under 6 years	Type of Program Total	Bacc	AD	Dipl	PN
Yes	13%	7%	18%	9%	20%
No	87	93	82	91	80
Total	100%	100%	100%	100%	100%
N	(6,214)	(1,150)	(1,650)	(1,956)	(1,458)

Source: DHEW, May 1975.

136

The Inactive R.N.

A survey by Margaret Sheehan and Josephine Fitzpatrick of 51,000 inactive registered nurses (sponsored by the Division of Nursing-1969) showed that 54% intended to return to work, 18% did not wish to do so and 29% were undecided. Of those planning to return to work, most were under 49 years of age (90% married). Approximately 64% of those planning to return wished to have refresher courses (17% of those who did not expect to return also indicated interest in refresher courses). Of those surveyed, the majority gave full-time family obligations as the primary reason for being inactive.

Another survey, reviewed the work attitudes held by 300 active nurses and 300 inactive nurses.*

Table 9-5 Disadvantages of returning to work as reported by inactive nurses

Response category	Inactive nurses percent	
Frustration associated with nursing	25.5	
Dissatisfactions of patients and staff		9.3
Too much responsibility without enough time and authority		10.0
Inadequate nursing knowledge		6.9
Tasks unrelated to nursing care		8.6
Indifference of personnel		2.8
Dissatisfactions with employment conditions	57.6	
Poor pay-cost differential		47.6
Hours, rotating shifts, floating		26.9
Poor personnel policies		6.5
Time competition—less time for	70.3	
Immediate family		63.5
Household activities		15.9
Social, community and personal activities		10.3
Health problems	13.1	
No response	4.5	

N = 290

*Source: V. Cleland et al., "Decision to Reactivate Nursing Career," *Nursing Research,* Sept.–Oct. 1970. ©American Journal of Nursing Company.

Table 9-6A Advantages of quitting work as reported by active nurses by percentage

Response category	Active nurses percent	
Avoid:		
Frustrations of nursing employment	6.0	
Poor pay-cost differential	3.0	
Time competition—more time for	72.9	
Immediate family		55.9
Household activities		40.8
Social, community and personal activities		48.8
Mental hygiene problems	11.4	
Physical health problems	7.7	
No response	4.1	

Table 9-6B Advantages of working as reported by active and inactive nurses

Response category	Active nurses percent	Inactive nurses percent
Nursing Factors	63.5	79.3
Professional maintenance	41.8	49.0
Personal fulfillment	16.4	36.9
Contribution to others	11.0	25.5
Interaction with health personnel	11.0	7.9
Professional advancement	8.0	7.9
Financial factors	68.9	70.7
Mental stimulation	51.5	39.3
Social contacts	15.7	22.4
No response	2.7	6.5
Note: Percentages do not sum to 100 since each nurse could make several responses.	N = 299	N = 290

Nurses Returning for Baccalaureate Degree

Admissions and enrollments of student bodies have been recently further swollen by students who have some previous education or experience in nursing or the health field.

The students involved are transfer and readmitted students to R.N. schools of nursing, registered nurses, licensed practical nurses, (as well as medical corpsmen and others). Such students are referred to as "open curriculum" students, to permit a distinction between them and basic students who enter freshmen classes for the first time. The admissions of students who transferred from other R.N. schools or were readmitted from R.N. schools represented 11% of all baccalaureate students admitted during the 1973–74 year. In addition 13% of all baccalaureate students admitted were already R.N.s with diplomas or associate degrees.

Table 9-7   Enrollments of open curriculum students in basic R.N. programs in nursing, Oct. 15, 1974

	Diploma	Associate degree	Bacca-laureate
Total Enrollments	64,083	85,452	104,532
Number of open curriculum students	4,707	7,785	16,581
Percent of open curriculum students	7	9	16

Table 9-8   Analysis of open curriculum students by educational background and type of program in which enrolled, Oct. 15, 1974.

Educational background	Diploma	Associate degree	Bacca-laureate
Registered nurses	—	—	7,511
Previously enrolled in R.N. school	636	1,020	1,311
L.P.N./L.V.N.s	680	2,659	355
Medical corpsmen	28	150	123
Aides, orderlies	71	255	139
Other health	52	71	146
Some college, not health	2,988	3,093	6,122
College completed, not health	339	448	874

Source: *Nursing Outlook,* Sept. 1975. ©American Journal of Nursing Company.

Nursing Uniforms

History of Nursing Uniforms*

The Augustinian Nuns of Hotel Dieu in Paris, established in 1155, was the first purely nursing order. These nuns set a precedent for unremitting toil: they nursed, scrubbed, cooked, sewed, and washed clothes in the River Seine, even in winter. Members of the order did this century after century with no rest or recreation, and their devotion has influenced the public's conception of nursing to the present day. The National Nursing Accrediting Service of the National League for Nursing has found this image of a selfless, night-and-day grind of dedication to the sick to be the greatest hindrance in developing schools of nursing.

The Sisters of Charity, established by St. Vincent de Paul, was the first nursing order to rise following the Reformation of 1517. At first its members wore the peasant dresses which they had brought with them from home, but they soon adopted a habit of grey-blue homespun woolen cloth, with a blue apron and the spreading headdress which is seen today.

The Deaconess Hospital at Kaiserswerth, Germany, was established in 1836 and is still a thriving institution. Its nurses wear a uniform of plain blue with a bibbed apron of white. The cap is hood-shaped, with a ruffle about the face, and is tied under the chin with a perky, distinctive bow.

Beginning in 1680, nurses at St. Bartholomew's Hospital in London were required to wear a uniform of dark-colored cloth. In others, for the most part, the dresses were of dark heavy material, as dark cluny, rough dark maroon cloth, black serge, black woolen dresses, black alpaca, and holland brown. These dresses were made with high collars, long sleeves, and a full skirt touching the ground, as it was considered a disgrace for a lady's neck, arms, and ankles to show. . . .

American Uniforms

The early uniforms of the American nurses, although strongly influenced by the prevailing fashion of women's dress, were copied from those worn by nurses in English hospitals. These uniforms were designed to be practical

*Source: Helena L. Dietz, *History of Modern Nursing* (Philadelphia; F. A. Davis, 1964).

but comfort was not considered and sanitation was unknown. The high collar, the long stiff cuffs and the skirt two inches from the floor could not have been comfortable.

An apron was part of the original uniform. It began as a length of white muslin gathered into a belt; a square of the muslin was sewed into the belt in front and pinned at the two upper corners as a bib.

The most conspicuous part of the apron was the utility bag which dangled from its belt. The early bag contained a pencil, scissors, and a tiny case containing matches to light the candles and kerosene lamps. As the clinical thermometer and the hypodermic syringe were invented, these, two, were added to the bag. The thermometer was encased in a tiny metal tube and the syringe in a small flat case. The student was required to purchase both of these instruments.

The early uniforms for both graduates and students were made from a dark material. Later students adopted an easily washable material of gingham and percale, but the director of nurses continued, as late as the early 1900s, to wear a black alpaca dress with a high white collar and stiff white cuffs.

The high-buttoned shoes worn by early nurses were not made with the support and comfort needed. At the Boston City Hospital "a physician was called upon to examine every nurse as to the condition of her feet before she was accepted as a member of the school, and in that way there came about the regulation shoe." (AJN, November 1931).

The change from black shoes to white shoes came slowly. The white uniform for graduates had been generally accepted, but both graduates and students continued to wear black shoes. The first white shoes were made of canvas; white leather came much later. As late as World War I the hair was never cut and it was often a prideful boast that a girl could sit on her hair. Hairwashing was an eventful undertaking and infrequently done. The dust-cap type of head covering served to make hairwashing less necessary and also satisfied the ascetic idea of plainness.

The cap of the early schools was designed to be functional. Although many of the caps did not cover the entire hair, all nurses were required to comb their long hair high upon the head in such a manner as to be completely covered by the cap. Many of these caps were

edged with ruching that added greatly to their attractiveness.

The cape, whose history began during the Crusades, still has considerable vogue in schools where the nurses' residence is some distance from the hospital.

History of Operating Room Attire*

Cleanliness Standards and Surgical Clothing

In the late nineteenth century, the nurse assisting in an operation was instructed to take a bath if possible before all cases and never to go into an operation without a clean apron and sleeves. Her hands and arms were to be thoroughly scrubbed and washed in soap and water, and carbolized, giving special attention to the fingernails.

In cases of laparotomy, the nurse was directed to take a carbolic bath, cleansing her hair well. She then put on clean clothes throughout and a new cap.

Any abrasions or cuts on her hands were covered with collodion before washing sponges, and she was always to wear silent shoes.

It was during the last quarter of that century that special surgical clothing, head coverings, gloves and masks were first introduced into the operating room to protect the patient from the germs of the surgeon and his assistants and prevent wound infection. A 1905 nurse's guide instructs the nurse, for an operation in a private home, to "wear a calico dress and over it an aseptic gown.... Microbes attach themselves more readily to woolen fabric than linen or calico," the guide cautions.

Amy Armour Smith, one of the first registered nurses to write a text on operating room nursing, stated in 1924: "The circulating nurse should be easily picked out, wearing an operating room cap, but no mask, and a gown with special pockets for pencil and pad." The scrub nurse, who is advised to silently mind her own business, is "instructed to don a mask before scrubbing and a gown after the scrub."

In the 1950s, colored scrub clothes were introduced primarily to reduce the glare, but a

*Source: Adapted from "From Apron to Gown: A History of OR Attire" by Elinor Shrader, ©AORN, July 1976.

welcome side effect was to brighten the operating room. Now scrub clothes are available in pastels and prints, and in durable press fabrics as well as cotton.

Pantsuits for OR nurses were first seen in the OR in the 1960s.

Pants have been accepted slowly. The scrub dress is probably still the preferred style.

With the development of nonwoven materials in the 1950s, disposable surgical gowns were introduced to the OR in the 1960s.

Linen or cotton gowns are still more widely used. It is estimated that only one out of three gowns in today's operating rooms is disposable.

Some of the most explicit standards for OR attire were established in 1975 by the Association of Operating Room Nurses.

The standards specify that "material for surgical gowns must establish an effective barrier eliminating the passage of microorganisms between the sterile and nonsterile areas." The standards state that street clothes shall not be worn in the restricted areas of the surgical suite.

Caps

Nurses traditionally wore caps to cover their hair and, according to early photographs, wore the same caps into the operating room. A photograph in 1900 shows the surgeon bareheaded; but a 1907 photograph shows the sterile nurse wearing a turban-style head covering and a 1908 photo reveals the nurse wearing a shower cap-style head covering.

The AORN standards prohibit nylon caps. In the 1960s, disposable head coverings were introduced, bringing to an end homemade, wash-at-home OR caps. But by the 1970s, disposable caps blossomed forth in colors and prints and different styles, all designed to give the OR nurse a more attractive image.

A more important trend of the 1970s has been the use of the hood by both surgeons and nurses.

Approximately 75% of all head coverings in the OR are disposable. The AORN standards for head covering specify that all hair must be completely covered by a clean, lint-free scrub hat or surgical hood.

Rubber Gloves

It was not unitl the 1890s that their use was popularized by a renowned Johns Hopkins surgeon William S. Halsted, M.D. The oft-told story of the introduction of gloves to the operating room is a romantic one involving an operating room nurse. Halsted gives his own account of his involvement:

In the winter of 1889 or 1890—I cannot recall the month—the nurse in charge of my operating room complained that the solution of mercuric chloride produced a dermatitis of her arms and hands. As she was an unusually efficient woman, I gave the matter my consideration, and one day in New York requested the Goodyear Rubber Company to make as an experiment two pairs of thin rubber gloves with gauntlets.

This "unusually efficient" nurse was Caroline Hampton, who soon after married Dr. Halsted. Halsted himself points out that "operating in gloves was an evolution rather than an inspiration or happy thought."

It was the nurse's job to take care of the rubber gloves, a job that, in 1905, started with washing and examining them for holes by carefully filling them with water. After boiling them for five minutes, they were dried and powdered, wrapped in a sterilized towel, placed in a glass jar and kept in a cool place until used. The first disposable gloves [were introduced] in 1958. [Today] 98% of all hospitals use disposable gloves.

Surgical Masks

By 1920, the use of masks became routine practice in the operating room, but it was not until the 1960s and the development of disposable masks that a comfortable, efficient mask was readily available.

From the earliest mask until the 1960s, almost all masks were gauze.

Early photographs show only the mouth covered by the mask, and it was not until 1937 that (it was) proven that wearing the mask only over the mouth was inadequate.

When antibiotics appeared in the 1940s, interest in masks decreased. When it became apparent, however, that wonder drugs were no substitute for asepsis, interest revived and the search for the ideal mask continued.

The first disposable masks were molded shells introduced in the early 1960s. In 1963, the first flat-fold design disposable mask was introduced. It opened into a pouch and had a somewhat beak-like appearance.

The AORN standards recommend a high filtration (95% or above) disposable mask at all times in the OR. Today, about 95% of all masks are disposable. The gauze and muslin masks have all but disappeared.

Shoes

Operating room foot attire, perhaps because it is the farthest removed from the patient, appears to have received the least attention. Even today, soiled and bloody shoes are seen in the OR, as well as inappropriate attire such as clogs, sandals, and tennis shoes.

Before the turn of the century, nurses in the operating room at the Hartford Training School were advised to wear silent shoes.

It was not until the 1950s that operating room personnel were required to change their shoes when they came into the OR, but cleaning shoes often was a problem.

Better were shoe covers, first made of cloth and later disposables. They eliminated the problem of bloody, pus-covered shoes and also served as an electrical ground. The AORN standards require all persons entering the restricted areas of the surgical suite to wear shoe coverings.

The Latest in Nursing Uniforms*

In the search for something to break the uniform monotony, the question nurses ask again and again is "So what's new?" An important question for manufacturers and retailers to consider in an industry that sells somewhere around $50 million worth of uniforms yearly.

The answer this year to what's new is twofold: fabrics and prices. First the good news: new fabrics are being created and blended to increase wearability, enhance their look and texture and to decrease their amount of care. Since 1968, there has been more than a 30% increase in the use of knit fabrics (as compared to wovens such as cotton). The trend is definitely continuing, with bolts of polyesters, synthetic blends and cotton/Dacron® combinations rolling off the production lines.

Now the bad news: prices have climbed, though in some cases only a few pennies. The

*Source: Adapted from "A Uniform Forecast" by Freda B. Friedman, *Journal of Practical Nursing*, January 1975.

average price of uniforms by one leading company in 1975 was $15–$16 for dresses and $20–$29 for pantsuits, about 7–8% higher than last year. Other manufacturers say average prices for uniforms used to be $11–$17 and will go up to $14–$20.

What there will be are more separates that *mix and match,* a concept of dressing that has become very popular in sportswear. Separates are tops and bottoms sold separately, instead of as a two-piece outfit.

Styles that are very trendy and modish are hard to come by in uniforms, because manufacturers and retailers have learned that it just doesn't pay to offer uniforms that people talk about but don't buy. A couple of years ago, for example, the culotte (split-legged skirt) was a big fashion headliner and was made into a nursing style. The style was never repeated because it didn't sell.

The styles that continue to be offered are geared to what nurses want, and according to studies on nursing apparel, the major criteria are: tailoring, styling, easy care, fabric selection, long wearability.

Wanted features in tailoring and styling are more dresses and tops with:

- Zippers and snaps rather than buttons.

- Pockets are a must, and hardly a uniform around these days lacks large functional ones, either sewn into the side seams or patched on to the front.

- This year, one pants outfit is expected to sell for every 1½ dresses.

- Back zippers are becoming more popular because they allow for more design interest in the front.

The demand for long-lasting and well-wearing fabrics seems to have rung a death knell for the disposable nursing uniforms which were considered a very salable item some years back. However, they have never become popular outside operating rooms and other specialty areas.

The standard tie-up oxford shoe has blossomed and is now available in variations of heeled and wedged types. Growing in popularity are slip-on shoes, either in the loafer style or the clog. Some hospitals restrict clogs; however, many nurses who are permitted them, prefer clogs in summer.

The fabrics that are getting the highest marks are those such as blends of 80% Dacron® and 20% cotton which wear well, look well and are priced well.

The most popular price range for shoes is between $15–$19, up a couple of dollars from two years ago. Multiply this by two or three, since most nurses have reported in studies that they buy two to three pairs yearly. The array of hosiery is growing with increasing variety in stockings, pantyhose and knee-highs. No nurse has to accept uncomfortable hosiery any longer. Stockings and pantyhose come in support styles as well. The source of all these goods is shifting from department stores to specialty stores.

Catalogue sales, buying services and mail order outlets are also becoming increasingly popular sources of uniforms and accessories for nurses.

Job Relocation

Which Areas Are Gaining and Which Losing Population

Table 9-9   Population change 1970–1975 (in thousands)

State	April 1, 1970 to July 1, 1975 Net increase	
	Number	Percent
United States	9,817	4.8
New England	352	3.0
Maine	66	6.6
New Hampshire	80	10.9
Vermont	26	5.9
Massachusetts	138	2.4
Rhode Island	−23	−2.4
Connecticut	63	2.1
Middle Atlantic	50	0.1
New York	−121	−0.7
New Jersey	145	2.0
Pennsylvania	26	0.2
East North Central	713	1.8
Ohio	102	1.0
Indiana	116	2.2
Illinois	32	0.3
Michigan	275	3.1
Wisconsin	180	4.3

Table 9-9   (continued)

State	April 1, 1970 to July 1, 1975 Net increase	
	Number	Percent
West North Central	362	2.2
Minnesota	120	3.1
Iowa	45	1.6
Missouri	85	1.8
North Dakota	17	2.7
South Dakota	17	2.6
Nebraska	61	4.1
Kansas	18	0.8
South Atlantic	3,036	9.9
Delaware	31	5.7
Maryland	174	4.4
District of Columbia	−41	−5.4
Virginia	315	6.8
West Virginia	59	3.4
North Carolina	367	7.2
South Carolina	227	8.8
Georgia	338	7.4
Florida	1,565	23.0
East South Central	736	5.7
Kentucky	175	5.4
Tennessee	262	6.7
Alabama	170	4.9
Mississippi	129	5.8
West South Central	1,530	7.9
Arkansas	192	10.0
Louisiana	148	4.1
Oklahoma	152	6.0
Texas	1,037	9.3
Mountain	1,354	16.3
Montana	53	7.7
Idaho	107	14.9
Wyoming	42	12.5
Colorado	324	14.7
New Mexico	130	12.7
Arizona	448	25.3
Utah	147	13.8
Nevada	103	21.1
Pacific	1,686	6.3
Washington	131	3.8
Oregon	197	9.4
California	1,214	6.1
Alaska	49	16.3
Hawaii	95	12.3

Source: *Statistical Abstracts, U.S.A.*, 1976.

Table 9-10   Population, urban and rural, by race. 1970 (An urbanized area comprises at least 1 city of 50,000 inhabitants (central city) plus contiguous, closely settled areas (urban fringe).)

Year and area	Total	White	Negro and other	Percent distribution		
				Total	White	Negro and other
1970, total population (in thousands)	203,212	177,749	25,463	100.0	100.0	100.0
Urban				73.5	72.4	80.7
Inside urbanized areas				58.3	56.8	68.7
Central cities				31.5	27.9	56.5
Urban fringe				26.8	28.9	12.3
Outside urbanized areas				15.2	15.7	12.0
Rural				26.5	27.6	19.3

The Costs of Moving*

Some states set intrastate rates as a function of weight and distance, while others base their tariffs on an hourly rate—which is typically higher for moving than for packing and unpacking.

When moving companies charge by the hour, they do so on a portal-to-portal basis, and this could add another one and a half to four hours to the bill for the round trip.

When you receive an estimate from a moving company, remember that it is a statement of probable cost rather than a binding statement of actual charges.

For interstate moves, you must pay for the actual charges immediately upon delivery of your household goods up to 10% beyond the estimate. Within each state, the regulations differ but requirements for immediate payment up to 25% beyond the estimate are not unusual.

Close to 20% of all shipments are delayed, while damage claims for $50 or more are filed with government agencies on 16% of all long-distance moves. It is important, therefore, to be aware of how rates are determined and what you can do when a problem arises. In both situations, the key factor is whether the move you are making is interstate or intrastate.

Interstate moves across state lines are regulated by the Interstate Commerce Commission, which authorizes moving companies to charge rates depending on the weight of the items and the distance they are moved. Loaded moving vehicles must be weighed by a certified weighmaster or on a certified scale—a process that should be observed by a member of your family in order to prevent overcharging.

Each state sets up its own procedures for establishing moving rate structures within its jurisdiction. Obtain three estimates from movers in your area before choosing a mover. Make a complete inventory of the items to be shipped. Do not pack money, jewelry or valuable papers and documents that may be needed quickly.

If you discover a loss or damage before the mover has left, notify him and write exactly what you found on the bill of lading before signing the receipt.

*Source: L. Sloane, "Watching Your Finance," American Journal of Nursing, April 1976. ©American Journal of Nursing Company.

Living Costs in Metropolitan Areas*

Table 9-11 Living costs in 40 metropolitan areas

The following figures show annual average budgets for a city family of four, as calculated by the Labor Department. These budgets are based on prices in autumn, 1976. Since then, living costs have climbed about 3% nationally.

	Minimum budget	Moderate comfort budget	Upper income budget
Northeast			
Boston	$11,104	$19,384	$29,187
Buffalo	$10,198	$17,175	$25,017
Hartford	$10,601	$17,238	$24,207
Lancaster, Pa.	$ 9,799	$15,685	$22,194
New York	$10,835	$18,866	$29,677
Philadelphia	$10,343	$16,836	$24,482
Pittsburgh	$ 9,697	$15,515	$22,418
Portland, Me.	$10,412	$16,633	$23,280
North Central			
Cedar Rapids	$ 9,702	$15,976	$23,198
Champaign–Urbana	$10,564	$16,578	$24,104
Chicago	$10,380	$16,561	$23,804
Cincinnati	$ 9,448	$15,708	$21,974
Cleveland	$10,023	$16,412	$23,486
Dayton	$ 9,466	$15,101	$22,022
Detroit	$ 9,865	$16,514	$24,226
Green Bay	$ 9,626	$16,008	$23,881
Indianapolis	$ 9,876	$15,911	$22,586
Kansas City	$ 9,677	$15,628	$22,968
Milwaukee	$10,306	$17,307	$25,221
Minneapolis–St. Paul	$10,085	$16,810	$24,556
St. Louis	$ 9,612	$15,623	$22,437
Wichita	$ 9,816	$15,102	$21,628
South			
Atlanta	$ 9,222	$14,830	$21,410
Austin	$ 8,887	$14,209	$20,628
Baltimore	$10,280	$16,195	$23,715
Baton Rouge	$ 8,914	$14,472	$21,334
Dallas	$ 9,114	$14,699	$21,393
Durham	$ 9,600	$15,525	$22,205
Houston	$ 9,532	$14,978	$21,482
Nashville	$ 9,102	$14,821	$21,307
Orlando	$ 9,271	$14,378	$20,878
Washington, D.C.	$10,650	$16,950	$24,769
West			
Anchorage	$16,492	$23,071	$33,273
Bakersfield	$ 9,599	$15,004	$21,214
Denver	$ 9,765	$15,906	$23,078
Honolulu	$12,711	$19,633	$30,086
Los Angeles–Long Beach	$10,523	$16,016	$23,977
San Diego	$10,007	$15,989	$23,687
San Francisco–Oakland	$10,920	$17,200	$25,315
Seattle	$10,770	$16,204	$22,935

(In 1976) the budget for comfortable family living for four had risen to an average of $16,236 a year—up $918, or 6%, from a year earlier.

- If the same family followed a "minimum but adequate" budget, it would have had to spend $10,041.

- The cost of a higher, more luxurious budget ran $23,759

As Table 9-11 points up, living costs vary widely.

Top category—Among the metropolitan areas included in the survey, the most expensive in which to live comfortably—aside from high-cost Anchorage and Honolulu—are Boston, New York, Milwaukee and Hartford.

More-luxurious living now costs most in Anchorage, Honolulu, New York, Boston, San Francisco and Milwaukee.

For those sticking to the low-cost budget, Boston has the highest minimum outside of Alaska and Hawaii.

In all three categories, the least-expensive cities are in the South.

Behind the wide variation between major U.S. cities are some big differences in the cost of individual items. Food is highest in New York, Boston and Milwaukee. Housing runs about $4,000 a year in the Northeast, but under $3,200 in Atlanta and Austin. Clothing bills are near $1,400 in Buffalo, but below $1,100 in Dallas. And medical costs vary from above $1,000 in West Coast cities to less than $800 in St. Louis.

What does it cost households of varying sizes to live? The survey found that on average a middle-income family of three could get by for $10,140, a single person under 35 for $4,330 and a single person 65 or older for $3,460.

*Source: Reprint from *U.S. News & World Report,* May 9, 1977. Copyright 1977 U.S. News & World Report, Inc.

Locations and Preferences*

Table 9-12   Willingness to work for high earnings in a small community and in a poor section of metropolitan area: marital status and training (percentage distribution)

Response by community type	Marital status			Type of RN education		
	Single	Married	Other	A.A.	Dip.	B.A.
Small community:						
Does not apply since already live in such a location	18.9	33.3	18.6	29.8	29.7	20.8
Yes, even if need to move	13.1	5.5	15.7	9.5	7.3	11.1
Yes, if move not necessary	11.6	13.7	10.8	13.5	13.0	13.7
Yes, but money not important	12.8	6.4	8.6	9.9	6.4	14.2
No (includes probably not)	43.6	41.1	46.2	37.2	43.6	40.2
Total	100.0	100.0	100.0	100.0	100.0	100.0
Poor section of metropolitan area:						
Does not apply since already live in such a location	9.6	3.8	7.1	5.9	5.0	8.1
Yes, even if need to move	5.2	2.3	3.5	3.6	2.3	6.3
Yes, if move not necessary	9.3	14.5	9.3	14.0	12.5	12.9
Yes, but money not important	10.1	4.9	6.4	7.9	5.0	10.3
No (includes probably not)	65.8	74.5	73.7	68.6	75.2	62.4
Total	100.0	100.0	100.0	100.0	100.0	100.0

Table 9-13   Willingness to work for higher earnings in a small community and in a poor section of a metropolitan area: income and dependents (percentage distribution)

Response by community type	Income and dependents									
	$0–5,000		$5,001–10,000		$10,001–15,000		$15,001–25,000		Over $25,000	
	No dep.	With dep.	No dep.	With dep.	No dep.	With dep.	No dep.	With dep.	No dep.	With dep.
Small community:										
Does not apply since already live in such a location	37.0	32.3	33.3	38.6	25.8	33.1	25.0	23.4	33.3	35.5
Yes, even if need to move	8.3	9.7	7.9	5.2	6.5	1.5	9.4	3.2	0.0	0.0
Yes, if move not necessary	10.2	11.3	15.5	13.6	21.8	15.4	15.6	13.3	0.0	6.5
Yes, but money not important	16.7	9.7	7.9	3.9	12.1	4.6	12.5	8.0	16.7	3.2
No (includes probably not)	27.8	37.1	35.4	38.6	33.9	45.4	37.5	52.1	50.0	54.8
Total	100.0	100.0	100.0	100.0	100.0	100.0	100.0	100.0	100.0	100.0
Poor section of metropolitan area:										
Does not apply since already live in such a location	5.9	2.0	1.9	2.9	6.3	2.4	18.8	1.8	0.0	3.7
Yes, even if need to move	4.0	3.9	3.5	1.8	3.6	0.3	0.0	1.2	0.0	0.0
Yes, if move not necessary	14.9	15.7	15.5	13.7	16.2	17.5	3.1	17.2	0.0	14.8
Yes, but money not important	14.9	5.9	5.8	1.8	7.2	3.3	6.3	3.7	33.3	7.4
No (includes probably not)	60.4	72.5	73.3	79.7	66.7	76.6	71.9	76.1	66.7	74.1
Total	100.0	100.0	100.0	100.0	100.0	100.0	100.0	100.0	100.0	100.0

*Source: DHEW, May, 1975.

Table 9-14   Willingness to work for higher earnings in small community and poor section of metropolitan area: ethnicity and birthplace (percentage distribution)

Response by community type	Ethnicity			New York New Jersey Pennsylvania		N. Carolina S. Carolina Georgia Florida		Iowa, Kansas Nebraska Missouri		Washington Oregon[2]	
	White	Black	Total[1]	White	Black	White	Black	White	Black	White	All
Small community:											
Does not apply since already live in such a location	29.5	9.4	28.5	27.8	7.7	26.8	7.4	31.9	0.0	37.5	28.4
Yes, even if need to move	8.1	11.3	8.2	8.5	15.4	9.5	7.4	8.1	100.0	3.8	8.4
Yes, if move not necessary	13.2	15.1	13.2	14.9	15.4	12.7	11.1	14.3	0.0	12.5	14.2
Yes, but money not important	8.2	6.6	8.2	6.7	23.1	5.9	3.7	6.6	0.0	17.5	7.3
No (includes probably not)	41.0	57.5	42.0	42.1	38.5	45.0	70.4	39.2	0.0	28.8	41.7
Total	100.0	100.0	100.0	100.0	100.0	100.0	100.0	100.0	100.0	100.0	100.0
Poor section of metropolitan area:											
Does not apply since already live in such a location	5.1	15.5	5.5	7.8	23.1	5.2	18.5	5.7	50.0	0.0	7.0
Yes, even if need to move	3.1	5.2	3.1	1.8	15.4	3.6	0.0	4.3	0.0	1.4	2.7
Yes, if move not necessary	13.0	14.4	12.9	9.2	15.4	16.5	14.8	12.6	0.0	24.7	12.2
Yes, but money not important	6.3	7.2	6.4	4.1	23.1	5.2	3.7	6.1	0.0	6.8	5.0
No (includes probably not)	72.5	57.7	72.1	77.0	23.1	69.6	63.0	71.3	50.0	67.1	73.1
Total	100.0	100.0	100.0	100.0	100.0	100.0	100.0	100.0	100.0	100.0	100.0

[1]Total includes R.N.s of American Indian, Oriental and Spanish American descent. These groups are excluded from the subtotals.
[2]There are no black R.N.s who were born in Washington or Oregon in the sample.

Far more black than white R.N.s would not consider employment in a small community, judging from the percentages answering "no" to their willingness to accept employment in this type of community.

Financial Matters

Comparative Income
Health Occupations Salaries (1971)

Table 9-15   Health workers and salaries

Most figures given represent the 1971 mean starting salary and the mean maximum salary.

Administrative Assistant	$ 8,266	11,220	Diagnostic X-ray		
Biochemist	10,800	(BS)	Technologist	6,612	8,268
	12,500	(Master's)	Dietitian	8,280	10,260
	15,800	(Ph.D.)[1]	Electrocardiograph		
Certified Laboratory			Technician	5,268	6,420
Assistant	5,604	7,080	Electroencephalograph		
Computer Operator	6,456	7,908	Technologist	5,664	7,080
Computer Programmer	8,484	10,860	Executive Housekeeper	6,396[4]	
Cytotechnologist	7,080	8,500	Food and Drug		
Dental Assistant	3,600[2]		Inspector and		
Dental Hygienist	7,000[1]		Analyst	8,098[2]	
Dental Laboratory			Food Service		
Technician	5,824[3]		Supervisor	5,252[4]	
Dentist	29,000[1]				(continued)

Table 9-15   (continued)

Most figures given represent the 1971 mean starting salary and the mean maximum salary.

Histologic Technician	6,396	7,968	Professional Nurse	7,900	9,700
Hospital Administrator	10,000	13,000[2]	Psychologist	9,600	(Master's)
Inhalation Therapist	7,176	8,676		10,900	(Ph.D.)[2]
Licensed Practical			Recreational Therapist	7,656	9,204
Nurse	5,700	7,140	Safety Engineer	9,732	11,400
Medical Assistant	6,500	8,320[1]	Sanitarian	7,000	7,500[2]
Medical Librarian	7,836	9,864	Speech Pathologist		
Medical Record			and Audiologist	9,144	12,588
Administrator	8,316	10,000	Sociologist	15,000[1]	
Medical Social Worker	9,264	11,600	Technical Writer	5,000	7,000[2]
Medical Technologist	7,900	9,900	Vocational Rehabilita-		
Nuclear Medical			tion Counselor	8,384	10,876[6]
Technologist	7,512	9,000			
Occupational Therapist	8,268	9,984			
Occupational Therapy					
Assistant	6,500	7,800[1]			
Optometrist	25,000[1]				
Osteopathic Physician	25,000	30,000[1]			
Pharmacist	10,600	13,000			
Physician	34,000	39,000[5]			
Physical Therapist	8,340	10,284			
Podiatrist	21,500[1]				

[1] Average income, 1970. [2] Starting salaries, 1970.
[3] Starting salaries in the federal government, 1970. [4] Average income, 1969.
[5] Estimated net income of physicians in patient care, 1970.
[6] Salary ranges of selected state classes, 1971, U.S. Civil Service Commission.

Source: U.S. Bureau of Labor Statistics

Comparative U.S. Employee Salaries

Table 9-16   Weekly earnings of full-time wage and salary workers 1975 (in 1967 dollars)

Characteristics	1975
All workers	$116
Male	139
16–24 years old	94
25 years and over	148
Female	86
16–24 years old	73
25 years and over	92
White	119
Male	141
Female	87
Negro and other races	98
Male	109
Female	82
Occupation:	
Professional and technical	154
Managers, administrators	172
Salesworkers	119
Clerical workers	94
Craft and foremen	140
Operatives	103
Operatives, except transport	99
Transport equip. operatives	124
Nonfarm laborers	97
Private household workers	34
Other service workers	77
Farmworkers	70

Source: U.S. Bureau of Labor Statistics

Table 9-17   Average annual wages and salaries and wage supplements per full-time equivalent employee

(In dollars. Wage and salary payments include executives' compensation, bonuses, tips, and payments in kind supplements to wages and salaries include employer contributions for social insurance, compensation for injuries, directors' fees, jury and witness fees, etc.)

Industry	Annual Wages and Salaries 1974	Annual Supplements 1974
All domestic industries	9,994	1,440
Agriculture, forestry, fisheries	5,756	594
Mining	12,935	2,281
Contract construction	12,206	1,467
Manufacturing	10,834	1,914
Transportation	12,616	2,055
Communication	12,353	3,497
Electric, gas, sanitary services	13,059	2,591
Wholesale and retail trade	8,749	1,051
Finance, insurance, real estate	9,854	1,670
Services	8,141	892
Government and gov't enterprises	10,632	1,323

Source: U.S. Bureau of Economic Analysis, *The National Income and Product Accounts of the United States 1923–1974.*

Table 9-18   Hourly and weekly earnings in private industry

(Data are for production workers in mining and manufacturing, construction workers in contract construction, and nonsupervisory employees in other industries.)

Industry Group	1976, Apr.	Industry Group	1976, Apr.
Total, gross hourly earnings	$4.76	Total, gross weekly earnings	$170
Manufacturing	5.05	Manufacturing	197
Mining	6.30	Mining	272
Contract construction	7.49	Contract construction	276
Transportation and public utilities	6.34	Transportation and public utilities	249
Wholesale trade	5.10	Wholesale trade	197
Retail trade	3.48	Retail trade	112
Finance, insurance, and real estate	4.31	Finance, insurance, and real estate	157
Services	4.29	Services	143

Source: U.S. Bureau of Labor Statistics.

Nurses' Total Income

Table 9-19   R.N. earnings and income from other sources (1973 Survey)

Number of years with current employer	Mean annual gross earnings	Mean hourly gross earnings	Mean annual spouse earnings (excl. single or widow)	Mean annual income from nonemployment sources
Under 1	$7,635	$4.50	$12,333	$477
1	7,828	4.50	12,040	486
2	7,979	4.75	12,714	512
3	7,791	4.72	13,107	567
4	7,856	4.75	14,120	525
5	7,243	4.60	14,717	414
6–10	7,728	4.83	14,731	519
11–15	7,562	4.77	14,681	669
Over 15	8,092	4.91	13,932	849

Source: DHEW, May 1975.

A 1972 U.S. Department of Health, Education, and Welfare publication, "The Present and Future Supply of Registered Nurses" by Stuart H. Altman, compared the earnings of general duty nurses in hospitals (R.N.s) with the earnings of secretaries and public school teachers in 13 selected cities. Dr. Altman reported that in 1960 the average registered nurse earned $4,193, which was only 61% of the earnings of the average public school teacher and 88% of the secretarial salaries. By 1969, the earnings of nurses had increased to $7,815 and they earned 83% of teachers' wages and 21% more than secretaries. Using the same method as Dr. Altman, we calculated comparable figures for 1972 and found that nurses' earnings averaged $9,990 per year, 81% of teachers' salaries and 26% more than secretaries.

Family Income Needs*

Table 9-20 Public response to question: "What is the smallest amount of money a family of four (husband, wife, and two children) needs each week to get along in this community?"

January 30–February 2, 1976

	Median averages
NATIONAL	$177
Sex	
Male	177
Female	180
Race	
White	190
Nonwhite	152
Education	
College	199
High School	177
Grade School	151
Region	
East	199
Midwest	176
South	152
West	198
Age	
Total Under 30	178
18–24 years	176
25–29 years	181
30–49 years	199
50 & older	161
Income	
$15,000 & over	200
$10,000–$14,999	175
$ 5,000–$ 9,999	152
Under $5,000	149
Politics	
Republican	175
Democrat	175
Independent	198
Occupation	
Professional & Business	200
Clerical & Sales	200
Manual Workers	176
Nonlabor Force	150
City Size	
1,000,000 & over	201
500,000–999,999	198
50,000–499,999	181
2,500–49,999	152
Under 2,500, Rural	151
Labor Union families	198
Nonlabor Union families	176

Family income needs (Non-farm families)	Median averages
1976 (Latest)	$177
1975	161
1974	152
1973	149
1971	127
1970	126
1969	120
1967	101
1966	99
1964	81
1961	84
1959	79
1957	72
1954	60
1953	60
1952	60
1951	50
1950	50
1949	50
1948	50
1947	43
1937	30

*Source: "Public's Cost of Living Estimate," Gallup Opinion Index (#129, April 1976), Princeton, N.J.

Comparative Employment Benefits
(all U.S. workers)

Table 9-21   Workers in establishments with formal provisions for selected supplementary wage benefits, 229 SMSAs: 1971–1974

Data based on sample of establishments with 50 or more employees, excludes administrative, executive and professional employees.

Type of Benefit	Percent	Type of Benefit	Percent
Health insurance and		Paid holidays (continued)	
pension plans:		8 or more days	78
Life insurance	97	9 or more days	59
Hospitalization	97	10 or more days	35
Surgical	98	11 or more days	20
Medical	94	12 or more days	9
Major medical	93	Paid vacations:	
Dental insurance	11	2 weeks or more:	
Sickness/accident insurance	46	After 1 year of service	80
Sick leave (full pay and no		After 5 years of service	99
waiting period)	65	3 weeks or more:	
Sick leave (partial pay		After 5 years of service	28
and/or waiting period)	9	After 10 years of service	87
Retirement pension	85	After 15 years of service	94
Paid holidays:		4 weeks or more:	
No paid holidays	—	After 15 years of service	29
6 or more days	97	After 20 years of service	71
7 or more days	88	After 25 years of service	76

Source: U.S. Bureau of Labor Statistics.

Table 9-22   Employee-Benefit Plans—Summary: 1950 to 1974 (Coverage data refer to all civilian wage and salary workers)

Item	1950	1955	1960	1965	1970	1972	1973	1974
Percent of workers covered								
All employees:								
Life insurance and death	38.8	50.8	57.8	63.7	69.3	71.6	71.4	74.2
Accidental death and dismemberment	16.2	28.2	35.3	43.1	51.5	52.4	52.7	53.7
Health benefits:								
Hospitalization	48.6	59.3	66.5	69.4	70.7	69.8	70.1	69.9
Surgical	35.4	54.6	63.3	65.9	68.6	68.1	68.4	68.1
Regular medical	16.4	36.6	47.7	58.0	63.9	63.6	66.3	66.5
Major medical	(x)	4.0	14.8	25.2	32.7	34.0	34.0	34.3
Private employees:								
Temporary disability	46.2	49.1	48.7	44.3	47.9	48.6	47.2	45.9
Long-term disability	(x)	(x)	(x)	3.4	11.2	12.8	15.9	16.4
Retirement	22.5	29.6	37.2	39.5	42.1	43.1	43.7	44.0

Source: *Statistical Abstracts, U.S.A.,* 1976.

Table 9-23   Workers in public and private employment with health insurance benefits, 1950–1970 (percents)

	Hospital Care	Surgical	Regular Medical	Major Medical
1950	48.7	35.5	16.4	—
1955	60.0	54.7	37.0	4.0
1960	68.9	65.5	50.2	16.5
1965	74.3	72.0	60.3	26.8
1970	80.2	79.2	71.1	35.8

Source: U.S. Department of Labor, 1975.

Credit and Women

The federal Equal Credit Opportunity Act (PL93-495) enacted in 19   was designed to end discrimination in extending credit and to lessen the problems women have faced in obtaining credit.

Under the act's regulations*:

- the use of sex or marital status is forbidden in determination of credit worthiness;
- if requested, the creditor must present reasons for denial of credit;
- creditors may not inquire into birth control practices or into child bearing capabilities or intentions, or assume from her age that an applicant or applicant's spouse may drop out of the labor force due to child bearing and thus have an interruption of income;
- part-time income must be counted in granting credit although the creditor may examine the probable continuity of the applicant's part-time job;
- creditors may ask about obligations to pay alimony, child support and maintenance payments if the applicant relies on such payment to obtain credit;
- creditors must keep on file credit applications and related information for 15 months after creditor gives notice of action;
- on or after November 1, 1976, creditors must be able to furnish credit information on accounts that both spouses may use, so that each spouse may utilize the credit history;
- by February 1, 1977, the creditor must inform holders of existing credit that the credit history can be reported in both names;

- creditors may not terminate credit on an existing account because of a change in marital status without evidence that the applicant will not pay;
- creditors may not use unfavorable information about a spouse, if credit is applied for independent of the spouse, and if applicant can show the unfavorable history should not apply;
- creditors may not refuse to grant credit in birth given and surnames.

Investments

(Note: The following investment categories are covered in greater detail under "Planning for Retirement.")

Stock investments can yield high returns but may involve more risk. Stock brokerage firms can often give you detailed studies on individual stocks or on a particular industry. The New York Stock Exchange will send you its Investors Information Kit for $2. Send a check or money order to the Investors Service Bureau, P.O. Box 252, Dept. G, Wall Street Station, New York, N.Y. 10005.

Women accounted for half of the nation's adults who owned stock in 1970. About 22% of women (21 years of age and over) owned stock, compared with about 25% of adult men. Women stockholders were nearly 30% of all shareholders of record.[1]

Women owned shares with an estimated market value of $172.1 billion, or 25% of the total owned by individuals. On the basis of a total of $1.1 trillion value of all shares owned by individuals, brokers and dealers, and various other institutions in 1970, women owned 16% and men owned 23% of the total value.

Mutual funds let you become a part-owner of a package of stocks and bonds, sometimes for as little as $25. A money manager invests for you, you get diversification and professional management.

Real estate ties up your capital but is a viable investment even if you are single and not possession-oriented. There are several kinds of mortgage plans, some requiring surprisingly low down payments.

Series E U.S. Savings Bonds offer small savers some of the tax shelter advantages normally available only to big investors.

*Source: Citizens' Advisory Council on the Status of Women, March, 1976.

[1] New York Stock Exchange: Shareownership 1970: Census of Shareowners.

The Individual Retirement Account and Keogh Plans are excellent ways to save for retirement and offer big tax advantages if you work for a firm without a pension plan or are self-employed.

Insurance*

Ownership by women: at the end of 1973, women owned about $270 billion, or 15% of the life insurance in this country. Their ownership of ordinary policies accounted for much of their total life insurance holdings. They are substantial holders of industrial life policies, and their ownership of group life insurance matches their participation in the business world.

Generally, adult women's lapse rates are lower than adult men's at every level of duration through the first fifteen policy years.

Table 9-24   Life insurance policies

	% of Policies		% of Amount	
	1965	1975	1965	1975
Male adults	62%	55%	86%	18%
Female adults	22	28	10	17
Children	16	17	4	5
Size of Policy				
under 10,000		42%		
10–25,000		37%		
25,000–over		21%		

Table 9-25   Attitudes toward life insurance

	Women 1974	Men 1974
Life insurance is as much a necessity as food, clothing, & shelter	69%	59%
Women should carry as much life insurance as men	37	40
When husband is bread winner support insuring of wife	64	72

---

*Source: American Council of Life Insurance.

Tax Benefits and Deductions for Nurses

There are a number of tax benefits and deductions, specifically available to nurses, which go unnoticed each year. For example, some nurses are free-lancers, (self-employed) part or full-time; all nurses require special professional clothing and shoes; some seek further education; some volunteer their specialized skills; most belong to professional associations and travel in the line of duty; a sizable number each year return to nursing, give up working or change jobs.

Each of these factors can entitle a nurse to income tax savings. Listed below are descriptions of selected deductions which nurses may be able to claim in completing their income tax forms.

Professional Work Factors

Deductions allowed

- *Employment agency* charges for a job assignment are deductible when itemized. Private duty nurses who frequently hire out through agencies use a different procedure.
- *Travel expenses:* daily costs are allowable deductions if accrued while in transit from a first to a second daily job or in the case of self-employed nurses, while in transit *between* patients' homes. Car allowances are based on mileage, currently 15 cents for the first 15,000 miles.

  Business travel expenses for out-of-town transportation, food and lodging are deductible if the trip is directly connected with your work and no reimbursement is supplied by your employer.
- *Uniform* cost and maintenance, from cap to shoes, can be claimed provided they are a condition of the job and not suitable apparel off the job. Keep receipts of purchases, as well as cleaning and repair bills.
- *Equipment* purchased for professional use is allowable when itemized. Deductions may include expenditures for nurse's bag, blood pressure equipment, scissors. Regularly employed nurses, with their equipment supplied by their employer-institution, would have a more difficult time justifying these deductions than self-employed nurses.
- *Professional expenses:* Dues and fees for membership in related professional associations (from local chapters to national level)

are deductible. Attendance at a professional workshop or convention must be firmly related to your professional needs before expenses can be justified as deductions. In addition the IRS makes careful distinction between the expenses attributed to the "work" and "holiday" aspects of those increasingly popular conventions held in resort areas.

- *Volunteering* for a charity may result in deductible expenses for gas, parking tolls, or meals away from home.

Treatment of special job-related income

- *Nurses* are frequently recipients of free lodging (e.g., at an institution, summer camp) or free meals (e.g., at a hospital) or both (e.g., on private duty). These "freebies" have an equivalent cash value which the IRS may determine as nontaxable or as taxable additional income, depending on the circumstance in which they are offered.
- *Considered non-taxable:* the value of the employer-supplied free lodging and/or free meals when they are a "required condition of employment" or for the "employer's convenience" (i.e., to keep on-duty staff instantly available).
- *Considered taxable:* the specific sum or equivalent value when a nurse is given a choice of a cash allowance for lodging or free lodging, whatever her choice.
- *Patient gratitude* at times is reflected in cash gifts in excess of the nurse's salary. The IRS may quibble and consider the money taxable income instead of a nontaxable gift.

Career Advancement Deductions

- *Educational expenses* are deductible when related to a nurse's current employment position; that is, if the courses are taken to maintain or improve skills on the job, to meet an employer's requirements or new regulations. The cost of training for a new career or occupation is not deductible, nor is a "brush-up" course taken by nurses returning to prior employment.
- *Subscriptions* to professional and technical journals are deductible expenses.

Personal Circumstance Factors

Relocation and moving costs can be claimed as deductions by those who have worked at least 39 weeks full-time (78 weeks for self-employed) in a new job at least 50 miles away from their old employment and home. The maximum for total moving deduction is $2,500 to cover the actual cost of moving personal effects as well as expenses for transporting the family and for preliminary house-hunting searches.

Child care cost can be claimed up to a limit of $400 a month if the children are under 15 years and the annual family income is under $18,000. (Acceptable costs are phased out as the annual income figure becomes higher.) This deduction can be related also to expenses for a spouse or any dependents unable to care for themselves. The definition of allowable services is wide, but the services are not deductible if performed by a relative or another dependent. In addition, to make the claim a worker has to be gainfully employed full-time, meaning at least three-quarters of the regular work week.

Retirement plans permit an annual withdrawal of a specified portion of income which is then entered into a fund held until retirement age, minimum 59½ years. These annual amounts and any interest income they earn are not taxed until the fund is drawn upon, at a point where it is reasoned, the individual is older and both tax burden and income would be less.

Nurses who are self-employed may use the Keogh Plan, which permits an annual deduction of up to 15% of self-employed earned income for contribution to the fund. In dollars, the maximum amount is $7,500 per year.

Nurses who are neither enrolled in an employer-sponsored retirement plan nor self-employed may set up an Individual Retirement Account, which permits deductible contributions of up to 15% of annual salary. In dollars, the maximum amount is $1,500.

For further information, obtain the free basic IRS guide *Your Federal Income Tax* plus other explanatory pamphlets on more complicated tax regulations.

For direct assistance, the IRS maintains toll-free numbers, listed in their instruction booklet, where quick questions will be answered.

Planning for Retirement*

Your retirement years will be an important part of your life. For instance, on the average, a man age 65 will live 13 additional years. For a

---

*Source: American Council of Life Insurance

woman of that age, it is 18 additional years. So you can see that your retirement is apt to be a long period of time.

Your way of life will change. You will not have the responsibilities that occupy your attention now. You will have a lot of free time.

Your financial situation will change. You won't have the same regular income. You'll have to look to other financial sources and quite likely you will have less money coming in.

The first step is to focus on your goals. Have you decided what you want to do with your retirement? Travel? Move to another part of the country? Stay where you are and perhaps move into a smaller home or apartment? Take up a new hobby? Start your own business? Or will you just relax and enjoy some recreational activities?

Next, have you thought about whether or not you will be able to *afford* to do these things? Have you estimated what your retirement income and expenses will be?

But first, let's look at those vital money considerations. Here are some possible financial resources for you:

- Social Security;
- a pension;
- life insurance, annuities;
- savings;
- investments;
- a house, other real estate;
- a part-time job;
- health insurance, Medicare.

Social Security

A monthly Social Security check provides basic income for the majority of retired people in this country.

You can start drawing full Social Security benefits at age 65. Or you can decide to retire as early as 62 and start collecting benefits then, but you will not get as much money each month.

A non-working wife is also eligible to start collecting an amount equal to 50% of her husband's benefit at age 62 or later. Again, she will get more money if she waits until 65 to start collecting. A wife who has worked and qualifies for Social Security in her own right may collect 100% of her own benefits, or 50% of her husband's, whichever is larger.

The benefits paid by Social Security are now increased automatically each year if the cost of living increases. You are permitted to earn up to a maximum amount a month without changing your benefit. If you earn more than this amount, your Social Security check will be reduced. After age 72, there is no limit to what you can earn and still get full benefits.

Social Security also provides a death benefit, usually $255, payable in a lump sum immediately after the death of a person who is covered by Social Security. Survivors' benefits are available to dependents of workers who die.

Pension Plans

Almost all pension plans have certain features in common. Here are some of the things you should find out about your plan.

- How long do you have to work for your employer or how old do you have to be to become eligible for a pension?
- How will the amount of money you get through your pension plan be determined?
- Does your plan provide for vested benefits? If so, when? (Vesting means that after a specified period of time on the job you will become entitled to a pension from that particular place at retirement even though you may leave that employer and work somewhere else—or not work at all. Through vesting, a person who works for several employers may eventually receive payments from more than one pension plan.)
- Will the payments you receive from your pension plan be reduced by the benefit payments you will receive from Social Security? By how much?
- Will there be a continuing benefit for the surviving spouse? Both husband and wife should check this out.

If you work for an employer who does not provide a pension plan, you can establish your own. Under the new federal law, you can set aside up to 15% of your salary or wages (up to a maximum of $1,500 a year) in an Individual Retirement Account for your use after you stop working. The amount you set aside may be deducted from your taxable income. You will need professional help to do this. Your lawyer, bank or life insurance agent can advise you.

If you are self-employed, you can set up a Keogh retirement program. The new federal law has increased the amount you can put into this, tax-free, to 15% of your income up to a maximum of $7,500 a year. It is taxed, however, when you start drawing it out as retirement income. Here, too, you should get professional guidance.

Life Insurance

The primary purpose of life insurance coverage, of course, is to provide income for your dependents if you should die prematurely. But if you have a whole life insurance policy (sometimes called straight life), you will find that there is money in your policy you can use at retirement time.

How can you use this cash value when you reach retirement age? In one of several ways: you can surrender your policy and take the cash value in a lump sum or in regular monthly payments; you can continue your life insurance protection, without having to pay any more premiums, by converting your policy to a paid-up policy for a reduced amount of insurance or converting to extended term coverage.

If you have the kind of life insurance policy that pays dividends, you can use these to add to the money you will have available later on. You can arrange to have the dividends accumulate at interest with the company or use them to purchase additional life insurance.

In case you have term life insurance, you probably know this does not ordinarily build up cash values. It is usually purchased by individuals for a specific number of years, say a five-year term. Term insurance is the kind of insurance used by most group plans.

Annuities

Annuities are sold by life insurance companies but have a different purpose: they provide a guaranteed income which you cannot outlive.

There are different kinds of annuities available. Some give you regular payments and stop at your death. Other types will continue to pay a certain remaining amount to a beneficiary. For a couple, there is a "joint and survivor" annuity. This provides an income to both and then to the survivor as long as he or she lives.

Annuities can be purchased in several ways. You can buy one with a lump sum at any given time. Some people do this at 65 with the cash value from their life insurance policy. You can also buy them by regular payments similar to your insurance premiums.

Your life insurance agent would be able to advise you on which annuity plan is the most suitable to your individual circumstances.

Savings Plans

There are many types of savings plans. There is a regular savings account that you can get at a commercial bank. Or you can get a savings account that gives you a higher rate of interest at either a savings bank or at a savings and loan association. In all three cases, this is money you can usually withdraw at any time—and you should have an adequate amount there, ready for emergencies.

There are also long-term savings plans. These give you an even higher rate of interest but the money must be left on deposit for specified periods of time to get this higher interest.

Since you will not be using your retirement savings for a while, you should look into these longer term accounts. And since safety is a primary concern in planning for the future, you will want to select a bank or savings and loan association where your savings are insured by the federal government. Interest or dividends on savings do vary, depending on the kind of bank you choose and the kind of accounts it has. It will pay you to do a little comparison shopping before you decide where to put your money.

Investments

Stocks are liquid—which means you can buy and sell easily without tying up your money. But there are also risks. The prices of stocks go down as well as up. The stocks of first-rate companies with long records or success are often better bets over the long haul than the stocks of lesser and more speculative companies. They will not go through the roof, but then they are not likely to go through the floor either. Talk to a few stock brokers and explain your objectives and pick the one who seems best attuned to your needs.

Corporate or municipal bonds are purchased primarily for income. Sold usually in units of $1,000, bonds pay a stated rate of interest. However, while the rate of interest remains constant, the value of a bond itself can fluctuate up and down just as a stock does. Investing in bonds requires a good deal of expertise and for this you need guidance also.

Mutual funds are aimed primarily at producing income and funds aimed primarily at increasing the value of your investment. These are available through stock brokers or directly from some of the funds themselves.

But you should remember that the time to think about stocks and bonds is only after you have constructed a solid foundation—Social Security, pension, life insurance, annuities, savings—on which to build a happy and secure retirement.

A house can be an important asset in your retirement planning. Chances are that by the time you do retire, the mortgage will be almost or entirely paid off and your expenses will be reduced almost entirely to taxes, maintenance and utilities.

On the other hand, if you decide to move to an apartment or another community, you will be able to sell your house and wind up with some money. A well-kept house in a good neighborhood is almost certain to increase in value in coming years. In fact, you can regard your house as an investment in real estate.

Health Insurance

Medical expenses can put a severe burden on the best of retirement budgets. So protection against them is a must.

First, there is Medicare. This is the government health insurance available through your local Social Security office. To qualify, you must be 65 years or over and have registered at the Social Security office; or, in some cases, under 65 and disabled. Medicare Part A pays for hospitalization and certain health services after you leave the hospital. You do not have to pay anything for this coverage, but it does not cover all your hospital bills. Medicare Part B helps pay for doctor bills and other medical services. You are automatically enrolled in Part B if you apply for Part A but you will have to pay a small monthly charge for Part B. To get a complete breakdown of what is and is not covered by Medicare, ask your Social Security office for a brochure.

It is important to understand that Medicare will not pay for all your medical expenses, and some it will not pay at all. So you may want to consider getting some supplementary private health insurance.

If you have group health insurance where you work, find out if your company extends its

benefits to cover retired employees. You might also be able to convert your group insurance to an individual policy when you retire.

Social Security*

In 1975 the percentage of salary deducted for Social Security tax was 5.85%, and the maximum taxable amount of your income was $14,100, making the maximum payment per year $824.85.

You become fully insured and eligible for these benefits if you work the required number of calendar quarters in which you were paid at least $50 each year. (This refers to the years after 1950 and before the year you become 62). If you retire in 1977 at age 62 for instance, you need 27 quarters . . . in 1978 you will need 28, and so on.

Receiving retirement benefits at 62 is possible although you will have to settle for reduced payments. Your benefits will be 80% of the primary insurance amount you would have received by waiting until 65 to apply for them.

To continue receiving full Social Security benefits, you cannot earn more than $2,520 a year—otherwise you lose $1 of benefits for every $2 you make. When you reach 72, however, there is no limit to your earnings while continuing to get full benefits.

Benefits depend on your average monthly wage. Dependents and survivors benefits are based on a percentage of your own retirement benefits. In finding your average wage, you can subtract the five years of lowest earnings from the total number of the years that you have worked.

Social Security benefits increase automatically as the cost of living rises.

Your retirement benefit will rise 1% a year during the period between ages 65 and 72 if you did not collect any benefits because you were working. And if you qualify for Social Security both on your own working record and as a dependent of your husband, you will get the larger of the two amounts.

As a final cheery note, Social Security checks are not subject to federal income taxes.

---

*Source: Adapted from "Watching Your Finances" by Leonard Sloane *American Journal of Nursing,* April 1975. ©American Journal of Nursing Company.

Table 9-26 Social Security—effective and scheduled contribution rates
(OASDHI: Old-age, survivors, disability and health insurance)

| Period or Year | Annual maximum taxable earnings | Contribution rates (percent) | | | | | | Monthly premium for supplementary medical insurance |
| | | Employers and employees (each) | | | Self-employed | | | |
		Total	OASDI	HI	Total	OASDI	HI	
1976	15,300	5.85	4.95	0.90	7.90	7.00	0.90	7.20
Future schedule:								
1977		5.85	4.95	0.90	7.90	7.00	0.90	(NA)
1978–1980		6.05	4.95	1.10	8.10	7.00	1.10	(NA)
1981–1985		6.30	4.95	1.35	8.35	7.00	1.35	(NA)
1986–1998		6.45	4.95	1.50	8.50	7.00	1.50	(NA)

NA Not available.

Source: U.S. Social Security Administration.

Nearly half of all female Social Security beneficiaries in 1973 were women who retired as workers in their own right. The other half were entitled to benefit payments based on their husband's record of earnings.

Pension Plans and Your Rights*

More than 30 million workers in the U.S. are covered by private pension plans.

Two areas of pension plans have been of particular concern to women workers. One was the typical exclusion of part-time and part-year workers. The other was the long period of unbroken service usually required in order to achieve "vesting," that is, a nonforfeitable right to retirement benefits. The work pattern of married women leaving the labor market temporarily because of family responsibilities or changing jobs when their husbands are transferred left a great many women unable to meet plan eligibility and vesting standards, and therefore no pension rights at all, even though at retirement age their total years of work and contributions to pension plans might be only slightly less than those of their male counterparts.

In addition, a great many workers—women and men—who had agreed to employer contributions toward a pension plan as a form of deferred wages realized little or no benefits

because, for example, the employer went bankrupt, the company was sold to or merged with another company which refused to continue the plan, or the fund was depleted due to imprudent action by trustees.

As protection, Congress passed the Employee Retirement Income Security Act of 1974 (commonly known as the Pension Reform Act) which sets standards for existing plans whose sponsors decide to continue them and for any new plans that may be established. These standards are in such areas as participation (eligibility), vesting, funding, fiduciary responsibility and reporting and disclosure. In addition, the Pension Reform Act establishes an insurance program for pension plans and liberalizes provisions for individual pension plans.

Generally, you cannot be excluded from a plan if you are at least 25 years old and have had at least one year of service (defined as a minimum of 1,000 hours of employment during a year). You may not be eligible for participation if you are within five years of normal retirement age when you are first employed. If your employer does not have a qualified pension, profit-sharing, or similar plan, you can set up your own plan by contributing up to 15% of your compensation or $1,500, whichever is less, to an individual retirement account, or for an individual annuity or individual retirement bond. An annuity is an amount payable yearly or at other regular intervals.

The law guarantees your right to your own contributions to a pension plan, as well as a nonforfeitable or "vested" right to all or part of

*Source: U.S. Dept. of Labor, 1975.

your retirement benefits contributed by your employer in one of the following three ways:

1. a right to all of your benefits after ten years of service;
2. a right to 25% of your benefits after five years of service, with 5% annual increases for the next five years and 10% annual increases thereafter;
3. a right to 50% of your benefits after five years when the sum of your age and years of service equals 45, with 10% increases in each of the next five years (however, regardless of age, if you have at least ten years of service you are entitled to 50% of your benefits, with an additional 10% for each of the next five years).

If the employer maintaining your plan goes bankrupt or does not have enough money to pay your benefits, a new Pension Benefit Guaranty Corporation will guarantee at least a portion of your benefits.

From your employer you are entitled to receive a copy of the statement of assets and liabilities of the plan and of receipts and disbursements during the preceding 12-month period, within 210 days after the close of the fiscal year of the plan. Once every 12 months you may request in writing—and you are entitled to receive—a statement indicating the total benefits you have accumulated, and the nonforfeitable benefits, if any, you have accumulated or the earliest date your benefits will become nonforfeitable.

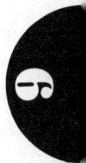

10

NURSING EDUCATION

Overview

Professional nursing schools fall into three general categories: junior or community college schools offering a two-year associate degree program; hospital schools of nursing offering a two and one-half- to three-year diploma program; and colleges offering a four-year baccalaureate program. All three types require graduation from high school, various pre-entrance examinations, plus a physical examination. Their programs cover the nursing arts and sciences which form an essential background for nursing practice.

The associate degree program (two years) will include general education courses, especially science, at the junior college level, in addition to nursing theory and practice. The diploma course (two and one-half- to three-years) may also involve general education subjects, including biological, physical and social sciences, and nursing theory and practice.

Graduates of either of these courses are fully prepared for bedside nursing in a hospital, nursing home, or private duty, but they are not prepared for supervisory or administrative positions in nursing. Some students who complete a two-year or three-year program may wish to go on to the four-year college program. This they can do, but should not count on getting transfer credit for the full two or three years of education they have had. Colleges may grant credit for some of the courses, or they may provide credit on the basis of examinations provided by the college.

The four-year baccalaureate program ("baccalaureate" and "bachelor's" are interchangeable terms) includes work in the arts, humanities, and sciences. The major is in nursing, including theory and practice. Graduates are prepared for general duty staff nursing, for beginning positions in public health agencies, for advancement to supervisory and administrative work in nursing, and for graduate study leading to a master's or doctor's degree.

A graduate degree, which would involve one to five years of study beyond the baccalaureate, is ordinarily required for advanced clinical practice, teaching, research, and other advanced positions.

Historical Perspective

Before the establishment of the New Training Schools in 1873, nursing had been largely a vocational skill, acquired in hospitals through short training periods and considerable on-the-job experience. As the hospital schools proliferated, so did the disparities in the training systems. In an effort to set forth acceptable standards for nursing education, the *Standard Curriculum for Schools of Nursing* was created in 1917.

In 1920 the Committee for the Study of Nursing Education was formed to review the application of the new curriculum. Their famous report, known as the Goldmark report, stressed the inadequacies and pointed out the conflicting dual role of the hospital nursing schools. The hospital schools were responsible for both educating nurses and providing nurse service to the patients. However, when the requirements for service predominated, the needs of education yielded.

Subsequent investigations continued to reveal inconsistent quality and content among hospital nursing schools. Even in 1968 one critic commented "The great bulk of nurses are still being trained in diploma schools associated with hospitals and largely on an apprenticeship basis, with unsystematic exposures to theoretical and tested knowledge."

The first steps to develop professional nursing programs within a college setting were undertaken in 1907, with the establishment of the Division of Hospital Economics at Teachers College, and in 1909, with the inauguration of the University of Minnesota School of Nursing. In 1916 degree programs in nursing were offered at Yale and Cincinnati. The increase has been steady; for example, from 1962–67 the number of collegiate schools rose from 170 to 214. Some critics of collegiate education complain that educators tend to consider nursing education as only "training" and give it low academic prestige in the college. Others feel collegiate educators have overly separated nursing education from the hospital and direct patient care.

Needs and Trends

Needs

A survey of 10,000 nurses conducted by *Nursing '77* in January produced the following suggestions for improving nurse education:

- Reintroduce basic nursing care techniques into collegiate nurse preparation; emphasize *nursing care* in all levels of nursing education;
- More psychological training—not basic Psych 101, but "interpersonal relations;"

- Internships for nurses;
- Standardization of nursing school programs;
- Required inservice education or continuing education;
- Compulsory educational upgrading of staff who need this because of years out of school;
- Less care left to aides and better training for them;
- LPNs should also get some kind of college credit for their experience.

Trends

- Increasing numbers of college graduates with baccalaureate, master's, and doctoral degrees in other disciplines are seeking admission into nursing education programs.
- More students of nursing, particularly at the graduate education level, are enrolled for part-time study.
- Many more students with previous experience in nursing are being admitted at appropriate levels in all educational programs in nursing based on evaluation by testing knowledge and by demonstrated competence in practice.
- The nursing education system has shifted from traditional preparation in the hospital

setting to academically based programs in junior and senior colleges and universities. This trend, while evident much earlier, accelerated during the past decade.

- The significant development of associate degree programs in the last few years and the smaller, but still sizable, increase in the number of baccalaureate programs, reflect the trend toward more academic education for young people and their preference for collegiate education.

Future*

If diploma programs continue to close down at the present rate, diploma programs in nursing may cease to exist. Associate degree programs will stabilize in numbers and will realize their goal to prepare highly efficient technical nurse practitioners. Baccalaureate degree programs will concentrate on general, cultural, scientific, and value education for all the professionals and will cease to offer the formal preparation in nursing. The master's degree programs in nursing will prepare the generalized professional nurse practitioner. Finally, the doctoral degree programs in nursing will prepare clinical nursing specialists, researchers, scholars, teachers, administrators, and consultants for nursing.

*Source: Dorothy Ozinek, *The Future of Nursing Education,* NLN Pub. No. 15-1581, 1975.

Education and Where Employed

Table 10-1   Estimated number of registered nurses practicing in various fields, by academic credential

Field of employment	Total	Percent			
		Master's or doctoral degree	Bacca-laureate	Nursing diploma	Associate degree
Total 1974	857,000	3.3	15.2	75.5	6.0
Total 1972	780,000	3.1	13.7	78.7	4.5
1972					
Hospital, nursing homes and related institutions	578,000	1.3	12.0	81.3	5.4
Public health and school	54,800	7.1	35.2	56.2	1.5
Nursing education	28,400	42.6	39.1	17.2	1.1
Occupational health	20,000	1.0	7.0	89.5	2.5
Private duty, doctors' offices and other fields	98,800	0.4	5.6	91.0	3.0

Sources: Interagency Conference on Nursing Statistics. Estimates by field of employment revised 1974. Estimates of educational preparation by U.S. Department of Health, Education and Welfare, Division of Nursing, 1974.

The figures in the preceding table reflect the fact that, until the 1950s, almost all nurses were trained in diploma programs and that associate degree programs were hardly a factor in nurse training.

Education and Salary Rewards

Baccalaureate and graduate training in nursing is subsequently reflected in higher wages, but the amount of the increase is small.

Using the averages obtained from this (*Nursing '74*) survey of nurses, the average pay differential between a starting salary for a three-year diploma graduate and a four-year baccalaureate graduate is about $312 per year—at the 42% of hospitals that give any differential at all. The costs involved in a diploma graduate receiving a B.S. can easily run up to $20,000—not to count the hours and lost wages, if she foregoes salaries. At that rate, it would take up to 65 years for her to recover her out-of-pocket expenses for further education.*

If your starting pay does vary, please supply your current average starting pay for the categories below.

A.D. graduate	$723/mo.
Diploma	$731/mo.
B.S. degree	$757/mo.
M.S. degree	$895/mo.

Where you work, are promotions related to educational level?

	All
Yes	31%
No	49%
Sometimes	4%
Don't know	16%

Does your nursing staff's pay scale vary according to the educational level of the nurse?

Yes	42%
No	58%

Do nurses with baccalaureate degrees start at a higher salary than nurses with diplomas?

Yes	38%
No	60%
No answer	2%

Nursing Education Programs

Summary Information

Number of Programs**

Overall, a virtual zero growth rate seems the likely forecast for the next few years in nursing education. The internal composition, however, is likely to change. In light of the more steady and somewhat higher growth rate in baccalaureate programs, it also seems likely that these programs will be producing increasingly larger proportions of R.N. graduates.

It must be remembered that the present leveling off in growth comes at the end of a marked expansion that began in the late 1960s in R.N. education.

The rates at which the number of programs and admissions of students were increasing could not be sustained for an indefinite period. Associate degree programs were advancing at 25% per year for several years. Baccalaureate programs increased from 8 to 10% per year for many years and were briefly propelled to 34% in one year (1971–72). Diploma programs, though declining in numbers, did not decline nearly as rapidly in terms of admissions and enrollments.

Table 10-2   Number of programs, by type

Year	Total	Bacca- laureate	Associate degree	Diploma
1962	1,136	173	84	874
1967	1,269	221	281	767
1972	1,377	293	541	543
1975	1,375	329	618	428

Source: DHEW, June 1976.

---

*Source: "Nursing '74 Probe: Further Education," *Nursing '74,* July. (Survey of 420 nurses.)

**Source: *Nursing Outlook,* June 1976. ©American Journal of Nursing Company.

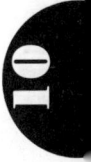

162

Table 10-3   Nursing programs—by state, 1975

Jurisdictions	Number of schools	All programs			Bac. Total	A.D. Total	Diploma Total
		Total	Accredited	Not Accredited			
Alabama	27	27	16	11	8	13	6
Alaska	2	2	0	2	1	1	0
Arizona	15	15	9	6	2	13	0
Arkansas	13	14	7	7	6	8	0
California	84	84	41	43	19	60	5
Colorado	11	11	7	4	3	6	2
Connecticut	25	25	18	7	7	7	11
Delaware	9	9	3	6	2	3	4
District of Columbia	7	7	6	1	5	1	1
Florida	28	28	10	18	6	21	1
Georgia	31	32	19	13	7	19	6
Guam	1	1	0	1	0	1	0
Hawaii	4	5	2	3	1	4	0
Idaho	6	6	5	1	1	5	0
Illinois	79	79	50	29	14	32	33
Indiana	26	28	26	2	9	12	7
Iowa	32	32	14	18	8	14	10
Kansas	21	21	16	5	6	8	7
Kentucky	26	27	17	10	5	18	4
Louisiana	16	16	11	5	7	6	3
Maine	9	9	5	4	2	2	5
Maryland	23	23	15	8	5	11	7
Massachusetts	58	59	46	13	10	19	30
Michigan	46	46	21	25	11	23	12
Minnesota	25	25	21	4	9	9	7
Mississippi	19	19	4	15	5	12	2
Missouri	34	34	21	13	7	14	13
Montana	5	5	2	3	2	2	1
Nebraska	13	14	13	1	4	2	8
Nevada	3	3	1	2	2	1	0
New Hampshire	9	9	6	3	2	1	6
New Jersey	41	41	32	9	7	13	21
New Mexico	9	9	5	4	1	8	0
New York	122	124	94	30	31	43	50
North Carolina	46	46	18	28	11	26	9
North Dakota	9	9	6	3	4	2	3
Ohio	68	68	56	12	11	24	33
Oklahoma	19	19	12	7	6	10	3
Oregon	12	12	9	3	2	9	1
Pennsylvania	108	108	83	25	21	18	69
Puerto Rico	9	11	7	4	3	8	0
Rhode Island	7	7	7	0	3	2	2
South Carolina	13	14	9	5	3	10	1
South Dakota	9	9	8	1	3	3	3
Tennessee	28	29	23	6	7	15	7
Texas	44	44	32	12	11	27	6
Utah	4	4	3	1	3	1	0
Vermont	3	4	3	1	1	3	0
Virgin Islands	1	1	1	0	0	1	0

Table 10-3   (continued)

Jurisdictions	Number of schools	All programs			Bac. Total	A.D. Total	Diploma Total
		Total	Accredited	Not Accredited			
Virginia	38	38	21	17	7	15	16
Washington	22	22	16	6	6	14	2
West Virginia	15	15	9	6	3	10	2
Wisconsin	24	24	17	7	8	7	9
Wyoming	2	2	1	1	1	1	0
Total	1,360	1,375	904	471	329	618	428

Source: *State Approved Schools of Nursing—RN, 1976,* N.Y.: National League for Nursing, 1976.

Geographic Differences
The high concentration of diploma programs in the East reflects the historical lead of the East in number of hospitals and thus the number of hospital schools, diploma programs and faculty.

The West has few diploma programs because its rapid population increase occurred in the last 30 years and by the time large hospitals became established the trend was away from diplomas and toward baccalaureate and associate degrees.

The South is relatively the most backward based on its disproportionately large number of faculty with only an associate or diploma degree teaching in L.P.N. programs.

Admissions Criteria

An applicant to a nursing program must be 17 or 18 years of age. The maximum age limit depends on the individual applicant and the school. Most schools admit men students as well as women. Opportunities for men in nursing are excellent.

Most schools of professional nursing will accept only applicants who are from the top half of their high school graduating class; and some will accept only those from the top third.

All schools of professional nursing require at least high school graduation for admission, and a few require college work. In addition, most require the completion of certain high school subjects.

The most frequently used selection criteria in 698 schools of nursing surveyed by E. E. Taylor (1966) were as follows:*

Table 10-4   School selection criteria

	Most important	Frequency of use
HSGPA	49%	91%
Application forms	23	90
Interview	18	92
Health forms	15	88
Biographical inventory	12	59
References	12	88
Test Battery:		
NLNPNG	47	41
Psych. Corp. Others not		
designed for nursing	48	46
Other procedures	26	17

The NLN reported in 1970 that the best achievement test predictors of performance on the licensing examination for students in baccalaureate and diploma programs were the three medical-surgical nursing achievement tests.
The NLN Achievement Tests are comprehensive tests designed to provide broader coverage of a field and to require greater depth and breadth of understanding.

*Source: Litwack, *Counseling Evaluation and Student Development,* (Saunders, 1972).

Admissions, Graduations and Enrollments

Table 10-5   Admissions, graduations, and enrollments in schools of nursing—R.N. by administrative control and type of program

Administrative control and type of program	Number of programs Oct. 16, 1974– Oct. 15, 1975		Number of students					
			Admissions Aug. 1, 1974– July 31, 1975		Graduations Aug. 1, 1974– July 31, 1975		Enrollments Oct. 15, 1975	
University or Senior college								
Baccalaureate	327		34,801		20,149		99,805	
Associate degree	152		11,979		7,465		22,698	
Diploma	0		0		0		0	
Total	479	33.9%	46,780	42.5%	27,614	37.1%	122,503	48.9%
Junior or Community college								
Associate degree	466		38,181		25,153		66,632	
Total	466	33.0%	38,181	34.7%	25,153	33.7%	66,632	26.6%
Hospital								
Diploma	446		23,917		20,816		58,454	
Total	446	31.6%	23,917	21.7%	20,816	27.9%	58,454	23.4%
Independent								
Baccalaureate	3		391		92		875	
Associate degree	3		20		4		162	
Diploma	15		779		857		1,759	
Total	21	1.5%	1,190	1.1%	953	1.3%	2,796	1.1%
Grand total	1,412[1]	100.0%	110,068	100.0%	74,536	100.0%	250,385	100.0%

[1]Includes 37 programs that closed between October 16, 1974 and October 15, 1975 but admitted 62 and graduated 1,553 students.

Source: *State Approved Schools of Nursing, RN—1976,* N.Y.: National League for Nursing, 1976.

Table 10-6   Admissions: by programs which prepare for state licensure in nursing

Academic year	Associate degree	Diploma	Baccalaureate	Total basic RN programs
1970–71	29,889	28,980	20,413	79,282
1971–72	36,996	29,801	27,357	94,154
1972–73	44,387	29,848	30,478	104,713
1973–74	48,596	26,943	32,672	108,210
1974–75	50,180	24,696	35,192	110,068

Source: *Nursing Outlook,* June 1976. © American Journal of Nursing Company.

Table 10-7   Graduations: from programs which prepare for state licensure in nursing

Academic year	Associate degree	Diploma	Baccalaureate	Total basic RN programs
1970–71	14,754	22,334	9,913	47,001
1971–72	19,165	21,592	11,027	51,784
1972–73	24,850	21,445	13,132	59,427
1973–74	29,299	21,280	17,049	67,628
1974–75	32,622	21,673	20,241	74,536

Source: *Nursing Outlook,* June 1976. © American Journal of Nursing Company.

Table 10-8   Graduations and enrollments in schools of nursing—R.N. by jurisdiction, 1974–75*

Jurisdictions†	Enrollments October 15, 1975				Graduations Aug. 1, 1974–July 31, 1975			
	Total	DE	AD	DI	Total	DE	AD	DI
Alabama	4,584	2,509	1,396	679	1,123	313	485	325
Alaska	133	77	56	0	40	15	25	0
Arizona	2,988	1,757	1,231	0	756	312	444	0
Arkansas	1,744	630	1,114	0	517	85	432	0
California	12,550	4,236	7,377	937	4,825	1,339	3,087	399
Colorado	1,937	993	661	283	555	207	289	59
Connecticut	3,741	1,655	815	1,271	1,182	282	249	651
Delaware	1,279	781	233	265	354	154	61	139
District of Columbia	1,967	1,519	275	173	338	239	37	62
Florida	5,437	1,305	3,650	482	2,221	418	1,687	116
Georgia	5,277	1,579	2,541	1,157	1,511	312	902	297
Guam	87	0	87	0	20	0	20	0
Hawaii	363	125	238	0	136	54	82	0
Idaho	655	177	478	0	247	42	205	0
Illinois	13,553	4,304	4,624	4,625	4,023	741	1,643	1,639
Indiana	6,694	2,986	2,446	1,262	1,982	548	1,029	405
Iowa	3,916	1,297	1,072	1,547	1,352	393	494	465
Kansas	2,205	779	561	865	895	288	220	387
Kentucky	4,572	1,942	2,263	367	1,273	305	771	197
Louisiana	4,507	2,811	950	746	812	354	212	246
Maine	1,240	509	230	501	353	94	92	167
Maryland	3,836	1,348	1,797	691	1,427	512	639	276
Massachusetts	10,591	3,993	2,474	4,124	3,227	853	893	1,481
Michigan	9,261	3,535	3,699	2,027	3,175	690	1,501	984
Minnesota	5,362	2,117	2,015	1,230	1,833	578	765	490
Mississippi	2,491	1,065	1,214	212	715	158	513	44
Missouri	5,792	1,664	1,376	2,752	1,899	342	629	928
Montana	1,220	892	186	142	280	170	58	52
Nebraska	2,443	644	487	1,312	769	200	144	425
Nevada	521	483	38	0	129	57	72	0
New Hampshire	1,293	562	150	581	307	105	45	157
New Jersey	7,873	2,459	2,701	2,713	2,125	303	1,041	781
New Mexico	911	338	573	0	281	100	181	0
New York	31,580	11,179	13,678	6,723	8,643	2,068	4,146	2,429
North Carolina	6,171	3,041	2,266	864	1,640	629	689	322
North Dakota	1,317	696	243	378	506	190	101	215
Ohio	12,684	3,484	3,741	5,459	3,988	744	1,400	1,844

(*continued*)

Table 10-8   (continued)

Jurisdictions†	Enrollments October 15, 1975				Graduations Aug. 1, 1974–July 31, 1975			
	Total	DE	AD	DI	Total	DE	AD	DI
Oklahoma	2,180	862	1,058	260	732	268	314	150
Oregon	1,885	747	805	333	717	228	306	183
Pennsylvania	16,103	5,194	2,596	8,313	5,181	983	968	3,230
Puerto Rico	2,076	843	1,233	0	585	71	403	111
Rhode Island	1,739	1,003	503	233	428	168	193	67
South Carolina	2,573	1,210	1,278	85	595	183	382	30
South Dakota	1,627	821	458	348	446	156	175	115
Tennessee	6,039	2,590	2,145	1,304	1,355	346	701	308
Texas	13,002	7,719	4,241	1,042	3,203	1,400	1,506	297
Utah	950	804	146	0	368	139	229	0
Vermont	680	339	341	0	213	71	142	0
Virgin Islands	51	0	51	0	16	0	16	0
Virginia	5,249	1,903	1,613	1,733	1,390	388	499	503
Washington	4,272	2,093	1,861	318	1,320	542	691	87
West Virginia	2,287	625	1,305	357	770	131	482	157
Wisconsin	6,590	4,224	847	1,519	1,690	937	300	453
Wyoming	307	232	75	0	68	36	32	0
Total	250,385	100,680	89,492	60,213	74,536	20,241	32,622	21,673

*Includes 62 admissions and 1,553 graduations from 37 programs closed between October 16, 1974 and October 15, 1975.

† No Schools of Nursing—R.N. in American Samoa and Canal Zone.

Source: *State Approved Schools of Nursing—RN, 1976,* N.Y. National League for Nursing, 1976.

Diploma Programs*

Diploma programs are conducted by hospitals, usually require two to three years to complete, and emphasize actual nursing experience. They have traditionally been highly "work oriented," and nursing students used to spend much of their time in on-the-job training. Although classroom work has been an important part of the program, it generally has tended to be closely connected to day-to-day nursing practice.

In the past, diploma programs were the most numerous within the nursing education system, but their predominance and numbers have declined markedly over the past 15 years. In 1975 they accounted for only about 30% of all nursing education programs, in comparison with over 80% in 1959–60.

**Note: One of the characteristic and sig-

nificant aspects of hospital nursing education has been and continues to be the emphasis upon clinical experience in the educational process. [As] a significant number of hospital schools of nursing have closed their doors, the education of nurses (has been left) to other institutions. This has placed hospitals in the position of being increasingly dependent upon less well-prepared nursing service personnel.

Many that have terminated their schools of nursing find that they have to rely more and more upon nursing personnel from nearby community colleges or to go farther afield for nurses prepared in a hospital school of nursing or in a baccalaureate program. Nurses generally are not mobile, and recruitment of staff from other parts of a state or from out of state is difficult. The competition for nurses in large urban areas is so keen that some hospitals already find that they have to rely more and more upon nursing personnel from nursing schools in countries outside the United States. In many instances, hospitals are turning to less experienced and less well-prepared personnel to fill their needs.

*Source: DHEW, December 1973
**Source: John A. Wilkinson, "Hospital Schools of Nursing Counterpoise Costs" *Hospitals, JAHA,* April 16, 1976. Reprinted with permission of the American Hospital Association.

Distinctive Aspects of Diploma Programs*

- The school offers a readily accessible clinical laboratory that promotes understanding of the hospital climate, resources and other health disciplines.
- The school may enter into cooperative relations with colleges or universities for educational courses and/or services. The school may also enter into cooperative relationships with health care institutions and agencies in order to provide learning experiences for students.
- The faculty are committed to the improvement of nursing education as it relates to nursing practice and the delivery of health care and have a unique opportunity to promote changes in nursing practice in hospitals and other health care agencies.
- Admission requirements include graduation from high school or its equivalent with successful completion of certain prerequisite courses, satisfactory achievement on preentrance examinations and satisfactory assessment of personal qualities and health status.
- Students are selected by the faculty and admitted directly to the program in nursing.
- The curriculum includes courses in the theory and practice of nursing and courses in the biological, physical and behavioral sciences. Learning is reinforced through the application of scientific and nursing principles in the care of individuals and groups with nursing and health needs.
- Early and substantial patient care experiences are provided in the hospital and in a variety of community agencies which serve to foster within the student a strong identification with nursing.

The graduates of diploma programs (1) are eligible to take the examination leading to licensure as a registered nurse; (2) plan, organize, implement and evaluate plans of nursing care for individuals and groups of patients; (3) have an understanding of the hospital climate and the community health resources necessary for extended care of patients; (4) understand the role of other health disciplines and are contributing members of the health team; (5)

adjust readily to the role of beginning registered nurse practitioners in hospitals and similar community institutions; and (6) are permitted initial freedom of choice in the provision of nursing service to people and subsequent academic and experiential alternatives.

Associate Degree Programs**

Although this type of program is relatively new, the first having been instituted in 1952, it is now multiplying at a rate faster than that of any other type of nursing program.

In 1959, the 48 associate degree programs comprised only 4% of the total number of programs. By 1975, the 618 associate degree programs accounted for nearly one half of all nursing education programs.

Associate degree programs emphasize course work directly relevant to nursing, but they usually are not as closely tied to day-to-day practice as diploma programs are.

- The majority are conducted and controlled by public junior or community colleges, some are in senior colleges or universities, some are in technical institutes and a few are in private institutions.
- The programs vary in length from two academic years to two calendar years.
- The program of study combines nursing courses and supportive college courses.
- Students must meet requirements of the college to be admitted to the nursing program.
- Costs and living arrangements for nursing students are comparable to those for students in other curriculums in the college. The costs are usually minimal for local students.
- The associate degree nursing program prepares students to be eligible to write the state licensure examination to become registered nurses.

Some of the college credits earned in the program can be applied toward a baccalaureate degree in nursing should a graduate decide later to pursue education for professional nursing. The amount of credit granted will depend on the policies of the senior college or university that offers the particular baccalaureate degree program.

---

*Note: A complete list of accredited programs "Diploma Programs in Nursing Accredited by the NLN" is published annually in the August issue of *Nursing Outlook* (a supplementary list appears in March).

**Source: "Associate Degree Education for Nursing, 1974–75," National League for Nursing, 1975.

168

High school graduation or a high school equivalency certificate is the minimum requirement for admission to an associate degree program in nursing. The programs are attractive to married women and others whose family responsibilities require them to live at home, to men who wish to pursue nursing careers and to older students.

Baccalaureate Programs

Baccalaureate programs for nurse education usually require four or five years for completion, are conducted by colleges and universities and emphasize course work in liberal arts, sciences and theoretical subjects related to nursing. These programs are generally affiliated with one or more hospitals for the clinical training requirements. Since the programs are conducted as part of a college or university's overall program, admissions standards are generally similar to those of the parent institution. Graduates are awarded bachelor's degrees, usually a Bachelor of Science. By 1975 there were 329 college baccalaureate programs comprising about 25% of the total number of nurse training programs.

Distinctive Features *

A number of distinctive qualities identify education for professional nursing in an NLN-accredited senior college or university program.

- Students majoring in nursing are college students (colleges and universities conduct and control the nursing programs); thus, they enjoy the advantages of college and campus life with men and women preparing for careers in many fields.
- Standards are high; nursing students must meet the same intellectual and academic requirements as students majoring in other fields.
- The preparation of the nursing faculty, who are qualified for college teaching by education and experience, insures high-quality nursing education.
- The course of study combines special education in the theory and the practice of nursing with general education in the humanities and the behavioral, biological and physical sciences.
- Studies progress from lower division (freshman and sophomore years) to upper

* Source: National League for Nursing

division (junior and senior years), with courses in the nursing major—both theory and practice—being given largely in the junior and senior years.

- Upper-division courses in nursing theory and nursing practice build on preceding and concurrent courses in the sciences and the humanities; thus, students achieve the broad understanding and the skills needed today in professional nursing.
- Graduates of accredited collegiate programs in professional nursing are prepared to give high-quality nursing care to patients and their families and to direct the nursing care given by other nursing team members working with them.
- Graduates are qualified for employment as professional nurse practitioners in a variety of settings: homes, community health agencies, hospitals, extended care facilities, the military and other federal nursing services, and others.
- Graduates have the educational background necessary for graduate study in nursing at the masters degree level; thus, if they wish, they may move more rapidly to the most challenging, demanding and rewarding opportunities in nursing—teaching, administration, expert practice or research—for which masters education is a requirement.

Admissions

Each college or university sets its own requirements for admission and for graduation and determines the curriculum patterns of the baccalaureate programs it offers. This applies to nursing as it does to other majors. Although requirements and curriculums in nursing vary, the undergraduate college student usually must complete specified liberal arts subjects in the freshman and sophomore years. These lower-division requirements build the foundation for the student's major, which is concentrated in the junior and senior years. The registered nurse student must expect to fulfill degree requirements of the college or university both in the liberal arts (usually lower division) and in the nursing major (upper division).

College or university policies regarding admission, evaluation of previous education, granting of advanced standing and placement will apply to you as to others majoring in nursing or in other fields. Some institutions give advanced standing by transfer of credit; some award credit for or exemption from specific courses by examination. Because of these variations, the amount of credit or advanced standing granted to you, if any, will depend entirely on the policies of the college or university you elect to attend.

Applicants

Unlike the other programs, the baccalaureate program attracts a variety of students:

- high school students and graduates who wish to enter professional nursing.
- college graduates, college students or persons with some college work who wish to enter professional nursing;
- already licensed (with diploma or associate degree) registered nurses or students about to graduate from diploma or associate degree programs.

For the majority of registered nurses who go to a senior college or university, completion of a baccalaureate program in nursing represents additional preparation for the job. For some, it is the first step toward fulfilling requirements for positions as teachers, clinical nursing specialists, administrators, supervisors, consultants or researchers.

College Graduates Choosing Nursing

The University of Massachusetts has had a separate admissions program for the growing number of students applying for a second baccalaureate degree since 1972. About 35% of these applicants apply for nursing. The male applicants for nursing increased from 18 to 23% between 1974 and 1975. Biological science majors represented about 20%.

Why they choose nursing:

11%   A desire for advancement, a lack of marketable skills or recognition of wider opportunities in the health field—influenced by practical considerations.
16%   A return to their original goal.
25%   Thought better of their initial career choice.
11%   Changing image of nursing.
34%   Interest in people and desire to help others.

R.N.s Entering Baccalaureate Programs*

One problem that has plagued nursing educators is the question of systematic procedures

---

*Source: Litwack, *Counseling, Evaluation and Student Development,* (Saunder, 1972).

for admitting graduates of A.D. and diploma programs into baccalaureate programs in nursing. The same problem occurs in admitting diploma graduates into A.D. programs, and L.P.N.s into any of the three main kinds of nursing schools. At one time some colleges such as Teachers College, Columbia University, gave two years' automatic credit to any graduate of a diploma program. But as time went by the trend seemed to shift away from automatic credit toward a more systematic way of evaluating the level of each applicant. This occurred as colleges found that graduate nurses had widely varying skills and knowledge, resulting from the wide variance in the quality of the nursing program from which they graduated. In an apparent effort to upgrade the profession of nursing, the new directions seemed to fall into two groups, the use of nationally standardized tests for proper placement and locally developed procedures.

In 1965 the NLN reported that the Graduate Nurse Examination (GNE) could be used for placement testing of graduates from other programs. In 1969 the NLN reported on the increasing use of proficiency examinations in admitting R.N.s to baccalaureate programs.

Today emphasis is being placed on systematic clinical evaluation in order to determine the proper placement for an individual student.

Nurse Preceptorships

The term "preceptorship" is being defined broadly to mean a course of study in which students receive part of their training in a health care setting outside the direct confines of the educational institution and under the supervision of a practicing professional who serves as a preceptor. These off-campus experiences are referred to by several terms—clerkships, clinical electives, field placements or preceptorships. Most preceptorships are only open to nurses enrolled in an undergraduate program, but a few are limited to students working on a graduate level.

The sites where the work is done tend to be in the vicinity of the sponsoring institution, but usually in deprived areas—inner cities, backward rural areas, etc. A few programs send students far afield in this country, and at least one sends students abroad. Lengths of service vary from three weeks to six months. Expenses are involved, though they vary according to assignment. Some financial assistance is often available.

For a list of universities offering preceptorship programs write to the National Health Council and ask for *A Directory of Preceptorship Programs in the Health Professions.*

Nursing Program Accreditation

Numbers Accredited

During 1976 NLN accredited only 904 of the 1,375 nursing programs being offered. Of the three types of programs, the associate degree programs were the most likely to have no accreditation. The reason may be that many of these programs are comparatively new, and new nursing programs are not eligible for NLN accreditation until the first class of students has completed or is near completion of its program.

California has 60 associate degree programs, but only 18 are accredited.

Table 10-9   Initial programs of nursing education *accredited* by the National League for Nursing

Type of program	All programs	1976	
		Accredited programs	
		No.	Percent
Total	1,375	904	65.7
Baccalaureate	329	254	77.2
Diploma	428	382	89.3
Associate degree	618	268	43.4

Source: National League for Nursing

Accrediting Agencies*

1. *State approval:* The practice of nursing is regulated in each state by law. Each state and territory appoints an authority—usually a board of nursing or of nurse examiners—to administer its particular nurse practice act. Approval by such an authority means that the program in nursing meets the minimum legal requirements set by the state for the preparation of nurses for licensure. Only graduates of a

*Source: National League for Nursing

school offering a program approved by a state board are eligible to take the state examination for licensure to practice nursing as a registered nurse.

2. *Professional (national) accreditation:* In the United States, institutions that offer educational programs in nursing and other professions are not regulated by a federal authority. Instead, an organization or an agency that is national in scope and represents the educational institutions and the profession is designated as the body responsible for conducting a program of voluntary national accreditation.

At present more than 30 national professional agencies are recognized by the Council on Postsecondary Accreditation as the official accrediting agencies responsible for the quality of professional education for their particular fields. These agencies grant specialized accreditation to professional schools or programs within colleges and universities. Professional accreditation is voluntary, national in scope and applies only to special fields of study.

The purpose of such a program is to ensure that education for the particular profession will continue to improve and that quality programs will be offered to students. This type of accreditation program serves as the means whereby the educational institutions themselves voluntarily formulate and apply criteria of excellence in education for the profession. The procedure for accreditation usually includes four steps: formulation of criteria; evaluation of the institution and the program of studies by competent educators; publication of a list of institutions meeting the criteria; and periodic reevaluations to determine whether or not institutions and programs continue to meet the criteria.

The National League for Nursing is officially recognized as the accrediting agency for masters, baccalaureate and associate degree programs by the Council on Postsecondary Accreditation. NLN is also approved for accreditiation of masters, baccalaureate and associate degree, diploma and practical nursing programs by the U.S. Office of Education. In addition, the NLN is recognized as the national accrediting agency for nursing education by the nursing profession itself.

Accredited programs must meet educational standards for faculty and curriculum *above* minimal standards set by state nursing boards.

Figure 10-1   Accrediting agencies

Occupation and field(s) accredited	Accrediting agency	Agencies selecting representatives
Nursing:		
Associate degree programs	Council of Associate Degree Programs, National League for Nursing	National League for Nursing
Baccalaureate and graduate degree programs	Council of Baccalaureate and Higher Degree Programs, National League for Nursing	National League for Nursing
Diploma programs	Council of Diploma Programs, National League for Nursing	National League for Nursing
Nurse-anesthetist	Board of Trustees, American Association of Nurse Anesthetists	American Association of Nurse Anesthetists
Nurse-midwife	Approval Committee, American College of Nurse-Midwives	American College of Nurse-Midwives
Practical nurse	Accrediting Review Board, National Association for Practical Nurse Education and Service	National Association for Practical Nurse Education and Service
	Council of Practical Nursing Programs, National League for Nursing	National League for Nursing
Public health:		
Graduate programs: public health; community health education	Executive Board, American Public Health Association	American Public Health Association

Allied medical occupation	Collaborating organizations with American Medical Association	Curriculum review boards and committees
Assistant to the primary care physician	American Academy of Family Physicians American Academy of Pediatrics American College of Physicians American Society of Internal Medicine Physician's assistant members at large	Joint Review Committee on Educational Programs for the Assistant to the Primary Care Physician
Orthopaedic physician's assistant	American Academy of Orthopaedic Surgeons	Committee on the Training of the Orthopaedic Physician's Assistant, American Academy of Orthopaedic Surgeons
Medical assistant	Accrediting Bureau of Medical Laboratory Schools	Accredited schools Accrediting bureau American Medical Technologists

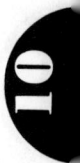

10

Students

Student Characteristics

In 1950, 7% of all female high schools graduates went into nursing schools. By 1966 the percentage had dropped to 5%. But with new federal funds going into associate degree programs and loan programs, the percentage has again risen to 7%.

Demographic Characteristics

Baccalaureate students tend to be drawn from higher income families than students in other types of programs, and a higher proportion of their parents are engaged in the health or other professions, characteristics frequently correlated with high quality job performance. The performance of students in baccalaureate—and diploma—programs appears to be somewhat better than that of students in associate programs.

Baccalaureate programs obtained over 65% of their students from the top quarter of high school graduating classes, while diploma schools obtained 49% of their students from the top quarter and associate degree programs obtained only 37%. Thus, as would be expected, baccalaureate students score higher than diploma or associate degree students on the Pre-Nursing and Guidance Examination, and diploma school students score slightly higher than do those in associate degree programs.

Psychological Counseling

The Association of American Medical Colleges estimates that from 65 to 85% of medical students seek some form of psychological counseling during their four years of study. This compares with estimates of 50 to 60% in nursing school, 30 to 40% in dental school and 15 to 20% at the undergraduate level.

Medical students feel they are confronted with a body of knowledge so vast as to defy mastery, yet they also worry that failure to learn may result in a patient's death.

Most, used to being near the top of their undergraduate classes, face unaccustomed and anxiety-producing competition for grades in medical school. They have money troubles. They feel that faculty members press them too hard at a time in their lives when they need emotional support.

In reviewing Table 10-10, note the older age and the larger number of marrieds among the associate degree students. Also note the better high school academic standing enjoyed by the baccalaureate students.

School and Work *

- Thirty-two percent of practical nurse students never worked before attending nursing school. However, 40% of practical nurses worked before but not while attending nursing school.

- Only one out of five newly licensed R.N.s and P.N.s plan to continue their education.

- Fifty-one percent work both before and while attending nursing school.

As can be seen from Table 10-11, the overwhelming majority of newly licensed diploma and baccalaureate nurses are under the age of 25 (88% and 87%, respectively). However practical nursing and A.D. programs had sizable percentages of student graduates over 25 years of age.

---

* Source: DHEW, May 1975.

Table 10-10   Characteristics of nursing students, by type of program

Characteristic	Diploma	Associate degree	Baccalaureate
		Type of program	
Sex			
Female	98.2%	95.5%	99.1%
Male	1.8	4.6	0.9
Marital status			
Single	96.5%	66.9%	96.6%
Married	2.7	26.9	2.1
Other	0.8	6.2	1.3
Race			
Caucasian	96.2%	90.6%	91.9%
Black	3.2	6.9	6.6
Other	0.4	2.2	1.3
Age (at admission)			
Under 20	90.4%	52.2%	87.0%
20–24	6.9	19.9	11.3
25–29	1.3	7.5	0.8
30–34	0.7	6.2	0.4
35–39	0.3	5.8	0.2
40–49	0.3	6.9	0.3
50 and over	0.1	1.4	0.0
Family income			
Below $5,000	17.6%	18.6%	14.4%
$5,000–$9,999	49.1	45.5	35.8
$10,000–$14,999	24.6	26.1	31.1
$15,000–$20,000	6.1	5.7	10.2
Over $20,000	2.7	5.0	8.6
High school academic standing			
Top quarter	49.4%	37.3%	65.1%
2nd quarter	39.7	44.2	27.2
3rd quarter	10.2	6.7	6.6
Bottom quarter	0.7	1.8	1.1
PNG mean percentile scores	69	65	78

Source: National Institutes of Health, 1972 (1969 data)

Age of Newly Licensed Nurses

Table 10-11   Newly licensed nurses by age and type of program

Age	All programs		Type of program			
	Number	Percent	Bacc.	A.D.	Dipl.	P.N.
Under 25	4,185	68%	87%	44%	88%	52%
25 years +	1,974	32	13	56	12	48
(unreported)	55					
Total		100%	100%	100%	100%	100%
Number	6,214		(1,150)	(1,650)	(1,956)	(1,458)

Source: DHEW, May 1975.

Pursuing A Career

Career Expectations of Student Nurses

Baccalaureate nurses have relatively high expectations of becoming head nurses, supervisors or public health nurses. This is consistent with the presumed program objectives of the three types of nursing education programs. The baccalaureate graduates also display stronger inclinations to work as staff nurses than do the graduates of the two programs designed primarily to produce staff nurses, but this may reflect a desire to provide professional bedside care, especially in the public health setting.

Where They End Up Working

Although hospitals and related institutions were the largest employer of nurses in 1970 (69% of the total), they attracted higher proportions of associate degree graduates (78%) and diploma school graduates (72%) and a smaller proportion of baccalaureate school graduates (54%).

A whopping 38% of baccalaureate nurses were employed in public health and nursing education, in comparison with 3% of associate degree graduates and 6% of diploma school graduates. It may be that these two fields provide more opportunity for independent activity and judgment and thus appeal to the better-educated nurse.

Table 10-12   Nursing field and position *expectations* of nurses 15 years after graduation, 1962

Field/position	Diploma	Associate degree	Baccalaureate
Nursing field			
General nursing	28.4%	22.5%	15.4%
Clinical specialties	49.3	50.1	39.7
Public health nursing	4.6	5.2	23.2
Education or administration	4.4	6.4	6.1
Two or more choices	2.7	3.6	4.2
Nonnursing	3.1	4.0	4.2
Undecided, no response	7.5	8.2	7.2
Total	100.0%	100.0%	100.0%
Position			
Staff nurse	17.7%	13.3%	23.6%
Head nurse or supervisor	26.6	29.4	41.3
Administrator	2.0	3.6	0.3
Educator/researcher	16.8	15.6	10.8
Private duty nurse	15.9	14.2	6.4
Other	13.0	12.2	10.3
Undecided, no response	8.0	11.7	7.3
Total	100.0%	100.0%	100.0%

Source: DHEW, 1972.

Important Factors in Career Choice*

Table 10-13   Important career factors to college freshmen, 1966

Factor in choice	All college students %	Career choice	
		Nurses %	Physicians %
Job openings are generally available	53.0	65.2	39.6
Rapid career advancement is possible	18.5	23.2	12.5
High anticipated earnings	41.3	37.5	34.8
It's a well respected or prestigious occupation	48.7	50.0	53.1
Provides a great deal of autonomy	35.9	28.2	58.9
Chance for steady progress	32.2	38.2	16.8
Chance for originality	38.2	36.9	37.5
Can make an important contribution to society	65.2	70.6	71.5
Can avoid pressure	11.5	7.9	8.7
Can work with ideas	45.0	44.8	40.5
Can be helpful to others	82.9	89.1	80.4
Have leadership opportunities	38.3	54.6	29.4
Able to work with people	77.0	85.6	73.2
Intrinsic interest in the field	61.7	58.3	71.9
Enjoyed my past experience in this occupation	47.4	63.6	32.0

Table 10-14   Important life goals to college freshmen, 1966

Life goal	All college students %	Career choice	
		Nurses %	Physicians %
Becoming accomplished in one of the performing arts (acting, dancing, etc.)	5.5	5.1	4.3
Becoming an authority on a special subject in my subject field	58.1	52.0	65.1
Obtaining recognition from my colleagues for contributions in my special field	35.2	29.8	37.8
Becoming an expert in finance and commerce	4.5	3.1	4.7
Having administrative responsibility for the work of others	23.1	32.6	12.5
Being very well off financially	28.6	24.5	20.9
Helping others who are in difficulty	81.0	83.5	89.3
Participating in an organization like the Peace Corps or Vista	15.0	15.2	16.4
Becoming an outstanding athlete	4.3	4.1	5.5
Becoming a community leader	19.0	12.4	27.7
Making a theoretical contribution to science	16.6	7.6	28.5
Writing original works (poems, novels, short stories, etc.)	7.4	6.5	9.0
Never being obligated to people	24.5	21.8	23.4

*Source: DHEW, November 1974.

Drop-Out Rate

Fully one of every three beginning students withdraws from a nursing program prior to completion. Only a small percentage of students who complete preparatory programs go on to advanced graduate study in nursing, and most of these are in programs designed to develop teachers or administrators rather than advanced clinical practitioners.

Drop-out rate of
student nurses

Program	Drop-out rate
A.D.	44%
Bac.	41%
Dip.	26%

Source: DHEW, 1976.

Do you wish your education had contained more of the following?

	Percent of respondents answering yes				
	AD	Diploma	BS orig. BS	BS orig. diploma	All
Bedside care	47%	6%	35%	7%	13%
Psychology	9%	25%	15%	27%	22%
Basic nursing theory	21%	13%	15%	13%	15%
Humanities	5%	29%	17%	20%	22%

Source: "Probe: Further Education," *Nursing '74,* August (survey of 420 nurses).

Student Views on Curriculum

A University of Oklahoma survey of student nurses who were just being exposed to clinical experiences found their interests changed 3 months and 15 months later.

Figure 10-2   Expressed preferences and interests of student nurses

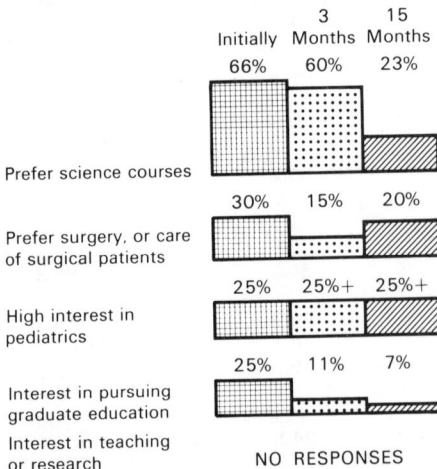

	3	15
Initially	Months	Months
66%	60%	23%

Prefer science courses

| 30% | 15% | 20% |

Prefer surgery, or care of surgical patients

| 25% | 25%+ | 25%+ |

High interest in pediatrics

| 25% | 11% | 7% |

Interest in pursuing graduate education

Interest in teaching or research   NO RESPONSES

Source: *Nursing Outlook,* July 1968. ©American Journal of Nursing Company.

Faculty

Number

In 1976 a total of 25,365 full-time and 5,221 part-time nurse-faculty members were employed in nursing programs. Over half of these faculty members had masters or doctoral level preparation.

While student enrollment in nurse education programs increased 24% between 1973 and 1975, faculty increased only 9%. Much of this discrepancy is due to associate degree programs, where student enrollment increased 40% with only a 15% increase in nurse-faculty.

Table 10-15   Number of nurse-faculty by nursing program

	Estimated total nurse-faculty	
Type of program	1972	1976
Baccalaureate and higher degree	6,157	9,834
Associate degree	4,067	6,560
Diploma	8,624	6,928
Total R.N.	18,848	23,322
Practical nursing	5,123	5,624
Grand total	23,971	28,946

Source: *Nurse Faculty Census, 1976,* National League for Nursing, Pub. No. 19–1650, 1977.

Education of Faculty

In the 1976 census of full-time nurse-faculty employed in all nursing programs by the highest credential earned: 52% were prepared at the master's or doctoral level, 36% at the baccalaureate level, 3% at the diploma level and 1.5% at the associate degree level.

Table 10-16   Full-time nurse-faculty by highest earned credential (as of January 1976)

| Highest earned credential | Total | | Type of program | | | | | | | |
| | | | Baccalaureate and higher degree | | Associate degree | | Diploma | | Practical nursing | |
	Number	Percent	Number	Percent	Number	Percent	Number	Percent	Number	Percent
Doctorate	892	3.5	817	9.5	57	1.0	13	0.2	5	0.1
Masters	12,246	48.3	6,737	78.7	3,304	58.2	1,646	26.0	559	11.7
Baccalaureate	9,149	36.1	984	11.5	2,147	37.8	3,844	60.8	2,174	45.4
Associate	384	1.5	19	0.2	63	1.1	56	0.9	246	5.1
Diploma	2,694	10.6	10	0.1	109	1.9	766	12.1	1,809	37.7
Total	25,365	100.0	8,567	100.0	5,680	100.0	6,325	100.0	4,793	100.0

Source: *Nurse Faculty Census 1976,* N.Y., NLN, Pub. No. 19–1650, 1977.

Faculty Salaries*

Table 10-17   Annual salaries and change in buying power by type of program and the educational level of faculty members, for 1968 and 1973

| Type of program and educational preparation level | Median salaries | | Percent change in buying power 1968–73 |
	1968	1973	
All programs—RN	$ 8,820	$11,880	2.2
Diploma programs	8,530	11,417	1.5
Less than baccalaureate	7,500	9,880	−0.1
Baccalaureate	8,435	11,076	−0.4
Master's and above	10,295	13,520	−0.4
Baccalaureate programs	9,200	12,075	−0.4
Baccalaureate	7,000	9,000	−2.5
Master's	9,380	12,100	−2.2
Doctorate	15,000	18,299	−7.6
Associate degree programs	9,300	12,065	−6.6
Baccalaureate	8,000	9,850	−7.1
Master's and above	10,500	13,557	−2.1

Administrators continue to receive higher salaries than nonadministrative faculty. The median salary for full professors in teaching positions was $18,947, while the median salary for full professors who were administrators was $22,452.

*Source: "Report on Survey of Salaries of Nurse Faculties and Administrators in Nursing Education Programs," ANA D-47, The American Nurses' Association, December 1973.

Fluctuations in median salary from state to state: California had the highest median, $14,192, followed by New York ($13,397), Maryland ($13,335), Florida ($12,400) and Massachusetts ($12,368). The lowest median salaries among the 44 states (plus the District of Columbia) with adequate returns in 1973 were found in: Arkansas ($9,260), Delaware ($9,523), New Mexico ($9,700), South Dakota ($9,750) and New Hampshire ($9,817).

10

Cost of Nursing Education

The High Costs at Nursing Schools

Studies have shown that the costs for professional nursing courses are roughly four times the cost of the general academic courses that comprise the remainder of a college level nurse education program. As a result, few colleges offered preparatory nurse education programs until the federal government decided that more nurses were needed.

Federal support for nursing education has shown a dramatic expansion. In 1950, nursing education was allotted about one quarter of a million dollars. By 1974, over 141 million dollars a year was provided for the various R.N. programs. Nursing scholarships and loans alone, amounted to more than 44 million dollars.

The early hospital schools of nursing quite simply offered training in return for service. This, combined with a pattern of low tuition payments from students, made the diploma school a particularly inexpensive form of education. In contrast, colleges in the early 20th century were less egalitarian than today and were perhaps surrounded by an aura of "expensiveness."

The early diploma school concept of student service in exchange for training has changed somewhat; however, some hospital schools still require up to ten weeks of service, plus weekend and night duty, over the course of the school year from each student.

Another problem faced by nursing schools more than other educational institutions is the lack of endowment or outside financial support. This, too, adds to the student's costs.

It is not possible to give any average figures for the cost of nursing education because there is considerable variation.

The two-year junior or community college nursing programs would be the least expensive. Some of these are public-supported, and tuition is free except for incidental expenses. In a hospital or nursing school offering a diploma program, costs are somewhat higher than at a community or junior college. Costs for a college degree nursing program are comparable to those for a regular college program.

Many nursing schools have scholarships and loan funds. Several states provide state funds for nursing education, and federal loans are also available in many nationally accredited schools. (See "Loans and Scholarships" for more specific information.)

Table 10-18   Average expenses for nursing school students (1973 est.)

Program	One year expenses (tuition, fees & books)	Total expenses through graduation (tuition, fees & books)
Diploma	$1,445	$ 4,334 (3 years)
Associate degree	2,175	4,349 (2 years)
Baccalaureate	2,558	10,231 (4 years)

Source: U.S. Health Resources Administration, DHEW.

Going Back to College for a Baccalaureate

For the nurse who must stop working, (especially if she must relocate to a new state) here are some estimated costs for a typical college requiring two full years of education:

Tuition	$ 1,940		
Books	550	Add if you go to a high-tuition	
Lab and other fees	200	school such as Columbia	
Add if you need dormitory		University	2,000
residence	2,000	Add if you must forego wages	
Add if you need board	2,000	during enrollment period	18,000
Add if you are nonresident of the			
state	1,800	Total	$28,490

How Students Pay for Their Education

Table 10-19   Student nurses' sources of funds for their expenses

Source	Amount (millions)	Percent of total
Earnings and savings	$ 82	30%
Contribution by spouse	46	17
Contribution by parents	75	27
Loans	28	10
Scholarships	26	9
Armed Services	6	2
Veterans benefits	4	2
Other	8	3
Total	$276	100%

Source: H. R. Saigh, *A Study Of Student Finance In Nursing Education,* 1970.

The proportion of students using the federal nursing loan program did not vary widely among programs. Students in baccalaureate programs made use of federal loan monies more than students in other types of programs: according to Saigh's data, 12% of baccalaureate students used loan monies.

Private vs. Public Funding of Schools

Note that associate degree (junior or community college) programs are publicly funded, whereas almost all hospital (diploma) programs are privately funded.

Table 10-20   Schools of nursing—R.N. 1975 by principal source of financial support and school administrative control

Administrative control	Number of schools by principal source of financial support	
	Public	Private
University or senior college	280	184
Junior or community college	442	22
Hospital	64	353
Independent	4	11
Total	790	570

Source: *State Approved Schools of Nursing: RN, 1975* National League for Nursing, 1976.

In-Service and Continuing Education*

Overview

Early efforts at staff education in hospitals parallel rather closely the efforts to upgrade teachers in the public school system through the provision of in-service training. A later impetus to the development of education provided by the employing agency follows the pattern of on-the-job training established in industry particularly during and immediately following World War II.

Another early development took place in Veteran's Administration hospitals. Initially programs were planned for all nurses who had no education or experience in psychiatric nursing, but content later also included tuberculosis nursing.

Early staff education programs for practicing nurses often were primarily lectures by phy-sicians. Additional content included reviewing nursing procedures, learning to operate new equipment, and studying the policies of the institution. From these early developments, the concept of in-service education for practicing nurses slowly evolved in hospitals and other health agencies.

There seems little doubt that the ineffectiveness of many in-service programs resulted from the inadequate preparation of the nursing staff responsible for the program. Many hospitals appear to have established in-service programs because it was the thing to do, without careful consideration of the many factors involved in providing an effective program.

Organization of In-Service Education

Today, in-service education is seen as an integral part of an effective nursing service, but

*Source: Jean McNally, *Continuing Education for Nurses,* American Nurses' Association 1972.

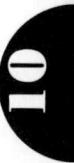

Table 10-21

Hospitals Offering Refresher and In-Service Courses

Variable	All hospi-tals	Size (beds)					Census area				Ownership		
		Under 50	50 to 99	100 to 199	200 to 399	400 and over	North-east	North central	South	West	Non-profit	Govern-ment	Proprie-tary
Personnel policies:													
Refresher courses:													
Offering (%)	29.9	24.5	26.8	35.4	31.9	37.5	36.2	27.1	31.3	25.9	30.6	29.5	27.3
Available from sources other than hospital (%)	76.9	87.0	79.2	68.8	69.8	73.1	63.4	80.6	78.7	81.2	73.9	79.3	85.0
Hospital subsidizes tuition costs	55.4	49.2	47.7	57.7	62.9	72.2	65.6	54.6	51.4	53.0	58.0	52.8	50.8
Inservice education:													
Offering (%)	87.0	73.8	84.4	91.7	97.4	99.9	94.7	88.6	78.6	90.4	91.1	83.5	77.3
Hospital budgets for inservice education (%)	72.3	48.5	70.1	76.5	87.6	87.5	83.1	72.9	63.2	72.7	77.1	65.9	67.3
Hospital not offering but sends R.N.s to other institutions for in-service education (%)	92.3	91.8	95.3	87.5	92.9	87.5	90.0	95.5	91.4	90.3	93.0	92.3	85.7

Source: DHEW, May 1975 (1973 data).

A poll of 10,000 nurses conducted by *Nursing '77* in January found that most nurses (90%) reported that their own institution had in-service education programs. Ratings of those programs, however, were not high—the majority (59%) said that their in-service education programs were fair, poor or, as indicated, nonexistent.

this has been a slow development. Emory University Hospitals in Atlanta established a separate division of in-service education in the nursing service department in 1952, and other institutions soon adopted this pattern. New patterns of organization are now emerging within institutions, but the agency's responsibility for providing its employees with opportunities for learning has been firmly established.

University Involvement in Continuing Education

Initial involvement of universities in continuing education for nurses began in the early 1920s. This interest was sporadic until 1959 when federal funds became available for short-term courses. The courses offered by colleges and universities varied from one- or two-day workshops to classes held weekly for an entire quarter or semester. The acceptance by university schools of nursing of their responsibility for the continuing education of nurses has evolved slowly.

The Staff Development Department of a Hospital Nursing Service*

Following is a summary of the major functions of a representative, well-organized staff development department (The Nursing Service Division of Tucson Medical Center Department of Staff Development and Research):

Organized under the administrative leadership of a director, the educational functions of the medical center's staff development department includes orientation as well as in-service and continuing education:

- *Orientation.* Each level of nursing personnel receives orientation classes as well as skill delineation and clinical supervision. Clinical supervision runs from a minimum of four weeks up to as long as six months' individualized supervision for particular specialty skills. The Department of Staff Development and Research has a full-time staff of seven nurse clinicians. Each nurse clinician is a staff specialist responsible for the development needs of nursing personnel organized as follows: medical nursing, surgical nursing, urgent nursing, maternity, pediatrics, ostomy therapy, and cardio-vascular nursing.

- *In-service* includes on-the-job training, counseling, and reviewing skills; introduction of new procedures, policies, and products is usually carried out at the unit or individual level of education or specialty area. Overall programs—such as a monthly Nursing Grand Rounds and multidiscplinary patient care programs every three months—are also presented.

- *Continuing education* coordinates attendance at approved programs locally as well as in the state, helps in the presentation of appropriately approved programs within our own facility, and furnishes opportunities for the sharing with other staff of things gleaned from attendance at such programs. Unit and departmental programs are coordinated by the nurse clinicians through the head nurses, with both nursing and educational department staff actually presenting such programs. Educational needs are determined by directors, head nurses and nursing staff itself in coordination with the nurse clinicians.

The Hospital In-Service Training Director**

- Twenty-seven percent of all institutions have independent training and education departments; 63.8% in-service sections within the nursing department; 9.2% training operations administered by personnel or other departments.

- Forty-one percent of training directors have responsibilities for hospitalwide education (the trend toward hospitalwide education continues); 49.5% are responsible for nursing in-service only; 9.5% operate out of nursing but with broader responsibilities.

- Eighty percent of training directors continue to come from nursing, but education experience looms larger; 64.5% of all trainers have teaching experience; 14% have education experience but no nursing experience.

- Sixty-one percent of all training directors have college degrees; 31% have graduate degrees and 76.5% are R.N.s.

- Men represent 30% of all hospital educators and 12.5% of nursing in-service directors.

- Average salary is $12,652 a year; it is

*Source: Adapted from "Four Approaches to Staff Development," National League for Nursing, Pub. No. 20-15781.

**Source: Survey conducted by *In-Service Training and Education,* May 1975.

10

higher for hospitalwide directors and for men, lower for nursing education and women.

- Eighty-six percent have funds specifically allotted for education and training, and 71.6% have their own budgets.
- The average training budget is $49,944 per year, 71.6% of which goes to salaries. The remaining discretionary budget is $13,900; 28.4% of this spendable amount is allotted for AV equipment, 18.1% for travel, 16.3% for books and periodicals.
- The average training director teaches an average of 25 subjects a year, with orientation and coronary care given most often.
- Eighteen percent of all the training programs now being offered feature self-paced learning, while 83% are based around classroom sessions. Nursing training, logically enough, uses more self-paced learning—close to 25%—mostly for night shifts and floaters. Thirty-three percent of the courses make use of packaged educational programs, and 50% use home-made materials.
- Continuing education continues to be a mainstay of the in-service calendar: 10% of respondents reported that CE for some health care professionals (chiefly nurses, dietitians and pharmacists) is now mandatory in their states; 73% believe that they give courses which would meet CE requirements if necessary; 44% give some form of credit other than contact hours: the most popular are certificates of attendance or completion, annotations to the employee's record and points toward merit raises or promotions.

Continuing Education

Among the major developments in the United States are: increasing learning opportunities provided by hospitals and other employing agencies and by educational institutions; the development of a variety of learning approaches suitable to the adult nurse learner, including independent and self-directed learning resources; formal recognition of continuing education by nursing organizations; experimentation with measurement of continuing education activities; and the promotion of continuing education as a condition for the relicensure of nurses, frequently identified as "mandatory continuing education."

Since the early 1920s, many colleges and universities have provided conferences and workshops for nurses. The number of these educational offerings steadily increased, particularly in the last decade. These offerings vary in length from one to five days, and usually do not include clinical practice. Offerings of this nature are frequently provided by professional associations, voluntary health organizations and other groups.

In contrast to the conference, workshop, or institute, the short-term course, which may be two weeks or longer, usually includes clinical practice. The short-term course provides an opportunity for intensive clinical study, and has been of particular value in helping nurses prepare for new responsibilities. Examples include intensive short-term courses designed to prepare nurses for coronary or intensive care.

Table 10-22 Continuing education course—by sponsor

Total number of courses sponsored	District or state nurses association	Hospital	League for nursing	Regional medical program	School of nursing	State health department	U.S. public health service	Voluntary health agency	Other
4,282	513	1,751	63	1,234	1,322	241	111	821	469

Sponsor	More popular courses
Schools of nursing:	Communication, community health nursing, drug abuse, emergency nursing, family dynamics, geriatric nursing, group dynamics, leadership and administration, medical-surgical nursing, nursing process, pediatric nursing, psychiatric nursing, school nursing and the teaching-learning process.
Hospitals:	Coronary care nursing, expanded health care, intensive care nursing, maternal-newborn nursing, rehabilitation.
Regional medical programs:	Health screening and assessment, long term nursing.

Table 10-23   Continuing education courses—by subject

Courses	Total number of courses		Credit given	
	Number	Percent	Number	Percent
Total	4,282	100.0	957	100.0
Communication	139	3.2	28	2.9
Community health	170	4.0	35	3.7
Coronary care	948	22.2	254	26.6
Drug abuse	36	.8	9	.9
Emergency	44	1.0	9	.9
Expanding health care	222	5.2	60	6.3
Family dynamics	68	1.6	2	.2
Geriatrics	78	1.8	10	1.0
Group dynamics	42	1.0	7	.7
Health screening & assessment	67	1.6	11	1.1
Intensive care	185	4.3	52	5.4
Leadership & administration	361	8.4	75	7.8
Long-term nursing	140	3.3	58	6.1
Maternal-newborn nursing	113	2.6	19	2.0
Medical-surgical	385	9.0	69	7.2
Nursing process: assessment & evaluation	256	6.0	62	6.5
Occupational health	48	1.1	20	2.1
Pediatric nursing	76	1.8	18	1.9
Psychiatric nursing	138	3.2	34	3.6
Refresher	42	1.0	20	2.1
Rehabilitation	80	1.9	8	.8
School nursing	36	.8	13	1.4
Teaching-learning process	211	4.9	17	1.8
Other	397	9.3	67	7.0

Continuing Education Courses*

A 1972 ANA survey of continuing education courses being offered discovered that there were some differences in the courses which were most popular when the sponsors were taken into account.

Over half of the courses reported used interdisciplinary or multidisciplinary planning.

A variety of learning strategies was used in these continuing education courses; however, 72% of the courses relied on the lecture method alone or in combination with other teaching methods. While the lecture method quickly provides information, its use is limited in continuing education. A minimum of instructional technology was used.

Mandated Continuing Education

In 1973, with professional obsolescence in nursing estimated at two and a half to five years, the HEW Medical Malpractice Com-

mission recommended that states revise their licensure laws, as appropriate to enable their licensing boards to require periodic re-registration of nurses and other health professionals, based upon proof of participation in approved continuing medical education programs.

To date, only one state, California, has passed legislation requiring continuing education for relicensure; but such legislation has been proposed in a number of other states. To meet the requirement, California nurses will need to acquire 60 hours of continuing education, or its equivalent, in the two-year license renewal period between 1976 and 1978. Nurses may substitute academic credit for continuing education with each semester credit being worth 15–18 contact hours. The California criteria also provide that nurses can earn a waiver through such activities as taking part in a panel discussion or publication of a book. While the ANA and the majority of states favor voluntary continuing education for nurses, there is considerable support for some mandatory scheme in Pennsylvania, New

*Source: Jean McNally, *Continuing Education for Nurses,* American Nurses' Association, 1972.

Mexico, New York, Minnesota, Missouri, Illinois and elsewhere. The CEU as a standardized tool for recording continuing education has wide acceptance.

CEU

Nurses—and others—who participate in formal continuing education offerings often voice a concern over the absence of records of their participation in these activities. The continuing education unit (CEU) was designed to provide a system for the measurement and recording of continuing education.

The CE unit is related to the college level instructional hour. It is intended for use in the measurement, recording, reporting, accumulating, recognition and transfer of the individual's record to employers, organizations and others who require evidence of continuing education.

One definition of a CEU is "ten hours of participation in an organized continuing education experience under responsible sponsorship, capable direction and qualified instruction."

Continuing Education Recognition Program (CERP)

When a sponsor for an educational experience, activity or program wants that offering approved/endorsed and/or awarded a CEU, the sponsor submits a completed application (and fee) to the responsible group at the state nurses association. The programs are referred to as "Continuing Education Recognition Programs."

Not all state nurses' associations have an established CERP agency. Many are in the process of developing criteria and guidelines and a mechanism for approving or accrediting continuing education offerings. Not all states use the uniform system of the CEU. Some other systems in use:

- a point system interchangeable with the CEU under which a set number of points is equal to one CEU;
- CERP's (continuing education recognition points);
- clock hours of participation;
- 1 point = 1 contact hour; 10 points = 1 CEU.

Some agencies have developed a transfer mechanism for accepting CEUs from other states. Some SNAs circulate information on CE offerings. Not all agencies maintain records for the nurses in the state.

Accreditation in Continuing Education Programs*

In 1970 a voluntary group composed of heads of continuing education programs in university schools of nursing met and formed the National Conference on Continuing Education in Nursing. This group in 1973 was influential in establishing the ANA Council on Continuing Education, which supports the principle of extended education as essential to nurse competency.

The ANA Council on Continuing Education:
- develops standards;
- provides a nationwide system for recording nurses' continuing education activities, to facilitate transfers between states;
- accredits sponsoring agencies;
- promotes a model plan for state continuing education programs.

In the following 12 states, the state nurses' association approves or accredits education offerings:

Arizona	Kansas	Montana
California	Kentucky	New Jersey
Colorado	Maine	North Dakota
Florida	Massachusetts	Texas

Twenty-two states are in the process of developing accreditation procedures.

Courses, Workshops and Seminars

A wide variety of short courses, seminars and workshops on an equally wide variety of topics of interest to nurses are given year-round by universities, hospital schools and private organizations. Most are one to three days long and cost between $40–$200. Many grant CEU credit; others certificates of attendence. Below is a representative sample of offerings available during 1975. A monthly listing is printed in major nursing publications.

Representative titles:
Courses, Seminars, Workshops, Symposiums and Conferences
Cancer, Chemotherapy, Communication, Care
Emotional Needs in Physical Illness—Perspectives for Nursing Assessment
Respiratory Therapy
Human Sexuality for Professional Nurses
Parenteral Nutrition (Hyperalimentation)
Conference on Emergency Medicine
Is Your Nursing Practice Legal?

*Source: *Outdate-Update; Continuing Education, Who What When Where and Why,* National League for Nursing, Pub. No. 52–1579, 1975.

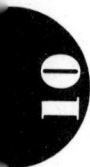

Trauma

Coping With Chronic Disease: Patient Needs and Nursing Intervention

Lungs—Young and Old

Preventive Nursing Skills

Spinal Cord Injury

Psychosocial Aspects of Physical Disability

Infection Control

Neurological, Neurosurgical Problems

Team Approach of the Urology Patient

Birth Defects and Genetic Counseling

Clinical Performance Evaluation

The Association of Operating Room Nurses Conference

American Association of Neurosurgical Nurses—Annual Scientific Meeting

Consumer Concerns for the Delivery of Health Care—Reality or Fantasy?

American Association of Nephrology Nurses and Technicians Conference

National Student Nurses Association Conference

In-service Education Methods and Techniques

Emergency Nursing

New Dimensions in Shock and the Implications for Nursing

Patient Care Planning

Nursing Audit/Quality Assurance

Symposium on Respiratory Care

Cancer Nursing for Professional Nurses

Infection Control

Legal Issues Every Nurse Ought to Know About

Patient Education—Staff Responsibilities

Nutritional Disorders of American Women

Creating a Climate for Care

Nursing Theory Development

National Nurse Practitioner Symposium

Assessment of the Newborn

Graduate Education

Overview

Many feel that there is great need for an increasing number of nurses with masters or doctoral degrees to fill positions such as:

- clinical nurses or master nurse clinicians capable of providing direct care while serving as model,
- instructors and professors,
- specialists in organization and delivery of episodic and distributive care,
- researchers.

In the United States in 1971, only 69 colleges offered master's degree programs for nurses and only a handfull offered doctoral programs.

Enrollments and Graduations

There is a tendency for students in graduate programs to attend part-time rather than full-time.

Table 10-24   Enrollments in nursing programs leading to masters and doctoral degrees, 1971-75

As of Oct. 15	Masters programs			Doctoral programs		
	Total	Full-time	Percent full-time	Total	Full-time	Percent full-time
1971	5,405	3,925	72.6	293	151	41.1
1972	6,342	4,324	68.1	402	180	44.8
1973	6,786	4,159	61.2	375	161	42.9
1974	7,924	4,462	56.3	482	192	39.3
1975	9,662	5,402	55.9	572	199	38.2

Source: *Nursing Outlook*, September 1976. ©American Journal of Nursing Company.

Table 10-25   Graduations from nursing programs leading to masters and doctoral degrees, 1970-71 through 1974-75

Academic year	Masters programs	Doctoral programs
1970-71	2,083	41
1971-72	2,135	27
1972-73	2,446	49
1973-74	2,643	46
1974-75	2,694	74

Source: *Nursing Outlook*, September 1976. ©American Journal of Nursing Company.

Graduate Nursing School Survey: Admission of Non-R.N.s to Graduate Programs for Nurses*

In response to the question, "Do you admit R.N.s with non-nursing baccalaureate degrees?", 54% of graduate schools said "yes," and 46% indicated they did not. Of the programs that reported admitting students with non-nursing baccalaureate degrees, 43% used challenge exams, 48% assessed past education and work experience, and 57% required some make-up of undergraduate nursing courses.

Of the master's programs that do not admit nurses with non-nursing baccalaureate degrees, 50% rationalized that only the baccalaureate degree in nursing includes the background information essential for master's study.

*Source: *Nursing Outlook*, October 1975. ©American Journal of Nursing Company.

Master's Programs

Enrollments

Table 10-26   Full-time enrollments in master's programs (Fall 1972)

| | | Functional purpose of curriculum | | | | | | |
| | | Administration | | | | | | |
Nursing focus	Total	Service and education	Service	Education	Supervision	Teaching	Advanced clinical practice	Not designated
Total	4,324	31	241	40	208	1,439	2,340	25
Medical-surgical	1,448	—	—	—	47	641	760	—
Medical-surgical	1,388	—	—	—	47	641	700	—
Specialties	60	—	—	—	—	—	60	—
Maternal-child	701	—	—	—	17	284	400	—
Maternal-child	381	—	—	—	8	185	188	—
Maternity	67	—	—	—	6	24	37	—
Pediatrics	253	—	—	—	3	75	175	—
Psychiatric-mental health	1,124	—	—	—	57	272	795	—
Public health nursing	553	—	70	—	87	155	241	—
Public health	552	—	70	—	87	155	240	—
School nursing	1	—	—	—	—	—	1	—
Other[1]	84	—	—	—	—	59	25	—
None	414	31	171	40	—	28	119	25

[1] Includes sciences, fundamentals, in-service, combined majors, rehabilitation.

Source: *Some Statistics on Baccalaureate and Higher Degree Programs in Nursing,* National League for Nursing 1972–73.

Graduations

Table 10-27   R.N. graduations from master's programs preparing for advanced practice, by nursing specialty

Nursing specialty	1966–67	1967–68	1968–69	1969–70	1970–71	1971–72
Total	323	367	438	771	885	966
Medical-surgical	92	131	111	236	293	313
Medical-surgical	81	117	87	200	260	288
Specialties	11	14	24	36	33	25
Maternal-child	48	92	80	154	180	187
Maternal-child	15	30	57	71	85	111
Maternity	14	23	6	28	34	13
Pediatrics	19	39	17	55	61	63
Psychiatric-mental health	145	121	214	265	306	331
Public health	36	23	32	76	98	98
Public health	18	16	24	61	90	89
School nursing	18	7	8	15	8	9
Other	—	—	—	16	6	11
None or not designated	2	—	1	24	2	26

Source: *Some Statistics on Baccalaureate and Higher Degree Programs in Nursing,* National League for Nursing, annual editions.

Area of Specialty for Nursing Master's Degree Graduate

Table 10-28

Year	Total gradua-tions	Percent of graduations by functional area[1]			
		Adminis-tration	Super-vision	Teach-ing	Advanced clinical practice
1972–73	2,446	6.3	4.5	31.1	55.2

[1] Percentages do not add to 100.0. The small difference is the percent in "other" functional areas. Graduates of the initial master's program are not included in the table.

Source: *Some Statistics on Baccalaureate and Higher Degrees in Nursing, 1973–74,* National League for Nursing. New York: The League, 1974, table 10.

Table 10-29   Typical educational preparation for teaching or supervisory positions

Position and field of employment	Educational preparation
Deans of collegiate programs, faculty of graduate programs, research investigators and nursing service directors of large hospital systems or health agency systems	Doctorate
Teachers in all nursing education programs	Master's
Directors and assistant directors of nursing service in hospitals, related institutions and health agencies	Master's
In-service education directors, supervisors, clinical specialists and consultants in all types of institutions and health agencies or services	Master's
Head nurses, team leaders, public health and school nurses and occupational health nurses at staff level	Baccalaureate
Directors of nursing service in nursing homes giving "skilled nursing care"	Baccalaureate

Source: DHEW, December 1974.

Doctoral Programs*

Nurse Doctorates

The nurse–doctorates earned their doctoral degrees in 115 universities in the United States. Columbia University has consistently

*Source: M. Pitel and J. Vian, "Analysis of Nurse Doctorates," *Nursing Research,* Sept.–Oct. 1975. ©American Journal of Nursing Company.

been the top producer of nurse–doctorates (21.5%). Many of the universities which rank high on the list of top producers of nurse–doctorates are located in high-density urban areas with a high percentage of nurses per population, have had long-established graduate programs in nursing, and have participated in the Nurse Scientist Training Program of the U.S. Public Health Service (Table 10-31).

10

Table 10-30   Major field of degree earned by nurse–doctorates in percent

Major field	Doctoral Degree	
	(%)	Number
Nursing	13.5	
Nursing education	6.9	
Nursing administration	0.7	
Education	50.6	
Behavioral/social sciences	17.5	
Natural sciences	9.0	
Humanities	1.9	
NI/NA[1]	0.0	
Total	100.0	1,020

[1] No information/not applicable.

Table 10-31   Universities granting doctoral degrees to nurses

University	Number of doctoral degrees
Columbia U—Teachers College	219
New York U	77
Boston U	62
Catholic U	49
U of Washington	29
U of Maryland—College Park	28
U of Pittsburgh	28
Indiana U	26
U of California—Los Angeles	26
U of California—Berkeley	25
U of Chicago	21

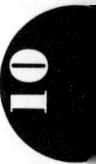

Employment—Eighty-four percent of nurse–doctorates were either completely or partially involved in nursing; 80.2% were faculty members; 8.1%, administrators; 3.7%, consultants; 3.5%, researchers; 3.1%, clinical practitioners; 1.3%, others, such as journal editors or medical librarians.

Profile—In a 1973 survey of nurses with doctoral degrees, the majority were single; most were employed in a university or college where they held either full or associate professorships; most considered themselves still to be in the field of nursing, although their doctoral studies frequently took them out of the discipline; their work responsibilities were heavily loaded with administrative duties. As compared with the holders of doctoral degrees in other fields, nurses earned their degrees later, but took no longer to complete them. Universities in the Mid-Atlantic states were the largest producers of nurse–doctorates. Universities in the Midwest were found to be the most frequent employers.

Table 10-32   Nurse–doctorates by race, marital status, sex*

Characteristic	Total N (%)	Male total N (%)
Race		
Caucasian	847 (85.8)	29 (90.6)
Black	38 (3.8)	2 (6.3)
Mongoloid	15 (1.5)	0 (0.0)
NI/NA[1]	88 (8.9)	1 (3.1)
Female total	988 (100.0)	
Male total		32 (100.0)
Marital status		
Single	550 (55.7)	11 (34.4)
Married	282 (28.6)	20 (62.5)
Widowed	32 (3.2)	0 (0.0)
Divorced	65 (6.5)	0 (0.0)
NI/NA[1]	59 (6.0)	1 (3.1)
Female total	988 (100.0)	
Male total		32 (100.0)

[1] No information/not applicable.
* Includes 55 from foreign countries.

Table 10-33   Sources of support for doctoral study by nurse–doctorates

Source	Doctoral study first source percentage
USPHS-Division of nursing	43.1%
American nurses' foundation	.4
Institutional scholarship	7.2
Sigma Theta Tau	.8
National fund	
Graduate nursing education	.9
Nurses' educational fund (or NLN)	6.6
Philanthropic foundation	.8
Self	24.5
Other	9.6
NI/NA[1]	6.2
Total	100

[1] No information/not applicable.

Sources of Information

Write to the National League for Nursing for lists of NLN-accredited programs in nursing education at the masters, baccalaureate, associate degree, diploma and practical nursing levels. NLN also publishes a list of universities that offer doctoral programs:

15–1448	Doctoral Programs in Nursing/Nurse Scientist Graduate Training Grants Program	$.50
15–1312	Masters Education in Nursing: Route to Opportunities in Contemporary Nursing—1975–76	$.50
15–1311	Baccalaureate Education in Nursing: Key to a Professional Career in Nursing	$.75
23–1309	Associate Degree Education for Nursing	$.75
16–1314	Education for Nursing: The Diploma Way	$.75
38–1328	Practical Nursing Career	$.75

11

LOANS, GRANTS AND SCHOLARSHIPS

Steps to Take in Seeking Funds*

The first place to consult in seeking financial help for study is the college or university you plan to enter, since the majority of student aid programs are administered by the schools. Recipients of financial aid are frequently selected several months before the beginning of the academic year, so it is important to make your approach to the school about available scholarships as soon as possible after you decide on the school to which you intend to apply for admission. Be sure to ascertain well in advance the deadlines for application for financial help.

Ask your state departments of health, mental health, education or social welfare or your state board of nursing about state and federal funds for preparation in such fields of nursing as public health, psychiatric and maternal and child health. Consult state and district nurses' associations, constituent leagues for nursing, committees on nursing careers and the alumnae association of your school of nursing. Some other possible sources of funds are: state or local lung associations, state cancer society units, women's auxiliaries to state or county medical societies, hospital auxiliaries, the American Legion and its auxiliaries. Many large industries also make scholarships available to graduate students. Many banks, businesses, and foundations as well as civic, fraternal, religious, and charitable organizations help deserving students preparing for careers in nursing.

Among the local organizations that may provide scholarships and loans (the list varies from one community to another) are men's service clubs such as the Rotary, Kiwanis, and Lions clubs; The American Legion; Forty and Eight; fraternal orders such as the Elks, the Knights of Pythias, the Odd Fellows, and the Loyal Order of Moose; B'nai B'rith; labor unions; women's organizations, including the city and county federations of women's clubs, the Business and Professional Women's Club, Daughters of the American Revolution, Altrusa, Zonta,

Quota, Pilot; women's auxiliaries of service and fraternal organizations; the Farm Bureau; health agencies; and foundations and charitable trusts.

Directories of such scholarships are compiled and published in many of the larger cities. Many high schools, too, collect similar information. Other files are kept by women's clubs and service organizations.

If your city has a chapter of the Citizens' Scholarship Foundation, ask your guidance counselor or principal about it. Each chapter raises and administers funds locally. Your high school can get information by writing to Citizens' Scholarship Foundation of America, Inc., One South Street, Concord, NH 03301.

Financial Aid for Education

Private Sources

Specific Programs**

1. **Nurses' Educational Funds**—The purpose of these funds is to increase the supply of nurses qualified for administrative, supervisory, teaching or research positions and clinical specialization in nursing. Scholarships and fellowships are available to registered nurses who seek further study in nursing. Men and women qualifying for these awards are expected to study in NLN-accredited nursing programs in colleges and universities of their choice. Awards may be made at the baccalaureate, masters or doctoral level. The amount and number of awards are determined each year on the basis of availability of funds and qualifications of applicants. Applicants are required to be citizens of the United States or to have declared official intention of becoming citizens. In addition, they must be members of the American Nurses' Association. The deadline for completion of all applications is January 15 preceding the academic year for which the awards are made.

Scholarships and fellowships vary in amount from $1,000 to $3,000. Scholarships under $1,000 have also been awarded. Total amount of support: $27,300 for the year 1974.

History of fund: The Isabel Hampton Robb Memorial Fund was established in 1910 for post-R.N. study in nursing and later was amal-

---

*Much of the information in this chapter (unless otherwise noted) has been drawn from two NLN publications: "Scholarships and Loans for Beginning Education in Nursing," Pub No 41-410; and "Scholarships, Fellowships, Educational Grants, and Loans for Registered Nurses." Pub No 41-408.

**Source: National League for Nursing.

gamated with other funds for nurses to become what is now Nurses' Educational Funds (NEF). Administered by The American Journal of Nursing Company, NEF is an independent, nonprofit, professionally endorsed organization governed by a board of directors consisting of nursing and business leaders and supported by contributions from foundations, business corporations, nurses, and persons interested in nursing. Although not designed specifically for research training, many of the past 564 recipients have qualified as nurse researchers and five of the 22 awards in 1975 were made for doctoral study. During the years of its and its predecessors' existence, NEF has given over a half million dollars in scholarships.

For more information, write to Nurses' Educational Funds, 10 Columbus Circle, New York, NY 10019. (212) 582-8820.

2. **NLN Fellowship Program**—The National League for Nursing Fellowship Program was initiated in 1955 through a grant from the Commonwealth Fund for the purpose of helping nurses with outstanding ability obtain advanced educational preparation. The first grants provided for full-time study for nurses already enrolled in graduate programs to complete requirements for the doctoral degree. Commonwealth terminated its support in 1963.

3. **American Nurses' Foundation**—Founded in 1955 by the American Nurses' Association (ANA) for the express purpose of promoting and supporting nursing research and the dissemination of research findings, ANF has been vitally concerned with helping nurses conduct research. To this end, in its 20 years of existence, ANF has awarded 89 grants for nursing research projects, totaling $529,000.

In 1959, nurses organized a nationwide fund-raising campaign for ANF and by the close of the campaign in 1964 had raised $750,000. Currently major contributions are made by the ANA and the American Journal of Nursing Company, with additions from corporations, foundations and individuals. ANF, incorporated separately from ANA, is a tax-exempt foundation.

4. **Allstate Foundation Nursing Scholarships**—These are awarded through constituent leagues for nursing. Consult your constituent league. (Addresses are available

from the National League for Nursing, 10 Columbus Circle, New York, NY 10019.)

5. **Hattie M. Strong Foundation**—Loans up to $2,000 for one year ($4,000 maximum) for entire period of schooling, without interest or collateral, are made to American college students who are within two years of their final degree. Loans of up to $2,000 are also made to residents of Metropolitan Washington, D.C., who are enrolled in vocational schools in the Washington area. For details, write Hattie M. Strong Foundation, 1625 Eye Street, N.W., #409, Washington, D.C. 20006.

6. **Independent Order of Odd Fellows**—Applicant must write personally, stating age and school classification. Maximum of $1,000 lent for any one year of study, except in the case of seniors, who may borrow $1,500 if they have no previous financial obligations. Maximum of $4,000 lent for a complete course of study (four years or more). Interest is charged at 4%; payment begins three months after graduation. To be eligible, nurses must have completed the probationary period of their training. For details and applications, write the Executive Secretary, Educational Foundation, Independent Order of Odd Fellows, P.O. Box 214, Connersville, Ind. 47331.

7. **Harry R. Kendall Scholarship Fund**—Scholarships are available for masters degree programs (with preference to black nurses). Amounts of grants are based on the educational and personal needs of the applicant. Apply to: Charles P. Kellogg, Kendall Scholarship Committee, Health and Welfare Ministries Division, General Board of Global Ministries, United Methodist Church, 1200 Davis St., Evanston, Ill. 60201.

8. **Eight and Forty Lung and Respiratory Nursing Scholarships Fund**—Scholarship awards are made in amounts of $1,500 each. These awards assist nurses to secure advanced preparation for positions in supervision, administration or teaching. Students must have prospects of employment in specific positions with a full-time, direct relationship to lung and respiratory disease prevention and treatment in hospitals, clinics or health departments upon completion of their study. Application deadline date on awards granted for a school year is June 1 of the calendar year in which the school year begins. Announcements of awards are made by July 15 of the same year. Application forms may be obtained from

the American Legion Education and Scholarship Program, Box 1055, Indianapolis, Ind. 46206. Attn: Eight and Forty Scholarships.

9. **American Lung Association**—1740 Broadway, New York, New York 10019. (212) 245-8000.

Nursing Fellowships in Respiratory Disease: fellowship awards are offered for the training of clinical nurse specialists, teachers, and researchers in the specialty of lung disease. Amount of support per award: $6,000 a year.

Other Sources

(For a full discussion of each of these aids refer to *Financial Aids for Higher Education* by Oreon Kesslar, 1974–5 Catalogue)

Nursing:
AAL Competitive Nursing Scholarship Program.
Arkansas Rural Endowment Fund Loan Program.
Army Registered Nurse Student Program.
California PTA Patient Nursing Scholarship.
Connecticut Prospective Nurses Program.
Daughters of the American Revolution Scholarships.
General Electric Company Employees Educational Fund.
Georgia State Scholarship Program.
Girls' Clubs of Boston.
Greater Youngstown AFL-CIO Council (Ohio).
Illinois Grant Program.
Independent Order of Odd Fellows Revolving Loan Fund.
Jewish Vocational Aid Society Loan Program.
Jones Truck Lines, Inc.
Ladies Garment Workers International (Fall River, Massachusetts).
Louie Le Flore Scholarships (Indian students).

Louisiana Higher Education Assistance Student Loan Program.
Massachusetts Medical, Dental and Nursing Scholarships.
Merrit Hospital School of Nursing (Indian students).
Minnesota Department of Public Welfare Nursing Scholarships.
Minnesota Higher Education Programs for Indian Students.
National Licensed Practical Nurses Educational Foundation.
Navy Nurse Corps Candidate Program.
New York State Regents Scholarships for Nursing.
New York State Scholar Incentive Awards.
North Dakota Nursing Scholarships.
Oregon State Scholarship Commission Need/Grant Program.
Nurses Training Incentive Scholarships.
Nursing Student Loans.
Pennsylvania Hospital School of Nursing (Indian students).
Pennsylvania State Scholarships.
PTA Student Loan Funds.
Rhode Island Nursing Education Scholarships.
St. John's Hospital School of Nursing (Indian students).
Spring City Truck Company (Waukesha, Wisconsin).
Texas Tuition Exemption Programs.
United Auto Workers Local 412 (Detroit).
United Methodist Student Loan Fund.
University of Arizona (Colonial Dames) Nursing Scholarships (Indian students).
Virginia State Nursing Scholarship Loans.
Walter Reed Army Institute of Nursing.
Westmoreland Coal Company, Stonega Division.

Foundation Support

Table 11-1   Private foundation support for nursing students by type of aid: 1971

	Total		Loans		Scholarships		Fellowships		Other	
Health profession category	Number of grants	Amount	Number of grants	Amount	Number of grants	Amount	Number of grants	Amount	Number of grants	Amount
Nursing education (R.N.)	69	907,817	1	5,000	58	646,651	2	28,000	8	228,166
Nursing education (Practical)	3	20,500	0	0	3	20,500	0	0	0	0

Source: DHEW, May 1974.

Table 11-2 Legislation enacted in states for scholarship aid to students of nursing education, 1973 and 1974

State[1]	Amounts appropriated				Agency administering program	Amount/year of individual grant or upper limit		Commitment to work in state	Commitment to work in particular field of nursing
	Basic nursing students		Graduate students			Basic nursing students	Graduate students		
	1973	1974	1973	1974					
Alaska	unknown	unknown	unknown	unknown	Department of Education	$1,400	$1,400	No	No
California	—	—	$30,000	$30,000	Manpower Development, State Dept. of Health	—	—	—	—
Florida	$ 13,000	$ 18,000	—	—	Department of Education	1,200	1,200	Yes	No
Guam	unknown	—	—	—	University of Guam	1,500	—	Yes	No
Massachusetts	unknown	—	—	—	Department of Education	260	—	No	No
Minnesota	125,000	125,000	—	—	State Board of Nursing	[2]2,000	—	[3]Yes	Yes
North Carolina	[4]217,500	[5]	[4]	[5]	Medical Care Commission	[6]1,000	2,000	Yes	Yes
North Dakota	—	—	[7]88,000	—	State Board of Nursing	[2]1,000	1,800	Yes	No
Tennessee	83,244	—	—	—	Tennessee Educational Loan Corporation	—	4,000	Yes	—
Vermont	2,00,505	2,000,692	—	—	Vermont Student Assistance Corporation	[8]1,300	—	No	No
Virginia	60,000	60,000	30,000	30,000	State Health Department	2,000	4,000	Yes	No
Virgin Islands	[9]64,800	[9]68,400	—	—	Health Scholarship Board	1,800	1,800	Yes	—

[1] States and territories not listed have no scholarship aid legislation specifically designated for nursing students.
[2] Total for duration of program.
[3] Applies for one year only.
[4] Includes appropriations for graduate students.
[5] $1,500,000 was allocated for 18 fields of study on health professions.
[6] Amount per year varies by type of program: $500 for diploma and $1,000 for associate degree and baccalaureate.
[7] Biennial appropriation for 1973–75.
[8] Amount per year varies: $1,300 for private and $1,150 for public funded programs.
[9] Includes students other than nursing students.

Source: American Nurses' Association, Statistics Department, "State Nurses Associations Report to American Nurses' Association as of March, 1974."

State Sources

A number of states have scholarship and loan programs for which the state appropriates funds. State departments of education keep a file of these and other scholarships open to residents of the state. Ask your state education department for a list of scholarships and loans for which you may apply.

Other agencies in your state that may help you locate scholarships and loans to aid you in financing your education in nursing are the state board of nursing, the state nurses' association, the women's auxiliary to the state medical association, the state organization of The American Legion and your constituent league for nursing. See also Table 11-2 on preceding page.

Example of One State's Programs—New York

New York State Education Department—99 Washington Avenue, Albany, New York 12210. (518) 474-5851

Nursing Expansion Program:

Type:
Contracts with institutions to aid nursing programs.
The grant carries a contractual amount. Total amount of support: $1,200,000 for the year 1973–74.
Number of applicants most recent year: 19.
Number of awards: 19 for the year ending March 1973.

Regents Scholarships for Basic Professional Education in Nursing:

Type:
Scholarships for full-time, matriculated study in New York State in an undergraduate program approved for the training of registered professional nurses in a college or in a hospital school. Amount of support per award: $250. Total amount of support: $600,000 for the academic year 1975–76.

Federal Aid Programs for Nurses

The nursing student loan and scholarship programs provide financial aid to needy students, particularly those from disadvantaged and minority groups. The traineeships program assists registered nurses to obtain the necessary knowledge and skills to become academically prepared for positions as teachers, administrators, supervisors and clinical specialists. These grants cover costs of tuition, stipends and dependency allowances. The Loan Repayment program provides for the repayment of outstanding educational loans for students who agree to practice in a shortage area and for those who are financially disadvantaged.

Loan and scholarship funds are awarded to participating schools of nursing on the basis of statutory formulas. The schools in turn award funds to students on the basis of individual needs and resources. Traineeships are awarded to participating schools which select trainees according to their individual needs. The Loan Repayment program provides repayment of education loans up to 85% to nurses who agree to serve in a shortage area or who fail to complete their education and are financially disadvantaged.

Table 11-3　Federal aid funds for nursing education

	1976 Revised President's Budget	1976 Appropriation	1977 Estimate
Nursing:			
1. Student assistance:			
Loans	9,000,000	21,000,000	5,000,000
Scholarships	4,000,000	6,000,000	2,000,000
Traineeships	—	13,000,000	—
Loan repayments	2,500,000	2,500,000	3,000,000
Subtotal	15,500,000	42,500,000	10,000,000
2. Institutional assistance:			
Capitation grants	—	44,000,000	—
Financial distress	—	—	1,000,000
Advanced nurse training	1,000,000	2,000,000	3,000,000
Nurse practitioner	2,000,000	3,000,000	7,000,000
Nursing special projects	15,000,000	15,000,000	15,000,000
Subtotal	18,000,000	64,000,000	26,000,000
Total, Nursing	33,500,000	106,500,000	36,000,000

194

Student Loans—Nurse Training

The program of low-cost loans for full- and half-time nursing students provides a maximum loan ceiling of $2,500 per student per year, or an aggregate of $10,000. Loans are repayable over a ten-year period following completion of training.

Federal student loans as a supplement to other types of student financial assistance has made nursing education possible for many students who could not otherwise go to school.

Table 11-4   Student loans

	1976 Estimate	1977 Estimate
Number of schools	1,190	1,230
Number of new loans supported	8,125	9,375
Average per student	$800	$800
Estimated repayments	$6,500,000	$7,500,000

Table 11-5   Loans for Nurse Training

Fiscal years 1965–75		Total amount of loans $1,000's	Number of students awarded loans						Mean average loan per student
					Type of program				
Fiscal year	Total no. of programs		Total	Diploma	Associate degree	Baccalaureate degree	Graduate degree		
		$154,175	259,179	92,954	55,885	107,975	2,365		$683
1965	426	3,090	3,645	1,868	38	1,707	32		848
1966	592	8,871	11,740	6,407	375	4,930	28		756
1967	656	12,677	17,218	9,667	1,060	6,426	65		736
1968	687	16,390	21,430	11,414	1,901	8,049	66		765
1969	694	16,008	25,055	12,361	2,901	9,699	94		639
1970	854	12,281	27,064	11,519	4,584	10,865	96		454
1971	902	17,091	27,900	9,696	6,589	11,532	83		613
1972	1,003	20,985	38,127	10,814	11,004	16,165	144		550
1973	1,093	20,982	26,250	6,540	8,051	11,238	421		799
1974	1,151	25,800	32,250	7,206	10,203	14,132	709		800
1975	1,185	22,800	28,500	5,462	9,179	13,232	627		800

Loan Forgiveness—The 1971 Nurse Training Act, currently in effect, allows the nursing student to borrow up to $2,500 per academic year and a total of $10,000 at a fixed interest rate of 3% per annum. It allows nursing students to secure loans from any source. Loan forgiveness provisions become effective when the nurse enters an agreement with the Secretary of the Department of Health, Education and Welfare. If the nurse agrees to serve in a private, nonprofit or public institution within specified shortage areas for at least two years, a maximum of 85% of educational loans plus interest may be forgiven at the rate of 30% for the first two years and 25% for the third. If the nurse is employed in a private, nonprofit or public institution, not designated to be within a shortage area, a maximum of 85% may be forgiven at a rate of 15% a year of full-time employment for the first three years and 20% for the next two years. As with the earlier loan forgiveness laws, nurses employed by proprietary hospitals are not eligible for loan forgiveness.

Table 11-6   Relationship between nurses in loan forgiveness program (LF) at time of graduation and current employer (percentage distribution)

% of all nurses	Year completed basic nursing education	Employed in specified loan hospital (LF debt)		Employed in non-specified loan forgiveness hospital (LF debt)		Employed in non-loan hospital (LF debt)	
		Owe	Paid	Owe	Paid	Owe	Paid
18.5	1969–1970	12.8	5.7	13.7	4.7	10.0	6.7
17.5	1971–1972	13.0	4.5	16.4	3.3	11.1	2.2
22.5	1973	21.1	1.4	14.8	0.7	30.8	0.0

(Note: A list of the shortage areas can be found in *The Federal Register,* June 24, 1976.)

Scholarships

In an effort to provide improved nursing care to underserved areas and to bring about a reduction in the then existing nursing shortage, special federal scholarship programs were initiated in 1968 to encourage young people in exceptional financial need to attend nursing schools. In 1977, this scholarship program continued to be deemphasized, intended to support students who were prior recipients of such scholarships.

Undergraduate nursing students now have access to the expanded Basic Opportunity Grants program in the Office of Education.

	1976 Estimate	1977 Estimate
Number of Schools	1,252	1,300
Number of Students Assisted	6,000	2,000
Average per Student	$1,000	$1,000

Table 11-7   Nursing scholarships by educational program

Fiscal year	Fiscal years 1968–75 Total no. of programs	Total amount of grants Total $1,000's	Number of students awarded scholarships Total	Diploma	Associate degree	Baccalaureate degree	Graduate degree	Mean average amount per student Mean all program
	255	**$96,571**	**135,799**	**38,051**	**40,146**	**56,402**	**1,200**	**$ 755**
1968	255	4,120	7,773	3,449	935	3,389	0	530
1969	337	4,322	8,142	2,854	1,653	3,635	0	531
1970	677	10,727	15,856	5,012	3,812	6,935	97	677
1971	918	16,971	24,655	7,600	7,331	9,612	112	688
1972	1,019	19,487	32,443	8,779	10,749	12,817	98	601
1973	1,141	19,474	19,474	4,521	6,468	8,157	328	1,000
1974	1,225	21,470	21,476	4,500	7,309	9,203	464	1,000
1975	1,198	8,000	6,000	1,356	1,889	2,654	101	1,000

Traineeships

This program provided financial assistance to registered nurses undertaking advanced education prepration for leadership positions. Traineeships provide stipend, tuition and dependence allowances which enable nurses to prepare for positions as teachers, administrators or supervisors for nursing services in institutional and community settings. In 1976, $13 million was available for this program. No funds were requested in 1977. Students needing financial assistance in the future will have access to the Guaranteed Loan Program in the Office of Education.

Table 11-8   Long-term trainees under the professional nurse traineeship program

| Fiscal year | Total trainees | Reappoint-ments | Trainees receiving first awards | | | |
			Total	Bacca-laureate	Master's	Post-master's
1972–73	3,875	—	—	—	—	—
1971–72	3,414	1,194	2,220	748	1,457	15

| Fiscal year | Total first awards | First awards by purpose of training | | | |
		Adminis-tration	Super-vision	Teaching	Clinical specialty
1972–73	2,720	337	386	1,218	779
1971–72	2,220	314	415	1,037	454

Source: DHEW, 1974.

Advanced Nurse Training

A new institutional support authority was added by the Nurse Training Act of 1975 for grants and contracts to collegiate schools of nursing to plan, develop, operate, significantly expand or maintain programs for the advanced training of professional nurses to be teachers, administrators, supervisors or nursing specialists. These funds will support projects to assist nursing education programs in meeting this need. It is expected that 250 students in 1976 and 350 in 1977 will be entering the training programs developed with these funds.

Nursing Special Projects

In order to provide care in shortage areas and in ambulatory and community settings, this program awards grants and contracts to assist in the establishment of nurse training programs in academic settings through cooperative merger efforts of hospitals and academic institutions; to develop continuing education and retraining opportunities; to increase the full utilization in nursing of individuals from disadvantaged backgrounds, who otherwise would be unable to pursue a nursing career; to upgrade the skills of licensed practical nurses and auxiliary nursing personnel; to effect a more equitable geographic distribution of nurses and specialty skills; and to assist in developing curricula and training programs of nurses for primary and specialized care in pediatrics and nursing homes, emphasizing the special problems of geriatric patients.

Nurse Practitioner

A new authority was added by the Nurse Training Act of 1975 for grants and contracts to schools of nursing, medicine, and public health, as well as hospitals and other public or nonprofit private entities to plan, develop and operate or significantly expand or maintain existing programs for the training of nurse practitioners. Emphasis is placed on training to meet the particular problems of geriatric and nursing home patients, as well as training to provide primary health care in home, ambulatory facilities, long-term care facilities and other health care institutions.

By expanding the activities and responsibilities of the R.N., the nurse practitioner can provide comprehensive health care to individuals, families and groups in a variety of settings, including homes, clinics, offices, institutions, industry, schools, nursing homes and others. The practitioner is prepared to assess the health status of individuals, to make decisions about treatment in collaboration with physicians and to provide routine care, counseling and teaching to patients and families. Nurse practitioners can substantially extend the delivery of health services in rural and other underserved areas and thus help alleviate the health professions maldistribution problem and bring needed health services to people who are not now getting them. It is expected that 240 students in 1976 and 560 students in 1977 will be entering the training programs developed with these funds.

Special Fellowships in Nursing Research *

Special fellowships in nursing research have been awarded since 1955. Their purpose is to increase the number of nurses prepared to do independent research and able to collaborate in interdisciplinary research. The fellowships are intended to stimulate and guide research of importance to nursing. Fellowship awards are for graduate, full-time study in the physical, biological and behavioral sciences and in such related fields as biometry, health organization, health economics and human development.

These fellowships may be granted for either predoctoral or postdoctoral work. They cover

---

* (*Note:* At publication date, it was doubtful that this program would be funded.)

living and educational costs. Applicants must have a baccalaureate degree. Fellowships are awarded by the Director of the National Institutes of Health upon recommendation of the Nurse Scientist Graduate Training Committee, which meets to review applications three times a year.

Awards are made on a competitive basis. Fellows are selected for their area of research interest, their demonstrated research potential, and their commitment to engage in nursing and other health-related research.

From five to six months are required for processing of applications, review by the Nurse Scientist Graduate Training Committee and disbursement of available fellowship funds. Candidates are notified of action on their applications approximately 30 days after date of review.

The number of applicants for Special Nurse Research Fellowships has steadily increased: 67 in 1969, 99 in 1970, 85 in 1971, 93 in 1972, and 144 in 1973.

Publications: An overwhelming majority of the applicants have published articles. Some have written chapters in books and/or have written nursing textbooks. Many have published articles in scientific journals including *Nursing Research, The American Journal of Nursing,* and *Nursing Outlook.*

Employment Opportunities for Nurses with Research Training—Qualified nurse researchers are in demand for challenging posts. Among the former fellows are principal investigators in nursing research projects, research directors in public health agencies, deans and research faculty in schools of nursing and the editor of a research journal.

Profile of Nurse Fellowship Winner—The average age of nurse fellows is 27 years. A large majority of those awarded fellowships already have a masters degree (M.S.) and/or special preparation in the clinical areas in which they function.

An increasing number of nurse fellows have presented a well-developed doctoral research proposal accompanied with a bibliography. Many of the doctoral research proposals have grown out of masters research and have been related to prior clinical nursing experience. Many fellows have also participated in formal and informal research.

An overwhelming majority of the applicants have published articles, written chapters in

198

books and/or written nursing textbooks. Four fellows published more than 18 articles each.

Graduate Record Examination: Scores on both verbal and qualitative tests are consistently high, and the majority of fellowship applicants hold total scores ranging from 1,000 to 1,350.

At both undergraduate and graduate levels, nurse fellows have achieved a grade point average of 3.50 to 4.00.

Nursing Research Projects*

This program, unfortunately, was being phased out in 1977. However, programs involving research are still being funded under the Nurse Training Act. In 1977 there were 92 master's programs and 12 Ph.D. programs directly concerned with research.

Studies supported by the original grant program deal with all aspects of patient care and closely related health problems involving nursing. The projects are directed toward improvement of patient care through research.

Research awards have been made to support clinical research studies in the various medical specialties as well as studies of patient care systems and health care technologies, including the organizational characteristics of health care systems. Other investigations have identified criteria of quality patient care, the nurse role and its impact on patient care systems and the factors associated with recruitment, selection and retention of students and practitioners.

Recent projects in the clinical area have focused on nursing care of the newborn, of patients undergoing renal dialysis and cardiac surgery and of severely retarded and physically handicapped children.

Investigators on other projects are developing methods of self-instruction in activities of daily living for stroke patients and are determining circulatory and postural factors associated with the development of pressure sores.

A number of projects have dealt with the expanded role of the nurse in institutional and community settings and with the effects on patient care of the use of highly skilled clinical nurse specialists.

Two other types of support are available, one for support of conferences on the communication of research findings, the other for research development awards that enable institutions to strengthen research efforts and overcome obstacles to research. With these grants institutions can meet emerging research opportunities, explore new and promising ideas, and recognize and support scientific talent.

Who Are the Investigators?—Of the principal investigators, about three-fourths are nurse researchers. A number of nursing research projects are conducted by interdisciplinary teams that include behavioral scientists, economists, industrial engineers and hospital administrators.

Awarding of Grants—The Director of the National Institutes of Health awards grants for nursing research on the recommendation of the National Advisory Council on Nurse Training. In turn, the council's recommendations are based on the recommendations of the scientific review panel charged with review of all nursing research grant applications—the Research in Nursing in Patient Care Review Committee. The review process usually takes six months from the time of submission of the application.

Selection for award is based on an applicant's qualifications for conducting independent research, on the scientific merit of a research proposal and on the adequacy of research resources at the proposed project site.

Nursing Research Grants (A Sampling of Topics and Projects*)—

Medical or clinical studies

Pain alleviation through nursing intervention
Nutrition as an aspect of nursing care
Crying as a physiological state of the newborn infant
Sensory deprivation and effective nurse intervention
Tracheostomy suctioning—an experimental study
Preoperative distress and postoperative recovery
Measurement of microcirculation in skin
A study of nurse action in relief of pain

---

*Source: Division of Nursing, DHEW, 1970.

---

*Source: Division of Nursing, DHEW.

Studies on advanced nurse specializations

Primary health care to the elderly by nurse practitioners

Primary care nursing in the emergency room

Primary care judgments of nurses and physicians

Development of the role of clinical nurse specialist

The professional nurse in public health

The potential role of the professional nurse

A study of an extendor role for professional nurses

Studies on nurse research, education, training and recruitment and conferences

Conference on teaching and guiding nursing research

Nursing research critique conferences

Conduct and utilization of clinical nursing research

Survey and assessment of areas and methods of research in nursing

Curriculum research and evaluation in basic nursing education

Faculty research development program

Reality shock and conflict resolution in neophyte nurses

Factors determining selection or rejection of nursing as a career

Study of cost of nursing education

Men who enter nursing: a sociological study

Maternity studies and psychiatric nursing

Psychophysiological correlates of progress in labor

Nursing in maternity and newborn care

Pilot study of teaching in maternity and infant care

Nursing with chronically ill psychiatric outpatients

Relationship of patient improvement to psychiatric nursing service time

Community nursing services for psychiatric patients

Intensive nursing care with the severly retarded

Studies on nurse-patient interaction and nurse functions

Nurse autonomy and patient welfare

Altering patients' response to threatening events

Ways of improving nursing service

The repersonalization of older patients

Hospital personnel, nursing care and dying patients

The dynamics of nursing in ambulatory patient care

Other studies

Community health education

Psychosocial factors in illness outcome

Study of the U.S. cadet nurse corps

Improving quality care through performance ratings

The role of the local public health nurse

Home care in comparison with continued hospitalization

Nurse Scientist Grants*

Nurse Scientist Graduate Training Grants have been awarded since 1962 to advance nursing and other health-related research by increasing the number of research scientists with a nursing background.

These training grants are usually made to graduate schools of nursing. The funds are used for two purposes: to expand doctoral programs in university departments of basic science and to provide training stipends to nurses who are studying *full-time* toward doctoral degrees in the biological, physical or behavioral sciences.

Role of the Nurse Scientist—A nurse scientist has preparation in depth in two discipliens: nursing and a basic science. She is, therefore, able to correlate nursing knowledge with knowledge in a health of health-related science and to conduct scientific inquiry in disciplines that have significance for nursing theory and practice. Nurse scientists are in a strategic position to develop foundations for a science of nursing.

Application for Grants—Graduate schools of nursing in universities with demonstrated research accomplishment and with the necessary resources for doctoral training in the basic sciences may apply directly to the Division of Nursing.

Application for Stipends—Applications for nurse scientist stipends should be made directly to the dean of a school of nursing that has received a Nurse Scientist Graduate Training grant.

---

*Source: Division of Nursing, DHEW, 1970.

Nurses who have baccalaureate or higher degrees and who meet the requirements of both the graduate school and a specific science department within the school may apply.

Awarding of Grants—Nurse Scientist Graduate Training Grants are awarded to qualifying institutions by the Director of the National Institutes of Health upon the advice of two separate scientific review committees: the Nurse Scientist Graduate Training Committee and the National Advisory Council on Nurse Training.

Institutions Providing Training*—The schools of nursing in universities that are participating in the Nurse Scientist Graduate Training Grants program, and the respective university science departments authorized to provide nurse scientist training, are listed below:

School or Department of Nursing	University Science Departments
Case Western Reserve University	Biology, Mathematics, Physiology, Psychology, Sociology
Boston University	Anthropology, Biology, Psychology, Sociology
Teachers College, Columbia University	Anthropology, Psychology, Sociology
The University of Arizona	Anthropology, Physiology, Sociology
University of Colorado	Anthropology, Physiology, Psychology, Sociology
University of Illinois	Anatomy, Microbiology, Physiology
University of Kansas Medical Center	Anatomy, Anthropology, Physiology, Psychology, Sociology, Human Development and Family Life, Communication and Human Relations
University of Washington	Anthropology, Microbiology, Physiology, Sociology

Psychiatric Mental Health Nursing—Trainees**

The NIMH program of support in nursing is designed to expand and improve training in the field of psychiatric-mental health nursing. Grants are made to colleges and universities for undergraduate training, graduate training, doctoral training in behavioral sciences related to mental health and for nursing training in special problem areas critically short of professional personnel, such as aging, delinquency, alcoholism and drug abuse. Individuals may obtain lists of participating institutions by writing directly to the Psychiatric Nursing Training Branch, Division of Manpower and Training Programs. Application for trainee support is made directly to the training institutions.

Undergraduate Training—Grants to fully accredited baccalaureate programs may include financial assistance for basic and registered nurse students interested in preparing for careers in mental health nursing. Students who plan to continue study in psychiatric-mental health nursing at the master's level upon completion of the baccalaureate program are eligible to receive an annual stipend of $1,800 plus tuition and fees during the final two years of prebaccalaureate study.

Graduate Training—Professional nurses who wish advanced preparation in psychiatric-mental health nursing may receive stipends, tuition and fees from participating institutions at the master's, post-master's, doctoral and postdoctoral levels in clinical practice, teaching, supervision, administration, research and consultation. Clinical training areas include adult and child psychiatricmental health nursing (includes nursing of the mentally retarded), community mental health and training for positions in public health.

Stipend support is available for up to six years of graduate training within a range of $2,400 to $4,700, and for a maximum of two years of postdoctoral clinical and research training at $6,000 to $7,000. (Graduate trainees may receive a dependency allowance for each eligible dependent.)

Nurses seeking support for studies leading to a doctorate in nursing or in a behavior science must have a master's degree with training in psychiatric-mental health nursing or in mental health nursing in public health.

Support to nurses for preparation in psychiatric-mental health nursing is provided through several National Institute of Mental Health programs. From academic year 1960–61 through 1971–72, 8,957 master's and predoctoral stipends, 2,698 baccalaureate stipends, 60 career teacher stipends and 5 senior stipends were awarded under the NIMH program.

---

*Source: Division of Nursing, DHEW, 1970.
**Source: Health Services and Mental Health Administration, DHEW 1972.

Table 11-9   National institute of mental health trainee stipends in psychiatric nursing

Academic year	Baccalaureate	Master's	Predoctoral	Career teacher	Senior stipend
1972–73	309	1,019	39	—	1
1971–72	333	1,014	60	1	—

Source: Division of Manpower and Training Programs, DHEW, 1974.

Special Areas Training—Grant support is available to institutions and agencies for training of nurses in special areas. The purposes of this program are (1) to provide mental health training in all areas of nursing confronted with mental health problems; e.g., school health, maternal and child health, industrial health, public health and medical-surgical nursing; and (2) to provide nurses with special training in community mental health and in specific mental health problems areas, such as geropsychiatry, juvenile delinquency, alcoholism and drug addiction and in poverty programs. Training support is available in either of two categories: (1) for the extension and adaptation of psychiatric-mental health nursing to other areas of nursing through programs of integrative teaching of behavioral science and psychiatric-mental health nursing content in established and developing graduate programs in the nonpsychiatric areas, and (2) for full-time training in the special mental health and social problem subspecialties. Training may be supported in academic or nonacademic settings and may include trainee-stipend support at the postbaccalaureate, master's, post-master's, and pre- and postdoctoral levels.

Short-Term Training—Under a new program, NIMH offers grant support for the training of nurses to meet immediate nursing needs arising out of the development of community mental health centers programs. Grants are available for programs of intensive, short-term preparation of nurses to work in specific community mental health services providing direct patient care. This training is intended for nurses who are either not interested in or are unable to undertake full training in psychiatric-mental health nursing. Courses of training may vary from three to nine months, depending upon training program goals.

Career Teaching—The career-teacher award recognizes the importance of teaching and educational leadership in psychiatric-mental health nursing, and is available to selected psychiatric nurses to broaden clinical training and further develop teaching skills. Support is provided for a maximum of two years through participating institutions.

Other Support—Senior stipends for special training needs are also available to advanced practitioners and teachers, and for research training.

Support for experimental and special training projects including conferences, workshops, demonstrations, etc., are available.

Other Federal Aid Programs Open to Nurses

General Student Aid

Federal funds support the National Direct Student Loan (NDSL), College Work-Study (CW-S) and Supplemental Educational Opportunity Grant (SEOG).

Educational institutions administer these "campus-based" financial aid programs, distributing the funds to students whose need is established according to family income.

The federal contribution provides 90% of the principal for the student loans, with education institutions making up the remaining 10%. A total of $2,500 may be borrowed for vocational study or the first two years of college and a total of $5,000 for all undergraduate work. The ceiling for graduate study is $10,000, including any NDSL funds the student received as an undergraduate.

Repayment begins nine months after the borrower leaves school and is made to the educational institution that issued the loan. The payments go into a revolving fund for further student loans. CW-S covers 80% of the salaries earned by undergraduate and graduate students in jobs on school and college campuses or with a public or private nonprofit agency—such as a hospital—which puts up the remaining 20% of the salary.

The SEOG program supports student grants ranging from $200 to $1,500 this year. Only undergraduate students in extreme financial need are eligible for these grants, which are supported entirely by the federal government. When the student receives an SEOG award, the educational institution must add to it an equal amount of financial aid from some other source of funding.

Maternal and Child Health Scholarships

Maternal and Child Health funds within the Bureau of Community Health Services, Public Health Service, HEW, support a variety of educational programs for all levels of registered nurses who provide nursing care to mothers, infants, children and their families.

Support is given to nondegree programs to prepare nurses for new roles in pediatrics, high risk perinatal and maternity care, including midwifery. Students accepted into these programs are eligible for stipends to cover tuition and limited living and travel expenses. Eligibility for stipends is determined by the school.

In fiscal year 1972–73, 253 fellowships were awarded by the Maternal and Child Health Service for advanced study in maternal and pediatric nursing. Of the 253 awards, 70 students were enrolled in pediatric nurse practitioner, maternity nurse practitioner, or nurse-midwifery programs. The majority of these students are postbaccalaureate, and some are post-R.N. In fiscal year 1973–74, 302 fellowships were awarded.

A brochure listing all programs is available from the Nursing Section, Division of Clinical Services, Bureau of Community Health Services, Dept. of Health, Education, and Welfare, 5600 Fishers Lane, Rockville, MD 20852.

Navy Nurse Corps:

Collegiate students receive full financial assistance and salary for the junior and senior year after enlisting in the Navy Nurse Candidate Program.

Contact: U.S. Navy Recruiting Office

Walter Reed Program:

Full financial aid is offered for students interested in pursuing a collegiate nursing program. The student spends two years at the college of his choice, then two years at the University of Maryland.

Contact: The Surgeon General, Attn: MEDPT-MP, Dept. of the Army, Washington, D.C. 20315.

Additional Information on Financial Aid for Education*

Scholarships and Loans for Beginning Education in Nursing, though designed primarily for students beginning a nursing education, may contain some additional suggestions of sources for nurses planning to enter baccalaureate programs. Copies are available from the National League for Nursing, 10 Columbus Circle, New York, N.Y. 10019. Publication No. 41-410. Price, $.50.

Scholarships, Fellowships, Educational Grants and Loans for Registered Nurses. Though designed primarily for R.N.s planning to work toward baccalaureate, masters or doctoral degrees, this publication may contain some suggestions for those interested in other programs. National League for Nursing, 10 Columbus Circle, New York, N.Y. 10019. Publication No. 41-408. $.50.

Helping Hands. Financing a Health Career. A brochure giving information on financial aid available to people in health careers. Copies available from Order Dept. OP-417, American Medical Association, 535 N. Dearborn St., Chicago, Ill. 60610. Price $.15.

Need A Lift? Published annually as part of the American Legion's Education and Scholarship Program. It contains information on scholarships, fellowships and loans and information relative to state laws offering educational benefits not only for veterans and their dependents, but for all students. Copies are available at $.50 per copy (prepaid), or in quantities of 100 or more at $.30 per copy from The American Legion, Dept. S, P.O. Box 1055, Indianapolis, Ind. 46206.

Nursing Outlook, official monthly magazine of the National League for Nursing, and *American Journal of Nursing,* professional monthly magazine of the American Nurses' Association, report new scholarships, fellowships and training grants.

------

* Source: National League for Nursing.

12
LICENSING AND ETHICS

Licensing

Overview

All states license professional nurses under the title of "Registered Nurse" (R.N.). Licensure requirements are set by state statute in most states.

Usually the law is administered by a board which functions independently. The number of board members ranges from 5 to 13, with over half of the boards consisting of 5 to 7 members. Nearly all state boards issue initial and renewal licenses. About one-half of the boards issue temporary licenses to qualified applicants pending examination or completion of endorsement procedures.* The boards also have the power to discipline members of the profession for breaches of professional standards by suspension or revocation or other varied means.

Eight states and the District of Columbia specify minimum periods of education. These range from one to three years. In the remaining states there is no minimum period, but curriculum requirements are specified. All states require successful completion of a written examination for initial licensure.

The scope of the examination is set by state boards in 46 states. All states have recently adopted the State Board Test Pool Examination (SBTPE) as their state examination although statutes, allowing oral or practical examinations at the board's option remain in effect. (The SBTPE is administered in February and July on the same dates throughout the country. Future dates are—1978: February 1–2 and July 11–12; 1979: February 6–7 and July 10–11; 1980: February 5–6 and July 9–10.) Seventeen states have biennial renewal of licenses, while all others are annual. Eight states have continuing education requirements.

All the states except Virginia offer reciprocity or endorsement to applicants from states with equivalent standards. Alabama requires the applicant to pass a special examination, and Pennsylvania has a five-year practice requirement.

Senior nursing students who haven't yet passed state boards but know definitely they'll be working in another state, should write the board of nursing in that state. The board may suggest they take the SBTPE there. Some states will allow you to work on a temporary basis until your license is issued.

Nurses licensed since 1950: Many boards now give a temporary permit that will allow you to nurse while your endorsement application is being processed.

Most states also offer reciprocity or endorsement to foreign-trained applicants. All state boards require the foreign-educated nurse to take the State Board Pool Test Examination. Most foreign nurses have had to take the test at least twice before they passed.

New Trends in Licensing**

Recently, the trend has been to broaden the scope of permissible practice of professional nurses. There are at least three different kinds of changes that states have made. The first trend, as exemplified by California's statute, is to allow nurses to perform, under standardized procedures, certain basic health care testing and prevention procedures, including such procedures as administering skin tests. The second trend, as exemplified by Vermont's statute, is to allow nurses to assess health care problems of individuals and groups for the purposes of preventing illness, caring for the ill and providing rehabilitation. Finally, the third change, as in New York, for example, is to allow nurses to diagnose human responses to health problems through such services as casefinding and health teaching. This diagnostic process is distinct from medical diagnosis.

---

*Upon graduation 85% of student nurses were able to find a job in nursing while awaiting licensure. (Source: DHEW, HRA, May 1975).

**Source: Health Resources Administration, DHEW, 1976.

Requirements

Table 12-1 **Requirements for initial state licensure of professional nurses**

State	Age	Citizen-ship	Good Character	Prelim-inary	Profes-sional	SBTPE Written	Profi-ciency	Number of times Candidate may be reexamined[8]
Alabama		x	x	H.S.	1 yr.	x^2		
Alaska			x	H.S.	x	x	350	
Arizona			x^4	H.S.	x	x^1	350	
Arkansas			x	H.S.	x	x		
California			x^7	H.S.	2 yrs.	x^1		
Colorado					x	x		
Connecticut			x		x	x		
Delaware			x	H.S.	x	x		
Florida	19	x^3	x	H.S.	x	x^1		4^5
Georgia	21		x		3 yrs.	x		
Hawaii				H.S.	x^2	x		
Idaho			x^4	H.S.	x	x^1		
Illinois	18	x^3	x	H.S.	2 yrs.	x^1		
Indiana			x	H.S.	x	x^1		
Iowa			x	H.S.	2 yrs.	x		3^5
Kansas			x	H.S.	x	x^1		
Kentucky			x	H.S.	x	x^1		
Louisiana			x	H.S.	x	x^1		
Maine			x	H.S.	2 yrs.	x		
Maryland			x	H.S.	x	x		
Massachusetts			x		x	x^1		
Michigan				H.S.	x	x		
Minnesota	19		x^4	H.S.	22 mos.	x^1		
Mississippi		x^3	x	H.S.	x	x	350	2^6
Missouri	19		x	H.S.	x	x^1		
Montana				H.S.	x	x^1		
Nebraska			x	H.S.	x	x		
Nevada			x^4		x	x^1		
New Hampshire			x^4		x	x		
New Jersey	18		x^4	H.S.	x	x^1		3^6
New Mexico			x	H.S.	x	x^1	350	
New York	18		x	x^2	x	x		
North Carolina			x	H.S.	x	x		3^5
North Dakota			x	H.S.	x	x		2^5
Ohio			x	H.S.	x	x^1		2^5
Oklahoma			x	H.S.	27 mos.	x	350	2^5
Oregon			x^4	H.S.	x	x^1	350	3
Pennsylvania			x	H.S.	x	x		
Rhode Island			x^4	H.S.	x	x^1		
South Carolina	18	x^3	x	H.S.	x	x^1		2^6
South Dakota		x^3	x	H.S.	x	x		
Tennessee			x^4	H.S.	x	x		
Texas			x^4		x	x	70%	

Table 12-1 (continued)

State	Age	Citizenship	Good Character	Preliminary	Professional	SBTPE Written	Proficiency	Number of times Candidate may be reexamined[8]
					Personal Qualifications / Education / Examination				

State	Age	Citizenship	Good Character	Preliminary	Professional	SBTPE Written	Proficiency	Number of times Candidate may be reexamined[8]
Utah			x		x	x		
Vermont			x	H.S.	x	x		
Virginia			x	H.S.	x	x		
Washington					x	x		
West Virginia			x	H.S.	x	x		2[5]
Wisconsin		x[3]	x	H.S.	x	x		
Wyoming					x	x		
District of Columbia	19				2 yrs.	x		

[1] At discretion of board may be supplemented by oral or practical examination.
[2] Determined by board.
[3] Or declared intent to become a citizen.
[4] Physical health and mental health also required.
[5] Reexamination exhausts original application.
[6] Additional education required before reexamination.
[7] Committed no act that would call for applicants disqualifications as a practitioner.
[8] If blank, not specified.

Source: Adapted from Aspen Systems Corp. Study of Nurse Licensure for HRA, DHEW, 1976.

Reciprocity

Table 12-2 Reciprocity/endorsement for professional nurses

	Fees for licensure or endorsement	Examination	Reciprocity/ endorsement [1,3]	Equivalent standards
Alabama	40		E	X[8]
Alaska	40		X[2]	X
Arizona	—		E[2]	X
Arkansas	30		E[2]	X
California	35		X	X
Colorado	30	40	E[2]	X
Connecticut	30		X	X
Delaware	30		E[2]	(4)
Florida	—		X[2]	(4)
Georgia	50	45	X[2]	X
Hawaii	30		E	X
Idaho	45	45	X[2,5]	X
Illinois	25		X[2,5]	X
Indiana	25	40	E[2,5]	(4)
Iowa	10	30	E[2]	(4)
Kansas	—		E[2,5]	X

(continued)

Table 12-2   (continued)

	Fees for licensure or endorsement	Exam-ination	Reciprocity/ endorsement [1,3]	Equivalent standards
Kentucky	15	40	X[2,5]	X
Louisiana	17	55	X[2]	[4]
Maine	25	40	E[2]	[4]
Maryland	30		E[2,5]	[4]
Massachusetts	50	30	X	X
Michigan	20		E[2]	X
Minnesota	35		E[2]	X
Mississippi	25		E[2]	[6]
Missouri	25		X[2]	X
Montana	35		X	[4]
Nebraska	25		X	[4]
Nevada	30	40	X[2]	X
New Hampshire	30		X	[4]
New Jersey	25	35	X	[4]
New Mexico	50		E[2]	[4]
New York	—		I[2]	[4]
North Carolina	30	25	E[2]	X
North Dakota	35		X	[4]
Ohio	30		E[2]	[4]
Oklahoma	20		E[2]	[4]
Oregon	35	45	X[7]	[4]
Pennsylvania	10		R	X
Rhode Island	30		X	[4]
South Carolina	50		X[2]	[4]
South Dakota	30		E	[4]
Tennessee	25		E	[6]
Texas	30		X	X
Utah	30		X	X
Vermont	25		E[2]	[4]
Virginia	30		—	—
Washington	25		X	X
West Virginia	30	40	X	X
Wisconsin	40	60	X	X
Wyoming	50		X	[4]
District of Columbia	45		X	X
Puerto Rico	—	5	—	—

[1] If licensed in another jurisdiction.
[2] Includes applicants licensed in foreign country.
[3] At board's discretion unless otherwise noted.
[4] Must meet state's requirements at time of licensure.
[5] If licensed by written examination.
[6] Must meet state's requirements at time of graduation.
[7] Must demonstrate competence and have five years experience.
[8] Requires equivalent standards & SBTPE exam.

Source: Aspen Systems Corp. Study of Nurse Licensure, HRA, DHEW, 1976.

Renewal

Table 12-3   Renewal of licenses and continued education for professional nurses

State	Renewal period (years)	Continuing education required	State	Renewal period (years)	Continuing education required
Alabama	1		Nebraska	1	X[3]
Alaska	1		Nevada	2	
Arizona	1		New Hampshire	2	
Arkansas	2		New Jersey	1	
California	2	X[1]	New Mexico	2	X[4]
Colorado	2	X[2]	New York	2	
Connecticut	1		North Carolina	2	
Delaware	1		North Dakota	1	
Florida	1	X[6]	Ohio	1	
Georgia	2		Oklahoma	1	
Hawaii	1		Oregon	2	X[1,2]
Idaho	1		Pennsylvania	2	
Illinois	1		Rhode Island	1	
Indiana	2		South Carolina	1	
Iowa	1		South Dakota	1	X[5]
Kansas	2		Tennessee	2	
Kentucky	1		Texas	1	
Louisiana	1		Utah	1	
Maine	1		Vermont	2	
Maryland	2		Virginia	1	
Massachusetts	2		Washington		
Michigan	1		West Virginia	1	
Minnesota	1	X[2]	Wisconsin	1	
Mississippi	1		Wyoming	1	
Missouri	1		District of Columbia	1	
Montana	1				

[1] Board approved continuing educational course. [2] May be determined by board. [3] As of 1980 continuing education will be required. [4] As of 1977, continuing education is required. [5] May be required at board's discretion. [6] 15-hours/year.

Source: Aspen Systems Corp. Study of Nurse Licensure, HRA, DHEW, 1976.

State Boards of Nursing

State Boards of Nursing—Addresses: (If you wish specific information about licensure requirements within individual states write to "State Board of Nursing" using the following addresses.)

ALABAMA, State Administrative Bldg., Montgomery 36130

ALASKA, Dept. of Commerce, Pouch D, Juneau 99811

ARIZONA, 1645 W. Jefferson, Phoenix 85007

ARKANSAS, 9107 Rodney Parkham Rd., Little Rock 77205

CALIFORNIA, Rm. 448, 1020 N St., Sacramento 95814

COLORADO, 1525 Sherman St., Denver 80203

CONNECTICUT, Rm. 101, 79 Elm St., Hartford 06115

DELAWARE, Rm. 234, Cooper Bldg., Dover 19901

DISTRICT OF COLUMBIA, Rm. 109, 614 H St., N.W., Washington 20001

FLORIDA, 6501 Arlington Expressway, Jacksonville 32211

GEORGIA, 166 Pryor St., S.W., Atlanta 30303

GUAM, P.O. Box 2816, Agana 96910

HAWAII, P.O. Box 3469, Honolulu 96801

IDAHO, 418 North Curtis Road, Boise 83704

ILLINOIS, 628 E. Adams St., 4th Floor, Springfield 62786

INDIANA, Rm. 1018, 100 N. Senate Ave., Indianapolis 46204

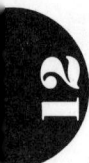

IOWA, 300 4th St., Des Moines 50319

KANSAS, Rm. 314, 701 Jackson St., Topeka 66603

KENTUCKY, 6100 Dutchmans Lane, Louisville 40205

LOUISIANA, Rm. 907, 150 Baronne St., New Orleans 70112

MAINE, 295 Water St., Augusta 04330

MARYLAND, 201 W. Preston St., Baltimore 21201

MASSACHUSETTS, Rm. 1509, 100 Cambridge St., Boston 02202

MICHIGAN, 1033 S. Washington Ave., Lansing 48926

MINNESOTA, 717 Delaware St., S.E., Minneapolis 55414

MISSISSIPPI, Suite 101, 135 Bounds St., Jackson 39206

MISSOURI, P.O. Box 650, Jefferson City 65101

MONTANA, Rm. 5, Lalonde Bldg., Helena 59601

NEBRASKA, Box 94703, State House Station, Lincoln 68509

NEVADA, Rm. 202, 100 Vassar St., Reno 89502

NEW HAMPSHIRE, 105 Loudon Rd., Concord 03301

NEW JERSEY, Rm. 319, 1100 Raymond Blvd., Newark 07102

NEW MEXICO, 505 Marquette Ave., N.W., Albuquerque 87102

NEW YORK, State Education Dept., Div. of Professional Education, 99 Washington Ave., Albany 12230

NORTH CAROLINA, Box 2129, Raleigh 27602

NORTH DAKOTA, Upper Suite 5, 219 N. 7th St., Bismarck 58501

OHIO, Suite 1130, 180 E. Broad St., Columbus 43215

OKLAHOMA, Suite 76, 4545 Lincoln Blvd., Oklahoma City 73105

OREGON, Rm. 574, 1400 S.W. Fifth Ave., Portland 97201

PENNSYLVANIA, Box 2649, Harrisburg 17120

PUERTO RICO, Box 3271, 261 Tanca St., San Juan 00904

RHODE ISLAND, Health Bldg., Davis Street, Providence 02908

SOUTH CAROLINA, 1777 St. Julian Pl., Columbia 29204

SOUTH DAKOTA, 132 South Dakota Ave., Sioux Falls 57102

TENNESSEE, Rm. 354, Capitol Hill Bldg., 301 7th Ave., N., Nashville 37219

TEXAS, 7600 Chevy Chase Dr., Suite 502, Austin 78752

UTAH, 330 E. 4th Ave. S., Salt Lake City 84111

VERMONT, 126 State St., Montpelier 05602

VIRGINIA, #305, 6 N. 6th St., Richmond 23219

VIRGIN ISLANDS, P.O. Box 1442, Charlotte Amalie, St. Thomas 00801

WASHINGTON, P.O. Box 649, Olympia 98504

WEST VIRGINIA, Rm. 416, 1800 Washington St. E., Charleston 25301

WISCONSIN, 201 E. Washington Ave., Madison 53802

WYOMING, Board of Nursing, Cheyenne 82002

Ethics

Nurses' Ethics Surveys*

When should you reveal a patient's confidences entrusted to you during the course of nursing care?

When I believe it's justified to protect the patient or community	68%
When I'm requested to do so by the law	20%
Never	10%
Whenever requested, unless told not to	1%
When requested to do so by the patient's family	0.4%

Some nurses have published books that reveal extensive details about famous patients in their care. Do you think this violates the patient-nurse bond of confidence?

Yes	90%
No	10%

*Sources: "Ethical Problems Survey," *Nursing '74,* September; "Nursing Ethics," *Nursing '74,* October; "Quality of Care," *Nursing '77,* January (surveys of 10,000 nurses).

Based on your personal experience, to what extent do nurses take supplies such as bandages, underpads, linens, etc., from hospitals for their own use?

Very commonly	30%
Occasionally	50%
Seldom	27%
Never	3%

Based on your personal experience, to what extent do nurses take *medication* (other than aspirin and antacids) from hospitals for their own use?

Very commonly	10%
Occasionally	40%
Seldom	40%
Never	10%

Nurse Sharon receives a letter with $100 from a former patient who was very pleased with Sharon's care and concern. If you were in Sharon's place, what would you do?

Highest nursing position	Would keep money
Staff nurse	28%
Team leader	27%
Asst. head nurse	31%
Head nurse	34%
Supervisor	34%
Nursing administrator	38%

Age	Would keep money
Under 22	23%
From 23 to 28	25%
From 29 to 34	31%
From 35 to 39	32%
From 40 to 49	43%
50 or over	46%

Apparently, higher-positioned and older nurses are more likely to keep a gift of money than lower-status and younger nurses.

What happens when a patient suffers a serious mishap inside the hospital and the family comes in seeking information? How much should a nurse reveal to the family when the patient's doctor is not available?

Would tell family full story—even if incriminating	8%
Would answer specific questions but not volunteer information	70%
Would tell family to ask the attending physician	19%
Would refuse to make any comment	2%

What would you do if a doctor insists that a patient be given an excessive dosage of a drug?

Refuse and tell him to give it himself	42%
Check with supervisor and follow her advice	53%
Give the drug	5%

What would you do if you went to your supervisor with documented proof of the incompetence of an emergency room doctor with whom you worked, only to have the supervisor brush you off with "don't make waves."

Drop the matter completely	1%
Ask for a transfer	4%
Go to the director of nurses	80%
Report the doctor to the medical director	9%
Confront the doctor himself	6%

When asked if they had ever reported a doctor or nurse for incompetence:

Had reported a doctor for incompetence	36%
Had reported a nurse for incompetence more than twice	20%
Had never reported other nurses for incompetence	33%

Making Ethical Decisions—A Procedure*

A course in medical ethics at the University of Colorado Medical Center offers a nine-step procedure for making ethical decisions; students have found them helpful in organizing their thinking on ethical issues and finding a common ground for discussion. When faced with an ethical decision, here's what you do:

1. Identify the health problem. This clearly must be at least brought to light, if not agreed upon, before any decision can be made.
2. Identify the ethical problem.
3. State who's involved in making the decision (the nurse, the doctor, the patient, the patient's family, etc.).
4. Identify your role. (Quite possibly, your role may not require a decision at all.)
5. Consider as many possible alternative decisions as you can.
6. Consider the long- and short-range consequences of each alternative decision.
7. Reach your decision.
8. Consider how this decision fits in with your general philosophy of patient care.
9. Follow the situation until you can see the actual results of your decision, and use this information to help in making future decisions.

Codes For Nurses

ANA Code For Nurses

1. The nurse provides services with respect for the dignity of man, unrestricted by considerations of nationality, race, creed, color, or status.
2. The nurse safeguards the individual's right to privacy by judiciously protecting information of a confidential nature, sharing only that information relevant to his care.
3. The nurse maintains individual competence in nursing practice, recognizing and accepting responsibility for individual actions and judgements.
4. The nurse acts to safeguard the patient when his care and safety are affected by

incompetent, unethical or illegal conduct of any person.
5. The nurse uses individual competence as a criterion in accepting delegated responsibilities and assigning nursing activities to others.
6. The nurse participates in research activities when assured that the rights of individual subjects are protected.
7. The nurse participates in the efforts of the profession to define and upgrade standards of nursing practice and education.
8. The nurse, acting through the professional organization, participates in establishing and maintaining conditions of employment conducive to high-quality nursing care.
9. The nurse works with members of health professions and other citizens in promoting efforts to meet health needs of the public.
10. The nurse refuses to give or imply endorsement to advertising, promotion, or sales for commercial products, services, or enterprises.

ICN Code for Nurses

(International Council for Nurses)

Adopted 1973

1. The fundamental responsibility of the nurse is fourfold: to promote health, to prevent illness, to restore health and to alleviate suffering.
2. The need for nursing is universal. Inherent in nursing is respect for life, dignity and rights of man. It is unrestricted by considerations of nationality, race, creed, color, age, sex, politics or social status.
3. Nurses render health services to the individual, the family and the community and coordinate their services with those of related groups.

Nurses and People

4. The nurse's primary responsibility is to those people who require nursing care.
5. The nurse, in providing care, promotes an environment in which the values, customs and spiritual beliefs of the individual are respected.
6. The nurse holds in confidence personal information and uses judgment in sharing this information.

---

*Source: Murphy & Murphy "Making Ethical Decisions Systematically," *Nursing '76,* May.

Nurses and Practice

7. The nurse carries personal responsibility for nursing practice and for maintaining competence by continual learning.
8. The nurse maintains the highest standards of nursing care possible within the reality of a specific situation.
9. The nurse uses judgment in relation to individual competence when accepting and delegating responsibilities.
10. The nurse when acting in a professional capacity should at all times maintain standards of personal conduct which reflect credit upon the profession.

Nurses and Society

11. The nurse shares with other citizens the responsibility for initiating and supporting action to meet the health and social needs of the public.

Nurses and Co-Workers

12. The nurse sustains a cooperative relationship with coworkers in nursing and other fields.
13. The nurse takes appropriate action to safeguard the individual when his care is endangered by a coworker or any other person.

Nurses and the Profession

14. The nurse plays the major role in determining and implementing dependable standards of nursing practice and nursing education.
15. The nurse is active in developing a core of professional knowledge.
16. The nurse, acting through the professional organization, participates in establishing and maintaining equitable social and economic working conditions in nursing.

12

13
FINDING A JOB

How to Find the Right Job

Preliminary Self-Assessment

To save time and avoid frustration for both yourself and a prospective employer, you should be forthright about your qualifications for and your expectations of a prospective new job. You might find it useful to check the following guidelines before answering any advertisement or filling out any application form.

Identify Your Skills and Special Interests

- In what areas of nursing have you accumulated experience? Do you have preferences in specific departments or functions where your skills and experience can best be utilized?
- Do you wish to explore career expansion possibilities in a particular field?
- Apply to those hospitals with openings in your selected specialty: medical-surgical; labor and delivery; nursery; emergency room; operating room; recovery room; medical, surgical and cardiac intensive care units; pediatrics; psychiatry; physical therapy; respiratory therapy; cardiovascular diagnosis and open heart surgery; teaching metabolic unit; obstetrics-gynecology; center for neurological sciences or ambulatory clinic.

Identify Your Personal Needs

- Establish acceptable geographical limits: consider whether you want a change of scenery (in another state or abroad); whether you find yourself restricted by a mate's job; whether the time and expense of daily commuting will be a factor.
- Review alternative shift schedules which are compatible with your home/family responsibilities or with additional educational pursuits.
- Keep in mind the opportunities for professional growth. Check out such features as: availability of in-service training courses, proximity of educational institutions, whether tuition or stipends are provided to encourage continuing education, whether staffing schedules are adjusted to accommodate schooling hours.

Procedure

- For jobs out of state, first contact the state Board of Nursing for detailed information on endorsement of your present license and other specific requirements. (See "Licensure" in Chapter 12 for brief summaries of state requirements.) For other sources of information contact the area nursing association or the local or state Chamber of Commerce.
- Review available hospital openings against your checklist of requirements. After making your selections arrange them in order of priority.
- Find out what you can about a prospective place of employment by talking informally with nurses who work or have worked there. Probe for the reasons behind their attitudes: one nurse may reject a hospital because of a particular philosophy or administrative policy that would be quite satisfactory to you. Be sure to use information offered in confidence with discretion.

Making Contact

Since you may be applying to several hospitals for slightly different reasons (their advertised need or your own special interest), your application letter should be personalized. That means that an original covering letter (freshly typed each time) should accompany your resumé. The resumé of course is the basic presentation of your qualifications and this can be duplicated by Xeroxing, mimeographing or offsetting.

The Application Letter—The application letter should be in proper business form, using the full name and title of the person addressed. It should immediately try to interest the reader with a personalized remark about the hospital or yourself. It should include the reason for the application, indicate that a resumé is enclosed, and offer available times for an interview.

The Resumé—The resumé should contain vital data about your education, experience and skills. It should be readable, clear in organization and as distinctive as possible in descriptions. Use 8 ½ x 11 inch white paper, set good margins, triple-space between each section. Place headings along the left margin. Chronological listings of education and experience should be in reverse order, the most recent education first and the most current position first. After titling the page and centering your name, address and telephone number, organize your data in the following sections.

1. *License information:* number, date and state in which registered.

2. *Employment experience:* for each position give the year, title of position held, employer and address, description of duties, skills utilized and responsibilities involved.

3. *Educational background:* give the certificate/degree attained, name and location of school and year you graduated. If you are engaged in advanced studies, list whatever credits have already been attained and what you are currently taking. In a separate bloc summarize any extracurricular educational efforts including in-service training, workshops, etc.

4. *Awards and prizes:* (include *only* if applicable) list any special recognition that you have received at work or in school.

5. *Additional skills and experience:* personalize yourself somewhat in this section by providing information on volunteer work, civic contributions, educational studies beyond nursing (e.g., psychology courses), special interests or skills that may be helpful in a particular unit.

6. *Professional membership:* list groups of which you are a member and include offices held, committee participation, etc.

7. *Professional and personal references.* Carefully select three references (request their permission to use their names first) and indicate their full names, titles, and business addresses.

Preparing for the Interview

Most interviewers will not only expect but welcome questions from you during the interview. You might concern yourself with questions about hospital policies, procedures and opportunities.

To cover all your concerns it might be well to group your questions into categories and then deal with one category at a time. If you receive vague answers, without being abrasive, you might ask for more specifics.

Following are some suggested categories and some questions in each category.

The Job

- Is the hospital accredited?
- What service specialties does it offer?
- What and who determines assignment in a specialty?
- What is the procedure for transferring to other units?

- Are there separate descriptions of duties and responsibilities in each staff job?
- What does the orientation for new staff members cover and how long does it last?
- What is the policy on performance evaluations? On promotions?

Administration of the Nursing Service

- Does each nursing unit conduct regular nursing care conferences?
- Does each nursing unit: update its plans? have written descriptions of care procedures? have guidelines on the responsibilities of each shift?
- Are there written procedures for grievances? for emergencies? for evacuation?

Pay Scales and Shifts

- What is the starting salary?
- Are increments automatic (how often?) or according to merit?
- Are there pay differentials or compensation for weekend service, holidays, overtime?
- How is the rotation shift arranged?
- Is sufficient advance notice given on time schedules?
- Will there be any flexibility to accommodate personal needs? to accommodate professional needs such as workshops, courses, special meetings, etc.?

Fringe Benefits

Most hospitals provide a written statement on personnel policies. This statement should answer all queries on policies and procedures covering vacations, holidays, sick leave, employee health services, promotion, transfer, retirement, leave of absence and other practices affecting employees. If there is such a booklet, you should review it before asking any further questions on benefits. You might have a specific interest in learning immediately, however, whether housing is provided and under what conditions.

Education Opportunity

- Is there an active in-service or continuing education program?
- Is it held during each shift?
- Does the hospital provide tuition assistance for nurses registered at a college or university in job-related studies?
- Will the hospital make scheduling arrangement to accommodate such studies?
- Will the college consider such studies in determining raises or promotions?

13

At the Interview

- Be punctual and dress conservatively.
- Bring along a copy of your resumé. It may prove helpful in filling out the data required on the hospital application form. Don't forget your Social Security number.
- Maintain eye-contact with the interviewer.
- Be direct in your answers, nonrepetitive in your questions, forthright in the discussion of your goals.
- If you are offered the position, request a tour of the facilities and the specific department you will probably be assigned to in order to arrive at a well-considered decision.

Sources of Assistance*

Among the sources are professional nurse placement offices, placement offices in educational institutions, announcements of Civil Service examinations, advertisements in professional periodicals, relatives, friends, acquaintances and direct contacts with employers, physicians, patients and others. If you desire a position in the Army, Air Force or Navy Nurse Corps, or in the PHS of the U.S. Department of Health, Education, and Welfare, write directly to the service of choice for information. The VA hospitals also employ a large number of nurses.

Nurse placement may be conducted by hospitals, other health institutions and educational institutions; national, state and district nurses' associations; other professional groups; employment centers operated by the state or local offices of the U.S. Employment Service; and by commercial agencies. Not all of these are professionally sponsored services.

The placement services that have seemed to be the most satisfactory for nurses are those sponsored and conducted by the professional nurses' associations.

Assistance from the Professional Association

Nurse placement services may be national, state or local. Professional registries for nurses in private practice are organized by, affiliated with and approved by district nurses' associations and approved by state nurses' associations.[1] The American Nurses' Association Professional Credentials and Personnel Service, Inc. (ANA PC&PS) is located at 10 Columbus Circle, New York, N.Y., 10019.

The functions of the ANA PC&PS is limited to professional record services. Counseling and placement assistance remains the responsibility of the state nurses' associations.

Service from State Nurses' Associations

State nurses' associations develop their own professional counseling and placement services with assistance from the ANA PC&PS. By 1968, 43 states provided services including:

1. Information about positions open in the state.
2. General information about employment opportunities and standards in the state, including salaries; license to practice; and names and addresses of principal hospitals, public health agencies, schools of nursing, professional registries, public schools and business and industrial organizations that employ nurses.
3. Information about cost of living, residence accommodations, climate and recreation facilities.
4. Assistance to nurses with plans for professional growth and development, including information about educational programs and financial aid for study and help with questions related to professional practice and employment conditions.

Employers of nurses are assisted by listing position openings and referral of openings to nurses interested in employment in the state. The state office also provides employers with current information about salaries and employment conditions, which will help to attract and hold qualified nurse personnel. Periodically, state associations send a list of position openings to the ANA PC&PS office for duplication and distribution to all states. This provides a method for distributing information about employment opportunities in all states to nurses throughout the country.

Employers also appreciate receiving the

---

*Source: Ruth Spalding, *Professional Nursing,* J. B. Lippincott, 1970.

[1] State approved registries are listed in the back of the May and November issues of the *American Journal of Nursing.*

professional biographies prepared for nurses by the ANA PC&PS. The value of reviewing professional credentials of candidates for positions prior to employment, and of retaining credentials of employees in confidential personnel files, is increasingly recognized.

Registries & Temporary Service Companies*

In the Yellow Pages of your phone book under "Nurses," [there is usually a list of] registries and temporary service companies.

A *registry,* like an employment agency, is a state-licensed referral agency. For a fee, the registry will give you the names of people or institutions that want to hire a nurse. But the registry *does not* employ you. If you accept a client from the registry list, you provide the care required as a self-employed nurse. That is, *you* bill the client. (Your fees are set by the registry or by state law.) And you pay your own liability insurance and Social Security.

A *temporary service company* is *not* a licensed agency. It's a business that employs nurses (and other professional, industrial and clerical workers). As a nurse employed by a TSC, you would be paid weekly for the actual hours you have worked. The TSC would bill the client-patient or institution, pay you, and perform the other payroll functions of an employer required by law. (These include Social Security deductions, worker's compensation, unemployment insurance and professional liability insurance.)

Temporary nurses have no job security. They rarely have any benefits such as hospitalization, in-service education, sick pay or holiday pay. And the unpredictable demand for temporary nurses makes financial planning difficult.

Most services pay their nurses a flat hourly rate which equals or slightly exceeds the starting salary for nurses in that area. But, re-member, hospital and industrial nurses also draw many benefits which may amount to 40% of their salary. Thus, the new hospital nurse may take home $4 an hour, but her full benefit package is worth $5.60 an hour. You, as a TSC employee, get only $4. (But the TSC will charge the hospital close to $5.60 an hour for your work.)

Unlike your hospital-based colleagues, you will not receive merit or longevity raises (with rare exceptions).

---

*Source: *Nursing '76,* September.

Service from the ANA PC&PS

The professional record service consists of compiling a cumulative record of professional education and experience, including references from previous employers; sending biographies; updating records and biographies as needed; and safe-keeping and storage of the records. Completion of the PC&PS application form provides the basis for compilation of a record. Confirmation of diplomas and degrees awarded, dates and titles of positions held, and evaluation of performance (references) are obtained by PC&PS directly from the schools and employing organizations. From two to six weeks are required to compile a new record, depending upon the speed with which references are returned. The PC&PS record remains on file throughout the nurse's professional career.

References are obtained by PC&PS from former employers and educational institutions, with the nurse's permission. Reference requests are automatically sent to the head of the department of nursing in the school or employing organization; it is important that the evaluation be supplied by someone to whom the nurse has been administratively responsible. Usually only one reference is obtained for each period of employment. PC&PS policy permits sharing a reference with the nurse on request. It is expected that references will be based on periodic evaluations of performance discussed by the supervisor and nurse during employment. It is suggested that the nurse, planning to leave a position, should ask her employer for a final evaluation before she leaves.

The PC&PS biography is a summary of the PC&PS record and contains the following information: a list of educational programs completed, including confirmation and evaluation of progress in these programs, date of diploma or degree awarded and major program of study; R.N. licenses and state certificates held; foreign language skills; professional activities, publications, workshops and institutes attended; titles of positions held, including confirmation of dates, clinical area where indicated, name and address of employing organizations and evaluation of performance. Unless otherwise indicated, only references covering the last ten years of employment and at least three employment periods are included in a biography. If desired, the nurse may supply a statement to be sent with the biography describing professional interests, expectations and goals.

Biographies are released only on authorization sent to PC&PS by the nurse; they are not released on request from the employer without prior permission from the nurse. The request to send a biography must include the name and title of the recipient, with his responsibility in the employing organization clearly indicated. Also needed is the title of the position for which the nurse is applying, or the reason for sending the biography.

A charge of $10.00 is made to begin a new record and to send one biography. A fee of $2.00 is required to send a biography at other times.

There is no charge to update a record already on file, and the compilation fee includes safe-keeping and storage of the record. Since assistance with counseling and placement is provided by SNA offices, there is no charge to send a biography to an SNA office for use in assisting the nurse.

Any ANA member or associate member can have her record compiled by the ANA PC&PS and receive counseling and assistance with placement. When requesting service from PC&PS you should:

1. Enclose your current ANA membership card (member or associate) in your letter requesting service from the ANA PC&PS or from a state nurses association (SNA) office.
2. Include your PC&PS file number (Social Security number), and former name, if name has changed since last contact with PC&PS.
3. When requesting assistance from an SNA office, be specific about interests in regard to type of position desired, preferred location within the state, minimum salary acceptable and date of availability.

4. Investigate positions carefully. Although the SNA office provides preliminary information about positions, detailed information should be obtained from the employing organization. If interested in a position, write a letter of application or further inquiry.
5. Send *written* request to the ANA PC&PS office to release your biography, and enclose a check for the required fee.
6. When your need for service is ended, inform the SNA offices that provided assistance.

Job Leads

Where Newly Licensed Nurses Get Job Leads

A survey of 6,000 newly licensed nurses, conducted by the National League for Nursing and the Department of Health, Education, and Welfare, indicates what sources of job information the nurses rate as good to excellent. Here is a summary of the study:

Source of information	% of nurses
Direct application	87%
Faculty	82
Friends	76
Recruiters	73
Professional journals	68
School placement bureau	61
Nurses' conventions	59
Newspapers	54
Civil Service listing	50
State nurses' association	48
State employment service	36
Commercial employment agency	35

Source: P. M. Nash, Ph.D. "Evaluation of Employment Opportunities for Newly Licensed Nurses." Division of Research, National League for Nursing, published by Health Resources Administration of HEW.

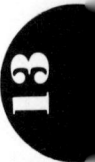

Job Leads That Produce Results

Table 13-1   Job lead sources that resulted in employment*

Sources utilized	Type of program				
	Total	Bacc.	A.D.	Dipl.	P.N.
Faculty	42%	46%	36%	47%	39%
Friends	51	61	47	57	39
Recruiter	12	19	12	13	4
Nurses convention	3	3	3	4	2

(*continued*)

Table 13-1 (continued)

Sources utilized	Type of program				
	Total	Bacc.	A.D.	Dipl.	P.N.
State Nurses Association	—	—	—	—	—
Placement service	2	2	2	2	2
State employment service	4	2	4	2	7
Commercial employ. agency	3	2	3	3	4
Placement bureau of school	6	9	4	5	5
Professional journals	18	28	15	24	4
Civil Service listings	5	6	5	4	5
Newspapers	23	22	24	23	23
Direct application	71	77	70	75	64

Source: DHEW, 1975.

Choosing a Place to Work

Factors Influencing Choice

When 11,000 nurses were asked in a *Nursing '75* survey how they went about choosing a place to work, "job satisfaction" was ranked the number one priority by 32% of nurses responding.

Salary was ranked first by 16%. Then came "appropriate working hours and shifts," with 15% putting that first, followed by "pleasant, convenient location," "reputation of employer" and "personal advancement opportunities." Just 1% considered fringe benefits the most important factor.

Table 13-2 Influential factors in nurses' choice of workplace

Rank	% ranked 1, 2 or 3	1	2	3	Rank	% ranked 1, 2 or 3	1	2	3
Salary	52%	16%	21%	15%	Physical working conditions	13	2	5	6
Job satisfaction	49	32	10	8	Inservice and continuing education opportunities	11	2	5	4
Appropriate hours/ shifts	36	15	11	10	Personal advancement opportunities	10	3	3	4
Fringe benefits	22	1	9	11	Written personnel policies	4	½	2	2
Convenient, pleasant location	19	9	5	5	Personal security/ safety	3	½	1	1
Adequate staffing	14	2	5	7	Housing availability	3	½	1	1
Reputation of employer	15	5	4	6	Recreational availability	½	—	—	½
Pleasant working associates	13	3	5	5					
Job security	13	3	4	5					
Job authority and responsibility	13	2	5	5					

Source: Marjorie Godfrey, "Your Fringe Benefits," *Nursing '75*, January.

Reasons for Difficulty in Finding a Job*

Nurses who reportedly had difficulty in obtaining the job they wanted were asked to indicate what might have contributed to this difficulty.

The reason most frequently reported by nurses who had difficulty finding the job they wanted was simply that there were no jobs in the area. The second most frequently reported reason was attributed to the employers' demands for nurses with more experience.

*Source: DHEW, May 1975.

Table 13-3   Reasons for difficulty in obtaining first position

Reason	By type of program				
	Total	Bacc.	A.D.	Dipl.	P.N.
Different education preparation wanted	4%	3%	5%	3%	5%
More experience wanted	22	19	34	17	20
Specialized skills wanted	1	1	2	1	2
Position not within reasonable distance	6	6	5	5	7
Unsatisfactory location	2	4	1	2	—
Salary too low	6	5	6	4	10
No jobs available in area	42	41	33	49	41
Other	17	21	14	19	15
Total	100%	100%	100%	100%	100%
N	(1,563)	(276)	(381)	(498)	(408)

Compromises Made

Table 13-4   Compromises made or considered in accepting first position

Compromises	By type of program				
	Total	Bacc.	A.D.	Dipl.	P.N.
Accept a position with a type of employer who was *not* initially your first preference	33%	33%	33%	32%	34%
Accept a position in a field in nursing which was *not* initially your first preference	34	19	26	34	20
Accept a position which made it necessary for you to move	21	34	14	27	11
Agree to work *less* acceptable hours	40	45	40	42	32
Accept a position in a type of neighborhood you did *not* like	14	16	13	14	11
Accept a position paying less than you would have preferred	35	37	34	31	40

Source: DHEW, May 1975.

Although there is very little differentiation among the four types of programs with regard to their accepting a position with a type of employer who was not initially their first preference (approximately 33% in each case), a different situation prevails with regard to compromising their preferred field of nursing. The most frequent compromise made concerned working less acceptable hours, followed by acceptance of a position paying less than you would have preferred.

Where Newly Licensed Nurses Work

Table 13-5   Where newly licensed nurses originally lived and where they now work

Town size before nursing school	Town size—first licensed job							
	Under 2,500	2,500– 10,000	10,000– 50,000	50,000– 75,000	75,000– million	Million and over	Other	Total
Under 2,500	106	180	225	195	33	63	65	867 (13.9%)
2,500–10,000	29	395	303	244	64	99	76	1,210 (19.5%)
10,000–50,000	21	86	805	316	97	143	90	1,558 (25.0%)

(continued)

Table 13-5   (continued)

Town size before nursing school	Town size—first licensed job							
	Under 2,500	2,500–10,000	10,000–50,000	50,000–75,000	75,000–million	Million and over	Other	Total
50,000–75,000	9	41	98	861	84	101	81	1,275 (20.5%)
75,000–million	5	8	19	30	160	31	23	276 (4.4%)
Million and over	7	13	34	40	21	583	40	738 (11.9%)
Other	8	20	38	54	11	35	133	299 (4.8%)
Total	185	743	1,522	1,740	470	1,055	508	6,223
	(3%)	(12%)	(24%)	(28%)	(8%)	(17%)	(8%)	(100.0%)

Source: DHEW, May 1975.

Note: 33.5% came from towns with less than 10,000 population but only 15% work in towns with less than 10,000 population. Obviously many nurses in larger cities and metropolitan areas are being drawn from smaller city backgrounds.

Table 13-6   Newly licensed nurses by type of current employer and type of program

Type of employer	Type of program				
	Total	Bacc.	A.D.	Dipl.	P.N.
Hospital—Public	57.3%	47.1%	57.8%	62.9%	57.2%
Hospital—Private	24.0	29.0	26.3	25.8	15.3
Nursing home	4.7	1.0	3.5	1.6	13.0
Official (Govt.) public health agency	2.4	5.0	2.5	1.6	1.4
Nonofficial (voluntary public health agency, e.g., VNA)	0.7	2.3	0.5	0.2	0.2
Combination official/nonofficial public health agency	0.4	1.0	0.1	0.4	0.1
Community health organization (e.g., Community Mental Health, HMO, etc.)	0.8	1.2	0.6	0.8	0.6
Board of education (school nurse)	0.2	0.2	0.2	0.2	0.1
School of nursing (teaching)	0.3	0.8	0.4	0.1	0.2
Industry	0.3	0.2	0.4	0.3	0.3
Private duty	0.5	0.3	0.4	0.2	1.1
Office nursing: doctor, dentist, etc.	2.4	1.0	2.7	1.8	4.0
Military	2.4	7.8	0.1	2.4	0.7
Another	1.2	1.7	1.3	0.7	1.4
Other	2.5	1.3	3.1	1.2	4.4
Total	100%	100%	100%	100%	100%
N	(6,214)	(1,150)	(1,650)	(1,956)	(1,458)

Source: DHEW, May 1975.

Mobility

Willingness to Move*

Nurses exhibit a substantial amount of mobility over a lifetime. A large proportion of moves are concentrated within the first few years after graduation from nursing school. Nurses generally take their first jobs in the same geographic area in which they completed their training. However, they are likely to move soon thereafter.

*Source: DHEW, May 1975.

Table 13-7   R.N. mobility: Interstate moves

Stage of movement	Remained in same state	Remained in same census division but changed states	Changed census divisions	Total
Nursing school graduation to first job				
Yr. R.N. grad.:				
1930–1939	87.2%	6.7%	6.1%	100.0%
1950–1959	85.0	6.5	8.5	100.0
1965–1969	83.2	5.4	11.4	100.0
First job to current job				
Yr. R.N. grad.:				
1930–1939	55.7	11.5	32.8	100.0
1950–1959	57.0	13.6	29.3	100.0
1965–1969	61.1	11.6	27.3	100.0

Although the majority of nurses do not want to move at all, nurses appear almost as willing to make interstate as intrastate moves.

Among the categories of R.N.s most willing to move are: the recently hired; male; single, separated, widowed or divorced nurses; and those with no children and relatively little income from sources other than R.N. employment. Married R.N.s, particularly those with children are highly immobile. For all practical purposes, this group should be treated as completely immobile. Single R.N.s, who as a group are relatively young, are willing to consider employment in other geographic areas; nonfinancial incentives provide more effective incentives for them than financial incentives. Though less willing to move as a group than single nurses, separated, widowed or divorced nurses who are willing to move are more likely to emphasize salary.

Table 13-8   Willingness to move to another state

R.N. group	Yes, for money	Yes, but not for money	No
Duration of current employment:			
Employed under 1 year	14.2%	16.5%	69.3%
Employed 1–5 years	13.9	13.9	72.2
Employed more than 5 years	6.5	6.1	87.3
Sex:			
Women	12.0	13.0	75.1
Men	30.6	23.6	45.8
Marital status:			
Single	21.6	27.2	51.3
Married, spouse present	7.7	9.0	83.3
Other (sep., wid., div.)	21.7	10.1	68.3
Children:			
Children ages 0–6 only	10.4	10.6	79.0
Children ages 7–18 only	9.8	5.3	84.9
Children ages 0–18	8.8	5.4	85.8
None	15.8	19.0	65.2
Spouse earnings and income from other sources (annual):			
$0–5,000	12.7	15.5	71.8
$5,001–10,000	8.9	9.3	81.8
$10,001–15,000	2.6	5.3	92.1
$15,001–25,000	5.1	7.8	87.1
Over $25,000	5.5	5.5	89.0

Table 13-9   Job changing: Education of those who stayed with their first employer

Current/First employer (since graduation)	Type of program				
	Total	Bacc.	A.D.	Dipl.	P.N.
Hospital—Public	81%	73%	80%	81%	84%
Hospital—Private	78	76	75	80	80
Nursing home	62	67	50	42	69
Official (Govt.) public health agency	65	54	71	66	80
Nonofficial (voluntary) public health agency (e.g., VNA)	64	59	88	50	67
Combination official/nonofficial public health agency	52	58	—	43	—
Community health organization (e.g., Community Mental Health, HMO, etc.)	58	50	80	40	78
Board of education (school nurse)	20	—	50	—	—
School of nursing (teaching)	48	22	71	—	33
Industry	25	50	29	33	—
Private duty	60	67	57	50	63
Office nursing: doctor, dentist, etc.	44	42	51	57	42
Military	62	69	—	44	80

Source: DHEW, May 1975.

13

Table 13-10   Job changing—Newly licensed nurses

Current/ Most recent employer	Remained with first employer (retention rate)[2]	New employer	
		Same employer type	New employer type
Hos—Pub	81.0	10.9[1]	8.1
Hos—Pvt	77.5	9.0	13.5
Nsg Home	62.1	8.6	29.3
Govt PH	64.9	3.3	31.8
Vol PH	64.3	0	35.7
PH MXD	52.2	0	47.8
Cmuty	58.3	2.1	39.6
Bd Ed	20.0	0	80.0
Sch Nsg	47.6	0	53.4
Indus	25.0	0	75.0
Pvt Duty	60.0	10.0	30.0
Ofc Nsg	43.7	2.0	54.3
Miltry	61.5	0	38.5

[1]Read: 10.9% of the newly licensed nurses currently employed by public hospitals had moved there from another public hospital where they had been first employed.

[2]The column labeled "retention rate" indicates that 81.0% of those currently employed by public hospitals had initially started working at that particular public hospital and were still currently employed there.

Source: DHEW, May 1975.

Table 13-11   Marital status of newly licensed nurses, by furthest application for job (in percentages)

Marital status	Furthest application for job			
	Total	Local	Requires move	Other
Single	42%	36%	58%	34%
Married	51	55	38	54
Separated/Divorced	6	8	4	10
Widowed	1	1	—	2
Total	100	68	26	6

Source: DHEW, May 1975.

Job Openings and Shortage Areas

Where the Jobs Are

In a recent survey of overall employment shortages across the country (*Changing Times,* May 1976), over half the states expressed a need for either registered nurses or practical nurses in the next few years.

Current job openings for R.N.s, as well as anticipated work opportunities over the next few years, were indicated in: Arizona, Arkansas, Iowa, Kansas (urban), Maine,

Table 13-12 Totals for employed R.N.s and ratio per 100,000 population, by state and region, 1972

State and region	Employed nurses[1] (adjusted figure)	Nurse-population ratio[2]	State and region	Employed nurses[1] (adjusted figure)	Nurse-population ratio[2]
United States	749,979	380	East north-central	152,089	370
			Illinois	44,783	397
New England	72,328	596	Indiana	15,841	298
Connecticut	17,887	579	Michigan	30,546	335
Maine	4,810	464	Ohio	42,032	389
Massachusetts	37,620	649	Wisconsin	18,887	416
New Hampshire	4,445	572			
Rhode Island	4,712	485	West north-central	68,044	406
Vermont	2,854	612	Iowa	11,959	413
			Kansas	9,098	400
Middle Atlantic	183,245	485	Minnesota	19,169	486
New Jersey	31,943	432	Missouri	14,982	312
New York	89,375	485	Nebraska	6,802	443
Pennsylvania	61,927	519	North Dakota	2,885	455
			South Dakota	3,149	462
South Atlantic	108,963	340			
Delaware	2,935	514	Mountain	35,322	393
District of Columbia	5,020	673	Arizona	8,513	428
Florida	26,202	353	Colorado	11,780	491
Georgia	12,492	263	Idaho	2,518	329
Maryland	14,847	363	Montana	3,261	451
North Carolina	16,649	318	Nevada	1,732	323
South Carolina	7,916	295	New Mexico	2,778	258
Virginia	16,647	348	Utah	3,260	285
West Virginia	6,255	350	Wyoming	1,480	425
East south-central	30,909	235	Pacific	96,443	352
Alabama	7,847	223	Alaska	1,399	422
Kentucky	8,487	256	California	68,668	334
Mississippi	5,129	226	Hawaii	3,110	380
Tennessee	9,446	233	Oregon	8,790	399
			Washington	14,476	420
West south-central	47,636	237			
Arkansas	3,776	190			
Louisiana	9,133	245			
Oklahoma	6,514	246			
Texas	28,213	240			

[1]Adjusted for nonresponse to questions on employment status and county of employment.
[2]Ratios based on 1972 population estimates, *Market Statistics,* N.Y., N.Y.

Source: *The Nation's Nurses: 1972 Inventory of Registered Nurses,* American Nurses' Association, Statistics Department.

Massachusetts, Missouri, Nevada, New Mexico (rural), Oklahoma (rural), South Carolina, South Dakota (rural), Texas (major cities), and Virginia.

Projected job openings for R.N.s during the next few years would be available in: Alabama, Alaska, California, Connecticut, Indiana, Louisiana, Michigan, Minnesota, New Hampshire (southern part), New Jersey, New York, North Dakota, Ohio, Pennsylvania, Tennessee, Utah, Washington, D.C., and West Virginia.

Projected openings for L.P.N.s over the next few years would be available in: Alabama,

Connecticut, Massachusetts, Nebraska, New Mexico (small town/rural), Ohio, Oklahoma, Pennsylvania and South Dakota (rural).

Nurse Shortages

It appears that the nearly universal shortage of nurses in the United States has been largely overcome, partly by the increase in practicing nurses in the past decade and the stabilization of hospital beds, partly through institutional reorganization and the substitution of other personnel for nurses, and partly by a retrench-

224

ment on the part of employers due to economic conditions. That there has been a reduction in the shortage of nurses *per se* does not, however, lead to the conclusion that shortages of particular kinds of nurses with particular skills and abilities have been reduced.

Maldistribution

Nurses are seriously maldistributed geographically in much the same pattern and for many of the same reasons as are physicians. As the following table indicates, the nurse–population ratio varies widely, from a high of 673 per 100,000 people in the District of Columbia to a low of 190 per 100,000 in Arkansas.

Survey of Hospital Nurse Supply*

The shortage seems to be easing—at least in terms of numbers of available R.N.s. About half the nation's short-term general hospitals no longer have any trouble filling vacancies on their R.N. staffs. The overriding need is for *experienced* R.N.s, particularly for nurses competent to work in specialty areas.

As might be expected, intensive care units are cited most often as the department having the most difficulty finding experienced nurses. OGN and OR also rank high as problem areas, with medical/surgical next.

The greatest problem is getting competent nurses willing to work evenings and nights. If all R.N.s who want to work in their profession would take the available shifts, the nurse shortage would recede still further.

Single nurses do not want to work nights because if they do they may always be single; the 11–7 can be very hard on social life. Married nurses, especially those with school-age children, also have an obvious preference for spending their evenings and nights with their families.

Hospitals are able to fill 79% of their R.N. vacancies from within the immediate area. Of the remaining openings, 19% are filled with applicants from within the same state and only 11% from out-of-state.

*Source: "R.N. Survey of the Hospital Nurse Supply," reprinted from *RN Magazine*, June 1974. Copyright © 1974 by Medical Economics Co., Oradell, N.J. 07649. All rights reserved.

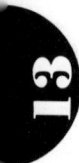

Table 13-13   Are there enough R.N.s available to meet your staffing needs?[1]

	Yes	No
Bed size		
Under 100	50%	50%
100–199	46	54
200–299	51	49
300–399	54	46
400 up	39	51
Region		
East	69	31
South	32	68
Midwest	54	46
West	57	43
Southwest	31	69
Averages	49%	51%

[1] Percentages based on 1,430 responses.

Table 13-14   Problems in filling vacancies

	% of responses[1]
Most common problems	
Lack of qualified R.N.s	42%
Filling nights, weekends	34
Rural or isolated locale	27
Inadequate salaries, benefits	11
Lack of specialized R.N.s	9
Getting full-time R.N.s	4
Getting part-time R.N.s	1
All other problems	4

	% of responses[2]
Departments having the most difficulty	
ICU, CCU, ICU/CCU	56%
OB/Gyn (OGN)	48
Operating room	44
Medical, surgical, med/surg	29
Emergency department	17
Pediatrics	9
General duty	5
Psychiatric	3
Geriatrics	3
Orthopedics	2
All others	9

[1] Based on 1,183 responses.
[2] Based on 1,049 responses. Tables add up to more than 100% because of multiple responses.

Job Market for Newly Licensed Nurses

Table 13-15   Job market by education

Availability of employment	Type of program				
	Total	Bacc.	A.D.	Dipl.	P.N.
Substantial number of good jobs available	27%	33%	27%	28%	20%
Substantial number of good jobs available but not interesting	9	13	7	9	7
Very few jobs available but some were good	15	13	15	16	16
Very few jobs available but those that were were uninteresting	5	4	4	5	7
Knew where nurse was going to work so did not look	38	32	40	38	40
Other	6	5	7	4	10
Total	100%	100%	100%	100%	100%
N	(6,214)	(1,150)	(1,650)	(1,956)	(1,458)

Source: DHEW, May 1975.

Thirty-eight percent of newly licensed nurses already had positions waiting for them. Those with baccalaureate degrees had more opportunities and thus were less inclined to pre-commit to a specific job. However, 46% of them indicated that there was a substantial number of good jobs available to them.

13

Table 13-16   Job market by region

Region[1]	N	Had job	Percent reporting					
			Sufficient number of good jobs	Sufficient but not interesting	Few jobs but good ones	Few jobs and most uninteresting	Other	Total
Boston	(492)	38%	25%	10%	15%	6%	6%	100%
New York	(829)	36	22	8	20	6	8	100
Philadelphia	(858)	37	27	9	17	5	5	100
Atlanta	(738)	43	32	9	8	3	5	100
Chicago	(1,470)	38	29	9	14	4	6	100
Dallas	(437)	45	28	9	7	3	8	100
Kansas City	(439)	39	25	12	15	5	4	100
Denver	(212)	32	25	8	22	6	7	100
San Francisco	(529)	32	26	8	19	6	9	100
Seattle	(210)	32	28	12	19	3	6	100
Total	(6,214)	38	27	9	15	5	6	100

[1]The city designated under "Region" refers not simply to that particular city but to a much larger geographic area. For example, Boston region includes the states of Conn., Maine, Mass., N.H., R.I., and Vt.

Source: DHEW, May 1975.

Table 13-17   Difficulty in getting the job they wanted

Region	N	Type of program				
		Total	Bacc.	A.D.	Dipl.	P.N.
Boston	(619)	26%	27%	15%	29%	28%
New York	(829)	30	27	31	26	40
Philadelphia	(858)	24	21	19	25	28
Atlanta	(738)	18	23	16	13	22
Chicago	(1,470)	24	21	22	27	25
Dallas	(437)	18	13	12	18	24
Kansas City	(439)	25	26	21	22	35
Denver	(212)	26	22	22	39	23
San Francisco	(529)	33	35	32	33	36
Seattle	(210)	27	30	29	22	23
Total	(6,214)	25	24	23	25	28

Source: DHEW, May 1975.

As we can see from Table 13-17, 25% of the respondents reported some difficulty in obtaining the job they wanted. This was more the case in the San Francisco and New York regions. However, regional differences also occur by type of program. In the San Francisco region difficulty in obtaining the desired job held at approximately one-third for each type of program. However, in the New York region, practical nurses were considerably more likely to report difficulty (40%) than either baccalaureate graduates (27%) or diploma graduates (26%).

Salaries

Overview

Occupational pay levels in private and state and local government hospitals usually were highest in the New York and San Francisco metropolitan areas and lowest in Houston and other Southern cities in August 1972.

Average weekly salaries of general duty nurses, one of the most populous jobs, ranged from $163.50 in Buffalo to $214 in San Francisco. Among the five registered professional nursing occupations studied, general duty nurses averaged the least per week in each area—typically 10% to 20% below head nurses and nursing instructors;

15% to 25% below supervisors of nurses; and 30% to 45% below directors of nursing.

Interarea ranges for the other professional nursing occupations studied were $180.50 to $246 for head nurses, $180.50 to $263 for nursing instructors, $203 to $267 for supervisors of nurses, and $247.50 to $364 for directors of nursing.

Licensed practical nurses and nursing aides—two numerically important nonprofessional occupations having direct contact with patients—typically earned about 25% and 40% less, respectively, than general duty nurses within the same area. Average weekly earnings for licensed practical nurses ranged from $164.50 in San Francisco to $110 in Dallas; for nursing aides, weekly averages ranged from $147 in San Francisco to $83 in Houston.

As increases varied in occupational averages, wage relationships changed in the industry, including a narrowing of wage advantages of general duty nurses over licensed practical nurses and nursing aides in most areas. In 1969, for example, licensed practical nurses in Philadelphia averaged 29% less and nursing aides, 44% less than general duty nurses. In August 1972, the corresponding differentials were 22% and 36%.

Workers in state and local government hospitals have enjoyed wage advantages over their counterparts in private hospitals, but the gaps are narrowing. Between the mid-1960 survey—when the bureau first developed separate occupational earnings data for private and government (nonfederal) hospitals—and this study, wage comparisons of workers in selected occupations indicate that earnings levels have usually risen at a faster pace for private than for government hospital workers.

Table 13-18   Median-city increase in average earnings between March 1969 and August 1972

Occupation	Percent increase
Supervisors of nurses	27.0
Head nurses	24.8
General duty nurses	23.9
Licensed practical nurses	27.9
Nursing aides	32.4
Psychiatric aides	37.9

Source: U.S. Bureau of Labor Statistics, 1974.

Table 13-19   Salary comparisons: special vs. short-term general hospitals

	% of special hospitals*	% of general hospitals
Percent of hospitals paying a top starting salary of $9,000 up	85	44
Percent of hospitals paying a top starting salary of $10,000 up	73	23
Composition of the R.N. working force:		
Full-time R.N.s	85	67
Associate degree R.N.s	12	13
Diploma R.N.s	67	76
Baccalaureate R.N.s	21	11

* Children's psychiatric and V.A.
Percentages given are the averages of all responses to each question regardless of hospital size and other classifications.

Source: "R.N. Survey of the Hospital Nurse Supply," reprinted from RN Magazine, June 1974. Copyright © 1974 by Medical Economics Co., Oradell, N.J. 07649. All rights reserved.

Starting Salaries of Newly Licensed Nurses

In 1973 the median salary of nursing seniors who accepted positions before graduation was in the $8,000 to $8,999 range.

For seniors attending schools in the South Atlantic and West South-Central regions the median was lower ($7,000 to $7,999 range) and in the Pacific region the median was higher ($9,000 to $9,999 range). Twenty-five percent of all the seniors responding accepted positions paying $9,000 or more.

Table 13-20   Starting salaries— nursing seniors—overview

Salary	No.	%
$0–4,000	2	*
$4,001–4,999	10	0.1
$5,000–5,999	32	0.5
$6,000–6,999	274	4.2
$7,000–7,999	1,886	28.7
$8,000–8,999	2,729	41.5
$9,000–9,999	1,206	18.3
$10,000–10,999	375	5.7
$11,000–11,999	56	0.9
$12,000–12,999	4	0.1
$13,000–13,999	2	*
Total reporting	6,576	100.0
Total nonreporting	1,233	

* Less than 0.1%.

Source: *Career Goals of Hospital School of Nursing Seniors,* 1975, (1973 Survey), reprinted by permission of the American Hospital Association.

Salaries by Experience and Type of Hospital

In Table 13-21 note that the financial return for experience in hospital nursing is small. The number of years spent in continuous employment with the nurse's current hospital employer has a larger impact on her hourly wage than does her general experience as a nurse.

Table 13-21 Salaries of staff R.N.s—0–10 years experience. (Note: salary refers to eight-hour day shifts.)

Variable	All hospitals	Size (beds)					Census area				Ownership		
		Under 50	50 to 99	100 to 199	200 to 399	400 and over	North-east	North central	South	West	Non-profit	Government	Proprietary
Staff R.N. monthly salary by years with hospital. No experience elsewhere:													
None:													
Diploma	$661	$628	$635	$668	$700	$718	$685	$644	$635	$702	$662	$652	$681
Associate	661	623	631	662	701	713	691	648	622	706	666	646	684
Baccalaureate	689	654	655	685	725	742	706	672	665	724	683	690	729
Two years:													
Diploma	716	665	690	721	763	792	742	692	688	770	717	713	725
Associate	723	674	695	719	759	790	746	708	682	772	724	717	737
Baccalaureate	751	701	721	742	787	814	769	728	724	795	741	759	794
Five years:													
Diploma	767	697	731	778	836	861	795	734	740	829	765	775	755
Associate	779	710	741	777	826	864	801	759	738	833	775	787	777
Baccalaureate	809	740	757	799	859	897	822	781	794	852	788	838	842
Ten years:													
Diploma	801	716	770	789	865	921	833	764	782	855	787	826	791
Associate	811	732	776	787	853	920	838	783	773	863	801	828	809
Baccalaureate	848	746	815	809	891	968	860	804	860	886	807	911	924
Staff R.N. monthly salary starting with hospital and fewer than 5 years experience:													
Diploma	691	650	664	698	732	768	713	669	668	738	689	690	703
Associate	697	655	665	691	732	768	721	680	661	742	698	691	708
Baccalaureate	721	670	687	718	751	800	735	698	705	755	711	729	759
Wage differential (% offering):													
Evening shift	77.4	58.7	77.5	89.6	89.7	82.5	89.4	74.9	74.5	74.3	81.5	72.8	72.1
Night shift	80.6	66.7	81.3	89.6	89.7	83.7	90.2	82.3	78.2	72.9	85.4	75.9	72.1

Source: DHEW, 1975.

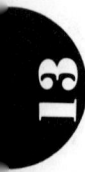

Salaries of Supervisory Nurses and General Duty Nurses*

Table 13-22   Salaries of hospital personnel by metropolitan area—All hospitals (except Federal)—(Number and average straight-time weekly or hourly earnings of full-time employees in selected occupations in nongovernment and government (non-Federal) hospitals, 21 selected areas, August 1972)

Average weekly earnings

Selected occupations	Atlanta	Baltimore	Boston	Buffalo	Chicago	Dallas	Denver	Detroit	Houston	Los Angeles–Long Beach and Anaheim–Santa Ana–Garden Grove	Memphis
Registered professional nurses:											
Directors of nursing	$302.00	$341.50	$333.50	$307.50	$335.50	$247.50	$295.50	$363.00	$249.00	$323.50	$252.50
Supervisors of nurses	206.00	241.50	242.00	232.50	243.00	210.00	223.50	248.50	206.00	258.00	203.00
Head nurses	190.00	217.50	219.00	201.00	221.00	186.50	188.00	226.50	180.50	234.00	186.00
General duty nurses	171.50	188.50	185.00	163.50	186.00	165.00	170.50	197.50	167.50	199.00	167.00
Nursing instructors	180.50	226.00	231.50	207.00	226.00	213.50	201.50	233.50	192.50	244.50	190.00
Licensed practical nurses	121.50	156.50	149.50	121.50	147.50	110.00	115.50	157.50	113.50	149.00	124.00
Nursing aides	94.00	119.50	114.50	99.50	119.50	86.50	95.00	117.00	83.00	117.00	95.50
Psychiatric aides	96.00	143.50	126.50	157.00	131.00	86.00	—	163.00	93.00	138.00	90.50
Surgical technicians	111.00	134.50	135.50	112.50	135.00	110.50	119.00	142.00	107.50	141.00	107.00

Average weekly earnings

Selected occupations	Miami	Milwaukee	Minneapolis–St. Paul	New York SMSA	New York City	Philadelphia	Portland	St. Louis	San Francisco–Oakland	Seattle–Everett	Washington
Registered professional nurses:											
Directors of nursing	$319.00	$317.00	$325.50	$364.00	$369.50	$301.00	$281.00	$273.00	$334.00	$315.50	$334.00
Supervisors of nurses	229.00	238.00	228.50	257.50	261.50	223.00	214.00	220.00	267.00	221.50	256.00
Head nurses	205.50	213.50	209.50	225.50	228.50	205.00	193.00	200.50	246.00	200.50	229.50
General duty nurses	180.00	179.00	180.00	207.50	211.00	172.50	175.00	173.00	214.00	177.00	182.50
Nursing instructors	223.00	201.50	204.50	263.00	269.50	216.50	211.50	203.50	256.50	216.00	234.50
Licensed practical nurses	126.50	132.50	132.00	156.50	157.00	134.50	135.50	128.00	164.50	121.00	139.50
Nursing aides	94.00	104.50	108.00	135.00	137.50	110.50	108.00	96.00	147.00	107.00	111.00
Psychiatric aides	—	149.00	123.50	153.50	153.50	134.50	—	105.50	161.00	108.00	116.50
Surgical technicians	111.50	128.00	126.00	152.50	155.00	128.50	133.00	111.50	166.00	119.50	139.00

*Source: U.S. Bureau of Labor Statistics, 1974.

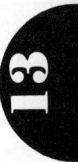

13

Table 13-23   Salaries of general duty nurses (distribution of full-time hospitals by straight-time weekly earnings,

Weekly earnings[1]	Atlanta	Balti-more	Boston	Buffalo	Chicago	Dallas	Denver	Detroit	Hous-ton
									All
Under $150	27	7	—	124	261	26	—	—	123
$150 and under $160	329	14	271	550	396	480	523	—	409
$160 and under $170	529	142	1,407	540	1,027	473	692	1	489
$170 and under $180	424	512	1,302	303	1,507	258	490	411	366
$180 and under $190	293	487	1,189	52	1,814	87	224	1,185	218
$190 and under $200	98	335	789	9	1,288	29	191	982	54
$200 and under $210	28	138	668	29	919	5	34	1,134	15
$210 and under $220	28	146	264	1	530	2	6	479	6
$220 and under $230	2	42	296	—	261	—	—	151	5
$230 and under $240	—	27	140	—	127	—	—	137	—
$240 and over	1	38	24	—	78	—	—	23	—
Number of employees	1,759	1,888	6,350	1,608	8,208	1,360	2,160	4,503	1,685
Average weekly earnings[1]	$171.50	$188.50	$185.00	$163.50	$186.00	$165.00	$168.00	$197.50	$167.50
									Nongovernment
Under $150	23	7	—	124	259	26	—	—	104
$150 and under $160	200	14	249	468	328	434	379	—	365
$160 and under $170	251	142	1,337	380	980	148	560	1	470
$170 and under $180	183	470	976	223	1,475	245	349	397	276
$180 and under $190	93	385	972	19	1,672	66	143	1,104	110
$190 and under $200	16	279	675	—	1,072	19	155	911	22
$200 and under $210	5	116	415	—	796	5	16	1,031	9
$210 and under $220	—	101	260	—	429	2	—	386	1
$220 and under $230	—	36	284	—	205	—	—	59	1
$230 and under $240	—	23	106	—	58	—	—	75	—
$240 and over	1	1	22	—	15	—	—	5	—
Number of employees	772	1,574	5,296	1,214	7,289	1,245	1,602	3,969	1,358
Average weekly earnings[1]	$167.00	$185.50	$184.00	$161.00	$184.50	$164.50	$170.00	$195.50	$165.00
									Government (non
Under $150	4	—	—	—	2	—	—	—	19
$150 and under $160	129	—	22	82	68	46	144	—	44
$160 and under $170	278	—	70	160	47	25	132	—	19
$170 and under $180	241	42	326	80	32	13	141	14	90
$180 and under $190	200	102	217	33	142	21	81	81	108
$190 and under $200	82	56	114	9	216	10	36	71	32
$200 and under $210	23	22	253	29	123	—	18	103	6
$210 and under $220	28	45	4	1	101	—	6	93	5
$220 and under $230	2	6	12	—	56	—	—	92	4
$230 and under $240	—	4	34	—	69	—	—	62	—
$240 and under $250	—	11	2	—	50	—	—	18	—
$250 and over	—	26	—	—	13	—	—	—	—
Number of employees	987	314	1,054	394	919	115	558	534	327
Average weekly earnings[1]	$175.00	$202.50	$188.00	$171.50	$199.50	$168.50	$171.00	$209.00	$178.00

[1] Earnings relate to standard salaries that are paid for standard work schedules and exclude extra pay for work on late shifts, as well as the value of room, board, or other prerequisites, if any, provided in addition to cash salaries. Average weekly earnings are rounded to the nearest half dollar.

[2] No data reported or data that do not meet publication criteria.

Source: U.S. Bureau of Labor Statistics, 1974.

general duty nurses in nongovernment and government (nonfederal)
21 selected areas, August 1972)

Los Angeles–Long Beach and Anaheim–Santa Ana–Garden Grove	Memphis	Miami	Milwaukee	Minneapolis–St. Paul	New York SMSA	Philadelphia	Portland	St. Louis	San Francisco–Oakland	Seattle–Everett	Washington
hospitals											
1	16	—	—	—	—	80	18	60	—	28	30
—	200	56	275	23	2	1,009	33	508	—	66	158
47	408	552	208	507	33	1,749	275	880	11	302	726
1,238	141	525	323	1,067	239	1,283	415	762	87	681	684
2,443	36	333	212	777	1,354	759	439	336	269	635	702
2,019	15	257	368	502	3,880	297	—	245	511	89	388
1,727	2	160	141	78	4,866	215	2	113	916	6	152
1,840	2	30	8	5	2,878	150	1	64	980	—	100
438	—	10	5	—	1,781	34	—	—	1,086	—	34
283	2	11	—	2	673	23	—	1	364	—	52
307	4	13	—	—	685	14	—	—	342	—	76
10,343	826	1,947	1,540	2,961	16,391	5,613	1,183	2,969	4,566	1,807	3,102
$199.00	$167.00	$180.00	$179.00	$180.00	$207.50	$172.50	$175.00	$173.00	$214.00	$177.00	$182.50
hospitals											
—	—	—	—	—	—	74	18	59	—	—	—
—	125	34	275	—	2	988	33	456	—	8	156
47	344	504	208	280	33	1,679	228	854	11	210	665
1,095	86	473	323	859	150	1,219	352	673	65	530	611
2,250	26	277	152	634	1,172	719	405	283	200	483	687
1,849	10	193	252	340	2,553	275	—	193	327	52	356
1,664	2	88	33	63	3,320	205	2	64	639	6	152
1,778	2	22	8	4	2,594	138	1	7	440	—	49
272	—	6	5	—	1,708	27	—	—	702	—	11
8	2	11	—	—	670	16	—	—	165	—	5
2	4	13	—	—	660	8	—	—	78	—	14
8,965	601	1,621	1,256	2,180	12,862	5,348	1,039	2,589	2,627	1,289	2,706
$196.50	$167.50	$179.00	$175.50	$180.50	$209.50	$172.50	$175.50	$171.00	$211.00	$178.00	$179.50
federal) hospitals											
1	16	—	—	—	—	6	—	1	—	28	30
—	75	—	—	23	—	21	—	52	—	58	2
—	64	—	—	227	—	70	—	26	—	92	61
143	55	—	—	208	89	64	—	89	22	151	73
193	10	—	60	143	182	40	—	53	69	152	15
170	5	—	116	162	1,327	22	—	52	184	37	32
63	—	—	108	15	1,546	10	—	49	277	—	—
62	—	—	—	1	284	12	—	57	540	—	51
166	—	—	—	—	73	7	—	—	384	—	23
275	—	—	—	2	3	7	—	1	199	—	47
277	—	—	—	—	25	6	—	—	201	—	25
28	—	—	—	—	—	—	—	—	63	—	37
1,378	225	(2)	284	781	3,529	265	(2)	380	1,939	518	396
$216.50	$165.50	(2)	$196.00	$179.00	$201.50	$180.50	(2)	$186.00	$218.00	$174.00	$200.00

13

13

Table 13-24 Salaries of newly-licensed nurses by type of educational degree held

Associate degree graduate

Salary	Total	Bos.	N.Y.	Phila.	Atla.	Chi.	Dal.	K.C.	Denver	S.F.	Seattle
Under $5,000	0%	1%	1%	1%	0%	0%	0%	0%	2%	1%	0%
$5,000–5,999	1	1	0	2	2	0	0	0	5	1	1
$6,000–6,999	5	2	3	5	10	2	8	13	12	3	4
$7,000–7,999	22	30	7	23	36	19	34	34	33	12	19
$8,000–8,999	26	27	21	32	27	29	28	21	21	18	33
$9,000–9,999	16	13	15	7	7	20	10	20	5	26	18
$10,000 +	11	9	31	9	2	12	2	1	0	14	2
Other	19	17	22	21	16	18	18	11	22	25	23
Total	100%	100%	100%	100%	100%	100%	100%	100%	100%	100%	100%

Diploma graduate

Salary	Total	Bos.	N.Y.	Phila.	Atla.	Chi.	Dal.	K.C.	Denver	S.F.	Seattle
Under $5,000	1%	0%	0%	1%	0%	1%	0%	1%	0%	2%	0%
$5,000–5,999	1	1	0	1	2	2	0	2	4	0	3
$6,000–6,999	6	4	3	7	8	6	5	14	7	6	0
$7,000–7,999	28	18	10	38	32	25	44	43	50	18	28
$8,000–8,999	30	39	28	31	34	30	14	21	22	16	22
$9,000–9,999	14	21	15	10	15	16	16	8	2	16	25
$10,000 +	10	8	34	3	3	9	5	3	0	27	11
Other	10	8	10	9	6	11	16	8	15	15	11
Total	100%	100%	100%	100%	100%	100%	100%	100%	100%	100%	100%

Baccalaureate degree graduate

Salary	Total	Bos.	N.Y.	Phila.	Atla.	Chi.	Dal.	K.C.	Denver	S.F.	Seattle
Under $5,000	1%	2%	1%	0%	0%	0%	1%	0%	2%	0%	2%
$5,000–5,999	1	0	0	0	1	0	0	0	7	2	2
$6,000–6,999	3	4	0	5	4	3	2	9	11	1	2
$7,000–7,999	17	13	8	16	30	12	26	27	37	14	14
$8,000–8,999	31	33	25	36	31	32	41	30	26	27	34
$9,000–9,999	20	22	14	19	16	27	16	20	4	24	18
$10,000 +	18	21	39	15	10	19	4	6	2	20	14
Other	9	5	13	9	8	7	10	8	11	12	14
Total	100%	100%	100%	100%	100%	100%	100%	100%	100%	100%	100%

Source: DHEW. May 1975.

Table 13-25 Starting salaries, by region

Salary	New England		Middle Atlantic		South Atlantic		East North Central		East South Central		West North Central		West South Central		Mountain		Pacific		Total	
	No.	%	No.	%	No.	%	No.	%	No.	%	No.	%	No.	%	No.	%	No.	%	No.	%
$0–4,000	0	0.0	0	0.0	0	0.0	1	0.1	0	0.0	1	0.1	0	0.0	0	0.0	0	0.0	2	*
$4,001–4,999	0	0.0	3	0.2	2	0.3	3	0.2	2	0.8	0	0.0	0	0.0	0	0.0	0	0.0	10	0.1
$5,000–5,999	1	0.1	3	0.2	12	1.8	8	0.4	1	0.4	5	0.5	1	0.4	0	0.0	1	0.7	32	0.5
$6,000–6,999	22	2.3	72	4.6	54	8.1	36	2.0	16	6.5	57	6.2	6	2.6	5	7.7	6	4.3	274	4.2
$7,000–7,999	190	20.3	396	25.1	297	44.8	370	20.7	102	41.5	332	35.8	145	61.7	38	58.5	16	11.4	1,886	28.7
$8,000–8,999	498	53.1	581	36.8	205	30.9	857	48.0	112	45.5	366	39.5	46	19.6	19	29.2	45	32.1	2,729	41.5
$9,000–9,999	200	21.3	247	15.7	82	12.4	425	23.8	13	5.3	157	17.0	33	14.0	3	4.6	46	32.9	1,206	18.3
$10,000–10,999	25	2.7	228	14.5	8	1.2	77	4.3	0	0.0	8	0.9	4	1.7	0	0.0	25	17.9	375	5.7
$11,000–11,999	1	0.1	42	2.7	3	0.4	9	0.5	0	0.0	0	0.0	0	0.0	0	0.0	1	0.7	56	0.9
$12,000–12,999	0	0.0	4	0.2	0	0.0	0	0.0	0	0.0	0	0.0	0	0.0	0	0.0	0	0.0	4	0.1
$13,000–13,999	0	0.0	1	0.1	0	0.0	1	0.1	0	0.0	0	0.0	0	0.0	0	0.0	0	0.0	2	*
Total reporting	937	100.0	1,577	100.0	663	100.0	1,787	100.0	246	100.0	926	100.0	235	100.0	65	100.0	140	100.0	6,576	100.0
Total nonreporting																			1,233	

Source: U.S. Bureau of Labor Statistics, 1974.

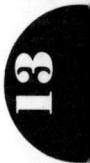

Table 13-26 Starting salaries, by type of employer

Employer	Under $4,000		$4,001–4,999		$5,000–5,999		$6,000–6,999		$7,000–7,999		$8,000–8,999		$9,000–9,999		$10,000–10,999		$11,000–11,999		$12,000–12,999		No response		Total	
	No.	%	No.	%	No.	%	No.	%	No.	%	No.	%	No.	%	No.	%	No.	%	No.	%	No.	%	No.	%
Hospital	10	100.0	29	93.5	232	91.0	1,764	97.8	2,557	98.1	1,107	95.6	351	97.8	53	98.1	4	100.0	2	100.0	601		6,710	96.1
Clinic	0	0.0	0	0.0	4	1.6	8	0.4	8	0.3	15	1.3	0	0.0	1	1.9	0	0.0	0	0.0	45		81	1.2
Military	0	0.0	0	0.0	6	2.3	2	0.1	15	0.6	15	1.3	4	1.1	0	0.0	0	0.0	0	0.0	23		65	0.9
Nursing home	0	0.0	0	0.0	6	2.3	15	0.8	10	0.4	8	0.7	1	0.3	0	0.0	0	0.0	0	0.0	13		53	0.8
Physician's office	0	0.0	2	6.5	6	2.3	8	0.4	1	*	2	0.2	1	0.3	0	0.0	0	0.0	0	0.0	13		33	0.5
Osteopathic	0	0.0	0	0.0	0	0.0	4	0.2	7	0.3	6	0.5	0	0.0	0	0.0	0	0.0	0	0.0	1		18	0.3
Prison	0	0.0	0	0.0	1	0.4	3	0.2	3	0.1	5	0.4	2	0.6	0	0.0	0	0.0	0	0.0	2		16	0.2
Industry	0	0.0	0	0.0	0	0.0	0	0.0	5	0.2	0	0.0	0	0.0	0	0.0	0	0.0	0	0.0	1		6	0.1
Total reporting†	10	100.0	31	100.0	255	100.0	1,804	100.0	2,606	100.0	1,158	100.0	359	100.0	54	100.0	4	100.0	2	100.0	699	100.0	6,982	100.0
Total nonreporting																							827	

* Less than 0.1 percent.
† Some percentages total more than 100 because students checked more than one answer; some percentages total less than 100 because some students did not answer the question.

Source: U.S. Bureau of Labor Statistics, 1974.

13

13

Table 13-27 Starting salaries, by specialty

Specialty	Under $4,000		$4,001– 4,999		$5,000– 5,999		$6,000– 6,999		$7,000– 7,999		$8,000– 8,999		$9,000– 9,999		$10,000– 10,999		$11,000– 11,999		$12,000– 12,999		No response	Total	
	No.	%	No.	%	No.	%	No.	%	No.	%	No.	%	No.	%	No.	%	No.	%	No.	%	No.	No.	%
Medical-surgical	4	36.4	12	48.0	110	49.8	743	44.9	1,087	45.1	498	45.9	145	41.9	20	42.6	2	50.0	0	0.0	281	2,902	45.1
Intensive care	2	18.2	1	4.0	25	11.3	185	11.2	276	11.4	131	12.1	33	9.5	8	12.8	0	0.0	2	100.0	71	732	11.4
Pediatrics	0	0.0	0	0.0	15	6.8	170	10.3	256	10.6	105	9.7	38	11.0	8	17.0	0	0.0	0	0.0	66	658	10.2
Obstetrics	2	18.2	3	12.0	22	10.0	159	9.6	175	7.3	79	7.3	31	9.0	6	12.8	0	0.0	0	0.0	42	519	8.1
Operating room	1	9.1	4	16.0	14	6.3	94	5.7	133	5.5	46	4.2	14	4.0	2	4.2	0	0.0	0	0.0	24	332	5.2
Emergency department	1	9.1	1	4.0	4	1.8	67	4.0	86	3.6	45	4.1	20	5.8	2	4.2	1	25.0	0	0.0	34	261	4.1
Coronary care	0	0.0	1	4.0	7	3.2	55	3.3	85	3.5	45	4.1	9	2.6	0	0.0	0	0.0	0	0.0	17	219	3.4
Orthopedics	0	0.0	0	0.0	1	0.4	37	2.2	77	3.2	30	2.8	6	1.7	0	0.0	0	0.0	0	0.0	13	164	2.5
Geriatrics	0	0.0	2	8.0	3	1.4	22	1.3	22	0.9	6	0.6	0	0.0	0	0.0	0	0.0	0	0.0	16	71	1.1
Rehabilitation	0	0.0	0	0.0	1	0.4	10	0.6	13	0.5	7	0.6	6	1.7	0	0.0	0	0.0	0	0.0	1	39	0.6
Burn care	0	0.0	0	0.0	0	0.0	5	0.3	7	0.3	1	0.1	2	0.6	0	0.0	0	0.0	0	0.0	2	16	0.2
Nursing	0	0.0	0	0.0	2	0.9	5	0.3	5	0.2	1	0.1	0	0.0	0	0.0	0	0.0	0	0.0	1	14	0.2
Public health	0	0.0	0	0.0	1	0.4	4	0.2	2	0.1	0	0.0	0	0.0	0	0.0	0	0.0	0	0.0	7	14	0.2
Midwife	0	0.0	0	0.0	0	0.0	5	0.3	3	0.1	1	0.1	1	0.3	0	0.0	0	0.0	0	0.0	3	13	0.2
Anesthesia	1	9.1	0	0.0	0	0.0	0	0.0	7	0.3	1	0.1	0	0.0	0	0.0	0	0.0	0	0.0	2	11	0.2
Clinician	0	0.0	1	4.0	0	0.0	1	0.1	1	*	1	0.1	0	0.0	0	0.0	0	0.0	0	0.0	0	4	0.1
Other	0	0.0	0	0.0	16	7.2	94	5.7	176	7.3	87	8.0	41	11.9	3	6.4	1	25.0	0	0.0	50	468	7.3
Total reporting	11	100.0	25	100.0	221	100.0	1,656	100.0	2,411	100.0	1,084	100.0	346	100.0	47	100.0	4	100.0	2	100.0	630	6,437	100.0
Total nonreporting																						1,372	

Source: U.S. Bureau of Labor Statistics, 1974.

Promotions*

A newly hired R.N. without previous experience elsewhere is estimated to spend about eight work weeks on the job before she is given the full responsibilities of her position. The estimate of the number of supervisory positions filled through internal promotion is 81.5%. In the vast majority of the hospitals, 84.4%, diploma R.N.s can frequently fill supervisory positions. This percentage decreases as bed size increases. By census area, it is highest in the South, and by ownership, highest in for-profit hospitals. See Tables 13-29 and 13-30 on following page.

Fringe Benefits*

Fringe Benefits Survey

A "typical" hospital offers its nurses the following benefits: a hospitalization plan such as Blue Cross, a major medical plan, life insurance, and retirement plans. A typical nurse receives 12 days of paid sick leave per year, six paid holidays (but probably not time off on the holiday itself), and two weeks of paid vacation after one year of employment. The typical hospital provides free (but not reserved) parking, has a reasonably priced cafeteria (but not free meals), and offers some discount on drugs and laboratory tests. The typical nurse does not have a long-term disability plan, paid maternity leave, a credit union, or a uniform allowance.

As a general rule, U.S. hospitals are more likely to provide health coverage for their nurses than are Canadian hospitals.

Putting a Dollar Value on Your Benefits

To realize the value of your fringe benefits, consider the typical figures below. They are based on dollars an employer spends on an employee whose base salary is $9,000 per year. Not every nurse, of course, will be receiving these benefits; but every nurse who is regularly employed will receive many of them. If you earn more or less than $9,000 per year, your benefits will vary upward or downward, accordingly, for the starred items.

*Source: Adapted from "Your Fringe Benefits" by Marjorie Godfrey and *Nursing '75,* May.

$526	Social Security payments employer makes for you
$9	Employer's contribution for Worker's Compensation protection for you
$84	Employer's contribution for your unemployment compensation
$123	Employer's contribution for your health insurance
$69	Employer's payments for your major medical insurance
$400	Aid for your tuition
$220	Free parking for you
$86	Employer's contribution for your disability insurance
$222	Your savings on low-cost cafeteria food
$100	Employer's payments for your life insurance
$183	Discount for your drugs
$382	Employer's contribution to pension plan for you
$433	Vacation pay
$567	Sick pay
$312	Holidays
$85	Savings on low-interest loans through credit union
$100	Uniform allowance
$2589	Total of additive items. Since these are tax-free dollars, their real value to you is approximately $3,000 ... or, if you are married and in a higher income bracket, $3,200 per year.
$1312	Pay you receive for not working (vacation, sick, and holiday time)
$3901	Total cost to your employer

Health Insurance

In the U.S., there are as many different kinds of health insurance plans as there are styles of uniforms. But most plans consist of hospitalization insurance, such as Blue Cross, offering protection against the cost of hospital care; a surgical plan offering basic protection against the cost of surgery and certain other medical services; and a major medical plan, which helps pay some of the expenses not covered in the other plans.

Major medical usually requires the employee to pay the initial costs—a specified deductible amount. After that, the carrier reimburses about 80% of the eligible charges remaining. Major medical is protection against catastrophic illness.

13

Table 13-28 Percent of promotions by institution

Variable	All hospitals	Size (beds)					Census area				Ownership		
		Under 50	50 to 99	100 to 199	200 to 399	400 and over	North-east	North Central	South	West	Non-profit	Government	Proprietary
Advancement:													
Mean days a new R.N. without experience works a job without full responsibility	39.1	28.2	35.5	42.4	48.2	53.6	45.9	38.0	37.0	37.2	41.0	38.9	30.5
Hospitals where diploma graduates can frequently fill supervisory positions	84.4	88.4	90.4	85.1	76.1	72.5	80.3	82.8	88.2	85.0	83.3	84.3	91.2
Mean percent of staff supervisory positions filled through internal promotion	81.5	70.7	82.8	85.6	86.1	84.7	83.4	81.7	82.1	78.5	81.3	82.4	79.3

Table 13-29 Opportunities for promotion to an R.N. supervisory position and R.N. professional advancement and development

Number of years with current employer	R.N. perception of percentage of full-time R.N. supervisory positions hired from outside						Hospital pays cost of tuition and related fees for continuing education					Hospital gives time off to participate in workshops, conferences				
	0–25%	26–50%	51–75%	Over 75%	Not sure	Total	Yes, and have taken advantage of this	Yes, but have not taken advantage	No	Not sure	Total	Yes, and have taken advantage of this	Yes, but have not taken advantage	No	Not sure	Total
Under 1	38.7	5.4	1.7	2.6	51.6	100.0	2.1	10.1	55.5	32.2	100.0	25.9	36.0	23.6	14.5	100.0
1	51.1	7.2	2.5	3.4	35.7	100.0	5.8	9.4	63.4	21.4	100.0	39.1	28.5	23.0	9.4	100.0
2	51.7	9.1	2.8	3.4	33.1	100.0	4.1	7.4	65.9	22.5	100.0	46.6	23.3	20.1	10.0	100.0
3	53.5	7.3	4.8	3.1	31.3	100.0	4.1	6.6	67.2	22.1	100.0	54.6	17.2	19.3	9.0	100.0
4	51.7	6.9	3.0	2.6	35.8	100.0	5.9	4.8	64.7	24.6	100.0	48.0	17.6	23.6	10.8	100.0
5	55.5	6.0	2.7	5.5	30.2	100.0	2.2	2.9	67.6	27.2	100.0	50.3	20.5	19.5	9.7	100.0
6–10	52.1	7.3	4.7	4.0	31.8	100.0	4.1	4.7	65.3	25.9	100.0	55.0	18.2	16.9	9.9	100.0
11–15	49.2	13.9	3.3	6.6	27.0	100.0	3.2	7.5	62.4	26.9	100.0	50.4	20.3	14.3	15.1	100.0
Over 15	45.1	7.1	3.5	8.8	35.4	100.0	4.1	5.2	74.2	16.5	100.0	52.3	19.5	22.7	5.4	100.0

* Source: DHEW, May 1975 (1973 data).

Health insurance of some kind is the most widely provided insurance benefit. Some 36% of U.S. nurses report contributing to the cost of such insurance, while 49% receive it free. Nine out of every ten U.S. hospitals surveyed reported providing hospitalization insurance, and some four out of every ten pay the entire premium. Major medical insurance is offered by roughly six out of ten U.S. hospitals.

Dental insurance is a relatively new idea and fairly costly to buy. About 3% of U.S. hospitals offer this protection to their employees.

Drug costs are covered by many major medical plans, but nurses get an extra break in this area; most hospitals give a discount on drugs to their employees (some 67% of the U.S. nurses).

More and more plans provide for payments covering maternity costs, abortions, and similar medical treatment for women, regardless of whether they are married or not.

Retirement Plans

These plans supplement Social Security and give regular monthly retirement income, usually beginning at age 65, although sometimes early retirement is possible at reduced benefits. The payout is based on earnings at the time of retirement and usually provides about 40% to 45% of base pay.

About three-fourths of all respondents reported having a pension plan of some kind. A third of the nurses contribute to the plan.

The larger the hospital, the more likely it is to offer a retirement plan. In the 6- to 50-bed category, 24% of the reporting hospitals had such a plan. In the 51- to 99-bed category, 61% had such plans. And in the over 100-bed category, 98% had some form of retirement plan. About one-fourth of those who offered such a plan ask nurses to contribute.

Life and Disability Insurance

Group life insurance is often made available to employees after a short waiting period, and in some cases the amount of insurance is based on salary earned by the employee.

About two-thirds of the responding U.S. nurses had hospital-provided life insurance plans. Most of the U.S. hospitals offering this coverage paid the premiums for the nurses.

Long-term disability insurance is a form of salary insurance that guarantees a monthly income to persons unable to perform their regular duties as a result of illness or injury.

(This is apart from injury sustained at or attributable to an employee's illness, which is covered by Worker's Compensation laws in both the U.S. and Canada.) Under long-term disability insurance, after a specified waiting period—which may run six months or so—the employees are paid some percentage of their regular salary.

About half of the U.S. nurses pay part of the costs themselves.

Educational Benefits

Over half of the U.S. nurses responding to the survey said they receive some financial assistance for education from their hospitals. Seven percent reported that the hospital pays all the costs, and another 45% get help.

When asked if their hospitals encourage them to seek more education, for example, by arranging work schedules so they can attend classes, almost 66% of the U.S. nurses replied they can count on their hospitals to help them in this way.

Paid Sick Leave

Twelve paid sick days a year is about standard for U.S. hospitals. Over half (57%) of the hospitals in the survey reported providing 12 paid sick days per year, accrued at the rate of one day a month.

Some hospitals reported insurance plans that take effect after a specified period of time—usually from three to five days—and which pay a percentage of salary in the neighborhood of 60% to 75%.

Maternity Benefits

Only two U.S. hospitals in the survey reported providing paid maternity leave—one in Nebraska, offering four weeks' paid leave and one in Idaho offering six weeks' leave. Many hospitals will permit employees to use accrued sick leave as paid maternity leave. Fifteen U.S. hospitals reported they give no maternity leave at all.

Hospitals were much more generous about granting unpaid maternity leave, the time varying from ten days to two years. In general, the larger the hospital, the longer the maternity leave. In hospitals of over 200 beds, almost half gave at least six months of unpaid maternity leave. Slightly less than a third of the medium-sized hospitals (51 to 199 beds) gave at least six months, and about 10% of the small (less than 50 beds) hospitals allowed at least six months. The type of hospital and its geographic location did not significantly affect the amount of maternity leave permitted, although hospitals in New York and New Jersey tend to allow a slightly longer leave time than the average.

Insurance Benefits Reported by U.S. Nurses

		U.S.
Health insurance of some kind		85%
Hospital pays all costs	49	
Nurse pays part	36	
Hospitalization insurance		91%
Hospital pays all	43	
Nurse pays part	48	
Major medical insurance		59
Hospital pays all	30	
Nurse pays part	29	
Disability insurance		53%
Hospital pays all	35	
Nurse pays part	18	
Retirement plan		74%
Hospital pays all	41	
Nurse pays part	33	
Life insurance		69%
Hospital pays all	53	
Nurse pays part	16	

Paid Time Off Reported by U.S. Nurses

Holidays	
5 days or less	11%
6 days	18
7 days	21
8 days	14
9 days	11
10 days	11
11 days	7
12 days	5
13 days	1
14 or more days	5
Average (mean) days	7.7 days
Median days	7.0
Sick Leave	
11 days or less	32%
12 days	57
13–15 days	3
16 days or more	8
Average (mean) days	14 days
Median days	12

Paid Vacation after One Year	
5 days or less	2.5%
6 to 9 days	5.5
10 days	73
11 to 14 days	6.5
15 days	7
16 to 19 days	1
20 days or more	4
Average (mean) days	10.7 days
Median days	10.0

Holidays

Only 25% of the U.S. hospitals give ten or more days. One-third of the U.S. hospitals give six or less holidays. Government hospitals tend to be more liberal than either private or non-profit hospitals. Geographically, the eastern U.S. coast hospitals observe more holidays, averaging nine paid holidays while the central sections of the U.S. range between five and seven paid holidays. The U.S. western coast is only slightly higher than average, with 7.9 paid holidays.

Most U.S. hospitals seem to pay time-and-a-half to those who work on the holiday, and straight time to those who get the day off. Some hospitals give double time to those who have to be on duty. And some hospitals just give another day off with pay to those who are scheduled to work on a holiday.

Vacation Plans

Which fringe benefit ranks highest on the worker's want list? Nurses, hospital administrators and personnel specialists all agree: it is vacation time.

Many women do, in fact, choose time off over money by choosing to work part-time, even though part-time work in the U.S. usually pays the lowest salary and rarely entitles them to the fringe benefits provided full-time workers.

Meal Allowances and Cafeteria

Almost all respondents reported availability of a cafeteria or snack shop in their hospital. Most were open 12 hours a day (45%), some open 24 hours a day (22%), and a few open only 8 hours a day (14%). A fortunate few (3%) of the nurses are provided free meals in the cafeteria, and most nurses (63%) feel the meals are reasonably priced. But a third of the nurses think the meals are too expensive.

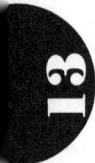

Of the hospitals surveyed, government hospitals and small hospitals were most likely to offer free or discounted meals. Some hospitals offer free meals to those on the night shift only, and at least one responding hospital gives a free cafeteria meal on the employee's birthday!

Uniform Allowance

Most nurses are on their own when it comes to buying uniforms. Only 11% of hospitals we surveyed give a uniform allowance. About $100 a year seems standard for the U.S. hospitals who make such allowance, but some pay much less.

Parking

Night nurses may sometimes get left out when it comes to cafeteria service. But they have an advantage in the parking lot, because there is plenty of space at night.

In general, most nurses appear to be content with the parking arrangements made for them. Over 80% of them have free parking and deem it to have safe accessibility. About 65% of all nurses rated "parking convenience" as either excellent or good, and only 35% found it fair or poor.

Credit Unions

Credit unions can be an enormous asset in these times of rising interest rates, since they are a source of low-cost personal loans. One nurse we talked with mentioned that she had just taken out a loan at her credit union at 8% interest.

(Of those surveyed) 64 of the 204 hospitals have credit unions—31%. As might be expected, the larger hospitals are more likely to have credit unions. More than half of the hospitals with more than 200 beds have credit unions, whereas only about a fifth of the hospitals under that size provide them. Some 36% of the nonprofit hospitals reported having a credit union; 7% of the for-profit hospitals; and rather surprisingly, only 26% of the government hospitals.

Housing

Twenty-six percent of the U.S. nurses had housing available to them, and 11% of the others could count on assistance in finding suitable housing.

Comparison of Nurses' Benefits with Others

Vacations after 1 year	Office workers receiving
Less than 1 week	Less than 0.5%
1 week	20%
1–2 weeks	1
2 weeks	76
More than 2 weeks	3

Holiday Benefits

The BLS found that office workers averaged 8.7 paid holidays in 1972. The national variations were as follows:

Continental U.S. average	8.7 days
Northeast	9.9 days
South	7.4 days
North Central	8.6 days
West	8.4 days

Differentials for Evening and Weekend Work

An earlier (*Nursing '74*) survey on salaries revealed that 84% of hospitals reporting paid differentials for evening work, with an average of 27 cents per hour more. Some 88% paid an average differential of 33 cents for night work. Only 8% of the hospitals compensated extra for weekend work, but when they did, it averaged 37 cents per hour. Large, nonprofit hospitals were the most likely to pay a differential; large, for-profit hospitals were the most generous.

Only about 30% of U.S. hospitals gave extra pay for additional training and responsibility required in specialty areas.

Hospitals' Weekend Policy for Nurses

Every weekend off	3%
Every other weekend off	51
Every third off	27
Every fourth off	5
No set policy	7

Hospital Fringe Benefits

Types of Fringe Benefits *

Work schedules: Work schedules of 40 hours a week were predominant. Major exceptions in private hospitals were Buffalo, where the typical workweek for each employment group was 37 ½ hours; and New York, where at least one-half of the employees were scheduled to work 35 or 37 ½ hours a week.

Shift differential: The proportions of registered professional nurses employed on second shifts in private hospitals ranged from slightly under one-fifth in Boston, Buffalo and Milwaukee to just over three-tenths in Dallas and Seattle. The corresponding range in government hospitals was from slightly more than one-eighth in Milwaukee, New York and Philadelphia to two-fifths in Dallas. (See tables 13-43 and 44) Between one- and two-tenths of the nurses in both hospital groups were employed on third or other late shifts at the time of the survey.

Nurses typically received extra pay for late-shift work. The amount and type of shift differential pay varied among the 21 areas. For example, in private hospitals in Boston, the typical differential for second-shift work was between 50 and 60 cents an hour above day-shift rates; in San Francisco, $15 to $20 per week; and in Miami, 10% to 15% above regular salaries.

Paid holidays: Private hospitals in Dallas commonly provided five paid holidays, compared with six days in Atlanta, Houston, and Memphis, seven days in eight areas; eight days in Chicago, Los Angeles, San Francisco, Seattle, and Washington, nine days in Baltimore, ten days in Boston and Buffalo, and twelve days in New York. In state and local government hospitals, typical provisions were usually more liberal and amounted to eleven paid holidays or more annually.

Paid vacations: Typical provisions were at least two weeks of vacation pay after one year of service, three weeks or more after five years, and at least four weeks after fifteen years. In private hospitals, provisions for more than five weeks of vacation were rare. Major exceptions were Baltimore, where about one-fifth of the

nurses received about six weeks of vacation pay after 20 years of service.

Health, insurance and retirement plans: Sick leave, usually at full pay and no waiting period, was provided to virtually all. Hospitalization, surgical, basic and major medical benefits were also provided (usually through insurance but in some instances, through care outside of insurance) to nine-tenths or more of the employees in most areas. Provisions for life insurance and accidental death and dismemberment benefits were also available to substantial proportions of nurses in a majority of areas. Government hospitals in Baltimore, Boston, Buffalo, Detroit, Memphis, Milwaukee, New York, Philadelphia, San Francisco, Seattle and Washington had hospitalization, surgical medical and major medical plans which generally provided for the extension of benefits to employees' dependents. This practice was less widespread in private hospitals.

Both private and state and local government hospitals usually provided some form of maternity benefit plan for workers. Although provisions for paid maternity leave were rare, nearly all hospitals allowed the use of paid vacation for maternity leave; similar provisions for the use of sick leave were less prevalent.

Nearly all employees in private hospitals were in establishments providing benefits under worker's compensation and unemployment insurance. Virtually all employees in government hospitals in most areas had worker's compensation benefits available. Provisions for unemployment insurance were considerably less common, ranging from all or nearly all workers in a few areas to approximately one-eighth or less in Atlanta and Los Angeles.

Some type of retirement plan applied to nearly all employees. Plans which combined private pensions with federal Social Security coverage were most common and applied to nine-tenths or more of the nurses in about one-half of the areas studied. Provisions for retirement severance pay were rare.

Education: A minority of hospitals offer refresher courses, but most state these courses are available from other sources (for example, through a state and/or regional hospital association). Slightly over half subsidize tuition costs for R.N. employees who enroll in refresher courses or courses to aid professional advancement. The vast majority of hospitals offer some form of in-service education.

---

* Source: U.S. Bureau of Labor Statistics, 1974.

Full-Time and Part-Time Employee Benefits in Hospitals

Table 13-30 Fringe benefits—full-time employees

Variable	All hospitals	Size (beds)					Census area				Ownership		
		Under 50	50 to 99	100 to 199	200 to 399	400 and over	North-east	North Central	South	West	Non-profit	Govern-ment	Proprie-tary
Fringe benefits:													
Mean days per year: full-time R.N.s													
Vacation:													
Employed 1 year	11.7	10.6	10.7	11.3	13.3	15.5	14.2	10.9	11.4	11.2	11.4	12.5	11.0
Employed 5 years	15.4	14.6	14.3	14.7	16.9	18.5	17.2	15.1	14.1	15.7	15.4	15.7	14.3
Sick leave:													
Employed 1 year	11.1	10.7	10.4	10.9	12.2	12.1	11.6	11.1	10.5	11.4	10.8	11.8	9.4
Employed 5 years	13.5	13.3	13.4	12.8	14.6	13.5	13.9	13.5	13.0	11.3	13.4	14.3	10.8
Maternity leaves:													
Providing (%)	90.8	78.3	92.5	97.0	95.7	98.7	94.7	90.2	87.7	92.9	93.1	88.9	85.3
Covering in part with sick leave (%)	34.9	30.2	35.8	34.3	30.8	51.2	31.1	29.8	41.4	36.4	28.6	46.0	27.9
Hospitals with "unsafe" parking areas (%)	0.6	0.0	1.1	0.8	0.0	1.3	0.8	0.9	0.9	0.7	0.5	1.2	1.5
Adequate or very adequate housing within walking distance (%)	42.6	36.1	40.2	52.3	44.6	42.0	50.9	42.6	36.5	43.4	47.0	36.2	40.8
Hospital housing:													
Providing (%)	10.6	5.3	6.6	7.7	17.2	27.5	25.4	5.2	9.7	6.5	12.6	10.1	1.5
Subsidizing if provided (%)													
Fully	9.0	57.1	0.0	22.2	0.0	0.0	6.5	0.0	21.1	0.0	6.8	13.6	0.0
Partially	44.8	14.3	54.5	44.2	42.1	52.4	45.2	55.6	36.8	50.0	50.0	36.4	0.0
Hospital transportation:													
Providing to parking areas (%)	2.3	1.1	0.0	0.8	5.2	1.0	3.8	2.4	1.9	1.5	1.5	2.0	1.6
Providing to other areas (%)	2.3	2.3	1.8	2.3	2.7	2.6	3.2	2.5	2.0	1.5	2.3	2.5	1.6
No distant parking areas	71.8	71.3	71.3	77.3	69.6	67.9	73.3	74.5	69.4	69.9	76.3	67.1	64.1
Day care:													
Providing (%)	2.8	0.5	3.0	3.0	9.4	5.0	1.5	2.3	5.5	0.7	3.7	1.9	1.5
Partially subsidized if provided	66.7	0.0	0.0	75.0	72.5	50.0	50.0	60.0	70.0	100.0	75.0	40.0	100.0
Life insurance:													
Providing (%)	70.1	55.9	60.7	75.2	85.3	94.9	74.4	63.8	74.0	69.8	70.2	68.9	74.6
If provided, % where													
Compulsory	31.3	20.0	25.8	34.1	39.8	39.1	42.0	28.1	29.2	29.4	37.6	19.6	38.8
Fully paid by hospital	59.6	50.5	63.1	64.6	60.4	59.2	79.6	61.7	42.1	65.2	73.0	33.3	79.2
Partially paid by hospital	26.5	32.3	20.4	21.9	30.2	28.2	16.1	25.0	36.8	21.7	19.8	38.2	20.8
Conversion to individual policy on termination is possible	74.8	73.7	71.7	72.6	77.8	80.3	72.9	74.4	79.6	69.6	74.1	75.8	75.6
Part-time R.N.s are eligible	46.7	51.0	50.5	36.2	43.3	53.6	47.1	51.2	38.0	53.3	39.3	57.3	49.0

(continued)

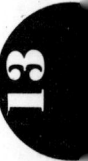

13

Table 13-30   (continued)

13

Variable	All hospitals	Size (beds)					Census area				Ownership		
		Under 50	50 to 99	100 to 199	200 to 399	400 and over	North-east	North Central	South	West	Non-profit	Govern-ment	Proprie-tary
Retirement:													
Percent of hospitals:													
All R.N.s have Social Security	92.3	95.7	96.2	93.2	90.6	76.3	91.7	93.4	90.3	94.3	98.9	80.9	98.5
Some R.N.s have Social Security	1.0	0.0	0.5	1.5	0.0	5.0	0.8	0.5	1.8	0.7	0.3	2.3	0.0
With a retirement plan	61.8	35.3	47.5	73.3	91.2	94.9	81.6	60.8	52.6	59.6	67.2	59.6	40.3
Plan is compulsory	55.3	49.1	41.9	57.0	55.8	72.7	58.2	52.5	60.4	49.3	46.7	70.1	40.0
Hospital's contribution is not lost on termination													
Regardless of employment time	17.3	22.0	16.7	25.0	13.0	9.4	15.6	20.9	18.2	13.0	15.0	22.6	8.3
Depending on employment time	38.8	33.9	38.5	36.4	40.2	45.3	45.6	36.5	33.3	41.6	46.4	24.1	54.2
Percent of time, where, after a period of time:													
All full-time R.N.s are eligible for retirement	55.9	31.2	43.9	65.7	82.9	86.3	69.7	54.9	49.5	54.3	61.4	53.6	33.8
Some part-time R.N.s are eligible for retirement	23.2	16.9	21.9	20.9	29.1	36.3	29.5	25.1	11.8	32.1	20.9	29.9	10.3
Health insurance:													
Percent of hospitals offering by type of plan:													
Basic only	27.1	30.6	28.8	32.8	19.8	16.5	27.5	34.8	24.0	20.3	28.1	27.4	20.9
Basic and major medical	58.2	49.2	55.4	56.5	64.7	78.5	57.3	51.7	63.6	60.1	56.7	58.7	64.2
Major medical only	10.1	9.3	12.5	6.9	14.7	5.1	11.5	7.2	8.3	15.9	11.8	7.5	10.4
No plan offered	4.6	10.9	3.3	3.8	0.9	0.0	3.8	6.3	4.1	3.6	3.5	6.3	4.5
Percent of hospitals with:													
A compulsory plan	15.8	12.6	14.2	14.8	18.8	23.4	15.8	17.8	38.6	27.7	48.5	34.7	16.8
A plan subsidized by hospital	86.8	81.3	84.8	89.2	91.8	90.8	92.4	79.9	85.4	93.6	87.9	82.4	96.7
Conversion to an individual policy on termination is possible	88.6	93.2	83.4	84.5	90.6	94.4	92.3	88.2	88.1	86.3	91.4	84.8	86.7
A family plan	98.9	98.7	99.4	98.4	99.1	98.7	98.4	100.0	99.0	97.7	98.6	99.1	100.0
Part-time R.N. eligibility	66.6	71.2	63.8	61.0	66.4	73.3	71.2	76.4	52.2	69.1	68.7	64.6	61.0
Sickness and disability insurance (other than worker's comp.):													
Percent of hospitals offering	35.5	27.0	26.1	41.5	48.7	48.7	53.1	33.2	29.0	32.8	41.4	27.2	34.8
If offered, percent of hospitals													
With compulsory coverage	43.5	32.6	41.3	41.2	52.8	50.0	69.8	27.9	23.3	58.5	48.6	25.4	60.9
With full subsidy	48.2	52.3	34.9	50.0	54.9	47.1	55.6	44.4	40.7	52.4	58.5	32.8	45.5
With partial subsidy	48.2	29.5	39.5	30.0	23.5	29.4	34.9	27.0	27.8	31.0	28.2	29.3	45.5
With part-time R.N. eligibility	57.2	56.8	63.0	44.0	56.9	68.4	73.8	46.2	39.3	72.1	56.8	61.7	47.6
Hospitals that subsidize moving costs (%):													
Always	3.3	5.6	4.6	0.0	2.8	1.3	1.7	1.0	6.8	3.0	2.0	5.8	1.5
Sometimes	7.7	9.0	8.1	6.3	7.4	6.5	5.0	6.8	9.8	8.3	7.3	8.6	6.2

Source: DHEW. May 1975 (1973 survey of Hospital Directors).

Table 13-31 Fringe benefits—part time employees

Variable	No. of obs.	All hospitals	Size (beds)					Census area				Ownership		
			Under 50	50 to 99	100 to 199	200 to 399	400 and over	North-east	North Central	South	West	Non-profit	Govern-ment	Proprie-tary
Part time, employed 1 year:														
Percentage of hospitals by vacation days policy:														
No vacation days	201	28.4	28.6	35.3	29.1	23.9	17.5	16.7	16.3	48.2	27.1	22.8	34.5	36.8
Fixed vacation days	177	25.0	22.2	24.1	28.4	25.6	27.5	31.1	27.9	20.5	22.1	29.6	19.2	22.1
Variable vacation days	0	0.0	0.0	0.0	0.0	0.0	0.0	0.0	0.0	0.0	0.0	0.0	0.0	0.0
No response	329	46.6	49.2	40.6	42.5	50.5	55.0	52.2	55.8	31.4	50.8	47.6	46.3	41.1
Mean vacation days if fixed days offered	177	7.6	6.7	7.1	6.3	9.5	10.1	7.9	7.6	7.9	7.0	7.0	9.4	5.7
Percentage of hospitals by sickness days policy:														
No sickness days	262	37.1	37.0	42.2	42.5	29.9	26.3	27.3	34.4	47.7	33.6	35.7	37.5	42.6
Fixed sickness days	126	17.8	16.4	15.0	19.4	22.2	18.8	25.8	15.3	15.5	17.9	21.2	13.0	17.6
Variable sickness days	127	18.0	13.8	15.0	17.9	21.4	30.0	26.5	23.3	6.4	20.0	19.0	17.6	13.2
No response	192	27.1	32.8	27.8	20.2	26.5	24.9	20.4	27.0	30.4	28.5	24.1	31.9	26.6
Mean sickness days if fixed days offered	126	7.7	7.6	7.8	7.5	7.2	9.0	7.3	7.8	7.5	8.6	7.4	9.5	5.1
Part time, employed 5 years:														
Percentage of hospitals by vacation days policy:														
No vacation days	191	27.0	27.0	33.2	29.1	21.4	17.5	15.9	17.3	45.5	26.4	20.6	34.1	35.3
Fixed vacation days	173	24.5	21.1	23.5	27.6	25.6	27.5	31.8	26.0	20.5	21.4	29.9	17.6	20.6
Variable vacation days	199	28.1	24.9	20.9	30.6	38.5	33.8	37.1	40.5	9.1	30.7	31.7	23.8	25.0
No response	144	20.4	27.0	22.4	12.7	14.5	21.2	15.2	18.2	24.9	21.5	17.8	24.5	19.1
Mean vacation days if fixed days offered	173	9.1	7.7	8.3	8.2	11.2	11.8	8.8	9.8	8.7	10.0	8.5	11.2	7.1
Percentage of hospitals by sickness days policy:														
No sickness days	250	35.4	35.4	40.6	42.5	25.6	25.0	26.5	32.1	45.4	32.9	33.3	36.8	41.2
Fixed sickness days	125	17.7	16.9	14.4	20.1	22.2	16.3	25.8	14.0	15.9	18.6	21.2	12.6	17.6
Variable sickness days	134	19.0	13.8	16.6	17.9	23.9	31.3	25.0	26.0	7.3	20.7	20.1	18.4	14.7
No response	198	27.9	33.9	28.4	19.5	28.3	27.4	22.7	27.9	31.3	27.8	25.4	32.2	26.5
Mean sickness days if fixed days offered	125	8.8	8.5	9.8	7.6	9.2	9.5	8.6	9.6	8.1	9.2	8.6	10.5	5.7

Source: DHEW. May 1975 (1973 survey of Hospital Directors).

13

Specific Benefits in Major Cities*

Table 13-32   Nongovernment hospitals: paid holidays (percent of with formal provisions for paid holidays,

Number of paid holidays	Atlanta	Balti-more	Boston	Buffalo	Chicago	Dallas	Denver	Detroit	Houston
									Registered
All employees	100	100	100	100	100	100	100	100	100
Employees in hospitals providing paid holidays	100	100	100	100	100	100	100	100	100
5 days	—	—	—	—	—	53	—	—	—
6 days	59	—	—	—	8	39	—	11	72
7 days	27	4	—	—	40	8	100	56	28
7 days plus 2 half days	—	—	—	—	—	—	—	5	—
8 days	15	15	—	8	45	—	—	15	—
9 days	—	81	—	30	7	—	—	13	—
10 days	—	—	86	63	—	—	—	—	—
10 days plus 2 half days	—	—	3	—	—	—	—	—	—
11 days	—	—	11	—	—	—	—	—	—
12 days	—	—	—	—	—	—	—	—	—
13 days	—	—	—	—	—	—	—	—	—
14 days	—	—	—	—	—	—	—	—	—

Table 13-33   Government (nonfederal) hospitals: paid holidays in hospitals with formal provisions for

Number of paid holidays	Atlanta	Balti-more	Boston	Buffalo	Chicago	Dallas	Denver	Detroit
								Registered
All employees	100	100	100	100	100	100	100	100
Employees in hospitals providing paid holidays	100	100	100	100	100	100	100	100
5 days	1	—	—	—	—	22	—	—
6 days	44	—	—	—	—	67	—	—
7 days	10	—	—	—	—	—	12	19
7 days plus 3 half days	—	—	—	—	—	—	—	—
8 days	35	—	—	—	—	—	28	10
8 days plus 1 half day	—	—	—	—	—	—	—	—
8 days plus 3 half days	—	—	—	—	—	—	—	1
9 days	—	—	—	—	—	—	—	—
9 days plus 1 half day	—	—	—	—	16	—	—	—
10 days	—	—	19	—	34	—	—	—
10 days plus 2 half days	—	—	3	—	—	—	—	18
11 days	—	—	10	59	50	—	44	3
11 days plus 1 half day	—	—	8	41	—	—	—	—
11 days plus 3 half days	—	—	—	—	—	—	—	24
12 days	10	—	60	—	—	—	17	—
12 days plus 1 half day	—	—	—	—	—	—	—	—
13 days	—	100	—	—	—	11	—	—
14 days	—	—	—	—	—	—	—	26
15 days	—	—	—	—	—	—	—	—

*Source: U.S. Bureau of Labor Statistics, 1974.

**full-time employees in selected occupational categories in hospitals
21 selected areas, August 1972)**

Los Angeles–Long Beach and Anaheim–Santa Ana–Garden Grove	Memphis	Miami	Mil-waukee	Minne-apolis–St. Paul	New York SMSA	Phila-delphia	Port-land	St. Louis	San Fran-cisco–Oakland	Seattle–Everett	Wash-ington
professional nurses											
100	100	100	100	100	100	100	100	100	100	100	100
100	100	100	100	100	100	100	100	100	100	100	100
—	—		—					—		—	—
2	49	15	28	—	—	—	4	13	—	—	—
22	51	51	49	100	—	28	96	44	—	4	21
—	—	—	—	—	—	1	—	—			
59	—	23	23	—	—	26	—	43	90	96	57
11	—	11	—	—	1	20	—	—	9	—	22
—	—	—	—	—	13	22	—	—	—	—	—
—					—						
4	—	—	—	—	29	2	—	—	—	—	—
2	—	—	—	—	53	—	—				
—	—	—	—	—	4	—	—	—	—	—	—
—	—	—	—	—	1	—	—	—	—	—	—

**(percent of full-time employees in selected occupational categories
paid holidays, 19 selected areas, August 1972)**

Houston	Los Angeles–Long Beach and Anaheim–Santa Ana–Garden Grove	Memphis	Mil-waukee	Minne-apolis–St. Paul	New York SMSA	Phila-delphia	St. Louis	San Fran-cisco–Oakland	Seattle–Everett	Wash-ington
professional nurses										
100	100	100	100	100	100	100	100	100	100	100
100	100	100	100	100	100	100	100	100	100	100
—	—	—	—	—	—	—	—	—	—	—
5	—	—	—	—	—	—	—	—	—	—
—	—	—	1	—	—	—	—	—	—	—
—	—	—	99	—	—	—	5	36	27	27
41	—	—	—	—	—	—	—	—	—	—
—	—	—	—	52	—	—	16	6	—	70
50	—	92	—	24	—	—	6	—	—	—
—	64	—	—	24	99	—	24	37	73	3
—	—	—	—	—	—	—	—	6	—	—
5	—	—	—	—	—	—	44	—	—	—
—	36	—	—	—	—	—	—	—	—	—
—	—	8	—	—	—	61	5	15	—	—
—	—	—	—	—	—	39	—	—	—	—
—	—	—	—	—	1	—	—	—	—	—

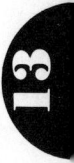

13

Table 13-34 Nongovernment hospitals: paid vacations (percent of full-time with formal provisions for paid vacations after selected

Vacation policy	Atlanta	Balti- more	Boston	Buffalo	Chicago	Dallas	Denver	Detroit	Houston
									Registered
All employees	100	100	100	100	100	100	100	100	100
Amount of vacation pay									
After 1 year of service:									
1 week	—	—	—	—	4	4	—	—	—
2 weeks	88	28	26	96	69	96	94	96	85
Over 2 and under 3 weeks	12	1	—	—	—	—	—	4	—
3 weeks	—	52	73	4	27	—	6	—	15
Over 3 and under 4 weeks	—	—	—	—	—	—	—	—	—
4 weeks	—	19	1	—	—	—	—	—	—
Over 4 weeks	—	—	—	—	—	—	—	—	—
After 2 years of service:									
1 week	—	—	—	—	4	—	—	—	—
2 weeks	81	28	19	34	69	100	34	86	85
Over 2 and under 3 weeks	12	1	—	—	—	—	5	6	—
3 weeks	7	24	80	62	25	—	61	—	15
Over 3 and under 4 weeks	—	18	—	4	3	—	—	7	—
4 weeks	—	29	1	—	—	—	—	—	—
Over 4 weeks	—	—	—	—	—	—	—	—	—
After 3 years of service:									
1 week	—	—	—	—	4	—	—	—	—
2 weeks	81	28	19	23	32	97	28	78	85
Over 2 and under 3 weeks	12	1	—	—	—	3	11	6	—
3 weeks	7	24	76	11	61	—	61	16	—
Over 3 and under 4 weeks	—	18	—	66	3	—	—	—	15
4 weeks	—	29	5	—	—	—	—	—	—
Over 4 weeks	—	—	—	—	—	—	—	—	—
After 5 years of service:									
1 week	—	—	—	—	4	—	—	—	—
2 weeks	15	7	6	5	2	42	—	5	35
Over 2 and under 3 weeks	—	—	—	—	—	3	—	2	8
3 weeks	73	36	69	19	76	56	95	89	43
Over 3 and under 4 weeks	—	—	—	4	3	—	5	—	15
4 weeks	12	39	25	72	15	—	—	4	—
Over 4 weeks	—	18	—	—	—	—	—	—	—
After 10 years of service:									
2 weeks	—	—	—	—	—	20	—	—	—
3 weeks	88	7	15	5	12	63	66	66	63
Over 3 and under 4 weeks	—	—	—	—	—	—	—	—	8
4 weeks	12	75	85	91	85	17	29	34	29
Over 4 and under 5 weeks	—	18	—	4	3	—	5	—	—
5 weeks and over	—	—	—	—	—	—	—	—	—
After 15 years of service:									
2 weeks	—	—	—	—	—	20	—	—	—
3 weeks	66	7	11	—	12	48	47	45	48
Over 3 and under 4 weeks	—	—	—	—	—	—	—	—	—
4 weeks	34	75	84	96	85	31	48	55	52
Over 4 and under 5 weeks	—	18	—	—	3	—	5	—	—
5 weeks	—	—	5	—	—	—	—	—	—
Over 5 and under 6 weeks	—	—	—	4	—	—	—	—	—
6 weeks	—	—	1	—	—	—	—	—	—
After 20 years of service:									
2 weeks	—	—	—	—	—	20	—	—	—
3 weeks	51	7	5	—	—	32	47	37	45
Over 3 and under 4 weeks	—	—	—	—	—	—	—	—	—
4 weeks	49	60	79	96	89	47	48	63	55
Over 4 and under 5 weeks	—	1	—	—	3	—	5	—	—
5 weeks	—	15	15	—	8	—	—	—	—
Over 5 and under 6 weeks	—	18	—	—	—	—	—	—	—
6 weeks	—	—	1	4	—	—	—	—	—

**employees in selected occupational categories in nongovernment hospitals
periods of service, 21 selected areas, August 1972)**

Los Angeles–Long Beach	Memphis	Miami	Milwaukee	Minneapolis–St. Paul	New York SMSA	New York City	Philadelphia	Portland	St. Louis	San Francisco–Oakland	Seattle–Everett	Washington
professional nurses												
100	100	100	100	100	100	100	100	100	100	100	100	100
95	93	72	94	100	3	—	47	100	87	97	100	70
—	—	—	—	—	—	—	—	—	—	—	—	19
5	7	28	6	—	4	—	44	—	13	3	—	4
—	—	—	—	—	—	—	—	—	—	—	—	7
—	—	—	—	—	84	89	9	—	—	—	—	—
—	—	—	—	—	8	11	—	—	—	—	—	—
85	93	53	80	—	—	—	37	100	82	9	100	46
—	—	19	—	—	—	—	—	—	5	—	—	43
15	7	28	20	100	—	—	51	—	13	91	—	4
—	—	—	—	—	—	—	—	—	—	—	—	7
—	—	—	—	—	92	89	12	—	—	—	—	—
—	—	—	—	—	8	11	—	—	—	—	—	—
84	93	30	72	—	—	—	33	100	74	6	100	35
—	—	23	—	—	—	—	—	—	5	—	—	28
16	7	47	28	100	—	—	54	—	21	94	—	25
—	—	—	—	—	—	—	—	—	—	—	—	7
—	—	—	—	—	92	89	12	—	—	—	—	4
—	—	—	—	—	8	11	—	—	—	—	—	—
6	64	7	9	—	—	—	18	4	26	—	4	10
—	—	12	—	—	—	—	8	7	10	—	—	—
93	30	60	85	—	—	—	45	—	64	16	96	71
—	—	11	—	—	—	—	—	89	—	—	—	15
1	7	11	6	100	82	76	29	—	—	84	—	4
—	—	—	—	—	18	24	—	—	—	—	—	—
—	—	2	—	—	—	—	7	4	—	—	—	—
29	93	72	75	—	—	—	48	92	81	—	4	59
4	—	—	—	—	—	—	3	—	8	—	96	8
66	7	22	25	100	79	71	39	4	11	97	—	11
—	—	—	—	—	7	9	—	—	—	—	—	14
—	—	5	—	—	15	20	3	—	—	3	—	7
15	74	63	34	—	—	—	28	7	57	—	4	34
—	3	5	—	—	—	—	3	—	—	—	—	—
81	23	21	66	100	73	71	63	85	43	14	96	44
4	—	—	—	—	7	9	—	—	—	—	—	14
—	—	5	—	—	19	19	6	4	—	85	—	—
—	—	5	—	—	1	1	—	—	—	—	—	7
—	—	2	—	—	—	—	1	4	—	—	—	—
13	74	63	14	—	—	—	28	7	35	—	4	34
—	—	5	—	—	—	—	3	—	—	—	—	—
81	26	21	86	100	68	64	63	85	60	14	96	40
4	—	—	—	—	7	9	—	—	—	—	—	14
1	—	5	—	—	25	26	6	4	5	85	—	—
—	—	—	—	—	—	—	—	—	—	—	—	12
—	—	5	—	—	1	1	—	—	—	—	—	—

Table 13-35   Government (nonfederal) hospitals: paid vacations (percent of (nonfederal) hospitals with formal provisions for paid vacations

Vacation policy	Atlanta	Baltimore	Boston	Buffalo	Chicago	Dallas	Denver	Detroit	Houston
									Registered
All employees	100	100	100	100	100	100	100	100	100
Amount of vacation pay									
After 1 year of service:									
Over 1 and under 2 weeks	7	—	—	—	—	—	—	—	—
2 weeks	83	30	58	58	37	100	12	64	50
Over 2 and under 3 weeks	—	12	—	42	—	—	17	26	—
3 weeks	10	—	42	—	4	—	72	10	50
Over 3 and under 4 weeks	—	—	—	—	—	—	—	—	—
4 weeks	—	—	—	—	43	—	—	—	—
Over 4 weeks	—	58	—	—	16	—	—	—	—
After 3 years of service:									
2 weeks	76	30	48	—	37	100	—	62	50
Over 2 and under 3 weeks	13	12	—	—	—	—	17	29	—
3 weeks	10	—	52	58	—	—	83	10	50
Over 3 and under 4 weeks	—	—	—	42	—	—	—	—	—
4 weeks	—	—	—	—	4	—	—	—	—
Over 4 and under 5 weeks	—	58	—	—	—	—	—	—	—
5 weeks and over	—	—	—	—	59	—	—	—	—
After 5 years of service:									
2 weeks	8	30	—	—	37	11	—	44	50
Over 2 and under 3 weeks	—	12	—	—	—	—	—	—	—
3 weeks	92	—	48	41	—	89	56	46	50
Over 3 and under 4 weeks	—	—	—	42	—	—	—	10	—
4 weeks	—	—	52	18	4	—	44	—	—
Over 4 and under 5 weeks	—	58	—	—	—	—	—	—	—
5 weeks and over	—	—	—	—	59	—	—	—	—
After 10 years of service:									
2 weeks	1	—	—	—	—	11	—	—	5
Over 2 and under 3 weeks	—	—	—	—	—	—	—	24	—
3 weeks	78	41	—	41	37	89	12	19	95
Over 3 and under 4 weeks	10	—	—	—	—	—	45	40	—
4 weeks	10	2	100	59	4	—	—	18	—
Over 4 and under 5 weeks	—	58	—	—	—	—	—	—	—
5 weeks	—	—	—	—	43	—	44	—	—
Over 5 and under 6 weeks	—	—	—	—	16	—	—	—	—
After 12 years of service:									
2 weeks	—	—	—	—	—	11	—	—	5
3 weeks	43	12	—	—	37	89	12	19	95
Over 3 and under 4 weeks	35	—	—	—	—	—	45	63	—
4 weeks	10	30	100	100	4	—	—	18	—
Over 4 and under 5 weeks	10	58	—	—	—	—	—	—	—
5 weeks	—	—	—	—	43	—	44	—	—
Over 5 and under 6 weeks	—	—	—	—	16	—	—	—	—
After 15 years of service:									
2 weeks	1	—	—	—	—	—	—	—	—
3 weeks	43	—	—	—	3	86	12	19	50
Over 3 and under 4 weeks	—	—	—	—	—	—	45	—	—
4 weeks	45	30	100	100	38	14	—	46	50
Over 4 and under 5 weeks	10	70	—	—	—	—	—	36	—
5 weeks	—	—	—	—	43	—	44	—	—
Over 5 and under 6 weeks	—	—	—	—	16	—	—	—	—
After 20 years of service:									
2 weeks	1	—	—	—	—	—	—	—	—
3 weeks	43	—	—	—	—	75	12	—	5
Over 3 and under 4 weeks	—	—	—	—	41	—	28	—	—
4 weeks	45	30	92	58	—	25	—	62	45
Over 4 and under 5 weeks	10	70	—	42	—	—	17	38	—
5 weeks	—	—	8	—	43	—	44	—	50
Over 5 and under 6 weeks	—	—	—	—	16	—	—	—	—
After 25 years of service:									
2 weeks	1	—	—	—	—	—	—	—	—
3 weeks	43	—	—	—	—	75	12	—	5
Over 3 and under 4 weeks	—	—	—	—	—	—	28	—	—
4 weeks	45	2	92	58	41	25	—	62	45
Over 4 and under 5 weeks	10	70	—	42	—	—	17	29	—
5 weeks	—	29	8	—	43	—	44	10	50
Over 5 and under 6 weeks	—	—	—	—	16	—	—	—	—

full-time employees in selected occupational categories in government after selected periods of service, 19 selected areas, August 1972)

Los Angeles–Long Beach	Memphis	Mil-waukee	Minne-apolis–St. Paul	New York SMSA	New York City	Phila-delphia	St. Louis	San Fran-cisco–Oakland	Seattle–Everett	Wash-ington
professional nurses										
100	100	100	100	100	100	100	100	100	100	100
—	—	—	—	—	—	—	—	—	—	—
100	84	100	8	—	—	69	27	80	27	—
—	16	—	48	19	11	14	—	4	73	100
—	—	—	—	4	—	18	73	17	—	—
—	—	—	45	—	—	—	—	—	—	—
—	—	—	—	72	89	—	—	—	—	—
—	—	—	—	5	—	—	—	—	—	—
96	—	100	—	—	—	41	12	43	27	—
—	16	—	55	—	—	14	—	4	73	30
4	84	—	—	5	—	45	88	39	—	—
—	—	—	—	18	11	—	—	—	—	—
—	—	—	45	72	89	—	—	14	—	70
—	—	—	—	5	—	—	—	—	—	—
—	—	1	—	—	—	41	6	—	—	—
—	—	—	—	—	—	14	—	—	—	—
100	84	99	48	4	—	45	94	64	100	30
—	16	—	8	19	11	—	—	—	—	—
—	—	—	—	72	89	—	—	36	—	70
—	—	—	45	5	—	—	—	—	—	—
—	—	—	—	—	—	—	—	—	—	—
—	—	—	—	—	—	12	—	—	—	—
2	84	1	48	4	—	88	100	38	—	—
82	—	—	—	1	—	—	—	20	73	3
17	—	99	—	17	11	—	—	42	27	97
—	16	—	8	5	—	—	—	—	—	—
—	—	—	—	72	89	—	—	—	—	—
—	—	—	45	—	—	—	—	—	—	—
—	84	1	24	4	—	100	100	38	—	—
83	—	—	—	—	—	—	—	20	73	3
17	—	99	24	18	11	—	—	42	10	97
—	16	—	8	5	—	—	—	—	17	—
—	—	—	—	72	89	—	—	—	—	—
—	—	—	45	—	—	—	—	—	—	—
—	—	1	—	4	—	14	50	—	—	—
4	—	—	—	—	—	—	24	4	4	3
96	84	99	48	18	11	86	—	74	10	27
—	16	—	8	5	—	—	26	17	86	—
—	—	—	—	—	—	—	—	6	—	—
—	—	—	45	72	89	—	—	—	—	70
—	—	—	—	—	—	—	5	—	—	—
4	—	—	—	—	—	—	—	—	—	3
96	84	1	48	4	—	98	71	74	14	27
—	16	—	8	23	11	—	24	20	70	—
—	—	99	—	—	—	2	—	6	17	—
—	—	—	45	72	89	—	—	—	—	70
—	—	—	—	—	—	—	5	—	—	—
—	—	—	—	—	—	—	—	—	—	3
100	—	1	48	4	—	98	71	74	10	27
—	16	—	8	23	11	—	24	20	73	—
—	84	99	—	1	—	2	—	6	17	—
—	—	—	45	72	89	—	—	—	—	70

13

Employer provisions for furnishing and cleaning uniforms	Atlanta	Balti-more	Boston	Buffalo	Chicago	Dallas	Denver	Detroit	Houston	Los Angeles
										General
Furnishes uniforms only	—	—	—	—	2	—	—	—	—	—
Cleans uniforms only	—	26	—	9	12	—	—	12	—	5
Furnishes and cleans uniforms	—	2	—	—	—	—	—	—	—	—
Cash allowance in lieu of furnishing and/or cleaning uniforms	17	5	—	—	—	3	—	—	—	—
										Nursing
Furnishes uniforms only	—	1	34	5	2	35	7	—	—	—
Cleans uniforms only	—	—	—	9	3	—	—	17	—	5
Furnishes and cleans uniforms	—	70	27	34	27	—	—	1	—	8
Cash allowance in lieu of furnishing and/or cleaning uniforms	17	7	—	—	—	15	—	—	—	—
										Licensed
Furnishes uniforms only	—	—	—	—	2	—	—	—	—	—
Cleans uniforms only	—	26	—	9	7	—	—	12	—	5
Furnishes and cleans uniforms	—	13	—	—	5	—	—	—	—	—
Cash allowance in lieu of furnishing and/or cleaning uniforms	17	7	—	—	—	3	—	—	—	—

Employer provisions for furnishing and cleaning uniforms	Atlanta	Balti-more	Boston	Buffalo	Chicago	Dallas	Denver	Detroit	Houston
									General
Furnishes uniforms only	—	—	—	—	—	—	—	17	—
Cleans uniforms only	54	59	8	61	—	—	—	9	43
Furnishes and cleans uniforms	—	—	—	—	—	—	—	—	—
Cash allowance in lieu of furnishing and/or cleaning uniforms	—	—	—	—	—	—	—	20	4
									Nursing
Furnishes uniforms only	—	—	7	—	1	—	—	47	—
Cleans uniforms only	54	25	8	61	—	—	—	9	43
Furnishes and cleans uniforms	—	72	9	—	11	—	—	—	—
Cash allowance in lieu of furnishing and/or cleaning uniforms	—	—	—	—	—	—	—	20	4
									Licensed
Furnishes uniforms only	—	—	—	—	1	—	—	47	—
Cleans uniforms only	54	59	8	61	—	—	—	9	43
Furnishes and cleans uniforms	—	—	—	—	—	—	—	—	—
Cash allowance in lieu of furnishing and/or cleaning uniforms	—	—	—	—	—	—	—	20	—

13

employees in hospitals with provisions for furnishing and cleaning uniforms
21 selected areas, August 1972)

Memphis	Miami	Mil-waukee	Minne-apolis–St. Paul	New York SMSA	New York City	Phila-delphia	Port-land	St. Louis	San Fran-cisco–Oakland	Seattle	Wash-ington
duty nurses											
3	—	—	—	17	21	2	—	—	3	—	—
—	—	—	—	—	—	2	—	—	—	—	—
—	—	—	—	36	43	—	—	—	8	6	6
aides											
—	4	—	4	—	1	14	—	—	—	—	—
3	—	—	—	2	—	4	—	—	3	—	—
—	—	—	14	71	79	12	—	—	25	—	27
—	—	—	70	15	15	—	—	—	—	6	14
practical nurses											
3	—	—	—	17	21	4	—	—	3	—	—
—	—	—	—	4	5	—	—	—	17	—	12
—	—	—	—	41	45	—	—	—	8	6	—

(percent of employees in hospitals with provisions for furnishing and
occupational groups, 19 selected areas, August 1972)

Los Angeles	Memphis	Mil-waukee	Minne-apolis–St. Paul	New York SMSA	New York City	Phila-delphia	St. Louis	San Fran-cisco–Oakland	Seattle	Wash-ington
duty nurses										
10	7	—	25	30	18	—	18	8	—	9
46	—	—	—	—	—	—	—	15	8	—
—	—	98	—	69	82	—	—	—	—	—
aides										
—	10	—	43	—	—	27	—	16	—	—
10	7	—	—	30	18	—	18	8	—	9
46	—	—	—	6	—	—	—	15	8	32
—	—	98	2	64	82	—	—	—	—	—
practical nurses										
10	7	—	25	30	18	—	18	8	—	9
46	—	—	—	—	—	—	—	15	8	—
—	—	98	—	69	82	—	—	—	—	—

13

Type of benefit and financing	Atlanta	Balti-more	Boston	Buffalo	Chicago	Dallas	Denver	Detroit	Houston
									Registered
All employees	100	100	100	100	100	100	100	100	100
Employees in hospitals providing:									
Life insurance	78	93	89	100	93	94	68	100	98
Noncontributory plans	78	88	80	100	86	54	57	79	67
Contributory plans	—	5	8	—	7	40	11	21	32
Accidental death and dis-memberment insurance	78	69	45	51	71	47	55	63	73
Noncontributory plans	78	64	42	51	66	26	44	44	39
Contributory plans	—	5	3	—	5	20	11	19	34
Sickness and accident in-surance or sick leave or both	100	100	100	100	100	95	100	100	100
Sickness and accident insurance	8	20	12	13	27	—	5	63	31
Noncontributory plans	8	20	6	13	19	—	5	43	27
Contributory plans	—	—	5	—	8	—	—	20	3
Sick leave (full pay, no waiting period)	100	100	100	91	71	87	100	96	84
Sick leave (partial pay or waiting period)	—	—	—	9	27	8	—	4	16
Hospitalization	100	100	100	100	97	100	93	100	100
Insurance	85	100	87	30	79	100	87	67	90
Noncontributory plans	34	100	48	7	49	10	5	67	62
Contributory plans	52	—	39	23	30	90	82	—	28
Care provided outside of insurance	15	—	—	—	—	—	6	—	2
Combination of insurance and care provided out-side of insurance	—	—	13	70	18	—	—	33	8
Surgical	100	93	100	100	91	100	93	100	100
Insurance	85	93	92	84	74	100	87	67	98
Noncontributory plans	34	93	43	53	47	10	5	67	70
Contributory plans	52	—	49	31	27	90	82	—	28
Care provided outside of insurance	15	—	—	—	—	—	6	—	2
Combination of insurance and care provided out-side of insurance	—	—	8	16	16	—	—	33	—
Medical	100	93	100	100	89	100	87	100	97
Insurance	85	93	92	49	69	100	87	67	95
Noncontributory plans	34	93	43	27	42	10	5	67	70
Contributory plans	52	—	49	23	27	90	82	—	24
Care provided outside of insurance	15	—	—	—	—	—	—	—	2
Combination of insurance and care provided out-side of insurance	—	—	8	51	20	—	—	33	—
Major medical	68	59	96	100	58	100	54	58	89
Insurance	54	59	88	40	49	100	54	24	81
Noncontributory plans	27	59	38	18	36	10	11	24	62
Contributory plans	27	—	50	23	13	90	42	—	18
Care provided outside of insurance	15	—	—	6	—	—	—	26	—
Combination of insurance and care provided out-side of insurance	—	—	8	54	10	—	—	7	8
Retirement plans:									
Retirement pension or Social Security or both	100	100	95	100	98	100	100	97	73
Pension (other than Social Security)	—	—	8	—	20	—	—	18	—
Noncontributory plans	—	—	4	—	17	—	—	18	—
Contributory plans	—	—	4	—	3	—	—	—	—
Social Security	7	4	—	5	7	15	19	—	6
Combination of pension and Social Security	93	96	87	95	72	85	81	79	67
Noncontributory plans	34	96	62	62	44	36	68	71	36
Contributory plans	59	—	25	33	28	49	13	8	31
Severance pay	—	—	1	—	7	—	6	4	—
Worker's compensation	100	100	100	100	98	100	100	100	100
Unemployment insurance	100	100	100	100	98	92	95	99	100

13

plans (percent of full-time employees in selected occupational categories and retirement plans, 21 selected areas, August 1972)

Los Angeles–Long Beach	Memphis	Miami	Milwaukee	Minneapolis–St. Paul	New York SMSA	Philadelphia	Portland	St. Louis	San Francisco–Oakland	Seattle–Everett	Washington
100	100	100	100	100	100	100	100	100	100	100	100
89	93	72	87	20	95	88	86	71	99	39	96
84	85	51	83	20	95	78	64	42	99	29	82
5	8	21	4	—	—	10	22	29	—	10	14
76	61	66	65	13	65	63	67	53	92	30	73
72	56	40	61	13	60	58	60	28	92	20	65
4	5	26	4	—	5	5	7	25	—	10	8
99	100	100	100	100	100	100	100	100	100	100	100
7	16	5	21	13	30	11	22	1	40	—	10
7	16	—	21	13	23	5	22	1	40	—	10
—	—	5	—	—	7	5	—	—	—	—	—
92	61	70	67	100	100	100	89	76	88	96	100
7	39	30	24	—	—	—	11	24	12	4	—
100	100	100	100	13	99	100	100	95	100	100	93
100	100	—	58	13	35	85	8	35	93	81	93
64	10	—	31	13	35	84	4	19	90	81	54
36	90	—	27	—	—	1	4	15	3	—	39
—	—	—	—	—	—	4	—	19	—	—	—
—	—	100	42	—	64	11	92	41	7	19	—
100	100	100	100	13	93	98	100	81	100	100	93
100	100	—	58	13	75	87	100	39	93	100	93
64	10	—	31	13	72	87	11	19	90	100	54
36	90	—	27	—	2	1	89	20	3	—	39
—	—	—	—	—	5	4	—	6	—	—	—
—	—	100	42	—	14	6	—	37	7	—	—
100	97	100	100	13	93	98	100	82	100	96	93
100	97	—	58	13	55	87	100	39	93	86	93
64	7	—	31	13	54	87	11	19	90	86	54
36	90	—	27	—	—	1	89	20	3	—	39
—	—	—	—	—	5	4	—	7	—	10	—
—	—	100	42	—	34	6	—	37	7	—	—
85	97	100	92	—	82	59	100	58	100	96	51
85	97	—	58	—	41	55	100	33	93	86	51
59	7	—	31	—	41	54	9	19	90	86	39
26	90	—	27	—	—	1	91	13	3	—	12
—	—	—	—	—	17	4	—	6	—	10	—
—	—	100	33	—	23	—	—	20	7	—	—
98	100	100	100	100	99	100	100	100	100	100	100
7	—	100	—	6	2	—	31	—	—	9	—
3	—	—	—	—	2	—	27	—	—	—	—
4	—	—	—	—	—	—	4	—	—	9	—
26	7	43	7	—	12	6	4	6	8	9	—
65	93	57	93	94	85	94	65	94	92	93	100
50	33	32	76	94	83	87	65	63	89	52	75
15	61	25	17	—	2	7	—	31	3	31	25
3	—	—	15	—	3	3	—	1	—	9	—
100	100	100	100	100	100	100	100	100	100	100	100
95	100	100	100	100	100	100	100	94	100	100	100

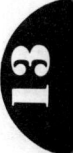

Table 13-39   Government (nonfederal) hospitals: health, insurance and categories in government (nonfederal) hospitals with specified health,

Type of benefit and insurance	Atlanta	Balti-more	Boston	Buffalo	Chicago	Dallas	Denver	Detroit
								Registered
All employees	100	100	100	100	100	100	100	100
Employees in hospitals providing:								
Life insurance	100	12	96	100	50	100	55	100
Noncontributory plans	53	12	3	100	50	89	55	43
Contributory plans	47	—	92	—	—	11	—	57
Accidental death and dismemberment insurance	69	—	96	—	—	93	12	22
Noncontributory plans	33	—	3	—	—	82	12	—
Contributory plans	36	—	92	—	—	11	—	22
Sickness and accident insurance or sick leave or both	100	100	100	100	100	100	100	100
Sickness and accident insurance	10	—	—	—	—	11	—	5
Noncontributory plans	—	—	—	—	—	11	—	—
Contributory plans	10	—	—	—	—	—	—	5
Sick leave (full pay, no waiting period)	100	100	100	100	100	93	100	100
Sick leave (partial pay or waiting period)	—	—	—	—	—	7	—	—
Hospitalization	100	100	100	100	100	100	100	100
Insurance	100	100	90	100	100	100	100	81
Noncontributory plans	58	—	—	100	100	89	—	48
Contributory plans	42	100	90	—	—	11	100	34
Care provided outside of insurance	—	—	—	—	—	—	—	—
Combination of insurance and care provided outside of insurance	—	—	10	—	—	—	—	19
Surgical	100	100	100	100	100	100	100	100
Insurance	100	100	90	100	100	100	100	81
Noncontributory plans	58	—	—	100	100	89	—	48
Contributory plans	42	100	90	—	—	11	100	34
Care provided outside of insurance	—	—	—	—	—	—	—	—
Combination of insurance and care provided outside of insurance	—	—	10	—	—	—	—	19
Medical	93	100	100	100	100	100	100	100
Insurance	93	100	90	100	100	100	100	81
Noncontributory plans	58	—	—	100	100	89	—	48
Contributory plans	35	100	90	—	—	11	100	34
Care provided outside of insurance	—	—	—	—	—	—	—	—
Combination of insurance and care provided outside of insurance	—	—	10	—	—	—	—	19
Major medical	93	100	100	100	100	100	100	57
Insurance	93	100	90	100	100	100	100	38
Noncontributory plans	23	—	—	100	100	89	—	29
Contributory plans	70	100	90	—	—	11	100	10
Care provided outside of insurance	—	—	—	—	—	—	—	19
Combination of insurance and care provided outside of insurance	—	—	10	—	—	—	—	—
Retirement plans:								
Retirement pension or Social Security or both	100	100	100	100	100	100	100	100
Pension (other than Social Security)	13	—	92	—	66	—	61	19
Noncontributory plans	13	—	—	—	—	—	—	—
Contributory plans	—	—	92	—	66	—	61	19
Social Security	11	—	—	—	—	22	12	—
Combination of pension and Social Security	76	100	8	100	34	78	28	81
Noncontributory plans	30	—	—	100	—	—	—	26
Contributory plans	45	100	8	—	34	78	28	55
Severance pay	—	—	—	—	—	—	—	—
Worker's compensation	65	100	99	100	100	25	100	100
Unemployment insurance	10	100	27	42	100	—	72	60

retirement plans (percent of full-time employees in selected occupational insurance and retirement plans, 19 selected areas, August 1972)

Houston	Los Angeles–Long Beach	Memphis	Milwaukee	Minneapolis–St. Paul	New York SMSA	Philadelphia	St. Louis	San Francisco–Oakland	Seattle–Everett	Washington
professional nurses										
100	100	100	100	100	100	100	100	100	100	100
50	82	100	100	100	94	100	56	68	86	30
5	82	84	100	100	90	100	56	45	17	27
45	—	16	—	—	4	—	—	22	70	3
10	2	16	1	100	4	86	—	36	17	30
5	2	—	1	100	—	86	—	36	17	27
5	—	16	—	—	4	—	—	—	—	3
100	100	100	100	100	100	100	100	100	100	100
—	17	—	—	—	4	20	—	—	70	—
—	17	—	—	—	4	20	—	—	—	—
—	—	—	—	—	—	—	—	—	70	—
100	100	100	100	100	100	100	100	100	100	100
50	100	100	100	100	100	100	76	100	100	100
50	100	100	100	100	100	100	76	100	100	100
46	35	—	100	100	100	100	71	61	14	3
5	65	100	—	—	—	—	5	39	86	97
—	—	—	—	—	—	—	—	—	—	—
50	100	100	100	100	100	100	76	100	100	100
50	100	100	100	100	100	100	76	100	100	100
46	35	—	100	100	100	100	71	61	14	3
5	65	100	—	—	—	—	5	39	86	97
—	—	—	—	—	—	—	—	—	—	—
50	100	100	100	100	94	100	76	100	100	100
50	100	100	100	100	94	100	56	100	100	100
46	35	—	100	100	94	100	56	61	14	3
5	65	100	—	—	—	—	—	39	86	97
—	—	—	—	—	—	—	—	—	—	—
—	—	—	—	—	—	—	21	—	—	—
45	100	100	100	100	100	100	76	100	100	100
45	100	100	100	100	100	100	76	100	100	100
41	35	—	100	100	100	100	71	61	14	3
5	65	100	—	—	—	—	5	39	86	97
—	—	—	—	—	—	—	—	—	—	—
—	—	—	—	—	—	—	—	—	—	—
100	100	100	100	100	100	100	100	100	100	100
—	34	84	—	—	—	—	—	17	—	70
—	—	—	—	—	—	—	—	—	—	—
—	34	84	—	—	—	—	—	—	—	70
—	—	—	—	—	—	—	5	—	—	—
100	66	16	100	100	100	100	95	83	100	30
41	—	—	100	48	14	88	—	42	27	—
59	66	16	—	52	86	12	95	41	73	30
—	—	—	—	—	86	—	—	—	—	—
50	100	100	100	100	100	100	35	100	100	100
54	4	100	99	52	8	57	35	54	83	73

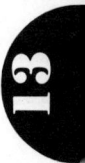

13

Table 13-40   Nongovernment hospitals: scheduled weekly hours
by scheduled weekly hours,

Weekly schedule	Atlanta	Balti-more	Boston	Buffalo	Chicago	Dallas	Denver	Detroit	Houston
									Registered
All employees	100	100	100	100	100	100	100	100	100
35 hours	—	—	—	—	—	—	—	—	—
37 ½ hours	—	8	3	95	2	—	—	—	—
Over 37 ½ and under 40 hours	—	—	5	—	—	—	—	—	—
40 hours	100	92	92	5	98	100	100	100	100

Table 13-41   Government (nonfederal) hospitals: scheduled weekly
categories by scheduled weekly hours,

Weekly schedule	Atlanta	Balti-more	Boston	Buffalo	Chicago	Dallas	Denver	Detroit	Houston
									Registered
All employees	100	100	100	100	100	100	100	100	100
35 hours	—	—	—	—	3	—	—	—	—
37 ½ hours	—	—	—	41	1	—	—	—	—
40 hours	100	100	100	59	96	100	100	100	100

**(percent of full-time employees in selected occupational categories
21 selected areas, August 1972)**

Los Angeles–Long Beach and Anaheim–Santa Ana–Garden Grove	Memphis	Miami	Milwaukee	Minneapolis–St. Paul	New York SMSA	New York City	Philadelphia	Portland	St. Louis	San Francisco–Oakland	Washington
professional nurses											
100	100	100	100	100	100	100	100	100	100	100	100
—	—	—	—	—	11	14	—	—	—	—	—
—	46	14	—	—	63	52	7	—	—	—	10
—	—	—	—	—	3	3	—	—	—	—	—
100	54	86	100	100	23	30	93	100	100	100	90

**hours (percent of full-time employees in selected occupational
19 selected areas, August 1972)**

Los Angeles–Long Beach and Anaheim–Santa Ana–Garden Grove	Memphis	Milwaukee	Minneapolis–St. Paul	New York SMSA	Philadelphia	St. Louis	San Francisco–Oakland	Seattle–Everett	Washington
professional nurses									
100	100	100	100	100	100	100	100	100	100
—	—	—	—	5	—	—	—	—	—
—	—	—	—	4	—	—	—	—	—
100	100	100	100	90	100	100	100	100	100

Table 13-42   Nongovernment hospitals: shift differential practices on late shifts by amount of pay differential,

Shift differential	Atlanta	Balti-more	Boston	Buffalo	Chicago	Dallas	Denver	Detroit	Houston
									Second
Workers employed on second shift	27.3	24.3	18.9	19.4	27.9	31.3	23.3	26.0	25.0
Receiving shift differential	23.6	22.0	18.9	16.9	27.5	29.2	23.3	26.0	23.9
Uniform cents per hour	14.3	12.5	13.9	8.0	19.1	13.7	23.0	17.5	5.1
Under 15 cents	—	—	—	1.3	1.3	—	—	1.2	—
15 and under 20 cents	—	.2	—	—	—	—	—	.4	—
20 and under 25 cents	1.8	—	—	1.6	.8	—	14.0	—	.2
25 and under 30 cents	—	.9	.2	.2	3.5	5.7	9.0	1.3	—
30 and under 40 cents	4.9	—	—	2.8	5.9	.5	—	1.1	—
40 and under 50 cents	7.7	—	1.1	—	4.0	7.4	—	.2	3.2
50 and under 60 cents	—	8.3	12.2	2.1	2.9	—	—	6.4	—
60 cents and over	—	3.1	.4	—	.8	—	—	6.9	1.7
Uniform dollars per week	9.3	—	.8	2.3	4.0	7.1	—	.7	16.4
Under $10	—	—	—	—	.7	—	—	.7	4.3
$10 and under $15	9.3	—	—	2.3	—	7.1	—	—	3.4
$15 and under $20	—	—	—	—	2.2	—	—	—	4.4
$20 and under $25	—	—	.8	—	1.0	—	—	—	4.3
$25 and over	—	—	—	—	—	—	—	—	—
Uniform percentage	—	7.5	3.6	3.9	4.4	8.4	—	4.1	.3
Under 10%	—	—	—	2.7	2.1	.5	—	2.6	.3
10 and under 15%	—	5.1	.4	1.2	2.3	.7	—	1.5	—
15% and over	—	2.4	3.3	—	—	7.2	—	—	—
Other formal paid differential	—	2.0	.5	2.7	—	—	.3	3.5	2.2
Receiving no shift differential	3.7	2.3	—	2.6	.4	2.0	—	—	1.1
									Third or
Workers employed on third or other late shift	12.0	16.2	11.3	14.2	17.7	18.9	17.6	18.8	16.7
Receiving shift differential	10.5	15.3	11.3	12.0	17.3	18.2	17.6	18.8	16.7
Uniform cents per hour	8.6	9.7	8.4	6.4	11.9	8.9	17.3	12.2	4.2
Under 15 cents	—	—	—	1.0	.5	—	—	1.1	.4
15 and under 20 cents	—	.1	—	—	—	—	—	.2	—
20 and under 25 cents	1.6	—	—	.8	.2	—	9.8	—	.2
25 and under 30 cents	—	.8	—	.5	1.7	4.3	7.4	.9	—
30 and under 40 cents	2.0	—	.1	—	3.2	.5	—	.8	—
40 and under 50 cents	5.0	.2	.7	4.1	2.7	4.0	—	.2	2.3
50 and under 60 cents	—	6.4	6.0	—	2.1	—	—	4.5	—
60 cents and over	—	2.3	1.6	—	1.4	—	—	4.6	1.4
Uniform dollars per week	1.8	—	.6	1.3	2.6	3.0	—	.5	11.0
Under $10	—	—	—	—	.6	—	—	.5	1.5
$10 and under $15	1.8	—	.5	1.3	—	3.0	—	—	3.4
$15 and under $20	—	—	—	—	1.1	—	—	—	3.7
$20 and under $25	—	—	.1	—	—	—	—	—	2.3
$25 and over	—	—	—	—	.9	—	—	—	—
Uniform percentage	—	4.5	2.0	2.8	2.5	6.3	—	4.0	.2
Under 10%	—	.4	—	2.1	.8	.1	—	2.7	—
10 and under 15%	—	1.4	.4	.6	.5	.6	—	1.2	.2
15% and over	—	2.7	1.6	—	1.2	5.6	—	—	—
Other formal paid differential	—	1.1	.3	1.6	.3	—	—	2.1	1.3
Receiving no shift differential	1.5	.9	—	2.1	.4	.7	.4	—	—

Note: Because of rounding, sums of individual items may not equal totals.

13

**for registered nurses (percent of full-time registered nurses employed
21 selected areas, August 1972)**

Los Angeles–Long Beach	Memphis	Miami	Mil-waukee	Minne-apolis–St. Paul	New York SMSA	New York City	Phila-delphia	Port-land	St. Louis	San Fran-cisco–Oakland	Seattle–Everett	Wash-ington
shift												
23.0	21.2	25.8	16.9	24.9	20.6	21.1	22.9	25.4	23.8	26.4	30.4	28.0
21.5	21.2	25.8	16.9	24.9	20.5	21.0	22.9	25.4	22.5	26.3	30.4	28.0
7.1	3.1	6.9	16.9	24.9	2.8	1.9	16.3	16.8	22.2	4.5	—	13.1
—	—	—	1.4	—	—	—	—	—	1.2	—	—	—
.1	—	.8	.6	—	—	—	1.6	1.8	1.5	—	—	—
2.0	—	.4	.9	—	—	—	2.2	—	.3	—	—	—
1.4	3.1	—	9.7	24.9	—	—	3.5	—	10.6	.1	—	—
1.1	—	—	4.3	—	—	—	4.6	15.0	8.7	—	—	—
1.2	—	1.9	—	—	—	—	1.6	—	—	4.4	—	11.2
—	—	3.8	—	—	—	—	1.8	—	—	—	—	2.0
1.3	—	—	—	—	2.8	1.9	1.0	—	—	—	—	—
10.8	11.2	7.5	—	—	15.5	16.4	2.6	8.6	—	20.0	30.4	3.1
3.2	10.2	—	—	—	—	—	.6	—	—	—	30.4	—
.7	1.0	—	—	—	—	—	1.4	7.7	—	2.0	—	—
4.0	—	—	—	—	.6	—	—	—	—	18.0	—	3.1
2.9	—	7.5	—	—	4.5	3.1	—	—	—	—	—	—
—	—	—	—	—	10.4	13.3	.6	.8	—	—	—	—
3.6	6.9	11.4	—	—	1.7	1.9	2.7	—	.2	1.8	—	6.5
1.6	4.9	—	—	—	—	—	—	—	—	1.8	—	1.8
2.0	—	11.4	—	—	.6	.8	2.7	—	.2	—	—	4.7
—	2.0	—	—	—	1.1	1.1	—	—	—	—	—	—
—	—	—	—	—	.6	.8	1.2	—	—	—	—	5.2
1.6	—	—	—	—	.1	.2	—	—	1.3	.1	—	—
late shift												
16.2	14.4	15.3	12.5	14.9	16.3	16.5	18.3	17.0	17.4	17.0	22.7	18.4
14.9	14.4	15.3	12.5	14.9	16.2	16.4	18.3	17.0	16.6	16.9	22.7	18.4
4.7	1.0	4.5	12.5	14.9	2.0	1.5	13.2	12.2	16.3	3.4	—	9.4
.3	—	—	.4	—	—	—	3.2	.9	1.2	—	—	—
—	—	—	.4	—	—	—	.4	—	1.0	—	—	—
1.5	—	.3	1.8	—	—	—	.2	—	.2	—	—	—
.6	—	.8	6.0	14.9	—	—	3.0	—	5.3	.1	—	—
.7	—	—	3.9	—	—	—	2.9	11.3	8.2	—	—	—
.7	—	1.2	—	—	—	—	.3	—	.4	3.3	—	7.9
—	1.0	2.2	—	—	—	—	2.0	—	—	—	—	1.4
.8	—	—	—	—	2.0	1.5	1.2	—	—	—	—	—
7.7	7.3	5.8	—	—	12.5	12.7	2.3	4.8	—	12.8	22.7	1.6
2.8	—	—	—	—	—	—	.3	—	—	—	22.7	—
.8	7.3	—	—	—	.6	—	1.4	3.9	—	.9	—	—
2.2	—	—	—	—	.4	.5	—	—	—	11.8	—	1.6
1.8	—	4.7	—	—	3.6	2.1	—	—	—	—	—	—
—	—	1.1	—	—	7.9	10.2	.6	.8	—	—	—	—
2.3	6.2	5.0	—	—	1.4	1.6	1.6	—	.2	.8	—	5.3
1.6	4.9	—	—	—	—	—	—	—	.2	.8	—	—
.7	—	4.0	—	—	.8	.8	1.6	—	—	—	—	5.3
—	1.2	.9	—	—	.6	.8	—	—	—	—	—	—
.2	—	—	—	—	.4	.6	1.2	—	—	—	—	2.2
1.3	—	—	—	—	.1	.1	—	—	.9	.1	—	—

13

Table 13-43   Government (nonfederal) hospitals: shift differential employed on late shifts by amount of pay

Shift differential	Atlanta	Balti-more	Boston	Buffalo	Chicago	Dallas	Denver	Detroit	Houston
									Second
Workers employed on second shift	27.6	25.4	21.8	18.7	22.9	42.4	24.9	21.3	25.4
Receiving shift differential	27.4	25.4	21.8	14.4	22.4	42.4	21.5	21.3	24.5
Uniform cents per hour	12.7	—	21.0	12.6	—	5.3	21.5	17.1	—
Under 25 cents	—	—	—	4.4	—	—	11.1	—	—
25 and under 30 cents	8.4	—	—	8.2	—	5.3	—	.4	—
30 and under 50 cents	4.2	—	2.1	—	—	—	10.4	8.0	—
50 cents and over	—	—	18.8	—	—	—	—	8.7	—
Uniform dollars per week	14.8	25.4	.8	1.8	22.4	1.2	—	3.6	12.4
Under $10	—	.3	—	1.8	4.4	1.2	—	3.6	—
$10 and under $20	14.8	4.1	.8	—	—	—	—	—	12.4
$20 and over	—	21.0	—	—	18.0	—	—	—	—
Uniform percentage	—	—	—	—	—	35.8	—	.6	12.2
5%	—	—	—	—	—	—	—	.6	—
10%	—	—	—	—	—	35.8	—	—	12.2
Other formal paid differential	—	—	—	—	—	—	—	—	—
Receiving no shift differential	.2	—	—	4.3	.5	—	3.4	—	.8
									Third or
Workers employed on third or other late shift	18.5	21.0	15.9	17.3	16.0	23.5	14.7	20.8	16.0
Receiving shift differential	18.4	21.0	15.9	9.9	15.5	23.5	13.1	20.8	15.4
Uniform cents per hour	8.9	—	15.3	7.6	—	4.5	13.1	13.0	—
Under 25 cents	—	—	—	—	—	—	6.3	—	—
25 and under 30 cents	2.7	—	—	7.6	—	4.5	—	.2	—
30 and under 50 cents	3.8	—	1.3	—	—	—	6.8	8.5	—
50 cents and over	2.5	—	14.0	—	—	—	—	4.3	—
Uniform dollars per week	9.5	21.0	.6	2.3	15.5	.8	—	3.6	6.3
Under $10	—	.2	—	2.3	3.7	.8	—	3.6	—
$10 and under $20	9.5	5.9	.6	—	—	—	—	—	6.3
$20 and over	—	15.0	—	—	11.8	—	—	—	—
Uniform percentage	—	—	—	—	—	18.1	—	.6	9.1
5%	—	—	—	—	—	—	—	.6	—
8%	—	—	—	—	—	—	—	—	—
10%	—	—	—	—	—	18.1	—	—	9.1
Other formal paid differential	—	—	—	—	—	—	—	3.6	—
Receiving no shift differential	.2	—	—	7.4	.4	—	1.7	—	.6

[1]Data for state and local government hospitals did not meet publication criteria in Miami and Portland.
Note: Because of rounding, sums of individual items may not equal totals.

13

practices for registered nurses (percent of full-time registered nurses differential, 19 selected areas,[1] August 1972)

Los Angeles–Long Beach	Memphis	Milwaukee	Minneapolis–St. Paul	New York SMSA	New York City	Philadelphia	St. Louis	San Francisco–Oakland	Seattle–Everett	Washington
shift										
26.1	27.8	14.3	28.0	13.7	12.8	13.9	21.0	23.9	26.0	25.2
26.1	27.8	14.3	13.3	11.0	11.2	6.0	18.2	23.9	26.0	25.2
22.5	—	14.3	13.3	—	—	1.5	—	8.5	1.0	21.1
.5	—	—	—	—	—	1.5	—	—	1.0	12.0
—	—	14.3	13.3	—	—	—	—	—	—	—
22.1	—	—	—	—	—	—	—	8.5	—	9.1
—	—	—	—	—	—	—	—	—	—	—
—	25.9	—	—	1.9	.2	—	—	7.3	25.1	—
—	1.0	—	—	.2	.2	—	—	—	25.1	—
—	24.9	—	—	1.1	—	—	—	7.3	—	—
—	—	—	—	.7	—	—	—	—	—	—
3.6	—	—	—	—	—	4.6	18.2	5.4	—	4.0
3.6	—	—	—	—	—	—	—	—	—	—
—	—	—	—	—	—	4.6	18.2	5.4	—	4.0
—	1.9	—	—	9.1	11.0	—	—	2.7	—	—
—	—	—	14.7	2.7	1.6	7.8	2.8	—	—	—
other late shift										
20.8	20.1	9.5	15.4	10.1	9.3	11.9	19.6	17.9	13.7	20.5
20.8	19.1	9.3	8.0	7.5	7.7	5.8	17.8	17.9	13.7	20.5
18.1	—	9.3	8.0	—	—	1.3	—	6.7	1.1	16.4
.4	—	—	—	—	—	1.3	—	—	1.1	12.0
—	—	9.3	8.0	—	—	—	—	—	—	—
17.7	—	—	—	—	—	—	—	6.7	—	4.4
—	—	—	—	—	—	—	—	—	—	—
—	17.2	—	—	1.3	.3	—	.7	3.0	12.6	—
—	—	—	—	.2	.3	—	—	—	12.6	—
—	1.3	—	—	.8	—	—	.7	3.0	—	—
—	15.9	—	—	.3	—	—	—	—	—	—
2.7	—	—	—	—	—	4.6	17.1	6.9	—	4.0
2.7	—	—	—	—	—	—	—	1.9	—	—
—	—	—	—	—	—	1.5	—	—	—	—
—	—	—	—	—	—	3.1	17.1	5.0	—	4.0
—	1.9	—	—	6.2	7.4	—	—	1.4	—	—
—	1.0	.2	7.3	2.6	1.5	6.0	1.7	—	—	—

13

262

The Value of Specific Fringe Benefits to Nurses*

To determine the relative value of specific fringe benefits to nurses a national survey was conducted by HEW in 1973.

Of all items in both lists, nurses appear to be most concerned about increases in patient load. Opportunities for professional advancement are valued second highest and are stressed particularly by blacks and baccalaureates. By contrast, recent hires place little emphasis on this, probably because they do not expect to remain with the hospital employer as long. Health insurance benefits rank third with nurses.

Many R.N.s do not know whether their hospitals pay the cost of tuition and related fees for continuing education, and very few have taken advantage of such an offering. This implied lack of interest suggests that these tuition payments are not highly valued by R.N.s. A week of vacation is generally valued, particularly among single nurses.

*Source: DHEW, May 1975.

A State Nurses' Association Recommended Minimum Standards for Professional Nurses**

Employment

A standard procedure for preemployment interviews should be established. When accepted for employment, a letter of confirmation including the title of the position and salary concepts should be given to the nurse with all terms of employment discussed and explained. Written copies of the personnel policies and job description should be provided for each new employee. The job description should include definition of the job and detailed responsibilities and qualifications required. Essential is an organized plan for orientation to the work setting and position responsibilities within that agency. Information regarding criteria for continued employment and promotional opportunities should be provided.

**Source: Virginia Nurses' Association, October 1976.

Table 13-44   Tradeoffs between wages, fringes and working conditions

Question	Mean equivalent monthly salary increase ($)		
	All R.N.s	R.N.s with young children	Black R.N.s
What raise in your salary would you regard as equivalent to one of these new fringe benefits?			
(Additional) term insurance on your life with death benefit of $25,000. Hospital pays the entire premium	18.48	19.43	26.31
An (additional) week of vacation	53.50	47.68	57.25
An (additional) week of sick leave	38.64	35.48	60.66
(Additional) $100 per month of retirement benefits at age 65. You pay nothing	29.80	26.08	33.70
Day care services for your children at no cost to you	24.64	51.91	36.09
Better parking facilities	8.78	7.86	22.61
What salary increases would compensate for the loss of these fringe benefits?			
Maternity leaves of absence removed	35.47	45.97	54.09
All opportunities for professional advancement with present employer removed	70.32	72.50	102.39
All in-service education benefits removed	40.54	41.04	53.88
All opportunities to determine your own scheduling removed	57.69	63.36	59.54
All health insurance benefits removed	64.58	57.58	91.99
Your patient load increased 25%	94.86	91.59	122.17

13

Personnel Policies

All employing agencies should have written personnel policies which are reviewed and upgraded annually in cooperation with the nursing staff. Recommendations for inclusion are:

- *Equal Opportunity:* Race, creed, color, sex or age should not be considered in hiring, placement, promotion, salary determination or other terms of employment.
- *Hours of Work:* A two-week work period should not exceed 80 hours. Nurses required to work overtime should be compensated according to provisions of the Fair Labor Standards Act, which includes compensatory time, if allowable and desired. Time schedules should be prepared in four-week blocks and posted at least two weeks in advance.
- *Salary Concepts:* Salary scales for each category of employment should be equivalent to salaries paid to comparable professionals. Education and experience of the nurse should be considered in selecting the appropriate step of the salary scale at the time of employment. (Refer to Recommended Salary Ranges attached.)
- *Differential for Shifts:* At least an additional 10% of the salary should be provided for evening and night tours of duty.
- *On Call Service:* One-fourth of the straight time hourly rate for "on call" emergency service should be provided, with time and one-half the straight time rate or compensatory time off for hours worked while on call.
- *Part-Time:* Salaries and fringe benefits should be provided in accordance with full-time employees for regularly scheduled part-time nurses in the same job title.
- *Temporary Assignment to Higher Position:* Temporary assignment is defined as filling the position of another who is on leave of absence, educational leave or long term illness, until such time as the absent employee returns to work or is permanently replaced. The appropriate rate of pay for the higher position should be provided.
- *Differentials for Position:* Each category of position should pay a sufficient differential to compensate for increasing complexity and level of responsibility.
- *Annual Job Performance and Salary Review:* A minimum of a 5½% increase based on professional growth and merit should be granted. Each nurse is entitled to an annual performance review with the im-

mediate supervisor. Cost of living adjustments should be considered separately.

- *Employee Grievance Procedure:* A grievance means any request or complaint which involves the interpretation or application of or compliance with the employment policies. A grievance may be initiated by one or more employees. Established written procedures which are given to all employees should be developed whereby employees may discuss concerns and dissatisfactions with the appropriate level of management. When properly implemented, this procedure will assist greatly in recruiting and retaining employees, establishing and maintaining a satisfying work situation.
- *Termination of Employment:*
  1. Staff Nurse:
     a. At least 14 days' written notice of resignation should be given by the nurse. Reason for resignation should be given.
     b. At least 14 days' written notice of dismissal or salary in lieu thereof would be given to the nurse by the employer. The employer should state the reasons for dismissal.
  2. Nurses in Supervisory or Administrative Positions:
     a. At least 30 days' written notice of resignation should be given by the nurse. Reasons for resignation should be given.
     b. At least 30 days' written notice of dismissal or salary in lieu thereof should be given by the employer. The employer should state the reasons for dismissal.
  3. There should be a termination interview which should become a part of the employee's permanent personnel record with the employer.
  4. Should it become necessary for an employer to immediately terminate a nurse's employment for a violation of the Nurse Practice Act, the employer should inform the Virginia State Board of Nursing (the legal body empowered to prosecute violators) documenting the circumstances necessitating the dismissal.

Benefits

Employee benefits constitute an essential part of the written personnel policies. Benefits should include:

13

- *Preemployment and Annual Health Examination* at no cost to the employee.
- *Social Security* coverage.
- *A Retirement Policy* with employer contributions.
- *Group Medical Insurances* paid by the employer for the employee.
- *Sick Leave:* One day of paid sick leave for each month of employment, to be accumulated indefinitely.
- *Holidays:* At least seven holidays per year plus one personal day with pay. If the holiday occurs on a regular day off or during a vacation period, one day should be added. If required to work on a recognized holiday, one compensatory day should be allowed.
- *Vacations:* One day per month for each month worked for employees with less than three years' service; one and one-quarter days for employees with more than three years' service; and one and one-half days for employees with five years' service. Accumulated vacation may be used after three continuous months of employment. If terminated after six months, employee should receive payment for accumulated leave. Vacation cumulative to 45 days.
- *Leave of Absence:* An approved leave of absence should be arranged in writing between the nurse and the employer and should not result in loss of tenure or accrued benefits.
- *Emergency Leave:* Up to three days with pay for critical illness or death in the immediate family should be granted.
- *Military Leave* should be granted to maintain status in the military forces.
- *Educational Leave:* Time off with half pay and at least 50% reimbursement of tuition should be provided after two years' employment, with a contractual agreement for continuing employment.
- *Jury Duty:* Supplemental pay to equal the nurse's regular rate should be provided for jury duty.
- *Expenses:* Reimbursement for travel and other predetermined, authorized expenses should be made when necessary to fulfill the responsibilities of employment.
- *Automobile Transportation:* If car ownership is a prerequisite for employment, then the nurse should be reimbursed as follows:

  To cover operating costs, a minimum of $90.00 flat monthly allowance, plus 17 cents per mile in excess of 400 miles driven in agency business.

If a nurse is required to use her personal car to transport others (students, clients, staff, etc.), the employing agency should assume responsibility for the liability insurance. If the nurse uses her car occasionally she should be reimbursed at 17 cents per mile.
- *Security Parking:* It is recommended that employers provide protected parking facilities for nurses.
- *Nursery:* Where conducive to recruitment and retention of nurses, it is recommended that employers provide nurseries.
- *Offices and Clerical Assistance:* Adequate office space and clerical assistance should be provided.

Job Satisfaction*

In a national survey of newly licensed nurses conducted by HEW in 1975 it was found that many nurses currently employed in one type of institution would actually prefer another type of employer.

Table 13-45   Job dissatisfaction

Present employer	% preferring another type of employer	1st choice of another employer
Public hospital	22%	Private hospital
Private hospital	33	Public hospital
Nursing home	67	Public hospital

Utilization of Skills

The majority (51%) of newly licensed nurses feel that their skills are adequately utilized. However, this is not a feeling mutually held by graduates of baccalaureate programs. While the majority of diploma (55%), A.D. (52%) and P.N.s (53%) report their skills are adequately utilized, a minority (42%) of baccalaureate graduates report this. Baccalaureate graduates (40%), more than the graduates from any other type of nursing program, report that their skills are underutilized. This finding is of particular interest in light of the fact that baccalaureate graduates had frequently complained about being "pushed into responsibilities too soon." In essence, baccalaureate graduates were, on one hand, complaining that their skills were underutilized, and on the other hand, complaining that they were getting too much responsibility.

---

*Source: DHEW, May 1975.

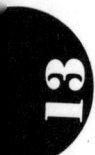

Table 13-46   Utilization of skills by type of program

Utilization	Type of program				
	Total	Bacc.	A.D.	Dipl.	P.N.
Underutilized	30%	40%	23%	29%	33%
Adequately utilized	51	42	52	55	53
Insufficient preparation	7	7	10	5	4
Insufficient background and experience	10	8	13	9	8
Other	2	3	2	2	2
Total	100%	100%	100%	100%	100%
N	(5,655)	(1,082)	(1,457)	(1,832)	(1,284)

Table 13-47   Comparison of types of employers by utilization of skills

Type of employer	N	Utilization of skills					
		Skills adeq. utilz.	Skills under- utilz.	Insuf. prep.	Insuf. bkkg. & exp.	Other	Total
Hos—Pub	(3,565)	50%	26%	7%	10%	7%	100%
Hos—Pvt	(1,496)	48	27	7	10	8	100
Nsg Home	(290)	38	42	3	6	11	100
Govt PH	(151)	39	36	7	7	11	100
Vol PH	(42)	50	33	—	10	7	100
PH MXD	(23)	57	26	9	4	4	100
Cmuty	(48)	38	44	—	6	12	100
Bd Ed	(10)	20	30	30	—	20	100
Sch Nsg	(21)	48	24	10	14	4	100
Indus	(20)	35	45	5	5	10	100
Pvt Duty	(30)	33	40	3	10	14	100
Ofc Nsg	(151)	37	38	7	5	13	100
Miltry	(148)	43	39	4	7	7	100
Other	(74)	34	37	2	5	22	100

Source: DHEW, May 1975.

13

14
NURSING PRACTICE

Whom to Serve?

Unlike most employees the nurse is beset by competing demands not only on her services but also for her priority concern. Aaron Levenstein in *Supervisor Nurse* speaks of:

1. The needs of the patient.
2. The needs of peers.
3. The needs of subordinates.
4. The needs of one's superior.
5. The needs of the department or unit.
6. The needs of support personnel.
7. The needs of the hospital as an entity in itself—its own economic and survival needs.
8. The needs of the physicians.
9. The needs of the community served by the hospital.
10. The needs of the patient's family.
11. The needs of the profession.
12. The needs of one's self.

American Nurses' Association Standards of Nursing Practice*

The ANA Standards focus on practice. However, they are not intended to imply that practice consists of a series of discrete steps, taken in strict sequence, beginning with assessment and ending with evaluation. The processes described are used concurrently and recurrently. These Standards for Nursing Practice apply to nursing practice in any setting.

Standard I

THE COLLECTION OF DATA ABOUT THE HEALTH STATUS OF THE CLIENT/PATIENT IS SYSTEMATIC AND CONTINUOUS. THE DATA ARE ACCESSIBLE, COMMUNICATED AND RECORDED.

Rationale—Comprehensive care requires complete and ongoing collection of data about the client/patient to determine the nursing care

---

*Source: American Nurses' Association, Publication Code NP-41, 1973.

needs of the client/patient. All health status data about the client/patient must be available for all members of the health care team.

Assessment Factors—

1. Health status data include:
   - Growth and development
   - Biophysical status
   - Emotional status
   - Cultural, religious, socioeconomic background
   - Performance of activities of daily living
   - Patterns of coping
   - Interaction patterns
   - Client's/patient's perception of and satisfaction with his health status
   - Client/patient health goals
   - Environment (physical, social, emotional, ecological)
   - Available and accessible human and material resources
2. Data are collected from:
   - Client/patient, family, significant others
   - Health care personnel
   - Individuals within the immediate environment and/or the community
3. Data are obtained by:
   - Interview
   - Examination
   - Observation
   - Reading records, reports, etc.
4. There is a format for the collection of data which:
   - Provides for a systematic collection of data
   - Facilitates the completeness of data collection
5. Continuous collection of data is evident by:
   - Frequent updating
   - Recording of changes in health status
6. The data are:
   - Accessible on the client/patient records
   - Retrievable from record-keeping systems
   - Confidential when appropriate

Standard II

NURSING DIAGNOSES ARE DERIVED FROM HEALTH STATUS DATA.

Rationale—The health status of the client/patient is the basis for determining the nursing care needs. The data are analyzed and compared to norms when possible.

Assessment Factors—

1. The client's/patient's health status is compared to the norm in order to determine if there is a deviation from the norm and the degree and direction of deviation.
2. The client's/patient's capabilities and limitations are identified.
3. The nursing diagnoses are related to and congruent with the diagnoses of all other professionals caring for the client/patient.

Standard III

THE PLAN OF NURSING CARE INCLUDES GOALS DERIVED FROM THE NURSING DIAGNOSES.
   Rationale—The determination of the results to be achieved is an essential part of planning care.
   Assessment Factors—

1. Goals are mutually set with the client/patient and pertinent others:
   - They are congruent with other planned therapies.
   - They are stated in realistic and measurable terms.
   - They are assigned a time period for achievement.
2. Goals are established to maximize functional capabilities and are congruent with:
   - Growth and development
   - Biophysical status
   - Behavioral patterns
   - Human and material resources

Standard IV

THE PLAN OF NURSING CARE INCLUDES PRIORITIES AND THE PRESCRIBED NURSING APPROACHES OR MEASURES TO ACHIEVE THE GOALS DERIVED FROM THE NURSING DIAGNOSES.
   Rationale—Nursing actions are planned to promote, maintain and restore the client's/patient's well-being.
   Assessment Factors—

1. Physiological measures are planned to manage (prevent or control) specific patient problems and are related to the nursing diagnoses and goals of care, e.g., ADL, use of self-help devices, etc.

2. Psychosocial measures are specific to the client's/patient's nursing care problem and to the nursing care goals, e.g., techniques to control aggression, motivation.
3. Teaching-learning principles are incorporated into the plan of care and objectives for learning stated in behavioral terms, e.g., specification of content for learner's level, reinforcement, readiness, etc.
4. Approaches are planned to provide for a therapeutic environment:
   - Physical environmental factors are used to influence the therapeutic environment, e.g., control of noise, control of temperature, etc.
   - Psychosocial measures are used to structure the environment for therapeutic ends, e.g., paternal participation in all phases of the maternity experience.
   - Group behaviors are used to structure interaction and influence the therapeutic environment, e.g., conformity, ethos, territorial rights, locomotion, etc.
5. Approaches are specified for orientation of the client/patient to:
   - New roles and relationships
   - Relevant health (human and material) resources.
   - Modifications in plan of nursing care
   - Relationship of modifications in nursing care plan to the total care plan
6. The plan of nursing care includes the utilization of available and appropriate resources:
   - Human resources—other health personnel
   - Material resources
   - Community
7. The plan includes an ordered sequence of nursing actions.
8. Nursing approaches are planned on the basis of current scientific knowledge.

Standard V

NURSING ACTIONS PROVIDE FOR CLIENT/PATIENT PARTICIPATION IN HEALTH PROMOTION, MAINTENANCE AND RESTORATION.
   Rationale—The client/patient and family are continually involved in nursing care.

Assessment Factors—

1. The client/patient and family are kept informed about:
   - Current health status
   - Changes in health status
   - Total health care plan
   - Nursing care plan
   - Roles of health care personnel
   - Health care resources
2. The client/patient and family are provided with the information needed to make decisions and choices about:
   - Promoting, maintaining and restoring health
   - Seeking and utilizing appropriate health care personnel
   - Maintaining and using health care resources

Standard VI

NURSING ACTIONS ASSIST THE CLIENT/PATIENT TO MAXIMIZE HIS HEALTH CAPABILITIES.

Rationale—Nursing actions are designed to promote, maintain and restore health.

Assessment Factors—

1. Nursing actions:
   - Are consistent with the plan of care.
   - Are based on scientific principles.
   - Are individualized to the specific situation.
   - Are used to provide a safe and therapeutic environment.
   - Employ teaching-learning opportunities for the client/patient.
   - Include utilization of appropriate resources.
2. Nursing actions are directed by the client's/patient's physical, physiological, psychological and social behavior associated with:
   - Ingestion of food, fluid and nutrients.
   - Elimination of body wastes and excesses in fluid.
   - Locomotion and exercise.
   - Regulatory mechanisms—body heat, metabolism.

- Relating to others.
- Self-actualization.

Standard VII

THE CLIENT'S/PATIENT'S PROGRESS OR LACK OF PROGRESS TOWARD GOAL ACHIEVEMENT IS DETERMINED BY THE CLIENT/PATIENT AND THE NURSE.

Rationale—The quality of nursing care depends upon comprehensive and intelligent determination of nursing's impact upon the health status of the client/patient. The client/patient is an essential part of this determination.

Assessment Factors—

1. Current data about the client/patient are used to measure his progress toward goal achievement.
2. Nursing actions are analyzed for their effectiveness in the goal achievement of the client/patient.
3. The client/patient evaluates nursing actions and goal achievement.
4. Provision is made for nursing follow-up of a particular client/patient to determine the long-term effects of nursing care.

Standard VIII

THE CLIENT'S/PATIENT'S PROGRESS OR LACK OF PROGRESS TOWARD GOAL ACHIEVEMENT DIRECTS REASSESSMENT, REORDERING OF PRIORITIES, NEW GOAL SETTING AND REVISION OF THE PLAN OF NURSING CARE.

Rationale—The nursing process remains the same, but the input of new information may dictate new or revised approaches.

Assessment Factors—

1. Reassessment is directed by goal achievement or lack of goal achievement.
2. New priorities and goals are determined and additional nursing approaches are prescribed appropriately.
3. New nursing actions are accurately and appropriately initiated.

14

Patient Care

Typical Nursing Functions

Table 14-1   Ten functions commonly performed by R.N.s

	% of hospitals by bed size					% of hospitals by geographic location				
	Under 100	100–199	200–299	300–399	400 up	East	South	Mid-west	West	South-west
Give IV medications	99%	97%	96%	91%	94%	91%	98%	99%	99%	98%
Transcribe doctors' orders	91	81	71	69	61	84	82	84	87	89
Do catheterizations	81	80	85	88	72	90	68	89	83	67
Check patients' input/output	53	60	68	69	51	72	45	59	61	44
Give mouth care	25	33	52	67	44	56	26	30	34	22
Give enemas	22	30	43	45	36	55	17	26	29	18
Take temperatures	21	28	36	43	32	47	20	24	26	17
Serve meal trays	22	23	29	31	31	31	14	26	29	20
Make beds	14	20	31	38	35	47	14	16	19	8
Clean discharge units	6	5	4	2	3	8	1	6	9	3

Based on 1,425 responses. Percentages add up to more than 100% because of multiple responses.

Source: "The Nurse Supply: Shortage or Surplus." Reprinted from *RN Magazine,* June 1974. Copyright © 1974 by Medical Economics Co., Oradell, N.J. 07649. All rights reserved.

In the relatively prosperous East, the largest percentages of hospitals use R.N.s for all ten functions. Hospitals in the West rank second in this respect.

Primary Care

Under a primary care nursing program, each patient coming into the hospital has a registered nurse assigned to his case to take overall responsibility for seeing that the patient gets all of the treatment, medication and tests scheduled for him, has all questions answered, and is generally cared for as a person, not just a body in a hospital room.

This program allows registered nurses to be involved directly in a patient's care, rather than merely acting as unit organizers who delegate care duties to practical nurses, aides and others.

It also means that the majority of a patient's care is provided by one nurse, not a new one every day. This fosters a relationship between nurse and patient which makes it more likely that patients will voice problems and fears and indicate when they need more information.

"Vital Signs"*

Merely recording the temperature, pulse, respiration and blood pressure is far from enough. The signs must be interpreted—their meaning and the measures to take. Taking and assessing vital signs is a serial process, not a one-time affair. Because variation, after all —variation from the norm, variation from the patient's norm, variation from the patient's last reading—that is what vital signs are all about. Know what's normal for your patient and learn his vital signs from the previous shift . . . gather vital signs as often as you think necessary . . . establish trends and compare changes.

Take your data on the patient's vital signs and put it together with his diagnosis, lab tests, history and charted records. Then analyze the information in terms of his complete health status. Do you see any relationships among the data? Do you see any trends evolving? Are any of the abnormal vital signs you've found to be expected because of the patient's condition?

---

*Source: C. M. Jarvis, RN, "Vital Signs," *Nursing '76,* April.

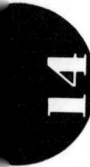

14

Temperature

As for the antiquated habit of waking your patients for a 6 a.m. check, one authority recommends this: take temperatures routinely between 4 and 8 p.m., and check early morning temperatures *only* on patients who had a fever above 99.5° F. the previous evening, or on those who have had surgery the day before or will have it that day.

The normal oral range in a resting patient is 97.7° to 99.5° F. (36.5° to 37.5° C.). Rectal temperatures register 1° F. higher. Both are usually 1° to 2° F. lower in early morning than in late afternoon.

A slight fever is normal for a day or two after surgery. Fever is commonest evidence of postoperative complications, usually (1) pulmonary, (2) wound infection, (3) urinary infection or (4) thrombophlebitis.

In the beginning, the fever patient may have cool limbs; this means his superficial blood vessels are constricted to conserve heat, and his skin may appear pale or mottled. He may complain of feeling cold; he may shiver and shake with chills. A light blanket keeps him comfortable without increasing his temperature. But once the production of heat brings the body temperature up to the hypothalamic thermostat setting, he will no longer complain of cold. Then he will have frankly feverish signs.

As a disease process stops, the hypothalamus setting returns to normal. Now the body's temperature is high enough for its own cooling mechanisms to be brought into play. General vasodilation reddens the skin and makes it hot to the touch. Intense sweating now cools the body by evaporation.

Pulse

Each beat of the heart pumps blood into an already full aorta, flaring its walls and generating a fluid wave through the arteries: this wave is the pulse. The heart normally beats about 70 times a minute to send 5 liters of blood through the adult body. This cardiac output equals the volume of blood in each systole—the stroke volume—times the rate per minute: $CO = SV \times R$. When the stroke volume lessens (as in shock), the rate increases, keeping the cardiac output constant.

You can normally see pulsations in the neck of a recumbent patient, either as the brisk localized throbbing of the carotid artery, or the diffuse undulant pulsation of the jugular vein. These pulsations ordinarily disappear as the patient is elevated to a sitting position, usually at 45°.

Next, palpate the peripheral artery, using the pads of the first three fingers. Completely occlude the artery and release it gradually. For routine signs, the radial artery is usually the most accessible and can be easily compressed against the radius. In small children, the temporal artery is useful.

You palpate the radial pulse not merely to determine its rate, but to assess the rhythm, force or amplitude and quality, as well as elasticity.

Rate. Count the pulse for 30 seconds and multiply by two. But if you find any irregularities, then check it for at least a minute. For the resting adult, 60 to 100 beats a minute are normal, slightly faster in women than men, faster still in infants and children. There is also a mild increase in old age.

Pain, as well as anger, fear and anxiety all increase the heart rate by stimulating the sympathetic nervous system. Congestive heart failure, anemia and fever all require greater oxygenation, therefore greater cardiac output. So does exercise.

Force or amplitude. The pulse pressure is the difference between systolic and diastolic pressure; amplitude is a reflection of pulse strength. Stroke volume increases with certain conditions such as anxiety, alcohol intake or exercise.

Respiration

The *quality* of normal relaxed breathing is effortless, automatic, regular and even and almost silent.

Rate and depth make up the type of respiration. The normal rate at rest is 12–18 breaths per minute in adults; more rapid rates are normal in infants and children. The ratio of pulse to respirations is fairly constant, about 5:1. Count the respiratory rate for at least 30 seconds, and for a full minute if you suspect any abnormality.

The depth is the volume of air moving in and out with each respiration. This *tidal volume* is normally about 500 cc in the adult, and should be constant with each breath.

The lungs' function is to maintain homeostasis of arterial blood. By retaining or venting

14

carbon dioxide, respiration, helped by the kidneys, maintains the pH of the blood.

Blood Pressure

Blood flows from heart to artery to capillary to vein by differences in their internal pressure, pressure being least in the veins. These vascular pressures are controlled by the vasomotor center in the medulla oblongata: this center signals for constriction or expansion of the muscular walls of the vessels. This alters pressure and, so, circulation—by shrinking or enlarging the container. Mostly the difference is temporary. Sometimes, by reason of physiologic change, it lasts.

Blood pressure climbs with age, as it does with weight gain, continued stress, or anxiety. Most likely to develop hypertension are people living in urban environments, those subjected to emotional distress, U.S. blacks, and women (two to one over men). Exercise drives blood pressure up temporarily, as does pain or rage. So, for a longer time, do several disease states.

Shock, myocardial infarction and hemorrhage are among the things that *drop* it, because through them, cardiac output or peripheral vessel resistance are reduced, or venous return is lessened after fluid loss.

You can expect the blood pressure to be an index to:

- elasticity of the arterial walls;
- peripheral vascular resistance;
- efficiency of the heart as a pump;
- blood volume.

When you take a blood pressure reading, you measure the *systolic* pressure, the *diastolic* pressure, and by subtraction, the *pulse pressure*, the difference between them. A reasonable systolic pressure—the maximum exertion against the arteries by the left ventricular systole—is a clue to the integrity of heart, arteries, and arterioles. The diastolic pressure, constantly present on the arterial walls, directly indicates blood vessel resistance. The pulse pressure tends to parallel the cardiac stroke volume.

But remember just the same, a single blood pressure reading is *almost always inaccurate*. You must know the average vital signs for your patient before you attach significance to one isolated figure.

The average blood pressure in a young adult—but often variable at that—is 120/80 mm Hg. The World Health Organization defines hypertension as a persistent elevation above 140/90; hypotension in adults is often given as below 95/60. Even so, hypotension in the healthy adult, shown as a persistent systolic pressure of 90 to 100 but without accompanying symptoms, is no cause for alarm.

Everybody's blood pressure is usually lowest in the early morning, after sleep. It rises after meals, during exercise, or with emotional upset. It is lower when lying down than when sitting or standing. And it is a little higher in the lower extremities. But whether you are going to take a sitting or supine reading, keep the patient in a stable, relaxed position for 5–10 minutes, and be sure he hasn't eaten or exercised for 30. Also be sure his arm is at heart level.

Taking the pressure. Put the center of the cuff over the brachial artery, and wrap the cuff evenly. Palpate the radial artery, inflate the cuff as rapidly as possible until the pulse you are feeling is gone, and then pump for an extra 20–30 mm Hg beyond that.

Place the diaphragm of your stethoscope over the brachial artery and release the cuff at a rate of 2 mm Hg per heartbeat. The systolic pressure is the reading at the *first return* of the sound.

As the cuff is released, you'll hear a damping or *muffling* of the sound. The American Heart Association accepts this as the most accurate index of diastolic pressure, but recommends recording both that and the *final distinct sound* as the complete record, so: 120/80/78.

Hypertension comes with such factors as kidney disease, coarctation of the aorta, viscous blood (such as that in polycythemia), or endocrine disorders, among them pheochromocytoma, an adrenal tumor causing headache, blurred vision, sweating, palpitations, and rapid heartbeat. There is a strong familial tendency for hypertension.

Hypotension occurs when the total blood volume is decreased, as it is in shock from hemorrhage, burns, vomiting, diarrhea, metabolic acidosis, heat exhaustion, or Addisonian crisis.

90-Second Emergency Patient Assessment*

The following outline was developed for the nurses at Illinois Masonic Medical Center in Chicago to aid them in performing systematic

*Source: Karen Eckstein, RN, "Initial Rapid Assessment," *JEN*, May–June 1976.

and thorough assessments [in emergency cases]. Once the nurse has committed this system to memory the complete evaluation can be done in minutes, hence it has been called the "90-second physical assessment."

Once the airway, breathing, and circulation of the emergency patient have been assessed, the nurse must make a complete (and rapid) evaluation of the patient's condition to determine if other problems exist which require medical attention.

1. Check for injuries. Ask patient to remain as he is until asked to move.
   A. Talk
      1. Introduction
         a. Alertness
         b. Orientation
      2. Reassure patient
      3. Make physical contact
      4. Check for medical tags
   B. Observe
      1. Complexion
         a. Flushed—may indicate hypertension, excitement, fever, poisoning
         b. Pale—circulatory problem
         c. Cyanotic—respiratory or ventilatory problem
         d. Jaundice
      2. Respiration: depth, sound, rate rhythm
         a. Airway obstruction
      3. Bleeding and/or other discharge
      4. Swelling or deformities
      5. Reactions: nervousness or restlessness
      6. Functional check—deep breath, cough (ability to follow simple commands)
   C. Feel
      1. Skin—diaphoretic or dry; warm or cold
      2. Surface check—skeletal integrity, evidence of bleeding
      3. Articulation check—passive and active
   D. Smell (presence or absence of)
      1. Stool and/or urine
      2. Alcohol
      3. Acetone
      4. Emesis
2. Systems Check
   A. Head
      1. Check scalp
         a. Feel, looking for indentations, bumps, lacerations
         b. Check hands for blood

2. Consider cervical injury
3. Check ears for:
   a. Bright red blood—look for local injury
   b. Thin watery fluid—cerebral spinal fluid
   c. Dark clotted blood
   d. Check ear lobes for color
4. Check nose
   a. Look for bright red blood
   b. Look for cerebral spinal fluid
5. Check mouth
   a. Look for broken teeth, dentures, partials
      i. Bring in any knocked out teeth
   b. Check patient's bite
   c. Look for fluid
      i. Bright red blood
      ii. Bright foamy blood
      iii. Coffee ground material
      iv. Cerebral spinal fluid
      v. Mucous
6. Check eyes
   a. Check pupils
   b. Check ability to follow and rotate eyes
   c. Remember possibility of glass eye and contacts
   d. Jaundice—present or absent in sclera
7. Check face
   a. Check cranial and facial nerves
      i. Ability to smile
      ii. Ability to wrinkle forehead
      iii. Ability to stick out tongue
      iv. Ability to see, hear, smell
   B. Check collarbone
      1. Feel for fractures
      2. Observe for bruises
   C. Arms
      1. Check from shoulder to hands—check pulse
      2. Feel and look for obvious deformities
      3. Check hands for blood
   D. Chest
      1. Observe for symmetry of movement, retraction; listen with stethoscope
      2. Depress sternum gently—observe for pain
      3. Place hands on lateral sides of ribs and gently push in—observe for pain
      4. Observe for crepitus (sub-g emphysema)
      5. Check hands for blood
   E. Abdomen
      1. Feel for softness or rigidity

14

2. Look for distention
3. Place hands on iliac crests, push in gently, checking for pain
4. Place hands on symphysis pubis and push down gently, checking for pain
5. Check for obvious injury and bruises

F. Legs
1. Begin at groin and check legs down to toes
2. Check for pulses—femoral, dorsalis pedis
3. Observe position of extremities
4. Check for color and temperature
5. Check hands for blood

G. Articulation check
1. Ask patient to move all extremities—compare movements of arms and legs

H. Vertebral check
1. Check vertebrae of entire spine, cervical to coccyx
   a. Avoid moving neck of suspect cervical injury
2. Check paravertebral areas for tightness and pain

Understanding the Patient

Patients' Reactions To Illness*

The Nature of Illness—The same illness can hold different meanings for different individuals. What one person dreads may not particularly frighten someone else.... The prognosis, severity and expected length of illness are additional concerns.

The Nature of the Patient—A patient's responses to illness are largely determined by his characteristic responses to anxiety.... One individual may calmly accept his fate and treatment, another with the same diagnosis may become disorganized, depressed, argumentative ... A person's ideas about himself will also determine his reaction to his illness.... For some people, illness is more a life pattern than health is.... Other things influence individual reactions: age, social class, general state of personal happiness, financial position and number of past illnesses.

The Attitude of Others—The attitudes of other people toward a patient's illness are ob-

*Source: Joan Luckmann and K. Sorenson, *Medical-Surgical Nursing: A Psychophysiological Approach* (W. B. Saunders Co., 1974) (Adapted from Chapters 10 and 11).

vious to him and will influence his self-image and his own reaction to his illness.... If the patient's illness is socially unacceptable—for example, venereal diseases—he may feel rejected, "dirty," and victimized. Communicable diseases such as tuberculosis and leprosy provoke fear in many people ... they may shun a patient with such illnesses.

The Patient's Own Attitudes—Illness disrupts a patient's normal living and disturbs his self-image.... He may try to solve his problem by using defensive patterns that worked for him in the past but are inappropriate now ... [such actions] may actually alienate him from those caring for him.

Anxiety— ... Any disease means the failure, more or less, of the organism. Complete failure, of course, is death. Anxious feelings, then, are actually feelings of concern for one's life and well-being.... The specific causes of anxiety vary from person to person, probably because they're associated with many unconscious thoughts and feelings that each person has repressed and inhibited up to that time.

Shock—Many people also experience a period of shock when they first learn of their diagnosis, particularly if the illness is serious. They feel immobilized; things seem unreal and dream-like.... Often, shock makes people incapable of thinking clearly or acting rationally ... they may act automatically, like robots.

Denial—Denial of illness ... often continues long after the initial shock has passed. "I'm not really sick" "How could I possibly have cancer?" "I don't believe it." ... the denying patient is not being stubborn ... [It] is generally a frightened attempt by the patient to fend off overwhelming threats.

Suspicion—The patient who is suspicious has not completely closed his mind to the truth. He tries ... to find many possible reasons for doubting his diagnosis.... Some patients will be suspicious if their diagnoses are serious, while others will be suspicious if they aren't serious.

Questioning—"Why me? Why did I have to get this? ..." People who are ill often scan their lives trying to find answers to such questions, believing that there must be a reason or purpose for their illness ... some find answers ... such as: illness is a punishment for sin; illness results from neglecting one's health; or illness is predestined and is in one's best interest.

Insignificance and Loneliness—Illness makes a patient feel insignificant ... also alone in facing his problems. Illness brings with it the realization that we all pass through life in separate orbits.

Regression and Dependency—Regression ... can be ... beneficial ... by allowing the patient to be more dependent than usual. By allowing himself to rest and be cared for, the patient can restore his strength and progress to health.... Regression often acts as a defensive device against stress. Under stress, all organisms tend to assume a less differentiated, more primitive way of life.... It is a kind of strategic retreat of the organism to mobilize new forces of resistance and regeneration.... Expect patients to regress to levels of behavior that are not as mature as usual.

Shame and Guilt—[Some] patients believe that their illnesses are a punishment for sin or wrongdoing.... Some people feel that they shame their families by having certain "unacceptable" conditions (such as mental disorders, epilepsy ...).

Rejection—Illness may precipitate feelings of being rejected. Illnesses ... such as communicable diseases, cause the patient to be rejected and isolated. Prolonged illnesses create many feelings of rejection in the patient's personal life, as family and friends may begin to take the illness for granted and proceed with their own lives.

Fear—Fears that accompany a dreaded disease ... *Fear of:*

- a strange place;
- equipment;
- pain, loss of body parts, or mutilation;
- being "experimented" on;
- being abused, neglected or treated impersonally;
- being left alone or isolated from loved ones;
- loss of function or loss of self-control;
- death;
- burdening others.

A fearful patient may be hostile to others; he is on the defensive and trying to protect himself.

Withdrawal and Depression—Withdrawal and depression commonly occur as reactions to diagnosis and illness ... Usually the depressed person looks sad or shows little expression. He may neglect personal hygiene ... [his] body appears to be slowed down or not working properly, appetite may be poor, apt to lose weight. He may attempt to take his life ... may show signs of sloth, weariness, exhaustion ... or may be hyperactive: pacing, moving about, picking rapidly at the bed clothing. A severely depressed patient longs for escape from his situation. ... His thoughts center

around despair, hopelessness, isolation ... he is apt to withdraw from others. Patients under the stress of serious or terminal illnesses frequently fear "losing their minds" because they can't endure their situations.

Paradoxical Reactions—[Patients] may joke about their condition, even though it is extremely serious. Patients with neurotic tendencies may appear relieved to learn that they are ill or that they require surgery.

Nurses' Reactions to Patient Suffering*

Many nurses speak about a shift from the idealism of school to the realism of practice, a shift from a kind of universal sympathy to more controlled and selective reactions. Some respond particularly to the young, some to the old, others to those who remind them of parents or friends.

The nature of the illness makes a tremendous difference in the nurse's reaction. She responds most strongly to those who are likely to die or be severely disabled. By and large, much less sympathy is felt for patients with minor illnesses, and those who don't have a "legitimate" complaint.

Sometimes the nurse's own personal experiences make a significant difference in her response to particular patients. Having gone through similar experiences, a nurse may be especially sensitive or "tuned in" to a patient's suffering.

Continuous complaints, if they are seen as unwarranted, are frustrating. For the nurse constantly faced with these complaints, irritation, annoyance and anger are not uncommon responses. In addition to feeling angry, the nurse typically avoids the complainer. Some nurses delay their responses; others respond, but don't hear what the patient says.

For some nurses not involved in psychiatric nursing, patients with emotional problems tend to elicit relatively little sympathy. Part of the nurse's difficulty in dealing with emotional problems is her feelings of helplessness or inadequacy in relieving this kind of suffering. She can administer medication to reduce physical pain, but she doesn't have similarly effective and efficient techniques for relieving psychological distress.

---

*Source: Lois J. and Joel R. Davitz, "How Do Nurses Feel When Patients Suffer?" *American Journal of Nursing,* September 1975. © American Journal of Nursing Company.

The effects of daily experience with the suffering of others is not only felt at work. Nurses often reported that they took patients' problems "home with them."

Frequently, the need for emotional distance developed as a result of experience with a patient for whom the nurse felt especially sympathetic and who subsequently died, leaving the nurse feeling drained, traumatized and ineffective.

Thus, to maintain their own emotional stability and remain effective in professional practice, nurses build psychological defenses against overinvolvement. These defenses typically involve establishing some emotional distance. But specific defensive reactions take many forms, including, for example, seemingly macabre but psychologically meaningful hospital humor.

Reactions to Death and Dying

Of all the daily problems encountered by nurses, the death of a patient is emotionally the most devastating. Even after years of professional experience, nurses described their reactions to the death of a patient with whom they have worked in terms of feelings of helplessness, depression, anger and despair. The death of young people is especially traumatic for many nurses.

When a patient with whom the nurse has been closely involved is dying, a common reaction reported is a desire to escape from the situation—though physical escape itself often does not relieve the nurse's own sense of emotional distress.

The trauma of death is reduced somewhat when the patient is elderly and the nurse senses that the person is "ready to die."

In addition to the nurse's immediate emotional reactions, the experience of the death of a patient also affects the nurse's thoughts and feelings about her own death and her reflections about herself and her life.

(This selection is based on a survey of 200 nurses in New York metropolitan hospitals.)

Psychological Aspects of Patient Care*

A patient's behavior during an illness is not always governed by the seriousness of the illness. Instead, it may be determined by the

---

* Source: Joanna Magda Polenz, "Psychological Aspects of Patient Care," *Nursing Care*, October 1975.

person's perception of the illness which, in turn, may be influenced not only by the present reality but also by past experiences. All patients have feelings about being ill and hospitalized; these feelings of anxiety, fear or sadness about being ill will always be present. Helping the patient accept and understand his feelings is part of good patient care.

Psychological factors are associated with all illnesses. Some patients come to the hospital suffering from conditions which have been largely caused by psychological factors. In some cases the actual stresses of the patient's life bring on the illness.

Stress contributes to the severity of asthma, ulcers, ulcerative colitis, high blood pressure, arthritic conditions, skin conditions, and many others. In the management of patients whose illnesses are caused or made worse by psychological factors, taking those factors into account is most important.

How Very Anxious Patients May Behave

The behavior of a patient influenced by feelings about being ill and being hospitalized may not be what it appears to be.

The quiet, uncomplaining patient from whom one hears very little is often viewed as a good, cooperative patient. Actually he may be immobilized by fear. Some patients are too afraid to ask when they don't understand instructions they are to follow. Such patients often do not exercise, do not move, are not noticed, and develop physical complications of hospitalization such as blood clots and pneumonia. These overly quiet patients are often people frozen with anxiety.

The overactive patient may not be a brave, vigorous person but one who is risking his chances for recovery by being too independent. He never asks for anything,' always takes care of himself, comes to the nurses' station for his medicine, takes care of his toilet needs. Often this person is so afraid of being sick or dependent that he denies his illness to the extent that he pushes himself too hard and jeopardizes his chances for recovery. This is particularly dangerous for patients who need rest: those with cardiac conditions or those recovering from cardiac infarctions.

Every nurse is familiar with the rude, hostile, aggressive patient who yells, swears and curses and is generally very unpleasant and uncooperative. These are often people who are terrified of being sick. They cannot tolerate being dependent and may have had unhappy experiences when they were small children. They equate their illness and being dependent with their childhood experiences.

The noisy, flirtatious, rambunctious patient is frequently responding to unconscious needs and fears which may also arise from childhood experiences. This is the person who feels his adulthood and his sexual identity threatened by being ill or hospitalized.

Special Groups With Special Problems

Children are not as verbal as adults so they communicate more by behavior than speech. It therefore becomes very important to understand the meaning of young children's behavior. Common signs of distress in children are regression and withdrawal. Regression means a return to more infantile behavior—whining, crying, soiling, demanding the bottle. These are signs of loneliness, anxiety and sadness. They are not necessarily signs of naughtiness and should not be handled as such. The young child needs support and reassurance, not scolding. Withdrawal and passivity are more serious signs of distress in young children. While these children are often easier to nurse because they allow things to be done to them and don't protest too much, this is a very bad psychological reaction in children. They need extra attention because they are showing signs of serious distress.

One frequently notices that when parents come to visit on the pediatric floor, the children are more difficult to manage. This is a normal reaction. Children feel more secure with their own parents and freer to express themselves. Since children express their feelings through behavior, they very often become more rambunctious when their parents are visiting. This makes nursing difficult, but frequently parental visits are the best thing for pediatric patients. Young children often misunderstand hospitalization and see it as abandonment. It can become a very serious psychological stress for them. They need to see their parents to feel reassured.

Adolescents are often very difficult patients, particularly when they suffer from chronic or potentially fatal illnesses. They often seem so rude and uncooperative that they appear stupid. They often behave in a daredevil manner, taking great chances. These patients are usually not rude or bad. Overwhelmed with anxiety, they are afraid of their illnesses, resentful of being sick, fearful that they will be mutilated or die. They are afraid they will be rejected by their families and friends because of their illnesses.

They become uncooperative and unwise about following instructions because they are using denial. They pretend they are not ill: they take risks to prove to themselves they are okay, and will not die.

The pregnant patient is influenced by the external reality: is it a wanted, planned and appropriate pregnancy or an unwanted and inappropriate one? The woman's internal psychological reality may also play a role: how does she see herself as a woman, as a mother?

Old age is often a sad time, a time of loneliness, a time of ill health and approaching death. When patients are helped to cope with their feelings about aging, much unpleasant behavior in old people becomes manageable. When elderly patients are more comfortable, happier and less afraid, they become less hostile and less quarrelsome.

Phobias

The following phobias may be observed among patients in the hospital environment.

air currents	aerophobia
alone, being	momophobia
bacilli	bacillophobia
bacteria	bacteriophobia
blood, sight of	hemophobia
bodies, dead	necrophobia
body, naked	gymnophobia
bound, being	merinthophobia
carcinoma	carcinophobia
childbirth	maieusiophobia
choking	pnigophobia
confined space	calustrophobia
contamination	molysmophobia
	mysophobia
darkness	achuluophobia
	nyctophobia
death	thanatophobia
disease	nosophobia
disorder	ataxiophobia
eating	sitiophobia
falling asleep	hypnophobia
filth	mysophobia
	rhypophobia
heart disease	cardiophobia
height	acrophobia
infection	molysmophobia

insane, becoming	lyssophobia
lice, infestation	pediculophobia
lightning	astraphobia
	keraunophobia
medicine, taking	pharmacophobia
needles	belonephobia
night	noctiphobia
noise	phonophobia
pain, seeing or feeling	algophobia
	odynophobia
physical contact	aphephobia
	haphephobia
people, deformed	teratophobia
poisoned, being	toxicophobia
sex	genophobia
silence, night	nyctophobia
sounds	acousticophobia
thunder	brontophobia
	tonitrophobia
uncleanliness, personal	automysophobia
vaccination	vaccinophobia
venereal infection	cypridophobia
	venereophobia
vomiting	emetophobia

improvement. Only 36% felt that fellow nurses gave good or excellent psychological support. One respondent suggested a reason for this: "The physical is stressed as all important. If we're found sitting in a patient's room offering support, we're not considered to be working—just talking."

Where you currently work, how would you rate the performance of your nurse coworkers (where applicable) in the following aspects of patient care?

	Excellent	Good	Fair	Poor
Physical care	20%	57%	20%	3%
Rehabilitation	9	38	40	13
Patient psychological support	8	28	42	22
Patient education	7	30	41	22
Discharge planning	7	26	38	29
Psychological support to relatives	7	23	40	30

Quality of Care

An Evaluation by 10,000 Nurses*

What is your opinion about the overall quality of care patients receive today?

Excellent	3%
Good	50%
Fair	42%
Poor	5%

The majority of the sample felt that not only were they very competent in delivering quality care, but that their nursing coworkers, as you'll see below, deserved high marks for the *physical care* they deliver.

Psychological support for patients and relatives, though, would seem to call for much

Doctors appear to be even more remiss when it comes to the patients' psychological needs. Only 23% of the respondents rated the doctors they work with as excellent or good in providing this.

Rate the doctors you work with.

	Very good	Good	Fair	Poor
Overall physical care	28%	53%	17%	2%

	Excellent	Good	Fair	Poor
Psychological support given to patients	4	19	45	32

How to explain? The more demanding specialties, such as ICU/CCU and emergency, require more technical skill—delivered under more pressure—and therefore create more opportunities for incompetence to manifest itself.

*Sources: G. R. Funkhouse & *Nursing '76,* "Quality of Care," *Nursing '76,* December; "Quality of Care," *Nursing '77,* January.

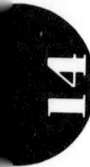

Differences in competence ratings from specialty to specialty

Respondents' specialty	% who feel they are presently working with an incompetent	
	Nurse	**Doctor**
Medical/Surgical	30%	36%
ICU/CCU	37	42
Geriatrics	33	27
Emergency	33	47
Ob/Gyn	41	32
Pediatrics	28	29
Psychiatric	28	37
Hospital administration	38	38
Other	30	29

Except for specialist M.D.s, none received very many "excellent" ratings either.

How would you rate the quality of care given to patients by the following?

	Excel- lent	Good	Fair	Poor
Doctors				
Specialist M.D.s	34%	57%	8%	1%
G.P.s	10	62	26	2
Foreign-trained doctors	8	42	40	10
Nurses				
L.P.N.s	15	65	19	1
Part-time nurses	12	68	19	1
Recent graduates	13	57	27	4
Private duty nurses	17	47	28	8
Float nurses	7	55	35	4
Aides and orderlies	6	50	37	6
Foreign-trained nurses	5	50	36	8
Nurses who return to work after several years of not practicing	4	43	47	6

Foreign-trained personnel. Foreign-trained doctors and nurses both received relatively low ratings. Language problems were the chief reason mentioned but other reasons were brought out as well.

Other departments. In rating the service provided by the different departments in their institutions, nurses gave their own department

by far the best rating—58% of the "best" votes and only 4% of the "worst" votes. Pharmacy was a distant second best.

The lowest rated departments were dietary and housekeeping, with laboratory, maintenance and radiology relatively ignored. This pattern probably emerges to some extent from the impact that incompetence in the dietary and housekeeping departments would have on the nurses' own job—i.e., make it harder.

Ratings of service in different departments

	% of "best" ratings	% "worst" ratings
Nursing	57%	4%
Pharmacy	17	8
Laboratory	8	16
Dietary	6	26
Housekeeping	5	24
Radiology	4	10
Maintenance	3	12

What percent of nurses would choose not to be patients in their own place of employment? More than a third (38%). And when it comes to nursing homes, more than half (55%) wouldn't want to be patients where they work.

Percentage of nurses who would choose to be a patient in the institution where employed, if seriously ill

	% who said "Yes"
Work Setting	
Hospital, more than 200 beds	68%
Hospital, fewer than 200 beds	52%
Nursing home or ECF	45%
Specialty	
Hospital administration	83%
Emergency	68%
Ob/Gyn	67%
ICU/CCU	63%
Pediatrics	62%
Medical/Surgical	60%
Psychiatric	48%
Geriatrics	44%

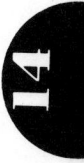

14

Physical care by both doctors and nurses is by far the most highly rated, however. In fact, even the *lowest* rated specialties in terms of *physical care* received more "excellent" and "good" ratings than the most highly rated specialties did on any of *the other aspects of health care.* For example, in geriatrics, psychiatry, pediatrics and Ob/Gyn, the role of the health care provider normally entails more *psychological support for the patient* than in emergency or ICU/CCU situations.

In pediatrics and geriatrics, where the patient's family is often directly involved with the patient's care, this shows up also. Both of these have higher ratings for *psychological support for relatives* than the other specialties.

Ob/Gyn and pediatrics would tend to involve more *patient education* than, say, emergency or ICU/CCU.

Table 14-2   Respondents' ratings of different aspects of health care provided by doctors and nurses. Percentage of ratings either "excellent" or "good"

| Respondents' specialty | Nurses | | | | | |
	Physical care	Psycho- logical support of patients	Psycho- logical support of relatives	Patient education	Rehabil- itation	Discharge planning
Ob/Gyn	82%	45%	28%	47%	46%	36%
Pediatrics	78	43	40	43	56	29
ICU/CCU	78	37	33	29	33	19
Emergency	73	36	25	29	23	23
Medical/Surgical	75	31	23	35	48	31
Psychiatric	59	50	31	30	51	35
Hospital admin.	80	29	25	29	29	30
Geriatrics	70	36	37	29	50	36
Other	77	39	32	47	49	37

14

Assistance with Nonnursing Duties

This issue received widespread attention in New York City in 1972 when the state nurses' association announced that the 5,500 members who worked in city hospitals would no longer perform nonnursing duties. The nurses calculated they had been spending 75% of their time serving meals, doing messenger work, housecleaning, and clerical jobs; they refused to continue. That demonstration lasted about ten days, and though no widespread reforms resulted, the action did make the issue visible.

The majority of nurses reported that they have the following kinds of assistance:

Table 14-3   Assistance for nurses

L.P.N.s/L.V.N.s	84%
Aides	66
Nurse assistants	43
Volunteers	35
Clerk/secretaries	9
Orderlies	3
Students	3
Technicians	2
None	2

Source: "Working Conditions," *Nursing '75,* May.

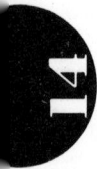

Episodic vs. Distributive Careers

The National Commission for the Study of Nursing and Nursing Education in 1976 recommended that two essentially related, but differing, career patterns be developed for nursing practice:

1. One career pattern, episodic, would emphasize the nursing practice that is essentially curative and restorative, generally acute or chronic in nature, and most frequently provided in the setting of the hospital or inpatient facility.
2. The second career pattern, distributive, would emphasize the nursing practice that is essentially designed for health maintenance and disease prevention. This is generally continuous in nature, seldom acute, and increasingly will take place in community or emergent institutional settings.

Interpersonal and Patient Relations

Who Is Important To A Nurse*

The patient seems to have very little power in the hospital setting. Usually, he has no voice in decisions which affect him: when he gets a bath, who will be his nurse and how his treatments will be administered. In part, he is at the mercy of the hospital, a leveling institution, which—if it is to operate efficiently—needs to standardize its policies, often to the detriment of patients' needs for individualized care.

What does all this tell us about the status of patients and their families in the power structure of a general hospital? We have found that nurses see the patients and their families as important but not very influential. Nurses cared a lot, they said, about evaluations of their work by patients, but they perceived patients as having minimal power over nurses' organizational rewards and penalties and, therefore, having little influence in the hospital system. Furthermore, that's the way it ought to be, the nurses seemed to think, thus supporting [the] theory that the professional believes that he, not the

consumer, is the best judge of services rendered.

Because patients' evaluations were found to be very or extremely important to the nurse, and yet patients are not an influential group of evaluators in the hospital, we would presume that there are other reasons for the importance of their evaluations to the nurse, ones probably rooted in the professional ideology of the nurse profession.

Table 14-4   Influence and importance of different evaluators to the nurse

Evaluators	Influence of the evaluator rank	Importance of evaluator
Head nurse	1	2
Supervisor	2	7
Director of nursing service	3	8
Members of nursing team	4	4
Doctors	6	3
Individual nurses	6	5
Patient	6	1
Patient's family	8	5

Getting Along with Aides**

There are a few basic principles which can be applied, perhaps, by anyone to improve his or her supervision.

First and perhaps most important, it appears that it's better to be firm than permissive. Studies have shown that permissive leaders (including those who have undergone "sensitivity training") usually either have no effect on group productivity . . . or even detract from group productivity and performance. Firm leaders tend to have more productive staffs. So, it'll usually pay you to be firm rather than permissive in dealing with subordinates.

Second, you should let subordinates know what's expected of them. Sound oversimplified? You'd be surprised how often subordinates *don't* know what they're expected to do. Lorane C. Kruse, R.N., Assistant Director of Continuing Education at Ohio State University's School of Nursing studied this

---

*Source: Gwen D. Marram, Ph.D., "Patients' Evaluation," *Nursing Outlook*, May 1973. © American Journal of Nursing Company (Survey of 194 Staff Nurses).

**Source: J. Wiley, "Getting Along Better with Those Aides," *Nursing '75*, June.

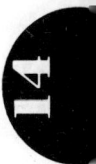

problem at four hospitals. She concluded: "If the supervisor *fails* to let followers know what they're expected to do (and not do), they remain in a constant state of indecision, uncertainty and unwillingness to act—except to carry out the minimum of routine duties. . . . On the other hand, group performance and loyalty to the hospital tend to be high when leaders let followers know what they're expected to do, have insight into what they're doing, and are nonpermissive."

Third, good management starts at the top. If the nursing administration is strong and sets a good example, that makes things easier all the way down the line. Even though the hospital may offer no formal training in supervision, it can help by providing good models for the R.N.s. to pattern their own supervision after. So, if you're a head nurse, nursing supervisor, or administrator, you can truly help others supervise by setting a good example. If you're a newcomer, try to find a model to pattern your behavior after. Even in a poorly run organization, there are usually several good leaders. Seek them out and try to imitate what they're doing.

Fourth, don't be afraid to experiment. There are no infallible principles when it comes to supervising. You'll find widely differing characteristics among effective leaders—some of them contradictory. Some good leaders are warm and outgoing; others are aloof and strictly business. Some good leaders have a strong sense of humor; others don't. You'll find that certain techniques work with certain subordinates; the same techniques won't work with others.

Fifth, don't be unrealistic in your expectations. In dealing with aides, you may find work mores that differ from your own, attitudes built up over a lifetime. Don't expect to change them very much. Don't even expect that your words will always mean the same to aides as to you.

Don't expect yourself to work well with everyone. Even leaders in the Army have met and arrived at a practical solution for this problem: they transfer the unmanageable soldier to another unit, to let someone else deal with him.

So in your own work, you may have to ask for a transfer—either of aides in your area or of yourself. If a situation seems unbearable, your best solution may be to quit and find another job where the supervisory climate is better.

And finally, if you're having trouble supervising, examine your technical competence. For as one aide said, people under you won't respect you as a leader if you don't know as much as they know, technically. If you honestly admit that you are technically deficient, then bone up, take crash courses, and do whatever you can to become competent in nursing technique. That may go a long way toward helping solve your supervisory problems.

Another aide summed it all up this way: "You'll win our respect when we feel the nurses are trying to do the best they can to do the job. If you want us to work hard, check the patients yourself, then sit down with us and tell us what we have to do. It's a lot easier if we all pull together . . . if we all feel everyone is doing the best she can."

14

15
EXPANDED ROLE FOR NURSES*

Perspective on Changes

Introduction**

One of the changes already in progress is that . . . nursing is moving away from the inpatient setting and into the community, with emphasis on primary care. Nurses are placing increasing emphasis on early detection of disease, and on efforts to predict and help control conditions that increase susceptibility to disease. They are moving to expand their responsibility for counseling people in sound health practices and prevention of illness, and fostering follow-up and administration to the health needs of the family and community, as well as the individual.

Every individual nurse will be affected by the forthcoming changes in nursing practice. As the continuing link between the client and the health care system, the individual nurse will influence the developing system and in turn will be affected by it. Nurses will have a markedly different philosophy regarding their roles in the health care system: that is, caring not only for the sick but for the well. They will be a vital part of the interdisciplinary health team, assessing the needs of patients, administering to some of these needs, and referring patients to other health professionals for other needs.

An expanded role for nurses includes both an increased range of independent responsibilities and an expanded set of functions in clinical areas.

The new concept is taking nurses far beyond the traditional nurse's role in health care. Certain medical decisions formerly exclusive to doctors are now being made by new types of nurses. Many R.N. baccalaureate programs already require students to conduct extensive health assessments, to make nursing diagnoses, and to prescribe treatment. In some programs, the prerequisite is that candidates already hold an R.N. or even a B.S.N. degree in order to function in an expanded role.

This enlarged role has been developing for some years now. In the 1950s a number of nurse leaders, concerned about nurses taking on more and more administrative functions,

began a movement to have nurses return to the patient's side. Francis Reiter coined the concept "nurse-clinician" and the movement had a label. Then in 1965, Loretta Ford and Henry Silver launched another new concept of nursing, the "nurse practitioner" movement.

Survey of Nurses' Attitudes

A *Nursing '77* survey of 10,000 nurses on expanding the role of the nurse (*Nursing '77,* Jan. "Quality of Care") found that:

- 60% of those polled thought that their responsibilities should be limited to nursing care without diagnosis or treatment.

- only 38% wanted greater responsibilities, including some responsibility for diagnosis and treatment.

Hospital department	% advocating greater responsibility
Psychiatry	55%
ICU/CCU	45
Emergency	43
Hospital administration	33
Geriatrics	27

- Most other departments averaged between 35% and 45%.

Those seeking greater responsibility were more likely to work in larger hospitals than in smaller ones. They were also more likely to have more education—50% of those with a bachelor's or master's degree as opposed to 15% for L.P.N.s.

---

*(Note: Information on specific programs designed to expand the role of the nurse is available in a joint American Nurses' Association Bureau of Health Resources Development publication. It may be obtained from the ANA, Inc., 2420 Pershing Rd., Kansas City, Missouri 64108, or from the Bureau of Health Resources Development, Health Resources Administration, Rm 5B-63, Bldg. 31, 9000 Rockville Pike, Bethesda, Maryland 20014.)

**Source: "Report to the Congress, Nurse Training," DHEW, 1974.

Schools Offering Programs for Expanded Roles for Nurses

Master's degree programs*

Broad nursing category	Area of concentration (occupational title)	Number of schools offering programs
Community Health	Community Health Nurse	7
	Community Health N.C.	10
	Family and Community N.C.	2
	Family Health N.C.	2
	Family Health Specialist	1
	Family N.P.	4
	Public Health C.S.	2
	Public Health N.C.	3
	Public Health Nurse	2
	Rural Health Specialist	1
	School Nurse	1
Maternal-Child	Child Health N.C.	2
	Child N.C.S.	2
	Child N.S.	2
	Maternal C.S.	1
	Maternal Health N.C.	1
	Maternal N.C.	1
	Maternal and Newborn N.C.	1
	Maternal-Child C.N.S.	2
	Maternal-Child N.C.	7
	Maternal-Child Nurse	5
	Maternal-Infant N.C.	3
	Maternity N.C.	1
	Nurse-Midwife	9
	Obstetrical N.C.	2
	Parent-Child N.C.	1
	Pediatric C.S.	3
	Pediatric N.A.	1
	Pediatric N.C.	4
	Pediatric N.P.	3
Medical-Surgical	Adult Health N.C.	2
	Adult Health N.P.	1
	Adult N.P.	7
	Adult N.S.	2
	Aging Specialist	1
	Biophysical-Pathology N.C.	1
	Burns N.C.	2
	Cardiac and Respiratory C.S.	1
	Geriatric Nurse Practitioners	1
	Cardiovascular N.C.	4
	Gerontology N.C.	5
	Health N.C.	1
	Medical C.S.	1
	Medical N.C.	1
	Medical Surgical C.N.S.	3
	Medical Surgical C.S.	1

Master's degree programs* (continued)

Broad nursing category	Area of concentration (occupational title)	Number of schools offering programs
	Medical Surgical N.C.	9
	Medical Surgical N.C.S.	1
	Medical Surgical Nurse	10
	Medical Surgical N.P.	1
Psychiatric/Mental Health	Adult Psychiatry C.S.	1
	Adult Psychiatric N.C.	1
	Biophysical N.C.	1
	Child Psychiatric C.S.	1
	Child Psychiatric N.C.	1
	Community Mental Health Nurse	5
	Psychiatric-Child N.C.	1
	Psychiatric Clinician	1
	Psychiatric C.N.S.	5
	Psychiatric C.S.	2
	Psychiatric N.C.	6
	Psychiatric Nurse	1
Rehabilitation	Chronic Illness and Rehabilitation C.S.	2
	Rehabilitation N.C.	4

*Source: American Nurses' Association, *A Directory of Programs Preparing Registered Nurses for Expanded Roles, 1974–5*, DHEW.

Clinical Nurse Specialist and Nurse Clinician

In the early 1950s, the master's programs in nursing began to place more emphasis on preparation for clinical specialty practice than on preparation for teaching, supervision, and nursing service administration. The clinical nurse specialist was to use her advanced theoretical knowledge to help nursing service personnel better assess and meet patient and family health needs.

Functions

Today the clinical nurse specialist plans, implements and evaluates, and most important, provides continuity in patient care. She engages in more specialized nursing practice such as cardiac, respiratory or neonatal, in hospitals and in other inpatient settings. She combines the laying-on-of-hands with formal and informal teaching.

The nurse clinician is likely to be demonstrating and teaching her role while the clinical nurse specialist frequently deals with entire organizations and institutions. The clinician may be involved in research as a participant; the specialist may well be the principal investigator. Among the clinical specialties:

- Pediatric nurses specialize in caring for children.
- Obstetric nurses care for mothers and new babies.
- Psychiatric and mental health nurses care for the mentally ill.
- Rehabilitation nurses care for patients with chronic and disabling conditions.
- Medical-surgical nurses care for patients before, during, and after surgery, and in most types of illness.

Other nursing specialties include the care of patients with particular diseases, such as cardiovascular illnesses, cancer, and pulmonary ailments.

Positions in advanced fields of nursing are open to nurses that have experience and have taken additional courses of study beyond the basic preparation, usually at the master's or doctoral level.

15

286

Education

The N.C., C.N.S., N.C.S., N.S., or C.S. is normally granted only to nurses with B.S. degrees completing a master's graduate program. The programs range from two semesters to two years, although most are scheduled for one year.

The following list of programs (as of 1974) suggests the large variety of subject areas as well as occupational titles that are available.

For the addresses of the specific schools offering these programs, write the Nursing Division, DHEW and ask for *A Directory of Programs Preparing Registered Nurses for Expanded Roles,* prepared by ANA and DHEW.

The Nurse Practitioner

Definitions

A nurse practitioner is an R.N. with additional education in a specialized area (such as geriatrics, family care or pediatrics, community or public health, nurse midwifery, nursing care of medical patients, and care of patients in physicians' offices) who can perform many patient services including examining, prescribing certain drugs and initiating tests. Nurse practitioners frequently work as part of a team with physicians and other health care professionals. Specialized training can range from several months of formal education and preceptorship experience to a master's or higher degree.

The American Nurses' Association defines a nurse practitioner as:

a licensed professional nurse who provides direct care to individuals, families and other groups in a variety of settings including homes, institutions, offices, industry, schools and other community agencies. The service provided by the nurse practitioner is aimed at the delivery of primary, acute or chronic care which focuses on the achievement, maintenance or restoration of optimal functions in the population. The nurse practitioner engages in independent decision making about the nursing care needs of clients and collaborates with other health professionals, such as physicians, social workers and nutritionists, in making decisions about other health care needs. The nurse practitioner plans and institutes

health care programs as a member of the health care team.

The acquisition of knowledge in depth and competence in skill performance in a particular field of practice enables this practitioner to:

1. Assess the physical and psychosocial health-illness status of individuals and families by health and developmental history taking and physical examinations.
2. Evaluate and interpret data in order to plan and execute appropriate nursing intervention.
3. Engage in decision making and implementation of therapeutic actions cooperatively with other members of the health care team.

This practitioner institutes and provides health care to patients within established regimens such as supervising and managing normal pregnancy and delivery, pediatric health supervision and diagnostic screening. The nurse practitioner provides counseling, health teaching and support to individuals and families.

The nurse practitioner is directly accountable and responsible to the recipient for the quality of care rendered.

Historical Background

The first nurse practitioner program was introduced in 1965 at the University of Colorado. The field was pediatrics. Public health nurses had traditionally been involved in the care of well babies. So it was logical for Dr. Henry Silver (University of Colorado, School of Medicine, Department of Pediatrics) and Dr. Loretta Ford (University of Colorado, School of Nursing) to think of extending the nurse's role in this area.

They developed a four month curriculum which was followed by 20 months in the field working with a pediatrician and practicing newly acquired skills under his supervision. Graduates of their program were called pediatric nurse practitioners.

Colorado still offers the original pediatric program through its Department of Continuing Education in the School of Nursing. The curriculum includes: history taking; physical examination; screening tests; common problems of childhood; well-child management;

and child growth and development. Lectures and seminars are led by nurses with assistance from physicians and other health professionals. Clinical experience is provided through hired patient models and by actual practice—under supervision of a nurse or physician preceptor—with patients in well-child care and management of minor illness.

Similar programs soon proliferated. In 1970 the University of Colorado's Continuing Education Services introduced a course to prepare school nurse practitioners. In 1972 a third program entitled "The Adult Health Nurse Practitioner Course" was developed. By 1973 there were 65 nurse-practitioner programs in pediatrics alone spread all over the country.

Between June 1973 and May 1974, 147 programs across the country graduated approximately 2000 nurse practitioners, granting them either certificates or master's degrees. Although pediatric nurse practitioners still lead the field in numbers, 38% of the teaching programs now concentrate on primary care, including the care of adults. Graduates are working in many settings: clinics, emergency rooms, neighborhood health centers, group practices and private offices throughout the country.

Over half of the academic medical centers recently surveyed by *Annals of Internal Medicine* supported nurse practitioner programs.

Education

A nurse practitioner receives a certificate, not a degree, and the training is often only 6 months, though many programs last a full year.

The majority of nurse practitioners function in ambulatory settings. Few work in hospitals. They come from a variety of formal educational programs, some holding diplomas after completing a nonacademic practitioner course, others having completed master's degrees in clinical specialties.

Problems

Doctors

Role conflict exists between the primary care physician, usually an internist or family physician, and one of his newest coworkers, the medical nurse practitioner. This conflict should be no surprise.

Table 15-1   Survey of nursing practitioner programs leading to certificate

	Number of programs
Acute Care Nurse Practitioner	1
Adult Health Nurse Practitioner	7
Ambulatory Care Nurse Practitioner	1
Ambulatory Child Health Care Nurse	1
College Health Nurse Practitioner	2
Critical Care Nurse Practitioner	1
Emergency Nurse Practitioner	2
Family Health Nurse Practitioner	20
Family Planning Nurse Practitioner	2
Geriatric Nurse Practitioner	7
Maternal-Child Nurse Practitioner	2
Maternity Nurse Practitioner	1
Medical Nurse Practitioner	4
Midwife and Family Nurse Practitioner	1
Neo-Natal Practitioner	1
Nurse Midwife	8
OB-Gyn Nurse Practitioner	4
Pediatric Nurse Practitioner	23
Primary Care Nurse Practitioner	3
School Nurse Practitioner	4

Source: American Nurses' Association, *A Directory of Programs Preparing Registered Nurses for Expanded Roles,* 1974–5, DHEW.

The nurse practitioner is usually a woman. In the past the nurse's role included care, comfort, counseling, guidance and helping the patient to cope. She was trained to assist the physician, to defer to him, to follow his orders.

But the nurse practitioner has an expanded role. It includes diagnosis and treatment in the less complex areas of traditional medicine. Working together with physicians, nurse practitioners have assumed new and significant responsibilities for patient care.

The average physician may have difficulty relinquishing any portion of his conventional role. Initially, he has trouble trusting the nurse's history and physical findings. In fact his teachers in medical school had specifically preached against this kind of behavior. "Any good consultant," he was warned, "does his

15

own history and physical." Even more difficult is sharing the decision-making process, accepting and trusting the judgments and decisions of others. The physician may also be reluctant to share the close personal relationship he has developed with his patients.

Patient Acceptance

If the nurse is seen as part of the therapeutic team, if her role is respected and legitimized by the physician, the patient will accept her counsel more readily. Without this, her efforts at intervention beyond the stereotyped nurse role may be unacceptable.

Hospital Coworkers

And for those who find themselves in a traditional hospital setting there are the problems with coworkers, including nurses and aides, who can sabotage the nurse practitioner, if they do not favor the change or feel that their own positions are in jeopardy. Then there are the questions of loyalty. Should practitioners remain a part of nursing service, be subject to nursing policies, schedules, staffing patterns, and budgets, or should they align themselves with medicine, risking professional isolation for apparent gain in freedom, excitement, and perhaps prestige?

Training*

It is generally accepted that nurse practitioner programs should be (1) affiliated with an accredited school of nursing and (2) held in conjunction with and in collaboration with a school of medicine.

Prerequisites range from being an R.N. with no previous experience to holding a baccalaureate degree with two years of specialized experience (usually in pediatric nursing). The length of the programs varies from four months to three years.

In some programs you're awarded a certificate upon completion; in others, you can earn a master's degree. The costs of the programs vary, too. Some examples of certificate program tuitions: no tuition for four months at the University of Colorado (the program is grant supported); $700 for eight months at the University of Michigan; $900 for one year at

Johns Hopkins University. Master's degree program tuitions: $6,000 for three semesters at the University of Pennsylvania: $2,800 to $3,500 per year for two years at the University of Rochester; $4,000 per year for two years at Yale University. Most schools offer some type of financial aid, such as scholarships, stipends, loans, and so forth.

Certification

A number of national organizations are considering the advantages of certification in a particular specialty area. For example, the American Academy of Pediatrics, the National Association of Pediatric Nurse Associates and Practitioners, the American Nurses' Association, the National Board of Medical Examiners, the National League for Nursing and the American Medical Association have been studying the certification of pediatric nurse practitioners.

Salary

The rewards of assuming increased responsibility as a nurse practitioner are many, but salary is not always one of them. In some areas, practitioners' salaries are almost identical to those of other nurses in the locale. A survey conducted by the ANA in 1974 revealed that the median annual salary of full-time practitioners was $12,195. In 1976 salaries in the Denver area ranged from $9,000 to $15,000.

Occasionally, a nurse practitioner is able to negotiate a higher salary on the basis that she's assuming more responsibility than the average nurse. Some pediatric nurse practitioners in private practices have been able to negotiate for a share of the profits based on the amount of added income they bring into the office.

Where Employed

Nurse practitioners are employed in a variety of situations—the majority being ambulatory settings such as physicians' offices, industrial settings, hospital outpatient departments, neighborhood health clinics, Health Maintenance Organizations and school systems in both urban and rural areas.

1. *In Institutions concerned with inpatient or ambulatory care.* As employees, they maintain professional autonomy and work collaboratively with other health

*Source: "Nursing is Coming of Age ... Through the Practitioner Movement," *American Journal of Nursing,* October 1975.

professionals with whom they jointly develop patient care objectives, plan and implement care and mutually evaluate outcomes.

2. *In self-employed, interdisciplinary groups.* Nurse practitioners function in incorporated ambulatory practices as partners or as employees of the corporation. They carry their own client load and practice collaboratively or interdependently with the others in the group. They also take their services to where patients are if this seems indicated.

3. *In solo practice, either self-employed, or as a member of a group of nurse-practitioners.* This practice has the greatest innovation potential. It could involve collaborative components with physician groups or other health care practitioners, or with institutions, through individual care delivery contracts. There could be consultation and teaching, relationships with community organizations and any number of other arrangements. This practice preserves direct access to clients and the reverse. It is the pinnacle of nursing autonomy. Yet, it should never embrace a concept of independence which runs counter to accepted principles, indeed to the very essence of the meaning of people care.

Characteristics of the Nurse-Practitioner

In a psychological study of female student nurses and nurse practitioners, published in *Nursing Outlook* (March 1975), regular nurses were found to score higher on nurturance, deference, order, abasement and endurance. Nurse practitioners scored low on these traits but were higher on such characteristics as autonomy, exhibition, dominance, change and heterosexuality. The practitioners' higher scores on "heterosexuality" were interpreted to mean that they were comfortable with men and that therefore they would be more likely to work well with male physicians.

When the female nurses and nurse practitioners were compared with college women in medical school or doing graduate social work, the practitioners were found to be more like the college women. Compared with nurses, practitioners were slightly more outgoing and higher in achievement orientation, intellectual efficiency and psychological-mindedness.

Expectation vs. Reality

Nursing Outlook (March 1975) published a survey of one-time nurses who had resumed work after recently graduating a nurse practitioner program in March of 1975. Among the findings were:

- Work had become more interesting, varied and creative.
- Work required greater independence, skill and responsibility.
- They felt their work was less secure, more stressful and risky.
- Salaries did not change much.
- Opportunities for promotion increased somewhat, but still remained low.
- Administrative responsibilities had not increased as much as they expected.
- Most problems with physician acceptance, support and supervision disappeared by the end of the first year.

Responsibilities
ANA Guides

The ANA offered the following tasks as suggestive of the range of responsibilities available to a nurse practitioner:

1. Obtaining a health history.
2. Assessing health-illness status.
3. Entering a person into the health care system.
4. Sustaining and supporting persons who are impaired, infirm, ill and during programs of diagnosis and therapy.
5. Managing a medical care regimen for acute and chronically ill patients within established, standing orders.
6. Aiding in restoring persons to wellness and maximum function.
7. Teaching and counseling persons about health and illness.
8. Supervising and managing care regimens of normal pregnant women.
9. Helping parents in guidance of children with a view to their optimal physical and emotional development.
10. Counseling and supporting persons with regard to the aging process.
11. Aiding people and their survivors during the dying process.
12. Supervising assistants to nurses.

DHEW Guides

A 1971 "blue-ribbon committee" established by the Secretary of HEW "to discuss and delineate the new responsibilities and the relationships of nurses in expanded roles" went further.

The committee concluded that expanding the roles of nurses will require "major adjustments in the orientation and practice" of both physicians and nurses. A substantial number of patient care functions were delineated in primary, acute and long-term care "for which many nurses are now prepared and others could be prepared." These included:

- Making physical and psychosocial assessments, recognizing the range of "normal" and the manifestations of common abnormalities.
- Interpreting selected laboratory findings.
- Making diagnoses, choosing, initiating and modifying selected therapies.
- Providing emergency treatment as appropriate, such as in cardiac arrest, shock, or hemorrhage.
- Providing appropriate information to the patient and the patient's family about a diagnosis or plan of therapy.

Physician and Nurse Attitudes toward Practitioner Functions

Medical Economics magazine conducted a survey of physicians and nurses to assess attitudes toward permitting nurses to assume duties usually performed by physicians.

The majority of physicians and nurses agreed that nurses could perform several functions which did not involve diagnosis or prescription, including routine prenatal visits, well-baby care, routine postpartum care, follow-up house calls, initial patient histories, and Pap smears. Nearly half of the hospital-based physicians and 70% of the nurses thought that nurses could handle normal deliveries. However, only 32% of the physicians in private practice were in agreement.

The majority of the nurses, but less than half of the physicians, thought that nurses could handle such tasks as prescribing medication for minor symptoms, screening new patients to decide whether they needed to see the doctor, handling post-operative visits, doing minor suturing, making referrals to psychiatrists, gynecologists, and other specialists, treating common childhood diseases, removing particles from eyes, treating sprains and strep throats, making house calls, performing initial routine physicals, and applying and removing casts. Nurses and physicians tended to agree that nurses should not make first house calls to diagnose, give and interpret ECGs, phonocardiograms or spirograms, order and read X-rays of injured limbs, do minor surgery, handle first post-operative visits, set minor fractures, or conduct diagnostic procedures such as arterial punctures, intravenous catheterizations, venous cutdowns, lumbar punctures, or thoracenteses.

A Yale University medical study of new health practitioners in October 1977 (NSF sponsored) found that patients in a group cared for by a nurse practitioner had "outcomes" similar to, or "better" than, those of patients cared for by a physician, judged by both process and outcome measures.

Legal Issues

Among the factors that limit the nurse practitioner are the state nurse practice acts. Most nurses practicing in "expanded roles" are functioning under standing orders, with legal authority delegated by physicians.

However, since 1971 there has been a rush to revise nurse practices acts. Thirty-nine states have amended their acts—and 33 of them have included "expanded nurses' roles."

State Nurse Practice Acts*

As indicated in Table 15-2 there are 30 states which have enacted amendments to their nurse practice acts in the last five years to facilitate nurses taking on diagnostic and treatment functions.

Ten other states do not include a prohibition of diagnosis and treatment in their nurse practice acts. However, 13 jurisdictions still have statutory prohibitions against nurses diagnosing and treating patients.

In some states nurses seeking to expand their activities to include acts of medical diagnosis or treatment are required to submit evidence to their agencies that they have obtained the necessary special education.

For example, nurses who give anesthesia must be certified by the American Association of Nurse Anesthetists, and nurses who write

---

*Source: *American Journal of Public Health,* March 1976.

Table 15-2   The state nurse practice acts and the legitimization of diagnosis and treatment by nurses (as of year-end 1975)

State	Amended since 1971 to facilitate role expansion	Diagnosis and treatment are not prohibited	Diagnosis and treatment prohibited under all circumstances
Alabama			Yes
Alaska	*		
Arizona	*		
Arkansas			Yes
California	*		
Colorado	*		
Connecticut	*		
Delaware			Yes
Florida	*		
Georgia			
Hawaii			Yes
Idaho	*		
Illinois	*		
Indiana	*		
Iowa		x	
Kansas			Yes
Kentucky			Yes
Louisiana			Yes
Maine	*		
Maryland	*		
Massachusetts		x	
Michigan			Yes
Minnesota	*		
Mississippi	*		
Missouri		x	
Montana	*		
Nebraska	*		
Nevada	*		
New Hampshire	*		
New Jersey	*		
New Mexico	*		
New York	*		
North Carolina	*		
North Dakota		x	
Ohio			Yes
Oklahoma			Yes
Oregon	*		
Pennsylvania	*		
Rhode Island		x	
South Carolina	*		
South Dakota	*		
Tennessee	*		
Texas			Yes
Utah	*		
Vermont	*		
Virginia		x	
Washington	*		
West Virginia		x	
Wisconsin		x	
Wyoming	*		
Washington, D.C.		x	
Guam			Yes
Puerto Rico			Yes
Virgin Isles		x	

prescriptions for controlled substances must be registered with the U.S. Bureau of Narcotics and Dangerous Drugs.

One approach to opening up the nursing role was first used by New York State in 1972 when it adopted the following definition of professional nursing:

> The practice of the profession of nursing as a registered professional nurse is defined as diagnosing and treating human responses to actual or potential health problems through such services as case-finding, health teaching, health counseling, and provision of care supportive to or restorative of life and well-being and executing medical regimens prescribed by a licensed or otherwise legally authorized physician or dentist. A nursing regimen shall not vary any existing medical regimen.

This basic approach also seems reasonable and may eventually emerge as the dominant one, as nurses become more confident and the public becomes more aware of their abilities.

The Question of Reimbursement for Nursing Services*

Third-party payers almost universally deny payment for nursing care when it is distinct and separate from physician care.

Access to (or reimbursement for) individual nursing care services is almost exclusively subject to physician authorization. In most hospital insurance plans, private duty nursing fees are reimbursable items only if the nursing care is "ordered" by a physician. New York State law authorizes reimbursement for home health services, including professional nursing services, only if the plan for home health services is approved in writing by a physician.

Many feel it makes little sense to train nurse practitioners skilled in ambulatory care and interested in the care of the poor and the aged, and then provide no reimbursement mechanisms through Medicaid and Medicare so that they can be paid for their services.

New York State law authorizes professional nurses to establish professional service cor-

porations and thereby engage in group practice. However, the absence of insurance provisions for reimbursement of such services renders this statutory opportunity practically meaningless.

The American Nurses' Association's Commission on Economic and General Welfare has denounced both the restricted access to nursing service by consumers and the economic disparity for the profession and exhorted third-party payers to broaden existing reimbursement practices. A few individual insurance companies, notably the Phoenix Mutual, have voluntarily modified policies to permit subscribers to seek nursing services at their own discretion.

In Washington, the state nurses association has for two consecutive years sought legislation to provide reimbursement for services in nurse clinics. Although twice defeated, the association believes eventual enactment is likely.

The Kennedy-Javits proposal to create a "National System of Health Security" does *not* include professional nurses among the groups cited as qualified professional providers. And, in any number of states as well as at the federal level, various proposals would confine reimbursement benefits to the services of only those nurses designated as "physician extender personnel."

Community Nurse Practitioner (C.N.P.)

The C.N.P. role emphasizes community self-help, rather than expanded one-to-one patient services. It focuses on the health of an entire community. A primary function is to discover with the community what its health priorities are, what resources are available, and what would be an effective and acceptable manner to approach the problem.

Increased emphasis is placed on disease prevention, health promotion, and improving communication, cooperation and collaboration among the various participants in the health services community.

History

Although Florence Nightingale initiated family health practice, community nursing was first established in the United States in 1877. By

---

*Source: C. A. Welch, "Health Care Distribution and 3rd Party Payment for Nurses' Services," *American Journal of Nursing,* October 1975. © American Journal of Nursing Company.

1893 "all the social, economic, and industrial conditions affecting the lives of those receiving services were considered integral to the practice of 'visiting nurses.'"

The first prenatal care in the Western world was initiated by the Instructive Nursing Association of Boston in 1901. Throughout the early 1900's "nurses on horseback" were the sole health providers to the mountain people of Kentucky. The first United States Public Health Service officer to be decorated by two foreign governments was a nurse.

C.N.P. Profile

A survey of C.N.P.s (*Nursing Outlook,* August 1976) revealed the following profile:

- 71% had master's degrees; 6% doctorates; 16% bachelor's degrees
- average age was 37
- 40% held some form of certification (most were family nurse practitioners or pediatric nurse practitioners; only 5% had certificates in public health nursing)
- 27% functioned in administrative or supervisory roles
- 77% were exclusively or partly involved in direct client services.

Responsibilities

The *Nursing Outlook* survey found that 70% of the C.N.P.s had responsibilities beyond direct patient care. These included teaching, supervising, and managing for the purpose of facilitating students' and staff members' delivery of direct client services; administering a school of nursing, working for a professional organization, serving as a lobbyist, being involved in community health planning, and doing research and service evaluations. These activities are all focused on the health care delivery system and have institutions, agencies, and organizations as clients.

On-the-Job*

The actual process of getting to know the community varies and depends on the C.N.P. and the nature of the community. Most become involved both as observers and as participants in various action groups, churches, community

centers, schools, and clinics. Various sources of reported data, e.g., census, vital statistics, clinic records, police reports, and school absenteeism, are utilized to complete the assessment process. As this process continues, certain health problems emerge as characteristic of a given community.

Examples of problems which have emerged thus far for C.N.P.s include: low immunization rates, poor nutrition in the young and elderly, high rat population, no street lights, raw sewage draining into open ditches, drug abuse in teenagers, and no feeling of community. The next step in the process is to understand the nature of a given health problem well enough to make meaningful inferences for possible interventions.

Activities in which the C.N.P.s have been involved thus far include setting up a telephone crisis intervention service, writing a grant proposal to set up a pretrial home for delinquents, securing street lights, setting up visits of mobile immunization clinics, and transporting children to the beach.

Curriculum

At the University of Texas School of Public Health the first C.N.P. seminar focuses upon community development, its philosophical base, and approaches to working with communities.

The second seminar, community assessment, focuses upon the use of secondary data sources (e.g., census publications, vital statistics), demographic concepts and methods relating to data gathering, organization, and analysis.

The third seminar is concerned with an in-depth analysis of at least one identified problem in order to plan for effective intervention directed at its amelioration.

Independent or Family Nurse Practitioner**

The family nurse practitioner is prepared to make independent judgments and to assume principal responsibility for primary health care of individuals and families. She assumes major

---

*Source: "Community Nurse Practitioner, an Emerging Role," *AJPH*, September 1974.

**Source: "Moral and Legal—Issues—Nursing Judgement." National League for Nurses, Pub. No. 16–1551, 1974.

professional responsibility for decision making in relation to health needs. She works with physicians and other members of the health team in the delivery of health services to individuals and families. Her practice is community-oriented, related to needs, concerns, and priorities of consumers. Unlike the community nurse practitioner she emphasizes one-to-one patient service.

Currently the remuneration of the independent practitioner is less than that of the salaried employee. The more financially successful depend in part on consultant fees to supplement fees received from clients. Rural areas in particular offer much opportunity for this work, owing to the marked scarcity of physicians, since the health needs of people living in such areas are great.

Whether nurses setting up an independent practice will become a trend in nursing is not certain. However, after 25 years in nursing, Lucille Kinlein, assistant professor, Georgetown University School of Nursing, Washington, D.C., established an independent practice in 1971 and set up her office in a residential section of College Park, Maryland. Her ultimate purpose was to provide and improve health care for persons somewhat lost in the present health care delivery system.

Here is how one family nurse described her start in the field and her current practice:*

When I started my solo practice, the term "nurse practitioner" was not well known. At that time, there were probably no more than eight independent, self-employed nurse practitioners in the country. After 3 years in practice my primary care calls had increased significantly. Those physicians who were neutral about my being in an independent practice were more cooperative and responsive to my communications and initiated contact with me more often. Most internists were willing to hospitalize a patient on my assessment data and recommendation. I no longer had problems in obtaining an immediate medical opinion related to action in a situation when a patient had no physician or his physician was not available. I even received a few referrals directly from [metropolitan health care centers].

My major activities are concerned with:**
1. Monitoring long-term illnesses—especially a variety of cardiovascular conditions.
2. Primary care calls—acute medical, some surgical.
3. Dressings—postoperative and severe infections—occasional minor first aid.
4. Terminal illness at home—emotional support for family and patient, care and/or supervision of care.
5. Consultation and counseling on individual problems—mental health, plus
6. Miscellaneous—removal of accumulated cerumen, removal of stitches, and so forth.

Throughout all categories, the role of patient advocate is strong. I have the advantage of being responsible only to the patient and my professional self.

Pediatric Nurse Practitioner (P.N.P.s)**
Role Definition

At present, the largest group of nurse practitioners consists of pediatric nurse practitioners who, in addition to providing comprehensive well-child care, identify, appraise, and manage many acute and chronic conditions of the sick child. Pediatric nurse practitioners obtain complete histories; perform extensive physical examinations; carry out necessary immunization and other preventive services; evaluate hearing, speech, and vision; and determine developmental status. They also perform laboratory tests; counsel parents; assist in managing emergencies; care for newborn infants; and provide health maintenance through personal contacts and telephone calls.

P.N.P.s can work in a private practice with a physician (pediatrician, or general or family practitioner) in a public health agency or in an outpatient clinic. Some work with hospitalized children and their families. Basically, they assume primary responsibility for well-child care.

Educational Programs

Since 1965, when the first pediatric nurse practitioner program was started, approximately 50 other pediatric nurse practi-

---

*Source: "Promoting an Independent Nurse Practice," *American Journal of Nursing,* August 1975. ©American Journal of Nursing Company.

**Source: "Nurse Practitioners for Children—Past and Future," *Pediatrics,* November 5, 1974.

tioner programs have been established in the United States. These programs have graduated more than 1,100 nurses.

Surveys and evaluation studies of the Colorado pediatric nurse practitioner program have shown that:

1. Pediatric nurse practitioners can, by themselves, care for approximately three-fourths of all children coming to ambulatory health care settings.
2. Pediatric nurse practitioners can provide almost total care to all well children and can evaluate and manage the problems of a majority of all sick and injured children seen in office settings.
3. Pediatric nurse practitioners are very well accepted by parents; 94% of parents expressed satisfaction with the combined care provided jointly by a pediatrician and a pediatric nurse practitioner in a private office, and more than one-half of the parents indicated that joint care was better than that which they had received from the same pediatrician alone.
4. Pediatric nurse practitioners and pediatricians exhibit a high degree of agreement in assessing the health status of children; significant differences in assessment occurred in only 1% of cases.

Table 15-3   Field of employment for P.N.P.'s

Total	100%
Hospital clinic/hospital	22
Schools of nursing	9
Self-employed or Joint practice }	1
Physician's office	19
Public/community health	42
Student health services	5
Other	2

Salary*

The median annual salary of full-time pediatric nurse practitioners surveyed was $12,195. Close to one-fourth of the pediatric nurse prac-

*Source: "Pediatric Nurse Practitioners," American Nursing Association, March 5, 1975.

titioners reported annual salaries of $14,000 or above. A few pediatric nurse practitioners reported receiving salaries in excess of $20,000.

School Nurse Practitioners

School nurse practitioners perform routine health assessments; provide extensive well-child care; evaluate and assist in managing children who are ill or injured; and assess and coordinate the evaluation of perceptual and other learning disorders, psychoeducational problems, and behavior disturbances.

Although practices vary according to the wishes of parents, schools and other health professionals in the community, a survey reported in *Nursing Outlook* (June, 1975) found that many S.N.P.'s also:

- conduct routine examinations of well children identified as non-users of traditional health facilities (evaluations are similar to those performed by private physicians).

- manage the treatment of such illnesses as anemia, constipation, minor allergies, dermatological conditions, minor upper respiratory conditions, bacterial infections, trauma and injury with emergency first-aid measures.

Another study comparing school nurse practitioners and regular school nurses discovered that the school nurse practitioner:

- spends twice as much time providing direct patient care.

- spends three times as much time with parents of students discussing emotional, physical, learning and other problems that students have.

- is less likely to refer pupils inappropriately to physicians or others for consultation or care.

16
NURSING AND THE LAW*

Malpractice

Definitions of Malpractice and Negligence

Malpractice is the term for negligence or carelessness of professional personnel. To determine what is and what is not careless, the law has developed a measuring scale called the standard of care. Usually the standard of care is determined by deciding what a reasonably prudent person acting under similar circumstances would do. A jury makes this determination.

This reasonably prudent person is a legal fiction—in other words, a hypothetical average person with average skills and training in the relevant field and with a hypothetically average amount of judgment and good sense. But if the defendant's actions fail to meet the standard, then there has been negligence, and the jury must make two determinations: First, was it foreseeable that harm would follow the failure to meet the standard of care? Second, was the

carelessness or negligence the proximate or immediate cause of the harm or injury to the plaintiff? A nurse who fails to meet the standard of care will be liable for negligence if that failure results in harm to another.

The four elements of negligence are: (1) a standard of due care under the circumstances; (2) a failure to meet the standard of due care; (3) the foreseeability of harm resulting from failure to meet the standard; and (4) the fact that the breach of this standard proximately causes the injury to the plaintiff.

A nurse may be negligent and still not incur liability if no injury results to another person. The term "injury" includes more than mere physical harm. In some states it may include mental anguish and other invasions of rights and privileges. For example, a wife whose husband has been hospitalized as a result of a third person's negligence may sue that third person for loss of marital services.

The accompanying guidelines on negligence summarize the concepts of negligence and malpractice and the standard of care to be met in a particular situation.

*Source: This entire section consists of excerpts from *Nursing and the Law* (The Health Law Center, Aspen Systems Corp., 1975) unless otherwise noted.

Table 16-1   Guidelines on negligence—professional negligence is malpractice

Elements of liability	Explanation	Example— giving medications
1. Duty to use due care (defined by the standard of care)	The care which should be given under the circumstances (what the reasonably prudent nurse would have done)	A nurse should give medications: • accurately and • completely and • on time
2. Failure to meet standard of care (breach of duty)	Not giving the care which should be given under the circumstances	A nurse fails to give medications: • accurately or • completely or • on time
3. Foreseeability of harm	Knowledge that not meeting the standard of care will cause harm to the patient	Giving the wrong medication or the wrong dosage or not on schedule will probably cause harm to the patient
4. Failure to meet standard of care (breach) *causes* injury	Patient is harmed because proper care is not given	Wrong medication causes patient to have a convulsion
5. Injury	Actual harm results to patient	Convulsion or other serious complication

298

Nurse Malpractice Cases*

In 1969 the Hollinger baby [was found to have a] severe croup or cough and ... sent to the hospital. The suit alleged that when the baby arrived at the hospital the nurse, without authorization, placed him in a steam room where his heart stopped beating for several minutes and as a result he suffered permanent brain damage and lost the use of his limbs. In 1974 the parents were awarded $1 million in damages in Circuit Court.

[In another case] the nurse allegedly falsified the hospital records to show that she had monitored the fetal heartbeat every half hour while the testimony of the mother was that the fetal heartbeat was not monitored for more than one hour and this could have been a substantial factor in leading to the child being stillborn. The Oregon state supreme court affirmed a jury verdict of $22,500 in favor of patient and against hospital.

[In still another case] a 73-year old female who was hospitalized for the treatment of rheumatoid arthritis and needed help while walking, fell and sustained a fracture of the hip while being transferred from a chair to a bed. According to the patient, she was standing next to the bed when the licensed vocational nurse who had assisted her from the chair let go of her.

Testifying as an expert for the patient, a registered nurse said that not to support the patient at all times during the transfer from chair to bed was below the standard of care. The patient received a settlement of $45,000 from the hospital.

Hospital Malpractice Suits

In a study of hospital malpractice suits eight major problem areas were identified: (1) suicide and "elopement;" (2) anesthesia; (3) surgical cardiac arrest; (4) emergency room and nursing floor cardiac arrest; (5) qualification of surgical assistants and surgical privileges; (6) infection control; (7) maternal and neonatal injury; and (8) injection injury.

The Biggest Win

In the case of *Niles v. City of San Rafael School District,* an eleven-year-old boy who was injured in a school-yard fight became a quadriplegic as a result of emergency room

*Source: Helen Creighton, "Law," *Supervisor Nurse,* December 1974.

negligence. He was awarded in excess of $4,000,000 in a malpractice action against a hospital pediatrician and the school district.

Hospital and Doctor Malpractice Pay Outs

A study by the National Association of Insurance Commissioners released in May 1976 made public the amount of money paid out by insurer, for malpractice claims. During the period July 1, 1975, to March 15, 1975, a total of $105 million was paid on medical malpractice cases that had been fully processed. The money was used to cover slightly more than 3,000 claims. Fifty percent of the claims were from California, New York, Florida, Illinois and Pennsylvania, with 35% arising in New York and California.

Of the $105 million paid out, there were 311 instances in which more than $50,000 was paid, representing 3% of total claims and 63% of all dollars paid.

The highest payment was $1.3 million for a diagnostic error that ended in nervous system injury and paralysis.

Central nervous system damage accounted for 31% of all dollars paid, and 29% of the money paid out was for death following treatment.

Malpractice Premiums

In 1976 the American Hospital Association put the premium outlay for doctors and hospitals at $1.5 billion per year, and asserted that hospitals alone spend $750 million annually for coverage. The average hospital, by AHA reckoning, spends about $100,000 per year.

Public Attitudes Toward Malpractice

A July 10, 1975 Harris survey reported that only 15% of the 1,448 adults participating said that they, or someone close to them, had ever had medical treatment they would consider malpractice. And among those who reported the alleged malpractice, only 6%, or less than 1% of all Americans, tried to sue the doctor involved, although of those who did, 71% say they collected damages.

The Nurse and the Law

Scope of Practice

The consequences to a nurse for exceeding the scope of practice can be severe. The nurse may be accused of a violation of licensure provisions or of performing tasks that are statutorily reserved for a physician.

Suspension and Revocation

All nurse licensing boards have the authority to suspend or revoke the license of a nurse who is found in violation of specified norms of conduct. Such violations may include procurement of a license by fraud; unprofessional, dishonorable, immoral, or illegal conduct; performance of specific actions prohibited by the act; and malpractice.

A nurse may believe that the assigned duties and functions imply that the nurse is being called upon to make medical diagnoses and select therapeutic measures, which are basic elements of medical practice. However, a nurse who engages in activities beyond the legally recognized scope of practice runs the risk of prosecution for violating the state medical practice act, and the hospital that employs the nurse could also be held criminally responsible for aiding and abetting the illegal practice of medicine.

In addition to the risk of criminal prosecution, the risk of civil liability for harm suffered by a patient may be enhanced in a suit alleging negligence if the nurse has exceeded the legal scope of nursing. The law in some states would allow a jury to infer that a nurse was negligent if the nurse performed functions restricted by law to physicians and harm was suffered by a patient.

Delegation of Authority

A nurse with supervisory responsibility is not liable merely because one of the persons to whom duties have been assigned or delegated is negligent and thereby causes harm to a patient. The supervisor is liable only for negligence in carrying out supervisory duties. The supervisor's liability should be clearly distinguished from the liability of the employer—the hospital—for negligence under the doctrine of *respondeat superior*. The nurse with supervisory responsibilities is not the employer; the hospital is the employer and the supervising nurse is another hospital employee who has administrative responsibility for the performance of subordinate personnel.

Thus if a nursing supervisor assigns a task to an individual who the supervisor knows or should have known is not competent to perform the particular task, and if a patient suffers injury because of incompetent performance of the task, the supervisor can be held personally liable for negligence as a supervisor.

A supervisor may ordinarily rely upon the fact that a subordinate is licensed or certified as an indication of the subordinate's capabilities in performing tasks within the ambit of the license or certificate. But where the individual's past actions have led the supervisor to believe that the person is likely to perform a task in an unsatisfactory manner, assigning the task to the person can lead to liability for negligence because the risk of harm to the patient is increased.

The Nurse as Employee

Respondeat superior is the term for a form of vicarious liability wherein an employer is held liable for the wrongful acts of an employee even though the employer's conduct is without fault.

The doctrine of *respondeat superior* does not absolve the employee of liability for wrongful acts. Not only may the injured party sue the employee directly, but the employer may also seek indemnification from the employee—that is, compensation for the financial loss occasioned by the employee's wrongful act. Since the employee is primarily responsible for the loss, the law does not relieve the employee of liability when the hospital is held liable through the application of *respondeat superior*.

The doctrine of *respondeat superior* may impose liability upon a hospital for a nurse's acts or omissions that result in injury to a hospital patient. Acts and omissions may constitute negligence on the part of a nurse and may render a hospital liable under the doctrine of *respondeat superior*. But some examples may illustrate the circumstances under which the doctrine will apply. Cases have involved the application of overheated hot water bottles, the administration of an enema of too high a temperature, the injection of incorrect medication, the failure to catheterize a patient at the intervals requested by the patient's physician, and the failure to warn a patient of the danger inherent in lowering a bed.

A hospital will also be held liable for the failure of nursing personnel to take action when a patient's personal physician is clearly unwilling or unable to cope with a situation that threatens the life or health of the patient.

16

Nursing Risk

A nurse who provides professional services to another person for pay may be legally responsible for any harm that the person suffers as a result of the nurse's negligence; furthermore, the nurse may be subject to a loss of money in the form of legally awarded damages. Many nurses protect themselves from the risk of a legal loss by acquiring a professional liability insurance policy.

The Law: Areas of Concern

Consent to Medical and Surgical Procedures

Before any medical or surgical procedure can be performed on a patient, even a procedure involving the simple movement of a patient's limb, the consent must be obtained from the patient or from someone authorized to consent on the patient's behalf. [The need for such consent is] separate and distinct from any question of negligence or malpractice in performing the procedure. Liability may be imposed even if the procedure improved the patient's health.

Proof of Consent

A written consent has one purpose only: to provide visible proof of consent. An oral consent, if proved, is just as binding as a written one, for there is no legal requirement that the patient's consent be in writing. However, an oral consent may be difficult to prove in court. A valid written consent must include these elements: it must be signed; it must show that the procedure was the one consented to; and it must show that the person consenting understood the nature of the procedure, the risks involved, and the probable consequences.

Who Must Consent?

Consent of the patient is ordinarily required before treatment. However, when the patient is either physically unable or legally incompetent to consent, and no emergency exists, consent must be obtained from a person who is empowered to consent on the patient's behalf. The person who gives consent for treatment of another must have enough information to make an intelligent judgment, and the physician must disclose risks involved in the procedure.

Most courts have held that, as a general proposition, the consent of a minor to medical or surgical treatment is ineffective, and the physician must secure the consent of the minor's parent or someone standing *in loco parentis,* or must risk liability. Parental consent is no longer needed in certain cases where the minor is married or is otherwise emancipated.

Many states have recognized by legislation that there are conditions—specifically pregnancy, veneral disease, and drug dependency—for which a minor is likely to seek medical assistance without the knowledge of a parent. To require parental consent for the treatment of these conditions is to increase the risk that the minor will delay or do without treatment in order to avoid explanation to the parents.

When a physician doubts a patient's capacity to consent, even though the patient has not been adjudged legally incompetent, the consent of the nearest relative should be obtained.

An emergency exists when immediate action is required to save a patient's life or to prevent permanent impairment of the patient's health. If it is impossible in an emergency to obtain the consent of the patient or someone legally authorized to give consent, the required procedure may be undertaken without any liability for failure to procure consent. In other words, an emergency removes the need for consent.

The Nurse's Consent

It is generally the nurse who has to fill in the consent form, take it to the patient, explain it in language that the patient can understand, and then get the patient's consent.

It is sometimes difficult to make the explanation clear, in order to satisfy the legal requirement that the patient understand, and at the same time avoid frightening the patient. At least as much discretion and care are needed for this as for any other nursing act in order to avoid overemphasis or underemphasis of risks. Thus it is preferable that the patient's consent be procured by the operating physician.

The patient may withdraw consent at any time, and the withdrawal may be oral even though the original consent was written.

The emergency room provides the nurse with additional problems of patient consent. Because most patients who are treated in a hospital emergency room need immediate care, it is unwise for a nurse on duty in an emergency room to withhold or delay treatment while a consent form is procured, filled out, and signed. The emergency room illustrates the situation in which presence and voluntary submission to treatment constitute consent. At no time should care be delayed for paperwork, whether patient information or consent form. In these situations, consent is implied, and the nurse should see to it that immediate help is provided.

Patient Rights*

What does informed consent include? Much the same as the AHA Bill of Rights. The basic elements are (1) an explanation of the condition; (2) a fair explanation of the procedures to be used and the consequences; (3) a description of alternative treatments or procedures; (4) a description of the benefits to be expected (not assured); (5) an offer to answer the patient's inquiries; and (6) an understanding that the patient is not being coerced to agree and may withdraw if he changes his mind.

It is generally agreed that nurses are not primarily responsible for explaining medical treatments. They should be alert, however, to signs that the patient does not clearly understand what is involved and bring this to the attention of the persons involved. If the patient is coaxed or coerced into signing without such an explanation, the consent is invalid. Moreover, if the patient withdraws consent, even verbally, the nurse is responsible for reporting this and seeing that the patient is not treated. This is her responsibility not only to the patient but also to the hospital, which can be held liable.

The nurse's own and specific responsibility is to explain nursing care, including the whys and hows. A warning has already been sounded by some attorneys in the health field that lack of clear, understandable instruction on how patients can care for themselves is possible grounds for malpractice suits. Without knowledge of his condition and how to care for himself for optimum health, the patient is possibly denied the right of self-determination.

If a terminally ill patient has not been told of his condition, and the doctor refuses to do so, does the nurse tell him? At what price? If a patient is being coerced into unwanted surgery, does the nurse inform the patient of dangers which have not been explained and

*Source: "The Patient's Right to Know," L. Y. Kelly, *Nursing Outlook,* January 1976. ©American Journal of Nursing Company.

encourage refusal? At what price? If a doctor wants his patient to have no teaching about his condition, does the nurse provide it, anyway? At what price?

There may indeed be a price to pay—medical and administrative displeasure and consequent subtle or not so subtle punishment, even loss of job. We have encouraged the nurse to be autonomous, to make independent decisions within her scope of practice, to consider herself as accountable to the patient. But, if she does indeed practice in this fashion and, as a result, finds herself in personal or professional difficulty, are there support systems available to her?

Medical Records

Proper recording of the facts of a patients illness, symptoms, diagnosis, and treatment is one of the most important functions in furnishing modern medical and hospital care. Nurses and physicians are primarily charged with the responsibility of keeping accurate and up-to-date medical records. All hospital personnel who have access to medical records have both a legal and an ethical obligation to protect the confidentiality of the information in the records.

Medical records are maintained primarily to provide accurate and complete information about the care and treatment of patients. They are also the principal means of communication between physician and nurse in matters relating to patient care, and they serve as a basis for planning the course of treatment. Because the nurse is in a position to keep constant watch over the patient's illness, response to medication, display of pain and discomfort, and general condition, the patient's care as well as the nurse's observations should be recorded fully, factually, and promptly. No nurse should attempt to make a diagnosis, even if the conclusions seem obvious. Also, the nurse should promptly and accurately comply with the orders the physician writes in the record and should check, in case of doubt, to make certain that the order is correct and that it has not already been completed.

Legislation and regulations concerning medical records vary from state to state. Some states detail the information to be recorded, other states specify the broad areas of information required concerning the patient's treatment, and some states simply declare that the medical record shall be adequate, accurate, or complete. State hospital licensure rules and regulations may also set out requirements and standards for the maintenance, handling, signing, filing, and retention of medical records.

The Medical Record in Legal Proceedings

The increasing incidence of personal injury suits and the expanding acceptance of life, accident, and health insurance have made medical records important evidence in legal proceedings. These records aid police investigations, provide information for determining the cause of death, and indicate the extent of injury in workmen's compensation or personal injury proceedings.

When nurses or physicians are called as witnesses in a proceeding, they are permitted to refresh their recollections of the facts and circumstances of a particular case by referring to the record. Courts recognize that it is impossible for a medical witness to remember the details of every patient's treatment, and the record may therefore be used as an aid in relating the facts. In this situation the record stimulates the recall of the witness who testifies under oath and is subject to cross-examination.

The medical record itself may be admitted into evidence in legal proceedings. In this situation, the record is not under oath and is not subject to cross-examination. In order for medical record information to be allowed in evidence, the court must be assured that the information is accurate, that it was recorded at the time the event took place, and that it was not recorded in anticipation of the particular legal proceeding. In short, while it is recognized that witnesses may refresh their memories and that records may be admitted into evidence, there is nevertheless a need for assurance that the information is trustworthy.

When a medical record is introduced, its custodian, usually the medical record librarian, must testify to the manner in which the record was made and the way in which it is protected from unauthorized handling and change. It is to be noted that whether such records and other documents are admitted or excluded is governed by the rules of evidence. Thus whether the records are admissible depends on the facts and circumstances of the particular case.

Whatever the situation, it is clear that the record must be complete, accurate, and timely. If it can be shown that the record is inaccurate or incomplete or that it was made long after the event it purports to record, it will not be accepted.

Confidential Communications

Medical information may be gained by examination, treatment, observation, or conversation. The nurse, as well as the physician, has a clear moral obligation to keep secret any information relating to a patient's illness or treatment which is learned during the course of professional duties, unless the nurse is authorized by the patient to disclose the information or is ordered by a court to do so.

The confidentiality of communications in a medical situation is a principal tenet of the nursing code of professional ethics. There are also state statutes that forbid physicians, dentists, and other health practitioners from disclosing, without the patient's consent, any information acquired during the course of caring for a patient. Some of the statutes expressly include disclosures made to a professional, registered, or trained nurse, which means the nurse cannot be forced to testify in a legal proceeding about information obtained while caring for the patient. However, in most pertinent state statutes, nurses are not subject to the restrictions concerning revelation of confidential communications. The courts of a few states have held that, by implication, these statutes include nurses who are assisting or acting under the direction of a physician who treats the patient.

Negligence

The medical record must be both accurate and complete. Failure to comply with the minimum record maintenance standards set out in state statutes may cause the revocation of medical personnel licenses or hospital accreditation.

A nurse is also responsible for making the proper inquiry if there is uncertainty about the accuracy of an order in the record.

Drugs & Medications

The nurse is also exempt from the prohibitions of the various pharmacy statutes when administering a medicine or a drug to a patient upon an oral or written order of a physician. Any nurse who administered a drug without an order from a physician would be in violation of the state's pharmacy statute.

Intentional Wrongs

Although most incidents raising issues of a nurses's liability concern harm allegedly resulting from negligence, a nurse may also be liable for intentional wrongs. Intentional tortious conduct (in other words, conduct implying a civil wrong) that may arise in the context of patient care includes assault, battery, false imprisonment, invasion of privacy, libel, and slander.

Battery

A battery is an intentional, unconsented touching of another's person. The principle upon which liability is based is an individual's right to be free from invasion of his person.

False Imprisonment

False imprisonment is the unlawful restraint of an individual's personal liberty or the unlawful detention of an individual. Actual physical force is not necessary to constitute a false imprisonment. All that is necessary is a reasonable fear that force, which may be implied by words, threats, or gestures, will be used to detain the individual.

Not allowing a patient to leave a hospital until all bills have been paid may constitute false imprisonment. However, hospitals or nurses are not liable for false imprisonment if they compel a patient with a contagious disease to stay in the hospital. Mentally ill patients may also be kept in the hospital if there is a danger that they will take their own lives or jeopardize the lives and property of others.

A patient of sound mind who needs further medical attention but wants to go home should not be detained merely because the medical staff believes the patient would benefit from further hospitalization. The nature of the patient's condition and its probable consequences should be explained. The insistence on leaving should be noted on the medical record, and the patient should be asked to sign a form releasing the hospital from liability for harm resulting from premature departure.

Invasion of Privacy

Nurses may become liable for invasion of privacy if they divulge information from a patient's medical record to improper sources or if they commit unwarranted intrusions into the patient's personal affairs.

There *are* occasions when a nurse has a legal obligation or duty to disclose information. The reporting of communicable diseases, gunshot wounds, child abuse, and other matters is required by law.

Nurses should not allow pictures to be taken without the patient's consent. Furthermore, every hospital should implement rules and policies outlining the freedom permitted visitors in the hospital. If any visitor should try to roam around, peeking into rooms or reading charts, nurses should prevent these invasions lest the hospital be held liable.

Defamation

Libel is the written form and slander the oral form of defamation.

There are four generally recognized exceptions when no proof of any actual harm to reputation is required in order to recover damages: accusing someone of a crime; accusing someone of having loathsome disease; using words which affect a person's profession or business; and calling a woman unchaste.

When a person has said something that is damaging to another person's reputation, the person making the statement will not be liable for dafamation if it can be shown that the statement was true.

The Law—Areas of Specific Concern

Abused Children

The physically abused or neglected child is a medical, social, and legal problem. What constitutes an abused child is difficult to determine because it is often impossible to ascertain whether a child was injured intentionally or accidentally. Even the legal definition of a child varies. In one state a 12-year-old is an adult in the eyes of the law; in another state an 18-year-old is legally still a child.

Today, however, all states and the District of Columbia have enacted laws to protect abused

16

children. Furthermore, almost all states protect the persons required to report cases of child abuse.

Most state laws require certain people to report suspected cases of abuse. In a few states, although not required to report instances of child abuse, certain identified individuals who do so are protected. The child abuse laws may or may not provide penalties for failure to report. The classification of individuals covered by the various statutes ranges from physicians to "any person." Many of the statutes specifically include nurses.

All abused child statutes provide protection from civil suit for anyone making or participating in a good faith report. Most states also provide immunity from criminal liability. Even in states that do not, it is extremely unlikely that anyone making a good faith report of suspected child abuse would be subject to criminal liability.

Reporting laws specify the nature and content of the report of child abuse. Almost all the statutes require that when a person covered by statute is attending a child as a staff member of a hospital or similar institution, and child abuse is suspected, the staff member must notify the person in charge of the institution, who in turn makes the necessary report.

Diseases in Newborns

Many states require anyone in attendance at birth to report, either to the physician in charge or to an appropriate health officer, all instances of diarrhea, staphylococcal disease, or other infections. Most states provide for penalizing any violator of these laws.

Communicable Diseases

Many states have enacted laws which require that actual or suspected cases of communicable disease be reported to the proper authorities. Although other persons are affected, the responsibility for reporting generally falls upon the public health nurse.

Births Out of Wedlock

The responsibility for reporting births out of wedlock falls primarily upon someone other

than the nurse. However, there are situations where a nurse may be the appropriate person to make the report.

Gunshot Wounds

Gunshot wound laws require reports where injuries are inflicted by lethal weapons or, in some cases, by unlawful acts. Some statutes even include automobile accidents within their definition of lethal weapons.

Criminal Acts

Besides the subjects specified by statute as reportable, the nurse may have a moral or legal duty to report to the police such acts as attempted suicide, assault, rape, or the unlawful dispensing or taking of narcotic drugs. Much of this information may be learned while caring for patients and would ordinarily be privileged communication. Therefore, care must be taken that only the police are given such information.

Refusal of Treatment in Terminal Cases*

The long line of cases upholding refusal of treatment based on religious principles—even at the risk of death—further strengthens the basic right of a competent individual to refuse treatment.

Several questions of fact must be resolved initially. It must be determined that the patient is a terminal case. Such a determination should be made and documented by the attending physician in consultation with the appropriate members of the hospital's medical staff. Secondly, it must be ascertained that the patient is indeed competent. Any questions of competence should be handled by the attending physician in consultation with at least one other physician. It must be ascertained that the patient is competent at the time of refusal of treatment. Next, it is extremely important—to preclude any informed consent problems—to assure that the patient understands the types of treatment he or she is refusing and, moreover, that the patient fully understands the consequences of refusal.

---

*Source: "Hospital Law Manual Newsletter," Aspen Systems Corp., August 1976.

MODEL HOSPITAL RELEASE FORM
FOR REFUSAL OF TREATMENT

I, _____ hereby refuse any and all treatment rendered by _____ Hospital for the purpose of merely extending my life processes.

I hereby release and forever discharge _____ Hospital, its agents, employees, successors and assigns, from any and all liability actions, cause of actions, claims and demands whatsoever, whether at law or in equity, which may be incurred by reason of _____ _____ Hospital admitting and treating _____

(patient's name)

related to the nonapplication of any or all of the below listed medical procedures: *

  1. Hyperalimentation
  2. Chemotherapy
  3. Radiotherapy
  4. Cardiac Resuscitation
  5. Use of Respirator or other life-support systems
  6. Antibiotics for unrelated complications
  7. Operating procedure
  8. Tests other than routine admission tests

I otherwise authorize the use of any procedures that will ensure my comfort during my hospitalization provided that such procedures are not used solely to sustain my life processes.

I agree that this release is being sought for the purpose of not needlessly prolonging my life. I understand that the probable outcome of the nonuse of these procedures will be the more rapid deterioration of my health and will probably accelerate the deterioration of my life processes.

I acknowledge that this release is being executed at my sole request and free will, that I intend this release to be binding on my heirs, executors and administrators.

I further acknowledge that I have read this release, fully understand the provisions contained in it, and that I am mentally competent to make such release.

(Patient) _____

(Attending Physician) _____

(Witness) _____

Dated: _____, 19 _____

*The listing herein is merely illustrative. The listing can be tailored to meet the needs of the individual situation.

Mercy Killing*

In 1975 Karen Ann Quinlan, in a comatose state, her prognosis for recovery poor, was being sustained by a respirator and other mechanical devices. The superior court denied Joseph Quinlan, Karen's adoptive father, the right to act to discontinue all extraordinary medical procedures sustaining her vital processes. The question was then taken to the New Jersey Supreme Court. On March 31, 1976, the supreme court decided that declaratory relief could be granted.

*Source: "Hospital Law Manual Newsletter," Aspen Systems Corporation, August 1976.

The court found that there is a real and determinative distinction between the unlawful taking of the life of another, e.g., homicide, and the ending of artificial life-support systems as a matter of self-determination, even when a third person makes the decision to terminate artificial life-support systems. Second, the court concluded that there is a right of privacy that would permit termination of treatment in the circumstances of this case.

Briefly summarizing the holding in this case, the court established the following criteria for discontinuing life-support measures for incompetent individuals:

1. the attending physicians must conclude that there is no *reasonable* possibility that

the patient will emerge into a *congnitive, sapient state;* and,

2. the patient's family and guardian must concur in the decision; and,
3. once the attending physician and the family have reached agreement, they must consult with the hospital's ethics committee or a similar committee of the institution in which the individual is a patient; and,
4. the committee must agree with the decision reached by the attending physician.

Good Samaritan Laws

Most states have enacted good samaritan laws which relieve physicians, nurses, and in some instances laymen from liability in certain emergency situations. Good samaritan legislation encourages health professionals to render assistance at the scene of emergencies. By offering immunity, the laws attempt to overcome the widespread notion that physicians, nurses, and others who render assistance in an emergency are likely to be held liable for negligence.

Whatever the limits on legal duty, the law does require that anyone who volunteers to aid another in distress assumes a legal responsibility to exercise reasonable care and skill in rendering such aid. Thus the fact that a good samaritan acts in good faith and for no payment is immaterial. It is the act of giving aid that creates a duty and subjects the good samaritan to liability if there is a lack of due care. However, one who is confronted with a medical emergency is not held to the same standard of care as normally is applied in a nonemergency situation.

Under most statutes, immunity is granted only in an emergency or for rendering emergency care.

Nurses are covered in the good samaritan statutes of 45 jurisdictions.

Table 16-2   State-by-state summary of good samaritan laws

	A. Date of act or last amended act	B. Covers any emergency or accident	C. Covers only roadside accidents	D. Covers everyone	E. Covers in-state physicians	F. Covers out-of-state physicians	G. Covers in-state nurses	H. Covers out-of-state nurses	I. Does not cover acts of gross negligence or willful misconduct	J. Covers only gratuitous services
Alabama	1966	X			X	X	X	X	X	X
Alaska	1967	X		X					X	X
Arizona	1967	X		X	X	X	X	X	X	X
Arkansas	1963	X		X	X				X	X
California	1963	X			X		X		X	
Colorado	1965	X			X	X	X	X	X	
Connecticut	1969	X			X	X	X	X	X	X
Delaware	1963	X			X		X		X	
District of Columbia	1966	X			X	X	X	X	X	X
Florida	1965	X		X					X	X
Georgia	1963	X		X					X	X
Hawaii	1969	X		X					X	X
Idaho	1965	X		X					X	
Illinois	1970			X					X	X
Indiana	1964	X			X		X		X	X
Iowa	1970	X		X					X	X
Kansas	1969	X			X	X	X	X	X	X
Kentucky										
Louisiana	1964	X			X	X	X	X	X	X

Table 16-2   (continued)

	A. Date of act or last amended act	B. Covers any emergency or accident	C. Covers only roadside accidents	D. Covers everyone	E. Covers in-state physicians	F. Covers out-of-state physicians	G. Covers in-state nurses	H. Covers out-of-state nurses	I. Does not cover acts of gross negligence or willful misconduct	J. Covers only gratuitous services
Maine	1961	X			X		X		X	
Maryland	1973	X			X		X		X	X
Massachusetts	1970	X			X	X	X	X	X	X
Michigan	1964	X			X	X	X	X	X	
Minnesota	1971	X		X					X	
Mississippi	1964	X			X	X	X	X	X	
Missouri										
Montana	1963	X		X					X	X
Nebraska	1963	X			X	X	X	X	X	X
Nevada	1965	X		X					X	X
New Hampshire	1967	X			X	X	X	X	X	X
New Jersey	1968	X		X					X	
New Mexico	1963	X		X					X	X
New York	1968	X			X	X			X	X
North Carolina	1965		X	X					X	
North Dakota	1963	X			X	X			X	
Ohio	1964	X		X					X	X
Oklahoma	1969	X			X	X	X	X	X	
Oregon	1968	X			X	X	X	X	X	X
Pennsylvania	1965	X			X	X	X	X	X	
Rhode Island	1963	X			X	X			X	X
South Carolina	1964	X		X					X	X
South Dakota	1963	X			X	X	X	X	X	
Tennessee	1964	X		X					X	X
Texas	1964	X		X					X	X
Utah	1967	X			X		X		X	
Vermont	1967	X		X					X	X
Virginia	1968	X		X					X	X
Washington	1971	X			X				X	
West Virginia	1967	X		X					X	X
Wisconsin	1964	X			X		X		X	X
Wyoming	1963	X		X					X	X

Eugenic Sterilization

The term "eugenic sterilization" refers to sterilization of persons within certain classes or categories described in statutes, without the need for consent by, or on behalf of, those subjected to the procedures. Persons classified as insane, mentally deficient, feebleminded, and, in some instances, epileptic are included within the scope of the statutes. Several states have also included certain sexual deviates and persons classified as habitual criminals.

Therapeutic Sterilization

If the life or health of a woman may be jeopardized in the event that she becomes pregnant, the danger may be avoided by terminating her ability to conceive or her husband's ability to impregnate. Such an operation is a therapeutic sterilization, one to preserve life or health. It is the medical necessity for sterilization which renders the procedure therapeutic.

Ordinarily, the patient's consent is sufficient authorization for an operation; however, since sterilization affects the procreative function, the patient's spouse has an interest that could be legally recognized. Therefore, when the operation is primarily to accomplish sterilization, it would seem advisable to obtain the spouse's consent. However, when the procedure is medically necessary and sterilization is an incidental result, the patient's consent alone is sufficient.

Where it is predictable that an operation needed to cure a condition will incidentally destroy the ability to procreate, it is imperative that the effect on the reproductive function be made clear to both patient and spouse.

Dead Bodies

Cases involving wrongful handling of dead bodies may be classified into four groups: mutilation of a body, unauthorized autopsy, wrongful detention, and miscellaneous wrongs such as unauthorized sale, refusal or neglect to bury, or unauthorized use of publication of photographs taken after death.

Autopsies

Approximately one-half of the autopsy consent statutes provide that the deceased may authorize an autopsy upon his remains.

The person upon whom the duty to bury the deceased is imposed has the right to custody of the body and the right to recover for mutilation of the corpse and is thus the person from whom authority to perform an autopsy should be obtained.

Where custody of the body has been assumed by the first person in the preference order, that person's consent is sufficient to authorize the autopsy and prevent liability for mutilation of the corpse.

Summary of the Uniform Anatomical Gift Act

Any individual who is of sound mind and 18 years of age or older is permitted to dispose of his own body or body parts by will or other written instrument for medical or dental education, research, advancement of medical or dental science, therapy, or transplantation. Among those eligible to receive such donations are any licensed, accredited, or approved hospital, accredited medical or dental school, surgeon or physician, tissue bank, or any specified individual who needs the donation for therapy or transplantation. The statute provides that when only a part of the body is donated, custody of the remaining parts of the body shall be transferred to the next of kin promptly following removal of the donated part.

In cases of a donation made by a written instrument other than a will, the instrument must be signed by the donor in the presence of two witnesses who, in turn, must sign the instrument in the donor's presence. If the donor cannot sign the instrument, the document may be signed at the donor's direction and in the presence of the donor and the two signing witnesses.

In the absence of a contrary intent evidenced by the decedent or of actual notice of opposition by a member of the same class or a prior class in the preference order, the decedent's body or body parts may be donated by the following persons in the order specified: surviving spouse, adult child, parent, adult brother or sister, decedent's guardian, or any other person or agency authorized to dispose of the body. A donation by a person other than the decedent may be made by written, telegraphic, recorded telephonic, or other recorded consent.

Unclaimed Dead Bodies

When there are no known relatives or friends of the family who can be contacted by the hospital to claim the body, the hospital has a responsibility to dispose of the body in accordance with law.

Unclaimed bodies are generally buried at public expense; a public official, usually a county official, has the duty to bury or otherwise dispose of such bodies. Most states have statutes providing for the disposal of unclaimed bodies by delivery to institutions for educational and scientific purposes. Thus unclaimed bodies in the custody of public officials, such as coroners or administrators of governmental hospitals, are subject to use for such purposes.

Research on Humans*

The formal human research requirements adopted by the American Medical Association are: voluntary consent, assessment of danger in animal experimentation, and performance of research under proper medical protection and management.

Where investigational drugs are administered primarily to acquire scientific knowledge, such as to study drug behavior, body processes, or the course of disease, the FDA regulations require consent to be obtained in writing from patients, or their representatives.

It frequently happens that the nurse in the large hospital becomes involved in such research without any choice because she cares for patients who are receiving experimental drugs or other experimental therapy as a part of medical treatment and investigation. In such situations, she must assess the patient and make specific observations; frequently she administers the investigational drug or other therapy that represents variations from the usual. Such duties are an expected part of her daily work, and no one seeks her consent to participate in the research.

At the same time, the nurse has a basic commitment to render quality nursing, including safety, to all patients entrusted to her care; to carry out this responsibility, she must know what is happening to them. She should be aware of the individual's rights and of her share in the responsibility of preserving them: privacy, self-determination, conservation of personal resources, freedom from arbitrary hurt and intrinsic risk of injury, and the special rights of minors and incompetent persons. As a nurse investigator, she assumes primary responsibility for preserving such rights. Guidelines have been delineated in the ANA publication, *The Nurse in Research: ANA Guidelines on Ethical Values.*

Both for her own protection and that of the patient, she needs sufficient knowledge of the research design to enable her to participate in the required activities in an informed, effective, and ethical manner.

When administering investigational drugs

---

*Source: Creighton and Armington, "Legal Consensus of Research and Nurse Researchers," *Issues in Research,* American Nurses Association, Pub. No. D-44.

which are potentially harmful to the patient, a nurse should have basic information about the drug including method of administration, strength available, action and use, side effects, symptoms of toxicity, and so on.

Professional Insurance

Professional Liability Insurance Policy

A nurse who is covered by a professional liability insurance policy must recognize the rights and duties inherent in the policy. The nurse should be able to identify the risks that are covered, the amount of coverage, and the conditions of the contract.

Although coverage may vary in the policies of different insurance companies, the standard policy usually says the insurance company will "pay on behalf of the insured all sums which the insured shall become legally obligated to pay as damages because of injury arising out of malpractice, error, or mistake in rendering or failing to render nursing services."

A standard liability insurance policy has five distinct parts: (1) the insurance agreement; (2) defense and settlement; (3) policy period; (4) amount payable; and (5) conditions.

Sample: If a jury determines that a nurse is liable to an injured person for $45,000, and the maximum coverage in the nurse's insurance policy is $40,000, the insurance company will pay only $40,000 to the injured party; the remaining $5,000 must be provided from other resources by the nurse.

Benefits

The cost of professional liability insurance is modest, especially if it is obtained through the state nurses' association or through the American Nurses' Association. At a time when the number of lawsuits against hospitals, physicians, and nurses is increasing, this type of insurance protection seems desirable. Three benefits to the policy holder are provided by such insurance: (1) in the event of an award of damages against the nurse, the insurance pays any sum within the specified limits of the policy; (2) it pays the cost of the lawyer

16

furnished to defend the person who is sued in a civil court for some alleged injury resulting from her professional work; and (3) it will pay for bond for a nurse in the event it is required during an appeal.

How Much Insurance?*

No one can predict whether he or she will ever be involved in a malpractice action—and, if so, what the judgment will be. Without that ability, no one can determine the adequate limits of liability. Today, limits of liability on a primary policy of $200,000 for each incident and $600,000 for each annual period are quite common. What do these figures mean?

In a policy which limits liability to $200,-000/600,000, the $200,000 indicates that the insurance company will provide payment for any individual claim up to $200,000. Defense coverage is usually provided in addition to the limit of liability. Thus, if a nurse were sued successfully for $400,000, the insurance company would provide defense and pay $200,000 of the judgment, leaving $200,-000 to be paid by the nurse out of her own pocket.

The $600,000 indicates that the company will pay judgments up to $600,000 total (on all claims) during the year.

Nurses should supplement their personal policy with an "umbrella" policy. Such a policy would provide liability coverage for any losses beyond those covered by the primary policy. For example, an "umbrella" policy with limits of $1,000,000 would pay up to $1,000,000 over the amount paid by the primary policy for a single incident or for all occurrences during the year.

Like the primary policy, the "umbrella" policy may also cover excess personal liabilities. That is, it may extend liability coverage over your homeowner's, major medical, and automobile liability insurance policies.

Premiums for a personal, professional liability policy for general nurses are usually less than $30 annually, depending on the limits of liability purchased. Premiums for nurse anesthetists and X-ray technicians are much more—from a few hundred dollars to over a thousand dollars a year.

The Emergency Dept. Nurse and Malpractice Insurance**

Many E.D. nurses mistakenly believe they are covered under the insurance policy of the hospital which employs them. This may or may not be true.

The professional E.D. nurse is liable for her or his own acts of negligence. The negligence may also make the hospital liable as their employer. The E.D. nurse should seek and obtain written verification of liability (malpractice) coverage from the hospital or the hospital's insurance agent or insurance company. This written confirmation is the only proof upon which the E.D. nurse should rely if he or she decides not to purchase a personal malpractice policy.

There are important reasons why the E.D. nurse should possess a personal malpractice insurance policy. The premium is very inexpensive for a sizeable amount of coverage. The E.D. nurse should carry approximately $200,-000 to $600,000 of coverage. Such a policy should include "umbrella protection" to cover personal as well as professional liability.

A personal nursing malpractice policy will also cover any liability arising outside of the hospital. The hospital's malpractice coverage of the nurse is generally limited to acts which occur within the confines of the hospital. Also, coverage for assault, battery, slander and libel may not be included in the hospital's policy.

Furthermore, nurses are now being sued individually as well as jointly with the hospital.

Also, the interests of the hospital may conflict with those of the nurses where they are both codefendants in the negligence suit. The hospital's defense attorney may have to sacrifice the interests of the nurse if they detract from the interests of the hospital.

Finally, if a hospital is sued for the negligence of one of its E.D. nurses and pays a claim, the hospital has the legal right to sue the negligent nurse for reimbursement to the hospital for the costs it has incurred on behalf of the nurse.

*Source: "Career Guides," *Nursing '76.*

Sample of a Professional Liability Policy

Figure 16-1   Nurse's professional liability policy.

Declaration of Contents

Insurer	THE X INSURANCE COMPANY 111 MAIN ST., CHICAGO, ILL.
Agent	SMITH & JONES CO., AGENTS 222 SOUTH ST., PITTSBURGH, PENNA.
Insured	MISS IDA GREEN 333 ELM ST., PITTSBURGH, PENNA.
Policy period	FROM JANUARY 1, 1978 TO JANUARY 1, 1979

Liability limits
each claim ....$ 40,000
aggregate...$120,000

Premium
yearly...$7.00

Pending actions
The named insured represents that no claims, demands, or legal actions are pending against the named insured arising out of any actual or alleged error, mistake, or malpractice.

The insurer named in the declaration of contents contracts with the named insured, named in the declaration of contents, in consideration of the paying of the stated premium and in reliance upon the statements made in the declaration and subject to all of the terms of this policy:

INSURING AGENT
1. Coverage
   A. Malpractice Liability—to pay on behalf of the insured all sums which the insured shall become legally obligated to pay as damages because of injury arising out of malpractice, error, or mistake in rendering or failing to render nursing services.

DEFENSE AND SETTLEMENT
The insurance company under this policy shall:
   A. Defend any suit against the named insured alleging injury to persons and/or property and which is seeking damages that are payable under this policy.
   B. Make any settlement of any claim or suit as it determines expedient.

POLICY PERIOD
This policy is applicable only to accidents occurring during the stated policy period.

CONDITIONS
1. Notice of Occurrence—When the insured knows of any alleged accident covered herein, he shall notify the company as soon as possible.
2. Notice of Claim—When any claim is instituted against the insured, he must immediately notify the company in writing and forward every notice or summons he or his representative has received.
3. Assistance—The insured must assist the company upon the company's request and such assistance shall include attending all hearings and trials and the giving of evidence. The insured must also assist in making settlements upon request of the company.
4. Other Insurance—If the insured has other insurance against a loss included under this policy's coverage, this company will pay its pro rata share of the loss.
5. Assignment—The insured cannot assign any interest in this policy, unless he receives written authorization from a properly authorized representative of the company. Every other attempt to assign the insured's interest shall not be effective.
6. Subrogation—Whenever the company makes any payment under this policy, the company will be subrogated to all of the rights of the insured to recover against any other person.
7. Changes—No agent of the company may change any section of this policy unless he receives written authorization from the company.
8. Cancellation—The insured may cancel this policy at any time by returning the policy to any agent of the company.
9. Limits of Liability—The liability of this policy shall be limited by the declaration applicable to "each claim" on each claim or suit. The liability of this policy shall be limited by the declaration applicable to "aggregate" for the total liability of the company.

_____   _____
Signature of Agent   Signature of Named Insured

_____
Witness

_____
Witness

17

L.P.N.s, L.V.N.s AND AIDES

LICENSED PRACTICAL NURSE (L.P.N.) OR LICENSED VOCATIONAL NURSE (L.V.N.)

Overview

Definitions

Serving as an important member of the nursing team in most hospitals and other nursing care settings is the licensed practical (or vocational) nurse, who works under the direction of a professional nurse or physician.

Chiefly concerned with the bedside care of patients, the licensed practical nurse helps feed and bathe patients; takes their temperature, pulse and blood pressure; observes and reports symptoms to the nurse or doctor; and, in some localities, gives prescribed medications and treatments.

Practical nurses sometimes have the direct responsibility of providing nursing service for patients who are not seriously ill. They often care for convalescent patients, those with long-term illness, and for new mothers and their babies. Practical nurses share in the care of patients who are seriously ill or otherwise require the more complex skills of professional nurses. They may also assist with the supervision of nursing aides, orderlies, and attendants.

Trends

Licensed practical nurses employed in the United States numbered about 492,000 as of January 1, 1973. About 60% of them worked in hospitals. The others were primarily employed in nursing homes and doctors' offices.

The growth in employment has been rapid, increasing from the census enumerations of 137,500 in 1950 and 206,000 in 1960.

The percentage of registered nurses who are inactive is greater than the proportion of licensed practical nurses who are inactive.

To characterize generally the entire population of licensed practical nurses (both the employed and inactive in nursing): they were predominantly female (about 3% were male); the majority were married (59%); 21% were widowed, divorced or separated; almost 14% were single; and the median age was 44.1 years.

Men L.P.N.s

There is an increasing demand for men as licensed practical nurses, especially in the area of psychiatric and rehabilitation nursing. In 1974 they represented 2.7% of all employed licensed practical nurses. The median age of employed, male, licensed practical nurses was 44.0 years. Only 22% of the employed male licensed practical nurses were single.

Functions

The L.P.N. or L.V.N. cares for ill, injured, convalescent, and handicapped persons in hospitals, clinics, private homes, sanitariums, and similar institutions. Takes and records temperature, blood pressure, and pulse and respiration rate. Dresses wounds, gives enemas, douches, alcohol rubs, and massages. Applies compresses, ice bags, and hot water bottles. Observes patients and reports adverse reactions to physician or nurse, general duty. Administers specified medication, and notes time and amount on patients' charts. Assembles and uses such equipment as catheters, tracheotomy tubes, and oxygen suppliers. Performs routine laboratory work, such as urinalysis. Sterilizes equipment and supplies, using germicides, sterilizer, or autoclave. Prepares food trays and feeds patients. Records food and fluid intake and output. Bathes, dresses, and assists patients in walking and turning. Cleans rooms, makes beds, and answers patients' calls. Washes and dresses bodies of deceased persons.

L.P.N. and Aide Task Overlap*

In a survey by Gilligan & Sherman of tasks performed by L.P.N.s and aides, a high degree of task overlap (see accompanying figure) was found between people with different job titles. Of the 346 nursing tasks in the survey, L.P.N.s perform 271 or 78%, N.A.s in hospitals perform 203 or 58%, N.A.s in nursing homes perform 153 or 44%, and H-H.H.A.s perform 113 or 33%. The level of agreement among job titles and among different types of health care institutions as to which tasks are performed in common is surprisingly high.

---

*Source: V. C. Sherman, "What Exactly Do Aides Do," *In-Service Training and Education,* November, 1974.

Figure 17-1   Overlap in nursing task performance as a percent of tasks performed by compared job titles

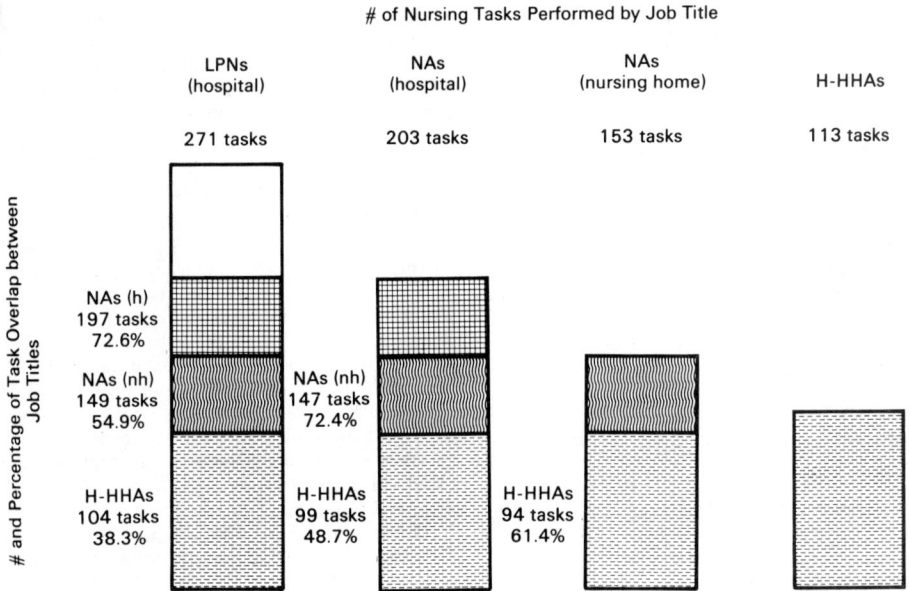

# of Nursing Tasks Performed by Job Title

LPNs (hospital)	NAs (hospital)	NAs (nursing home)	H-HHAs
271 tasks	203 tasks	153 tasks	113 tasks

and Percentage of Task Overlap between Job Titles

NAs (h)
197 tasks
72.6%

NAs (nh)
149 tasks
54.9%

NAs (nh)
147 tasks
72.4%

H-HHAs
104 tasks
38.3%

H-HHAs
99 tasks
48.7%

H-HHAs
94 tasks
61.4%

Typical Tasks Performed

Hospital L.P.N.s only

- Oxygen Procedures II
- Administering Blood
- Enterostomy
- Medications

Hospital L.P.N.s
Hospital Aides

- Assist Physician in Exams
- Application of Heat. Cold
- Pre/Post-Operative Care
- Oxygen Procedures

Hospital L.P.N.s   Nursing Home Aides
Hospital Aides

- Admitting and Discharging Patient
- Skin Care
- Basic Catheter Care
- Applying Restraints
- Isolation Techniques
- Housekeeping Role of Facility Based Personnel

Hospital L.P.N.s   Nursing Home Aides
Hospital Aides   Homemaker-Home Health Aides

- Orientation
- Handwashing
- Making the Bed
- Cleanliness of Patient's Surroundings
- Elements of Asepsis
- Human Interaction
- Dressing and Undressing the Patient
- General Grooming
- Normal Mouth Feeding
- Elimination
- Collecting and Testing Urine Specimens
- Vital Signs
- Charting
- Oral Communication
- Assist Patient in Movement
- Decubiti Care
- Observing Patient's Condition
- Transport Patient in Wheel Chair
- Evaluate Patient Care
- Bandages
- Health Education

Employment

Employment Outlook

The employment outlook for licensed practical nurses is expected to be very good through the mid-1980s. Employment is expected to continue to rise very rapidly through the mid-1980s in response to a growing population, the increasing ability of persons to pay for health care, and the continuing expansion of public and private health insurance plans. Jobs will be created also as licensed practical nurses take over duties previously performed by registered nurses. Also, thousands of newly licensed practical nurses will be needed each year to replace those who die, retire, or leave the occupation for other reasons.

Current Employment Status

Table 17-1   Employment status of practical nurses after graduation

| | Time after graduation | | |
Employment status	One year (%)	Five years (%)	Ten years (%)
Full-time L.P.N./L.V.N.	74.4	52.7	38.6
Part-time L.P.N./L.V.N.	8.1	13.1	18.6
Working as R.N.	—	1.9	4.7
Not employed	14.0	25.7	29.5
Non-nursing work	1.1	4.8	8.4
No response	2.4	1.8	0.2
Total	100.0	100.0	100.0

Ten years after graduation only 38.6% of the practical nurses indicated that they were employed as full time practical nurses (Table 17-1.) But there was an increase over the years of the proportion employed in practical nursing part-time.

Combining full-time and part-time work in practical nursing and work as a registered nurse, 61.9% of the respondents were engaged in nursing work ten years after graduation.

Those who were not employed said most frequently they would seek nursing work but at present they had children to care for at home (40% of the non-employed, Table 17-2.)

For more than half not working ten years after graduation, caring for their children made

employment unlikely. The next largest group, 10.2%, said they would seek nursing work if they needed the money.

Table 17-2   For those not employed and those not working in nursing, circumstances under which they would seek nursing employment

Would seek employment in Nursing:	Not employed (%)	
But have children to care for	40.0	
Children and other reason	17.5	62.4%
But have family responsibility	4.9	
If health were better	6.6	
If needed the money	10.2	
If could get job, hours, or job and hours wanted	7.0	
Other reason	13.7	

Source: "Practical Nurses in the Health Labor Force," *Nursing Care*, March 1975.

Earnings and Working Conditions

The average starting salary of licensed practical nurses who worked in hospitals and medical schools was about $120 a week in 1972, according to a national survey conducted by the University of Texas Medical Branch.

Public health agencies paid licensed practical nurses salaries that averaged about $6,600 a year in 1972. Federal hospitals offered beginning licensed practical nurses annual salaries ranging from $6,128 to $6,882 in early 1973, according to personal qualifications and the geographical area.

Many hospitals give periodic pay increases after specific periods of satisfactory service. Some hospitals provide free lodging and laundering of uniforms. Practical nurses generally work 40 hours a week, but often this workweek includes some work at night and on weekends and holidays. Many hospitals provide paid holidays and vacations, health insurance, and pension plans.

In private homes, licensed practical nurses usually work 8 to 12 hours a day and go home at night.

Turnover

High turnover of aides is a problem nationwide. For example, in metropolitan Washington, the annual turnover rate of aides in hospitals is 60%; in nursing homes, 75%. A nursing home can expect 100% turnover every 16 months—a hospital every 20 months.

Regional Comparison of Salaries

Table 17-3   Salaries of newly licensed L.P.N.s

Salary	Total	Bos.	N.Y.	Phila.	Atla.	Chi.	Dal.	K.C.	Denver	S.F.	Seattle
Under $5,000	18%	10%	11%	14%	31%	11%	35%	24%	25%	6%	17%
$5,000–5,999	26	10	16	33	35	25	31	30	40	10	30
$6,000–6,999	20	31	19	18	11	27	10	13	5	31	19
$7,000–7,999	8	17	18	7	2	11	3	3	0	12	2
$8,000–8,999	2	4	7	2	1	2	1	0	0	8	0
$9,000–9,999	1	1	3	0	0	0	0	0	0	3	0
$10,000+	1	1	1	0	1	0	0	1	0	1	2
Other	24	26	25	26	19	24	20	29	30	29	30
Total	100%	100%	100%	100%	100%	100%	100%	100%	100%	100%	100%

Source: DHEW, May 1975.

Where Employed: Job Description and L.P.N. Profile

The majority of licensed practical nurses work in hospitals, clinics, homes for the aged, and nursing homes. In 1972, some 196,000 full-time L.P.N.s were employed in hospitals.

An additional 54,000 were employed in nursing and related homes and 6,000 in other inpatient health facilities. Many others are employed in private homes. Most of the remainder work in doctors' offices, schools, and public health agencies. In 1972 an estimated 4,000 licensed practical nurses were employed in public health work under the supervision of public health staff nurses.

Hospitals

In hospitals, licensed practical nurses provide much of the bedside care needed by patients. They take and record temperatures and blood pressures, change dressings, administer certain prescribed medicines, and help bed patients with bathing and other personal hygiene. They assist physicians and registered nurses in examining patients and in carrying out nursing procedures. They also assist in the delivery, care, and feeding of infants, and help registered nurses in recovery rooms by reporting any adverse changes in patients. Some licensed practical nurses help supervise hospital attendants.

Licensed practical nurses in hospitals had a median age of 41.4 years. One-quarter of them were 28.6 years or younger and one-quarter were over 52.2 years. Licensed practical nurses in hospitals and those working in offices were younger on the average than those working in other employment settings. The median age of licensed practical nurses in offices was 40.1 years.

Three-fourths of the single nurses worked in hospitals, a far greater proportion in hospitals than was found for all employed licensed practical nurses. The median age of single licensed practical nurses in hospitals was 24.8 years.

The proportion of licensed practical nurses in hospitals who received their original licenses by waiver was comparatively low (19.5%) compared to all other fields in which large numbers of licensed practical nurses were found. The exceptions were the physicians' or dentists' offices where only 19.9% of licensed practical nurses received their first licenses by waiver.

Private Homes

Licensed practical nurses who work in private homes provide mainly day-to-day patient care that seldom involves highly technical procedures or complicated equipment. In addition to providing nursing care, they may prepare meals and care for the patient's comfort and morale. They also teach family members how to perform simple nursing tasks.

Private nursing is the second largest field of employment for licensed practical nurses. These nurses are older on the average than licensed practical nurses in any other employment setting; the median age is 54.9 years. Because of their age level, they show, as a group, significantly higher proportions of widowed, divorced and separated persons than all licensed practical nurses. Forty-three percent of licensed practical nurses doing private nursing reported receiving their original licenses by waiver, the highest percentage of any field in which licensed practical nurses were working.

Nursing Homes

Nursing homes employ the third largest number of licensed practical nurses among the various employment settings. These nurses also tend to be older, on the average, with a median age of 48.2 years. A significantly higher proportion are married and widowed than are found for all licensed practical nurses.

As a group, licensed practical nurses in nursing homes have a high proportion (32.9%) of waivered licenses.

Medical and Dental Offices

In doctors' offices and in clinics, licensed practical nurses prepare patients for examination and treatment. They also may make appointments and record information about patients.

Physicians and dentists employ the fourth largest group of licensed practical nurses to work in their offices. Insofar as age and basis of obtaining original license is concerned, they are similar to the group of licensed practical nurses in hospitals. The marital status distribution of each group is, however, quite different: 69% of those employed in offices are married while 58.6% of those employed in hospitals are married.

Selected Data on Employment Fields

Figure 17-2 Median age of single and married L.P.N.s in selected fields of nursing

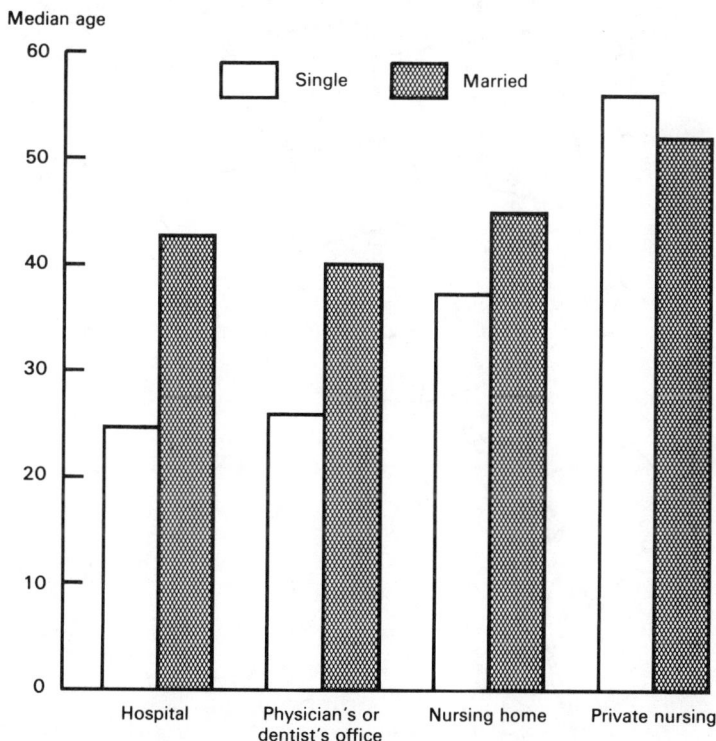

Source: National Institutes of Health, DHEW, 1970.

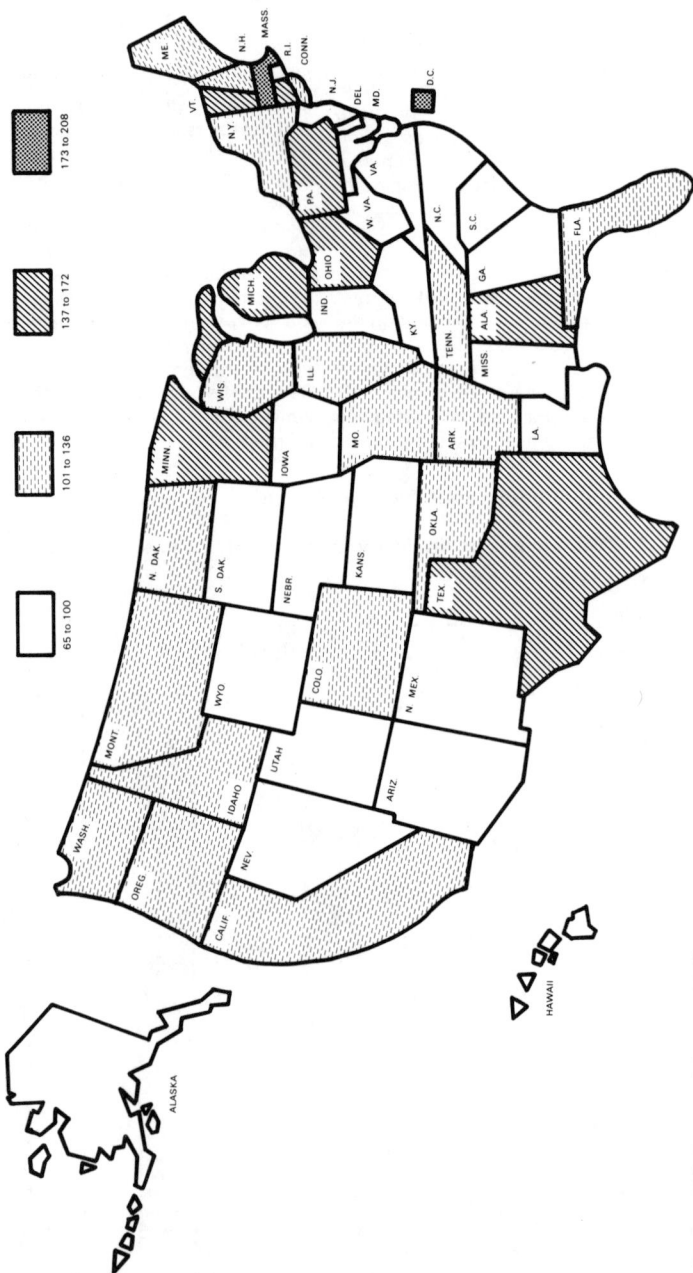

Figure 17-3 Practical nurses per 100,000 resident population, by state: United States, 1970

173 to 208

137 to 172

101 to 136

65 to 100

Source: U.S. Bureau of Census, 1970.

Figure 17-4   Licensed practical nurses by field of employment, 1972, N = 427,000

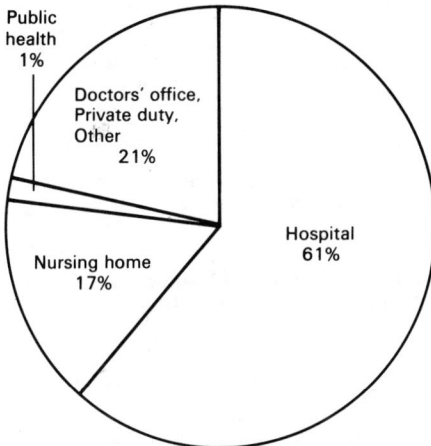

Public health 1%

Doctors' office, Private duty, Other 21%

Hospital 61%

Nursing home 17%

Source: Division of Nursing, DHEW, 1973.

Education Overview

Most practical nursing programs require full-time attendance. This will include classes, practice of nursing procedures, and supervised learning experiences with real patients in a hospital, extended care facility, or nursing home.

Instruction and nursing practice include the care of medical, surgical, and obstetric patients, and special care required for infants, children, the elderly, and the chronically ill. They also include some selected background information in the behavioral and biological sciences.

Requirements for admission to a practical nursing school program vary. The age limits for admission to a school of practical nursing are generally from 17 or 18 to 50.

In most states the applicants are required to have completed at least two years of high school; a few states require a high school diploma. The program is usually 12 to 18 months and may be obtained in trade, technical, or vocational schools operated by public school systems or in private schools controlled by hospitals, health agencies, or colleges. By October 1972, 1,310 programs in

1,220 schools of practical nursing education were approved by the state agencies. There were 61,680 admissions and 44,446 graduates in academic year 1971–72.

The National Association for Practical Nurse Education and Service is the accrediting body for schools and programs of practical nursing.

Costs

Total costs for a practical nursing course, in 1971, ranged from $50 to $1,280. If the course is offered by a public education system for high school students as a part of its vocational education program, there is usually no charge, but there may be minimum fees and incidental expenses. Tuition free courses are also sponsored under the Manpower Development and Training Act (MDTA), and some of these may provide a stipend. (For more details contact the local state employment service office.) Scholarships are available in some schools of practical nursing to cover the cost of the program.

Educational Programs for Practical Nursing

Although there were 5,655 L.P.N. and L.V.N. programs operating in 1975, only 1,364 of them were state approved. (For a complete list of schools write to National League for Nursing and ask for the booklet: "State-Approved Schools of Nursing L.P.N./L.V.N., New York. It is published annually.)

Table 17-4   Faculty education level

	Diploma	B.N.	M.N.	Ph.D.
Practical nursing programs (1972)				
Education of administrators	24.5%	43.6%	31.5%	0.5%
Education of faculty members	46.9	42.0	7.8	0.1

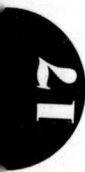

Table 17-5 Schools, enrollments and graduations, in practical and vocational nursing. By jurisdiction, 1974–1975

Jurisdictions	Number of schools	Enroll- ments	Gradua- tions
Alabama	26	1,214	860
Alaska	1	29	21
American Samoa	1	17	17
Arizona	11	437	436
Arkansas	27	929	630
California	94	4,335	3,364
Colorado	17	577	482
Connecticut	10	593	531
Delaware	4	185	102
District of Columbia	3	244	101
Florida	31	2,213	1,686
Georgia	53	1,689	1,468
Guam	1	0	20
Hawaii	4	121	70
Idaho	13	201	197
Illinois	35	2,621	1,972
Indiana	12	1,079	989
Iowa	16	918	933
Kansas	14	619	590
Kentucky	14	610	520
Louisiana	28	1,367	864
Maine	5	201	180
Maryland	24	886	531
Massachusetts	34	1,446	1,237
Michigan	35	2,182	1,888
Minnesota	27	1,132	1,223
Mississippi	14	674	709
Missouri	31	1,226	1,070
Montana	7	228	146
Nebraska	9	549	493
Nevada	6	89	109
New Hampshire	4	169	121
New Jersey	38	2,032	1,442
New Mexico	11	231	274
New York	82	7,086	3,768
North Carolina	41	1,312	963
North Dakota	3	224	273
Ohio	39	2,576	2,188
Oklahoma	22	786	630
Oregon	12	288	298
Pennsylvania	51	2,654	2,567
Puerto Rico	20	976	668
Rhode Island	2	185	225
South Carolina	30	1,150	553
South Dakota	6	253	218
Tennessee	7	1,074	1,034
Texas	151	4,541	3,538
Utah	6	298	205
Vermont	3	200	207
Virginia	55	2,000	999

Table 17-5 (continued)

Jurisdictions	Number of schools	Enroll- ments	Gradua- tions
Washington	27	877	937
West Virginia	16	488	431
Wisconsin	14	1,160	1,037
Wyoming	3	82	65
Total	1,250	59,453	46,080

Source: National League for Nursing *State Approved Schools of Nursing LPN/VN,* 1976.

Table 17-6 Financial support of L.P.N./L.V.N. programs 1974–75

Principal source of financial support	Total			
	Programs		Admissions	
	Num- ber	Per- cent	Num- ber	Per- cent
Public funds	1,233	90.4	56,157	91.2
Private funds	131	9.6	5,400	8.8
Total	1,364	100.0	61,557	100.0

Source: National League for Nursing *State Approved Schools of Nursing LPN/VN,* 1976.

Table 17-7 Graduations according to control program 1974–75

Administrative control of program	Total			
	Programs		Graduations	
	Num- ber	Per- cent	Num- ber	Per- cent
Secondary school	91	6.7	2,005	4.4
Trade, technical or vocational school	701	51.4	25,806	56.0
Senior college or university	17	1.2	541	1.2
Junior or community college	358	26.2	12,036	26.1
Hospital	152	11.2	3,898	8.4
Independent agency	8	0.6	311	0.7
Government agency	37	2.7	1,483	3.2
Total	1,364	100.0	46,080	100.0

Source: National League for Nursing *State Approved Schools of Nursing LPN/VN,* 1976.

Table 17-8   L.P.N./L.V.N. Nurse education data and requirements by state

State	Practical nursing Students	Programs	Gr.	4 yr. H.S.	G.E.D. 2 yr.	G.E.D. 4 yr.	Mos.	Wks.	Hrs.	Pharm.	Time, hrs./wks.	Mental hlth.	Time, hrs./wks.	OB	Time, hrs./wks.	Peds.	Time, hrs./wks.	Other
Alabama	1203	26		X		X	NS	NS	1320	—	NS	—	NS	X	220 hr.	X	160 hr.	—
Alaska	21	1	10			X	NS	NS		X	NS	X	NS	X	NS	X	NS	NS‡
Arizona	391	11		X	25 y.o.		1 Year—R.S.			X	S/I	X		X	NS	X	NS	
Arkansas	689	29		X	X	X	12			X	S/I	X	S/I	X	NS	X	NS	NS
California	NA	95	10			X	12	46	1530	—	NS	O		X	NS	X	NS	NR
Colorado		20		X		X												
Connecticut	NA	10		20 y.o.	20 y.o.		12			X	45 hr.	X	4 wks	X	3 wks.	X	3 wks.	OB/Ped = 10 wks.
Delaware	125	4		X		X	12			6 day	45 hr.	SEP	SEP	X		X		Individualized
D.C.	Survey not returned																	
Florida	2149	31		X		X			1300	X		X		X	NS	X	NS	NS
Georgia	92	58	10	X	X		12 / 30 Units			X	30 hr.	If Avail.	If Avail.	X	60 hr.	X	60 hr.	
Hawaii		4																
Idaho	181	13		X	X		12		1400	X	—	X	—	X	→	X	→	
Illinois	NR	36		X			9			X	—	X	—	24th	4–6 wks.	X	4–6 wks.	30–40 hr., 8 wks.
Indiana	1088	18		X		X	12		1535	—	NS	X		X	6 wks.	16th	4 wks.	
Iowa	NR	NR		X		X	1 Acad. yr.			X	NS	X	NS	X	NS	X	NS	All S/I
Kansas	Survey not returned																	
Kentucky	651	14		X		X		48	1440	NS	—	NS	—	NS	40/4	NS	20/3	NS
Lousiana				X		X	NS	NS	NS	X		X		X		X		
Maine	NR	5		X		X				X		X		X		X		
Maryland	Survey not returned																	
Massachusetts	1464	32	8	X		X	12	48	1200	S/I	50 hr.	X		X	150 hr.	X	150 hr.	
Michigan	NR	NR		X		X		R.S.		X	NS	X		X	4 wks.	X	4 wks.	
Minnesota	1160	23		X		X				—	NS			NS	NS		NS	
Mississippi	NR	12		X		X	12			S/I	30 hr. +	S/I	10 hr.	30 hr.	6–8 wks.	20 hr.	4–6 wks.	
Missouri	1125	31				X	1 Year			X	—	X	SEP.	X	OB/Peds = 10 Units = 150–180 Hrs.	X	OB/Peds = 150–180 Hrs.	
Montana	200	7		X			12			X	SEP.	X	—					
Nebraska	Survey not returned																	
Nevada	119	7	10			X	12	42		—	NS	X	NS	X	120 hr.	X	NS	NS
New Hampshire	155	4		X						X	—	X	—	X	120 hr.	X	120 hr.	
New Jersey	NA	38	10	X	X		12	52	1700	NS	NS	NS	NS	4 wks.	40 hr.	4 wks.	40 hr.	
New Mexico	394	11		X	X		11–12			—	NS	I-15		X	NS	X	NS	As needed
New York	3700	80	8				9	44	1200	—	NS	I-15	45 Cl	30th	90 Cl	15th	45 Cl	
North Carolina	1272	37	9							X		X		X	X	X		
North Dakota	340	4	•	•			9–12			—	NS	NS	NS	NS	NS		NS	NS

(continued)

17

Table 17-8 (continued)

State	Practical nursing — Students	Programs	Min. ed. — Gr.	4 yr. H.S.	G.E.D. 2 yr.	G.E.D. 4 yr.	Length — Mos.	Wks.	Hrs.	Pharm.	Time, hrs./wks.	Mental hlth.	Time, hrs./wks.	OB	Time, hrs./wks.	Peds.	Time, hrs./wks.	Other
Ohio	2552	42		X		X	1 year		600		NS	Concepts		X	NS	X	NS	
Oklahoma	NR	22	10				12				S/I	X	S/I	X	NS	X	NR	
Oregon	444	12		X			9			X				X	NS	X	NS	
Pennsylvania	3794	53		X		X	1 year		1500	X	NS			X	NS	X	NS	
Puerto Rico	Survey not returned																	
Rhode Island	185	2		X			10	40			S/I		S/I	X	8 wks.	X	4 wks.	NR
South Carolina	824	30	10		X		10	(Most 12)			S/I			X		X		••
South Dakota	254	6		X		X	••	•• ••		X								
Tennessee	NR	7	10		X		12	†		NS		May have		X	6–8 wks.	X	Not required	
Texas	4500	150	10		X		12	††		X	40/8	X	20 hr.	X	6–8 wks.	X	Not required	
Utah	NA	7		X			12	#		SEP	60 hr.	SEP	50 hr.	20th	72 CI	20th	72 CI	
Vermont	149	3		X		X	1 year academic				NS		NS	45+	NS	45+	NS	NS
Virginia	NR	55	10		X		12			S/I	65 hr.	S/I	30 hr.+	45+	4–6 wks.	45+	4–6 wks.	
V.I.	Survey not returned																	
Washington	1011	26			X		9	40		Statewide performance objectives								
West Virginia	490	16	10		X		12		1300	S/I	80 hr.	S/I	80 hr.	X	80 hr.	X	80 hr.	
Wisconsin	1281	14	10		X			36		S/I	24–36 hr.	S/I	96 hr.	X	48 hr.	X	48 hr.	
Wyoming	52	3		X		X	12	52		School plans curriculum								Hrs. clinical

* "As required by program."
** Meet program objectives.
† 550 hours theory + clinical.
†† 550 hours theory + 1250 hours clinical.
# 650 hours theory + 950 hours clinical.
‡ Each curriculum evaluated individually.

Source: National Association for Practical Nurse Education and Service, Inc.

Aid for Education

National licensed practical nurses educational foundation—Applicants must have been accepted for admission to a state-approved school of practical nursing in the state where they live, and give evidence of physical, academic and character fitness. Further information is available from the National Licensed Practical Nurses Educational Foundation, Inc., 250 West 57th Street, New York, N.Y. 10019.

Sources of Additional Information

The National Federation of Licensed Practical Nurses, with about 35,200 members in 1972, is the association for licensed practical or vocational nurses.

A list of state-approved training programs and information about practical nursing is available from:

● ANA Committee on Nursing Careers, American Nurses' Association, 2420 Pershing Rd., Kansas City, Mo. 64108.
● National Association for Practical Nurse Education and Service, Inc., 122 East 42nd St., Suite 800, New York, N.Y. 10017.
● National Federation of Licensed Practical Nurses, Inc., 250 West 57th St., New York, N.Y. 10019.

Information about employment opportunities in U.S. Veterans Administration hospitals is available from your local Veterans Administration hospital, as well as:

● Department of Medicine and Surgery, Veterans Administration, Washington, D.C. 20420.

Licensure

Licensure and School Accreditation

Licensure of practical nurses is provided for by law in the 50 states and the District of Columbia. To be licensed as a licensed practical nurse (L.P.N.) or licensed vocational nurse (L.V.N. in California and Texas), an appli-

cant must have graduated from a state-approved school of practical nursing and passed a state board examination.

Graduates from correspondence schools are not eligible to take the licensing examination.

Schools may be accredited by the National League for Nursing (NLN) or by the National Association for Practical Nurse Education and Service (NAPNES). The standards set by these organizations for accreditation are generally higher than those required for state approval.

How Practical Nurses are Licensed*

Practical nurses are licensed in all the states and the District of Columbia.** The licensing body is a board of practical nurse examiners in seven states and the District of Columbia, while the board of nursing licenses the profession in the other 43 states. In five instances the boards contain no L.P.N. members.

All states renew licenses, 15 of them biennially, the rest annually. In addition, about half of the boards issue temporary licenses. All states except Virginia offer some form of reciprocity or endorsement to applicants who are licensed in another state.

In 20 states a minimum age requirement of 17 to 20 years must be met. High school graduation is also required in 24 states. Applicants must also pass a written examination in 47 states after completing a course of professional education. At the present time, all state boards have chosen to utilize the State Board Test Pool Examination as their written examination.

All state boards, except four, have the power to issue licenses initially. They also generally have the power to revoke or suspend licenses, or in some cases take other disciplinary action, to maintain professional standards.

Four states have provisions for continuing education for practical nurses.

Forty-three states will license foreign-trained practical nurses, generally under the same provisions that they offer reciprocity or endorsement.

---

*Source: Health Resources Administration, DHEW, 1977.
**For addresses of the State Boards of Nursing see Chapter 12.

21

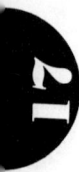

Table 17-9 LP/VN Licensure summary: state by state

State[1]	Approved upgrading opportunities — Aide L.P./V.N. program	Approved upgrading opportunities — L.P./V.N. to R.N. program	License renewed — Yearly frequency	License renewed — Date/month	License law — Mandatory or permission	Access — Graduates from other states	Access — Drop-out R.N. program	Access — Student R.N. program	SBTP	Minimum pass score	Total L.P./V.N. in state	Total taking exam 1975	Total pass exam 1975	Mean scores (all pass)
Alabama		X	2	10 & 12	M	X	X		X	350	11,041	871	781	N/A
Alaska		X	1	6	M	X			X	350	612	33	29	557
Arizona	X	X	1	1	M	R/S			X	350	4,761	546	517	501.8
Arkansas	X	X	2	1 & 5	M	X	R/S		X	350	8,772	757	658	N/A
California	X	none	2	B/D	P	X		R/S	NO	Var.	50,000[2]	6,600[2]	6,600[2]	N/A
Colorado	X	N/A	2	7	M	R/S			X	350	6,700	524	475	N/A
Connecticut		X	1	1	M	X			X	350	9,987	613	602	N/A
Delaware		XO	2	12	M	X			X	350	1,595	118	108	441
Florida		X	1	3	M	X			X	350	29,752	1,687	1,570	N/A
Georgia	X		2	12	P	X	X	X	Xt	350	21,970	2,005	124	N/A
Hawaii	X	X	1	6	M	X	X	X	X	375	2,860	180	193	N/A
Idaho		·	1	6	M	X	X	X	X	350	3,333	209	95%	536.3
Illinois	X-all		2	5	M	X			X	350	27,619	1,500	976	350
Indiana	X	X	2	12	P	R/S	X		X	350	8,555	1,024	N/R	N/A
Iowa	X	X	1	7	M	X	X	X	X	350	13,460	N/R	909	N/R
Kentucky	X	X	1	10	M	X			X	350	8,500	600	237	N/A
Louisiana			1	1	M	X		R/S	X	350	10,246	1,031	1,271	N/R
Maine		X	1	7	M	X	R/S	R/S	X	350	3,340	250	1,888	N/A
Massachusetts		X	2	B/D	M	X	X		X	350	34,950	1,307	1,185	graduates
Michigan		X	1	3	M	X			X	350	31,576	1,993	510	N/A
Minnesota			1	1	M	X			X	400	14,000	1,344	897	N/R
Mississippi			1	5 & 6	M	X	R/S	R/S	X	350	5,481	672	164	N/A
Missouri		·	1	7	P	X	R/S		X	350	13,041	948	151	N/R
Montana	X		1	1	M	X			X	350	1,976	178	154	N/A
Nevada		·	2	2	M	X			X	350	1,582	177	1,800	528.5*
New Hampshire			2	B/D	M	X			X	350	2,159	163	310	N/A
New Jersey			2	1	M	R/S	R/S	R/S	X	375	20,154	2,657	7,075	N/A
New Mexico	X		2	B	M	X	X		X	350	6,521	350	1,374	536.3
New York	X	X	2	9	M	X			X	350	67,126	9,646	247	N/A
North Carolina		X	2	12	M	X			X	350	N/R	1,653	2,347	N/A
North Dakota	X	X	2	12	M	X			X	350	2,136	252		516
Ohio		X	1	9	M	X			X	350	36,954	2,466		N/A

Table 17-9 (continued)

| State[1] | Approved upgrading opportunities | | License renewed | | License law | Access to P/V nursing licensing exam | | | SBTP | Mini-mum pass score | Total L.P./V.N. in state | Total taking exam 1975 | Total pass exam 1975 | Mean scores (all pass) |
	Aide L.P./V.N. program	L.P./V.N. to R.N. program	Yearly fre-quency	Date/month	Man-datory or per-mission	Grad-uates from other states	Drop-out R.N. pro-gram	Stu-dent R.N. pro-gram						
Oklahoma	N/R	N/R	1	6	P	N/R	N/R	N/R	X	350	N/R	N/R	N/R	N/R
Oregon	X	X	2	3	M	X			X	350	5,727	401	387	540
Pennsylvania	X	X	2	7	M	X			X	350	N/R	3,570	2,674	N/A
Rhode Island			1	3	M	X	X	O	X	350	3,363	191	191	N/A
South Carolina		X	1	10 & 12	M	X	X	X	X	350	5,492	550	486	N/A
South Dakota		X	1	1	M	X	X	X	X	350	4,039	236	227	N/A
Tennessee		X	2	12	M	X	R/S		X	350	N/R	N/R	N/R	N/R
Texas		X	1	5 & 8	P	X	X	X	X	350	66,656	3,919	3,073	N/A
Utah		X	1	1	*M	X	R/S	R/S	X	350	3,299	307	302	N/A
Vermont			2	4	M	X			X	350	2,649	130	130	533.6
Virginia	X		1	12	M	X	R/S		X	350	15,000	1,189	1,013	N/A
Washington	X	X	1	B/D	P	X	R/S	R/S	X	400	12,000	997	937	N/R
West Virginia			1	7	M	X			X	350	8,601	395	360	N/A
Wisconsin		X	1	7	P	X	X	O	X	Var.	N/A	1,100	N/A	N/A
Wyoming			1	6	M	X			X	350	747	59	58	N/A

[1] The following seven areas did not return survey answers: Kansas, Maryland, Nebraska, Wisconsin, Washington, D.C., Puerto Rico, and Virgin Islands.
[2] Approximate.

Summary of Symbols

A—Academic year.
B/D—Birthday.
C—Calendar year.
C/E—Continuing education.
Cl—Clinical.
I—Integrated.
M—Mandatory.
N/A—Not available; not computed.
N/R—No response: incomplete response.
N/S—Not specified.
O—No.

P—Permissive.
R/S—Requirements/stipulations.
S/I—Separate or integrated.
Th—Theory.
Var—Variable or varies.
Wk—Weeks.
X—Yes.
?—Not yet determined, questionable.
$—Fee required.
*—See below for that state.
+—Own exam in addition to SBTP.

Source: National Association for Practical Nurse Education and Services.

Renewal

Table 17-10   Continuing education and reciprocity on renewal of license

	Continuing education required	Reciprocity or endorsement*		Continuing education required	Reciprocity or endorsement*
Alabama		E[2,7]	North Dakota		X[2]
Alaska		X	Ohio		E[2]
Arizona		E[2]	Oklahoma		E[2]
Arkansas		E[2]	Oregon	X[AC]	X[7,8]
California	X[AC]	X	Pennsylvania		R
Colorado		E[2]	Rhode Island		X
Connecticut		X .	South Carolina		X[2]
Delaware		E[2]	South Dakota	X[A]	E
Florida		X[2]	Tennessee		X
Georgia		X[2]	Texas		X
Hawaii		E	Utah		X
Idaho		X[2,5]	Vermont		E[2]
Illinois		X[2,5]	Virginia		X
Indiana		X[2,5]	Washington		X
Iowa		E[2]	West Virginia		X
Kansas		E[2,5]	Wisconsin		X
Kentucky		X[2,5]	Wyoming		X
Louisiana		X[5]	District of		
Maine		E[2]	Columbia		X
Maryland		E[2]			
Massachusetts		X			
Michigan		E[2]			
Minnesota		E[2]			
Mississippi		E[2]			
Missouri		X[2]			
Montana		X			
Nebraska		X			
Nevada		X[2]			
New Hampshire		X			
New Jersey		X			
New Mexico	X[B]	E[2]			
New York		E[2]			
North Carolina		E[2]			

[A] Board approved Continuing Education Course.
[B] As of 1977 Continuing Education is required.
[C] Determined by Board.
*[1] If licensed in another jurisdiction.
[2] Includes applicants licensed in a foreign country.
*[3] At Board's discretion unless otherwise noted.
[4] Must meet state's requirements (at time of licensure).
[5] If licensed by written examination.
[6] Must meet state's requirements at time of graduation.
[7] Requires SBTPE exam also.
[8] Also requirement of school of practice.

Source: Health Resources Administration, DHEW, 1977.

Moonlighting*

Profile of Hospital Moonlighters

All hospital employees in this survey worked on some type of schedule other than the traditional 8-hour pattern; these schedules are primarily of the 10-hour and 12-hour types. The total sample size was 853 employees of which 6.1% held second jobs compared with a U.S. moonlighting rate of 5.1%. The male moonlighting rate for the sample, 19.3%, is much higher than the U.S. male figure of 6.7%.

In the study, the following percentage of people held second jobs:

Charge nurse	2.6%
Staff Nurse (R.N.)	1.8%
Licensed Practical Nurse	
(female)	8.3%
(male)	16.7%

● Few registered nurses hold a second job in

*Source: W. C. Johnson, *A Review and Analysis of Changed Work Schedules in Hospitals* (Manpower Administration of D. of L., May 1975).

this sample—perhaps because they can work as many extra hours as they wish at their primary jobs, they feel no need to seek a second job.

- 86% of the male moonlighters are married, while only 43% of the female moonlighters are married.
- Most of the moonlighters have children under the age of 18 to support, implying some economic necessity in the second job.
- Moonlighters are typically young.
- Moonlighting is highest for those aged 25–44 years.
- Moonlighting is inversely related to earnings on the primary job.

U.S. Data on All Workers

Only 19% of the four million moonlighters are women. The rate of male moonlighting, 6.7%, is more than twice the female rate, 2.6% (Bureau of Labor Statistics, 1971).

Employee Strategy in Collective Bargaining*

Prior to negotiations, you (L.P./V.N.s) must select a negotiating committee to act with your agent on behalf of L.P./V.N.s in the preparation of proposals for a contract and in negotiation with your employer. Usually the basis for these proposals is all of your current employment policies and benefits and any other items or issues that you would like to have implemented or added as part of the conditions of your employment. After the committee has formulated its proposals, a general meeting of all L.P./V.N.s in the unit should be held to discuss these proposals, to make suggestions, and to make additions or deletions. Upon approval by the members, the committee can then meet with the employer to negotiate a contract or written agreement. It is important that the membership give the negotiating committee the authority to make decisive commitments in the course of negotiations.

*Source: Ruth Bloem, "Collective Bargaining Part III," *Journal of Practical Nursing,* May 1975.

Table 17-11   Ways to do a better job at the bargaining table.

1. "Win" by negotiating a settlement that gives the other side just enough to make it willing to agree, but no more.
2. Approach each situation as being unique.
3. Don't let personality differences interfere.
4. Learn to sense when you are approaching a critical point.
5. Don't defend obvious errors or weak positions.
6. Know when your opponent is putting you on through nonverbal communication.
7. Always ask for more than you expect to get.
8. Never make demands that have no real advantage.
9. Be realistic when presenting demands.
10. Avoid last minute concessions that give your opponent a foot in the door.
11. Never say "never" unless you can fully support your position.
12. Don't be in too much of a rush to settle, but try to speed up ratification after settlement has been reached.
13. Hold each meeting for a purpose, not just a get together.

Table 17-12   Issues negotiated by NAPNES State Associations

1. Representation on Nursing Care Committees.
2. The Status of the L.P./L.V.N.
3. Paid released time for attendance at educational meetings and conventions.
4. In-service training programs.
5. Tuition refunds.
6. Use of facilities for meetings.
7. Released time for attendance at special conferences to settle disputes regarding grievances, matters concerning working conditions, scheduling, and nursing care.
8. Incorporation of a Code of Ethics for L.P./V.N.s Frequently, the NAPNES Code of Ethics is utilized.

NURSING AIDES, ORDERLIES, AND ATTENDANTS

Overview

Nursing aides, orderlies, and attendants perform a variety of duties to care for sick and injured people. Women usually are called nursing aides and men generally are known as orderlies. Other job titles include *hospital attendant, nursing assistant, auxiliary nursing worker, home health aide,* and (in mental institutions) *psychiatric aide.*

The total number of aides, orderlies, and attendants employed in 1973 was estimated at 910,000 by the U.S. Public Health Service Division of Nursing, 35,000 more than in 1972. (This estimate excludes home health aides.) More than four-fifths were women. Most of them work in hospitals. Others work primarily in nursing homes and other institutions that provide facilities for care and recuperation. A small number give supportive services to patients in their homes.

Functions

The duties of nursing aides depend on the policies of the institutions where they work, the type of patient being cared for, and—equally important—the capacities and resourcefulness of the nursing aide or orderly. In some hospitals, they may clean patients' rooms and do other household tasks. In others, under the supervision of registered nurses and licensed practical nurses, they may assist in the care of patients. The tasks performed for patients differ considerably, and depend on whether the patient is confined to his bed following major surgery, is recovering after a disabling accident or illness, or needs assistance with daily activities because of infirmity caused by advanced age.

Hospital Nurse Aide

The hospital nurse aide assists in care of hospital patients, under direction of nursing and medical staff. Answers signal lights and bells to determine patients' needs. Bathes, dresses, and undresses patients. Serves and collects food trays and feeds patients requiring help. Transports patients to treatment units, using wheelchair or wheeled carriage, or assists them to walk. Drapes patients for examina-tions and treatments, and remains with patients, performing such duties as holding instruments and adjusting lights. Dusts and cleans patients' rooms. Changes bed linens, runs errands, directs visitors, and answers telephone. Takes and records temperature, pulse and respiration rates, and food and liquid intake and output, as directed. May apply compresses and hot water bottles. May clean, sterilize, store, prepare, and issue dressing packs, treatment trays, and other supplies and be designated as nurse aide, central supply. May prepare patients for delivery and clean delivery rooms. May bathe, weigh, dress, and feed newborn babies and be designated as nurse aide, nursery. May clean, sterilize, and assemble into packs supplies and instruments used in surgery, and maintain cleanliness and order of operating rooms and be designated as nurse aide, surgery.

Psychiatric Aide

Charge attendant; ward attendant; psychiatric technician, psychiatric nursing assistant: The psychiatric aide assists mentally ill patients, working under the direction of nursing and medical staff. Performs several of the following patient care services: accompanies patients to shower room and assists them in bathing, dressing, and grooming; accompanies patients to and from wards for examination and treatment and administers prescribed medications; assists patients in becoming accustomed to hospital routine and encourages them to participate in various activities to promote rehabilitation; observes patients to insure that none wanders from the grounds; feeds patients or attempts to persuade them to eat, noting reasons for rejection of food; observes patients to detect unusual behavior; and aids or restrains them to prevent injury to themselves or other patients. May escort patients off the grounds when necessary.

Training, Other Qualifications, and Advancement

Although some employers prefer high school graduates, many, such as Veterans Administration hospitals, hire non-graduates. Many employers accept applicants 17 or 18 years of

Time Spent on Hospital Tasks

Figure 17-5   Nurse's Aide: percent of time spent in various functions in typical hospital

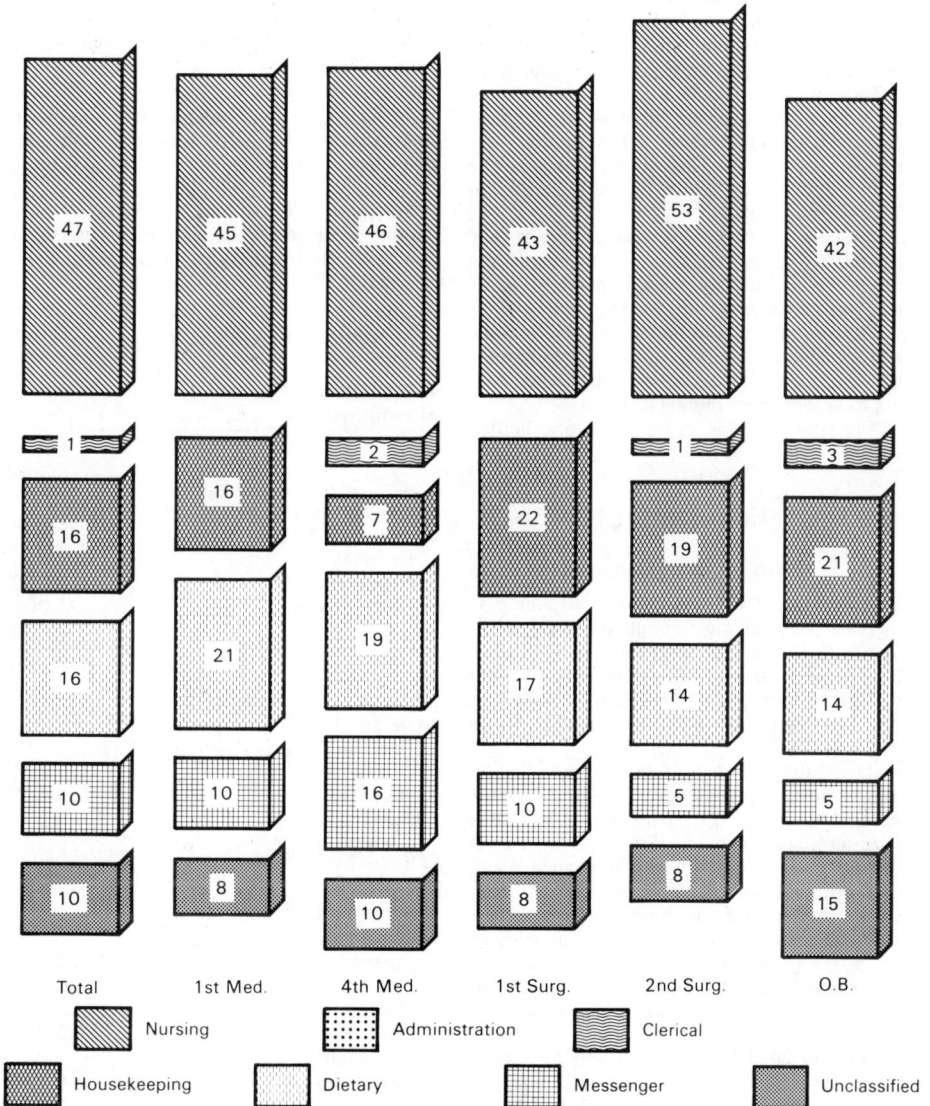

47	45	46	43	53	42
1	16	2	22	1	3
16		7		19	21
16	21	19	17	14	14
10	10	16	10	5	5
10	8	10	8	8	15

Total   1st Med.   4th Med.   1st Surg.   2nd Surg.   O.B.

Nursing   Administration   Clerical

Housekeeping   Dietary   Messenger   Unclassified

Source: DHEW, 1964.

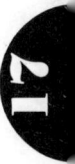

age. Others—particularly nursing homes and mental hospitals—prefer to hire more mature men and women who are at least in their mid-twenties.

Nursing aides generally are trained after they are hired. Some institutions combine on-the-job training, under the close supervision of registered or licensed practical nurses, with classroom instruction. Students learn to take and record temperatures, bathe patients, change linens on beds that are occupied by patients, and move and lift patients. Training may last several days or a few months, depending on the policies of the hospital, the complexity of the duties and the aide's aptitude for the work.

Courses in home nursing and first aid, offered by many public school systems and other community agencies, provide a useful background of knowledge for the work.

Nursing aides, like other health workers, should have a genuine desire to help people, be able to work as part of a team, and be willing to accept some menial tasks.

Opportunities for promotions are limited without further training.

Employment

Employment Outlook

Employment of nursing aides is expected to increase very rapidly through the mid-1980s. In addition to those needed because of occupational growth, many thousands of new aides will be needed each year to replace workers who die, retire or leave the occupation for other reasons.

Most jobs for nursing aides and orderlies are in hospitals, but many new openings will be in nursing homes, convalescent homes, and other long-term care facilities, because of the growth of public and private health insurance plans, and the expanded medical services of Medicare and Medicaid. Employment opportunities also will arise as hospitals continue to delegate to nursing aides tasks which, although associated with patient care, do not require the training of registered and licensed practical nurses.

Nursing aides employed full-time by nursing homes and related facilities earn considerably less than those in hospitals. Depending on the experience of the applicant, salaries of inexperienced nursing aides in Veterans

Administration hospitals ranged from $92 to $102 a week in early 1973.

With few exceptions, the scheduled work-week of attendants in hospitals is 40 hours or less. Because nursing care must be available to patients on a 24-hour-a-day basis, scheduled hours include night work and work on weekends and holidays.

Attendants in hospitals and similar institutions generally receive paid vacations which, after one year of service, may be a week or more in length. Paid holidays and sick leave, hospitalization and medical benefits, and pension plans also are available to many hospital employees.

For more information on Auxiliary Nursing Careers write to: American Hospital Association, 840 North Lake Shore Drive, Chicago, Illinois 60611.

Where Aides Are Employed

Table 17-13   Number of aides and place of employment

	No. employed
Employed aides, orderlies and attendants (1973)	
Hospitals	597,000
Nursing homes	280,000
Public health	21,000
Other	12,000
Total	910,000
Employment in non-federal hospitals (1970)	
Short-term general and other special	377,504
Psychiatric	119,103
Tuberculosis	3,291
Other long-term	19,384
Total	519,282
Hospital departments in which employed (1970)	
Inpatient unit	473,150
Operating room	20,117
Outpatient and emergency unit	15,685
Administrative unit	3,949
Central service and other areas	46,170
Total	559,071

Source: DHEW data.

Table 17-14   All employed nursing aides, orderlies, and attendants aged 16 years and over by characteristics and state, 1970

	All employed nursing aides, orderlies, and attendants, 16 years and over			Place of residence							
				Urban		Rural				Negro	
						Farm		Nonfarm			
Area	Both sexes	Male	Fe-male	Male	Fe-male	Male	Fe-male	Male	Fe-male	Male	Fe-male
United States	717,968	108,946	609,022	83,022	448,615	2,726	22,311	23,198	138,096	29,962	150,666
Alabama	11,438	2,890	8,548	1,831	5,366	83	289	976	2,893	1,619	3,296
Alaska	420	73	347	40	141	—	—	33	206	15	13
Arizona	4,741	700	4,041	632	3,472	13	11	55	558	42	381
Arkansas	7,519	1,076	6,443	748	3,661	45	353	283	2,429	272	1,523
California	59,294	8,908	50,386	8,004	45,563	54	324	850	4,499	1,702	9,581
Colorado	8,136	1,191	6,945	1,043	5,596	19	188	129	1,161	37	548
Connecticut	10,904	1,543	9,361	1,158	7,336	4	28	381	1,997	123	1,533
Delaware	1,614	113	1,501	77	1,001	—	34	36	466	38	676
District of Columbia	3,178	739	2,439	739	2,439	—	—	—	—	696	2,335
Florida	21,592	3,294	18,298	2,393	14,428	96	169	805	3,701	1,198	7,851
Georgia	13,487	3,062	10,425	2,033	7,013	106	267	923	3,145	1,674	5,066
Hawaii	1,240	242	998	201	764	—	—	41	234	—	6
Idaho	1,844	200	1,644	145	981	13	158	42	505	—	19
Illinois	37,669	3,889	33,780	3,232	26,539	97	1,303	560	5,938	988	8,154
Indiana	21,085	2,177	18,908	1,598	12,671	102	1,072	477	5,165	310	3,680
Iowa	15,541	1,223	14,318	866	8,235	85	1,993	272	4,090	31	378
Kansas	13,205	1,136	12,069	834	7,504	57	1,188	245	3,377	170	1,140
Kentucky	10,371	1,692	8,679	1,167	5,138	113	727	412	2,814	291	1,400
Louisiana	12,239	1,890	10,349	1,390	7,013	32	239	468	3,097	1,120	5,148
Maine	3,883	486	3,397	300	1,834	4	46	182	1,517	—	8
Maryland	11,786	2,071	9,715	1,601	7,702	16	118	454	1,895	1,134	5,686
Massachusetts	22,702	3,541	19,161	3,115	16,581	8	57	418	2,523	255	1,660
Michigan	33,396	4,161	29,235	3,182	21,685	105	718	874	6,832	985	8,683
Minnesota	21,304	2,474	18,830	1,955	12,098	123	1,969	396	4,763	56	296
Misisippi	6,903	1,236	5,667	691	2,970	60	374	485	2,323	540	2,395
Missouri	20,687	2,649	18,038	2,041	13,035	138	1,202	470	3,801	511	5,079
Montana	2,962	321	2,641	175	1,591	5	114	141	936	—	1
Nebraska	8,643	856	7,787	710	4,809	25	751	121	2,227	39	328
Nevada	993	216	777	197	619	—	4	19	154	19	110
New Hampshire	2,655	365	2,290	246	1,388	4	47	115	855	10	9
New Jersey	18,197	2,434	15,763	2,133	13,886	3	69	298	1,808	1,110	6,844
New Mexico	2,685	530	2,155	374	1,646	10	62	146	447	10	74
New York	70,992	14,683	56,309	12,197	47,158	51	584	2,435	8,567	4,706	22,515
North Carolina	14,356	3,604	10,752	2,024	5,732	120	567	1,460	4,453	2,053	4,065
North Dakota	3,776	388	3,388	255	1,885	48	411	85	1,092	—	12
Ohio	35,285	4,586	30,699	3,304	23,328	155	803	1,127	6,568	1,022	9,050
Oklahoma	13,936	1,220	12,716	884	8,064	64	812	272	3,840	143	1,742
Oregon	8,711	982	7,729	720	5,180	35	266	227	2,283	40	204
Pennsylvania	34,339	6,119	28,220	4,495	20,032	51	479	1,573	7,709	1,585	6,618
Rhode Island	3,724	645	3,079	545	2,661	—	—	100	418	21	172
South Carolina	6,774	1,463	5,311	977	3,102	44	154	442	2,055	967	2,972
South Dakota	4,415	594	3,821	430	1,920	28	463	136	1,438	—	4
Tennessee	13,078	2,878	10,200	1,845	6,974	145	602	888	2,624	851	3,204
Texas	34,675	5,184	29,491	4,264	23,033	191	907	729	5,551	1,515	9,305
Utah	2,587	446	2,141	420	1,834	—	34	26	273	4	24
Vermont	1,656	211	1,445	112	571	4	47	95	827	—	—
Virginia	14,095	3,099	10,996	2,034	7,229	117	276	948	3,491	1,605	4,315
Washington	9,957	1,290	8,667	1,108	6,421	32	200	150	2,046	87	379
West Virginia	6,101	1,211	4,890	528	2,248	35	129	648	2,513	222	297
Wisconsin	25,963	2,810	23,153	1,904	15,758	186	1,677	720	5,718	146	1,867
Wyoming	1,235	155	1,080	125	780	—	26	30	274	—	20

Source: Division of Nursing, DHEW, 1972.

332

Other Jobs

Home Health Aide and Homemaker

Nursing agencies and social service agencies concerned with assistance to the homebound have come to rely with increasing frequency on two relatively new categories of worker—the home health aide and the homemaker.

Although the duties of the two often overlap, the home health aide, sometimes called home aide or visiting health aide, is more involved with the physical and simple health needs of the homebound or disabled person, while the homemaker concerns herself mainly with the standard housekeeping services.

The homemaker and home health aide are recruited primarily from mature women who have had experience in bringing up their own families, and from among young people seeking job training.

In 1973, there were 30,700 home health aides and homemakers employed. Of these, approximately 13,200 were employed on a full-time basis. More than 1,700 home health aide and homemaker service programs are in public and voluntary agencies now.

For the home health aide, typical assignments might include bathing or exercising a convalescent person, or semi-invalid; seeing to it that the patient takes medicine; keeping in touch with the nurse or doctors as to the patient's condition. She would also assist in the preparation of meals and help feed the patient.

The homemaker would do the cleaning, shopping, and cooking for an invalid or a handicapped person. She might take care of the children and keep house while the mother is in the hospital or is sick at home and unable to take care of the family.

The agencies most likely to employ and assign these workers are local health departments, welfare dependents, private social work agencies, hospitals, or community voluntary agencies.

The employing agency is responsible for on-the-job training, with a nurse providing the basic and ongoing training in personal care services, and with other health personnel involved in their appropriate aspects. Standardized statewide certificate programs for home health aides are conducted in some states. A state license is not required for persons providing homemaker services.

Training courses range from 40 to 120 hours, and combine instruction in homemaking and home health care. These are generally provided by local schools (adult education), the Manpower Development and Training Act program of the federal government, and hospitals and voluntary agencies. The courses include training in household management, nutrition, infant and child care, and personal care. On completion of class work, trainees receive on-the-spot training, working under the supervision of a public health nurse, social worker, occupational therapist, nutritionist, or other professional. A few states, including New Jersey and California, require certification, obtained after a training course of specified minimum length, for home health aide positions.

Opportunities exist for advancement to occupational and physical therapist assistants and aides in hospitals and visiting nurses services.

For further information write to: National Council for Homemaker-Home Health Aide Services, Inc., 1740 Broadway, New York, New York 10019.

Nursing Clerk*

The nursing clerk is becoming an increasingly valuable worker in nursing service. If carefully selected and properly trained, the nursing clerk can greatly relieve other personnel prepared to give patient care to do their work. Job descriptions of nursing clerks vary greatly but could easily include such responsibilities as control of all communications into and out of a busy nursing station, coordination of patient services, record keeping, and maintenance of environment and supplies. She can be trained to answer patient and intensive care intercommunications systems properly. She can provide telephone service, including answering incoming calls, taking messages, giving information within the scope of her specified responsibility, making requests for services, and assisting with the transportation of messages. She may

---

*Source: Robert M. Sloane & Beverly LeBon Sloane, *A Guide to Health Facilities Personnel & Management* (V. Mosby Company, 1971).

receive, sign for, and deliver mail and flowers and other messages to patients. She can act as a receptionist for patients' relatives, visitors, clergy, and other hospital personnel. She can post schedules and notices, maintain the area bulletin boards, and provide continuity of unit desk operations by holding interval reports with oncoming nursing clerks. She can be taught to prepare daily diet changes and nourishment lists and can check to see that all patient menus are submitted to the dietary department. She can notify such departments as inhalation therapy, laboratory, and x-ray of specific orders for services. Well trained clerks can accurately transcribe doctors' orders for treatment, medication, and laboratory services.

Other nursing personnel involved in caring for patients include nursing aides, attendants, orderlies, messengers, and various specialized technicians.

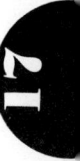

18
DOCTORS

Doctor and Nurse Relations

Survey*

How often have you felt used as a servant by a doctor?

Almost always	2%
Frequently	13%
Often with some, not with others	48%
Occasionally	18%
Seldom or never	19%

Nurses who rate their professional relations with physicians as very satisfactory also tend to rate their *personal* relations with physicians as very satisfactory, seldom feel that they are used as servants by physicians, and tend to rate their own ethical standards as about the same as those of physicians.

The less satisfactory a nurse's professional relations with physicians, the less satisfactory are her *personal* relations with them and the more likely is a feeling of being used as a servant; she also tends to feel her ethical standards are higher than physicians'.

*Source: "Ethical Problems Survey," *Nursing '74* September (Survey of 11,000 nurses.)

Nurses' Evaluation of Physicians

Table 18-1   Specific physician behaviors, and ratings

	Rank		
Physician behaviors	Importance to nurse	Descriptiveness of the typical physician	Deficiency of physician performance
Direction			
Gives orders which are correct, clear, sufficiently detailed	1	3	13
Gives adequate orders so nurses may act	2	15	15
Puts his orders in writing	3	16	16
On own initiative, discontinues unnecessary orders	14	14	5
Communication			
On own initiative gives information to nurse about:			
Treatment plan, anticipated procedure, or need for equipment	4	5	14
Something he has done in patient care, e.g. changing IV flow rate or filling out requisition	5	8	6
Patient's medical condition needs	7	9	10
Patient's emotional problems needs	10	13	1
Anticipated patient arrival	15	12	11
Which physician is in charge of patient	16	16	7
Patient's family, social situation	17	18	3
When he expects to see patient	18	17	8
Participation and Decision Making			
Seeks nurse's observations	6	6	12
Plans with nurse for patient management	8	11	4
Responds to nurse's observations	9	4	17
Includes nurse in physician nurse-patient discussion	11	15	2
Seeks nurse's suggestions	12	10	9
Responds to nurse's suggestions	13	7	18

Source: Barbara Bates and Robert W. Chamberlin, "Physician Leadership as Perceived by Nurses," *Nursing Research,* Nov.–Dec. 1970. (Survey of 312 nurses covering interns (54%), residents or fellows (32%) and attending physicians (12%).) © American Journal of Nursing Company.

18

Doctor-Nurse Differences*

The trends in nursing toward baccalaureate education and graduate training may, in time, bring about considerable reduction in the educational gap between physicians and nurses. Less difficulty in communication should be one of the end results.

Physicians tend to emphasize the subordinate qualities of the nurse rather than her patient-supportive qualities. More attention is paid to her relationship with the physician as an assistant than to her work with patients.

A study exploring differences between college-and hospital-trained nurses revealed that nursing students in hospital schools of nursing were prone to select nurse-doctor interactions rather than nurse-patient interactions as the situations from which they obtained most personal gratification. For students in college schools of nursing, preference was in reverse order. A possible conclusion from this study is that hospital education fosters greater dependence on the medical profession.

Also, because nurses are better rewarded for utilizing their skills on organizational problems than for clinical competence, those desiring advancement address themselves to promotion through the organizational hierarchy. Therefore, nurses who might well become the best clinicians (and communicate most effectively with physicians) are being drained away from direct patient care.

Socioeconomic-Class Differences—The pronounced difference in the economic rewards of physicians and nurses produces a different style of life for the members of both professions. By comparison with nurses, physicians are well paid. No one disputes the justice of additional preparation commanding more salary. Nevertheless, the resulting economic class differences trigger off an entirely different style of life. Very little social interaction occurs except in the usually highly prescribed fashion of the work situation. Physicians and nurses customarily do not have the opportunity to know each other as persons, to understand each other's viewpoints, and to build interpersonal trust.

Physicians traditionally come from families with professional and business backgrounds.

Nurses, on the other hand, most often come from working-class and lower-middle-class families. Both groups take their social perspectives into training with them. Both groups tend to reflect the attitudes of their socioeconomic class.

Autonomy Differences

Physicians, with a disregard for hospital routine yet with the power to disturb it, often place great strain on nurses because nurses are primarily responsible for maintaining this routine. Nurses are likely to perceive this action as an irrational use of power.

Physicians also have many conflicting demands on their time. However, they have the opportunity for much more self-direction. If physicians assume that nurses have this same privilege, it may lead to considerable misunderstanding.

Physicians are usually self-employed and self-directing. Essentially, they are responsible only to their peers. Most nurses are employees—and employees in an unusual position. Nurses are subject to the control of three departments of the hospital: the medical staff, hospital administration, and nursing administration. All three can and do intervene in the daily work schedule of nurses.

A physician is a power unto himself in his own office. Nevertheless, when he enters the hospital, he must work in an organizational pattern in which there is a complex division of labor and one in which he shares power. However, he frequently appears to be acting on the same set of power expectations that he displays in his own office. His intense preoccupation with the clinical problems of his patients probably accounts for much of this attitude. When several physicians in the course of a day display this same behavior and the demands of each cannot equally be met, a power squeeze is on and nurses are apt to use coping tactics which can easily inhibit communication.

The Doctor-Nurse Game**

The object of the game is as follows: The nurse is to be bold, have initiative, and be responsible for making significant recommendations, while

---

*Source: L. P. Christman, Ph.D., "Nurse—Physician Communications in the Hospital," *Journal of the American Medical Association*, November 1, 1965.

**Source: L. I. Stein, "The Doctor Nurse Game," *American Journal of Nursing*, January 1968. © American Journal of Nursing Company.

at the same time she must appear passive. This must be done in such a manner as though to make her recommendations appear to be initiated by the physician. . . . The cardinal rule of the game is that open disagreement between the players must be avoided at all cost. Thus, the nurse must communicate her recommendations without appearing to be making a recommendation statement. The physician, in requesting a recommendation from the nurse, must do so without appearing to be asking for it. . . . The nurse who . . . see(s) herself as a consultant, but refuses to follow the rules of the game in making her recommendations, has hell to pay. The outspoken nurse is labeled a "bitch" by the surgeon. The psychiatrist describes her as unconsciously suffering from penis envy and her behavior as the acting out of her hostility toward men. Loosely translated, the psychiatrist is saying she is a bitch. The employment of the unbright, outspoken nurse is soon terminated. The outspoken bright nurse whose recommendations are worthwhile remains employed. She is, however, constantly reminded in a hundred ways that she is not loved. . . .

The following example is not subtle, but happens frequently. The medical resident on hospital call is awakened by telephone at 1:00 A.M. because a patient on a ward, not his own, has not been able to fall asleep. Dr. Jones answers the telephone and the dialogue goes like this.

This is Dr. Jones.
(An open and direct communication.)
Dr. Jones, this is Miss Smith on 2W—Mrs. Brown, who learned today of her father's death, is unable to fall asleep.
(This message has two levels. Openly, it describes a set of circumstances, a woman who is unable to sleep and who that morning received word of her father's death. Less openly, but just as directly, it is a diagnostic and recommendation statement; Mrs. Brown is unable to sleep because of her grief, and she should be given a sedative. Dr. Jones, accepting the diagnostic statement and replying to the recommendation statement, answers.)
What sleeping medication has been helpful to Mrs. Brown in the past?
(Dr. Jones, not knowing the patient, is asking for a recommendation from the nurse, who does know the patient, about what sleeping medication should be prescribed. Note,

however, his question does not appear to be asking her for a recommendation. Miss Smith replies.)
Pentobarbital mg. 100 was quite effective night before last.
(A disguised recommendation statement. Dr. Jones replies with a note of authority in his voice.)
Pentobarbital mg. 100 before bedtime as needed for sleep, got it?
(Miss Smith ends the conversation with the tone of a grateful supplicant.)
Yes I have, and thank you very much doctor.

To understand how the game evolved, we must comprehend the nature of the doctors' and nurses' training which shaped the attitudes necessary for the game.

Nursing students' begin to learn to play the game early in their training. They are taught how to relate to physicians. They are told the physician has infinitely more knowledge than they, and thus he should be shown the utmost respect. In addition, it was not many years ago when nurses were instructed to stand whenever a physician entered a room. When he would come in for a conference the nurse was expected to offer him her chair, and when both entered a room the nurse would open the door for him and allow him to enter first. Although these practices are no longer rigidly adhered to, the premise upon which they were based is still promulgated. One nurse described that premise as, "He's God almighty and your job is to wait on him."

Medical Students*

Marital Status

Table 18-2 Married medical students, 1971

Medical school class	All schools
Total	47%
Freshman	35
Sophomore	41
Junior	51
Senior	65

* Source: *How Medical Students Finance Their Education,* DHEW, June 1974.

Source of Income

Table 18-3   Medical students—source of income

Source of income	All students[1]	Single	Married no children
Total income	100%	100%	100%
Total non-refundable funds	81	75	88
Own earnings and savings	18	24	13
Spouse's earnings	30	(2)	55
Gifts/loans from family	20	36	11
Federal Health Professions Scholarship	3	4	1
NIH-supported research grants, etc.	1	1	1
Other Federal research grants, etc.	1	1	1
Stage government scholarship	1	1	1
Other non-refundable funds	7	8	5
Total refundable funds	19	25	12
Federal Health Professions loan	5	6	3
Federal Office of Education guaranteed loan	2	3	2
Own professional school loan	2	4	1
State government loan	3	4	2
Private bank loan	2	2	2
Other loans	5	6	2

[1] Includes students who were widowed, divorced, or separated.

[2] Less than 0.5%.

Among single students, parents' contributions were the principal source of income—accounting for 36% of the income reported. Married students reported that only 11% of their income came from parents or other relatives. Spouse's contributions accounted for 55% of married medical students' income.

Physician Specialties

Physician Specialty Certification

There are 22 specialty boards which grant certification to physicians who have the required additional, professional and educational qualifications in a specialized field. The earliest board was established in 1917 in the field of ophthalmology; the two most recent ones in 1971, in allergy and immunology and in nu-clear medicine. Board certifications can be verified in the *American Medical Directory;* the certificate is also displayed in the doctor's office. At times, initials which begin with an *F.A.C.* are displayed after the traditional *M.D.* These initials indicate that the physician is a "Fellow of American College ..." of radiology (*FACR*), of surgeons (*FACS*) or of anesthesiologists (*FACAn*). While this designation confirms that the physician has received specialized training to the satisfaction of the particular college, it is no guarantee that he has also received his board-certification in the specialty.

Titles and Abbreviations

Following are the board-certified titles for specialties:

Specialty Board	Abbreviation of certification
Medical Specialties:	
Allergy and Immunology	D–AI
Dermatology	D–D
Family Practice	D–FP
Internal Medicine	D–IM
Pediatrics	D–P
Surgical Specialties:	
Surgery	D–S
Neurological Surgery	D–NS
Obstetrics and Gynecology	D–OG
Ophthalmology	D–O
Orthopedic Surgery	D–OS
Otolaryngology	D–OL
Plastic Surgery	D–PS
Colon and Rectal Surgery	D–CRS
Thoracic Surgery	D–TS
Urology	D–U
Other Specialities:	
Anesthesiology	D–A
Pathology	D–PA
Preventive Medicine	D–PM
Psychiatry and Neurology	D–PN
Nuclear Medicine	D–NUM
Physical Medicine and Rehabilitation	D–PMR
Radiology	D–R

Number of Specialists—by Field

Table 18-4   Active physicians by specialty: actual and projected

	1970	1980	1990
Total Active Physicians (M.D. only)	100.0% (311,210)	100.0% (430,240)	100.0% (571,030)
General Practice	18.1	11.0	6.4
Medical Specialties	21.3	27.0	30.6
Dermatology	1.3	1.3	1.3
Family Practice	0.5	1.5	2.2
Internal Medicine	13.5	16.7	18.7
Pediatrics	6.0	7.5	8.4
Surgical Specialties	27.4	30.0	31.7
General Surgery	9.6	12.2	13.8
Neurological Surgery	0.8	0.8	0.8
Obstetrics and Gynecology	6.1	6.1	6.1
Ophthalmology	3.2	3.0	2.9
Orthopedic Surgery	3.1	3.1	3.2
Otolaryngology	1.7	1.6	1.5
Plastic Surgery	0.5	0.7	0.8
Thoracic Surgery	0.6	0.7	0.8
Urology	1.9	1.9	1.9
Other Specialties	33.2	32.1	31.3
Anesthesiology	3.5	4.0	4.3
Child Psychiatry	0.7	1.0	1.2
Neurology	1.0	1.5	1.9
Psychiatry	6.8	7.6	8.2
Pathology	3.3	3.9	4.2
Physical Medicine	0.5	0.6	0.7
Radiology	3.4	3.4	3.5
Therapeutic Radiology	0.3	0.4	0.5
Miscellaneous	13.8	9.6	7.0

Source: DHEW, December 1974.

Public Attitudes Toward Doctors

Honesty and Ethics

Table 18-5   Public ratings on honesty/ethics of doctors and other professionals

	(Ratings of total sample)					
	Very high	High	Average	Low	Very low	No opinion
Medical doctors	17%	39%	35%	6%	3%	(¹)
Engineers	10	39	43	3	1	4%
College teachers	9	35	44	7	2	3
Journalists	7	26	49	13	3	2
Lawyers	6	19	48	18	8	1
Building contractors	5	18	54	18	3	2
Business executives	3	17	58	16	4	2
Senators	3	16	51	22	7	1
Congressmen	3	11	47	27	11	1
Labor union leaders	2	10	38	31	17	2
Advertising practitioners	2	9	43	29	15	2

¹ Less than 1%.

Source: *Gallup Opinion Index* (134, September 1976), Princeton, N.J.

Public Confidence in Doctors vs. Other Leaders

Confidence levels in the leadership of most major American institutions continued to drop in 1974.

Doctors, educators and those running television news stand at the head of the list in generating public confidence, while Congress, the executive branch of the federal government and leaders of organized labor finish at the bottom.

Perhaps the most striking single result is that eight of the 12 institutions asked about

Table 18-6   Confidence in key institutions

	Great deal of confidence (%)		Great deal of confidence (%)
Medicine			
1975	43	1972	35
1974	50	1966	62
1973	57	Major Companies	
1972	48	1975	19
1966	72	1974	21
Colleges		1973	29
1975	36	1972	27
1974	40	1966	55
1973	44	Law Firms	
1972	33	1975	16
1966	61	1974	18
Television News		1973	24
1975	35	1972	XX
1974	31	1966	XX
1973	41	Organized Labor	
1972	17	1975	14
1966	25	1974	18
Organized Religion		1973	20
1975	32	1972	15
1974	32	1966	22
1973	36	Congress	
1972	30	1975	13
1966	41	1974	18
U.S. Supreme Court		1973	29
1975	28	1972	21
1974	40	1966	42
1973	33	Executive Branch of	
1972	28	Federal Government	
1966	51	1975	13
The Press		1974	28
1975	26	1973	19
1974	25	1972	27
1973	30	1966	41
1972	18	XX Not Asked	
1966	29		
The Military			
1975	24		
1974	33		
1973	40		

Source: "Confidence in Key Institutions," *The Harris Survey,* October 1975.

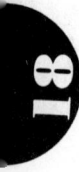

have hit all-time lows since the Harris Survey first began asking about them in 1966: doctors, the U.S. Supreme Court, the military, major companies, law firms, organized labor, the executive branch of the federal government, and Congress.

Recently, the Harris Survey asked a cross section of 1,579 adults nationwide: "As far as people in charge of running (READ LIST) are concerned, would you say you have a great deal of confidence, only some confidence or hardly any confidence at all in them?"

Patients Visiting Physicians*

Overview

There were an estimated one billion physician visits during 1974. Female patients accounted for three of every five visits.

The average person made five visits during the one year period. (However, note the sharp

decline in physician visits *to the patient's home* in Table 18-8.)

- General and family practitioners accounted for 40.4% of all visits; medical specialties, 26.3%; and surgical specialties, 28.5%.
- Pediatricians had an average of 139 office patient visits per week. General and family practitioners averaged 118 visits while the average for all office-based physicians was 91 office visits per week.
- More than 60% of all visits were by patients seen previously for the same problem; and about 20% were for problems considered serious or very serious by the physician.
- During 63% of all visits, the patient expressed a "symptomatic" problem or complaint as the major reason for the visit. "Nonsymptomatic" problems accounted for 18% of all visits.
- Either a disease of the respiratory system or a disease of the circulatory system was the diagnosis in about one of every four visits.

(Note the sharp decline in home visits from 1957 to 1971.)

*Source: *National Ambulatory Medical Care Survey, May 1973–April 1974,* DHEW, October 1975.

Age and Sex of Patients

Table 18-7   Physician visits by age and sex: U.S. 1974

Sex	All ages	Under 17 years	17–24 years	25–44 years	45–64 years	65–74 years	75 years and over
Number of physician visits in thousands							
Both sexes	1,025,340	260,689	133,706	254,839	236,503	90,373	49,230
Male	427,042	137,456	45,416	87,490	99,540	38,998	18,142
Female	598,298	123,233	88,290	167,349	136,963	51,375	31,088
Number of physician visits per person per year							
Both sexes	4.9	4.1	4.5	5.0	5.5	6.9	6.5
Male	4.3	4.3	3.2	3.5	4.9	6.8	6.3
Female	5.6	4.0	5.8	6.3	6.1	6.9	6.6

Source: *Current Estimates from the Health Interview Survey, U.S., 1974,* DHEW Pub. No. (HRA) 76–1527.

Where Patients Visit

Table 18-8   Physician visits by place of examination: selected years

Place of visit	July 1957– June 1958	1971
All visits	100.0%	100.0%
Office	65.0	69.6
Home	10.2	1.7
Hospital clinic	10.0	10.2
Company or industry health unit	1.1	1.0
Telephone	10.4	13.3
Other and unknown	3.2	4.2

Source: *Vital and Health Statistics,* DHEW, 1975.

Who Patients Visit

Table 18-9   Office visits by physician type of practice: May 1973–April 1974

Physician specialty and type of practice	Number of visits in thousands
All specialties	644,893
General and family practice	260,310
Medical specialties	169,316
Internal medicine	74,693
Pediatrics	53,659
Other	40,964
Surgical specialties	183,787
General surgery	44,846
Obstetrics and gynecology	50,715
Other	88,227
Other specialties	31,481
Psychiatry	20,300
Other	11,180
Type of practice	
Solo	386,208
Other	258,685

Source: *National Ambulatory Medical Care Survey, May 1973–April 1974,* DHEW, October 1975.

Patient Problems

Table 18-10   Visits to office-based physicians most frequent patient problems: U.S. May 1973–April 1974

Patient's principal problem classified by NAMCS symptom classification[1]		Number of visits in thousands	Percent of visits
Total, all problems		644,893	100.0
1. Progress visits	980,985	75,673	11.7
2. Problems of lower extremity	400	25,944	4.0
3. Pregnancy examination	905	25,942	4.0
4. Throat soreness	520	20,726	3.2
5. Problems of upper extremity	405	18,956	2.9
6. Problems of back	415	18,824	2.9
7. Cough	311	18,347	2.8
8. Abdominal pain	540	16,418	2.5
9. General physical examination	900	15,022	2.3
10. Cold	312	13,460	2.1
11. Gynecologic examination	904	13,154	2.0
12. Visit for medication	910	13,103	2.0
13. None	997	13,043	2.0
14. Headache	056	12,314	1.9
15. Fatigue	004	11,768	1.8
16. Pain in chest	322	11,350	1.8
17. Required physical examination	901	11,095	1.7

18

Table 18-10   (continued)

Patient's principal problem classified by NAMCS symptom classification[1]		Number of visits in thousands	Percent of visits
18. Well-baby examination	906	10,699	1.7
19. Fever	002	9,822	1.5
20. Allergic skin reaction	112	9,458	1.5
21. Problems of face, neck	410	9,327	1.4
22. Vision dysfunction, except blindness	701	9,219	1.4
23. Weight gain	010	8,999	1.4
24. Vertigo	069	7,606	1.2
25. Earache	735	7,466	1.2
26. Wounds	116	7,391	1.1
27. High blood pressure	205	7,014	1.1
28. Shortness of breath	306	6,858	1.1
29. Nasal congestion	301	6,675	1.0
30. Swelling, mass of skin	115	6,158	1.0
31. Skin irritation (nonallergic)	113	6,144	1.0
32. Anus, rectal problems	560	5,254	0.8
33. Symptoms of nervousness	810	4,767	0.7
34. Symptoms of depression	807	4,761	0.7
35. Vaginal discharge	662	4,687	0.7
36. Nausea	572	4,269	0.7
37. Pain, irritation of eye	705	4,182	0.7
38. Menstrual disorders	653	4,178	0.7
39. Acne	100	4,061	0.6
40. Painful urination	604	3,582	0.6
41. Diarrhea	555	3,092	0.5
42. Hearing dysfunction, except deafness	731	2,954	0.5
43. Menopausal symptoms	650	2,729	0.4
44. Situational problems	941	2,488	0.4
45. Symptoms of anxiety	800	2,369	0.4
46. Nocturia	601	2,309	0.4
47. Laboratory testing	920	2,279	0.4
48. Swelling or mass, site unspecified	015	2,234	0.4
49. Stomach upset	570	2,212	0.3
50. Pain, site unspecified	013	2,150	0.3
51. Lump in breast	680	2,146	0.3
52. Skin moles	109	2,026	0.3
53. Irregular heartbeat	200	1,971	0.3
54. Warts	111	1,891	0.3
55. Sinus problem	304	1,814	0.3
56. Pelvic disorder	660	1,712	0.3
57. Weakness, numbness of extremity	420	1,652	0.3
58. Hoarseness	325	1,643	0.3
59. Blocked feeling of ear	737	1,559	0.2
60. Vulvar disorder	663	1,503	0.2
61. All other problems	Residual	114,445	17.7

[1] Symptomatic groupings and code number inclusions are based on a symptom classification developed for use in the NAMCS.

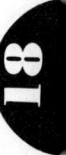

Source: *National Ambulatory Medical Care Survey, May 1973–April 1974,* DHEW, October 1975.

344

18

Tips For Selecting a Doctor:

Whether transferred to a new community or confronted by a sudden illness, most people find the selection of a physician a confusing dilemma. Consider the sources commonly relied upon for recommendations: a neighbor or family friend, whose information may be juicy—or scandalous—but also biased, unreliable and incomplete; a doctor from the last neighborhood, who may be unfamiliar with physicians in the new locale; or a hospital, which will simply name doctors on its staff without further background details. Even if a doctor refers a patient to another medical specialist, there are details a patient might want to check out before making a final decision.

Factors to Check:

- medical school attended and year of M.D. degree
- state licensure and year acquired
- specialty and type of practice
- certification by specialty board
- hospital affiliation
- level of hospital affiliation; whether an active or associate staff member or simply courtesy privileges
- office fees and hours
- participation in health plans
- association with a medical group practice

Sources of Information on Doctors' Training and Licensure

- *American Medical Directory*, published by AMA, lists doctors, according to city location, in separate volumes for each state. Training background, licensure and specialty credential information is given for each doctor in a numerical code which is explained at the front of the book.
- The Health Research Group, a division of Nader's Public Citizen Inc., which concentrates on health-related affairs, will provide a list of communities where citizen-interest groups have printed background information on cooperating local doctors.

The directories usually contain most of the check-factors listed above. For further assistance you might contact the director, Dr. Sidney Wolfe, at Health Research Group, 2000 P Street N.W., Washington, D.C. 20036.

Other Information:

- Hospitals will usually answer inquiries about the type of affiliation a selected physician has with it. They will also provide, on request, a list of associated doctors qualified in a specific specialty. These can then be checked out in the directory.
- Most physicians' secretaries will answer questions on fees, hours, participation in health plans, and association with hospitals or medical groups.

19

THE PHYSICIAN'S ASSISTANT

Overview

The AMA House of Delegates in December 1970 adopted the following working definition of the "Physician's Assistant"—"A skilled person qualified by academic and practical on-the-job training to provide patient services under the supervision and direction of a licensed physician, who is responsible for the performance of that assistant."

The assistant to the primary care physician is not intended to supplant the doctor in the sphere of the decision making required to establish a diagnosis and plan therapy. He or she will assist in gathering the data necessary to reach decisions and implement the therapeutic plan for the patient.

Dr. E. A. Stead of Duke University was the first to start a program for the training of physician's assistants.

Then, in 1970, Dr. Ernest Howard announced a plan for the American Medical Association to make 100,000 nurses into physician's assistants. The tart but understandable response of the American Nurses' Association to this event was that it was not the prerogative of the medical profession to decide what nurses should do—then, or in the future.

Controversy

The status of P.A.'s is still controversial. The program has ardent supporters who believe that in addition to solving the physician shortage, it will also result in improved patient care. Its detractors believe the P.A.'s are unnecessary and will cause a double standard of care (physicians for the rich and P.A.'s for the poor).

In addition, some members of professions, such as nursing, feel that functions assigned to P.A.'s overlap their responsibility and that the program is an attempt to advance males over the predominantly female nursing profession.

Traditionally, the physician-nurse relationship has been one of superordination-subordination to the point that, when the need for some type of middle medical worker emerged, many physicians simply did not think of nurses as being capable of independent or cooperative decision making, turning instead to physician's assistants. The mind set of the physicians, however, was only part of the problem; the more important psychological barrier consisted of the feelings which nurses held about themselves. Many nurses experienced difficulty in seeing themselves as decision makers in the diagnostic and treatment process. They had, of course, been making diagnostic decisions for years but had protected themselves with elaborate games which cast the physician in a decision-making role even when the decision had been made by nurses.

Giving Orders to Nurses*

The problem of whether a nurse must carry out an order written by a physician's assistant has been and is a troublesome one. At present, there appears to be legal protection only for the nurse who carries out the orders of a licensed doctor or dentist. Hence nurses, such as those in the New York area, have adopted the policy of not complying with an order unless it is given by a licensed physician or dentist. Elsewhere, nurses who question the correctness of a physician's assistant's order are endeavoring to check its accuracy or validity with the physician who is to countersign the assistant's order.

To better cope with the problem, individual hospitals are adopting bylaws that establish requirements for physician's assistants who work in their hospitals and specifically define the respective responsibilities of physicians, physicians' assistants and nurses. Under the bylaws, only after a review of his qualifications would a physician's assistant be allowed to practice in the hospital. Such schemes savor strongly of institutional licensure. Whether the rights of patients to high quality care or the rights of nurses and nursing would be adequately protected under such schemes is open to serious question. Likewise, it is not known whether nurses and nursing service would have adequate input and voice in the formulation of such hospital bylaws or whether they would be given only meaningless, token representation.

Profile of the Physician's Assistant

- Young white male: Average age 29, only 7% black. Ophthalmologic assistants and pediatric assistants are the only specialties in which women predominate.

---

*Source: Helen Creighton, *NLN Review*, #16–1551, 1974.

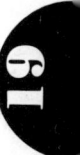

- 3.4 years of prior experience (before P.A. training) in health care field
- attended 2 years of college (before P.A. training)
- living in Southeast
- working primarily in private medical practice and in hospital inpatient facilities
- working in same geographic areas in which they were trained

On-the-Job Functions

Job Titles

- Anesthetic assistant.
- Assistant to the primary care physician.
- Child health associate.
- Clinical associate.
- Community health medic.
- MEDEX.
- Orthop(a)edic physician's assistant.
- Orthopedic assistant.
- Pediatric associate.
- Physician's associate.
- Surgeon's assistant.
- Surgical assistant.
- Urological physician's assistant.

Types of Tasks Performed*

The tasks performed by the assistant include but need not be limited to the following:

1. The initial approach to a patient of any age group in any setting to elicit a detailed and accurate history, perform an appropriate physical examination, and record and present pertinent data in a manner meaningful to the physician;
2. Performance and/or assistance in performance of routine laboratory and related studies as appropriate for a specific practice setting, such as the drawing of blood sam-

---

*Source: *Educational Programs for the Physician's Assistant,* American Medical Association, Division of Medical Education, Summer 1974.

ples, performance of urinalyses, and the taking of electrocardiographic tracings;

3. Performance of such routine therapeutic procedures as injections, immunizations, and the suturing and care of wounds;

4. Instruction and counseling of patients regarding physical and mental health on matters such as diets, disease, therapy, and normal growth and development;

5. Assisting the physician in the hospital setting by making patient rounds, recording patient progress notes, accurately and appropriately transcribing and/or executing standing orders and other specific orders at the direction of the supervising physician, and compiling and recording detailed narrative case summaries;

6. Providing assistance in the delivery of services to patients requiring continuing care (home, nursing home, extended care facilities, etc.) including the review and monitoring of treatment and therapy plans;

7. Independent performance of evaluative and treatment procedures essential to provide an appropriate response to life-threatening, emergency situations; and

8. Facilitation of the physician's referral of appropriate patients by maintenance of an awareness of the community's various health facilities, agencies, and resources.

Time Spent at Various Tasks

Physician's assistants spend the greater part of their work day caring for patients under the direct or indirect supervision of a physician and engage only peripherally in technical and supervisory tasks.

Physician's Assistant specialties needing more intensive physician supervision or a closer working relation with the physician include cardiology, orthopedic general surgery, and urology. On the other hand, more independence from close physician supervision is the practice in the specialties of anesthesiology, ophthalmology, pediatrics, radiology, and general medicine.

Table 19-1   Physician's assistant: task time distribution during an average work day

| Specialty of the P.A. | Patient care | | Type of task | | | | |
	Directly Super-vised by M.D.	Indirect Surveil-lance by M.D.	Tech-nical or Lab-oratory	Clerical or Secre-tarial	Adminis-trative or Super-visory	Teaching in a Health Profession	Other
General medicine	27%	45%	10%	4%	12%	5%	3%
Anesthesiology	14%	48%	14%	2%	10%	11%	1%
Cardiology	38%	18%	23%	2%	9%	8%	2%
Ophthalmology	29%	43%	11%	8%	6%	3%	0%
Orthopaedics	48%	27%	7%	2%	8%	8%	0%
Pathology	11%	3%	22%	6%	25%	19%	13%
Pediatrics	26%	44%	0%	5%	8%	10%	7%
Radiology	2%	58%	3%	0%	35%	2%	0%
General surgery	53%	27%	8%	3%	6%	2%	1%
Urology	46%	20%	7%	12%	3%	2%	12%
Column Total (average over entire population)	32%	37%	10%	4%	10%	5%	3%

Source: R. M. Schieffer & D. D. Stinson, "Characteristics of Physician's Assistants," *Medical Care,* December 1974.

On-the-Job Performance

A Yale University Medical School survey in 1974 of research on Expanded Roles of Health Workers found that physician assistants are:

- Able to manage at least ⅔ of the patients assigned to them without consulting the supervising physician.

- Able to manage without the physician actually examining the patient in about ½ the cases where patients sought physician consultation.

- Able to perform as well as the physicians with whom they were compared and to provide continuity of care.

- Responsible for increased physician productivity.

- Accepted as practitioners by consumers.

What Physician Extenders Do*

Extensive studies of what physician extenders do in practice are only beginning to be published. The American Society of Internal Medicine (ASIM) obtained data on 3,425 members in 1969 concerning their attitudes toward anticipated task delegation to physician extenders.

The ASIM survey used was concerned with (1) physicians current (1969) practices in task delegation, and (2) their attitude (as expressed in 1969) about what specific tasks *could and should* be delegated to "... an appropriately trained person (male or female)" ... "under direct supervision of an internist" ... "directly responsible to him" where "legal and liability problems are covered." These reported results are shown in Table 19-2.

---

*Source: Glenn & Goldman, "Task Delegation to Physician Extenders." *American Journal of Public Health,* January 1976.

Table 19-2   Doctors' views on task delegation, 1969

Laboratory and related tasks	Could & should be delegated to non-MD ASIM survey (% MDs)	Task is currently being delegated to non-MD ASIM survey (% MDs)
Obtain and mount electrocardiogram tracings	—	94
Obtain venous blood samples for lab	94	72
Procure urine sample for lab	—	96
Perform urinalysis (glucose, protein)	97	94
Prepare urine for microanalysis	97	91
Determine hemoglobin	98	91
Determine hematocrit	98	93
Perform blood cell counts, smears or both	97	91
Perform pulmonary function studies	89	58
Perform Master's two-step exercise test	67	62
Perform skin tests (allergic, fungi, tuberculosis (Tbc))	77	47
Therapy		
Administer immunizations	90	63
Administer medications intramuscularly	90	61
Administer medications intravenously	42	12
Perform ear irrigations	67	26
Remove sutures	69	18
Give diet instruction for obesity, diabetes, etc.	71	20
Clerical and Office Tasks		
Fill out insurance forms	—	86
Do billing	—	98
Order refills of prescriptions with physician authorization	83	84
Schedule appointments for X-ray and lab work	97	94
Schedule admissions to hospital	87	66
Schedule appointments on referral cases after conferring with MD	96	92
Type progress notes on chart	—	70
Physical Examination Tasks		
Obtain height and weight	—	81
Take blood pressure on initial visit	—	17
Take blood pressure in following hypertensive patient	—	21
Take temperature	—	76
Administer screening tests for hearing	93	47
Administer screening tests for vision	94	69
Perform tonometry	51	15
Perform proctoscopic examination	9	1
Perform pelvic examination and do Pap smear	6	1
Perform Pap smear only	34	3
History and Patient Contact Tasks		
Take and record routine elements of history (family, operations, injuries, etc.)	60	13
Take and record history of present illness	28	4
Take and record elements of systemic review	37	5
Provide telephone advice on routine medical questions	61	43
Provide (a) telephone advice on routine minor medical problems and (b) schedule patient for examination at office if necessary	67(a) 77(b)	76
Visit nursing homes for routine medical rechecks	43	3
Visit patients' homes to determine necessity of physicians' exam at home	65	15

— = Not Applicable or No Response

Education

Overview

The first P.A. training program in the U.S. was started at Duke University in 1965 to (1) meet the need for highly skilled technical personnel to staff special diagnostic and treatment units within the hospital and (2) provide more broadly trained individuals to work with the practicing physician, primarily in the rural areas of North Carolina where the physician/patient ratio was one-third the national average.

Today, the typical specialty care program is a two-year program sponsored by a junior college. (Some run for just 12 months.)

It is likely to require only a high school diploma for admission, yet about one-fourth of its enrollees will have had previous military or civilian medical experience.

It accepts 11 new enrollees each year from among the 40 applications it receives, and produces 8 or 9 graduates per year.

On the average, it costs about $3,400 to train each graduate.

Graduates of specialty care programs are likely to receive either an associate degree or a certificate. They usually work in hospitals and private offices in urban areas. The tasks they perform depend on the type of specialist they assist and are likely to be more specialized than those performed by the primary care PA.

Curriculum

Table 19-3   Tasks P.A.'s have been trained to perform (from a broad sample of physician's assistant training programs)

Tasks graduates trained to perform	% of students trained in this task	Tasks graduates trained to perform	% of students trained in this task
Take medical histories	(71%)	Assist in Operating Room	
		Administer some anesthesia	(17%)
Laboratory Procedures		Provide preoperative care	(60%)
Blood analysis	(57%)	Provide postoperative care	(60%)
Urinanalysis	(61%)	Assist physician with major	
Bacteriology tests	(57%)	surgery	(53%)
Pulmonary function studies	(39%)	Assist physician with minor	
Skin tests (allergy, tuber-		surgery	(73%)
culosis, etc.)	(48%)		
EKG	(64%)	Injection Procedures	
EEG	(16%)	Intramuscular	(64%)
X-Ray	(31%)	Draw blood	(71%)
		Start and monitor IVs	(68%)
Physical Examination Tasks		Vaccination	(57%)
Obtain physical measure-			
ments	(69%)	Bandages and Casts	
Measure vital signs	(80%)	Apply and remove bandages	
Administer hearing and		and casts	(73%)
vision tests	(53%)	Set simple fractures	(24%)
Perform tonometry	(45%)	Remove casts	(65%)
Perform proctoscopic exams	(31%)	Other Tasks	
Perform physical exam—		Suture wounds	(65%)
adults	(61%)	Perform irrigations	(67%)
Perform physical exam—		Make home visits	(51%)
children	(53%)	Order medication (standing	
Perform physical exam—		order)	(53%)
pregnant women	(41%)	Monitor patients	(61%)
Perform pelvic examination	(45%)	Disease management	(45%)
Order tests	(60%)		
Patient instruction and			
counseling	(69%)		

Source: T. W. Dobmeyer, et al., "A Report on a 1972 Survey on Physician's Assistant Training Programs," *Medical Care,* April 1975.

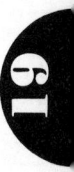

Requirements for State Licensure

Table 19-4   Analysis of physician extender legislation (37 states), 1974[1]

State	Category of Legislation	Type A Assistant						Physician Supervisor				
		Approval	Educational program approval	Equivalent training accepted	Job description	Restriction on activities	Periodic review	Approval	Supervision defined	No. of Type A assistants/physician	Rules and Regulations by Regulatory Agency	Report to Legislature
Alabama	Approval job description (1971)	+	+	+	+	+		+			+	
Alaska	Exception (1972)											
Arizona	Exception (1969)											
	Approval (1972)	+				+					+	
Arkansas	Exception (1971)					+						
California	Approval job description (1970)	+	+	+	+	+	(1)	+		2	+	1972
Colorado	Exception (1963)											
	License category (1969)	+	+			+	(1)	+		1	+	1977
Connecticut	Exception (1971)					+						
Delaware	Exception (1971)					+						
	Approval job description (1973)	+	+	+	+		(1)	+	Not PP	2	+	(1)
Florida	Exception (1970)											
	Approval job description (1971)	+	+	+	+		(1)	+	PP	2	+	1973
Georgia	Approval job description (1972)	+	+		+	+	(1)	+		2	+	
Hawaii	Exception (1973)		+			+			Not PP			
Idaho	Approval (1972)	+	+			+		+			+	
Iowa	Approval job description (1971)	+	+	+	+	+	(1)	+	Not PP	2	+ AC	1973
Kansas	Exception (1964)											
Maine	Exception (1973)		+			+			Not PP			
Maryland	Exception (1972)										+	
Massachusetts	Exception (1973)		+			+	(1)		Not PP	2	+	
Michigan	Exception (1973)		+	+							+ AC	(1)
Montana	Exception (1970)											
Nebraska	Approval job description (1973)	+	+	+	+		(1)	+	PP	2	+	(1)
Nevada	Approval (1973)	+	+			+		+		1	+	
New Hampshire	Approval (1971)	+	+								+	
New Mexico	Approval (1973)	+	+			+	(1)			2	+	
New York	Approval (1971)	+	+	+			(2)			2	+ AC	
North Carolina	Approval (1971)	+	+							2	+	
Oklahoma	Exception (1968)											
	Approval (1972)	+	+		+						+	
Oregon	Approval job description (1971)	+	+		+		(1)	+			+	1973
South Carolina	Approval (1974)	+			+						+	
South Dakota	Approval job description (1973)	+	+	+	+	+	(1)		Not PP		+	1981
Tennessee	Exception (1973)											
Utah	Exception (1971)		+									
Vermont	Approval (1972)	+									+	1975
Virginia	Approval job description (1973)	+	+		+	+	(1)	+			+	
Washington	Approval job description (1971)	+	+		+	+	(1)	+	Not PP		+	

Table 19-4 (continued)

State	Category of Legislation	Type A Assistant						Physician Supervisor				
		Approval	Educational program approval	Equivalent training accepted	Job description	Restriction on activities	Periodic review	Approval	Supervision defined	No. of Type A assistants/physician	Rules and Regulations by Regulatory Agency	Report to Legislature
West Virginia	Job description (1971)				+	+	(1)	+			+	
Wisconsin	Approval (1973)	+	+	+		+	(1)				+AC	1974
Wyoming	Approval job description (1973)	+	+	+	+	+	(1)	+			+AC	1975

[1](1), Annual, (2), biennial; PP, supervision requires physical presence of physician; Not PP, supervision does not require physical presence of physician; AC, Advisory Committee established.

Source: Roger M. Barkan, M.D., "Directions for Statutory Change—The Physician Extender." *AJPH,* December 1974.

Additional Information

For those interested in additional information about physician support personnel training programs, contact:

Association of Physician's Assistant Programs
2120 L St., N.W., Suite 210.
Washington, D.C. 20037

Council of MEDEX Programs
C/O Medex/Seattle Program
444 N.E. Ravenna Boulevard
Seattle, Washington 98115.

M.E.D.I.H.C. (Military Education Directed into Health Careers) a guidance service for ex-military personnel, organized through state agencies:

Miss Alice B. Frazier, Program Coordinator, MEDIHC
Division of Associated Health Professions
Bureau of Health Resources Development
Health Resources Administration
Federal Building
7550 Wisconsin Avenue
Bethesda, Maryland 20014

Pediatric Associate, Assistant, and Aide training programs:

Director, Office of Allied Health Manpower
American Academy of Pediatrics
1801 Hinman Avenue
Evanston, Illinois 60204

Veterans Administration participation in training programs for physician's assistant and other allied health occupations:

Mrs. Martha Long Phillips, Coordinator
Allied Health Training Program
Veterans Administration
Vermont Avenue at "H" Street, N.W.
Washington, D.C. 20420

For a list of accredited educational programs throughout the nation for the Assistant to the Primary Care Physician write to: AMA (American Medical Association), Department of Allied Medical Professions and Services, 535 North Dearborn St., Chicago, Illinois 60610.

A listing is published (and revised) each January and April. It contains information on the school and program, the directory, length of course, class size, starting date, tuition (if any), stipends and scholarships when offered.

Legal Limits and Licensure

The Physician's Assistant (the Type A assistant as defined by the National Academy of Sciences) has duties that include collecting historical and physical data, integrating and interpreting these findings, and exercising a degree of independent judgment, whether the

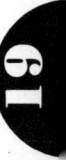

19

individual is a nurse or a nonnurse with special training.

Thirty-seven states have enacted statutory changes that legitimate the assistant. Over 80% of these laws have been enacted within the last four years. (See Table 19-4.)

Type A assistants may be subject to both personal and program approval and periodic reapproval. Several states have specified that attention be directed toward developing criteria for the acceptance of training equivalent to formal programs. Job descriptions are required by 14 statutes and 22 states place restrictions upon activities of Type A assistants in the areas of optometry, dentistry, and/or pharmacy.

Physician's Assistant—Certification*

The National Commission on Certification of Physician's Assistants certifies Assistants to the Primary Care Physician who successfully complete the proficiency examination administered by the National Board of Medical Examiners, and who meet other criteria established by the Commission.

The second annual examination was administered on December 11, 1974 at approximately 50 test centers throughout the country. An individual enrolled in a formal educational program was eligible to register for the

---

*Source: State Licensing of Health Occupations, Health Resources Administration, PHS. (Study by Aspen Systems Corporation, 1977)

examination if he/she had been graduated or would have been graduated by April 30, 1975 from:

1. A program that has been approved by the AMA Council on Medical Education for training Assistants to the Primary Care Physician.
2. A program that has received preliminary approval by the AMA Council on Medical Education for training Assistants to the Primary Care Physician.
3. A program that has been funded by the Bureau of Health Resources Development (not included in the above categories) that trains Assistants to the Primary Care Physician.
4. A program of at least four month's duration within a nationally accredited school of medicine or nursing that trains Pediatric or Family Nurse Practitioners.

An individual not enrolled in a formal educational program was eligible to register for this examination if he/she met all of the following requirements:

1. Has a high school diploma or an equivalency certificate.
2. Has had four years of medical, clinical experience in primary care as a Physician's Assistant or Nurse Practitioner since January 1, 1970.
3. Has met specific criteria concerning the nature of work experience. The details of an applicant's employment history will be verified by contacting the employing physician(s) and will then be evaluated in relation to specific criteria for eligibility.

20
HOSPITALS

Overview

History of Hospitals*

The first hospitals in the United States were established more than 200 years ago.

There is no record of hospitals in the early days of the American colonies. The first efforts for the care of the sick were incidental to shelter for the poor and unfortunate through almshouses. The first of these was founded in Philadelphia by William Penn in 1713, followed soon by others in New York City and Charleston, S.C. The famous Charity Hospital in New Orleans, dating from 1737, was originally both a hospital and an asylum for the indigent. The first bona fide hospital in the United States solely for the physically and mentally ill, without regard to economic status, race or creed, was established in 1751 and was known as the Pennsylvania Hospital. Other early hospitals grew out of a need to provide a place for clinical practice for medical schools, in New York and Massachusetts, and Connecticut. These early hospitals were chiefly of voluntary sponsorship, outside of public or church sponsorship.

Federal government participation in health care commenced with the establishment of the Public Health Service hospital program for merchant seamen in 1798. State government participation in health care was mainly confined to the mental health field, with construction of large state institutions between 1825 and 1850.

The first count of hospitals was compiled by the U.S. Bureau of Education in 1873; only 178 hospitals were listed. In 1909, the Bureau of the Census survey of hospitals showed 4,359 hospitals of all types, with a total of 421,000 beds. Subsequent surveys indicated that the number of hospitals and beds increased to 5,047 and 532,400 in 1914, and to 6,852 and 893,000 in 1928. By 1938, the number of hospitals had decreased to 6,166

but the number of beds had increased to 1,161,380. In 1963, the number again increased to almost 8,200 hospitals, with 1.5 million beds. By 1975, the estimated number had fallen to 7,156 hospitals.

Recent Trends

Although in the last few years the number of hospitals actually decreased, the number of beds available remained pretty much level (1,466,000 beds in 1975), and the occupancy rate actually fell from 86% to 76.7%, other indices of hospital manpower and expenses continued to soar. Between 1950 and 1975 admissions doubled, from 18 million to 36 million. In addition, the talley from 1970 to 1975 shows an upsurge of outpatient visits from 181 million to 255 million.

The tripling of personnel in the 25-year period from 1,058,000 to 3,023,000 was outmatched by a corresponding zoom in payroll expenses from $2.2 billion to $27.1 billion. An even sharper rise is reflected in total hospital expenses, from $3.7 billion to $48.7 billion. When these expenses are calculated along the lines of a per inpatient day figure there is nearly a 15 times greater cost, from $7.98 per inpatient day expense in 1950 to $118.69 in 1975.

Medical Costs: Who Pays and Who Receives*

The hospital is the scientific and technological hub of the medical care system and in 1974 accounted for the largest single portion ($40.9 billion or 39%) of the dollars spent on health care. Of the $104 billion spent on health care in 1974, $41.3 billion or approximately 39.6% was from public funds. Hospital expenditures accounted for 71% of government payments under the Medicare program ... and 37% under Medicaid. Fifty eight (58%) per cent of all public outlays for health services financed hospital care.

---

*Source: DHEW.

*Source: "Issues in National Financing of Health Care," House Report, November 1976.

Figure 20-1   Medical payment source

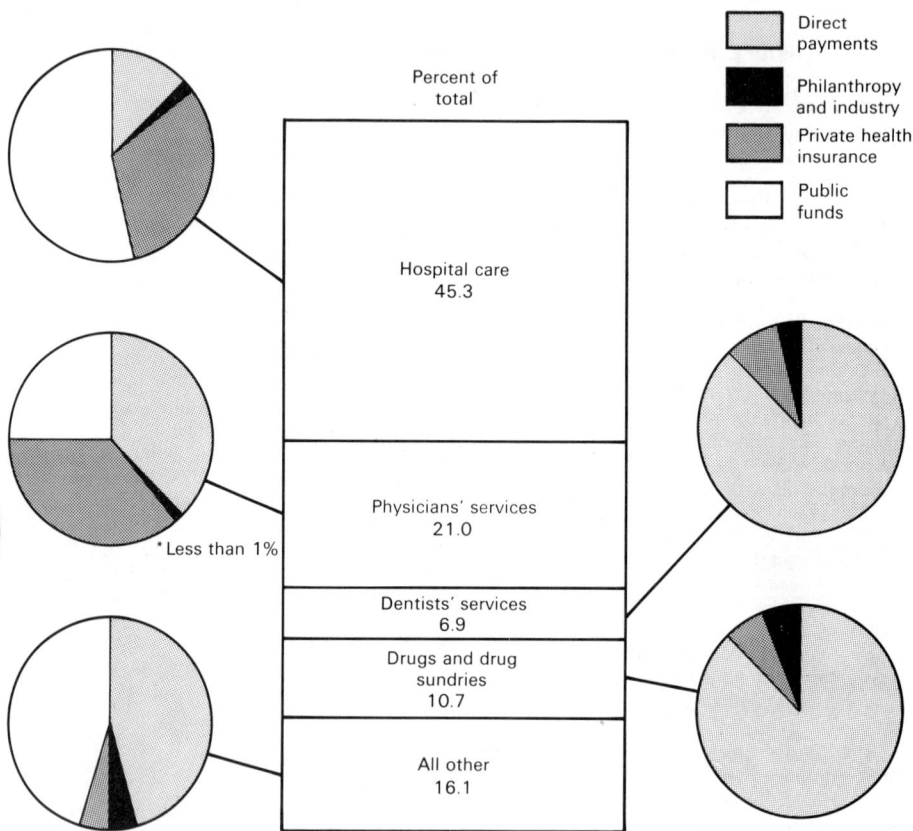

Direct payments

Philanthropy and industry

Private health insurance

Public funds

Percent of total

Hospital care
45.3

Physicians' services
21.0

Dentists' services
6.9

Drugs and drug sundries
10.7

All other
16.1

*Less than 1%

Source: U.S. Social Security Administration, 1976.

Licensing and Accreditation*

Although each state (except Ohio, which does not license general hospitals) requires that hospitals be licensed in order to operate, the requirements and standards for licensure vary considerably from state to state. State agencies—in most states, the health department—have the responsibility for the licensing of these facilities.

Accreditation standards, unlike licensure, do not vary by state; participation in the accreditation program is purely voluntary on the part

of the hospital. Hospital accreditation by the Joint Commission on the Accreditation of Hospitals (JCAH) may be granted for one or two years, or it may be withheld if the hospital does not meet specific standards. At the end of the accreditation period, the hospital requests a resurvey to redetermine its accreditation status. A hospital that has been refused accreditation may apply for another survey to determine its accreditation status, usually after six months have elapsed since the initial survey. As of January 1975, approximately 5,000 hospitals in the United States were accredited by the Hospital Accreditation Program

*Source: DHEW, 1976.

of the Joint Commission on Accreditation of Hospitals. The remaining hospitals either failed to apply or were rejected for accreditation.

Another accreditation program of JCAH, the Accreditation Council for Psychiatric Facilities, was formed in 1970. As of January 1975, approximately 425 psychiatric facilities were listed as being accredited.

Hospital Data

Number of Hospitals by State

Table 20-1   Distribution of hospitals by state, 1973

State	Total hospitals	General medical and surgical	State	Total hospitals	General medical and surgical
United States	7,438	6,458	Missouri	179	160
Alabama	151	138	Montana	69	67
Alaska	26	25	Nebraska	116	111
Arizona	83	79	Nevada	27	25
Arkansas	104	101	New Hampshire	35	32
California	655	583	New Jersey	143	111
Colorado	101	87	New Mexico	64	56
Connecticut	69	47	New York	419	333
Delaware	14	9	North Carolina	168	143
District of Columbia	21	16	North Dakota	61	60
Florida	234	214	Ohio	253	214
Georgia	200	178	Oklahoma	153	142
Hawaii	31	23	Oregon	88	80
Idaho	51	48	Pennsylvania	327	254
Illinois	297	255	Rhode Island	22	17
Indiana	136	117	South Carolina	94	84
Iowa	153	143	South Dakota	71	68
Kansas	169	158	Tennessee	175	149
Kentucky	133	116	Texas	583	531
Louisiana	165	151	Utah	42	39
Maine	59	55	Vermont	20	18
Maryland	80	55	Virginia	134	110
Massachusetts	211	136	Washington	134	121
Michigan	265	232	West Virginia	91	80
Minnesota	193	179	Wisconsin	206	153
Mississippi	132	126	Wyoming	31	29

Source: DHEW, 1976.

Hospital Expenditures*

In 1975, for the ninth consecutive year, total hospital expenditures increased at an annual rate of more than 10% (see Table 20-2). Total expenditures were $48.7 billion—17.6% higher than in 1974.** This represented the largest one-year increase of the decade from 1965 to 1975.

*Source: *Hospital Statistics, 1976 Edition.* Reprinted by permission of American Hospital Association, 1975 Annual Survey.

**Note: In 1975 hospitals received 45.3% of all health care expenditures. Physicians received only 21%.

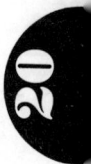

356

Table 20-2 Hospital expenditures and the gross national product, 1965–75

Year	GNP Amount (in billions)	GNP Percent change from previous year	Hospital expenditures Amount (in millions)	Hospital expenditures Percent change from previous year	Percentage of GNP
1965	$ 688.1	8.24	$12,948	7.62	1.88
1966	753.0	9.43	14,198	9.65	1.89
1967	796.3	5.75	16,395	15.47	2.06
1968	868.5	9.07	19,061	16.26	2.19
1969	935.5	7.71	22,103	15.96	2.36
1970	982.4	5.01	25,556	15.62	2.60
1971	1,063.4	8.25	28,812	12.74	2.71
1972	1,171.1	10.13	32,667	13.38	2.79
1973	1,306.3	11.54	36,290	11.09	2.78
1974	1,406.9	7.70	41,406	14.10	2.94
1975	1,498.9	6.54	48,706	17.63	3.25

Of the $6.3 billion increase in community hospital expenditures in 1975, $2.8 billion, or 43.8%, was attributable to inflation. Next in importance were nonpayroll expenses ($1.9 billion) and payroll expenses ($1.2 billion). Population growth ($0.2 billion) and utilization ($0.2 billion) had the least impact.

Over the ten-year period from 1965 to 1975, community hospital expenditures increased by $29.8 billion.

Adjusted expenses per inpatient day in community hospitals increased by 17.8% in 1975 to $133.81. This was larger than any one-year increase in the previous ten years.

Community Hospital Statistics*

The average cost to community hospitals to treat a person in 1975 amounted to $151.20 per patient day, an 87% increase since 1970. On a state-by-state basis the average cost per day in 1975 varied considerably, from a low of $98.50 in North and South Dakota to a high of $225.50 in Alaska.

In 1975, the average length of time a patient remained in a community hospital was 7.7 days compared with 8.2 days in 1970. In recent years there has been a steady decline in average hospital stays, due to more sophisticated medical techniques and increased number of persons convalescing at home.

Although the length of the average hospital stay declined over the five-year period, the cost

*Source: *Source Book of Health Insurance Data,* Health Insurance Institute.

for the average stay went up, climbing 75% to reach $1,164.20 per patient.

The average length of stay varied by area, from a low of 5.0 days in Alaska, to a high of 9.9 days in New York. Some factors that contribute to the substantial variations in length of stay are the incidence of different diseases, age distribution of the population, income levels and postponement of elective admissions.

A 1972 National Center for Health Statistics survey of Short-Stay Hospital Utilization reported the average length of stay was 8.3 days for males and 7.4 days for females. Length of stay increased with age from 4.5 days for children under 15 to 12.2 days for persons 65 and over.

Total operating costs of community hospitals increased to $39.0 billion in 1975, nearly two times the $19.6 billion in 1970.

The American Hospital Association reports that much of the increase in hospital operating costs was due to the continued rise in wages paid to hospital personnel, as such wages moved toward parity with other wage scales in the community. The 1975 payroll for hospitals amounted to $20.7 billion, almost double the $11.4 billion total in 1970. Additional expenditures for improvement in services and facilities also contributed to increases in hospital costs.

Hospital Construction

Since 1958 nearly $12 billion has been spent nationally on hospital construction and modernization of which approximately $3.6 billion came from the federal government.

Table 20-3 Community hospital statistics, by state—1975

State	Average cost to hospital per patient day	Average length of hospital stay (days)	Average cost to hospital per patient stay
Alabama	$113.90	7.3	$ 831.50
Alaska	225.50	5.0	1,127.50
Arizona	175.20	7.4	1,296.50
Arkansas	102.20	6.5	664.30
California	217.40	6.6	1,434.80
Colorado	148.90	6.6	982.70
Connecticut	188.60	7.5	1,414.50
Delaware	162.70	8.3	1,350.40
D.C.	207.60	7.9	1,640.00
Florida	151.10	7.4	1,118.10
Georgia	138.90	6.4	889.00
Hawaii	152.10	6.9	1,049.50
Idaho	121.50	6.3	765.50
Illinois	160.10	8.0	1,280.80
Indiana	127.10	7.9	1,004.10
Iowa	109.80	7.8	856.40
Kansas	113.00	7.8	881.40
Kentucky	109.70	7.1	778.90
Louisiana	136.80	6.5	889.20
Maine	137.50	7.4	1,017.50
Maryland	181.00	8.3	1,502.30
Massachusetts	205.30	8.5	1,745.05
Michigan	166.10	8.2	1,362.00
Minnesota	121.90	8.8	1,072.70
Mississippi	102.20	6.9	705.20
Missouri	129.10	8.2	1,058.60
Montana	111.10	6.4	711.00
Nebraska	116.70	8.1	945.30
Nevada	182.50	6.5	1,186.30
New Hampshire	129.50	7.1	919.50
New Jersey	142.40	8.7	1,238.90
New Mexico	142.20	5.9	839.00
New York	189.40	9.9	1,875.10
North Carolina	114.80	7.6	872.50
North Dakota	98.50	8.3	817.60
Ohio	139.00	8.2	1,139.80
Oklahoma	128.60	6.7	861.60
Oregon	158.80	6.3	1,000.40
Pennsylvania	142.80	8.5	1,213.80
Rhode Island	188.20	8.0	1,505.60
South Carolina	113.80	7.3	830.70
South Dakota	98.50	7.0	689.50
Tennessee	113.80	7.5	853.50
Texas	128.80	6.8	875.80
Utah	148.20	5.6	829.90
Vermont	131.10	7.8	1,022.60
Virginia	122.40	8.0	979.20
Washington	171.60	5.6	961.00
West Virginia	109.50	7.6	832.20
Wisconsin	127.70	8.2	1,047.10
Wyoming	116.90	5.5	643.00
United States	$151.20	7.7	$1,164.20

Source: Health Insurance Institute.

Despite a shifting emphasis in recent years from construction and expansion to modernization of existing facilities, current expenditures are approximately $4 billion annually and will probably reach $5 billion by 1980.[*]

The construction of hospitals has been largely a matter of local initiative by either voluntary bodies or units of state or local government, as suggested above. The mental and tuberculosis facilities, built mainly by state governments, followed plans developed by each of the 50 states to meet the estimated requirements, and the same was true of the federal hospitals serving mariners, veterans, or American Indians. General hospitals open to the average person, however, have been constructed in the past on the basis of local recognition of needs without any overall planning.

This policy was partially changed in 1946 with the enactment of the National Hospital Survey and Construction Act and later the Hill-Burton program. These laws provided, for the first time, federal grants to help finance the construction of local hospitals (either voluntary or government), but these grants were conditional on a "master plan for hospitals" being developed by the state government. In accordance with this state plan, hospitals in areas of greatest hospital bed deficiency (in relation to a stipulated standard of 4.5 general beds per 1000 population) received priority rating for construction subsidy. This policy helped to raise the number of hospital beds in areas of shortage, but over the last 20 years only about one-fourth of the new beds established have been provided under this subsidy program. The other beds have been provided entirely through local initiative.[**]

The basic goal of the federal program (the Hill-Burton program)—to improve the supply of health facilities in shortage areas—has been largely accomplished. Hill-Burton program expenditures have declined from 13% of the total $1.5 billion national medical facility construction expenditures in 1963 to 2.4% of the total estimated $4.6 billion construction expenditures in 1975. The vast majority of medical facility construction is now financed through long-term debt service of loans from the private capital markets.

---

[*] Source: *Issues in National Financing of Health,* House Report, November 1976.
[**] Source: World Health Organization, *Public Health and Population Statistics.*

Organization of the Hospital

Types of Hospitals*

Hospitals have been classified in many different ways. The most commonly accepted classifications, however, are those based on the types of patients treated (clinical) or on the type of ownership and control (government or nongovernment). Clinical hospitals include the general ones that treat a variety of illnesses and special ones that treat only one or several types of illnesses. Included in special hospitals are psychiatric, tuberculosis, pediatric, and maternity hospitals, as well as those in which catastrophic diseases are treated.

The classification of hospitals based on ownership and control means that either they are supported by the government or they are not. Under the government category are the federal hospitals such as the military hospitals, the Veterans Administration hospitals, and the United States Public Health Service hospitals. Other types of government hospitals are those run by the state, county, or city. All government hospitals are supported by tax funds and may be general or special.

Nongovernment hospitals vary in ownership and control. Church hospitals are owned by one of the church organizations. Catholic hospitals are usually under the organization of the Order, whereas in non-Catholic hospitals there is usually a separate governing body. Fraternal hospitals are owned by a fraternal order. The largest group of nongovernmental hospitals are called community hospitals because they are owned and maintained by the community, although they are incorporated under a separate charter. The governing board is representative of the community and relates the community needs and requirements to the hospital. These community hospitals are often spoken of as voluntary institutions, in contrast to government hospitals.

Many hospitals are privately owned and operated for profit and are called "for-profit" or proprietary instruments. They are owned either by a small, closed group or by corporations with stockholders. Many proprietary hospitals belong to large corporation chains.

---

*Source: From Sloane, Robert M., and Sloane, Beverly LeBov: *A Guide to Health Facilities,* 2nd ed., St. Louis, 1977, The C. V. Mosby Co.

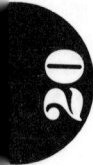

Hospital types

General hospital	(General medical and surgical) hospital.
	Short-stay hospital.
	Short-term (care) hospital.
Specialty hospital	Alcoholism hospital.
	Chronic disease hospital.
	Epileptic hospital.
	Eye, ear, nose, and throat (or, EENT) hospital.
	Long-stay hospital.
	Long-term (care) hospital.
	Maternity hospital.
	Narcotic hospital.
	Orthopedic hospital.
	(Physical) rehabilitation hospital.
	Psychiatric hospital.
	Tuberculosis (or TB) hospital.

The Hospital Governing Board

The policy-making responsibility for the operation and maintenance of a health facility lies with the governing council or board of directors. Board members are chosen for their ability as leaders within representative segments of the community and for their willingness to contribute their services. Outside of the traditional officer positions, the number of additional board members varies. The work of the governing body involves review and approval of major plans, programs and institutional policies; selection of the chief hospital administrator; appointment of medical staff members; evaluation of the hospital's efficiency; and alignment of the facility's health services with community need.

Administration

The chief administrator implements the policies established by the governing board, develops procedures and directs the day-to-day operations of the hospital. His administration coordinates the delivery of services to patients through supervising the organization of the health care team, the provision of equipment, the maintenance of a suitable environment and the operation of an efficient plant. The administrator is directly accountable to the governing board.

Hospital Organization—Departments

Figure 20-2   Prototype hospital organization chart

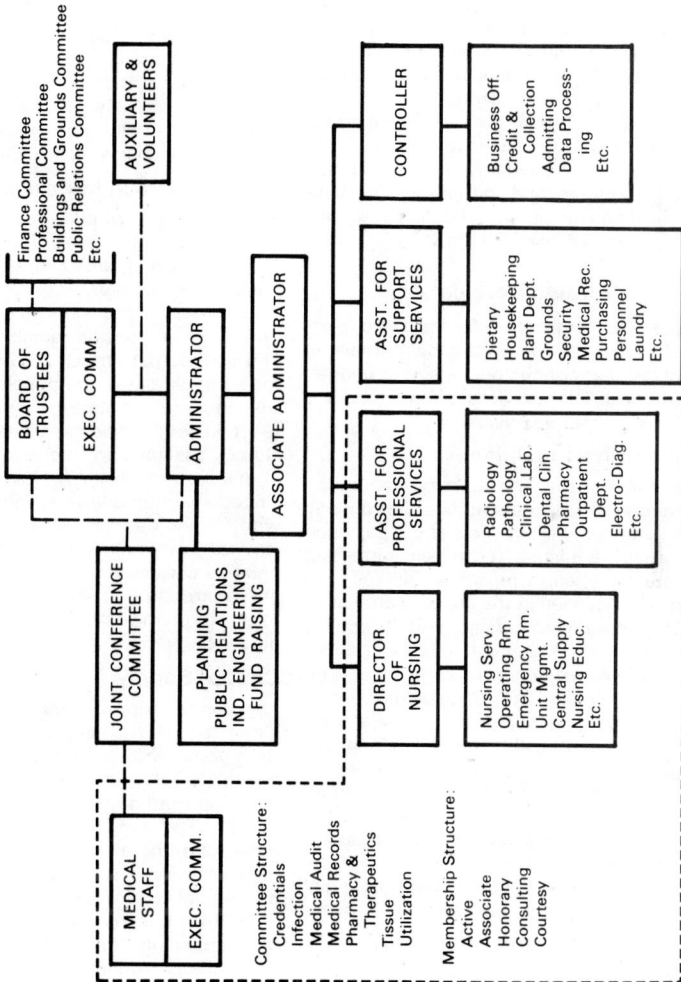

BOARD OF TRUSTEES

Finance Committee
Professional Committee
Buildings and Grounds Committee
Public Relations Committee
Etc.

EXEC. COMM.

AUXILIARY & VOLUNTEERS

ADMINISTRATOR

ASSOCIATE ADMINISTRATOR

JOINT CONFERENCE COMMITTEE

PLANNING
PUBLIC RELATIONS
IND. ENGINEERING
FUND RAISING

MEDICAL STAFF

EXEC. COMM.

Committee Structure:
Credentials
Infection
Medical Audit
Medical Records
Pharmacy & Therapeutics
Tissue
Utilization

Membership Structure:
Active
Associate
Honorary
Consulting
Courtesy

DIRECTOR OF NURSING

Nursing Serv.
Operating Rm.
Emergency Rm.
Unit Mgmt.
Central Supply
Nursing Educ.
Etc.

ASST. FOR PROFESSIONAL SERVICES

Radiology
Pathology
Clinical Lab.
Dental Clin.
Pharmacy
Outpatient Dept.
Electro-Diag.
Etc.

ASST. FOR SUPPORT SERVICES

Dietary
Housekeeping
Plant Dept.
Grounds
Security
Medical Rec.
Purchasing
Personnel
Laundry
Etc.

CONTROLLER

Business Off.
Credit & Collection
Admitting
Data Processing
Etc.

Source: "A Primer for Hospital Trustees," Chamber of Commerce of the United States, 1974.

20

Medical Staff

Appointment to a hospital medical staff is made by the governing body upon recommendation from the existing medical staff whose bylaws have defined requirements and the mechanism for selection. Most of the patient care in a hospital is delivered by physicians entitled "active staff members;" they have the privilege of voting, holding office and planning medical policy in alliance with the governing board and administrator, in addition to participating in the hospital's educational program. Other categories of staff membership include the associate level, a prior level for those who may achieve active member status, consulting, honorary and courtesy levels. There may be further distinctions in larger institutions according to specific service areas.

Nursing Service*

In almost every health care facility, the department of nursing is the largest department in terms of numbers of personnel, size of budget, types of specialized services offered, and variety of health workers utilized.

Administrative Personnel

The standards of the Joint Commission on the Accreditation of Hospitals require that nursing service be under the direction of a legally and professionally qualified, registered nurse and that there be enough registered nurses who are currently licensed in the state on duty at all times to give patients nursing care. It requires that, using their judgment and specialized skills, they plan, assign, supervise, and evaluate the nursing care of patients. Almost every nursing service has an administrative head who is responsible for organizing the nursing service. In a large institution she may employ other administrative nurses who function in a line relationship subordinate to her, such as associate directors of nursing, supervisors of various departments within the department of nursing, head nurses, assistant head nurses and charge nurses.

Nursing Service in the Outpatient Department

In an outpatient department a clinic is a subdivision in which a single disease or closely allied diseases are diagnosed and treated. For example, an outpatient department may have clinics specializing in cardiac, dental, dermatologic, gynecologic, neurologic, and psychiatric problems. In highly specialized outpatient departments, there may be a number of medical clinics dealing with specific medical problems, such as diabetes, arthritis, hematology, metabolism, and allergies. Regardless of the kind of outpatient department or clinic, daily nursing services are essential. Nursing personnel are usually responsible for the physical environment, such as keeping an adequate amount of supplies available in individual examining rooms to carry on the daily work scheduled there.

Nursing Care in Intensive Care Units

The intensive care unit provides a specialized, highly controlled environment designed to offer life-saving and life-sustaining supplies, equipment, and personnel resources. Emphasis is placed on the presence of professional nurses with specific qualifications, training, and staffing pattern. Often there is a necessity for a one-nurse-to-one-patient ratio to provide the necessary minute-by-minute observation, reaction, and response-and-action processes. Nurses assigned to intensive care units carry immense responsibility for patient welfare, since they often deal in an independent fashion with life and death matters. In the larger health centers, one is likely to find such special care units as coronary care, burn care, cardiac surgery care and artificial kidney care units, respiratory and stroke centers, and special nurseries.

Central Supply

The central supply department ... dispenses clean or sterile equipment and supplies throughout the nursing department. In some health care facilities, it services and receives direction from departments other than nursing service. The supervisor may be a registered nurse, but there is a distinct trend to utilize nonprofessional supervisory, clerical, and departmental employees.

In order to carry out their essential function of maintaining adequate supplies and equipment, the personnel order and store a vast array of supplies, clean, prepare, and sterilize equipment as needed, and repair and replace equipment. Increasing use of disposable items for providing patient care is changing the manner in which central supply rooms are staffed and the kind of work carried on by the employees.

*Source: From Sloane, Robert M., and Sloane, Beverly LeBov: *A Guide to Health Facilities,* 2nd ed., St. Louis, 1977, The C. V. Mosby Co.

The Health Care Team

Table 20-4   Characteristics of health care team members

Profession	Total length of professional training beyond H.S.	Basic curriculum structure	Indicator of academic achievement	Certifying bodies	Geographical location of training	Basic skills
Dietitian	5 yr	4 yr academic training 1 yr dietetic internship	B.S.—Foods and nutrition certificate for internship completion	American Dietetic Assn. (ADA)—registry exam (trend toward state licensure)	University setting Hospital, nursing homes, etc.	1 Determination of appropriate diet content for treatment of specific diseases 2 Source of information and advice to physicians
Inhalation therapy or respiratory therapy	Usually 2 yr, one summer	1st yr: 70-80% didactic training; 20-30% clinical training 2nd yr: 70-80% clinical training; 20-30% didactic training	Associate degree, inhalation therapy	American Assn. of Inhalation Therapists (AAIT)—registry board AMA-AAIT—review and approval of schools, state and local educational rules and regulations	Vocational technical school Hospital	1 Performs selected tests used in diagnosis of pulmonary diseases 2 Performs selected treatments for patients having pulmonary diseases
Laboratory assistant	12 mo	20% didactic training 80% clinical experience in affiliated lab	Diploma and certification	Amer. Society of Clinical Pathologists (ASCP) Amer. Medical Tech. Assoc. State and local educational rules and regulations	Vocational technical school Hospital	1 ECG techniques 2 Hematology 3 Urinalysis 4 Bacteriology 5 Serology 6 Chemistry
Medical technologist	4 yr	3 yr (90 credits) (basic sciences, liberal arts, etc.) 1 yr: 60% didactic training. 40% clinical experience in lab. (includes 3 mo. internship)	B.S. in med. technology Certificate upon completion of internship	AMA ASCP University approval	University setting Hospital affiliated lab.	Laboratory practice and theory: Chemistry Immunology Bacteriology Hematology

(continued)

20

Table 20-4 (continued)

Profession	Total length of professional training beyond H.S.	Basic curriculum structure	Indicator of academic achievement	Certifying bodies	Geographical location of training	Basic skills
Occupational therapy	4 yr 10 mo	4 yr academic (liberal arts and professional subjects)—some "preclinical" experience, 10 mo. clinical experience	B.S. occupational therapy Certificate for completion of clinical experience (trend toward master's degree in O.T.)	Americ. Occ. Therapy Assn. AMA—university approval	University setting Hospital	Manual arts and crafts, practice in functional prevocational and homemaking skills and activities of daily living. Sensorimotor, educational, recreational and social activities for patients
Pharmacy technician	1 mo	On-the-job training under supervision of trained technician and pharmacist	None	None	Hospital	1 Drug dispensation 2 Preparation of selected drugs 3 Maintenance of records
Pharmacist-B.S.	5 yr plus usually 1 yr internship	1st 2 yr: liberal arts; 3rd thru 5th yr: professional courses & basic sciences	B.S. pharmacy	University standards & state licensure	University setting	1 Knowledge of drug action & human physiology 2 Responsibility for drug dispensing 3 Source of information to physician, nurse, patient
Doctor of Pharmacy (Referred to as Pharm D.)	6 yr plus 1 yr internship	3rd thru 6th yr: professional courses	Doctor of Pharmacy	University standards and state licensure	University setting	Same as B.S. but more depth
Pharmacist-M.S. hospital pharmacy or Pharm. D.	2-3 yr beyond B.S.	1 yr academic 1 yr residency or combination of the above in 2-3 yrs.	M.S. hospital pharmacy or Doctor of Pharmacy	University standards and state licensure	University setting Hospital	1 More highly developed understanding of clinical implication of drug use or 2 Improved development of management skills in hospital pharmacy

Occupation	Length of training	Type of training	Degree	Standards	Certifying agency	Setting	Functions
Physical therapist	4-6 yr: 4 mo. internship	4 yr academic 4 mo clinical experience	B.S., physical therapy	University standards	Amer. Registry of Physical Therapists (certification) AMA	University setting; Certificate for completion of clinical experience	Therapy programs for patients involving physical means, e.g., exercise, heat, massage
Radiological (x-ray) technician	24 concurrent months 1 New trends: 4 yr programs leading to B.S. in radiological technology 2 2 yr training programs in vocational technical schools	Combinations of didactic training (physics, electronics, etc.) and clinical experience: 1/8 didactic training; 7/8 clinical experience	Certificate from hospital		Amer. Registry of Radiological Technologists (ARRT) AMA Amer. College of Radiologists	Hospital	Performance of radiographic examination
Social worker, B.S.	4 yr	4 yr didactic training—small amount of "field" experience	B.S., social work	University standards		University; Selected agencies	1 Knowledge of human behavior (small groups and organizational life) 2 Structure and function of community agencies 3 Understanding of development of social policy 4 Planning and evaluation of treatment using above knowledge (casework, group work, and community organizations)
Social worker, M.S.	1 to 2 yr beyond B.S.	Didactic training 50%: clinical experience 50%	M.S., social work	University standards		University; hospital or health agency	1 More depth knowledge practitioners 2 Supervisor of social work practitioners

20

Source: *Medical Care Chart Book*, 5th ed., Department of Medical Care Organization, School of Public Health, University of Michigan, Ann Arbor, 1972.

Patient Services

Admitting Department

Patients are admitted to hospitals upon the recommendation of their physician. The initial procedure is the accumulation of data by the admitting department staff: patient health information to be used by the medical care team and health insurance information or other financial statements to confirm credit arrangements. Assignments are then made for specific bed space and storage of valuables. During the patient's stay, the admitting department coordinates arrangements with the medical and nursing staff, operating room, if necessary, records department and business office.

At the end of a patient's stay, the admitting department arranges for the patient's proper disposition—discharge, transfer or post-mortem procedures. The department is also in charge of releasing patient information to authorized persons.

Medical Records

All clinical background and information, staff observations and data on the progression of a patient's illness are noted on separate records for each and every person receiving medical care in the hospital. This medical document is kept for an amount of time not less than the Statute of Limitations of the state in which the hospital is located. The Joint Commission on the Accreditation of Hospitals established that the following information should be contained in each medical record: identification data, complaint, present illness, past history, family history, physical examination, provisional diagnosis, clinical laboratory reports, x-ray reports, consultations, medical and surgical treatment, tissue report, progress notes, final diagnosis, discharge summary and autopsy findings.

Radiology*

A department of radiology is involved in the use of ionizing radiation for the treatment of disease, radioactive isotopes for both the diagnosis and treatment of disease, and fluoroscopic and radiographic x-ray equipment in the diagnosis of disease. The medical staff of a department of radiology is made up of physicians who have specialized in the use of radiant energy, radioactive isotopes, radium, cesium, and cobalt. A radiation therapist is a radiologist who has specialized basically in the use of radium, cobalt, and high voltage x-ray equipment

for the purpose of treating disease, particularly cancer and various types of tumors. A radiologist is a physician who is qualified in the use of x-ray, radium and radioactive materials for the treatment and diagnosis of disease. A diagnostic roentgenologist is one who is qualified in the use of x-ray films only for diagnostic purposes.

Electrocardiography*

The department of electrocardiography is another highly specialized department in the diagnostic service of the health facility. The electrocardiograph (also known as ECG, or EKG) records the electric current produced by the contraction of the heart muscle and is used to help diagnose heart disease or record the progress of patients with heart disease. A vectorcardiograph, which provides a graphic record of the magnitude and direction of the electrical forces of the heart, and a phonocardiograph, which aids in diagnosis by showing heart sounds, are also used.

Basically under the direction of a physician, the ECG technician contacts the patient, sets up the machine, and obtains the graphic results.

Occupational Therapy*

Occupational therapy is designed to help the patient, through the use of selected activities, to become as independently active as possible within the limitations of his physical, mental, or emotional problems. The occupational therapist works in collaboration with other members of the health team to plan a therapeutic activity program for a particular patient.

Physical Therapy*

Physical medicine and rehabilitation have been developing as a service program to all medical specialties. The program should not be considered as limited to the orthopedic or paraplegic patient.

Medical rehabilitation . . . involves the entire health team: the physician, the nurse, the social worker, the physical therapist, and other closely allied personnel. The objective is either to eliminate the patient's disability or restore as fully as possible his mental, social, or physical abilities that have been impaired by

*Source: From Sloane, Robert M., and Sloane, Beverly LeBov: *A Guide to Health Facilities*, 2nd ed., St. Louis, 1977, The C. V. Mosby Co.

disease or injury. The role of the physical therapy department in rehabilitation is the use of heat, cold, water, electricity, exercise, ultrasound, and other methods in restoring useful activity.

Social Service Department

The medical social worker acts as part of the immediate health team assisting the patient in adjusting to those personal difficulties, whether emotional or environmental, brought about by his medical circumstance. Initially, observations are made of the patient's situation and ability to cope; later, the social service department acts as a liaison with the appropriate community agencies to assist the patient toward a complete recovery or rehabilitation.

Dietary Department

The dietary department supplies patients with high quality diets, suitable to their individual health needs and requirements. Hospitals should have on staff a qualified dietitian assisted by competent administrative and technical personnel. The JCAH recommends that an accurate record of diets be correlated with the medical records. When diet therapy is part of the health treatment, instruction is given to the patient.

Business Services Department

The financial principle behind any large business organization is not at all unlike that of a health care institution: incoming revenues have to be balanced against outgoing expenditures.

Budget Expenditures

Expenses for a health facility consist of departmental payroll costs and supplies, equipment maintenance, projected replacement due to depreciation, and other capital requirements. The prepared budget reflects the anticipated expenditures for the forthcoming year in comparison with the anticipated revenue. The revenue, derived from pateints' fees, is flexible and may be increased by raising charges in order to meet the facility's operating expenses.

Credit and Collection

Around 60% of the health care revenue is supplied by third party payments from the government and private health insurance companies. The balance has to be collected from private individuals who frequently are financially unprepared to meet the high medical expenses of a sudden illness, accident or operation. To help the patient meet his obligations, the credit and collection department helps work out a feasible payment plan after a review of the patient's specific financial circumstances. Through the extension of credit, the health facility hopes to be fully reimbursed for its services to the patient.

Plant Management and Maintenance

Personnel

Personnel departments serve an important role in answering the diverse labor needs of a health institution. In a large institution, there may be as many as 300 different types of jobs, all of which must be filled appropriately.

Purchasing Department

The function of this department is to review available information on pertinent products, research new items, make purchases and handle the supplies in stock.

Housekeeping Department

The housekeeping department is responsible for those domestic chores essential to maintain the level of cleanliness expected in a health facility: general cleaning, mopping, garbage disposal, washing of windows, walls and woodwork, for example. In addition, the department is responsible for the sanitary precautions and care necessary for the control of infection.

Laundry and Linen Department

All linens used in patient care or for other divisions within the health facility are collected, processed and distributed by this department.

Physical Plant

The smooth running of utility services and machinery is essential in a health facility, where sudden breakdowns can be disastrous. A properly trained staff's function is to assure continuing operation by checking, repairing and maintaining the plant's equipment.

20

The Emergency Department
AMA Recommendations for a General Hospital Emergency Service*

Emergency Department—*Essential Staff:* The emergency department shall be staffed by a physician on-call from in-house 24 hours a day, and in addition, a registered nurse supported by other allied health personnel, all with special training in emergency lifesaving procedures.

Essential Capabilities and Equipment: The emergency department shall have a capability adequate for the care of all direct admissions. It is essential that the department be equipped with airway control and ventilation equipment, suction devices, electrocardiograph-defibrillator, apparatus to establish central venous pressure monitoring, surgical and intravenous administration sets, emergency resuscitative intravenous fluids, gastric lavage equipment, and emergency drugs and supplies.

Hospital—*Essential Staff:* The hospital staff shall be available 24 hours each day. A physician shall be on-call from in-house 24 hours a day. He shall be trained in emergency lifesaving procedures.

Blood Bank: Blood storage shall be in-hospital and contain conventional types of blood for immediate needs. In addition, there shall be ready access to a supplemental supply.

Laboratory Services: The laboratory service shall be capable of performing analyses of blood gases, pH, and electrolyte determinations, and staffed by a technician in-hospital or on-call 24 hours a day from outside the hospital.

Radiological Services: Radiological service, utilizing either fixed or mobile equipment as needed, shall be staffed by qualified personnel in-house or on-call 24 hours a day from outside the hospital.

Operating Room(s): The operating room(s) staffed by operating room personnel, including an anesthesiologist or experienced nurse anesthetist, shall be readily available from in-house or on-call from outside the hospital at all hours for emergency surgical procedures.

Postoperative Recovery Unit(s): The postoperative recovery unit shall be in or adjacent to the operating suite and staffed by trained personnel when the unit has patients. Other

special care areas may be utilized at other times.

Intensive Care Units: The intensive care units for surgical and medical patients shall have adequate monitoring and therapeutic equipment and be staffed at all hours by specially trained personnel.

Communications Equipment: Communications equipment shall be available and operating for in-hospital coordination. In addition, direct two-way radio service available between hospital, ambulances, and other appropriate emergency service personnel is required.

Reasons for Increased Use of Hospital Emergency Departments**

A. *Population Factors:* (sociomedical, socioeconomic, and demographic)

1. population increase of about two per cent per annum,
2. the aging of the population,
3. increasing prevalence of chronic diseases,
4. the rise in accident rates,
5. large concentrations of low income groups in metropolitan areas with few physicians,
6. inability to afford private medical care,
7. the high level of geographic mobility with substantial numbers of patients without a regular family doctor,
8. persons who are no longer housebound and can visit a hospital outpatient facility for minor conditions previously treated at home.

B. *The Physician Factors:* (availability and accessibility of primary care)

1. the decrease in the number of general practitioners who function as the primary care physician of first contact,
2. private physicians are leaving the inner-city areas by relocation or death and are not being replaced,
3. physicians are increasingly unavailable at night or on weekends or holidays,
4. physicians are reluctant to make house calls,
5. patients often do not like to incon-

---

*Source: *Categorization of Hospital Emergency Capabilities,* American Medical Association, 1971.

**Source: M. L. Webb, M.D., D.P.H., "The Emergency Medical Care System in a Metropolitan Area." (A study of Baltimore emergency services, 1969 thesis for doctorate in public health at the Johns Hopkins University School of Hygiene and Public Health.)

venience their private physician outside of office hours,
6. increasing physician specialization has resulted in:
   the patient not knowing which specialist to call, arrangement of office hours by appointment only, physician unwillingness to accept responsibility for a patient's problem outside his field of interest,
7. the independent capacity of the physician to treat emergency conditions optimally in his office may well have decreased with the increase in medical science and technology.

C. *Institutional Factors:* (the institutionalization of medical care in hospitals)
1. the role of the hospital in medical care has changed from the last resort of the dying to the workshop of the physician for all serious sickness to the functional community health center,
2. the availability of complex and costly equipment operated by highly skilled personnel,
3. physician acceptance of the emergency facility as a place, preferable to his office, for treatment of the injured and acute illnesses and, at times, nonacute conditions,
4. increased public awareness, expectations, and confidence in the hospital as an appropriate place to seek care,
5. informal, nonappointment, casual

medical care has been relinquished to the hospital,
6. availability of round-the-clock medical care at the hospital which is often legally required to provide it,
7. accessibility of hospitals to the highly concentrated urban population.

D. *External Factors:*
1. a number of health insurance plans extend benefits for services rendered in emergency departments but not for those rendered on office visits or house calls,
2. the growing tendency for industries, schools, and police to refer patients to the emergency facility,
3. an increasing sophistication of the public concerning symptoms and the immediacy with which they should be treated by a physician,
4. the absence of effective "triage" or screening at the various entry points to the emergency medical system so that many nonurgent patients are entering.

Emergency Department Utilization

About 196 million outpatient visits were made to community hospitals in 1975 of which 69 million (34.5%) were to the emergency department. In 1955 only 15 million visits were made to the emergency departments of all hospitals as compared to 73 million in 1975—almost a 500% increase.

Table 20-5   Emergency department utilization—outpatient visits

	Emergency	Clinic	Referred	Total
U.S. hospitals				
Total 1975	73,448,051	94,190,865	87,205,427	254,844,343
Non-federal short-term general hospitals and other special hospitals				
1975				
No. of outpatient visits	69,242,557	55,394,725	71,673,754	196,311,036
% of outpatient visits	35.3%	28.2%	36.5%	100%
1974				
No. of outpatient visits	67,056,890	59,761,704	68,019,720	194,838,314
% of outpatient visits	34.5%	30.7%	34.8%	100%

Source: Data based upon *Hospital Statistics,* 1975 and 1976 Editions. Reprinted by permission of the American Hospital Association.

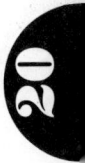

A U.S. Public Health Survey in 1971 found that the nation's hospitals have neither the physical facilities, the equipment, the trained personnel, nor the organization to cope with the tremendous increase in the emergency patient load of recent years.

- Only 12% of 727 hospitals surveyed had a physician present in the hospital 24 hours a day.
- Only about 17% had x-ray and laboratory services available around-the-clock.
- Less than 20% had a plan for the training and orientation of staff responsible for making initial contacts with emergency patients.

Only 15% of the hospital administrators believed their emergency departments were adequate in terms of space, traffic flow, and location.

The Emergency Room Nurse and the Law *

CPR—The Joint Commission on the Accreditation of Hospitals says all emergency department personnel should be trained to perform CPR (cardio-pulmonary resuscitation). All enlightened emergency medical technician training courses require first aid, ambulance and rescue squad personnel to be capable of performing CPR. Many police and fire departments require CPR training for their people.

Acute Cardiac Care—Although the ICU/CCU nurse possesses a high degree of cardiology training and skill, he or she still does not institute action until the physician has been summoned.

The same procedure is applicable to the emergency department situation. Although the emergency department nurse is capable of diagnosing and treating cardiac emergencies, such as ventricular tachycardia or fibrillation, the physician should always be called before a standing order procedure for dealing with the acute cardiac problem is instituted. With a standing order procedure for dealing with this problem, the implementation of acute cardiac or other intensive care activities is appropriate and can be assumed to be authorized nursing

---

*Source: This article was written by James E. George, M.D., J.D., and first published in the *Emergency Nurse Legal Bulletin,* copyright 1975, 1976, 1977 by Med/Law Publishers, Inc., P.O. Box 293, Westville, New Jersey 08093 all rights reserved.

procedure for the properly trained emergency department nurse.

Intravenous Procedures—As the use of intravenous infusion increased and it became impossible for physicians to perform the volume of procedures required . . . the nurse became involved in this activity. Today, in view of customary medical and nursing practice, and the opinions such as that of the New York attorney general, it is clear that intravenous infusion and the administration of intravenous medications are within the scope of emergency nursing activities.

The emergency department nurse, of course, must be qualified to take on this added responsibility and must know the mechanics of starting and maintaining an open intravenous line as well as how various intravenous medications are administered, and the possible complications associated with the use of the various medications.

Suturing and Other Wound Treatment—After a wound (e.g. laceration, puncture, abrasion, etc.) has been inspected by the emergency physician, it is appropriate for the trained emergency department nurse to locally anesthetize and cleanse the wound. Regional blocks (e.g., digital metacarpal, etc.) should be performed by the emergency physician. Whether an emergency department nurse should suture a laceration depends on size, location, and characteristics. Since hand lacerations are a constant source of litigation for emergency physicians, due to undiagnosed tendon and nerve injuries, these should not be sutured by the emergency department nurse. Also, lacerations which require reconstruction and layer closure should be performed by the emergency physician.

Puncture wounds and abrasions with embedded foreign material may be anesthetized, debrided, and cleansed by the emergency department nurse. However, these wounds and lacerations should always be inspected, before and after, by the emergency physician for retained foreign material. This oversight is a constant source of litigation for the emergency physician. Suture and drain removal is another function which the trained emergency department nurse can feel safe in performing, provided caution and supervision are exercised. If the emergency physician first examines the healing wound and instructs the nurse to remove the sutures or drain, this activity has appropriate supervision; however, if the decision to remove sutures or drain is made by the emergency department nurse alone, the procedure has become an independent nursing function. The safest course to follow is to have the emergency physician render a clinical judgment before pursuing some action.

Applying Casts, Splints, or Dressings—The splinting of suspected fractures or dislocations in trauma cases is also an appropriate function for the emergency department nurse. These procedures are basic first aid and should be elementary skills in which the emergency department nurse is proficient. Other splinting procedures which the emergency department nurse should feel comfortable in performing include the application of plaster or other splints for minor contusions, sprains, and strains of the upper and lower extremities. These generally should be done after examination by, and on instructions of, the emergency physician.

Emergency Equipment, Supplies, and Pharmaceuticals*

The emergency equipment listed here has been found to be essential and should be kept within the department or be promptly available. The list of categories of drugs contains those frequently stocked in emergency departments and is adapted from the *Hospital Formulary* published by the American Society of Hospital Pharmacists.

Equipment—Major
Cart, orthopedic, with cast equipment
Defibrillator
Ophthalmoscope-otoscope, combination set
Oxygen, piped, with masks
Oxygen tanks with positive pressure and masks
Resuscitation equipment, positive pressure
Stretchers, recovery type with accessories**

---

*Source: *Emergency Services; The Hospital Emergency Department in an Emergency Care System,* 1972. Reprinted by permission of the American Hospital Association.

**A type of stretcher that requires the least handling of the patient is desirable. Suggested features are: a. Side rails; b. Locking conductive wheels; c. Mechanism for Fowler's or Trendelenburg position; d. Radiolucent mattress and space for x-ray cassettes beneath the mattress. The stretcher must be of sufficient height and width to fit over the existing x-ray tables; e. Provision for intravenous solution standards and small oxygen tanks if portable resuscitation equipment is not used.

Stretchers, portable
Suction apparatus, if centralized suction system is not provided
Sphygmomanometers
Wheelchairs

Equipment—Minor
Airways, including all sizes
Applicators, ENT, metal
Cap, ice, rubber
Cast cutters, manual and electric
Cot, finger, rubber
Crutches and canes
Culture tubes
Depressor, tongue, metal
Droppers
Esophageal balloon
Flashlights; bulbs; batteries
Glass, medicine
Gloves, rubber, assorted sizes
Heels, walking, assorted lengths and sizes
Lamp, alcohol
Razors, safety or reusable
Scissors, bandage
Sheets, fenestration, sterile
Splints, Thomas
Splints, other
Stethoscopes
Syringes and needles: irrigating; catheter tip; disposable; hypodermic; locking hub; insulin; tuberculin
Thermometers
Towels, surgical, sterile
Tourniquets, pneumatic
Tracheotomy tubes, including children's sizes
Tube, esophageal
Tube, Cantor
Tube, Miller Abbott
Tubes and other bottles for collecting serum for chemical analysis
Tubes, Levine and gastric lavage
Tubing, for tourniquets

Supplies
Adhesive solvent
Adhesive tape, assorted cuts
Applicators, wood, and cotton-tipped
Bandages, adhesive prepared
Bandages, elastic
Bandages, flannel
Bandages, gauze, assorted
Bandages, muslin
Bandages, plaster of paris, all sizes
Basins
Blades, surgical, sterile, assorted (handles included with sterile sets)

20

Cellulose, oxidized
Closures, butterfly
Cotton, absorbent
Cotton, balls
Drains, rubber
Dressings, pressure
Dressings, surgical
Felt
Gauze, packing, assorted
Gauze, petrolatum, sterile
Packing, all sizes, plain and petrolatum
Pads, combination
Pads, sanitary
Pharmaceuticals for emergency use
Spatulas, wooden
Splints, plaster, all sizes
Sponge, gelatin absorbable
Stockinet
Suture materials, all sizes and needle types
Syringe administration set, disposable, assorted
Venoclysis set, disposable, assorted
Venoclysis set, series hook-up, disposable
Wadding, surgical

Prepared Trays
Blood culture sets
Catheterization, male and female
Chest suction
Cutdown, venous
Endotracheal intubation set with cuffed endotracheal tubes of all sizes (including children's), laryngoscope, syringe, and adapters for delivery of positive pressure oxygen
Irrigation sets and syringes
Lumbar puncture
Paracentesis
Poison tray with a list of antidotes for specific poisons, stomach tubes, syringes, and oral airways
Scalp vein infusion
Surgical suture*
Thoracocentesis
Thoracotomy equipment for cardiac massage
Tracheotomy sets with tubes of all sizes (including children's)
Venesection
Venous pressure sets

---

*Surgical suture sets may include: a. Curved and straight hemostats, large or small; b. Needle holders, large or small; c. Forceps, rat-toothed, large or small; d. Scissors, curved and straight, large or small; e. Scalpel blades and handles, various sizes; f. Probes; g. Self-retaining retractors.

Pharmaceuticals
Examples of Selected Categories of Drugs
Antihistaminics
Autonomic drugs
Blood derivatives and plasma expanders
Blood coagulation
  Anticoagulants
  Antiheparin agents
  Hemostatics
Cardiovascular drugs
Central nervous system drugs
  Analgesics
  Anticonvulsants
  Narcotic antagonists
  Psychotherapeutic agents
  Respiratory and cerebral stimulants
  Sedatives and hypnotics
Electrolytic, caloric, and water balance
  Replacement solutions
Enzymes
Expectorants
Eye, ear, nose, and throat preparations
  Antibiotics
  Sulfonamides
  Anti-infectives
  Anti-inflammatory agents
  Local anesthetics
  Mouth washes and gargles
  Vasoconstrictors
  Unclassified agents
Gastrointestinal drugs
  Antacids and absorbents
  Antidiarrhea agents
  Cathartics
  Emetics
Heavy metal antagonists
Hormones and synthetic substitutes
Local anesthetics
Oxytocics
Serum, toxoids, and vaccines
Skin and mucous membrane preparations
Spasmolytics
Vitamins

List of Emergency Conditions
Emergency Resuscitation Measures
- Respiratory Resuscitation
- Cardiac Arrest and Cardiopulmonary Resuscitation
- Emergency Endotracheal Intubation
Control of Hemorrhage
Control of Shock
Injuries
- Intra-abdominal Injuries
- Crush Injuries
- Multiple Injuries

- Thoracic Injuries
- Craniocerebral Injuries
- Spinal Cord Injury
- Eye Injuries

Fractures

Burns

Heat Stroke

Cold Injuries

Anaphylactic Reactions

Poisoning
- Swallowed Poisons
- Inhaled Poisons
- Skin Contamination Poisons
- Injected Poisons
- Food Poisoning

Alcoholism

Drug Abuse

Psychiatric Emergency

Rape

Nursing in Disaster Conditions

The Emergency Department Nurses' Association

EDNA has been granted full accreditation by the National Accreditation Board of the American Nurses' Association. This action, announced April 14, 1976, identifies EDNA as an agent for conducting evaluation and approval not only of its own programs, such as the Scientific Assembly, but also for constituent programs, such as EDNA chapter and state meetings.

The most important benefit will be transferability of credits for continuing education activities. Nurses moving from one location or attending a meeting in one part of the country can receive credit for this activity in another part of the country, especially in states which require continuing education credits for relicensure.

Hospital Laboratories

The largest group of laboratories (outside of doctors' offices) is in the hospital setting. Hospital laboratories, with their expanded procedures and sophisticated equipment, have added an invaluable dimension to the diagnosis, prognosis, and treatment of disease.

These laboratories employ methods and precise instruments for the examination of tissues, secretions, and excretions to diagnose disease or ascertain the cause of disease. It is customary to separate the laboratory functions of the clinical laboratory and the anatomical laboratory, sometimes by having the ana-

tomical laboratory and morgue located in a different part of the facility.

The clinical laboratory performs studies on urine, blood, gastric contents, bacteria, parasites, and chemical changes in the body to aid in prognosis. The study of tissue, either with the naked eye (gross pathology) or with the microscope, distinguishes the anatomical laboratory from the clinical laboratory. Typical tests include blood chemical determinations, white blood cell count, blood grouping, hemoglobin, urinalysis, and others, all of them important in diagnosis and measuring patient progress, particularly in connection with chronic illness. Comprehensive hospital laboratory services include microbiologic testing (for diagnosis and management of infections); immunohematology (e.g., for testing transfusion and related incompatibilities); clinical physiology (medical physics—e.g., electrocardiograms, electroencephalograms); morphologic hematology (e.g., bleeding time and coagulation time determinations); immunoserology (e.g., standard blood tests for syphilis); and anatomic pathology (e.g., for examination of tissue removed in surgery).

Hospital Outpatient Services

Ancillary Department
Abortion service outpatient unit.
Burn care unit.
Cobalt therapy unit.
Dental service.
Electroencephalography department.
Extended care unit.
Genetic counseling department.
Inhalation therapy department.
Occupational therapy department.
Pathology laboratory.
Physical therapy department.
Podiatrist service.
Radioisotope facility.
Radiology department.
Radium therapy department.
Rehabilitation outpatient unit.
Renal dialysis outpatient unit.
Social work department.
Speech therapy service.

Emergency Department
Emergency care service.
Emergency (outpatient) unit.
Emergency room.

Outpatient Department
Ambulatory care department.
Outpatient care unit.

Hospital Drug Distribution*

PHASES OF HOSPITAL DRUG DISTRIBUTION

Phase I

Initiation of the Medication Order by the Physician.

The physician writes the order on the page of the patient's chart entitled "Doctor's Order Sheet"; this includes not only the medications but all orders for the individual patient.

Phase II

Obtaining the Medication Specified in the Physician's Order.

Some drugs are ordered for the individual patient from the central pharmacy, others from floor stock.

Drugs ordered for an individual patient are kept in some type of compartment labeled with the patient's name and/or room number.

Narcotics are used from a floor supply with records of those used returned to the pharmacy when the supply is exhausted.

Emergency drugs are used from floor supply and reordered as used.

Phase III

Planning for Administration of Medication—Advance.

In planning for the administration of the medication the nurse transcribes the order to the Kardex and a medicine card. In so doing, she is responsible to note whether the patient has been reported to have allergies or other conditions which contraindicate receiving the medication. She is also expected to note the dosage ordered and to check with the physician if it is outside normal limits.

The time at which medications are scheduled to be given follows the routine hours used by the individual hospital. This schedule may be adjusted when the medication is first ordered.

New medication cards are given to the team leader and then placed in the progressive card file. The team leader is responsible to remove cards for temporary holds and return them to the active file as indicated.

Medicine cards are made for all medications but stat orders may not appear on the Kardex.

Conditional medications are given on the judgment of the team leader responsible for medications.

Medicine cards are checked with the Kardex each shift.

The ward clerk makes out medicine cards and the Kardex but the registered nurse is always responsible for review of this work.

Phase IV

Actual Administration of Medication

Medicine cards for medications to be given at any hour are removed from the progressive card file and checked with the Kardex. As the nurse prepares the medication, she checks the label on the bottle of medicine with the medicine card (3 checks) and "pours" the medicine.

The medications are prepared in the medication area usually adjacent to the nursing station and carried to the patient's room by medicine tray.

At the patient's room, the patient is positively identified (by checking the Identiband, asking patient's name) and the medication is administered.

Selected medications (i.e., insulin) are checked by a second nurse.

Phase V

Recording after Administration of Medication

In the traditional system, medications were recorded on the page of "Nurse's Notes" and a few irregular medications continue to be recorded in this way.

The most common practice today is to use a page called the Medication Record on which medications given over a 4-7 day period are recorded. The name of the medication, dosage, and route are entered before administration and when the medication has been given, the nurse records the time (or checks it off) and signs her initials.

Narcotics are charted in the narcotic book when they have been given and a count of narcotics remaining in the supply is made each shift.

Additional recordings of medications given may be made for preoperative checklists, discharge, etc.

Once the medication has been given and appropriately recorded on the patient's chart, the medicine card is returned to the progressive card file in the hour slot for the next time of administration.

*Source: "A Nurse Looks at Hospital Drug Distribution Systems," E. Price, from *American Journal of Hospital Pharmacy*, March 1967, Vol. 24, pp. 104–11.

The Hospital Pharmacy

In 1976 approximately 13,000 pharmacists were employed in hospital pharmacies. Few hospitals where pharmacotherapy is of any volume are without at least one pharmacist. Approximately two-thirds of the hospitals in the United States maintain hospital pharmacies with registered pharmacists generally serving both inpatients and outpatients.

There were, in 1973, approximately 133,000 registered pharmacists in active practice, 74 schools of pharmacy in 45 states and about 21,000 students enrolled and 5,800 graduates. Licensure to practice pharmacy requires graduation from an accredited pharmacy college, completion of a one-year internship (required in most states), and passing a state board examination. Customary degrees in pharmacy normally require five years of college study, resulting in the bachelor of science in pharmacy (B.S.) or the bachelor of pharmacy (B. Pharm.).

Among the criteria set for the hospital pharmacy by the Joint Commission on the Accreditation of Hospitals are:

- There shall be a pharmacy directed by a registered pharmacist or drug room under competent supervision.
- Records shall be kept of the transactions of the pharmacy and correlated with other hospital records where indicated. Such special records shall be kept as are required by law.
- Drugs dispensed shall meet the standards established by the United States Pharmacopeia, National Formulary, or New and Non-official Drugs.
- Policies must be established to control the administration of toxic or dangerous drugs with specific reference to the duration of the order and the dosage.

The previous page outlines the phases of a hospital's drug distribution plan.

Medical Library

The JCAH criteria for a hospital medical library include:

- The hospital must maintain a medical library according to the needs of the hospital.
- Facilities should be provided to meet the requirements of the services in the hospital.
- Basic textbooks and current periodicals should be available and catalogued according to the needs of the hospital.

The American Hospital Association statement is more specific:

The modern health science library must go beyond the hospital walls and extend its service through participation in library systems and in local, regional, and national communication networks. It is more than a warehouse of stored information. It is an essential source of knowledge, capable of generating information economically and efficiently. The modern health science library represents all the interests of the hospital, including patient care, public health, education, research, and administration.

Special Facilities and Services Summary

Hospitals are frequently gauged on the quantity of specialized services they provide.

In a 1976 survey of hospitals by the American Hospital Association the following specialized facilities and services were reported as being available.

Table 20-6   Special facilities/services

Percent of hospitals	Provide facility/service
78.0	emergency department
75.0	postoperative recovery room
74.4	physical therapy department
69.8	respiratory therapy department
66.8	hospital auxiliary
66.5	pharmacy/registered pharmacist (full-time)
63.1	intensive care unit (mixed)
59.5	blood bank
58.3	social work department
47.8	histopathology laboratory
46.8	diagnostic radioisotope facility
46.6	electro-encephalography
45.3	volunteer services department
40.4	dental services
31.9	intensive care unit (cardiac only)
31.3	premature nursery
29.2	organized outpatient department
28.4	x-ray therapy
28.3	occupational therapy department
24.2	speech pathology services
22.8	pharmacy/part-time pharmacist
21.7	therapeutic radioisotope facility
21.5	radium therapy
20.8	podiatric services
18.5	abortion outpatient service
14.7	patient representative services

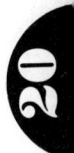

(continued)

Table 20-6   (continued)

Percent of hospitals	Provide facility/service	Percent of hospitals	Provide facility/service
13.0	skilled nursing/long-term care unit	3.8	self-care unit
12.6	cobalt therapy	2.6	chemical dependency inpatient
12.3	hemodialysis inpatient	2.5	organ bank
11.2	rehabilitation outpatient services		

		In psychiatric/ psychology services	
10.3	hemodialysis outpatient		
8.7	abortion outpatient service	23.4	clinical psychology services
8.7	open-heart surgery facilities	21.8	emergency services
8.1	alcoholism outpatient unit	18.0	outpatient services
8.1	family planning service	17.8	inpatient unit
7.6	alcoholism inpatient unit	11.6	partial hospitalization program
6.8	home care department	3.0	foster and/or home care
6.4	rehabilitation inpatient service		
4.0	chemical dependency outpatient		
4.0	genetic counseling service		
3.9	TB & other respiratory disease units		

Hospitals have tended to increase the scope of their services even to the point of duplicating expensive services.

Figure 20-3   Community hospitals reporting selected facilities and services, by bed-size category, 1975.

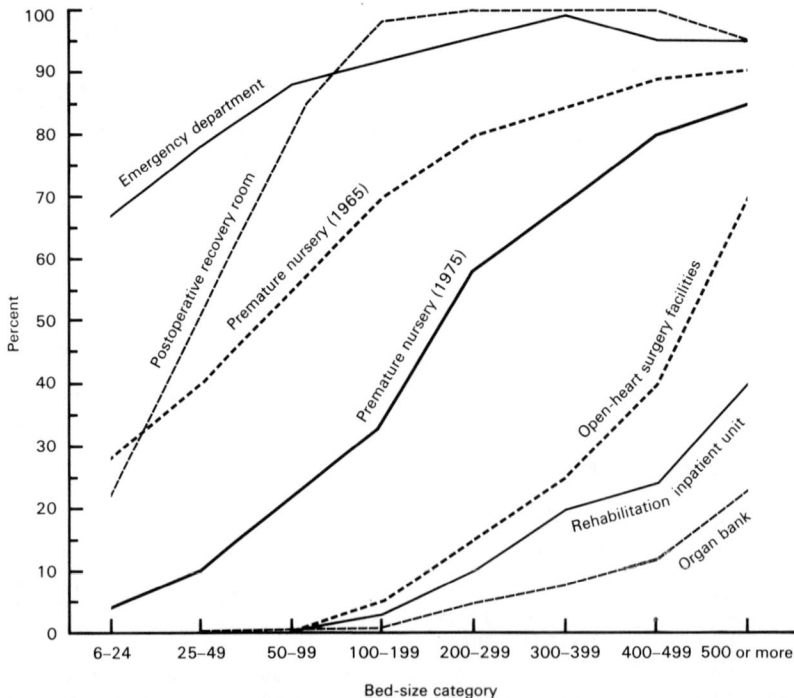

Bed-size category

Source: *Hospital Statistics, 1976 Edition.* Reprinted by permission of The American Hospital Association.

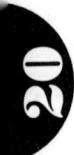

Manpower

Hospital Employment of R.N.s, L.P.N.s & Aides

Table 20-7   Percentage of nursing personnel (by type) in short-term hospitals, 1972

Type of hospital	R.N.s percentage	L.P.N.s percentage	Aides, orderlies, and attendants percentage	Other percentage
Short-term general and other special	39	19	32	10
Hospital units of institutions	54	9	30	7
Community	39	19	32	10
Nongovernment, not-for-profit	41	18	31	10
Investor-owned	35	21	37	7
State and local	34	21	35	10

Source: DHEW, 1974.

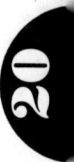

Table 20-8   Nursing personnel employed in U.S. hospitals by position, 1972.

Position	Total	Full-time (FT)	Part-time (PT)
Totals			
Registered nurses	529,677	386,846	142,831
Licensed practical nurses	237,346	198,771	38,575
Aides, orderlies, attendants	543,871	475,092	68,779
Department of nursing service			
Director and assistant	13,295	12,453	842
Inservice education personnel	8,398	6,899	1,499
All other administrative personnel	9,697	7,205	2,492
Supervisor and assistant	37,872	32,118	5,754
Head nurse and assistant	71,497	65,920	5,577
Staff nurse: R.N.	357,113	235,486	121,627
Licensed practical nurse	231,585	193,671	37,914
Aide, orderly, attendant	506,238	441,521	64,717
Other departments			
Administrator and assistant	1,449	1,359	90
Nurse anesthetist	10,802	8,738	2,064
Nursing school faculty	10,714	9,249	1,465
Research nurse	592	500	92
Central service: R.N.	2,534	2,143	391
All other areas: R.N.	5,714	4,776	938
Licensed practical nurse	5,761	5,100	661
Aide, orderly, attendant	37,633	33,571	4,062

Source: Division of Nursing, DHEW, 1974.

Table 20-9   R.N.s employed in hospitals:

Type and ownership of hospital	Total all hospitals			Administrative			
				Director & asst. dir.		Inservice training	
	Number	Beds	Census	FT	PT	FT	PT
Grand Total, U.S.	7,035	1,486,315	1,172,104	12,453	842	6,899	1,499
Federal Total	400	143,576	114,757	773	7	611	25
Long-term	61	53,549	45,801	168	6	191	7
Short-term	339	90,027	68,956	605	1	420	18
Nonfederal Total	6,635	1,342,739	1,057,347	11,680	835	6,288	1,474
Psychiatric	500	382,214	329,046	943	22	786	95
Tuberculosis	75	11,927	8,214	119	9	25	8
Other long-term	228	56,450	48,807	401	20	165	37
S-T Gen. & Oth. spec.	5,832	892,148	671,280	10,217	784	5,312	1,334
Under 25 beds	355	6,513	3,296	229	49	8	21
25–49	1,322	47,626	27,917	1,158	95	106	193
50–99	1,460	103,508	67,973	1,729	83	413	343
100–199	1,242	174,472	125,813	2,184	169	1,005	258
200–299	623	152,020	117,071	1,539	147	1,031	170
300–399	362	123,782	98,325	1,121	127	818	126
400–499	206	90,687	73,439	755	54	591	86
500 & over	262	193,540	157,446	1,502	60	1,340	137
Voluntary Total	3,329	614,163	473,299	6,590	604	3,968	903
Under 25 beds	129	2,443	1,179	74	18	0	4
25–49	521	18,624	10,844	460	60	35	102
50–99	697	50,665	33,636	837	51	221	167
100–199	817	115,593	84,570	1,434	123	702	181
200–299	504	122,921	95,055	1,249	140	851	149
300–399	304	104,030	83,497	920	118	702	112
400–499	169	74,421	60,819	620	47	497	74
500 & over	188	125,466	103,699	996	47	960	114
Proprietary Total	726	56,460	38,574	841	59	222	115
Under 25 beds	79	1,326	761	59	19	2	8
25–49	241	8,799	5,515	190	12	11	20
50–99	223	15,914	10,657	271	12	63	49
100–199	141	19,415	13,291	231	15	98	30
200–299	31	7,143	5,729	67	1	32	5
300–399	8	2,555	1,607	17	0	9	2
400–499	2	800	600	4	0	6	1
500 & over	1	508	414	2	0	1	0
State & Local Total	1,777	221,525	159,407	2,786	121	1,122	316
Under 25 beds	147	2,744	1,356	96	12	6	9
25–49	560	20,203	11,558	508	23	60	71
50–99	540	36,929	23,680	621	20	129	127
100–199	284	39,464	27,952	519	31	205	47
200–299	88	21,956	16,287	223	6	148	16
300–399	50	17,197	13,221	184	9	107	12
400–499	35	15,466	12,020	131	7	88	11
500 & over	73	67,566	53,333	504	13	379	23

20

nursing service administrative and inpatient units

personnel		Inpatient Unit					
All other personnel		Supervisor & asst.		Head nurse & asst.		Staff nurse	
FT	PT	FT	PT	FT	PT	FT	PT
7,205	2,492	23,847	4,922	57,277	5,020	198,488	107,639
469	33	1,222	49	3,897	4	19,676	1,686
133	3	275	13	957	0	4,253	576
336	30	947	36	2,940	4	15,423	1,110
6,736	2,459	22,625	4,873	53,380	5,016	178,812	105,953
576	64	3,425	204	5,188	540	4,727	1,165
38	6	204	24	298	59	342	89
91	33	930	175	1,411	219	2,040	1,012
6,031	2,356	18,066	4,470	46,483	4,198	171,703	103,687
26	6	157	84	291	132	660	767
58	26	1,231	529	1,830	834	3,545	3,810
411	220	3,281	1,100	4,633	1,289	9,874	9,365
1,514	840	3,837	1,266	9,568	1,097	28,613	21,447
1,348	528	2,597	588	8,320	369	34,046	23,189
983	327	2,085	342	6,481	132	28,868	17,931
685	210	1,420	184	5,168	153	21,421	11,832
1,006	199	3,458	377	10,192	192	44,676	15,346
4,487	1,805	11,757	2,962	32,653	2,380	132,872	84,561
6	1	34	18	111	47	263	389
18	8	421	201	769	358	1,606	1,947
208	114	1,545	567	2,504	635	5,835	5,917
1,055	622	2,492	866	6,270	686	20,472	16,092
1,109	437	2,085	509	6,605	299	28,313	20,496
826	285	1,709	320	5,426	101	24,500	16,142
563	195	1,077	138	4,102	130	18,250	10,920
702	143	2,394	343	6,866	124	33,633	12,658
348	167	1,576	550	2,998	569	6,801	4,845
10	2	54	24	48	26	117	92
12	2	306	100	336	149	573	481
95	48	562	179	706	197	1,423	1,114
142	67	483	212	1,196	157	2,761	1,893
54	44	113	32	481	20	1,333	859
16	3	35	3	125	19	339	291
17	0	14	0	88	1	148	51
2	1	9	0	18	0	107	64
1,196	384	4,733	958	10,832	1,249	32,030	14,281
10	3	69	42	132	59	280	286
28	16	504	228	725	327	1,366	1,382
108	58	1,174	354	1,423	457	2,616	2,334
317	151	862	188	2,102	254	5,380	3,462
185	47	399	47	1,234	50	4,400	1,834
141	39	341	19	930	12	4,029	1,498
105	15	329	46	978	22	3,023	861
302	55	1,055	34	3,308	68	10,936	2,624

Source: DHEW, December 1974 (1972 data).

Table 20-10   RN's employed in hospitals, by state:

State	Total all hospitals			Administrative			
				Director & asst. dir.		Inservice training	
	Number	Beds	Census	FT	PT	FT	PT
Total U.S.	7,035	1,486,315	1,172,104	12,453	842	6,899	1,499
Alabama	148	26,480	21,703	237	10	93	32
Alaska	25	1,682	1,107	33	2	7	1
Arizona	82	10,375	7,513	131	4	64	8
Arkansas	94	10,902	8,265	131	1	52	16
California	631	119,642	84,868	1,206	75	666	100
Colorado	94	14,049	10,599	135	6	62	16
Connecticut	67	20,399	15,768	159	11	96	28
Delaware	14	4,894	4,148	35	0	27	0
District of Columbia	21	12,077	9,947	86	10	71	1
Florida	206	49,455	38,689	382	12	249	26
Georgia	171	32,863	26,537	272	18	129	40
Hawaii	31	5,449	3,572	41	5	20	1
Idaho	52	3,534	2,338	60	4	18	6
Illinois	299	79,830	63,604	658	52	428	73
Indiana	135	36,211	28,794	280	19	157	38
Iowa	147	20,746	14,298	208	39	86	51
Kansas	159	18,113	13,181	188	8	59	23
Kentucky	131	19,430	15,582	183	12	76	16
Louisiana	151	25,677	19,607	211	10	93	16
Maine	52	7,904	6,351	81	4	31	17
Maryland	82	29,706	24,688	217	19	179	25
Massachusetts	206	52,301	42,570	420	20	319	69
Michigan	246	56,469	46,832	455	38	322	96
Minnesota	194	29,627	21,935	258	38	158	62
Mississippi	109	17,467	14,043	166	2	53	12
Missouri	152	36,201	28,456	308	32	193	52
Montana	66	4,568	3,047	76	14	16	11
Nebraska	106	10,980	7,680	134	12	57	21
Nevada	23	2,602	1,787	30	2	13	4
New Hampshire	35	6,332	5,036	45	4	28	8
New Jersey	136	48,002	39,310	337	24	216	31
New Mexico	59	5,693	3,764	86	8	23	9
New York	418	171,035	147,514	1,080	34	750	119
North Carolina	162	32,731	26,960	285	13	141	26
North Dakota	63	5,546	3,571	59	8	22	16
Ohio	241	76,479	62,493	524	28	357	74
Oklahoma	143	17,658	12,619	218	14	70	21
Oregon	85	11,557	8,283	115	8	55	25
Pennsylvania	317	98,836	80,959	634	26	453	61
Rhode Island	22	8,065	6,810	51	1	42	13
South Carolina	85	18,621	14,873	137	6	58	13
South Dakota	64	5,895	4,227	60	9	19	8
Tennessee	156	31,269	25,494	237	11	112	23
Texas	543	74,015	55,394	814	55	266	58
Utah	37	4,878	3,572	61	6	20	6
Vermont	21	3,937	3,149	32	1	19	3
Virginia	126	37,089	29,507	271	21	163	20
Washington	128	17,484	12,018	210	20	102	19
West Virginia	84	15,834	12,845	105	8	59	7
Wisconsin	185	32,964	24,383	273	51	123	73
Wyoming	31	2,762	1,814	38	7	7	5

20

nursing service administrative and inpatient units

personnel		Inpatient unit					
All other personnel		Supervisor & asst.		Head nurse & asst.		Staff nurse	
FT	PT	FT	PT	FT	PT	FT	PT
7,205	2,492	23,847	4,922	57,277	5,020	198,488	107,639
98	20	379	59	747	57	2,395	700
14	9	16	3	75	1	366	109
67	14	239	15	563	30	2,351	758
21	3	250	70	464	63	786	280
743	206	2,020	298	5,434	414	22,092	7,832
116	32	216	36	678	77	3,193	1,500
134	50	316	86	843	56	2,825	2,604
15	3	76	11	164	6	502	357
100	20	153	13	454	9	1,930	544
202	39	800	83	2,204	87	7,426	2,419
141	23	528	86	1,141	73	3,335	1,127
12	2	85	0	212	6	1,097	60
32	18	65	25	151	51	550	337
367	143	1,271	236	2,890	161	13,049	7,266
188	59	458	109	1,210	151	3,747	2,606
89	66	276	108	643	132	2,803	2,195
71	21	325	116	573	115	2,037	1,279
95	25	383	68	690	80	2,389	989
86	15	448	52	716	61	2,175	830
33	14	155	40	331	82	871	713
177	56	474	56	1,007	32	3,339	2,414
276	104	1,146	297	2,591	280	7,824	7,031
271	105	838	288	1,999	279	7,069	4,658
167	132	334	206	1,089	168	4,473	3,844
43	12	285	70	493	50	1,190	364
137	45	505	122	1,155	110	3,819	2,016
15	20	72	23	128	18	673	536
37	19	130	77	443	22	1,671	1,131
21	8	53	1	157	10	435	145
27	13	130	40	312	47	819	626
268	96	740	118	1,702	67	7,022	4,922
39	14	86	13	184	18	920	273
799	284	2,857	432	7,937	405	23,272	10,232
195	34	636	61	1,336	83	4,057	1,430
39	28	61	26	173	31	638	463
428	161	888	209	2,694	204	9,298	7,651
55	17	342	80	620	107	1,404	588
53	19	152	47	654	97	1,892	1,275
506	156	1,575	265	3,474	236	14,462	8,359
19	10	162	35	364	31	1,012	1,051
96	13	219	19	582	28	1,683	714
20	13	64	23	134	31	673	453
107	17	515	108	896	118	2,732	828
286	65	1,497	307	3,082	444	7,458	2,284
37	23	63	35	215	17	947	593
10	3	73	24	134	18	546	323
144	48	509	115	1,260	57	4,049	2,096
124	63	256	60	800	132	3,326	1,862
55	21	253	34	448	21	1,560	683
120	108	433	207	961	146	3,944	4,049
10	3	40	10	70	1	362	240

Source: DHEW, December 1974 (1972 data).

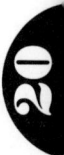

20

Table 20-11   Registered nurses employed in hospitals:

Type and ownership of hospital	Total all hospitals			Operating			
				Supervisor & asst.		Head nurse & asst.	
	Number	Beds	Census	FT	PT	FT	PT
Grand Total, U.S.	7,035	1,486,315	1,172,104	5,109	439	3,934	236
Federal Total	400	143,576	114,757	318	2	154	0
Long-term	61	53,549	45,801	28	0	22	0
Short-term	339	90,027	68,956	290	2	132	0
Nonfederal Total	6,635	1,342,739	1,057,347	4,791	437	3,780	236
Psychiatric	500	382,214	329,046	73	6	87	5
Tuberculosis	75	11,927	8,214	28	4	10	0
Other long-term	228	56,450	48,807	42	1	20	4
S-T Gen. & Other Spec.	5,832	892,148	671,280	4,648	426	3,663	227
Under 25 beds	355	6,513	3,296	26	29	11	8
25–49	1,322	47,626	27,917	404	172	117	62
50–99	1,460	103,508	67,973	1,079	120	345	51
100–199	1,242	174,472	125,813	1,195	58	710	36
200–299	623	152,020	117,071	671	9	612	15
300–399	362	123,782	98,325	450	11	467	10
400–499	206	90,687	73,439	273	13	372	10
500 & over	262	193,540	157,446	550	14	1,029	35
Voluntary Total	3,329	614,163	473,299	3,087	218	2,592	152
Under 25 beds	129	2,443	1,179	4	13	3	5
25–49	521	18,624	10,844	159	82	38	38
50–99	697	50,665	33,636	546	48	184	26
100–199	817	115,593	84,570	786	41	491	26
000–299	504	122,921	95,055	549	9	486	13
300–399	304	104,030	83,497	393	10	391	9
400–499	169	74,421	60,819	219	4	304	7
500 & over	188	125,466	103,699	431	11	695	28
Proprietary Total	726	56,460	38,574	533	68	200	25
Under 25 beds	79	1,326	761	15	7	5	1
25–49	241	8,799	5,515	97	31	29	10
50–99	223	15,914	10,657	197	23	53	12
100–199	141	19,415	13,291	178	7	77	2
200–299	31	7,143	5,729	33	0	25	0
300–399	8	2,555	1,607	11	0	9	0
400–499	2	800	600	1	0	1	0
500 & over	1	508	414	1	0	1	0
State & Local Total	1,777	221,525	159,407	1,028	140	871	50
Under 25 beds	147	2,744	1,356	7	9	3	2
25–49	560	20,203	11,558	148	59	50	14
50–99	540	36,929	23,680	336	49	108	13
100–199	284	39,464	27,952	231	10	142	8
200–299	88	21,956	16,287	89	0	101	2
300–399	50	17,197	13,221	46	1	67	1
400–499	35	15,466	12,020	53	9	67	3
500 & over	73	67,566	53,333	118	3	333	7

outpatient and emergency units and in operating room

room		Outpatient & emergency					
Staff nurse		Supervisor & asst.		Head nurse & asst.		Staff nurse	
FT	PT	FT	PT	FT	PT	FT	PT
22,217	6,705	3,162	393	4,709	321	14,781	7,283
1,189	33	497	9	364	1	936	28
151	6	77	1	47	0	152	7
1,038	27	420	8	317	1	784	21
21,028	6,672	2,665	384	4,345	320	13,845	7,255
58	10	180	14	188	14	149	18
4	2	26	2	7	0	7	1
28	18	39	3	38	5	49	10
20,938	6,642	2,420	365	4,112	301	13,640	7,226
20	39	29	9	9	0	51	29
237	290	122	50	56	33	202	174
1,378	547	304	88	265	74	574	585
4,202	1,303	511	115	778	88	1,902	1,650
4,529	1,483	399	33	763	51	2,709	1,718
3,545	1,193	320	23	605	15	2,403	1,286
2,510	799	205	17	457	10	1,622	764
4,517	988	530	30	1,179	30	4,177	1,020
16,505	5,438	1,629	236	2,714	232	9,762	5,802
5	15	6	4	3	0	8	13
102	141	61	26	27	22	64	95
817	342	168	52	170	52	337	391
2,944	961	342	79	543	62	1,419	1,250
3,771	1,298	334	30	587	47	2,178	1,511
3,103	1,078	264	15	432	14	1,885	1,138
2,147	756	151	15	333	8	1,240	649
3,616	847	303	15	619	27	2,631	755
1,168	363	103	19	117	22	337	249
9	9	5	3	1	0	9	0
79	48	12	2	2	5	33	19
262	77	37	9	22	9	72	52
517	153	31	3	60	7	117	112
208	54	15	1	24	1	60	51
52	11	2	1	5	0	26	9
30	5	0	0	3	0	14	1
11	6	1	0	0	0	6	5
3,265	841	688	110	1,281	47	3,541	1,175
6	15	18	2	5	0	34	16
56	101	49	22	27	6	105	60
299	128	99	27	73	13	165	142
741	189	138	33	175	19	366	288
550	131	50	2	152	3	471	156
390	104	54	7	168	1	492	139
333	38	54	2	121	2	368	114
890	135	226	15	560	3	1,540	260

Source: DHEW, December 1974 (1972 data).

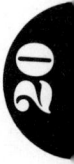

			Table 20-12	**Registered nurses employed in hospitals:**			
Type and ownership of hospital	Total all hospitals			Hosp. admin. or asst.		Nursing sch. faculty	
	Number	Beds	Census	FT	PT	FT	PT
Grand Total, U.S.	7,035	1,486,315	1,172,104	1,359	90	9,249	1,465
Federal Total	400	143,576	114,757	22	1	62	0
Long-term	61	53,549	45,801	2	0	19	0
Short-term	339	90,027	68,956	20	1	43	0
Nonfederal Total	6,635	1,342,739	1,057,347	1,337	89	9,187	1,465
Psychiatric	500	382,214	329,046	77	7	343	20
Tuberculosis	75	11,927	8,214	5	0	0	0
Other long-term	228	56,450	48,807	40	9	54	5
S-T Gen. & Oth. Spec.	5,832	892,148	671,280	1,215	73	8,790	1,440
Under 25 beds	355	6,513	3,296	66	7	3	0
25–49	1,322	47,626	27,917	183	8	26	2
50–99	1,460	103,508	67,973	201	37	96	18
100–199	1,242	174,472	125,813	220	6	654	139
200–299	623	152,020	117,071	170	2	1,514	315
300–399	362	123,782	98,325	132	4	1,907	314
400–499	206	90,687	73,439	92	2	1,465	255
500 & over	262	193,540	157,446	151	7	3,125	397
Voluntary Total	3,329	614,163	473,299	908	45	7,250	1,268
Under 25 beds	129	2,443	1,179	29	2	1	0
25–49	521	18,624	10,844	91	4	10	0
50–99	697	50,665	33,636	110	18	52	10
100–199	817	115,593	84,570	182	6	508	114
200–299	504	122,921	95,055	158	2	1,410	302
300–399	304	104,030	83,497	125	4	1,644	280
400–499	169	74,421	60,819	82	2	1,356	245
500 & over	188	125,466	103,699	131	7	2,269	317
Proprietary Total	726	56,460	38,574	72	15	63	15
Under 25 beds	79	1,326	761	10	3	0	0
25–49	241	8,799	5,515	19	2	2	0
50–99	223	15,914	10,657	25	10	18	3
100–199	141	19,415	13,291	15	0	21	2
200–299	31	7,143	5,729	2	0	0	0
300–399	8	2,555	1,607	0	0	22	10
400–499	2	800	600	1	0	0	0
500 & over	1	508	414	0	0	0	0
State & Local Total	1,777	221,525	159,407	235	13	1,477	157
Under 25 beds	147	2,744	1,356	27	2	2	0
25–49	560	20,203	11,558	73	2	14	2
50–99	540	36,929	23,680	66	9	26	5
100–199	284	39,464	27,952	23	0	125	23
200–299	88	21,956	16,287	10	0	104	13
300–399	50	17,197	13,221	7	0	241	24
400–499	35	15,466	12,020	9	0	109	10
500 & over	73	67,566	53,333	20	0	856	80

20

outside the department of nursing service

Nurse anesthetist		Research nurse		Central service		All others areas	
FT	PT	FT	PT	FT	PT	FT	PT
8,738	2,064	500	92	2,143	391	4,776	938
800	18	46	2	78	3	138	10
81	3	11	0	7	0	28	1
719	15	35	2	71	3	110	9
7,938	2,046	454	90	2,065	388	4,638	928
42	31	50	5	107	23	200	20
3	10	1	0	17	2	10	1
8	10	5	2	51	13	74	18
7,885	1,995	398	83	1,890	350	4,354	889
34	130	0	2	9	24	25	22
390	437	1	1	106	86	111	37
1,058	337	2	0	225	96	195	71
1,752	286	12	9	450	64	486	131
1,493	254	92	19	415	29	656	165
1,019	158	66	11	320	20	789	182
765	156	41	4	152	8	745	107
1,374	237	184	37	213	23	1,347	174
5,682	1,290	279	58	1,351	225	3,392	728
9	63	0	0	1	14	9	5
158	163	0	0	31	46	42	14
545	147	0	0	124	49	134	46
1,256	214	10	5	310	44	380	102
1,238	223	75	15	347	24	539	149
832	142	40	11	262	19	713	163
621	149	25	3	122	7	636	103
1,023	189	129	24	154	22	939	146
401	192	0	4	157	40	82	33
15	23	0	0	5	3	10	11
67	68	0	0	33	11	8	4
133	61	0	0	45	17	11	4
129	30	0	4	45	8	32	11
31	7	0	0	18	1	13	3
20	3	0	0	9	0	2	0
3	0	0	0	2	0	6	0
3	0	0	0	0	0	0	0
1,802	513	119	21	382	85	880	128
10	44	0	2	3	7	6	6
165	206	1	1	42	29	61	19
380	129	2	0	56	30	50	21
367	42	2	0	95	12	74	18
224	24	17	4	50	4	104	13
167	13	26	0	49	1	74	19
141	7	16	1	28	1	103	4
348	48	55	13	59	1	408	28

Source: DHEW, December 1974 (1972 data).

Table 20-13 Registered nurses employed in hospitals, by state:

State	Total all hospitals			Hosp. admin. or asst.		Nursing sch. faculty	
	Number	Beds	Census	FT	PT	FT	PT
Total U.S.	7,035	1,486,315	1,172,104	1,359	90	9,249	1,465
Alabama	148	26,480	21,703	14	0	140	13
Alaska	25	1,682	1,107	4	1	0	0
Arizona	82	10,375	7,513	16	0	20	1
Arkansas	94	10,902	8,265	34	4	44	2
California	631	119,642	84,868	103	4	274	18
Colorado	94	14,049	10,599	9	0	116	16
Connecticut	67	20,399	15,768	35	4	275	48
Delaware	14	4,894	4,148	0	0	38	3
District of Columbia	21	12,077	9,947	6	0	47	2
Florida	206	49,455	38,689	21	0	48	2
Georgia	171	32,863	26,537	17	0	176	14
Hawaii	31	5,449	3,572	8	0	1	0
Idaho	52	3,534	2,338	18	1	3	0
Illinois	299	79,830	63,604	74	2	479	66
Indiana	135	36,211	28,794	30	1	145	28
Iowa	147	20,746	14,298	25	0	181	53
Kansas	159	18,113	13,181	23	1	143	17
Kentucky	131	19,430	15,582	33	0	62	2
Louisiana	151	25,677	19,607	17	0	105	2
Maine	52	7,904	6,351	8	0	52	5
Maryland	82	29,706	24,688	21	0	310	43
Massachusetts	206	52,301	42,570	50	2	679	104
Michigan	246	56,469	46,832	52	10	375	93
Minnesota	194	29,627	21,935	42	7	198	76
Mississippi	109	17,467	14,043	7	0	26	1
Missouri	152	36,201	28,456	32	1	317	47
Montana	66	4,568	3,047	10	2	15	0
Nebraska	106	10,980	7,680	20	1	151	46
Nevada	23	2,602	1,787	9	0	3	0
New Hampshire	35	6,332	5,036	6	0	84	12
New Jersey	136	48,002	39,310	33	1	347	40
New Mexico	59	5,693	3,764	4	1	11	7
New York	418	171,035	147,514	119	5	1,079	144
North Carolina	162	32,731	26,960	13	0	160	35
North Dakota	63	5,546	62,493	12	1	60	6
Ohio	241	76,479	62,493	57	5	717	116
Oklahoma	143	17,658	12,619	15	5	59	8
Oregon	85	11,557	8,283	15	1	62	10
Pennsylvania	317	98,836	80,959	92	2	1,264	184
Rhode Island	22	8,065	6,810	3	0	41	14
South Carolina	85	18,621	14,873	8	0	48	3
South Dakota	64	5,895	4,227	8	1	44	9
Tennessee	156	31,269	25,494	19	0	122	6
Texas	543	74,015	55,394	93	9	195	19
Utah	37	4,878	3,572	18	4	1	0
Vermont	21	3,937	3,149	4	0	0	0
Virginia	126	37,089	29,507	18	1	267	53
Washington	128	17,484	12,018	21	1	51	4
West Virginia	84	15,834	12,845	7	1	56	32
Wisconsin	185	32,964	24,383	50	11	156	61
Wyoming	31	2,762	1,814	6	0	2	0

outside the department of nursing service

Nurse anesthetist		Research nurse		Central service		All other areas	
FT	PT	FT	PT	FT	PT	FT	PT
8,738	2,064	500	92	2,143	391	4,776	938
186	56	2	0	30	6	38	9
20	3	0	0	5	0	5	0
65	6	0	0	26	5	67	9
60	26	2	0	11	5	16	5
415	80	70	13	263	51	689	75
72	20	15	0	32	11	43	18
109	9	16	2	35	3	117	46
34	4	1	0	11	1	37	10
47	10	23	0	14	0	18	0
365	49	8	2	88	4	121	21
155	47	8	0	54	3	80	13
60	4	3	1	9	0	28	2
40	11	0	0	9	6	12	0
490	114	19	6	104	20	270	36
55	25	5	2	47	8	58	13
105	30	1	1	18	11	27	11
53	34	1	1	36	11	49	10
102	18	2	1	30	1	27	2
247	59	0	1	48	1	81	4
54	3	0	1	14	7	22	3
115	23	9	0	50	7	130	13
219	53	11	1	78	10	286	92
476	110	7	0	45	19	87	41
373	169	7	3	45	22	44	28
131	33	3	0	18	4	13	1
187	80	13	1	24	6	78	13
41	13	0	0	12	8	29	10
104	46	3	0	13	12	22	6
15	3	0	0	7	1	10	0
20	1	2	0	15	3	21	7
161	32	10	3	58	2	144	23
59	8	0	1	10	1	10	2
478	107	102	15	233	32	534	72
422	52	5	1	41	5	102	16
67	24	0	0	2	10	14	3
241	59	48	15	98	9	236	76
83	29	7	1	22	12	22	1
101	28	0	0	19	8	41	6
940	153	36	10	152	25	485	79
17	1	6	0	7	0	11	2
129	28	1	0	18	5	37	11
57	20	0	0	3	3	9	2
173	36	17	3	25	1	67	8
578	179	21	2	113	8	221	23
30	8	1	2	2	1	51	26
13	2	1	0	2	0	38	5
261	43	2	1	36	2	74	12
130	37	6	1	51	8	70	35
134	9	0	0	16	3	20	5
235	59	5	1	39	6	60	30
14	11	1	0	5	4	5	3

Source: DHEW, December 1974 (1972 data).

Table 20-14   Licensed practical nurses and aides employed in hospitals:

Type and ownership of hospital	Total all hospitals			Administrative	
				Practical nurse	
	Number	Beds	Census	FT	PT
Grand Total, U.S.	7,035	1,486,315	1,172,104	496	41
Federal Total	400	143,576	114,757	106	1
Long-term	61	53,549	45,801	27	0
Short-term	339	90,027	68,956	79	1
Non-federal Total	6,635	1,342,739	1,057,347	390	40
Psychiatric	500	382,214	329,046	287	1
Tuberculosis	75	11,927	8,214	1	0
Other long-term	228	56,450	48,807	2	0
S-T Gen. & Oth. Spec.	5,832	892,148	671,280	100	39
Under 25 beds	355	6,513	3,296	21	1
25–49	1,322	47,626	27,917	4	7
50–99	1,460	103,508	67,973	17	1
100–199	1,242	174,472	125,813	14	7
200–299	623	152,020	117,071	9	0
300–399	362	123,782	98,325	10	14
400–499	206	90,687	73,439	7	2
500 & over	262	193,540	157,446	18	7
Voluntary Total	3,329	614,163	473,299	51	28
Under 25 beds	129	2,443	1,179	0	1
25–49	521	18,624	10,844	2	7
50–99	697	50,665	33,636	4	1
100–199	817	115,593	84,570	12	7
200–299	504	122,921	95,055	6	0
300–399	304	104,030	83,497	6	6
400–499	169	74,421	60,819	6	2
500 & over	188	125,466	103,699	15	4
Proprietary Total	726	56,460	38,574	29	0
Under 25 beds	79	1,326	761	21	0
25–49	241	8,799	5,515	1	0
50–99	223	15,914	10,657	5	0
100–199	141	19,415	13,291	1	0
200–299	31	7,143	5,729	1	0
300–399	8	2,555	1,607	0	0
400–499	2	800	600	0	0
500 & over	1	508	414	0	0
State & Local Total	1,777	221,525	159,407	20	11
Under 25 beds	147	2,744	1,356	0	0
25–49	560	20,203	11,558	1	0
50–99	540	36,929	23,680	8	0
100–199	284	39,464	27,952	1	0
200–299	88	21,956	16,287	2	0
300–399	50	17,197	13,221	4	8
400–499	35	15,466	12,020	1	0
500 & over	73	67,566	53,333	3	3

20

nursing administrative and inpatient units

| personnel | | Inpatient unit | | | |
| Aides, ord. & attend. | | Practical nurse | | Aides, ord. & attend. | |
FT	PT	FT	PT	FT	PT
629	61	175,766	35,168	405,005	59,955
172	0	8,982	186	33,290	267
3	0	2,325	43	12,901	77
169	0	6,657	143	20,389	190
457	61	166,784	34,982	371,713	59,688
262	2	13,563	355	100,239	1,815
5	0	1,028	34	2,399	115
7	0	3,963	435	17,089	1,170
183	59	148,230	34,158	251,986	56,588
18	1	685	259	1,863	996
4	0	6,373	1,936	14,041	5,714
17	0	16,426	4,545	31,128	10,295
28	1	30,824	7,846	49,971	13,103
24	7	25,487	6,506	41,613	9,292
35	20	20,337	4,885	33,363	6,532
14	2	16,094	3,242	25,749	4,678
43	28	32,004	4,939	54,258	5,978
95	44	100,873	25,863	165,934	40,760
0	1	210	107	643	436
0	0	2,015	837	5,122	2,746
0	0	7,647	2,475	14,180	5,454
13	0	19,889	5,486	31,169	9,075
7	5	20,026	5,576	32,952	8,066
28	18	16,929	4,364	27,998	5,882
12	2	12,361	2,884	20,391	4,358
35	18	21,796	4,134	33,479	4,743
41	3	9,109	2,141	16,936	3,705
18	0	198	32	360	128
0	0	1,434	301	2,626	596
15	0	2,528	583	4,660	1,236
2	1	3,292	774	5,891	1,297
6	2	1,159	341	2,346	365
0	0	338	84	589	61
0	0	108	16	283	14
0	0	52	10	181	8
47	12	38,248	6,154	69,116	12,123
0	0	277	120	860	432
4	0	2,924	798	6,293	2,372
2	0	6,251	1,487	12,288	3,605
13	0	7,643	1,586	12,911	2,731
11	0	4,302	589	6,315	861
7	2	3,070	437	4,776	589
2	0	3,625	342	5,075	306
8	10	10,156	795	20,598	1,227

Source: DHEW, December 1974 (1972 data).

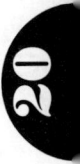

Volunteers*

The person responsible for planning, administering, and coordinating the volunteer services in a health care institution is the Director of Volunteer Services. Like other department managers, the director of volunteer services, who may be a man or a woman, reports to the administrator of the health care institution. His main function is to assist the institution in the delivery of health care by obtaining and retaining an adequate, competent, and satisfied volunteer staff to augment the services of personnel. In carrying out this function, he serves as an adviser to administration on the use of volunteers, on trends in volunteer work, and on policies and procedures relating to the volunteer services department.

Recruiting people to serve as volunteers is one of the director's major responsibilities. Before he initiates recruitment activities, he determines with each department head the specific needs for volunteer services, considering every department's operations, objectives, and relationships with other departments. Once he has obtained sufficient information, the director develops a job description for each volunteer position.

Hospital Auxiliaries

Membership and Membership Policies—At the end of 1973, auxiliary membership totaled 972,525 adults nationally, 97% of whom were women. The average membership size was 339 auxilians.

In-service volunteer activities: In-service volunteer activities were reported by 2,208 auxiliaries (77.0%).

Fund-raising activities: Fund-raising activities were reported by 2,622 auxiliaries (91.3%).

Legislative activities: Through education and organized activities, hospital auxiliaries and their one million members can have a bearing on the health care decisions made at many governmental levels. Of the total, 1,224

auxiliaries (42.7%) had undertaken to inform and educate their members on current health care legislation.

Blood donation activities: During 1973, one of three auxiliaries (32.1%) was active in programs promoting the voluntary donation of blood.

Consumer Health Education—Only 652 auxiliaries (22.7%) had been active in this area during the preceding year.

Volunteers: Language Banks

Harborview Medical Center in Seattle makes use of a language bank, consisting of more than 100 volunteers, on call 24 hours a day. They serve as friends and interpreters for patients who do not speak English.

About 80% of the language bank interpreters are recruited from the hospital's own staff, so they often are on the premises when their services are needed. Other interpreters include professors from Seattle's two universities and from private and community colleges, students and housewives. Those who do not work in the hospital may be summoned, or they may speak with a patient and the hospital staff by telephone.

Names of available interpreters and the language they speak are maintained and updated by the community relations department. More than 40 languages are listed in the hospital's current file, among the more exotic of which are Bengali, Haitian-Creole, Malayan, sign language, and Tamil.

Gloria Peel, a Spanish-speaking member of the hospital's housekeeping staff, was asked to interpret for a Mexican woman who needed a tonsillectomy. She found that the woman had no money, that she had come to Seattle to locate the body of her son, who had drowned in a fishing accident, and that she had been tricked out of her life savings. The Mexican woman received her operation and offers of housing, money and legal assistance when the press heard of her plight.

The most prevalent foreign languages among the staff are Spanish, Italian, French, German, Polish, Yiddish, Greek, Hungarian, Filipino and Russian.

---

*Source: "Survey of Auxiliaries 1974" *Hospitals, JAHA,* June 1, 1975. Reprinted by permission of the American Hospital Association.

Caring for the Hospital Patient

Nursing Hours per Patient Day*

Total nursing hours per adjusted patient day vary from a high of 7.17 in Arizona to a low of

---

*Source: DHEW, February 1975.

5.25 in Utah. Total nursing hours per civilian resident population vary from a high of 11.50 in the District of Columbia to a low of 4.29 in Utah.

Table 20-15   Total nursing hours per average patient day

	Bedsize class	Average hours per patient day
Nonprofit, nonteaching hospitals		
Government control	0– 20	7.962
	21– 40	6.943
	41– 60	6.731
	61– 80	6.417
	81–100	6.435
	101–140	6.320
	141–200	6.608
	201–300	6.769
Nongovernment control	21– 40	6.271
	41– 60	6.575
	61– 80	6.267
	81–100	6.428
	101–140	6.611
	141–200	6.720
	201–300	6.549
	301–400	6.254
	401 +	6.180
Total		6.553
Teaching hospitals		
Government control	401 +	6.264
Nongovernment control	141–200	6.303
	201–300	6.438
	301–400	6.111
	401 +	6.173
Total		6.232
For-profit, nonteaching hospitals		
For-profit	21– 40	6.348
	41– 60	6.553
	61– 80	7.178
	81–100	7.594
	101–140	6.958
Total		6.811

Source: DHEW, February 1975.

Table 20-16   Average staffing levels and patterns

Category	Hours per adjusted patient day		
	Non-profit hospital	Teaching hospital	For profit hospital
Total nursing personnel	6.6	6.2	6.8
Registered nurses	2.4	3.0	2.3
Licensed practical nurses	1.4	1.2	1.5
Aides, orderlies and/or attendants	2.9	2.1	3.0
General duty nurses	1.4	2.2	1.1
General duty and head nurses	1.9	2.7	1.7

Source: DHEW, February 1975.

For teaching hospitals, the ratio among R.N.s, L.P.N.s and ancilliary personnel is roughly 3.0:1.2:2.1. This group has the highest proportion of R.N.s and the lowest of ancillary personnel. Teaching hospitals have more advanced technology facilities and generally handle more complex cases. These features probably explain the need for more professionals among the nursing staff.

For nonprofit, nonteaching hospitals, the ratio is roughly 2.4:1.4:2.9. This group of hospitals has a lower proportion of R.N.s and a higher one of ancillary personnel than teaching hospitals.

For-profit hospitals' ratio is roughly 2.3:1.5:3.0. Notice that this hospital group has the lowest proportion of R.N.s and the highest of ancillary personnel.

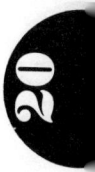

Patient Classification*

Table 20-17   Elements of physical care and levels of intensity**

Category	Criterion	Intensity level points assessed
Diet	Feeds self without supervision, or parent feeds patient.	1
	Feeds self with supervision by staff.	2
	Feeds self but needs constant presence of staff, or gastrostomy feeding q4h.	4
	Total feeding by personnel, instructing the parent, continuous I.V., or blood transfusion.	8
	Tube feedings more frequently than q4h.	12
Toileting—output	Toilets without supervision.	1
	Toilets with supervision, specimen to be collected, or uses bedpan.	2
	Up to toilet with stand-by supervision, or output measurement every hour, or daily colostomy irrigation.	4
	Incontinent, average output.	8
	Incontinent with diarrhea, or immediate postoperative colostomy or urethrostomy, or drainage with frequent dressing change.	12
Vital signs and measurements	Routine—daily temperature, pulse, and respiration.	1
	Vital signs q4h, or night observation q1h.	2
	Vital signs monitored, or hypothermia, or vital signs q2h.	4
	Vital signs and observation every hour, or vital signs monitored plus hypothermia and neurologic evaluation.	8
	BP, pulse, respirations, and neurologic evaluation q½h.	12
Respiratory aids	Bedside humidifier, or "blow bottle."	1
	Mist or Croupette when sleeping, or cough and deep breathe q2h, or IPPB without supervision q4h.	2
	Continuous oxygen, or cough and deep breathe q1h, or continuous assisted ventilation.	4
	Mechanical respiratory aid, or IPPB with supervision q4h.	8
	PPB continuously with intermittent Ambu "bagging."	12
Suction	Routine postoperative standby.	1
	Nasopharyngeal or oral suction prn.	2
	Tracheostomy suction every hour, or nasogastric tube irrigation q2h.	4
	Tracheostomy suction q½h, patient responsive.	8
	Tracheostomy suction q½h, patient not responsive.	12
Cleanliness	Bathes self, bed straightened.	1
	Bathes self with help or supervision, daily change of bed.	2
	Bathed and dressed by personnel, or partial bath given, daily change of linen.	4
	Bathed and dressed by personnel, special skin care, occupied bed.	8
Turning and/or assisted activity	Up in chair with assistance once in 8 hours.	1
	Up in chair with assistance twice in 8 hours, or walking with assistance.	2
	Bedfast with assistance in turning q2h, or up walking with assistance of two people twice in 8 hours.	4
	Bedfast with assistance in turning q1h.	8
	Turning on Foster frame or CircOlectric bed q1h.	12

**Time conversion guide.

Points	PCUs	Hours	Points	PCUs	Hours
4–11	1	1	44–51	6	6
12–19	2	2	52–59	7	7
20–27	3	3	60–67	8	8
28–35	4	4	68–75	9	9
36–43	5	5	76–80	10	10

To arrive at an intensity of care for a patient, add the appropriate points from each category and use this total to find the PCUs (patient care units in hours) from the conversion table. Point assessment was worked out from a time study, and flexibility was built in by rounding out minutes to the hour to allow for intangibles and unplanned incidents.

*Source: Poland, English, *et al.,* "PETO," *American Journal of Nursing* July 1970. ©American Journal of Nursing Company. (Used at Eugene Talmadge Memorial Hospital in Georgia.)

The Staff Nurse's Day

Figure 20-4   Staff Nurse: Percent of time spent at various activities—A.M. shift. Typical hospital.

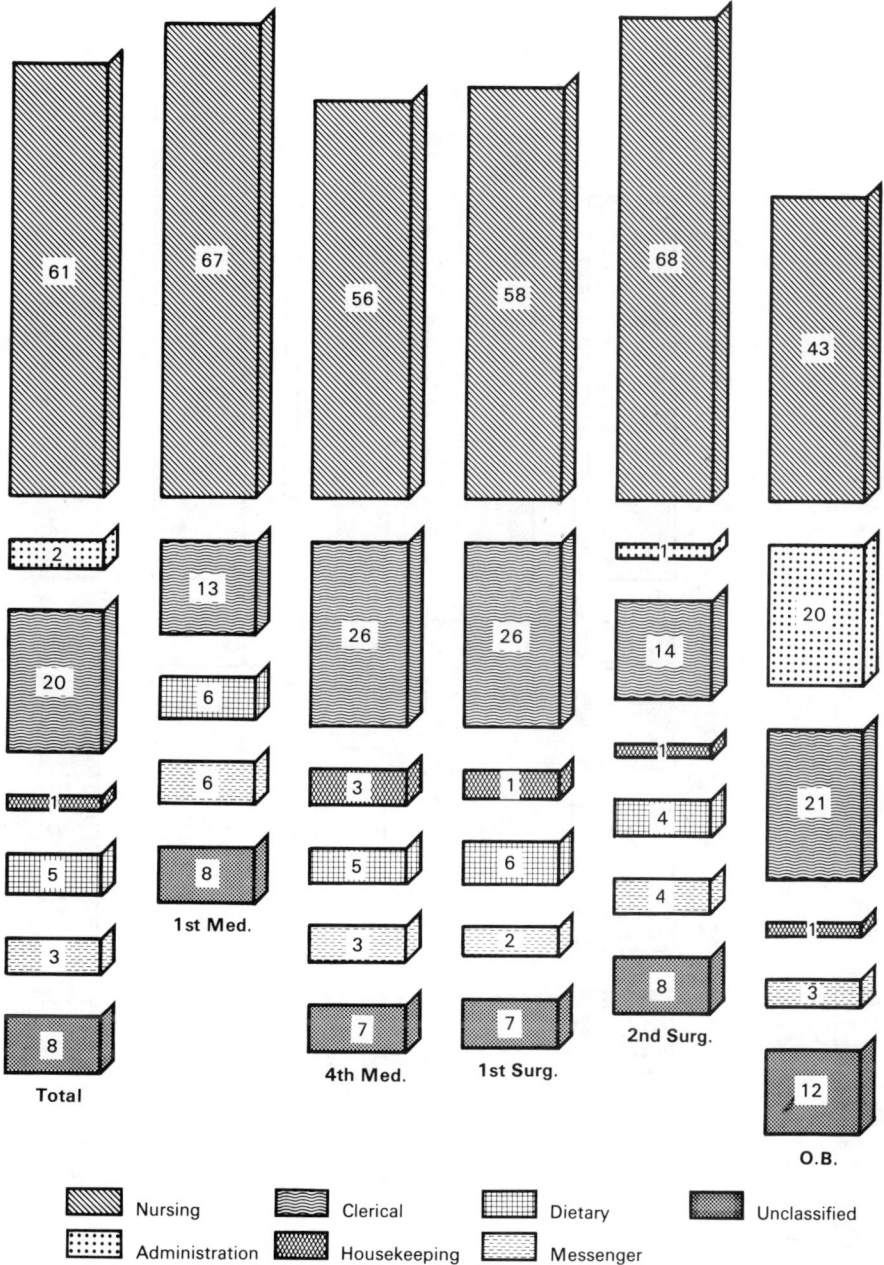

	Nursing		Clerical		Dietary		Unclassified
	Administration		Housekeeping		Messenger		

Source: DHEW.

The Practical Nurse's Day

Figure 20-5   Practical nurse: Percent of time spent at various activities—A.M. shift. Typical hospital.

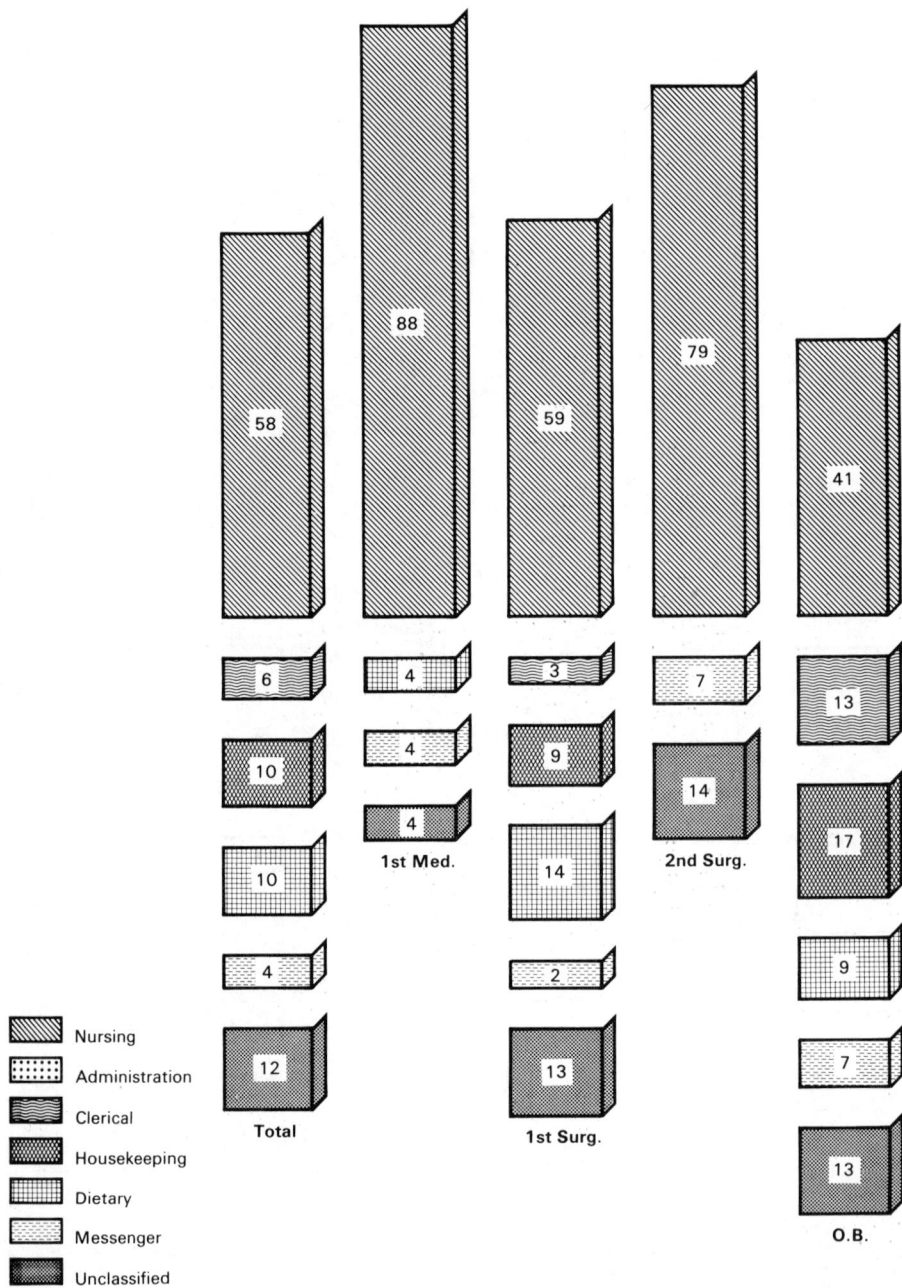

Nursing
Administration
Clerical
Housekeeping
Dietary
Messenger
Unclassified

Source: DHEW.

The Hospital Nurse's Shifts and Activities

Table 20-18   Shifts and stations in U.S. hospitals

Shifts and stations	All hospitals	Size (beds)					Census area				Ownership		
		Under 50	50 to 99	100 to 199	200 to 399	400 and over	North-east	North Central	South	West	Non-profit	Government	Proprietary
Mean percent of part-time R.N.s on regular shifts (not on call)	82.7	78.3	80.1	82.3	87.5	88.9	85.1	87.6	78.2	78.5	83.8	80.6	80.5
Hospitals where the majority of part-time R.N.s work regular M-F shifts (%)	8.8	9.5	8.6	10.4	5.1	10.0	7.6	5.6	15.0	5.0	8.7	8.0	11.8
Mean percent of full-time R.N.s who are regularly assigned to:													
One shift	70.3	65.8	79.1	84.4	64.5	44.6	67.7	67.5	67.8	81.1	71.2	63.1	88.0
One station	82.8	86.8	75.7	83.0	85.9	85.2	84.2	81.6	82.5	83.6	85.0	80.1	80.4
Mean days notice given to R.N.s regularly assigned to one shift before assignment to a new shift	16.2	16.1	13.5	16.7	17.5	18.5	18.8	14.3	15.1	17.5	16.2	15.9	17.2
Mean days R.N.s *not* assigned one regular shift work on any assigned shift	7.9	6.2	7.8	7.1	9.1	10.1	10.0	7.1	7.2	8.0	7.8	8.0	7.9
Hospitals where R.N.s frequently determine their own schedules (%)	50.1	54.5	61.0	44.0	37.6	42.5	47.7	50.2	48.2	55.0	50.0	48.7	55.9

Source: DHEW, May 1975 (1973 survey).

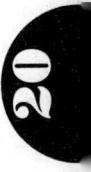

394

L.P.N.s Doing R.N.s Work

Table 20-19   Percentage of hospitals using non-R.N.s to do R.N. work

Hospital group	Total	
	All shifts only	Evening and night shifts
Size (beds)		
Under 50	11.7%	9.0%
50–99	17.3	20.1
100–199	16.1	23.3
200–399	14.1	17.8
400 and over	9.2	14.4
All hospitals	14.1	16.6
Loan forgiveness status		
Loan forgiveness	19.2	19.2
Non-loan forgiveness	8.0	8.5
Census Area		
Northeast	11.9	12.7
North Central	13.2	12.3
South	20.7	23.9
West	7.2	14.5

Source: DHEW, May 1975 (1973 data).

Hospital Patient Ailments

Overview

Among the most frequent hospital discharge diagnoses were diseases of the circulatory system (4.1 million discharges); diseases of the digestive system (4.0 million); complications of pregnancy, childbirth, and the puerperium (4.0 million); diseases of the respiratory system (3.4 million); diseases of the genitourinary system (3.4 million); and accidents, poisonings, and violence (3.4 million discharges). By class, the average length of stay ranged from 3.3 days for complications of pregnancy, childbirth, and the puerperium to 16.1 for arteriosclerosis.

For males, the highest rates were for diseases of the circulatory system (210.4 per 10,000 population), diseases of the digestive system (195.8), and accidents, poisonings, and violence (197.7). For females, complications of pregnancy, childbirth, and the puerperium had the highest discharge rate (372.7 per 10,000 population), followed by diseases of the genitourinary system (223.7) and diseases of the digestive system (192.6).

The diagnostic grouping with the largest number of discharges was heart and hypertensive diseases, with 2.6 million discharges.

For children under 15 years, the highest number of discharges by class was for diseases of the respiratory system, which had an estimated 1.4 million discharges and a rate of 256.0 per 10,000 population. Hypertrophy of tonsils and adenoids accounted for 46% of the children discharged in this diagnostic class and 17% of all discharges in this age group. The next highest classes were accidents, poisonings, and violence, with 557,000 discharges, and diseases of the digestive system, with 386,000. The discharge rates were 100.2 and 60.5 per 10,000 population, respectively. These three classes accounted for 60% of all discharged patients in this age group.

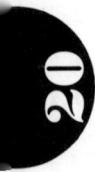

Diagnoses of Hospital Inpatients

Table 20-20   Diagnoses of inpatients discharged from short-stay hospitals—1974. (Excludes newborn infants and inpatients in federal hospitals.)

Diagnostic category	ICDA code	All discharges	Male	Female
All conditions		32,125	12,835	19,266
Excluding obstetrical conditions		28,154	12,835	15,295
Infective and parasitic diseases	000-136	790	379	409
Neoplasms	140-239	2,162	797	1,364
Malignant neoplasms	140-209	1,388	643	743
Benign neoplasms and neoplasms of unspecified nature	210-239	774	154	621
Endocrine, nutritional, and metabolic diseases	240-279	817	287	529
Diabetes mellitus	250	501	191	310
Diseases of the blood and blood-forming organs	280-289	274	116	157
Mental disorders	290-315	1,227	575	650
Diseases of the nervous system and sense organs	320-389	1,283	587	695
Diseases of the nervous system	320-358	455	199	256
Cataract	374	276	117	159
Other conditions and diseases of eye	360-373, 375-379	255	125	130
Diseases of ear and mastoid process	380-389	296	146	150
Diseases of the circulatory system	390-458	4,110	2,089	2,017
Heart and hypertensive disease:				
Acute myocardial infarction	410	354	233	121
Other ischemic heart disease	411-414	1,353	749	603
All other heart and hypertensive disease	390-404, 420-429	897	410	486
Cerebrovascular disease	430-438	602	282	320
Diseases of the respiratory system	460-519	3,427	1,725	1,699
Acute respiratory infections, except influenza	460-466	586	296	289
Pneumonia, all forms	480-486	726	396	330
Hypertrophy, of tonsils and adenoids	500	898	404	493
Diseases of the digestive system	520-577	3,999	1,945	2,052
Ulcer of stomach, duodenum, and gastrojejunal ulcer	531-534	405	240	165
Appendicitis	540-543	305	171	134
Inguinal hernia	550, 552	497	442	55
Cholelithiasis, cholecystitis, and cholangitis	574, 575	558	139	418
Diseases of the genitourinary system	580-629	3,390	1,006	2,383
Diseases of urinary system	580-599	1,205	527	678
Hyperplasia of prostate	600	232	232	—
Disorders of menstruation	626	551	—	551
Complications of pregnancy, childbirth, and the puerperium	630-678	3,971	—	3,971
Diseases of the skin and subcutaneous tissue	680-709	514	243	270
Diseases of the musculoskeletal system and connective tissue	710-738	1,548	666	881
Arthritis, all forms	710-718	448	173	275
Displacement of intervertebral disc	725	335	186	148
Congenital anomalies	740-759	322	172	150
Certain causes of perinatal morbidity and mortality	772, 774-778	19	10	8
Symptoms and ill-defined conditions	780-792, 794-796	586	277	306
Accidents, poisonings, and violence	800-999	3,351	1,864	1,483
Fractures, all sites	800-829	1,150	597	552
Intracranial injury (excluding those with skull fracture)	850-854	303	196	107
Laceration and open wound	870-907	388	279	108
Special conditions and examinations without sickness or tests with negative findings	793, Y00-Y13	337	97	240

Source: National Center for Health Statistics, June 10, 1975.

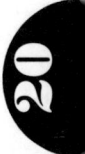

Table 20-21   Hospital patients: length of stay by ailment

Condition	All patients	<15	15–44	45–64	65+	White	Nonwhite	Male	Female
Total, all conditions	7.8	4.7	5.8	9.1	13.3	7.8	8.1	8.3	7.8
Infective and parasitic disease	9.1	6.2	9.2	11.3	12.2	8.2	14.8	9.7	8.6
Neoplasms	10.5	7.1	7.1	9.7	14.6	10.5	11.3	11.4	10.0
A. Malignant	14.1	11.0	11.1	12.1	15.5	14.1	16.1	13.9	14.3
1. Sex-specific	10.6	—	8.0	9.6	12.9	10.3	12.5	13.2	9.4
a. male	13.2	—	—	10.8	13.6	13.1	16.7	13.2	—
b. female	9.4	—	8.0	9.4	11.8	9.0	10.9	—	9.4
2. Not sex-specific	14.9	11.0	12.5	12.6	16.0	14.8	17.6	14.0	15.7
B. Benign	6.2	5.4	5.9	6.6	8.7	6.2	7.0	5.3	6.5
1. Sex-specific	7.3	5.9	7.3	7.2	7.4	7.2	8.0	—	7.3
a. male	—	—	—	—	—	—	—	—	—
b. female	7.3	5.9	7.3	7.2	7.4	7.2	8.0	—	7.3
2. Not sex-specific	6.2	5.4	4.4	5.9	8.9	5.4	5.8	5.3	6.5
Allergic, endocrine, metabolic and nutritional condition	9.6	6.8	7.0	9.3	13.1	9.3	11.4	9.9	9.4
A. Hay fever, asthma	7.6	6.1	5.7	7.3	12.4	7.6	8.4	8.6	6.9
B. Diabetes mellitus	11.2	7.1	8.4	10.9	13.3	10.9	13.7	10.9	11.5
C. Other	8.1	7.6	6.5	7.8	11.8	7.8	11.2	10.6	7.7
Conditions of blood and blood-forming organs	9.8	6.3	9.9	10.1	14.9	9.8	12.1	9.1	10.5
Mental, psychoneurotic, and personality disorders	11.2	11.2	10.7	4.3	7.5	10.9	12.9	10.5	11.9
Conditions of the nervous system and sense organs	10.1	4.7	8.8	10.1	14.9	10.1	13.2	9.8	10.6
A. Conditions of ear and mastoid process	4.0	2.9	4.2	4.3	7.5	4.0	6.8	3.5	4.6
B. Cataract and other conditions of eye	6.4	2.9	5.7	4.4	7.7	6.4	7.1	6.1	6.6
C. Other	13.6	10.4	11.6	13.7	18.6	13.4	16.0	13.1	14.0
Conditions of the circulatory system	11.7	5.9	9.7	11.1	13.7	11.7	13.2	11.5	12.0
A. Congestive heart failure	12.6	6.5	10.8	10.8	13.2	12.8	12.5	11.7	13.4
B. Arteriosclerosis	16.1	—	12.0	13.4	17.2	15.8	25.4	15.7	16.6
C. Other	12.4	5.7	9.7	11.1	13.6	11.5	12.9	11.4	13.4
Conditions of the respiratory system	5.8	3.4	5.4	8.2	12.0	5.8	6.2	5.9	5.6
A. Upper respiratory infection, acute	4.8	4.1	4.3	5.6	8.8	4.9	4.6	4.4	5.2
B. Pneumonia	9.0	6.2	7.5	9.1	14.1	9.3	8.1	8.3	9.8
C. Bronchitis, acute	6.3	4.4	5.2	8.0	9.1	6.3	6.2	6.4	6.3
D. Other	4.7	2.4	5.2	8.2	11.3	4.7	6.7	4.7	4.6
Conditions of the digestive system	7.5	4.2	6.1	8.4	10.8	7.5	8.2	7.3	7.9
A. Ulcers of stomach, duodenum, jejunum	9.8	7.8	7.9	9.8	12.8	9.6	10.4	9.4	10.5
B. Appendicitis	6.3	5.3	5.5	8.6	11.1	6.3	6.8	6.0	6.6
C. Inguinal hernia	6.6	3.2	6.3	7.5	9.9	6.7	6.6	6.7	5.4
D. Cholelithiasis and cholecystitis	10.1	11.1	8.3	9.9	12.6	10.2	10.9	11.0	9.8
E. Other	7.0	4.1	5.4	7.8	10.1	7.0	8.0	6.6	7.3
Conditions of the genitourinary system	6.6	4.3	5.3	6.8	11.6	6.6	7.4	7.8	6.0
A. Cystitis	5.7	3.7	4.6	5.5	9.1	5.5	6.3	6.3	5.6
B. Sex-specific	6.7	3.4	5.5	6.6	12.4	6.8	6.5	8.8	5.9
1. male	8.8	3.2	5.2	8.0	13.2	9.0	7.7	8.8	—
2. female	5.9	4.6	5.5	6.0	10.3	6.0	6.1	—	5.9
C. Other	6.7	5.0	5.1	7.3	11.0	7.1	9.1	7.1	6.4
Deliveries and complications of pregnancy, childbirth, and puerperium	3.8	3.5	3.8	3.7	—	3.8	3.8	—	3.8
A. Abortion	3.5	2.9	3.5	2.8	—	3.1	5.9	—	3.5
B. Normal delivery	3.8	3.4	3.8	3.8	—	3.9	3.3	—	3.8
C. Delivery with complications	4.7	4.3	4.7	5.3	—	4.8	4.5	—	4.7
D. Other	2.9	2.8	2.9	—	—	2.9	3.7	—	2.9

20

Table 20-21 **(continued)**

Condition	All patients	<15	15–44	45–64	65+	White	Nonwhite	Male	Female
Conditions of skin and cellular tissues	7.7	4.9	5.7	9.4	13.1	7.5	8.9	7.4	7.9
Diseases of bones and organs of movement	10.5	6.6	8.3	9.8	12.8	7.5	10.1	9.2	11.4
A. Osteoarthritis	11.3	—	7.6	10.8	12.7	11.3	11.8	10.8	11.7
B. Other	10.2	6.6	8.3	9.6	12.9	6.9	9.9	8.9	11.4
Congenital malformation	8.6	8.5	7.0	10.3	15.6	8.4	13.7	8.7	8.4
Certain conditions of early infancy	9.9	10.8	—	—	—	9.7	13.2	9.0	11.0
Miscellaneous or ill-defined symptoms or conditions	6.2	4.0	4.9	6.4	10.3	6.1	7.0	5.8	6.5
Injuries and adverse external effects	8.6	5.7	7.3	9.2	18.6	8.7	8.6	7.5	10.1
A. Fractures	12.5	7.8	11.2	11.7	23.9	12.8	11.6	10.6	14.7
B. Sprains, strains of back and neck	7.3	5.2	6.9	7.6	9.3	7.3	7.6	6.7	7.9
C. Lacerations	5.2	4.3	5.1	6.4	5.6	5.3	5.4	5.1	5.5
D. Other	6.6	4.6	6.1	8.1	10.6	6.5	8.3	6.3	7.1

Source: National Center for Health Statistics, March 1973.

Patients Hospitalized—By Age, Sex and Length of Stay

Table 20-22 **Number and rate of inpatients discharged and average length of stay: U.S. 1973 (short-stay hospitals—excludes newborn infants and federal hospitals)**

Age	Both sexes[1]	Male	Female Including deliveries	Female Excluding deliveries
Number of discharges in thousands				
All ages	32,125	12,835	19,266	16,173
Under 15 years	3,933	2,231	1,700	1,685
15–44 years	13,482	3,873	9,598	6,524
45–64 years	7,772	3,637	4,131	4,126
65 years and over	6,937	3,094	3,837	3,837
Rate of discharges per 1,000 population				
All ages	156.1	129.2	180.9	151.8
Under 15 years	70.8	78.8	62.4	61.8
15–44 years	154.4	91.7	212.9	144.7
45–64 years	182.2	179.1	185.0	184.8
65 years and over	341.8	367.0	323.5	323.5
Average length of stay in days				
All ages	7.8	8.3	7.4	8.1
Under 15 years	4.5	4.5	4.6	4.6
15–44 years	5.7	6.8	5.2	5.8
45–64 years	9.1	9.3	9.0	9.0
65 years and over	12.1	11.6	12.5	12.5

[1]Figures include data for sex not stated.

Source: National Center for Health Statistics, August 1975.

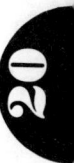

398

Hospital Patients—Frequency of Hospitalization

Table 20-23   Distribution of persons by number of hospital episodes according to sex and age (short-stay hospitals), 1974

Sex and age	Popu- lation	Number of hospital episodes				Popu- lation	Number of hospital episodes			
		None	1	2	3+		None	1	2	3+
Both sexes	**Number of persons in thousands**					**Percent distribution**				
All ages	207,344	185,162	18,434	2,790	958	100.0	89.3	8.9	1.3	0.5
Under 17 years	62,957	59,383	3,164	320	90	100.0	94.3	5.0	0.5	0.1
17–24 years	29,564	26,218	2,938	314	94	100.0	88.7	9.9	1.1	0.3
25–34 years	28,866	25,034	3,312	417	102	100.0	86.7	11.5	1.4	0.4
35–44 years	22,352	19,858	2,048	306	141	100.0	88.8	9.2	1.4	0.6
45–64 years	42,864	37,413	4,343	826	282	100.0	87.3	10.1	1.9	0.7
65 years and over	20,741	17,255	2,629	607	250	100.0	83.2	12.7	2.9	1.2
Male	**Number of persons in thousands**					**Percent distribution**				
All ages	100,030	91,212	7,179	1,202	436	100.0	91.2	7.2	1.2	0.4
Under 17 years	32,080	30,178	1,663	188	50	100.0	94.1	5.2	0.6	0.2
17–24 years	14,254	13,366	771	91		100.0	93.8	5.4	0.6	
25–34 years	13,959	12,972	840	110	37	100.0	92.9	6.0	0.8	0.3
35–44 years	10,740	9,866	708	109	57	100.0	91.9	6.6	1.0	0.5
45–64 years	20,420	17,796	2,064	406	155	100.0	87.1	10.1	2.0	0.8
65 years and over	8,578	7,033	1,134	300	111	100.0	82.0	13.2	3.5	1.3
Female	**Number of persons in thousands**					**Percent distribution**				
All ages	107,314	93,950	11,254	1,588	522	100.0	87.5	10.5	1.5	0.5
Under 17 years	30,878	29,205	1,501	132	39	100.0	94.6	4.9	0.4	0.1
17–24 years	15,310	12,852	2,167	224	68	100.0	83.9	14.2	1.5	0.4
25–34 years	14,907	12,062	2,472	307	65	100.0	80.9	16.6	2.1	0.4
35–44 years	11,612	9,991	1,340	197	84	100.0	86.0	11.5	1.7	0.7
45–64 years	22,444	19,617	2,279	420	127	100.0	87.4	10.2	1.9	0.6
65 years and over	12,163	10,222	1,495	307	139	100.0	84.0	12.3	2.5	1.1

Source: DHEW, 1976.

20

Surgical Operations

By Hospital Type

Hospitals with fewer than 100 beds show a progressive decline since 1970 in the importance of the surgical component of their services, in relation to the number of patients admitted.

Table 20-24   Surgical operations by hospital type

Hospital classification	Number of hospitals	Surgical operations	Admissions	Surgical operations as percentage of admissions
United States	7,156	17,418,335	36,156,516	48.1
6–24 beds	382	61,259	215,218	
25–49	1,363	446,933	1,588,789	
50–99	1,720	1,426,499	3,927,043	
100–199	1,552	3,439,284	7,297,493	
200–299	786	3,401,476	6,435,715	
300–399	441	2,627,451	4,980,536	
400–499	298	2,110,717	3,969,905	
500 or more	614	3,904,717	7,741,817	
Psychiatric	570	27,071	678,849	
Hospitals	505	22,213	664,775	
Institutions for mentally retarded	65	4,858	14,074	
General	6,230	17,112,796	35,019,313	
Hospitals	6,095	17,085,076	34,923,884	
Hospital units of institutions	135	27,720	95,429	
TB and other respiratory diseases	36	5,094	16,898	
Obstetrics and gynecology	24	41,158	71,034	
Eye, ear, nose, and throat	22	79,212	80,798	
Rehabilitation	69	8,243	47,665	
Orthopedic	34	32,859	44,556	
Chronic disease	63	3,465	23,819	
All other	108	108,438	173,584	
Federal	382	671,501	1,913,227	
Psychiatric	26	4,384	74,722	
General and other special	356	667,117	1,838,505	
Nonfederal	6,774	16,746,835	34,243,289	
Psychiatric	544	22,687	604,127	
Hospitals	479	17,829	590,053	
Institutions for mentally retarded	65	4,858	14,074	
TB and other respiratory diseases	36	5,094	16,898	
Long-term general and other special	215	31,170	103,084	
Short-term general and other special	5,979	16,687,884	33,519,180	
Hospital units of institutions	104	24,038	84,521	
Community hospitals	5,875	16,663,846	33,434,659	
6–24 beds	299	49,965	173,983	28.7
25–49	1,155	398,945	1,431,306	27.9
50–99	1,481	1,358,750	3,674,859	37.0
100–199	1,363	3,366,015	7,016,749	40.0
200–299	678	3,328,238	6,173,824	53.7
300–399	378	2,540,855	4,738,735	53.6
400–499	230	2,027,376	3,688,645	54.9
500 or more	291	3,593,702	6,536,558	54.9
Nongovernment not-for-profit	3,339	12,578,929	23,721,535	53.0
Investor-owned (for-profit)	775	1,320,092	2,645,812	49.9
State and local government	1,761	2,764,825	7,067,312	39.1

Source: *Hospital Statistics, 1976 Edition.* Reprinted by permission of the American Hospital Association Annual Survey.

By Type of Operation

Table 20-25 Number of surgical operations for discharged inpatients by surgery class and operations, sex, and age—U.S. 1973. (Short-stay hospitals—excludes newborn infants and federal hospitals)

Surgical class, operation	All-listed operations	All ages		15 years and over
		Male	Female	
	Number of operations in thousands			
All operations	18,426	6,936	11,480	16,100
Neurosurgery	310	157	152	282
Ophthalmology	655	295	358	542
Extraction of lens	279	116	162	278
Otorhinolaryngology	1,835	903	930	840
Myringotomy	215	122	92	17
Tonsillectomy with or without adenoidectomy	884	398	486	237
Operations on thyroid, parathyroid, thymus and adrenals	80	17	64	77
Thyroidectomy	64	10	54	64
Vascular and cardiac surgery	718	410	308	670
Excision and ligation of varicose veins	98	24	74	98
Thoracic surgery	240	138	102	224
Abdominal surgery	2,747	1,357	1,389	2,431
Repair of inguinal hernia	525	464	61	409
Appendectomy[1]	339	175	163	236
Cholecystectomy	411	94	318	410
Resection of small intestine or colon	146	65	81	141
Proctological surgery	565	303	262	555
Local excision and destruction of lesion of rectum and anus	140	76	65	138
Hemorrhoidectomy	218	111	107	218
Urological surgery	1,453	1,032	420	1,205
Dilation of urethra	227	82	145	169
Prostatectomy	249	249	—	248
Breast surgery	336	19	317	331
Mastectomy	290	11	279	286
Gynecological surgery	3,565	—	3,565	3,544
Oophorectomy; salpingo-oophorectomy	425	—	425	424
Ligation and division of fallopian tubes (bilateral)	299	—	299	299
Hysterectomy	690	—	690	688
Dilation and curettage of uterus, diagnostic	934	—	934	931
Obstetrical procedures[2]	1,077	—	1,077	1,066
Cesarian section	246	—	246	245
Dilation and curettage after delivery or abortion	273	—	273	271
Repair of laceration	182	—	182	180
Orthopedic surgery	2,351	1,217	1,133	2,081
Excision of bone, partial	157	64	93	145
Closed reduction of fracture without fixation	321	174	147	218
Reduction of fracture with fixation	284	119	164	269
Excision of intervertebral cartilage (prolapsed disk)	147	86	61	146
Operations on muscles, tendons, fascia, and bursa	307	169	138	261
Plastic surgery	1,041	543	497	891
Oral and maxillofacial surgery	174	92	82	150
Dental surgery	358	153	204	323
Biopsy	919	300	618	888

[1]Limited to estimated number of appendectomies excluding those performed incidental to other abdominal surgery.
[2]Excludes certain obstetrical procedures for inducing or assisting delivery.

Source: National Center for Health Statistics, May 30, 1975.

By Patients' Having or Not Having Operation

Table 20-26   Number of inpatients discharged from hospitals with and without surgery, 1973. (Short stay hospitals—excludes newborn infants and federal hospitals)

Number of operations	All discharges	Without surgery	With surgery	Percent with surgery
	Number of inpatients discharged in thousands			
Total	32,125	18,859	13,266	41.3
1 operation			9,230	
2 operations			2,912	
3 operations			1,124	

Outpatient Surgery

Surgery on an Outpatient Basis *

The evidence suggests that up to one-fourth of surgical procedures now performed in hospitals might be performed without hospitalization. If up to 25% of surgical procedures can be performed with equal safety on an ambulatory basis, this would mean substantial savings for both consumers and taxpayers.

At least three factors contributing to this excess hospitalization include:

1. Consumers receive little, if any, insurance reimbursement if the surgery is not done on an inpatient basis.
2. Hospitals receive no compensation for unfilled beds and unused operating rooms.
3. Physician fee-for-service reimbursement discourages use of the ambulatory mode for minor surgical procedures.

Surgicenter—Phoenix, Arizona

When Surgicenter opened in 1970, charging an average of $70 for an operation ($120 average now), four hospitals in the Phoenix area lowered outpatient surgery fees 30 to 50%. The center then charged $95 for a D and C (with an additional $10 charge made by the pathologist for laboratory fees). The usual charge for the same operation, with a two-day stay in a Phoenix hospital, was about $300 at

that time. (Surgicenter has recently raised its fees, and a D and C now costs $121.)

The center has had an impact not only on the cost of ambulatory surgical care in Phoenix but also on the way such care is delivered. It is forcing hospital administrators to take a closer look at the high cost of their inpatient ambulatory surgery. If it is assumed that at least 75% of Surgicenter's patients would have been hospitalized for two days if the facility had not been available, then it follows that Surgicenter allowed Phoenix to use 34,500 fewer hospital days, from February, 1970, to September, 1974.

Unnecessary Surgery **

Number of Patients Undergoing Operations

The Commission on Professional and Hospital Activities (CPHA) found that 7.6 million patients were operated on during the first six months of 1975—an annualized estimate of 15.2 million.

Number of Unnecessary Operations

A House Subcommittee on Health used 17% as the rate of unnecessary surgical procedures. The primary source for this estimate was an HEW-funded study conducted by Dr. McCarthy Professor of Public Health, Cornell University Medical School. He found that 24% of all surgical procedures recommended were not confirmed. The proportion not confirmed in each surgical specialty, in descending order of frequency utilization, were:

	Percent
General surgery	16.4
Gynecology	16.4
Orthopedic	40.3
Ear, nose, and throat	16.3
Ophthalmology	28.2
Urology	35.8

Utilizing 17% of the procedures as unnecessary and 14 million as the total number of elective surgeries, the Subcommittee concluded that approximately 2,380,000 surgeries were unnecessarily performed in 1974. The Subcommittee determined that the American public spent *$3.92 billion* in 1974 on unnecessary surgery.

---

* Source: "Unnecessary Surgery," House Committee on Interstate & Foreign Commerce, January 1976.

** Source: "Unnecessary Surgery," House Committee on Interstate and Foreign Commerce, January 1976.

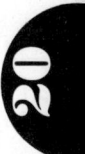

Second Opinions

Another study dealt with case histories of union employees in New York who had received an original opinion to operate and a second opinion arranged through the union. The voluntary program permitted a consumer to request a second consultation. The mandatory program required a second opinion prior to hospital admission for elective surgery.

Forty-six percent of the recommendations for hysterectomies were not confirmed under the voluntary program; 26% were not confirmed under the mandatory program.

Professional Competence

The chief of surgery at Johns Hopkins School of Medicine testified that 40% of operations performed in this country were performed by non-certified individuals who come from two groups:

1. non-certified specialist (two-thirds of whom have taken their certification examinations and failed them) and
2. general practitioners.

Mortality Due to Unnecessary Surgery

Another expert estimated that the mortality rate for elective surgery is 0.5% (it is higher for emergency surgery). If this rate is applied to unnecessary operations, the U.S. mortality due to unnecessary surgery may be 16,000 deaths per year.

This estimate of 16,000 deaths was based upon the 3.2 million surgical procedures deemed to be unnecessary.

HEW's Office of Research and Statistics published in 1975 an extensive study of Medicare recipients demonstrating a much higher mortality rate. This study, using 1967 data on hospital discharges, found that of 1,609,539 discharges with surgery, 85,222 patients were discharged dead representing a mortality rate of 5.2%.

Tonsillectomies

National data substantiates a major shift in the rates of tonsillectomies. In 1965, the rate per 100,000 population was 635.9 in the United States. In 1973, the rate per 100,000 population was 400.9, a drop of 23 out of every 100 people. The data also point out wide variations. John E. Wennberg, physician, Waterbury Center, Vermont, documented in his Vermont study that "for the tonsil, the probability of removal by age 26 ranges from 8% to 62% across 13 Vermont areas."

Data from 22 states providing complete information on tonsillectomies under their state Medicaid programs show a rate of 599 tonsillectomies per 100,000 population, with a total of 39,621 procedures reported for an eligible population of 6,609,684. The rates of tonsillectomies vary greatly among the states, ranging from 1,709 per 100,000 population in Nevada to 78 per 100,000 population in Mississippi. The following table details the rates of tonsillectomies in states with the highest rates, states with the lowest rates, and states closest to the national average under Medicaid:

Table 20-27   Select states' rates of tonsillectomies

	Tonsillectomies per 100,000 population
States with the highest rates:	
Nevada	1,709
Maine	1,324
Kansas	963
States with the lowest rates:	
Mississippi	78
Arkansas	179
Alabama	212
States with rates closest to the national average:	
Alaska	592
New Jersey	594
National average (22 states reporting)	599

Hysterectomies

Information on hysterectomies was provided by 22 states. A total of 20,016 procedures were reported for an eligible population of 6,609,684, for a rate of 303 hysterectomies per 100,000 population. The rates of hysterectomies varied greatly among the State medicaid programs, ranging from 2,488 per 100,000 population in Nevada to 34 per 100,000 population in Mississippi. The following data detail the rates of hysterectomies in states with the highest rates, states with the lowest rates, and states closest to the national average under Medicaid:

Table 20-28   Select states' rates of hysterectomies

	Hysterectomies per 100,000 population
States with the highest rates:	
Nevada	2,488
North Carolina	1,277
Louisiana	619
States with the lowest rates:	
Mississippi	34
Ohio	101
Arkansas	156
States with rates closest to the national average:	
Montana	305
Nebraska	306
National average (22 states reporting)	303

Hospital Infection Control*

Many of the thousands upon thousands of patients who go to the hospital every year do not recover. Some die because their illnesses are terminal. But every year, 50 to 100 thousand Americans who should have lived die from infections acquired in the hospital. (Bacteria can be transmitted through food or a contaminated water supply; some infections are airborne; spitting can cause "droplet" infection.)

A recent study in South Florida showed the prevalence of these infections: 1 out of 20 to 30 patients admitted to hospitals developed a hospital related infection.

Dr. Larry Edwards, an epidemiologist at Chicago's Presbyterian-St. Lukes Hospital, in charge of a four-year study (1969–1973) of 6000 cases each year, says hospital infections were the primary cause of death in 3 to 4% of the patients and a contributing factor in another 6 to 7%.

High risk cases (babies and young children, the elderly and debilitated, new post-operative

*Source: L. J. Carbary, "Hospital Acquired Infections," *Nursing Care,* Dec. 1975.

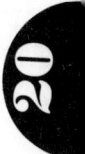

and postpartum patients, and those suffering from malnutrition, burns, or long-term illnesses like cancer or leukemia) are especially susceptible to infection because of poor germ immunity.

The growth of certain microorganisms is encouraged when such medicines as antibiotics and adrenal cortical hormones upset the immunization mechanism or the bacterial interrelations. The resulting superinfection, difficult to control, can be severe enough to cause death.

Viruses, bacteria, Rickettsiae, fungi, and animal parasites are the principal infection-causing agents. Infections can be transmitted by contact with someone afflicted with a communicable or infectious disease. Even utensils, linens, and instruments can carry infections.

JCAH Recommendations

The Joint Commission on the Accreditation of Hospitals recommended that the following measures for the control of infections be established through a committee made up of representatives of the medical staff, the administration, the microbiology laboratory, and the nursing service:

- Develop written standards for hospital sanitation and medical asepsis. These standards should include a definition of infection for the purpose of surveillance, as well as specific indications of the need for and the procedures to be used in isolation. Copies of the standards should be distributed and made readily available to all appropriate personnel.

- Develop, evaluate and revise on a continuing basis the procedures and techniques for meeting established sanitation and asepsis standards. This should include the routine evaluation of materials used in the hospital's sanitation program. The evaluation may be based upon data supplied from reputable sources or upon in-use tests performed within the hospital.

- Develop a practical system for reporting, evaluating and keeping records of infections among patients and personnel in order to provide an indication of the endemic level of all nosocomial infections, to trace the sources of infection and to identify epidemic or potential epidemic situations. Such a program is important not only for the pro-

tection of the patient, but also for the protection of the medical staff, of hospital employees, and of visitors.

- Review periodically the use of antibiotics as

they relate to patient care within the hospital.

- Provide assistance in the development of
the hospital's employee health program.

Table 20-29 Hospital-related infections, 1976

Hospital	Jan.	Feb.	Mar.	Apr.	May	June	July	Aug.	Sept.	Oct.	Nov.	Dec.
Rate of infection/100 discharged												
Community	2.6	2.8	2.8	2.5	2.6	2.5	2.7	2.5	2.5	2.4	2.5	2.5
Federal	5.2	5.1	4.5	4.2	4.5	4.5	5.8	5.5	4.1	5.2	4.7	4.8
Municipal	5.6	5.6	4.7	5.3	5.4	5.4	5.2	5.1	5.2	5.8	5.2	5.4
Community-teaching	3.7	4.0	3.8	3.3	3.3	3.5	3.7	3.6	3.5	3.5	3.7	3.4
University	5.0	4.6	4.6	4.1	3.8	3.7	3.6	3.5	3.9	3.4	3.5	3.7
Percentage of infections causing or contributing to death												
Community	3.8	2.8	3.0	3.6	3.8	2.7	3.3	2.2	2.3	3.0	2.0	2.6
Federal	7.0	5.6	5.4	2.5	3.5	2.5	4.5	4.9	2.0	4.8	.0	5.9
Municipal	8.2	7.6	6.4	8.7	4.0	7.6	7.9	2.3	9.6	6.9	9.0	3.4
Community-teaching	3.3	3.3	2.4	2.8	.8	3.1	1.9	1.8	2.3	2.7	2.8	1.6
University	2.2	.9	1.4	1.4	.3	3.0	2.7	1.4	2.4	2.2	3.9	1.2

Source: U.S. Center for Disease Control, January–December 1976.

Occupational Health and Safety in Hospitals*

Overview

Hospitals are now the third largest employer in
the United States, with approximately three
million employees working full and part-time.

Because the accident frequency rate for
hospitals has increased alarmingly during the
past ten years, the National Institute for Occupational Safety and Health conceived and implemented the Hospital Occupational Health
Services Study in 1972—the first such major
study ever conducted.

Among its findings were the following:

- Most hospitals provide some form of
general occupational health and safety
orientation for new employees.
- About half of the hospitals reported having a
formally organized program for employee
safety and health education. Again, analyzed
results showed that more of the large hospitals (70%), about half of the medium, and
only one-third of the small had formally organized programs.

*Source: National Institute of Occupational Safety
and Health, 1976.

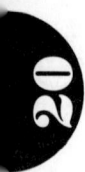

- Routine in-service training programs on
radiation exposure were *not* provided to employees in about 90% of the small hospitals,
75% of the medium and 60% of the large
hospitals. While this topic shows the highest
percentage with no training, other topics are
almost as high. For all hospitals, 55% have
no training for chemical exposures, 50%
have *no* training programs for infectious
disease exposure, 60% have *no* training for
safe use of equipment, 50% have *no* training
for use of personal protective equipment,
and 70% have *no* training for teaching
proper lifting and body mechanics. As expected, small hospitals had higher
percentages and large hospitals lower.
- Upon inquiry most hospitals indicated that
their safety committee had been assigned
the responsibility for managing their hospital's health and safety program.
- Respiratory problems ranked first as the
most frequent occupational health problem,
exclusive of injuries. Other infections ranked
second and dermatitis ranked third.
- Strains and sprains were the most
frequently reported types of occupational injuries listed by the total of all hospitals.
Puncture wounds were the second ranking
type of injury reported. Abrasions and
contusions took third place.

- In 80% of the hospitals, injuries and illnesses of employees on the job were treated in the Emergency Room. About 10% of all hospitals reported using an Employee Health Unit, and these were predominantly among large hospitals. Only a third of those hospitals which had separate facilities for employee health care reported use of the Emergency Room in addition to an employee health unit for treatment of employee illness or injury.
- In general, the findings reveal that nearly 50% of all hospitals stated that the Emergency Room Staff provided the day-to-day health care services for hospital workers. About 10% named the Occupational Health Nurse or the Floor Nurse. In 40% of the large hospitals, an Occupational Health Nurse was specified as the primary source of employee health care.

Hospital Employee Health Care Services*

Table 20-30   Estimated day-to-day employee health care services by service source and hospital size

Primary source of service	Total	Small	Medium	Large
Total	100.0	100.0	100.0	100.0
Occupational health nurse	11.0	1.4	13.2	39.8
Floor nurse	10.0	18.5	1.7	0.1
House physician	7.9	8.1	8.1	6.8
Outpatient department staff	7.0	8.0	5.3	7.1
Emergency room staff	45.7	39.8	61.3	29.1
Other	14.5	18.7	7.8	15.4
None	3.9	5.5	2.5	1.7

Percent / Hospital size[1]

[1]Hospital size based upon number of beds: (Small: 25–99) (Medium: 100–299) (Large: 300 +).

It is interesting to note that over 70% of small hospitals delegated employee medical treatment to the Employee's Family Physician.

It was found that applicants for full-time employment were given physical examinations by more reporting hospitals than were applicants for part-time employment. About 85% of

the hospitals conducted physical examinations on former groups, and 75% on the latter. Only about one-third of all hospitals required a physical examination for employees returning from illness or absence, while the study indicated that almost no hospitals required terminating employees to have physical examinations.

Only about 10% of all hospitals (7.7%) reported they had no formal policy with respect to pregnancy. However, less than 40% of the hospitals required early reporting of pregnancy, and less than 15% reassigned pregnant workers to safer working conditions. Very few hospitals (4.8%) provided for pre- and post-natal counseling of pregnant hospital employees. Medical clearance to continue employment while pregnant was a requirement in almost two-thirds of the hospitals, and almost 90% granted maternity leave.

Disasters

Hospital Disaster Plan Provisions**

The disaster plan should be developed in conjunction with other emergency facilities in the community so that adequate logistical provisions are made for the expansion of the hospital's activities in coordination with the activities of these facilities. Planning should include consultation with local civil authorities and with representatives of other medical agencies in order to establish an effective chain of command and to make appropriate jurisdictional provisions. Such planning should result in disaster site triage and distribution of patients that make most efficient use of available facilities and services.

The disaster plan should make provision, within the hospital, for:

- Availability of adequate basic utilities and supplies, including gas, water, food and essential medical and supportive materials.
- An efficient system of notifying and assigning personnel.
- Unified medical command.
- Conversion of all usable space into clearly

*Source: National Institute of Occupational Safety and Health, 1976.

**Source: "Hospital Disaster Plan," *Accreditation Manual for Hospitals*, Joint Commission on Accreditation of Hospitals, DHEW Pub. No. DEH-7.

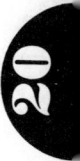

defined areas for efficient triage, for patient observation and for immediate care.

- Prompt transfer of casualties when necessary and after preliminary medical or surgical services have been rendered, to the facility most appropriate for administering definitive care.
- A special disaster medical record, such as an appropriately designed tag, that accompanies the casualty as he is moved.
- Procedures for the prompt discharge or transfer of patients in the hospital who can be moved without jeopardy.
- Maintaining security in order to keep relatives and curious persons out of the triage area.
- Preestablishment of a public information center and assignment of public relations liaison duties to a qualified individual. Advance arrangements with communications media will help to provide organized dissemination of information.

Patient Reactions to Disaster

The American Psychiatric Association Committee on Civil Defense has identified five types of reactions to disaster.

1. Normal—Some obvious signs of disturbance are shown, such as trembling, profuse perspiring, feeling weak and even nauseated. Composure is gained fairly soon after the first impact of a trying experience.

2. Individual panic—Judgment seems to disappear and to be supplanted by an unreasoning attempt to flee. This type of reaction occurs in a very few individuals; its danger lies in the fact that it can excite others and may result in mass panic.

3. Depressed reactions—These individuals react as though they were numbed; they are unable to help themselves without guidance.

4. Overly active responses—These responses are poorly directed, because the individual is easily distracted as he jumps from one task to another. Often he is intolerant of any ideas other than his own and may cause disturbances.

5. Bodily reactions—Severe nausea and vomiting, hysteria.

21
NURSING HOMES

Historical and Legislative Background*

At the turn of the 20th century, nursing homes, as they are known today, were virtually non-existent in the United States. Older Americans who were sick or disabled usually looked to their families or close friends to provide them with personal needs and assistance. Only the most destitute aged who were in need of institutional care became wards of the public and often residents of the Nation's almshouses or county poorfarms.

Over the next 30 years, dramatic increases in the number of persons reaching old age, and a complex series of social and economic changes in our society, led to increasing numbers of dependent older Americans without any private means of providing for themselves during their later years. In response to these developments, some of the states adopted and financed programs of cash assistance for the needy aged. By 1931, 18 states had established such programs. However, with the collapse of the economy during the Depression, increased numbers of persons sought public assistance. At the same time, state tax revenues used to finance public aid declined. The states turned to the federal government for financial relief. Congress responded by enacting the Social Security Act of 1935. Title I of this Act established a program of Old-Age Assistance (OAA), authorizing limited federal matching of state expenditures for cash assistance grants to the needy aged.

Of special importance in the development of the nation's system of nursing home care was a provision of Title I prohibiting federal matching of assistance payments made to persons residing in "public institutions." This prohibition was intended to discourage the states from using the pre-Depression poorhouse system as a means for dealing with the growing problems of aged dependency. However, cash grants could be paid those residing in private homes or facilities. Within a few years, proprietary homes, some of which offered limited medical care, began to appear throughout the United States.

During the 1950s other important changes were made:

- the prohibition against payments to persons in public institutions was removed for those who resided in public *medical* institutions
- states which provided federally matched cash assistance to institutionalized persons (including nursing home patients) were required to establish state standards for such facilities.

In 1960, amendments to the Act provided for an expansion of the federal role in financing the medical care of the aged; the amendments, known as the Kerr-Mills amendments, provided for:

- more favorable federal matching for states making improvements in their medical vendor payment programs for OAA recipients
- a new federal matching program, titled Medical Assistance for the Aged (MAA), for the medically indigent. Skilled nursing services were among the services for which federal matching was available, if covered by a state MAA program.

The 1965 amendments to the Social Security Act (Medicare) provided for financing of up to 100 days of extended care services for persons 65 and over in a certified facility during a single spell of illness. The Act covers specifically post-hospital extended care for continuation of necessary medical treatment (following discharge after a minimum stay of three days in a hospital) in an institution (or distinct part thereof) that provides a level of care distinguished from the level of intensive care ordinarily furnished by a hospital.

The enactment of Title XIX of the Social Security Act in 1965 (Medicaid) also had a marked effect on the provision of nursing home care in this country. The law and subsequent amendments specify that, among the services, states administering medical assistance programs under Title XIX must offer skilled nursing services and home health services to individuals over 21 who qualify for benefits under the program.

The 1972 amendments to the Social Security Act established a new name to reflect the common set of standards for institutions formerly identified as extended care facilities under Medicare and as skilled nursing homes

---

*Source: *Nursing Home Care in the United States,* Senate Special Subcommittee on Aging, November 1974.

under Medicaid. The name of these institutions is now *skilled nursing facilities.*

Title XIX of the Social Security Act also recognized another level of institutional care called "intermediate care." This is care in an *intermediate care facility* (ICF). Intermediate care facilities provide health-related care and services to those who do not need care in skilled nursing facilities but require institutional care beyond room and board. Under new regulations, institutions for the mentally retarded and institutions for victims of cerebral palsy, epilepsy, or other neurological conditions defined under the Developmental Disabilities Act could qualify as ICFs if they provided health and rehabilitative services. Recognition of ICFs became necessary because many elderly persons needed long-term institutional care, although they did not need the level and degree of care available in skilled nursing facilities under Titles XVIII and XIX.*

The Nursing Home Industry

Growth of the Nursing Home Industry**

One of the first inventories of the nation's nursing home industry was a 1939 study on institutional mortality by the Bureau of the Census, which counted 1,200 facilities and 25,000 beds. By 1960, there were 9,582 homes and 33,000 beds. Between 1960 and 1970, the number of nursing homes and related facilities increased 140% to 23,000.

Nursing homes can be classified by the level of care they provide. In 1972, there were 9,244 skilled nursing facilities with 643,403 beds; there were 4,455 intermediate care facilities with 217,922 beds and 9,292 related facilities with 238,087 beds.

In 1974, some 7,300 facilities qualified for Medicaid benefits as skilled nursing facilities. About 4,000 were also certified to participate as extended care facilities under Medicare. A few hundred qualified only for Medicare. About 8,500 participate in the Medicaid intermediate care program.

● There are more nursing home beds (1,235,-404) in the United States than general and surgical hospital beds (1,006,951).

---

*Source: *Health Resources Statistics*, DHEW, 1976.
**Source: *Nursing Home Care in the United States*, Senate Special Subcommittee on Aging, November 1974.

● There are more than three times as many nursing homes (23,000) than hospitals (6,-630).
● More inpatient days of care were given in long-term care facilities (384.2 million) than in short-term general hospitals (262.7 million).
● Expenditures for long-term care increased 640% from $500 million in 1960 to $3.7 billion in 1973 (less conservative estimates place the nursing home industry's total operating outlays at $6.2 billion).
● For the first time, Medicaid expenditures in 1972 for nursing home care exceeded payments to general and surgical hospitals: $1.6 billion (34%) as compared to $1.5 billion (31%).

Characteristics of the Industry

Growing government involvement—Public funds account for about $2 out of every $3 in nursing home revenues. There are few industries so dependent on government.

Average size—In 1971, 53 beds; 59% had fewer than 50 beds.

Seventy-seven percent of the nursing homes in the United States are operated for profit—and these proprietary homes control 67% of the beds. Fifteen percent of the U.S. nursing homes are philanthropic, accounting for 25% of the beds. Eight percent of the homes and beds are government controlled.

There is very little agreement as to the average cost of nursing home care in the United States—There are great variations from study to study. The range is $200 to $1,200 per month. HEW studies are underway to determine more definitive cost data.

Many studies confuse average charges with costs. Charges reflect what nursing homes bill private paying patients. There is some agreement that the average monthly charge for U.S. nursing homes is now about $600. Cost relates to how much operators must spend to provide quality care; many provide it for far less than $600 a month.

There is also very little agreement as to the number of nursing home beds that are needed—No firm national data are available. The few studies available indicate a national vacancy rate of 13.2%. Others suggest a need of 173,797 beds in 1973. Many locales will have a relatively high number of empty beds, but an acute shortage of beds for welfare or Medicaid patients.

The growth in both size and number of

nursing homes is startling—It can be seen in the increase in the number of patients. There were 290,000 patients in 1960 and 900,000 in 1970, for a 210% increase. By 1973 there were more than 1 million patients.

Characteristics by Ownership *

Of the nursing homes represented in the 1973–74 survey, an estimated 75% were operated under proprietary auspices while 25% were operated under nonprofit (nonproprietary and government) auspices (Table 21-1). Proprietary homes had the greater proportion of all beds (71%) and residents (70%), although the average size of these homes (70 beds) was smaller than that for the nonprofit homes (88 beds).

In addition to being larger, the nonprofit homes had a substantially larger number of FTE employees per 100 beds (83.5) than did the proprietary homes (57.4).

For the period of August 1973 to April 1974, the national estimates projected from the sample indicated some 15,700 nursing homes in the United States had a total of

*Source: DHEW, December 1975.

1,174,800 beds and served 1,075,800 residents. The average facility had available 63.9 FTEs (full-time employees) per 100 beds, of whom about 61% were employed as part of the nursing staff. Seventy-four percent of those on the nursing staff were classified as nurse's aides. During the 1973–74 period, the average monthly charge per resident for all aspects of care was $479. Almost 46% of the homes had average monthly charges of less than $400 and fully 71% had charges under $500.

In 1972 these nursing homes provided around 369 million resident days of care and experienced an average occupancy rate of 88.2%.

A survey made in 1973–74 by the Senate Special Subcommittee on Aging found that 106 publicly held corporations controlled 18% of the industry's beds and accounted for one-third of the industry's $3.2 billion in revenue (as of 1972). Between 1969 and 1972 these corporations experienced the following growth:

- 122.6% in total assets;
- 149.5% in gross revenues; and
- 116% in average net income.

Table 21-1   Financial and operating characteristics of U.S. nursing homes by ownership and size of facility, 1973

Operating and financial characteristics	Total	Proprietary	Nonprofit	Less than 50 beds	50–99 beds	100–199 beds	200 beds or more
Operating characteristics							
Number of homes (1973–1974)	15,700	11,900	3,900	6,400	5,500	3,200	600
Number of beds (1973–1974)	1,174,800	830,700	344,300	179,400	392,800	414,500	188,100
Average bed size (1973–1974)	75	70	88	28	71	130	314
Average total FTE employees per 100 beds	63.9	57.4	83.5	69.0	60.0	60.2	64.1
Nursing FTE employees per 100 beds	38.7	36.7	44.1	39.6	37.8	38.6	37.9
Administrative, medical, and therapeutic FTE employees per 100 beds	4.6	4.9	3.8	6.6	3.4	2.9	3.3
All other FTE employees per 100 beds	20.6	15.6	35.5	22.8	18.8	18.7	22.9
Number of residents (1973–1974)	1,075,800	756,200	319,700	162,600	367,700	386,100	159,300
Number of resident days of care (1972)	368,906,000	260,449,600	108,456,400	58,611,900	126,359,600	129,437,700	54,496,800
Average occupancy rate (1972)	88.2	88.8	86.5	88.5	89.1	86.3	83.9

Source: DHEW, December 1975.

Nursing Home Residents, Beds and Employees

Table 21-2   Nursing homes by type

	All homes	Nursing care homes	Personal care and other homes
Nursing home residents/1000 U.S. citizens 65 years and over	56.1	47.4	8.7
Nursing home beds/1000 U.S. citizens 65 years and over	62.3	51.9	10.3
Nursing home full-time-equivalent employees/1000 beds:			
R.N.s	4.4		
L.P.N.s	5.7		
Aides	28.6		

Source: DHEW, May 1976.

Patient turnover*—Admissions per bed. Nationally, the number of admissions per bed was 0.86. In other words, 86 out of every 100 beds "turned over" when a current resident was discharged and a new resident admitted. Homes certified by both Medicare and Medicaid had the highest turnover rate—1.27 admissions per bed. Beds in other types of homes turned over less frequently than once a year; rates ranged from 0.55 to 0.71.

This high turnover for homes certified by both Medicare and Medicaid was probably due to two factors influencing length of stay. The first was the short-term nature of the care needed by the Medicare resident. Since Medicare residents are admitted to ECFs (Extended Care Facilities) following discharge from a hospital stay, many of these residents were recuperating from an operation or illness and were discharged upon recovery. The second factor was the Title XVIII limit on length of stay due to the provision that Medicare will pay for *up to* 100 days of skilled nursing care in a Medicare-approved home.

*Source: DHEW, September 5, 1974.

Number of Residents in Nursing Homes by State

Table 21-3   Nursing care and related homes by type, number of residents and state, 1973

State	Total homes	Nursing care	Personal care and other homes	Total residence	Nursing care	Personal care and other homes[1]
United States	21,834	14,873	6,961	1,197,517	1,011,092	186,425
Alabama	197	188	9	14,138	13,350	788
Alaska	8	8	—	477	477	—
Arizona	88	75	13	5,671	5,332	339
Arkansas	211	199	12	16,179	15,404	775
California	4,145	1,618	2,527	130,278	100,742	29,536
Colorado	214	179	35	15,181	13,783	1,398
Connecticut	365	261	104	22,124	18,553	3,571
Delaware	36	34	2	2,081	2,071	10
District of Columbia	72	43	29	2,711	2,434	277
Florida	360	297	63	29,666	25,069	4,597
Georgia	306	285	21	24,518	23,174	1,344
Hawaii	142	41	101	2,490	1,967	523
Idaho	64	58	6	3,825	3,693	132
Illinois	1,039	786	253	72,319	60,998	11,321
Indiana	495	417	78	30,755	26,798	3,957
Iowa	678	464	214	31,906	24,591	7,315
Kansas	468	305	163	21,126	16,460	4,666
Kentucky	312	187	125	16,169	11,865	4,304

Table 21-3   (continued)

State	Total homes	Nursing care	Personal care and other homes	Total residence	Nursing care	Personal care and other homes[1]
Louisiana	212	202	10	16,040	15,666	374
Maine	341	168	173	8,679	7,315	1,364
Maryland	204	175	29	16,660	15,187	1,473
Massachusetts	945	754	191	50,197	43,271	6,926
Michigan	577	444	133	43,082	36,860	6,222
Minnesota	589	441	148	41,107	34,786	6,321
Mississippi	143	126	17	7,423	7,086	337
Missouri	502	415	87	30,819	26,827	3,992
Montana	105	79	26	4,511	3,765	746
Nebraska	251	195	56	15,834	13,325	2,509
Nevada	41	23	18	1,292	1,031	261
New Hampshire	130	106	24	5,480	4,925	555
New Jersey	549	356	193	31,569	25,857	5,712
New Mexico	66	43	23	2,828	2,268	560
New York	1,083	691	392	86,151	63,439	22,712
North Carolina	838	231	607	19,788	12,693	7,095
North Dakota	107	63	44	6,268	4,338	1,930
Ohio	1,163	1,015	148	59,243	53,305	5,938
Oklahoma	417	386	31	26,365	25,270	1,095
Oregon	312	218	94	16,945	13,135	3,810
Pennsylvania	768	666	102	60,895	53,724	7,171
Rhode Island	159	113	46	6,163	5,326	837
South Carolina	123	110	13	7,586	7,062	524
South Dakota	160	114	46	7,294	6,212	1,082
Tennessee	244	213	31	13,675	11,997	1,678
Texas	967	873	94	71,235	65,882	5,353
Utah	120	92	28	4,245	3,674	571
Vermont	101	71	30	3,441	2,974	467
Virginia	348	198	150	14,965	12,479	2,486
Washington	382	327	55	28,291	25,475	2,816
West Virginia	137	75	62	4,329	3,290	1,039
Wisconsin	516	421	95	41,791	34,484	7,307
Wyoming	34	24	10	1,712	1,403	309
Total beds				1,327,704	1,107,358	220,346

[1]Includes personal care homes with nursing, personal care homes without nursing and domiciliary care homes.

Source: DHEW, 1975.

Financing

Public and Private Sources of Income*

Approximately $9 billion was spent on nursing home care in the United States in fiscal year 1975; of this amount, $5.2 billion came from public sources. In fiscal year 1974 the average nursing home charges in the United States were about $600 a month. Average Social Security benefits for a retired couple amount to $310 a month.

*Sources: House Subcommittee on Oversight and Investigations, July 1975; Senate Special Subcommittee on Aging, November 1974.

Table 21-4 Expenditures and source of funds, 1950 to 1975

	Total expenditures	Source of funds Private	Source of funds Public	Public expenditures as percent of total expenditures
1950	$178	$167	$11	6.2
1955	291	244	47	16.2
1960	480	353	127	26.5
1965	1,271	822	449	35.3
1970	3,818	2,145	1,673	43.8
1971	4,890	2,919	1,971	40.3
1972	5,860	3,395	2,465	42.1
1973	6,650	3,386	3,264	49.1
1974	7,450	3,504	3,946	53.0
1975	9,000	3,799	5,209	57.8

Source: Social Security.

Table 21-5 Nursing home expenditures, by source, fiscal year 1974

Source	Amount (millions)	Percent
Public assistance	$3,597	48
Patients or family	3,474	47
Medicare	224	3
Veterans' program	125	2
Other	30	—
Total	7,450	100

Source: Social Security.

The great majority of the payments made by patients and their families are paid out of their own incomes, savings, or other personal resources without help from private insurance. Private insurance has provided little coverage because of the difficulty of distinguishing between medically oriented care and custodial care and the high costs that can result unless coverage is carefully limited. For example, Blue Cross plans, which underwrite 88% of the private insurance plans with nursing home benefits that are held by the aged, paid out only one-quarter of one percent of the nation's FY 1973 nursing home bill. Thus, of the total paid for nursing home care, about half is paid by public assistance and a slightly smaller portion is paid out of individuals' incomes and savings.

Table 21-6 Distribution of nursing home residents (for one month or more) by age and sex, according to primary source of payment for care, 1973-74

		Residents in nursing home for 1 month or more					
			Age			Sex	
Primary source of payment	Total	Under 65 years	65–74 years	75–84 years	85 years and over	Male	Female
All residents of 1 month or more	1,010,700	107,400	151,800	359,000	392,500	294,500	716,200
		Percent distribution					
Total	100.0	100.0	100.0	100.0	100.0	100.0	100.0
Primary source of payment							
Self & family resources	36.7	18.1	30.8	41.6	39.7	35.9	37.1
Medicare	1.2		1.6	1.5	0.9	1.0	1.2
Medicaid	49.1	55.9	53.2	46.5	48.1	47.9	49.6
Public assistance/welfare	10.0	20.1	11.9	7.4	8.9	10.8	9.7
All other sources	3.0	5.6	2.5	3.0	2.4	4.4	2.4

Source: National Center for Health Statistics.

Charges and Costs*

Table 21-7   Resident charges and facility costs, by type and size of nursing home

Financial characteristics	Proprietary	Non-profit	Less than 50 beds	50–99 beds	100–199 beds	200 beds or more	Total
1973–1974 resident charges:							
Average total monthly charge per resident	$489	$456	$397	$448	$502	$576	$479
Percent of homes by average total monthly charge per resident:							
Less than $299	16.2	22.4	32.2	9.3	6.2	7.9	17.8
$300–$399	27.4	30.2	27.8	33.1	23.0	12.0	28.1
$400–$499	26.1	22.9	20.2	27.6	30.0	31.9	25.3
$500–$599	16.5	10.0	10.5	16.9	18.9	20.9	14.9
$600 or more	13.8	14.4	9.2	13.2	21.9	27.3	13.9
1972 facility costs:							
Average total costs per resident day	$14.86	$17.71	$14.29	$15.77	$17.12	$20.31	$15.63
Labor costs per resident day	8.53	10.90	8.59	9.00	9.87	12.90	9.17
Nursing staff costs per resident day	5.10	6.06	5.21	5 22	5.64	6.70	5.36
Operating, fixed, and miscellaneous costs per resident day	6.33	6.81	5.69	6.77	7.25	7.42	6.44

In 1972 the average total cost per resident day in the nation's nursing homes was $15.63, about 59% of which went for labor expenses ($9.17). The average total cost per resident day was notably higher in nonprofit homes ($17.71) than in proprietary homes ($14.86). The apparent cause of this substantial difference in costs is the greater use of labor by the nonprofit homes.

The wages paid the nursing staff made up 63% of total wages and slightly more than a third of total expenses. Operating costs (at $3.41) were the second largest major cost component, accounting for about 22% of total costs. Fixed costs ($2.37) accounted for about 15% of the total, and miscellaneous costs ($0.68) for about 4%.

Medicare and Medicaid**

Medicare and Medicaid standards for skilled nursing facilities were unified in 1972. Some 7,300 of the 23,000 U.S. nursing homes par-

ticipate in one or both programs offering skilled nursing care. A second level of care called intermediate care is offered under the Medicaid program where some 8,500 homes participate. The remaining 7,200 homes are largely personal care homes offering minimal nursing services.

Nurse Coverage Requirements

1. **Skilled Nursing Facility Standards**—Every Skilled Nursing Facility (whether participating in Medicare or Medicaid) must have the minimum of one registered nurse in charge of nursing on the day shift, eight hours a day, seven days a week. In addition, a minimum of one licensed practical nurse must be in charge of nursing on the 3 p.m. to 11 p.m. (afternoon) shift and the 11 p.m. to 7 a.m. (evening) shift. The law allows the Secretary of HEW to make exceptions in rural areas where there is a shortage of nurses; there, registered nurse coverage is required only five days a week.

2. **Intermediate Care Facility Nursing Standards**—Nursing homes participating in the Medicaid program as Intermediate Care Facilities are required to have one L.P.N. in charge of nursing on the morning shift, seven

*Source: DHEW, December 1975.
**Source: Senate Special Subcommittee on Aging, November 1974.

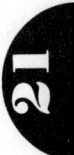

days a week. In addition, such facilities must make arrangements for consultation with an R.N. four hours per week.

3. **Resident/Personal Care Facility Standards**—There is no precise definition for homes providing a lesser degree of care. These may be called Resident Care, Personal Care, or even Domiciliary Care Facilities. They may provide regular, but not continuous nursing care, or they may simply provide clean, sheltered living conditions for patients incapable of fully caring for themselves, with no organized system for medical attention.

Current Nursing Home Benefits*

1. **Medicare Post-Hospital Extended Care Service Benefit**—Under provisions of the Hospital Insurance (Part A) portion of the Medicare program, persons over age 65 and disabled persons eligible for Medicare are entitled to 100 days of care during a benefit period in a skilled nursing facility (SNF) if their condition requires skilled nursing or skilled rehabilitation care on a daily basis. The benefit is available only after a patient has been hospitalized for a minimum of three consecutive days and transfers to a skilled nursing facility within 14 days (with certain exceptions) following hospital discharge. Cost of care is fully covered for the first 20 days of care with a copayment required (copayment rate is $11.50 per day during 1975) by the patient for the remaining 80 days.

2. **Medicaid Skilled Nursing Facility Service Benefit**—Under Medicaid, all states must provide skilled nursing facility (SNF) services for individuals over 21 years of age who are "categorically needy." If state programs cover the "medically needy," these persons are also eligible for SNF services. While the durational limits of skilled nursing care are determined by each state, almost all states provide SNF services as long as a medical need exists as certified by a physician. Prior hospitalization is *not* required under Medicaid as it is under Medicare. Many persons who have eligibility under both the Medicare and Medicaid programs and who exhaust their benefits under Medicare, may have additional SNF care paid for under the Medicaid program. In addition, many persons who are not eligible for Medicaid when they

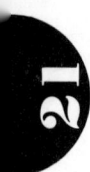

enter the institution achieve eligibility after a period of residence because they exhaust their personal resources.

While the individual is not required to share in the cost of nursing facility care under Medicaid, under a combination of federal and state laws the patient is required to turn over to the state or the operator of the nursing facility income received through Old Age, Survivors and Disability Insurance programs, the Supplemental Security Income program of the Social Security Administration or any state-sponsored income supplementation program. However, the Medicaid patient receives a "personal needs allowance" of $25 each month.

3. **Intermediate Care Facility Service Benefit**—Current law authorizes federal matching payments under Medicaid for care in an intermediate care facility (ICF) if a state chooses to include such care within its medical assistance program. Payments are authorized for (1) categorically needy recipients, (2) medically needy recipients and (3) residents in public institutions for the mentally retarded.

Medicaid and Nursing Homes

Medicaid payments in 1972 reached $5.2 billion; expenditures for nursing home care ($1.639 billion or 34%) exceeded expenditures for general and surgical hospital care ($1.518 billion or 31%). About 60% of the nation's nursing home bill is now paid by Medicaid.

Medicaid's Growing Role—Medicaid, a welfare program, remains virtually the only hope for most older Americans needing nursing home care. Medicare is of little help because its coverage is limited to "skilled nursing" which is narrowly defined. Since very few can afford to pay for their own care, senior citizens are left with no choice but to turn to welfare and apply for Medicaid.

In its early years, Medicaid, like Medicare, paid only for "skilled nursing care." But as thousands of elderly were forced to turn to Medicaid for assistance, the cost of the program skyrocketed. Critics of the program then emphasized that many patients did not need the intensive nursing services characterized as "skilled care." Consequently, Congress authorized a second, less intensive level of nursing home services, known as intermediate care. Consumer advocates, while conceding the need for a second level of care, expressed grave concern about possible consequences. They predicted that cost considera-

---

*Source: Senate Special Subcommittee on Aging, November 1974.

tions would override patient needs, leading to:

1. A restrictive definition of "skilled care."
2. Widespread reclassification of both facilities and patients into intermediate care.

Levels of Medicaid Reimbursement—Medicaid is a federal grants-in-aid program administered by HEW in which the federal government pays from 50 to 83% of the costs incurred by the states in providing medical assistance to the indigent, including nursing home care for qualifying individuals.

There has been no uniform reimbursement formula. Some states have paid nursing homes a flat fee, perhaps $14 per patient per day for skilled care. Other states reimburse nursing homes for reasonable costs expended. Section 249 of H.R. 1 mandated that all states reimburse nursing homes on a reasonable cost-related basis by January 1977.

Skilled Nursing—Until 1972, Medicaid provided only "skilled nursing," or that level of nursing home care nearest to hospital care. The definition of "skilled nursing" varied widely among the states. Some states employed the Medicare definition of "skilled nursing," but most did not. Today, this is changed because section 246 of H.R. 1 unifies Medicare and Medicaid standards, and section 247 mandates a single definition of "skilled nursing care" for facilities in both programs.

Intermediate Care—Intermediate care facilities (ICFs) are—as the name suggests—intended to help those who do not need round-the-clock nursing care and other mandatory services provided by a "skilled nursing" home.

The demand for ICFs arose when surveys indicated that many patients in nursing homes did not need such high-level care. They needed, first, a roof over their heads, and, second, some help from medical and other personnel to get them through each day. They were not well enough for "independent living"; they were not ill enough for expensive, round-the-clock nursing care.

Medicare and Nursing Homes*

In the early years, Medicare provided significant assistance to the nation's infirm elderly. However, the role of Medicare was sharply

*Source: Senate Special Subcommittee on Aging, November 1974.

curtailed in 1969. There were two reasons for this:

1. A decision by the Nixon administration to reduce costs, which took the form of new retroactive regulations for Medicare providers; and
2. Hearings and a followup report by the Senate Finance Committee calling attention to excessive costs, profiteering, abuses, and inefficiency in the Medicare program.

Regulations imposed on the Medicare ECF program by the Nixon administration were announced in April 1969. Former requirements were continued: prehospitalization for 3 days, transfer within 14 days to a certified facility, and physician's verification of the need for "skilled nursing" in continuation of care.

But a new condition was added requiring a patient to have "rehabilitative potential," effectively excluding coverage for terminal patients.

The second part of these April directives was the most devastating. It was a revised and narrowed definition of the term "skilled nursing," which by statute was a precondition to coverage.

Today, Medicare still pays for only 6.7% of the nation's total nursing home bill. Only 70,000 patients on any given day out of the 1 million who are in U.S. nursing homes have their care paid by Medicare. Of the $12.1 billion in Medicare reimbursement, only 1.67% or $200 million, went for nursing home care in 1973. Moreover, Medicare remains tied to a narrow and restrictive definition of skilled care which greatly limits coverage for the elderly. In short, Medicare is of little help to those who need nursing home care; those who need assistance must look elsewhere.

Nursing Home Personnel

The Governing Body

Federal regulations say that every nursing home must have an identifiable authority holding full legal and moral responsibility for all aspects of facility operations.

HEW's "Long Term Care Facility Improvement Study" (July, 1975) found:

● The governing body frequently does not discharge its obligations in a consistently effective manner.

- The administrator's overall direction for the operation of the facility is not always consonant with his professional status and responsibilities.
- Policies of the facility are in most instances documented but often not implemented.
- Patient care policies often lack input from health care professionals other than physicians and nurses.
- Personnel management practices do not appear to contribute to personnel resources that enhance the quality of patient care rendered.
- Management does not consistently provide the opportunity for or encourage staff to develop new skills and update existing ones.
- Outside resources are often not utilized, and when they are, management frequently fails to act upon their findings and recommendations.

The Industry Association

The American Health Care Association (AHCA) is the major spokesman for long-term care in the United States. Its representation extends to all areas including standards, regulations, legislation, and categories of care pertaining to long-term care. In speaking out for providers, AHCA interacts with governmental officials, other industry and trade associations, and consumer groups.

The Nursing Home Administrator

Nursing Home Administrator Responsibilities

The administrator is fully responsible for the day-to-day operation of the nursing home and is accountable to the governing body alone. Appointed by the governing body, the administrator is delegated in writing the responsibility for operating the home in accordance with policies, rules, regulations, and operating procedures adopted by the governing body.

The administrator evaluates and implements recommendations from the facility's committees, and maintains liaison with the governing body, medical staff, and other professional and supervisory staff. The administrator usually establishes the overall atmosphere of the home.

The HEW study found that administrative policies were in writing in 93.8% (6,179) of the facilities. In 19.5% (1,284) of these facilities, however, these policies had not been adopted by the governing body and in 29.1% (1,915) of

facilities, the policies had not been implemented.

State Requirements for Administrators

A report issued by a Ralph Nader study group supplies some specifics on state requirements for nursing home administrators:

> The regulations of 13 states in 1967 did not even mention the administrator, and those of 10 others did nothing more than refer to him by title. Twenty-eight states had no educational training or experience requirements for the person holding this critical position. Only 14 states required the administrator to be over 21 years of age, only 22 specified that he be in good physical health, and only 19 made the point that he be in good mental health. Only 9 required the administrator to be at least a high school graduate or the equivalent. Only 21 mentioned that he be of good moral character and only 9 indicated that he should have an interest in the welfare of the patients.

Nursing Home Administrators' Experience *

In 1969, there were about 18,390 nursing home administrators in the United States. Their median age was 53. Some 47% were employees; 44% were self employed; and 9% were both owners and administrators.

Some 91% were administrators of only one facility. Median experience for these individuals was 8 years in a hospital or nursing home.

About 71% of administrators had worked 4 years or more as an administrator in a nursing or personal care home, home for the aged, hospital, or similar facility. The median years of experience as an administrator in the current nursing or personal care home were 5.3 years. About 59% had worked in the current nursing or personal care home 4 years or more.

Salaries are even more uncertain. Studies show $8,500 in 1969 and $15,000 in 1972.

All administrative personnel had a turnover rate of 21% in 1970.

Administrators generally worked long hours, the mean hours worked being 57 during the week prior to the survey. Only 11% worked less than 40 hours; 31%, 40–49 hours; and the remainder, 50 hours or more.

---

* Source: DHEW, March 1973.

About 98% of the administrators spent some time the week prior to the survey performing professional services in the facilities; whereas only 60% spent time performing subprofessional services. Administrators were involved most frequently in administration, clerical work, kitchen or dietary work, housekeeping, and nursing care. The greatest proportion (59%) of their time was spent in administration of the facility.

Education and Training*

About 79% had completed high school, and 51% had some training thereafter. However, 72% had no undergraduate or graduate degree, and 65% had never taken a course in nursing home administration.

The associate's and bachelor's degrees were the most commonly held degrees; 28% of the administrators held one or both of these degrees. The master's and/or doctor's degree was held by 4% of the administrators.

A course in nursing home administration had been taken by 35% of nursing and personal care home administrators. The modal number of courses taken was one. About 88% of those who took a course in nursing home administration had completed at least 12th grade. Furthermore, 47% of those who had attended a course in nursing home administration had some college background.

Other than formal training, some administrators (39%) had received on-the-job training and 23% had received other training or education in nursing home administration. A good proportion of those who had received on-the-job training or other training or education in nurs-

ing home administration had a college background.

Nursing Home Employees**

More than three out of four employees in nursing homes are classified as service workers; most of these are health service workers. On the other hand, only about one employee in ten is a professional or technical worker, since the care provided in nursing homes generally consists of more routine tasks for which professional training is not required.

Nursing care homes employed 560,000 persons in 1973. By 1980 they are expected to employ 873,000 persons, and by 1985 the nursing home employment may reach 1,036,-000. The majority of full-time employees (FTE) (62%) were members of the nursing staff. As the level of education and training of the nursing staff increased from nurse's aide to licensed practical nurse (L.P.N.) to registered nurse (R.N.), the percentage of each group employed in nursing homes decreased from 46.5% for nurse's aides, to 8.3% for L.P.N.s, to 7.5% for R.N.s.

Professional and semiprofessional employees (including administrators, physicians, dentists, pharmacists, therapists, therapist assistants, dietitians, medical record administrators, and social workers) comprised the smallest portion of total FTE staff—6%.

A crude measure of the workload as well as the availability of staff to provide care is the rate of FTE employees per 100 residents. Overall there were 65.7 FTEs per 100 residents, which means that the average employee provided care for about 1.5 residents.

*Source: DHEW, February 1973.

**Source: DHEW, May 1976.

Table 21-8   Provisional distribution of full-time equivalent employees, by occupation category: certified nursing homes, United States, 1973–74. (Figures may not add to totals due to rounding.)

| | | Occupation category | | | | |
| | | Nursing staff | | | | |
All employees	Professional and semiprofessional	Total	R.N.	L.P.N.	Nurse's aide	Non-professional
Number of full-time equivalent employees						
722,200	41,500	450,600	54,500	60,300	335,900	230,100
Percent distribution of full-time equivalent employees						
100.0	5.7	62.4	7.5	8.3	46.5	31.9

Source: DHEW, September 5, 1974.

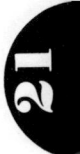

418

In 1964 there were 47.4 full-time employees per 100 nursing home residents. By 1973–74 the number had risen to 65.7 per 100 residents.

Table 21-9   Provisional number of full-time equivalent employees per 100 residents, by occupation category: certified nursing homes, United States, 1973–74. (Figures may not add to totals due to rounding.)

		Full-time equivalent employees per 100 residents				
		Nursing staff				
All employees	Professional and semiprofessional[1]	Total	R.N.	L.P.N.	Nurse's aide	Non-professional
65.7	3.8	41.0	5.0	5.5	30.6	20.9

[1]Includes administrators, physicians, dentists, pharmacists, therapists, therapist assistants, dietitians, medical record administrators, social workers, and other professional and semiprofessional occupations.

Source: DHEW, September 5, 1974.

The Nursing Supervisor: Duties and Responsibilities*

1. Development and maintenance of nursing service objectives.
2. Standards of nursing practice.
3. Nursing policy and procedure manuals.
4. Written job descriptions of each level of nursing personnel.
5. Methods for coordination of nursing services with other patient services.
6. Recommending number and levels of nursing personnel to be employed.
7. Dispensing medications and rendering treatments.
8. Supervising nursing personnel.
9. Hiring and terminating nursing personnel.
10. Indoctrination lectures.
11. In-service training.
12. Making out time card and assignment sheets.
13. Checking housekeeping and dietary personnel.
14. Maintaining patients' records.
15. Consulting with:
    Physicians
    Patients
    Patient's families
    Administrator
    Dietician
    Dentist
    Podiatrist

Social workers
Program directors
Bookkeepers
Speech therapist
Physical therapist
Community services
Outside professional groups
16. Member of:
    Utilization Review Committee
    Pharmacy Committee
    Patient Care Policies Committee
    Social Services Committee
    Restorative Services Group
    Infection Control Committee
    In-Service Training Committee
17. Documenting all the above.

These heavy burdens place in proper perspective the present federal Medicare and Medicaid requirement which requires only one registered nurse for every participating nursing home on the day shift and the minimum of an L.P.N. on each of the other two shifts.

Role of Licensed Practical Nurses and Nurses' Aides

The nursing team includes the registered professional nurse, the licensed practical nurse, and the nurse's aide. Licensed practical nurses assist the professional nurse to carry out nursing functions which require special technical skills. But the inventory of nursing home personnel clearly indicates the heaviest reliance is on the unlicensed aides and orderlies in U.S. nursing homes.

*Source: Senate Special Subcommittee on Aging, November 1974.

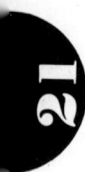

The number of nursing home employees increased by 405% from 1960 to 1970. In 1970, some 215,000, or 43% were aides and orderlies (280,000 in 1972); 7% were professional nurses; and 8% were licensed practical nurses. Nursing home employees have an average yearly turnover rate of 60%.

In terms of the total U.S. health industry, nursing homes have a disproportionate number of aides (26% of the 830,000 total). They account for few L.P.N.s (10% of 370,000) and for a miniscule number of the nation's R.N.s.

Licensed Practical Nurses—L.P.N.s often function in the stead of the R.N. They are in charge of nursing in the absence of an R.N. They must perform all the supervisory functions listed above, the care-giving and the administrative function. It is important to re-emphasize that L.P.N.s are generally in charge of the 3 p.m. to 11 p.m. afternoon shift and the 11 p.m. to 7 a.m. evening shift.

In addition to these functions, nurses are often asked to perform administrative duties such as ordering supplies, answering the telephone, and showing relatives or visitors around the nursing home.

There were some 40,000 licensed practical nurses employed in nursing homes in the United States in 1970. Twenty-five percent were licensed by waiver (that is, by past experience rather than on the basis of formal education). Licensed practical nurses received about $2.60 an hour for their work. They had a vacancy rate of 14% and a turnover rate of 35%.

Aides and Orderlies—Aides and orderlies work under the direction of an R.N. or an L.P.N. They are responsible for helping patients get out of bed and dress in the morning; they help wash the patient, make the beds, and clean the rooms; they bring meals to the patients and feed them if they are unable to feed themselves. They are often called upon to help administer treatments, or distribute medications. (Senate reports have detailed some of the disastrous results caused by untrained aides providing treatments and in being allowed to set up and pass medications.)

Unlicensed personnel comprise 43% of the staff, and most are women. The 215,000 aides and orderlies received an average of $1.70 an hour in 1970 for their work. They had a job vacancy rate of 4% and a turnover rate of 75% a year.

Nurse Shortages

Table 21-10 Nursing homes with charge persons on duty for three shifts, by level of skill

Level of skill of charge persons[1]	Homes with charge persons for three shifts[2]	
	Number	Percent
All levels of skill	12,600	100.0
R.N.s in charge for three shifts	3,600	28.7
Combination of R.N.s and L.P.N.s in charge for three shifts	4,300	34.2
L.P.N.s in charge for three shifts	—	—
Nurse's aides in charge for three shifts	—	—
Other combinations of skills in charge for three shifts	3,500	28.2

[1]A person in charge of a shift is on duty, awake, dressed, and routinely serving the residents.

[2]Excludes 3,600 homes having a charge person on duty less than three shifts a day.

Source: *Monthly Vital Statistics Report,* DHEW, September 5, 1974.

Unions

In a 1974 survey conducted by DOE, establishments having collective bargaining contracts covering at least a majority of their full-time R.N.s were found in only six metropolitan areas, whereas such unionization for full-time service and maintenance workers was reported in 17 areas.

New York had the largest proportion of union workers among service and maintenance employees and by far the largest number among R.N.s. Most homes in the survey had either a majority or none of the specified employee groups unionized; few homes had only a minority of either group unionized.

Wages and Benefits

Overview

New York stood alone as the pay leader among the 20 metropolitan areas covered by a 1973 DHEW study of nursing home employees. Registered professional nurses (R.N.s) in New

York averaged $6.07 an hour in May 1973, compared with the next highest average of $4.87 in the Los Angeles area. The two highest averages for licensed practical nurses (L.P.N.s) were $4.70 in New York and $3.77 in Los Angeles. The lowest averages for R.N.s ($3.76) and L.P.N.s ($2.80) were recorded in Denver and Atlanta, respectively.

Dallas hourly pay levels were lowest among

Hourly

Table 21-11   Nursing home average hourly wages for R.N.s, L.P.N.s and aides in nonsupervisory workers in selected occupations in nursing homes

Occupation	Northeast				South				
	Boston	Buffalo	New York	Phila-delphia	Atlanta	Balti-more	Dallas	Miami	Wash-ington, D.C.
Nursing employees									
Registered professional nurses	$4.50	$4.14	$6.07	$4.09	$4.05	$4.38	$4.04	$4.20	$4.38
Licensed practical nurses	3.60	3.07	4.72	2.86	2.81	3.57	2.87	3.35	3.35
Nursing aides (orderlies)	2.31	2.19	3.46	2.10	1.84	2.23	1.72	2.04	2.17

Source: DHEW, 1975.

21

Wages of R.N.s and L.P.N.s

Table 21-12   Occupational pay relationships, nursing homes (Nursing aides' average earnings

Area	R.N.s		L.P.N.s	
	Nursing homes	Nongovernment hospitals	Nursing homes	Nongovernment hospitals
Atlanta	217	177	152	126
Baltimore	195	162	160	128
Boston	188	169	151	135
Buffalo	191	176	140	119
Chicago	203	160	144	126
Dallas	241	198	167	129
Denver	212	179	160	122
Detroit	241	175	194	138
Los Angeles–Long Beach and Anaheim–Santa Ana– Garden Grove	251	178	194	130

Source: U.S. Bureau of Labor Statistics, 1975.

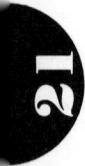

the area averages for nursing aides ($1.72), kitchen helpers ($1.72), and maids or porters ($1.73)—all numerically important jobs.

A large majority of the workers were employed in nursing homes that provided paid holidays (commonly six or seven days annually) and paid vacations after qualifying periods of service. The incidence of life, hospitalization, surgical, and medical insurance, and financial protection in case of sickness or accident, was not as common as paid holidays and vacations. Only in New York did retirement plans apply to at least one-half of the work force.

Wages

selected metropolitan areas. (Number and average straight-time hourly earnings of and related facilities, 20 metropolitan areas, May 1973)

| | North Central | | | | | West | | | | |
| | | | | | | | | | | |
Chicago	Cincin-nati	Cleve-land	Detroit	Minne-apolis–St. Paul	St. Louis	Denver	Los Angeles–Long Beach and Anaheim–Santa Ana–Garden Grove	Port-land	San Fran-cisco–Oakland	Seattle–Everett
$4.37	$4.17	$4.09	$4.50	$4.14	$4.16	$3.72	$4.87	$4.25	$4.31	$3.98
3.21	3.06	3.04	3.66	3.16	3.09	2.79	3.77	3.14	3.26	2.90
2.20	1.88	1.92	1.91	2.06	1.89	1.76	1.92	1.82	2.20	1.85

Compared with Wages of Aides

(May 1973) and nongovernment hospitals (August 1972). in each industry = 100)

| | R.N.s | | L.P.N.s | |
Area	Nursing homes	Nongovernment hospitals	Nursing homes	Nongovernment hospitals
Miami	208	191	167	138
Minneapolis–St. Paul	196	168	151	123
New York	174	155	135	123
Philadelphia	196	162	138	124
Portland	231	163	170	126
St. Louis	220	183	161	136
San Francisco–Oakland	193	145	145	114
Seattle–Everett	214	165	156	113
Washington	203	160	152	121

Nursing Home Employee Benefits*

Table 21-13   Percent of registered professional nurses and service and maintenance workers in nursing homes with provisions for selected perquisites, May 1973

Area	R.N.s		Service and maintenance workers	
	At least 1 free meal	Uniforms and/or laundering[1]	At least 1 free meal	Uniforms and/or laundering[1]
Northeast:				
Boston	32	11	37	8
Buffalo	21	28	29	24
New York	77	86	78	89
Philadelphia	48	10	43	20
South:				
Atlanta	31	44	18	51
Baltimore	39	7	18	11
Dallas	15	48	23	66
Miami	61	6	55	4
Washington, D.C.	32	31	37	23
North Central:				
Chicago	75	4	78	14
Cincinnati	58	20	48	30
Cleveland	41	—	39	15
Detroit	45	5	20	5
Minneapolis–St. Paul	21	8	24	15
St. Louis	20	7	19	21
West:				
Denver	44	17	48	24
Los Angeles–Long Beach and Anaheim–Santa Ana– Garden Grove	20	—	9	1
Portland	7	—	10	1
San Francisco–Oakland	16	—	16	3
Seattle–Everett	15	—	16	—

[1]Includes homes that provided a monetary allowance for uniforms and/or laundering.

Table 21-14   Scheduled weekly hours (Percent of registered professional nurses in

Weekly hours	Northeast				South				
	Boston	Buffalo	New York	Phila- delphia	Atlanta	Balti- more	Dallas	Miami	Wash- ington, D.C.
									Registered
All registered professional nurses	100	100	100	100	100	100	100	100	100
35 hours	—	—	37	—	—	—	—	—	—
Over 35 and under 37 ½ hours	—	—	1	—	—	—	—	—	—
37 ½ hours	7	20	48	9	5	18	—	15	—
40 hours	93	80	13	87	55	76	96	71	100
Over 40 and under 48 hours	—	—	—	3	37	—	4	4	—
48 hours and over	—	—	—	1	3	7	—	10	—

*Source: U.S. Bureau of Labor Statistics, 1975.

Scheduled Weekly Hours

Work schedules of 40 hours a week applied to at least seven-tenths of the R.N.s in all except two areas; 35 to 37½ hour schedules applied to seven-eighths of the R.N.s in New York and schedules exceeding 40 hours applied to two-fifths in Atlanta (Table 21-14). Approximately two-thirds or more of the service and maintenance workers in all but Atlanta, Baltimore, and New York were on 40-hour schedules. In Atlanta, schedules for about two-fifths of such workers were more than 40 hours, whereas in Baltimore and New York, a majority were scheduled to work fewer than 40 hours.

Slightly over 10% of the full-time R.N.s in the survey were employed by facilities that required them to be "on call" beyond their regular hours of work, but usually not on a 24-hour basis. The proportions in homes with "on-call" provisions were 72% in Dallas, 42% in Baltimore, 36% in Detroit, and 5% or less in Buffalo, Philadelphia, Miami, Cincinnati, San Francisco–Oakland, St. Louis, and Seattle–Everett.

Paid Holidays

Paid holidays were provided annually to a large majority of the R.N.s and service and maintenance workers in the survey (Table 21-15). The number of paid holidays for both groups varied considerably by area, but 6 or 7 days were most commonly provided. A major exception to this pattern was New York, where seven-eighths of both groups received 10 to 14 days.

Paid Vacations

Paid vacations, after qualifying periods of service, were provided to over nine-tenths of the workers in both groups (Table 21-17). Typically, workers received at least 1 week of vacation pay after 1 year of service and a minimum of two weeks after two years. More liberal vacation policies, such as three weeks or more after 10 years, were common in many areas. Four weeks or more of vacation pay after 15 years were available to at least one-half of both groups in Buffalo, New York, and San Francisco–Oakland.

Health, Insurance, and Retirement Plans

The extent to which nursing homes provided their employees with at least part of the cost of various health and life insurance benefits varied considerably by area (Table 21-16). At least one-half of the R.N.s were provided life insurance and major medical coverage in 10 areas; basic medical insurance in 13 areas; hospitalization and surgical insurance in 15 areas; and sickness and accident insurance or sick leave in 18 areas. Within the same areas, these benefit plans commonly applied to similar proportions of the service and maintenance workers.

Retirement plans, excluding social security, were available to a majority of the workers only in New York, where approximately seven-tenths in both groups were covered. The next highest proportions were between one-third and two-fifths of the R.N.s in Baltimore, Washington, and Cincinnati, and about two-fifths of

nursing homes and related facilities by scheduled weekly hours, May 1973)

| | North Central | | | | | West | | | | |
	Chicago	Cincin-nati	Cleve-land	Detroit	Minne-apolis–St. Paul	St. Louis	Denver	Los Angeles–Long Beach and Anaheim–Santa Ana–Garden Grove	Port-land	San Fran-cisco–Oakland	Seattle–Everett
professional nurses											
	100	100	100	100	100	100	100	100	100	100	100
	2	—	—	—	—	—	—	—	7	—	—
	—	—	—	—	—	—	—	3	—	—	3
	5	12	6	2	3	1	—	3	—	2	—
	93	86	90	98	97	99	100	94	93	98	97
	—	2	1	—	—	—	—	—	—	—	—
	—	—	2	—	—	—	—	—	—	—	—

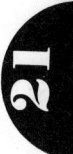

Table 21-15 Paid holidays (Percent of registered professional nurses in nursing homes

	Northeast				South				
Number of paid holidays	Boston	Buffalo	New York	Phila-delphia	Atlanta	Balti-more	Dallas	Miami	Wash-ington, D.C.
									Registered
All registered professional nurses	100	100	100	100	100	100	100	100	100
Workers in establishments providing paid holidays	94	94	100	84	94	99	70	100	91
Under 4 days	—	—	2	8	—	7	4	—	—
4 days	2	—	—	—	13	—	2	—	1
5 days	4	1	—	4	15	—	43	6	11
6 days	21	3	1	17	36	12	20	17	24
7 days	21	34	6	25	10	7	—	35	29
8 days	6	25	4	14	19	14	—	14	7
9 days	28	8	1	7	—	22	—	28	18
10 days	12	4	6	4	—	35	—	—	—
Over 10 days	—	18	81	4	—	2	—	—	—
Workers in establishments providing no paid holidays	6	6	—	16	6	1	30	—	9

Table 21-16 Health, insurance, and retirement plans (Percent of registered professional

	Northeast				South				
Type of plan	Boston	Buffalo	New York	Phila-delphia	Atlanta	Balti-more	Dallas	Miami	Wash-ington, D.C.
									Registered
All registered professional nurses	100	100	100	100	100	100	100	100	100
Workers in establishments providing:									
Life insurance	63	36	82	33	24	85	54	68	51
Noncontributory plans	40	36	82	28	1	81	9	37	39
Accidental death and dismemberment insurance	54	1	80	24	8	57	30	34	30
Noncontributory plans	36	1	80	18	8	54	4	18	18
Sickness and accident insurance or sick leave or both[3]	94	90	97	83	35	100	72	90	92
Sickness and accident insurance	57	—	46	16	—	60	4	—	11
Noncontributory plans	38	—	46	13	—	60	4	—	6
Sick leave (full pay, no waiting period)	80	88	97	66	33	98	57	84	91
Sick leave (partial pay or waiting period)	—	1	—	7	1	—	11	6	1
Hospitalization insurance	82	45	99	64	60	68	57	70	62
Noncontributory plans	36	35	96	53	60	64	20	39	34
Surgical insurance	84	45	99	61	60	68	57	70	58
Noncontributory plans	36	35	96	50	60	64	20	39	34
Medical insurance	84	31	89	59	47	68	57	56	58
Noncontributory plans	36	27	87	45	47	64	20	25	34
Major medical insurance	81	10	79	39	24	67	52	56	54
Noncontributory plans	35	8	77	31	24	64	20	25	32
Retirement plans	14	17	69	13	14	39	22	—	37
Pensions	14	17	69	13	14	39	22	—	37
Noncontributory plans	11	16	69	11	—	21	—	—	36
Severance pay	—	—	—	—	—	—	—	—	—
No plans	2	9	—	9	22	1	20	—	8

21

	North Central						West			
Chicago	Cincin-nati	Cleve-land	Detroit	Minne-apolis–St. Paul	St. Louis	Denver	Los Angeles–Long Beach and Anaheim–Santa Ana–Garden Grove	Port-land	San Fran-cisco–Oakland	Seattle–Everett
professional nurses										
100	100	100	100	100	100	100	100	100	100	100
82	88	93	99	83	90	58	93	78	98	88
—	—	5	1	2	5	6	6	1	—	4
1	2	—	—	1	—	3	7	7	—	12
5	—	7	6	1	—	3	14	6	—	10
34	16	53	53	27	29	39	40	44	10	14
35	50	10	26	45	46	7	22	19	35	31
2	7	8	13	8	10	—	3	—	34	13
4	14	10	—	—	—	—	1	—	18	4
—	—	—	—	—	—	—	—	—	—	—
—	—	—	—	—	—	—	—	—	—	—
18	12	7	1	17	10	42	7	22	2	12

	North Central						West			
Chicago	Cincin-nati	Cleve-land	Detroit	Minne-apolis–St. Paul	St. Louis	Denver	Los Angeles–Long Beach and Anaheim–Santa Ana–Garden Grove	Port-land	San Fran-cisco–Oakland	Seattle–Everett
professional nurses										
100	100	100	100	100	100	100	100	100	100	100
50	43	53	69	15	46	20	63	26	28	28
42	38	49	64	13	26	7	27	25	17	19
34	39	21	53	14	40	13	51	26	27	28
25	37	21	48	11	25	—	18	25	16	19
67	68	77	80	75	64	35	63	56	88	60
9	8	17	11	8	1	5	1	19	2	22
6	8	17	11	8	1	—	1	4	2	14
57	46	67	70	75	52	26	39	42	69	55
4	14	—	3	—	11	4	24	10	19	—
65	85	47	61	20	42	21	72	83	87	79
52	53	17	48	10	12	—	34	38	43	54
62	85	46	61	20	42	21	72	83	87	79
50	53	16	48	10	12	—	34	38	43	54
61	47	43	61	17	38	21	72	82	87	79
49	17	16	47	7	12	—	34	38	43	54
48	44	8	40	16	28	21	69	72	60	66
38	31	1	36	9	5	—	31	38	25	41
15	33	21	14	13	15	—	8	20	13	16
15	33	21	14	13	15	—	8	20	13	16
8	33	16	13	13	15	—	6	19	8	11
1	—	—	—	—	—	—	—	—	—	—
23	9	7	5	23	21	46	16	12	6	17

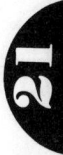

21

Table 21-17　Paid vacations (percent of registered professional nurses in

	Northeast				South				
Vacation policy	Boston	Buffalo	New York	Phila-delphia	Atlanta	Balti-more	Dallas	Miami	Wash-ington, D.C.
									Registered
All registered professional nurses	100	100	100	100	100	100	100	100	100
Method of payment									
Workers in establishments									
providing paid vacations	100	96	98	100	100	100	96	100	100
Length-of-time payment	100	96	98	99	100	100	96	100	100
Percentage payment	—	—	—	1	—	—	—	—	—
Workers in establishments									
providing no paid vacations	—	4	2	—	—	—	4	—	—
Amount of vacation pay[2]									
After 1 year of service:									
1 week	49	45	—	52	37	30	37	40	39
Over 1 and under 2 weeks	—	—	—	—	—	7	13	—	—
2 weeks	46	49	9	41	40	51	46	53	32
Over 2 and under 3 weeks	—	—	—	—	23	—	—	—	28
3 weeks	4	1	4	5	—	10	—	—	1
4 weeks or more	1	—	85	2	—	3	—	7	—
After 2 years of service:									
1 week	12	22	—	23	4	—	37	8	5
Over 1 and under 2 weeks	2	1	—	1	—	7	4	—	8
2 weeks	80	54	6	62	73	74	54	67	57
Over 2 and under 3 weeks	—	15	—	2	23	—	—	—	29
3 weeks	4	4	5	10	—	16	—	18	—
4 weeks	1	—	84	2	—	3	—	7	1
Over 4 weeks	—	—	4	—	—	—	—	—	—
After 3 years of service:									
1 week	11	7	—	9	4	—	33	6	3
Over 1 and under 2 weeks	2	1	—	1	—	7	—	—	8
2 weeks	76	69	6	70	68	46	59	69	45
Over 2 and under 3 weeks	—	15	—	2	28	—	4	—	24
3 weeks	10	4	2	14	—	37	—	18	19
4 weeks	1	—	87	4	—	10	—	7	1
Over 4 weeks	—	—	4	—	—	—	—	—	—
After 5 years of service:									
1 week	6	—	—	7	4	—	22	6	3
Over 1 and under 2 weeks	—	—	—	—	—	—	—	—	8
2 weeks	33	12	1	41	54	12	70	20	23
Over 2 and under 3 weeks	—	—	—	5	28	7	4	—	24
3 weeks	59	74	3	38	14	71	—	68	36
Over 3 and under 4 weeks	—	—	—	—	—	—	—	—	—
4 weeks	1	9	40	7	—	10	—	7	6

the service and maintenance workers in Baltimore and Buffalo. Retirement plans in all areas were nearly always in the form of pensions, rather than severance pay, and were typically paid for entirely by the employers.

Licensed Practical Nurse Benefits

The above discussion and tabulations of supplementary benefits do not include data for L.P.N.s. About one-fourth of the full-time L.P.N.s had supplementary benefits similar to

R.N.s within the same establishment; another fourth were employed in homes that provided the same benefits to L.P.N.s as to service and maintenance workers; and nearly one-half of the 11,700 full-time L.P.N.s had the same benefits that were granted to both R.N.s and service and maintenance workers. Fewer than 100 L.P.N.s were employed in homes that did not provide paid holidays, paid vacations, or health, insurance, and retirement plans. Nearly all L.P.N.s in the 20 areas combined were pro-

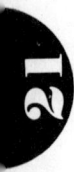

nursing homes with formal provisions for paid vacations, May 1973)

	North Central					West				
Chicago	Cincin-nati	Cleve-land	Detroit	Minne-apolis-St. Paul	St. Louis	Denver	Los Angeles–Long Beach and Anaheim–Santa Ana–Garden Grove	Port-land	San Fran-cisco–Oakland	Seattle–Everett
professional nurses										
100	100	100	100	100	100	100	100	100	100	100
97	100	100	100	100	99	100	100	92	100	100
97	100	100	99	100	99	100	100	92	100	100
—	—	—	1	—	—	—	—	—	—	—
3	—	—	—	—	1	—	—	8	—	—
58	23	41	61	58	55	17	68	50	58	43
2	—	—	3	1	—	—	1	—	—	—
27	77	55	32	39	44	33	31	42	39	57
—	—	—	—	2	—	—	—	—	—	—
4	—	4	—	—	—	—	—	—	3	—
4	—	—	3	—	—	—	—	—	—	—
15	16	23	26	6	30	25	27	19	2	22
—	—	—	3	1	1	4	1	4	—	—
72	84	71	61	83	65	71	68	68	91	77
2	—	—	—	2	—	—	4	1	—	1
4	—	6	6	8	3	—	—	—	7	—
2	—	—	3	—	—	—	—	—	—	—
3	—	—	—	—	—	—	—	—	—	—
10	9	16	2	—	8	8	11	6	1	6
—	—	—	—	1	—	5	1	—	—	—
74	79	76	84	76	88	81	78	85	89	85
2	5	2	3	10	—	—	4	1	—	2
6	7	6	8	13	3	6	6	—	10	7
3	—	—	3	—	—	—	—	—	—	—
3	—	—	—	—	—	—	—	—	—	—
9	6	11	—	—	2	5	8	3	1	5
—	—	—	—	—	—	4	—	—	—	—
14	72	54	33	41	60	68	42	48	6	44
3	5	—	—	3	—	—	4	1	—	6
65	10	35	60	47	36	22	41	40	87	42
—	—	—	—	—	—	—	—	—	—	—
4	7	—	3	10	—	—	4	—	6	2
3	—	—	3	—	—	—	—	—	—	—
—	—	—	—	—	—	—	—	—	—	—

(Continued)

vided paid holidays and paid vacations; about three-fourths were employed in homes that provided at least part of the cost of some health and life insurance; and one-fourth were provided pension plans.

Perquisites

As indicated previously, earnings data in this report relate to cash salaries and do not include the value of room, board, or other perquisites. New York also led the other areas in such perquisites for R.N.s and service and maintenance workers; in that area, more than three-fourths of both groups were granted free meals and uniform/laundry benefits. Free lodging for these two groups was virtually nonexistent in the survey. Perquisites for L.P.N.s were not studied.

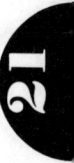

Table 21-17   (continued)

	Northeast				South				
Vacation policy	Boston	Buffalo	New York	Phila-delphia	Atlanta	Balti-more	Dallas	Miami	Wash-ington, D.C.
									Registered
Over 4 and under 5 weeks	—	—	—	—	—	—	—	—	—
5 weeks or more	—	—	54	1	—	—	—	—	—
After 10 years of service:									
1 week	6	—	—	7	4	—	22	6	3
2 weeks	20	3	1	26	54	9	52	18	29
Over 2 and under 3 weeks	—	—	—	2	23	7	4	—	25
3 weeks	67	42	(3)	51	19	37	17	56	36
Over 3 and under 4 weeks	—	—	—	1	—	—	—	—	—
4 weeks	7	50	43	11	—	41	—	21	7
Over 4 and under 5 weeks	—	—	—	—	—	7	—	—	—
5 weeks	—	—	4	1	—	—	—	—	—
6 weeks or more	—	—	50	—	—	—	—	—	—
After 15 years of service:									
1 week	6	—	—	7	4	—	22	6	3
2 weeks	20	1	1	26	46	9	52	18	29
Over 2 and under 3 weeks	—	—	—	2	23	7	4	—	24
3 weeks	66	38	—	51	27	37	7	56	36
Over 3 and under 4 weeks	—	—	—	—	—	—	—	—	—
4 weeks	9	56	43	12	—	41	11	21	9
Over 4 and under 5 weeks	—	—	—	—	—	7	—	—	—
5 weeks	—	—	4	2	—	—	—	—	—
6 weeks	—	—	49	—	—	—	—	—	—
Over 6 weeks	—	—	1	—	—	—	—	—	—
After 20 years of service:[4]									
1 week	6	—	—	7	4	—	22	6	3
2 weeks	20	1	1	26	46	9	52	18	29
Over 2 and under 3 weeks	—	—	—	2	23	7	4	—	24
3 weeks	65	38	—	50	27	37	7	56	36
Over 3 and under 4 weeks	—	—	—	—	—	—	—	—	—
4 weeks	10	56	43	13	—	41	11	21	9
Over 4 and under 5 weeks	—	—	—	—	—	7	—	—	—
5 weeks	—	—	4	2	—	—	—	—	—
6 weeks	—	—	49	—	—	—	—	—	—
Over 6 weeks	—	—	1	—	—	—	—	—	—

The Nursing Home Patient

Portrait of the Nursing Home Population*

Overview

One million older Americans are in nursing homes. What are they like? The following summary discusses facts which must be considered in any evaluation of long-term care in this nation:

They are very old. The average age of

patients is 82; 95% are over 65 and 70% over 70.

Most of them are female. Women outnumber men two to one in pre-1970 studies and three to one in more recent tabulations.

Most of them are widows. Sixty-three percent are widowed; 22% never married; about 5% were divorced and only 10% are married.

They are alone. Since most nursing home patients are in their 70's and 80's they may well have outlived their own children. Almost 50% have no viable relationship with a close relative, and another 30% have only collateral relatives near their own age.

The great majority are white. Ninety-six percent of nursing home patients are white,

*Source: Senate Special Subcommittee on Aging, November 1974.

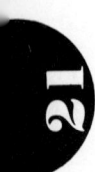

	North Central					West				
Chicago	Cincin-nati	Cleve-land	Detroit	Minne-apolis-St. Paul	St. Louis	Denver	Los Angeles–Long Beach and Anaheim–Santa Ana–Garden Grove	Port-land	San Fran-cisco–Oakland	Seattle–Everett
professional nurses										
9	6	11	—	—	2	5	8	3	1	5
9	43	22	19	22	25	63	30	33	4	44
—	—	7	—	—	—	4	2	—	1	—
61	43	53	60	52	72	27	44	54	38	46
—	—	—	—	1	—	—	3	—	—	—
16	9	7	18	25	—	—	13	2	55	5
3	—	—	3	—	—	—	—	—	—	—
—	—	—	—	—	—	—	—	—	—	—
—	—	—	—	—	—	—	—	—	—	—
9	6	11	—	—	2	5	8	3	1	5
9	43	19	19	15	25	59	30	33	4	40
—	—	—	—	—	—	—	2	—	—	—
54	39	47	58	56	65	36	42	40	38	47
—	—	—	—	1	—	—	—	—	—	—
23	12	23	18	27	7	—	17	16	54	8
3	—	—	3	—	—	—	—	—	—	—
—	—	—	1	—	—	—	—	—	3	—
—	—	—	—	—	—	—	—	—	—	—
—	—	—	—	—	—	—	—	—	—	—
9	6	11	—	—	2	5	8	3	1	5
9	43	19	19	15	25	59	30	31	4	40
—	—	—	—	—	—	—	2	—	—	—
53	32	31	58	55	62	36	42	41	38	47
—	—	—	—	1	—	—	—	—	—	—
22	20	39	18	28	10	—	17	16	54	8
3	—	—	3	—	—	—	—	—	—	—
2	—	—	—	—	—	—	—	—	3	—
—	—	—	1	—	—	—	—	—	—	—
—	—	—	—	—	—	—	—	—	—	—

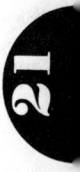

21

with blacks accounting for an additional 2%. The remainder includes diverse groups such as Mexican-Americans, elderly Asians or Indians, etc.

Most of them come to the nursing home from their private homes. More than 55% of patients came to the long-term care facility from their own or relatives' homes; 32% came from hospitals (22% from general and 10% from state mental hospitals); 13% came from other nursing homes or homes for the aged, boarding homes, or other housing.

Most nursing home patients are placed in facilities close to their homes. Five out of six nursing home patients are housed in facilities less than 25 miles away from their community home. Proximity is the major consideration to families of nursing home patients.

Some have visitors, but most do not. Estimates vary, but there is agreement that most nursing home patients do not have visitors. This is because a third or more have no relatives. A comprehensive New Hampshire study disclosed that 42% had visitors weekly.

Most of them could expect to be in a nursing home well over a year. But many studies indicate that the length of stay in a nursing home is two or more years.

Most patients entering a nursing home will die there. There is great variation in statistics on this subject. Some studies indicate that 87% of patients died in the nursing home;

others reveal that only 4% of nursing home patients can ever be returned to the community. The more conservative figures indicate that 50% of nursing home patients die in nursing homes; 21% are returned to hospitals; 19% are sent home (or to their relatives' homes) and 10% are placed in other accommodations.

Nursing home patients generally have about four chronic or crippling disabilities. Authoritative studies reveal that nursing home patients have 3.8 disabilities. Cardiovascular disease ranks first, experienced by 65% of the patients. What is loosely termed senility is generally found among 20% of the patients; fractures are third most prevalent at 11%, followed by arthritis at 10%.

A majority of patients are mentally impaired. Widely supported data establishes that 55% or more of long-term care patients are mentally impaired. One study, however, put the figure at 80%.

Less than half of the patients can walk. About 55% require assistance in bathing; 47% need help in dressing; 11% in eating and 33% are incontinent.

They take large quantities of drugs. The average nursing home patient takes 4.4 different drugs per day, some taken two and three times; 70% take five or more drugs per day. Some recent studies average seven different drugs a day. The average cost of drugs per patient is $300 per year.

They regard the nursing home with fear and hostility, and there are sharp increases in the death rate associated with transfer to nursing homes. Much evidence clearly indicates that old people look upon a nursing home with fear and hostility. It has been documented that old people believe entry into a home is a prelude to death, and that there is a negative relationship between survival and institutionalization. Substantially higher death rates were recorded among those admitted to nursing homes than among control groups, generally those on a list waiting admission.

This phenomenon has been termed "transplantation shock" by one researcher, who recorded a 42% death rate for those admitted to institutional facilities and 28% for those waiting admission.

Patients: Where They Come From and Where They Go

Table 21-18   Distribution of admissions to and discharges from homes for the aged and chronically ill, U.S.A. 1967 (excludes Alaska and Hawaii)

Type of service	Number	Percent	Mental hospital	General hospital	Other hospital	Patient's home	Another nursing home	Other places	Personal care or domiciliary home
			Patient's former place of residence Percent distribution						
Admissions to nursing home	801,013	100.0	3.5	53.9	5.0	25.9	9.4	2.4	
			Place patient discharged to Percent distribution						
Live discharges from nursing home	602,192	100.0	1.7	25.1	1.8	39.6	11.0	17.0	3.8

Source: DHEW, January 1974.

Patient Ailments

Medical Conditions

Patients' most common primary and secondary diagnoses when admitted to skilled nursing facilities are: heart disease, 38%; chronic brain disease, 29%; generalized arteriosclerosis and hypertension, 23%; diseases of the musculoskeletal system, 20%; stroke, 18%; fractures, 16%; neurological disease, 15%.

Other Impairments—Impaired vision is suffered by 68%; 3% more are legally blind; 33% have at least some hearing loss; 32% have some degree of speech impairment; 92%

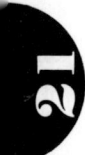

21

are missing some or all natural teeth, and 38% lack compensating restorations or dentures; 54% show some confusion as to time, place, or their own identity (27% occasionally and 27% continuously); 41% display inappropriate behavior—typically wandering or disruptiveness.

In What Daily Activities Do Patients Need Help?*—They cannot bathe without difficulty: 60% need some help, and 33% more cannot bathe themselves at all; 72% require help in dressing; 34% need some help in eating, and 16% must be fed by others; 45% must be helped in using the toilet, 29% cannot use it at all; 50% experience some degree of incontinence—from occasional to total; 87% are not fully ambulatory; 9% suffer pressure sores because of reduced ability to move in bed.

Note: Harris Survey results indicate that despite many die-hard myths about the elderly—which a majority of people under 65 still believe—people 65 and over may not be much different than people under 65. Older people feel they are alert, able to work and function well, and are not living wasted lives. And on the evidence, the similarities between people over 65 and under 65 are far more numerous than their differences.**

Table 21-20　Chronic conditions or impairments in nursing home residents. (Prevalence per 100 population of nursing home residents age 65 or older)

Conditions or impairments	Prevalence per 100
Mental and nervous disorders	44
Vascular lesions affecting the central nervous system	36
Diseases of the heart	31
Arthritis and rheumatism	24
Hearing impairments	20
Visual impairments; inability to read newspaper with glasses	19
Paralysis, palsy due to stroke	16
Orthopedic impairments	15
Chronic conditions of the digestive system	14
Conditions of the genitourinary system	9
Diabetes mellitus	8
Hypertension	5
Malignant neoplasms	4

Source: DHEW.

Table 21-19　Classification of patients according to visual perception

Visual state(s)	Patients	
	Number	Percent
All	283,912	100.0
No impairment	83,907	29.6
Impairment one eye (with glasses)	3,787	1.3
Impairment both eyes (with glasses)	145,895	51.4
Impairment one eye (no glasses)	3,010	1.1
Impairment both eyes (no glasses)	39,872	14.0
Legally blind	7,441	2.6

Source: DHEW, July 1975.

Table 21-21　Classification of patients according to hearing acuity

Hearing state(s)	Patients	
	Number	Percent
All	283,913	100.0
No impairment	190,407	67.1
Impairment one or both ears	89,212	31.4
(a) Hears loud voice no shouting	(60,286)	(21.2)
(b) Hears normal and loud voice with hearing aid	(9,543)	(3.4)
(c) Hears only shouting no hearing aid	(16,019)	(5.6)
(d) Hears only shouting with hearing aid	(3,364)	(1.2)
Does not hear	4,294	1.5

Source: DHEW, July 1975.

*Source: Monthly Vital Statistics Report—Fact Sheet, DHEW, 1974.

**Source: Harris Survey. (Copyright: 1975 *Chicago Tribune*.)

Table 21-22   Classification of patients according to speaking ability

Speaking state(s)	Patients		Speaking state(s)	Patients	
	Number	Percent		Number	Percent
All	283,913	100.0	Aphasic (conveys thoughts)	9,485	3.3
Normal speech	192,957	68.0			
Stuttering (not dysarthria)	7,423	2.6	Speaks (makes no sense)	24,317	8.6
Dysarthria (with intelligible speech)	25,002	8.8	Does not speak	24,729	8.7

Source: DHEW, July 1975.

Patient Admissions, Discharges and Deaths

Table 21-23   Percentage & number of admissions, discharges, and deaths in nursing homes during 1962, 1968, 1973 (United States)

All	Admissions number	Discharges & death number	Discharges percentage	Deaths percentage
Nursing Homes				
1962	402,896	378,326	60.9	39.1
1968	968,750	900,521	66.9	33.1
1973	1,118,553	1,040,880	73.9	26.1
Nursing Care Homes				
1962	264,955	253,156	59.6	40.4
1968	876,645	803,365	66.1	33.9
1973	994,999	931,639	73.5	26.5
Personal Care and Other Homes				
1962	137,941	125,170	63.5	36.5
1968	92,105	97,156	72.8	27.2
1973	123,554	109,241	77.5	22.5

Source: DHEW.

Patient Concerns

Overview*

The aging adult, in assignment to a nursing home, is experiencing his first major loss of autonomy and self-direction, consequent to this current act against his will. His severe losses, the traumatic shock of rejection and separation from the world, the sense of his ultimate aloneness, and the beginning realization of his changed and lessened final status in life, place the entrant in a state of jeopardy with acute ego damage.

*Source: DHEW, 1970.

The attitudes and behavior of patients vary widely. Many feel that no one cares about them, not even God. Others feel they have lost their usefulness to society and there is no longer a purpose in living. Still others want to die and even discuss suicidal method. Others feel if they do work hard to improve their functioning there will be no purpose, as they will never leave the nursing home or will die soon anyway. Others view their dilemma as a punishment for some earlier behavior in life which they felt to be unethical. Some feel everything meaningful in life has been taken away (personal belongings, their way of life, social relationships with others, personal freedom and rights to go and come at will) and as a result there is a preoccupation with death. There is also a preoccupation with self and a turning away from the outside world.

Nursing homes are regimented with rules and regulations which consequently mean losses of freedom and choices for the patient. In the usual nursing home a patient has a roommate which means a loss of privacy as there is almost no place the patient can go and be alone. Furthermore, there is at best, a loss of consistent family and social relationships, as usually there are regimented visiting hours. There also is a loss of freedom surrounding social activities, or freedom to move around in the community as they might choose. They are not allowed to attend club meetings, to attend the church of their choice or visit friends or even to walk down to the corner grocery store. Neither can they putter around in their garden, fish or continue other former activities as they choose, and in many instances they cannot even look at the TV program of their choice, as there are other people to be considered in choosing a program. There is usually a loss of meaningful possessions such as pieces of furniture, linens, china, pets, silver, pictures, paintings, homes, property.

Many patients refuse to get out of bed, perform selfcare functions or eat and become chronic complainers and demanders. These are the only remaining areas in which they can assert themselves.

Symbolically, then, the nursing home becomes a "prison" to which the patient feels sentenced for life. Even the civil right to vote is many times not feasible.

In many nursing homes there is very little verbal interaction or communication between patients. Many patients' complaints or demands to nursing personnel are believed to be methods to maintain communication with someone "adequate and independent" in counteracting the feelings of isolation which are so predominant in the nursing home patient.

Patient's Bill of Rights

(Conditions of Participation Medicare/Medicaid Skilled Nursing Facility) *

The governing body of the facility establishes written policies regarding the rights and

* Source: Health Services Administration, DHEW, May 18, 1976.

responsibilities of patients and, through the administrator, is responsible for development of and adherence to procedures implementing such policies. These policies and procedures are made available to patients, to any guardians, next of kin, sponsoring agency(ies), or representative payees selected pursuant to section 205(j) of the Social Security Act, and Subpart Q of Part 404 of this chapter, and to the public. The staff of the facility is trained and involved in the implementation of these policies and procedures.

These patients' rights policies and procedures ensure that at least each patient admitted to the facility:

1. Is fully informed, as evidenced by the patient's written acknowledgment, prior to or at the time of admission and during stay, of these rights and of all rules and regulations governing patient conduct and responsibilities;

2. Is fully informed, prior to or at the time of admission and during stay, of services available in the facility, and of related charges including any charges for services not covered under titles XVIII or XIX of the Social Security Act, or not covered by the facility's basic per diem rate;

3. Is fully informed, by a physician, of his medical condition unless medically contraindicated (as documented, by a physician, in his medical record), and is afforded the opportunity to participate in the planning of his medical treatment and to refuse to participate in experimental research;

4. Is transferred or discharged only for medical reasons, or for his welfare or that of other patients, or for non-payment for his stay (except as prohibited by Titles XVIII or XIX of the Social Security Act), and is given reasonable advance notice to ensure orderly transfer or discharge, and such actions are documented in his medical record;

5. Is encouraged and assisted, throughout his period of stay, to exercise his rights as a patient and as a citizen, and to this end may voice grievances and recommend changes in policies and services to facility staff and/or to outside representatives of his choice, free from restraint, interference, coercion, discrimination or reprisal;

6. May manage his personal financial affairs or be given, at least quarterly, an accounting of financial transactions made on his behalf should the facility accept his written delegation of this responsibility for any period of time, in conformance with State law;

7. Is free from mental and physical abuse, and free from chemical and (except in emergencies) physical restraints except as authorized in writing by a physician for a specified and limited period of time, or when necessary to protect the patient from injury to himself or to others;

8. Is assured confidential treatment of his personal and medical records, and may approve or refuse their release to any individual outside the facility, except, in case of his transfer to another health care institution, or as required by law or third-party payment contract;

9. Is treated with consideration, respect, and full recognition of his dignity and individuality, including privacy in treatment and in care for his personal needs;

10. Is not required to perform services for the facility that are not included for therapeutic purposes in his plan of care;

11. May associate and communicate privately with persons of his choice, and send and receive his personal mail unopened, unless medically contraindicated (as documented by his physician in his medical record);

12. May meet with, and participate in activities of social, religious, and community groups at his discretion, unless medically contraindicated (as documented by his physician in his medical record);

13. May retain and use his personal clothing and possessions as space permits, unless to do so would infringe upon rights of other patients, and unless medically contraindicated (as documented by his physician in his medical record); and

14. If married, is assured privacy for visits by his/her spouse; if both are inpatients in the facility, they are permitted to share a room, unless medically contraindicated (as documented by the attending physician in the medical record).

(All rights and responsibilities specified in paragraphs (k) (1) through (4) of this section as they pertain to (a) a patient adjudicated incompetent in accordance with State law, (b) a patient who is found, by his physician, to be medically incapable of understanding these rights, or (c) a patient who exhibits a communication barrier—devolve to such patient's guardian, next of kin, sponsoring agency(ies), or representative payee (except when the facility itself is representative payee) selected pursuant to section 205(j) of the Social Security Act and Subpart Q of Part 404 of this chapter.)

Patient Care

Overview*

What Physician Services Are Provided?

Of the patients who have been in a nursing home less than four months, 90% are reviewed by a physician at least every 30 days. For long-term patients, the proportion reviewed monthly by a physician drops to 75%. Of the physicians who review their cases monthly, 90% actually see their patients and 80% examine the overall care plans.

How Reliable Are Pharmaceutical Services?

Pharmacists are not able to work directly from a physician's written drug order 76% of the time. Twenty-eight percent of the time, physicians do not confirm their drug orders in writing within a two-day period.

Drugs are administered only by licensed personnel 93% of the time. Pharmacists make at least monthly reviews of patients' overall drug profiles in 68% of cases. Sixty-nine percent of facilities do not have separate rooms for drug storage. Controlled drugs are properly inventoried in 79% of all facilities.

How Are Social and Psychological Needs Met?

The proportion of facilities employing staff for social work is 49% (26% full-time). Sixty-two

*Source: DHEW, 1974.

percent of the time, patients' psychosocial needs are evaluated as part of the admitting process. In those facilities with social work staff, 70% of patients have written plans for psychosocial care. Family counseling is carried on 66% of the time.

In 72% of all facilities, social activity programs are conducted by qualified staff (working part-time in 28% of cases). About 50% of medical records note patients' needs for activities and their responses to them. Seventy-five percent of all facilities have space available for activities, and 71% have equipment available.

How Are Patients' Nutritional Needs Met?

Most facilities have the services of a dietician (part-time, in 90% of all cases). Dieticians spend anywhere from half a day to 20 days at a facility each month. Dietetic service supervisors are also retained (60% part-time). In 29% of facilities, too few nutrition staff are on duty in any 12-hour period to permit preparation of meals immediately prior to serving. Sixty percent of all patients' overall care plans lack dietary information.

More than 14 hours between major meals are allowed by 20% of facilities. Twenty-eight percent do not offer an appropriate snack at bedtime. Seventy-three percent of patients who reject half or more of a meal are not offered an appropriate substitute. Nineteen percent of patients who need help in feeding themselves do not receive it promptly at each meal. Thirty-four percent who need mechanical devices to help them eat do not receive them.

What Efforts At Rehabilitation Are Made?

Of the patients who need physical therapy 31% receive it; 11% of those needing occupational therapy get it; and 11% who could benefit from speech therapy get it.

Skilled physical therapists are retained by 72% of all facilities. Forty percent retain occupational therapists, and 32% have speech therapists. Of facilities offering physical therapy, 56% have it at least daily and 29% offer it two or three times a week. For 33% of patients undergoing therapy, there is no written therapy plan. And 84% of patient records do not contain baseline data for use in determining therapy needs.

Types of Therapy Received by Residents

Table 21-24 Nursing home residents receiving types of therapy by age and sex (U.S. 1973–74)

Type of therapy received	All residents	Age				Sex	
		Under 65 years	65–74 years	75–84 years	85 years and over	Male	Female
Number of residents	1,074,500	114,200	162,900	384,400	413,000	317,800	756,600
Percent receiving therapy[1]							
Physical therapy	9.9	11.2	13.4	10.6	7.5	9.5	10.1
Recreational therapy	15.2	17.0	17.3	15.3	13.8	14.1	15.7
Occupational therapy	5.7	8.6	6.7	5.7	4.4	5.1	5.9
Speech therapy	0.5	1.4	1.0	*	*	0.6	0.4
Professional counseling	8.0	11.7	9.3	7.6	7.0	8.7	7.8

[1]Percentages do not add to 100.0 because residents may receive more than one type of therapy.

Source: National Center for Health Statistics.

436

Level of Care Received by Residents

Table 21-25   Distribution of nursing home residents, according to level of nursing care received (U.S. 1973–74)

Level of nursing care received[1]	All residents	Age				Sex	
		Under 65 years	65–74 years	75–84 years	85 years and over	Male	Female
Number of residents	1,074,500	114,200	162,900	384,400	413,000	317,800	756,600
Percent distribution							
All levels	100.0	100.0	100.0	100.0	100.0	100.0	100.0
Intensive nursing care	41.0	35.5	37.0	41.1	44.1	37.6	42.5
Limited nursing care	9.8	9.5	11.0	10.2	9.1	10.1	9.7
Routine nursing care	32.3	30.0	33.8	33.2	31.5	33.6	31.7
Personal nursing care	16.0	24.1	17.1	14.5	14.7	17.5	15.4
No nursing care	0.9	*	1.0	1.0	0.6	1.1	0.8

[1]*Intensive nursing care* includes: full bed bath, catheterization, oxygen therapy, intravenous injections, tube feeding, or bowel/bladder training; *limited nursing care* includes sterile dressings, irrigation, or hypodermic injections; *routine nursing care* includes enemas, blood pressures, and temperature, pulse, or respiration checks; and *personal nursing care* includes a rub or massage, a special diet, medication or other treatment, or assistance in personal hygiene or eating. A resident receiving multiple types of services, was classified at the higher level of nursing care.

Source: National Center for Health Statistics.

Rehabilitative and Psychosocial Services*

Review of patient records indicate that a progressive decline occurs in many patients' mental and physical functioning after admission. Physical and emotional rehabilitation or maintaining patients at a given level is stated as a goal in policies. But relatively few facilities surveyed had qualified rehabilitative or social services staff needed to achieve these goals for the SNF patients.

Surveyors noted that in a large number of facilities, patients' dependency attitudes were reinforced continuously by the manner in which staff addressed them by first name and often as though speaking to a child. This prevalent attitude contrasts sharply with survey data which shows that two-thirds of the patients (66.1% or 187,920) had maintained themselves in the community within the previous 24 months. It underscores again the importance for staff to be aware of the need to strengthen and maintain the capacity of patients to make decisions and retain their dignity.

*Source: DHEW, July 1975.

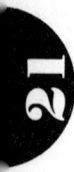

Staffing. While 49.1% of the facilities surveyed were reported as having social services program staff, in only 26.3% were they employed full time. For the part-time staff the time devoted to direct patient services was very limited, except for crisis situations. Hours of work reported for such staff ranged from 6–14 hours per week. In the greater number of facilities, there was very limited understanding of the importance of psychosocial services to assist in maintaining patient physical, social, and mental health. In these facilities staff/patient and patient/patient interaction was minimal. Many patients were found sitting in rows in the facility lobby and halls, not communicating, and waiting for the next meal one or two hours ahead of time. The activities or social programs were directed primarily toward the active resident.

The survey substantiates that there are many patients in skilled nursing facilities who need specialized rehabilitative services that are not receiving them.

The survey further substantiates that there is a significant lack of other critical elements in the specialized rehabilitation services of facilities:

1. Many facilities are not observing the prin-

ciples of electrical safety, particularly with occupational therapy and speech therapy equipment.

2. Preventive maintenance policies and procedure for rehabilitative equipment are absent in many facilities.

3. Many rehabilitative plans of care do not include treatment objectives.

4. There is a lack of documentation of baseline data from initial rehabilitative tests and measurements in patients' medical records.

5. Many specialized rehabilitation plans of care are not being coordinated with patient's total plans of care.

6. Frequently, nursing personnel do not participate in patient's rehabilitative programs.

Drugs in Nursing Homes*

- The average nursing home patient takes from four to seven different drugs a day (many taken twice or three times daily). Each patient's drug bill comes to $300 a year as compared with $87 a year for senior citizens who are not institutionalized. In 1972, $300 million was spent for drugs, 10% of the nation's total nursing home bill.

- Almost 40% of the drugs in nursing homes are central nervous system drugs, painkillers, sedatives or tranquilizers.

- Tranquilizers themselves constitute almost 20% of total drugs—far and away the largest category of nursing home drugs.

- Perhaps most disturbing is the ample evidence that nursing home patients are tranquilized to keep them quiet and to make them easier to take care of. Tragically, recent research suggests that those most likely to be tranquilized sometimes may have the best chance for effective rehabilitation.

- Not surprisingly, 20 to 40% of nursing home drugs are administered in error.

- Kickbacks are widespread. The average kickback is 25% of total prescription charges; over 60% of 4,400 pharmacists surveyed in California reported that they had either been approached for a kickback or had a positive belief that kickbacks were widespread.

Table 21-26   The nursing home prescription market and percent share of manufacturers' dollars (new and refilled prescriptions)

Drug category	Percent
Tranquilizers	21.0
Cardiovasculars	15.2
Diuretics	7.8
Analgesics	6.1
Vitamins	5.3
Sedatives and hypnotics	5.3
Diabetes therapy	5.3
Laxatives	2.9
Psychostimulants	2.7
Hormones	2.6
Antibacterials	2.6
Antispasmodics	1.7
Hematinics	1.7
Other drug categories	14.5
Total	100.0

Inadequate Physician Care*

Physicians have shunned their responsibility for nursing home patients. With the exception of a small minority, doctors are infrequent visitors to nursing homes.

Doctors avoid nursing homes for many reasons:

- Increasing specialization has left smaller numbers of general practitioners, the physicians most likely to care for nursing home patients.

- Most U.S. medical schools do not emphasize geriatrics to any significant degree in their curricula. This is contrasted with Europe and Scandinavia where geriatrics has developed as a specialty.

- Current regulations for the 16,000 facilities participating in Medicare or Medicaid require comparatively infrequent visits by physicians. The some 7,200 long-term care facilities not participating in these programs have virtually no requirements.

- Medicare and Medicaid regulations constitute a disincentive to physician visits; rules constantly change, pay for nursing home visits is comparatively low, and both programs are bogged down in redtape and endless forms which must be completed.

- Doctors claim that they get too depressed in

---

*Source: *Nursing Home Care in the U.S.,* Senate Special Subcommittee on Aging, November 1974.

21

nursing homes, that nursing homes are unpleasant places to visit, that they are reminded of their own mortality.

- Physicians complain that there are few trained personnel in nursing homes that they can count on to carry out their orders.
- Physicians claim they prefer to spend their limited time tending to the younger members of society; they assert there is little they can do for the infirm elderly. Geriatricians ridicule this premise. Others have described this attitude as the "Marcus Welby Syndrome."

The absence of the physician from the nursing home setting leads to poor patient care. It means placing a heavy burden on the nurses who are asked to perform many diagnostic and therapeutic activities for which they have little training. But there are few registered nurses (53,000) in the nation's 23,000 nursing homes. These nurses are increasingly tied up with administrative duties such as ordering supplies and filling out Medicare and Medicaid forms. The end result is that unlicensed aides and orderlies with little or no training provide 80 to 90% of the care in nursing homes.

It is obvious that the physician's absence results in poor medical and to some degree in poor nursing care. Poor care has many dimensions, it means:

No visits, infrequent, or perfunctory visits.
- The telephone has become a more important medical instrument in nursing homes than the stethoscope.
- No physical examinations, pro forma or infrequent examinations.
- Some patients receive insulin with no diagnosis of diabetes.
- Significant numbers of patients receive digitalis who have no diagnosis of heart disease.
- Large numbers of patients taking heart medication or drugs which might dangerously lower the blood pressure do not receive blood pressure readings even once a year.
- Some 20 to 50% of the medication in U.S. nursing homes is given in error.
- Less than 1% of all infectious diseases in the United States is reported—a special problem in nursing homes where patients have advanced age and lessened resistance. This fact was graphically proven in 1970 when 36 patients died in a salmonella epidemic in a Baltimore, Md., nursing home.

- Physicians do not view the bodies of patients who have died in nursing homes before signing death certificates.
- Over one-half of patients transferred from outside of institutional settings were not examined by the attending physician within 48 hours of admission; only three in ten had recorded medical findings; and four in ten immediate physician's orders for care.

Summary—The hard, cold fact is that nursing homes suffer from the lack of medical care and supervision. What patient care exists, is given by nurses. Even then it must be admitted that professional nurses are few and far between (only 53,000 out of some 583,000 nursing home employees). In the end, 80 to 90% of the care is given by untrained aides and orderlies, paid the minimum wage, and showing a turnover rate of 75% a year. Until physicians accept greater responsibility for the care of nursing home patients, the endless stories of negligence, poor care and abuse will continue.

Other Patient Care Abuses

In a 1971 study of 75 nursing homes conducted by the Department of Health, Education, and Welfare, it was found that:

- 37% of the patients taking cardiovascular drugs (digitalis or diuretics or both) *had not had a blood pressure reading in over a year;* and for 25% of these there was no diagnosis of heart disease on the chart.
- 35% of the patients on phenothiazines *had not had a blood pressure recorded in more than a year.*
- A third of the patients being treated for diabetes mellitus *had no diagnosis of diabetes on their charts;* and over 10% of those receiving insulin or oral hypoglycemic agents were not on diabetic diets; and a large number of these *had not had a fasting blood/sugar test in more than a year.*
- *Revised treatment or medication orders* had been written in the past 30 days for only 18% of the patients.
- *40% had not been seen by a physician for over three months.*
- 8% of the patients *had decubitus ulcers;* and 15% *were visibly unclean.*
- 39% of the patients reviewed were inappropriately classified and placed.

- Aides and orderlies provide 80 to 90% of the care in nursing homes.

- Only one-half of the 280,000 aides and orderlies are high school graduates. Most have no training and no previous experience. They are grossly overworked and paid the minimum wage. It is little wonder that they show a turnover rate of 75% a year.

Role of the Nurse

Overview*

Many of the problems of the aged are pathophysiologically complex and require complex pharmacologic and prosthetic interventions. They require careful supervision and monitoring, time-consuming patient education and supportive care. Many other needs have fallen traditionally within the direct purview of nursing, for example, problems with mobility, ambulation, feeding, skin care, bladder and bowel function. Also, such patients have enormous psychosocial needs. Through death or geographic isolation they have often lost the significant interpersonal relationships that previously sustained them. These relationships, or some substitute for them, are essential if the person is to retain his will to live and his capacity to enjoy life. Continuity between patient and provider is needed to sustain such meaningful relationships. It also is important to the efficiency of the care system itself. Significant amounts of time and energy must be spent in grasping the problems and the care plans and the personal idiosyncrasies of each individual patient. Every change in a provider introduces an inefficiency, or worse, an inadequacy into the system.

If these are the needs of chronically ill patients, logic dictates that nurses must play an important, and indeed a critical role in meeting them. Although the intent is not to belittle the importance of physicians, social workers, dietitians and other members of the health care team, it is believed that nurses are in the key position to meet many or most of the patients' needs, whether physical, functional or psychosocial. It is not an accident that facilities for such patients are called nursing homes.

The Emerging Role**

The emerging roles of the registered nurse need to be more widely utilized in long-term care. In the profession, these emerging roles are referred to as the expanded role of the nurse and/or the extended role.

The commitment and contribution of nursing to the large number of chronically ill and elderly persons includes assessment of the patient's health status and identification of his specific nursing problems, formulating a nursing diagnosis, planning with him and his family for his care and implementation, and evaluation of the plan with appropriate modifications when indicated to meet this patient's needs. Nursing's commitments and contributions also include teaching health care principles and practices to the patient and his family, assuming accountability for defining and validating all levels of nursing activity in terms of therapeutic effectiveness, increasing the sophistication of personal care services as health delivery systems expand, and accepting management responsibilities in providing nursing care to the patients.

Nursing contributes an understanding of the developmental stages of the life cycle, the effects of varying settings upon a person's life style, and the effects of chronicity upon a person. Nursing likewise attempts to decrease the regimentation imposed by health care in any setting, and to prevent, diminish, or restore the numerous losses associated with chronicity.

Contributions

Specifically, the commitment and contribution of nursing to promoting delivery of quality health care services to chronically ill and elderly persons include:

- Active nursing participation at the planning level in both the determination and the systematic evaluation of the delivery of health services for these persons.
- Delineation and assumption of appropriate nursing responsibilities for coordinating health services within the health care systems and subsystems so that chronically ill and older patients may have accessible movement into the system and receive continuing, high quality care.

---

*Source: DHEW, March 1976.

**Source: Senate Special Subcommittee on Aging, November 1974.

- Provision of direct, humanistic nursing care services which are based on the personal health needs of chronically ill and older patients. This includes health assessment, health maintenance, and consultative and restorative nursing care in primary acute and long-term care circumstances both in and out of the hospital environment.
- Demonstration of accountability for appropriate and effective use of human and material resources in the nursing management of patient care services in the home and in institutional and other community health care facilities.

Functions

Some of the functions which R.N.s perform include:

- Dressings of all kinds
- Clysis
- Catheter insertion and changes
- Impactions
- Tube feeding
- Oxygen therapy
- Intravenous injections
- Intramuscular injections
- Dispensing medications
- Subcutaneous injections
- Ostomy irrigations—all kinds
- Ostomy care
- Urological irrigations—all kinds
- Ear and eye irrigations
- Lavage and gavage
- Isolation
- Assistance with thoracentesis and paracentesis
- Suctions

Registered nurses are quick to stress that some of the functions mentioned above should be performed only by a professional nurse; they should not be performed by aides and orderlies. They also stress that nurses have considerable room for independent decisions with respect to patient care.

Patient Care Plan*

A nursing assessment is a method of learning enough about the patient, his problems and his strengths so that his nursing care can be tailored to meet his needs. It is composed of three integral parts: nursing history, nursing diagnosis and nursing therapy.

*Source: J. S. Rothberg, "Nursing Assessment of the Aged Person," October 28, 1968. (Speech at Boston College.)

Nursing History

A nursing history is the collection of pertinent information about the patient as a person. One part will yield knowledge about the person's normal life style and his pattern of daily living. This would include questions such as what his normal waking time is; what he likes to eat; his usual meal times; does he sleep well and uninterruptedly; whether he showers or bathes, and in the morning or at night, etc.

... The nursing history should identify the patient's perceptions and expectations related to his illness, hospitalization and care. Further, it focuses on the meaning of illness and hospitalization for the patient and his family. The nurse inquires about what is wrong with him, why he sought care, what he understands to be the cause of his illness, what he expects the outcome of treatment to be, etc.

We seek further information regarding the patient's condition—the relative state of health in physical, functional and behavioral areas. We are looking for both strengths and weaknesses in these areas and for both overt and covert problems.

Nursing Diagnosis

The next step in the progression is the nursing diagnosis. Nursing diagnosis consists of:

1. An evaluation of the patient's condition as a person including physical, physiologic, and behavioral aspects.
2. Development of a clearly defined set of goals for patient care. (One such goal, in the physical realm, might be to obtain the maximum possible improvement in the patient's condition, for instance, total cure. Another goal might have to be more modest—such as maintenance of his present condition without further deterioration. A different kind of goal might be one which aimed at an increase of the patient's verbal interaction with his roommates.) Goals include physical, functional and behavioral areas. The patient must be consulted in any goal-setting; he must be enlisted as a partner in his care or the care will not be effective.
3. A determination of which of the identified care needs are amenable to nursing interventions.

Nursing Therapy

Once the nursing care needs have been defined clearly by the history and diagnosis, a course of nursing activities purposefully

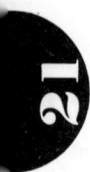

directed toward increasing the positive health of the patient can be initiated. The nurse selects the appropriate methods, resources, and personnel to meet the identified needs. Those needs which are beyond the scope of nursing are referred to the appropriate health workers. Nursing therapy is knowledgeable intervention in the form of nursing activities, based on the nursing diagnosis, and directed at moving the individual toward positive health.

There is a further step required. The nurse follows through on her actions to determine whether the need was met. She explores with the patient and makes observations to validate that her nursing therapy did achieve its purpose in helping him. She will be available to respond to his changing needs and to modify her actions in terms of his response.

The Nurse Practitioner*

The practitioner should use these principles:

1. Understand the interrelatedness of the aged person and his environment.
2. Look at the whole person—medically, psychologically, socially—and not just at symptoms.
3. Establish goals—to restore the sick to health, to help the individual function at his best. These goals are not only needed for the aged individual; they are necessary to the practitioner who otherwise will feel frustrated and futile.
4. Establish different goals for different individuals in different situations.
5. Treat specific diseases as well as health maintenance and promotion.
6. Utilize the full range of the community's health and social services in an integrated approach. Recognize that every health practitioner may have a contribution to make.

Problems and Answers

Nursing Home Abuses

The Senate Special Subcommittee on Aging identified what it considered to be the most important nursing home abuses in 1975:

- Negligence leading to death and injury
- Unsanitary conditions

- Poor food or poor preparation
- Hazards to life or limb
- Lack of dental care, eye care or podiatry
- Misappropriation and theft
- Inadequate control of drugs
- Reprisals against those who complain
- Assault on human dignity
- Profiteering and "cheating the system."

The report stated that "such abuses are far from isolated instances. They are widespread. Estimates of the number of substandard homes (that is, those in violation of one or more standards causing a life-threatening situation) vary from 30 to 80 percent." The subcommittee estimates at least 50% were substandard with one or more life threatening conditions.

Why Nurses Avoid Nursing Homes**

There are few nurses in the nation's 23,000 nursing homes. Of the 815,000 employed registered nurses (R.N.s) in the nation, only 65,235 can be found in U.S. long-term care facilities.

There are many reasons to explain the limited number of professional nurses in nursing homes. To begin with, federal regulations require registered nurses only in America's 7,300 skilled nursing facilities; even then only one R.N. is required seven days a week (exceptions are made in rural areas). Some nursing home operators, intent on limiting costs and increasing profits, have refused to hire more than the minimum number of nurses required by law. Instead they seek to "make do" with unlicensed aides and orderlies whom they need pay only the minimum wage. The 8,200 Intermediate Care Facilities are required to have only a licensed practical nurse in charge—again only during the day shift. The remaining 7,500 facilities need have no "licensed" nursing officer at all. To make matters worse, there are no requirements for ratios between nurses and patients in federal regulations. By contrast the state of Connecticut requires one R.N. for every 30 patients on the day shift, one for every 45 on the afternoon and one for every 60 in the evening.

- Nurses have little training in geriatrics and the needs of nursing home patients and are

21

*Source: DHEW, 1974.

**Source: Senate Special Subcommittee on Aging, November 1974.

442

therefore unprepared to work in long-term care facilities. Of the over 1,000 schools of nursing surveyed by the subcommittee, only 27 responded that they had a program wherein geriatrics was treated as a specialty.

● There are no graduate programs in geriatric or gerontology nursing. Federal government programs likewise neglect geriatrics. In 1970 there were 144 programs for the training of nurses and health care personnel administered by 13 agencies. None of these programs emphasized geriatrics.

Other reasons more directly explain the comparative absence of nurses. These include: the poor image of nursing homes, poor working conditions, low job satisfaction, low wages, and few fringe benefits. There is also a general dissatisfaction with the role of nurses in the nursing home setting. (1) They are saddled with more and more administrative responsibilities, cutting down on the time they can devote to actual patient care. (2) Scandals and persistent reports of abuses discourage even dedicated nurses who have committed themselves to long-term care. (3) They must struggle against negative attitudes toward nursing home care. The general public and fellow professionals tend to regard their work as uninteresting, depressing, and even second-rate.

In testimony before the Senate Subcommittee on Aging in November 1974, the American Nurses' Association explained why registered nurses bypass nursing homes:

1. Nursing homes have a poor image as far as nurses are concerned.
2. The average nurse is ill-prepared to meet the needs of elderly people with long-term, complex, medical problems without supplementary training.
3. The difficulties of practicing safe nursing care according to accepted standards of practice are very great because of restricted policies or lack of policies in many of these institutions.
4. The lack of authority vested in the nursing service department makes it very difficult to carry out the kind of care that is required.
5. The isolation of the nursing home from other health facilities makes it an unpopular place to practice.
6. There is a lack of stimulation and support

from nurses, physicians, and other health workers.
7. The overall administration of many of the facilities is very poor. An important factor in the high turnover of nurses was the scanty provision of services in proprietary homes.

Although all the homes retained a staff physician, many lacked provision for dental care, radiologic services, and a dietitian or a clinical librarian. Only half of the proprietaries had an occupational or speech therapist, and only three of ten a physical therapy program. Less than half had a recreational area and only 12% had a library. All of these shortages, detrimental as they are to the level of care that can be provided, meant that the nurses had to carry a heavier load. "It may be that the nurses' indication upon leaving employment that the pay is too low does not present the entire picture . . . What they may really mean is that the pay is too low considering the conditions in which work must be performed."

Training Nurses for Geriatrics
What's To Be Taught*

The Senate Special Subcommittee on Aging recommended in 1974 that all professionals and workers being prepared for long-term health care in any setting should have exposure to the following basic concepts (to be taught at the educational level of the worker and in the depth and detail he understood and used):

● Process of normal aging—biological, psychological, and sociological
● Attitude toward aging, including respecting the value and dignity of each individual and the patient's rights
● Concepts of disease prevention and maintenance of health
● Concepts of rehabilitation, both mental and physical, to the highest functioning level, to include remotivation and reality orientation
● Chronic diseases and the meaning of chronicity
● Nutrition as applied to long-term care
● Pharmacology and long-term care
● Administrative environment or climate in which care is given

*Source: Senate Special Subcommittee on Aging, November 1974.

- Death and dying
- Interaction with families
- Human sexuality—sexual needs of aged and long-term patients
- Mental health

In-service education and ongoing staff development programs should be an essential requirement for all long-term care agencies. There should be more adequate enforcement of the requirements in licensing rules and regulations. The option of a consortium approach and shared services of an in-service educator should be implemented by smaller agencies.

Federal Aid for Training*

In 1974, to further the Department of Health, Education, and Welfare's efforts toward upgrading the quality of care in nursing homes by improving the skills of those responsible for providing that care, 16 contracts for state and national training programs were awarded, totaling almost $1.3 million. These programs were designed to include: (1) the instruction of nurse aides employed in long-term care facilities in rural areas of four states; (2) the nationwide training of medical directors in skilled nursing facilities (to achieve compliance with legislative mandates, mandatory by December 1975); (3) nationwide seminars and workshops for dietitians and other food service personnel; and (4) a national training system for medical record consultants employed by long-term care facilities.

What Makes a Good Nursing Home?**

Good nursing homes are a matter of motivation. Of paramount importance is the administrator's ability to stimulate his staff, to create an intangible kind of harmony, unity of purpose, and spirit, rooted in competence and compassion.

A. Positive Approaches to Therapy and Rehabilitation

Many of the best nursing homes in the United States feature innovative approaches to therapy and rehabilitation. A variety of tech-

---

*Source: DHEW, July 1975.

**Source: Senate Special Subcommittee on Aging, November 1974.

niques are used to upgrade the mental and physical functioning of patients.

Two examples of good nursing homes are St. Joseph's Manor in Trumbell, Conn., and Golden Acres in Dallas, Tex. At Golden Acres the team spirit concept is expressed as the LIFE program (love, interest, fulfillment, and enrichment). Personnel at Golden Acres and St. Joseph's Manor begin with the premise that the disabled adult can be rehabilitated. It is assumed that much lost function can be restored. Likewise, the Crystal Springs Rehabilitation Center in San Mateo County, Calif., dedicates each and every staff member to the goal of rehabilitation of patients.

Reality Orientation—This is a term for a program developed by Dr. James Folsom. The basic aim is to put a regressed patient into renewed contact with the world around him. The program can be conducted in a class or through informal interaction. Orientation is begun at the most basic level. If a patient does not know his own name, he is taught.

If he does not know where he is from, he is told. Then, the patient is taught the day, the week, the month, the year, his age, etc. Typically, patients may exhibit confusion for many weeks. Yet, once a patient is able to grasp any bit of information such as his name, the name of his spouse, his birthday, he begins to recall and use ever-increasing amounts of previously known material.

Sensory Training—Sensory training supplements basic reality orientation by stimulating the patient's sensory sensitivity. As implemented at the White Plains Center for Nursing Care, N.Y., patients are gathered together in small groups and asked to identify objects by smell, taste, hearing, touch, and sight.

Remotivation—Remotivation is a technique which was developed in mental hospitals some years ago. Essentially, it is an effort to find out what activities the patient enjoyed doing in earlier life or would have liked to have done, and directing him to those same goals.

Remotivation can involve the use of rewards of many different types. Allowing a patient to participate in activities he enjoys is one form of reward. Certain foods can be given as a reward along with the verbal feedback and reinforcement given for increased effort and motivation.

B. Improvements in Physical Structure

Some homes boast improvements in the physical structure which facilitate better

21

21

patient care and greater patient comfort. Innovations in this area run the gamut from "campuses" for senior citizens, which provide the broad range of health care services in one location, to the use of color and design to make nursing homes more appealing and better suited to the needs of the infirm aged.

C. Positive and Innovative Approaches to the Education and Utilization of Employees

One of the most important series of positive and innovative programs relates to the education and utilization of employees. Nursing homes presently offer a variety of such techniques, including:

- Employee sensitivity training is the practice of requiring prospective employees to assume the role of patients for 24 hours before their employment. By this experience the employees are "sensitized" to the needs of the aged patients.
- Accident prevention programs reduce injury.
- In-service training programs and continuing education programs help employees perform their jobs. Some schools of nursing have established programs whereby student nurses work in nursing homes as part of their training. Some homes use computers to monitor patient care and for staff education.
- A novel program in St. Paul, Minn., trains able-bodied senior citizens to work in nursing homes. Under the direction of Dr. Lucille Poor, able-bodied senior citizens complete three-week training programs and are paid $1.65 an hour as they train. When the course is completed, the senior joins the staff of a nursing home at regular wages. The program emphasizes food nutrition in health and illness. Menu planning, food service, the psychological meaning of food and diet, as well as the special feeding of stroke patients, are given attention. The program may present a model for a wider program of employing able-bodied older Americans in nursing homes.

D. Innovative Activities or Services

Many of the best nursing homes in the nation feature comprehensive activity programs. Activity programs range from residents' councils (self-government by patients) to senior citizens' olympic games. Activity programs generally are inexpensive but they can have a

dramatic effect on the patient's sense of dignity and comfort in the nursing home environment.

Unfortunately, television in many nursing homes is the primary form of therapy, as well as diversion.

Recommendations*

1. Educational programs for nursing home administrators should be expanded. Nursing home administrators should make an effort to stimulate their employees, rewarding them for dedication and enthusiasm in the care of nursing home residents.
2. Activities and recreation should become a way of life, rather than a treat, in nursing homes.
3. Interpersonal techniques for dealing with the disturbed elderly (such as reality orientation, sensory training, and remotivation) should be implemented in nursing homes. Whenever possible, such techniques should be substituted for the excess reliance on tranquilizing drugs.
4. The physical design of homes should accommodate the unique problems of the infirm elderly. Special attention should be given to color schemes, warmth, texture, and to promoting maximum use of common areas.
5. All nursing homes should regularly offer in-service training programs and participate in extramural continuing education.
6. Schools of nursing, medicine, social work, public health, and other health professions should provide education in the specialty of gerontology and geriatrics.
7. Nursing homes and schools of nursing should cooperate to exchange information and expertise.
8. Nursing homes should offer outreach programs to the underserved elderly population in their community through senior citizen centers, meals-on-wheels, telephone reassurance, and other services.
9. Legislation should be enacted to pay able-bodied senior citizens for working in nurs-

---

*Source: Senate Special Subcommittee on Aging, November 1974.

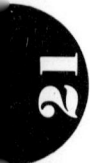

ing homes. Earnings under this program should be exempt from the Social Security retirement test which presently requires seniors to forfeit some of their Social Security checks if they earn more than $2,-520 a year.

10. All states should establish ombudsman projects to investigate nursing home complaints and monitor the quality of nursing home care. (See S. 1569, introduced by Senator Moss.)

11. Senior citizen groups and community leaders should publish nursing home directories and nursing home ratings. They should establish referral services to aid consumers in shopping for a nursing home.*

12. Local civic organizations should make an effort to "adopt" a nursing home, schedul-

---

*Those who would like to become involved in the effort to bring about a better quality of nursing home care will benefit from the report, *Citizens Action Guide: Nursing Home Reform,* prepared by Elma Griesel and Linda Horn for the Gray Panthers of Philadelphia, Pa., April 1975.

ing daily visits and providing other assistance to nursing home residents.

13. Nursing home administrators should actively seek and participate in peer review activity.

14. Nursing homes should consider incorporating telecommunications systems. Such systems used in conjunction with nursing practitioners can be particularly helpful in providing quality health care to every resident 24 hours a day.

15. Residents' councils should be established in nursing homes to provide residents with a real voice in the operation of their environment.

16. A model nursing home should be created within the National Institute on Aging incorporating the broad range of health care services including skilled nursing and intermediate care as well as day care and various kinds of outreach services—especially home health care. The model facility should serve as a focus for further research into the techniques and procedures which will improve the quality of care in U.S. nursing homes. The model facility should implement procedures found to be effective, and serve as an educational and consulting center for providers.

21

22
MENTAL HEALTH

The Decline of the Mental Hospital*

A quarter of a century ago and earlier, state and county mental hospitals were the primary resource for the treatment and care of mentally ill persons and were continuing to grow annually in the number of resident patients.

However, beginning in 1956 and in each succeeding year through 1974, the number of resident patients was lower than the previous year. Between 1955 and 1974 the number of resident patients declined from 558,922 to 215,573, a decrease of 61%. The decrease is due to a combination of medical, social, economic, and political factors. The first year of the decline (1956) coincided with the large-scale introduction of psychotropic drugs, medicines credited in numerous quarters for the abrupt reverse in the upward trend in the number of resident patients.

Other factors influencing the reduction in state mental hospital residents included more efficient admission and discharge procedures; more effective utilization review procedures; an increase in the availability and use of alternative resources in the community, including nursing homes, halfway houses, community mental health centers, and general hospital psychiatric services; affiliation of community mental health centers with state mental hospitals; administrative changes such as the introduction of the geographic unit system; and a gradual reduction in the average length of stay.

However, most observers share the view of H. Dingman (1974) who stated that "rising costs more than any other factor have finally made it obvious that support of the state mental hospitals is politically unfeasible and . . . this is the principal factor behind the present push to get rid of state mental hospitals."

Several studies have supported the belief that the majority of patients in state mental hospitals could be discharged if suitable alternatives were available in the community.

Two federal programs, the Community Mental Health Services Act and the Social Security Act, have had a significant impact on the shift of emphasis from services in large state hospitals to local community services. The Community Mental Health Services Act has provided funds to local communities for construction and staffing of local mental health facilities. Major changes in the subsections of the Social Security Act—Medicare, Medicaid, and increased public assistance—have provided a funding base for mental health services within the local community.

Mental Health Facilities

Mental Health Facilities, Admissions and Utilization*

Between 1972 and 1974 there was a 17% decrease in the number of beds available in mental hospitals—continuing a trend away from institutionalization of the mentally ill.

There were over 2.7 million admission episodes to the 3,200 mental health facilities in the United States in 1971, an admission rate of 1.3 per 100 population. About two out of every three admissions were to public mental health facilities, even though only about half (46.3%) of the facilities were operated under public auspices. This is due to the larger size of public vs. private facilities.

Of the total admissions, 47% were to inpatient services, 50% to outpatient services; and 3% were to day treatment services. Of the total admissions to inpatient and outpatient services combined, 36% were under 24 years of age, 38% were 25–44 years of age, 22% were 45–64 years old, and 5% were 65 or older. Males accounted for 52% of the total admissions. Nonwhite admissions constituted 17% of the total, with an admission rate (1,696 per 100,000 population) 45% higher than the white rate (1,173 per 100,000 population).

State and county mental hospitals account for only 17% of the total number of inpatient services, but they account for 32% of the admissions and 78% of the resident patients at the end of the year in inpatient services. This is because the state mental hospitals have a large resident population (an average of over 1,000 per hospital) relative to other types of inpatient facilities.

---

*Source: National Institutes of Mental Health,

448

Types of Facilities

Table 22-1   Mental health facilities by type of facility, 1975

Type of facility	Number of facilities	Number of beds	Percentage of beds
Total, all facilities	(3,200)[1]	393,394	100.0
Psychiatric hospitals	508	335,881	85.4
State & county	294	280,277	71.3
Proprietary	187	15,369	3.9
Veterans administration hospitals	27	40,235	10.2
General hospital psychiatric services	(770)	24,518	6.2
Public	(158)	6,374	1.6
Nonpublic	(612)	18,144	4.6
Residential treatment center for emotionally disturbed children	(344)	19,023	4.9
Federally funded community mental health centers	(295)	12,391	3.1
Day hospitals—free-standing	(34)		
Outpatient clinics—free-standing	(1,123)		
Public	(588)		
Nonpublic	(535)		
Other multi-service facilities	(33)	1,581	0.4

[1]All numbers in parentheses from 1971.

Patient Admissions

Table 22-2   Admission episodes by service and facility, 1971

	Number of annual admissions to:		
Type of facility	Inpatient services	Outpatient services	Day treatment services
Total, all facilities	1,269,029	1,378,822	75,545
Psychiatric hospitals	494,640	147,383	18,448
State & county	407,640	129,133	16,554
Proprietary	87,000	18,250	1,894
Veterans Administration hospitals	134,065	51,645	4,023
General hospital psychiatric services	519,926	282,677	11,563
Public	215,158	139,077	4,291
Nonpublic	304,768	143,600	7,272
Residential treatment centers for emotionally disturbed children	11,148	10,156	994
Federally funded community mental health center	75,900	335,648	21,092
Day hospitals—free-standing	—	—	1,514
Outpatient clinics free-standing	—	484,677	10,642
Public	—	273,358	7,737
Nonpublic	—	211,319	2,905
Other multi-service facilities	33,350	66,636	7,269

Utilization of Inpatient Services

Table 22-3   Utilization of inpatient services, mental health facilities

Type of facility	Number of inpatient services 1971	Resident population end of 1970	Patient care episodes[1] 1971
	Number		
All inpatient services	1,917	433,786	1,755,816
Psychiatric hospitals	482	348,296	843,222
State & county	324	337,619	745,259
Proprietary	158	10,677	97,963
Veterans Administration hospital	110	42,735	176,800
General hospitals	653	18,093	542,642
Public	141	4,899	223,551
Nonpublic	512	13,194	319,091

[1] Patient care episodes are defined as the number of residents in inpatient facilities at the beginning of the year (or the number of persons on the rolls of noninpatient facilities) plus the total additions to these facilities during the year.

State and County Mental Health Facilities

Types of Facilities*

1. **Psychiatric Hospital**—A public or private mental hospital in which the primary concern is to provide inpatient care and treatment to the mentally ill.

2. **General Hospital**—

a. *With separate psychiatric service(s):* A hospital that knowingly and routinely admits patients to a separate psychiatric service for the express purpose of diagnosing and treating psychiatric illness. A separate psychiatric unit is an organizational or administrative entity within a facility which provides one or more treatments or other clinical services for patients with a known or suspected psychiatric diagnosis and is specifically established and staffed for use by patients served in this unit.

b. *Without separate psychiatric service(s):* General hospitals accepting psychiatric patients for treatment but with no separate psychiatric services.

3. **Residential Treatment Center for Emotionally Disturbed Children**—A residential institution that primarily serves children who by clinical diagnosis are moderately or seriously disturbed emotionally,

*Source: *NIMH Mental Health Directory,* 1975.

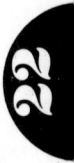

and provides treatment services usually under the supervision of a psychiatrist.

4. **Outpatient Psychiatric Clinic**—An administratively distinct facility whose primary purpose is to provide nonresidential mental health service and in which a psychiatrist assumes medical responsibility for all patients and/or directs the mental health program.

5. **Mental Health Day/Night Facility**—A separate facility designed for nonresidential patients who spend only part of a 24-hour period in the facility.

6. **Federally Funded Comprehensive Community Mental Health Center (CMHC)**—A legal entity through which comprehensive mental health services are provided to a delineated catchment area. This mental health delivery system may be implemented by a single facility (with or without subunits) or by a group of affiliated facilities which make available at least the following essential mental health services: inpatient, partial, outpatient, emergency care, and consultation and education. Further, one of the component facilities of the center is the recipient of Federal funds under P.L. 88-164 (construction) and/or P.L. 89-105 (staffing).

State and County Mental Hospitals

Despite a 36% decrease between 1969 and 1974 in the number of beds in state and county mental health hospitals, these beds still

450

comprised 71% of inpatient psychiatric beds in all types of mental health facilities in the United States.

Distribution of Hospitals and Beds—As of January 1974 the 324 state and county mental hospitals maintained 280,277 inpatient beds, or an average of 865 beds per hospital. The hospitals were all relatively large, as they have been historically, with 20%

maintaining 1,500 beds and over, 54% maintaining 200–1,499 beds, and 26% maintaining less than 200 beds.

In January 1974 there were only 135 beds in state mental hospitals per 100,000 population as compared with a rate of 221 beds per 100,000 population in January 1969. The percent decrease in the rates ranged from 7% in South Carolina to 67% for Maine.

Facilities

Table 22-4   Hospitals and inpatient beds, state and county mental hospitals, U.S.

	Jan. 69	Jan. 74	% change 69–74
Number of hospitals	314	324	+ 3.2%
Number of inpatient beds	441,551	280,277	−36.5%
Beds per 100,000 Civ. Res. Pop.	221.1	134.7	−39.1%

Source: National Institute of Mental Health, 1976.

Patients

Table 22-5   Resident patients by age, state and county mental hospitals

	All ages						
	1973	1972	1971	1970	1969	1968	1967
Total U.S.	248,518	274,837	308,983	337,619	369,969	399,152	426,309
Under 18	10,576	11,269	12,519	12,844	12,841	12,062	12,056
18–64	167,327	185,089	208,082	225,688	245,708	266,950	285,916
Over 65	70,615	78,479	88,382	99,087	111,420	120,140	128,337

Length of Stay

Table 22-6   Time intervals between admission and release—state and county mental hospitals, U.S., 1971 (Excludes state hospitals for the criminally insane)

Number of admissions	Cumulative percent released live within:					Median days of stay— all admissions
	Less than 8 days	8–30 days	31–60 days	61–90 days	91–182 days	
407,640	13.1	38.7	61.1	74.7	86.9	41

Community Mental Health Center

It was during the mid-twentieth century that significant developments began to take place in relation to community health services in this country. In 1956, Congress established the Joint Commission on Mental Illness and Health. The Commission's final report stimu-

lated the growth of community mental health services by recommending that the construction of large mental hospitals be ended and a flexible array of services be provided for the mentally ill in the community. In response, Congress passed the Mental Retardation

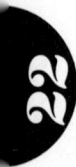

Facilities and Community Mental Health Centers Construction Act of 1963 (P.L. 88-164). This act and subsequent amendments provided financial assistance to public and nonprofit facilities for the construction and staffing of mental health centers. More than 500 comprehensive mental health centers have been established in this country since then.

In order to be considered a comprehensive mental health center, a center must provide at least five essential services: inpatient service, outpatient service, day care service, 24-hour emergency service, and consultation and educational services available to community agencies and professional personnel.

The community mental health center may consist of several types of health facilities joined by administrative arrangement to form a comprehensive program that provides a continuity of care.

Additional services such as rehabilitation, training, research and evaluation, central administrative services, and special services for specific patient groups are provided by many centers. Each center serves a distinct community ranging in size from 75,000 to 200,-000 persons.

In 1973 the number of people receiving care at centers increased to 1,094,430, and many more were reached by the indirect services provided.

Psychiatric Outpatient Services

In 1909 the first community psychiatric clinic was established at the Institute for Juvenile Research in Chicago and in the same year, the first guidance clinic was set up as a traveling clinic from the St. Lawrence State Hospital in New York State. In 1910 traveling clinics were established in Massachusetts and soon after outpatient clinics were set up in some state hospitals in other states. The high incidence of shock and other psychiatric disorders found among American soldiers during World War I gave strong impetus to further development of psychiatric clinics. The period following World War II extended the outpatient clinic movement as services were organized in communities to meet the needs of returning veterans with psychiatric problems.

In recent years a number of different types of outpatient mental health services and programs have been developed: outpatient services affiliated with psychiatric hospitals, public and private, and outpatient psychiatric services of other mental health facilities, such as residential treatment centers for emotionally disturbed children.

The National Institute of Mental Health (NIMH) classifies psychiatric clinics broadly as follows:

1. *Free-standing outpatient psychiatric clinic*—an administratively distinct facility whose primary purpose is to provide non-residential mental health services and in which a psychiatrist assumes medical responsibility for all patients and/or directs the mental health program.

2. *Hospital-affiliated outpatient psychiatric service*—an administrative subunit of a mental health facility. The primary purpose of this subunit is to provide nonresidential mental health services for which a psychiatrist assumes medical responsibility for all patients and/or directs the mental health program, that is, the outpatient service of a psychiatric hospital or a general hospital.

There were approximately 2,200 outpatient mental health services in the United States in 1974 (excluding 454 outpatient services of federally funded community health centers). Almost a third of these were located in the Northeast region of the United States. New York led the nation in the number of such facilities, with 272, followed by California (176) and Pennsylvania (131).

In 1973, 1.2 million persons entered outpatient psychiatric services for a ratio of 576 admissions per 100,000 population.

Of the 324 state and county hospitals, 169 (53%) provided outpatient treatment, 11% maintained halfway houses, 26% reported having some type of psychiatric emergency walk-in service (22% provided this service 24 hours, 7 days a week and 4% provided this service less than 7 days a week and/or less than 24 hours a day).

Of the 1,092 free-standing clinics in operation during 1974, 47% were operated by state or local governments. Services in clinics include: diagnosis, the provision of treatment, and related services for persons with mental and emotional disorders, as well as a variety of mental health services for the community.

Table 22-7   Changes in outpatient treatment by state and county mental hospitals, 1973

	Total patient additions	Average additions per hospital
Outpatient treatment	167,647	992
Day treatment	16,793	123
Halfway house	2,353	69

Table 22-8   Outpatient psychiatric services, 1974

No. of outpatient psychiatric services	2,217
Admissions	1,209,271
Admissions per 1,000 population	5.8

Personnel in Mental Health Facilities

Number of Personnel in Each Facility

Table 22-9   Personnel in state and county mental (psychiatric) hospitals, 1974

	Number	Percentage		Number	Percentage
Total all staff	236,599	100.0%	Mental health workers (less than B.A.)	93,182	39.4
Psychiatrists	5,881	2.5			
Other physicians	3,018	1.3			
Total psychologists	3,385	1.4	Physical health prof. & asst. (e.g., dentists, dental techs.,		
Psychologists—M.A. & above	2,745	1.2	pharmacists, dieticians, etc.)	6,434	2.7
Other psychologists	640	0.2			
Total social workers	6,248	2.6	Total patient care staff	153,585	64.9
Social workers—M.S.W. (or M.A.) and above	3,232	1.4	Total prof. patient care staff	51,182	21.6
Other social workers	3,016	1.2			
Registered nurses	15,422	6.5	Administrative & other prof. (nonhealth) staff (e.g., accts.,		
Licensed practical or voc. nurses	9,221	3.9	business administrators, etc.)	3,649	1.5
Other mental health prof., B.A. & above (e.g., vocational rehab. counselors, occupational			All other staff (clerical,		
therapists, teachers)	10,794	4.6	maintenance, etc.)	79,365	33.6

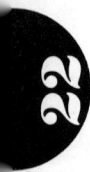

Table 22-10   Personnel in all mental health facilities, 1974

	All personnel		R.N.s		L.P.N.s		Social workers	
	Number	Percent	Number	Percent	Number	Percent	Number	Percent
Total all facilities	454,056	100.0%	39,228	100.0%	18,307	100.0%	27,042	100.0%
Total psychiatric hospitals	263,609	58.0	18,891	48.1	10,505	57.4	6,942	25.7
State and county	236,599	52.1	15,422	39.3	9,221	50.4	6,248	23.1
Private mental hospitals	27,010	5.9	3,469	8.8	1,284	7.0	694	2.6
Total VA psychiatric services	44,880	9.9	4,958	12.6	2,166	11.8	1,681	6.2
Neuropsychiatric hospital	28,600	6.3	2,777	7.1	926	5.0	737	2.7
Gen'l. hospital inpatient units	14,067	3.1	2,031	5.1	1,207	6.6	564	2.1
Gen'l. hospital outpatient units	2,213	0.5	150	0.4	33	0.2	380	1.4
Total nonfederal gen'l. hospital psychiatric services	43,968	9.7	9,419	24.0	3,695	20.2	3,169	11.7
Inpatient units	32,700	7.2	8,981	22.9	3,619	19.8	1,222	4.5
Outpatient units	11,268	2.5	438	1.1	76	0.4	1,947	7.2
Residential treatment center for emotionally disturbed children	20,907	4.6	337	0.9	158	0.9	1,919	7.1
Free-standing outpatient clinics	29,483	6.5	976	2.5	101	0.5	7,210	26.7
Community mental health centers	45,205	10.0	4,148	10.6	1,524	8.3	5,251	19.4
Other	6,004	1.3	499	1.3	158	0.9	870	3.2
Free-standing day/night fac.	1,246	0.3	48	0.1	3		120	0.4
Other multi-service facilities	4,758	1.0	451	1.2	155	0.8	750	2.8

Table 22-11   Personnel in federally funded community mental health centers (February 1974)

Category of personnel	Total employees	Full-time employees (more than 35 hours)	Part-time employees (less than 35 hours)	Trainees	Volunteers
Total professional and technical	45,205	30,343	7,443	3,097	4,322
Medical services:					
Psychiatrists	872	1,023	1,327	481	41
Other physicians	622	74	380	160	8
Nursing services:					
Nurses—R.N.	4,148	2,983	707	389	69
Licensed practical or vocational nurses	1,524	1,258	190	63	13
Therapeutic services:					
Mental health workers[1]	3,066	1,577	327	201	961
Other mental health professionals[2]	5,463	3,811	618	327	707
Other mental health workers[3]	7,735	4,881	897	296	1,661
Psychologists	3,781	2,515	702	489	75
Social workers	5,251	3,874	655	627	95
All other professional and technical	10,743	8,347	1,640	64	692

[1]Less than bachelor's degree.
[2]Bachelor's degree and above.
[3]Less than associate degree.

Source: National Institute of Mental Health, January 1974.

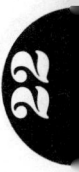

454

R.N.s

R.N.s represent the largest proportion of professional patient care staff in mental health facilities. R.N. positions account for 9% of the total positions and 25% of the professional patient care staff positions in mental health facilities.

Of the 39,228 R.N. positions, 77% were full-time, 14% part-time, and 9% trainee positions. R.N. positions were largely concentrated in mental health facilities providing inpatient psychiatric care. Only 2% of the full-time R.N. positions were located in outpatient psychiatric clinics.

Table 22-12 Registered nurse positions in mental health facilities, by status (January 1974)

	Status			
Type of facility	Total U.S.	Full-time	Part-time	Trainee
All facilities	100.0%	100.0%	100.0%	100.0%
State and county	39.3	43.9	18.8	32.4
Private mental hospitals	8.8	7.6	16.0	8.1
VA psychiatric services	12.6	13.9	8.3	8.9
Nonfederal general hospital psychiatric services	24.0	21.1	35.5	30.8
Residential treatment center for emotionally disturbed children	0.9	0.6	2.3	1.2
Free-standing outpatient clinics	2.5	1.7	4.5	6.0
Community mental health center	10.6	9.9	14.0	10.9
Other	1.3	1.3	0.6	1.7

L.P.N.s, L.V.N.s, and Mental Health Workers

There were 154,786 total L.P.N.s, L.V.N.s and mental health worker positions in mental health facilities in January 1974 (18,307 L.P.N.s or L.V.N.s and 136,479 mental health workers). Combined, these positions accounted for 34% of the total staff positions in mental health facilities. The number of L.P.N.s, L.V.N.s, and mental health workers was about equal to the number of professional staff. This is largely affected by the state and county mental hospitals, however, in which the number of L.P.N.s, L.V.N.s, and mental health workers exceeded the number of professional patient care staff by 200% and VA psychiatric services where the number of L.P.N.s, L.V.N.s, and mental health workers slightly exceed the number of professional patient care staff. In all other types of facilities, the number of professional patient care staff exceeds the number of L.P.N.s, L.V.N.s, and mental health workers.

Over two-thirds of the L.P.N.s, L.V.N.s, and mental health worker positions are located in state and county mental hospitals. The majority of these positions are full-time positions: 89% of the L.P.N.s and L.V.N.s, and 91% of the mental health workers. Between 1972 and 1974 there was a 4% increase in the number of L.P.N., L.V.N. and mental health worker positions.

Changes in Staffing Patterns

The total number of personnel in state and county mental health facilities increased only 1.5% from 1972–74. All disciplines but three experienced increases. Among the largest increases were "other mental health professionals" (e.g., vocational rehabilitation counselors, activity therapists, or school-teachers), psychologists (23%), social workers (12%) and R.N.s (8%). Nonpsychiatric physicians, L.P.N.s and administrative and maintenance staff decreased.

22

Table 22-13   Changes in the staffing patterns of state and county mental hospitals, U.S.

Selected staff categories	Estimated number of full-time equivalent staff				Average FTE staff per 100 resident patients			
	1968	1972	1974	% change 72–74	1968	1972	1974	% change 72–74
Total all categories	238,211	223,886	227,282	+1.5%	57.7	76.7	88.3	+15.0%
Total professional patient care staff	39,944	38,516	46,584	+20.9	9.7	13.2	18.1	+37.1
Psychiatrists	4,967	4,389	4,714	+7.4	1.2	1.5	1.8	+20.0
Physicians, nonpsych.	2,337	2,440	2,286	−6.3	0.6	0.8	0.9	+11.1
Psychologists	1,974	2,484	3,045	+22.6	0.5	0.9	1.2	+33.3
Social workers	4,519	5,324	5,934	+11.5	1.1	1.8	2.3	+27.8
Registered nurses	17,625	13,353	14,398	+7.8	4.2	4.6	5.6	+21.7
Other professionals	8,522	10,526	16,207	+54.0	2.1	3.6	6.3	+75.0
Other patient care staff	119,191	99,791	100,354	+0.6	28.8	34.2	39.0	+14.0
L.P.N., L.V.N.	5,443	12,277	8,971	−26.9	1.3	4.2	3.5	−16.7
Other	113,748	87,514	91,383	+4.4	27.5	30.0	35.5	+18.3
Maintenance & adm. staff	79,076	85,579	80,344	−6.1	19.2	29.3	31.2	+6.5

Source: National Institute of Mental Health, 1976.

Patients

Patient Residences

Table 22-14   Patients with mental disorders resident in selected long-term institutions, 1963 and 1969

Age and sex	Total	State & county mental hospitals	Private mental hospitals	VA hospitals	Nursing homes
1963					
No. of patients	792,827	504,604	9,998	56,504	221,721
%	100.0%	63.6%	1.3%	7.1%	28.0%
1969					
No. of patients	851,029	369,969	10,963	43,385	426,712
%	100.0%	43.5%	1.3%	5.1%	50.1%

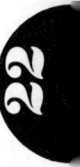

Patient Disorders by Age and Sex

Table 22-15   Residents in nursing and personal care homes by "mental disorder" (June–August, 1969)

		Residents with:		
Age and sex	All residents	Advanced senility	Senility not psychotic	Other mental disorder
		Number of residents		
U.S. total residents	815,130	279,007	180,665	147,705
Under 65	92,866	7,836	6,497	51,290
65 and over	722,264	271,171	174,168	96,415
Males	100.0%	30.2	21.7	21.5
Under 65	100.0%	9.2	6.6	52.3
65 and over	100.0%	34.7	24.9	14.8
Females	100.0%	36.0	22.4	16.6
Under 65	100.0%	7.7	7.3	57.9
65 and over	100.0%	38.7	23.8	12.8

Profile of Patient Disorders by Psychiatric Inpatient Facilities

Table 22-16   Mental patient disorders, by diagnoses and facility

	Type of facility			
Diagnostic category	General hospital separate inpatient services[1]	State and county mental hospitals	Private mental hospitals	Community mental health center inpatient services
All diagnoses	100.0%	100.0%	100.0%	100.0%
Alcohol disorders	8.3	17.8	10.7	13.7
Drug disorders	6.3	2.9	2.6	3.0
Depressive disorders	33.7	10.2	36.7	7.0
Schizophrenic reactions	17.2	29.9	19.0	22.0
Other psychotic disorders	1.7	1.9	1.8	2.2
Psychoneurotic disorders	12.0	2.7	7.2	21.5
Personality disorders	6.8	6.9	4.9	8.1
Transient situational personality disorders	3.6	2.5	0.8	5.7
Organic brain syndromes	6.5	11.0	4.4	4.8
All other disorders	3.9	14.2	11.9	12.0

[1]Excludes data from VA hospitals.

Source: National Institute of Mental Health, 1972 (1969 study).

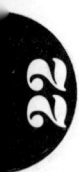

Care of Elderly Mental Patients*

- Some 2 ½ million elderly are going without the mental health services they need.
- Current programs designed to assist the mentally impaired elderly are ineffective and poorly administered.
- Responsibility for mental health programs is fragmented among dozens of federal, state, and local agencies.
- Some patients continue to be housed in state mental hospitals for the single reason that they have no place else to go.
- At the same time, thousands of individuals who need the intensive services which can only be offered at a state hospital have been precipitously discharged into smaller community based facilities.

Nursing homes are one category of such community based facilities receiving large numbers of former patients. Unfortunately, nursing homes are poorly equipped to meet the needs of ex-inmates. There are generally no psychiatric services available, no plans to rehabilitate patients; there are insufficient numbers of trained staff people to care for their needs, and a distinct absence of followup on the part of state hospitals to see that patients are appropriately placed. There are few recreation services, and a heavy and perhaps unwise use of tranquilizers to manage patients. Finally, the effect of mixing the physically infirm patients with the mentally impaired is often deleterious. "Normal" sick patients quite often manifest the behavioral patterns of the disturbed patients they see around them.

Given these facts, experts such as Dr. Jack Weinberg and Dr. Robert Butler have concluded that in most cases the mentally impaired are better off in state mental institutions (as bad as they are) than in nursing homes. However, there is a growing effort on the part of many state and nursing home operators to learn how to manage ex-inmates. Vermont is an excellent example of what is possible when nursing homes work closely with officials of the State Department of Mental Health.

If nursing homes are poorly prepared to meet the needs of the discharged mental patients, boarding homes are even less capable

*Source: Senate Special Subcommittee on Aging, 1975.

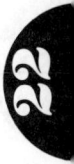

of doing so. More and more patients are being moved from state hospitals into such facilities which go by many names such as "foster care homes," "board and care homes," "domiciliary care facilities," "shelter care facilities," and "personal care homes." They may be greatly dissimilar in physical appearance. Most often, they are converted residences but they may also be new high-rise buildings or converted hotels, in some cases they may be converted mobile homes or renovated chicken coops. What they have in common is that they offer board and room but no nursing care and that most states do not license such facilities.

Between 1969 and 1974, the number of in-patients in state mental hospitals dropped 44%, from 427,799 to 237,692 remaining on an average day at the end of 1974. At the same time, the ranks of the elderly inmates were reduced by 56%, from 135,322 to 59,685. This sharp reduction in the number of in-patients was caused by four factors:

1. Humanitarian motives, the idea that mental hospitals are snakepits, and that patients are better off almost anywhere else.
2. The impact of recent court decisions, which have established that involuntarily committed patients have a constitutional right to treatment and that they must be released if such treatment is not forthcoming.
3. Cost. It costs the average state about $12,000 a year to care for a patient in a state mental hospital. Costs are much higher in some states. At St. Elizabeths Mental Hospital in Washington, D.C., the per patient, per year cost is now $24,000.
4. The impact of the Supplementary Security Income (SSI) program. SSI is a 100% federal welfare program for the aged. It pays $157 per recipient per month in most states. Some states, such as New York, supplement these welfare patients with their own money (New York adds $229 per month for a total SSI payment of $386).

All of these factors come together to push residents out of state hospitals and into boarding homes.

Many states including California, New Mexico, Pennsylvania, Ohio, Michigan, New York, the District of Columbia, and Illinois are beginning to feel the effect of this mass dumping into boarding homes. The reports of poor care, no care, poor food and unspeakable conditions are increasing daily. So many discharged patients have been deposited in the slums of major U.S. cities that instant "psychiatric ghettos" have been created including Chicago's Uptown and the Ontario Road, NW., section of Washington, D.C.

Through the enactment of SSI, the Congress created the beginnings of a for-profit boarding home industry just as it created the for-profit nursing home industry in 1935. In 1935, Congress enacted Social Security but barred payments to inmates in public institutions because of the widespread public reaction condemning conditions in public "poor houses" maintained by most states. However, funds were available to individuals living alone or with unrelated individuals in "boarding homes." Such boarding homes soon added nursing care and became known as nursing homes. In 1972, Congress barred the receipt of SSI funds by "inmates in public institutions" and required that SSI funds be reduced if SSI recipients were living with related individuals. Once again, however, SSI funds could be received in full by residents in boarding homes living with unrelated individuals.

It is obvious that if federal SSI funds are going to be used by the states to care for discharged mental patients, the federal government must step in and require that such facilities be licensed by the states and meet certain federal minimum standards. The alternative would be to permit thousands of mentally impaired Americans to vegetate in unspeakable conditions.

The Aged: Mental Hospitals vs. Nursing Homes*

Between 1960 and 1970 the percentage of institutionalized elderly persons in state and county mental hospitals decreased from about 30% to 12%, whereas the proportion in homes for the aged and dependent increased from 63% to 82%.

Of the total 815,130 residents in nursing and personal care homes in 1969, a little over one-half were identified as having a mental disorder; 279,000 or 34% were diagnosed with advanced senility; and 148,000 or 18% were diagnosed with other mental disorders.

---

*Source: *Statistical Notes,* NIMH, 1975.

Another 181,000 or 22% of the residents were designated as having a condition of senility without psychosis. If this latter group of conditions is included with the others, about three-quarters of the nursing home residents in 1969 had some form of mental disorder or mental disturbance. Since almost all of the residents in these homes are 65 years of age or over the corresponding proportions of this age group with these "mental" conditions are approximately the same.

Over a five year period (1969–1974) there was a 56% drop in the number of older Americans in state institutions on any given day, from 135,322 aged inmates in 1969, to only 59,685 at the end of 1974.

Where Have All the Mental Patients Gone?

Some have been returned to their own families or placed with foster families. Small numbers have found assistance from community mental health centers. However, most of the patients have been placed in for-profit nursing homes or boarding homes which are generally ill equipped to meet their needs.

In the case of nursing homes, severe problems exist because of the limited numbers of nursing personnel, particularly registered nurses, and the general lack of training or experience of these employees in handling psychiatric patients.

There are 5.3 nursing home employees for every 10 patients. The great majority of the employees are aides and orderlies, most of whom have no prior experience or training, some literally hired off the street and most paid the minimum wage. There is a turnover rate of 75% a year among such employees. At the same time there are comparatively few registered nurses in nursing homes (about 65,000 for 23,000 homes). Few of these nurses have psychiatric training, spending more than 50% of their time with administrative duties. They show a turnover rate of 71% a year.

The admission of a few mental patients to a nursing home (whose traditional orientation has been chronic physical disease) can be most disruptive. It places a heavy burden on the already overworked nursing staff. In spite of these shortcomings, it is clear that nursing homes are increasingly making an effort to care for the mentally impaired. There is evidence that some homes handle such patients very well. This is a hopeful sign. It is evident

Table 22-17   Reduction of inpatients in state mental institutions

Year	Total in-patients	Percentage of reduction 1969 base	Total over age 65	Percentage of reduction 1969 base	Percentage of in-patients over age 65
1969	427,799	—	135,322	—	32
1973	304,233	29	84,959	37	28
1974	237,692	44	59,685	56	25

Source: Senate Special Subcommittee on Aging, November 1974.

that with some assistance in terms of training and followup from state hospitals, nursing homes may be able to provide an acceptable alternative to hospital placement.

In some cases mental patients have been placed in the slums of our major cities in such numbers that their presence could scarcely remain unnoticed. This is the case in Uptown, an area of Chicago, where residents now speak of the "geriatric ghetto," a reference to the some 13,000 former mental patients that have been placed in this area of the city. The Ontario Road section of Washington, D.C., provides another example.

Costs

The Costs of Mental Illness*

The cost of mental illness in the United States, measured conservatively, was approximately $36.786 billion in 1974. Of this amount 40%, or $14.5 billion was expended for direct care alone. (This expenditure represented roughly 15% of all direct health expenditures in the U.S. and 1% of the gross national product.)

Nursing homes, together with public mental hospitals, accounted for slightly over 50% of all direct care expenditures in 1974. The remainder of the cost of mental illness was attributable to supportive activities (research, training and fellowships, facilities development, management expenses) and to indirect costs.

Indirect costs are the income or income-equivalent losses which result from deaths due to mental illness, total disability due to mental illness, and loss of productive time to those individuals who are institutionalized or who utilize outpatient therapy for mental illness.

*Source: DHEW, August 1975.

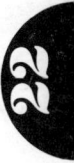

Table 22-18   Costs of mental illness

Type of cost	Cost (in thousands)
A. Direct care	$14,506,028
State & county mental hospitals	2,756,442
Other public mental hospitals	555,506
Private mental hospitals	427,352
General hospitals	1,700,560
Community mental health centers	602,054
Free-standing outpatient clinics	661,467
General medical services	508,049
Nursing homes	4,242,905
Rehabilitation facilities and halfway houses	444,024
Children's programs	497,970
Private practice psychiatrists	1,252,084
Private practice psychologists	122,706
Psychoactive drugs	734,909
B. Research	607,003
C. Training and fellowships	284,841
D. Facilities development	385,230
E. Management expenses	1,167,298
F. Unallocated expenditures of NIMH	22,658
G. Indirect costs	19,812,768
Due to death	4,942,320
Due to disability	10,345,951
Due to patient care activities	4,524,497
Total cost	$36,785,827

Hospital Expenditures

State mental hospitals spent nearly $2.6 billion during 1973. Approximately 80% of total expenditures was allocated to salaries. However, the proportion of total expenditures allocated to salaries ranged from 58% in Wisconsin county hospitals to 86% each in children's and security mental hospitals.

In other hospitals, the proportions of total expenditures allocated to salaries during 1973 were as follows: (1) for-profit psychiatric hospitals (54%), nonprofit psychiatric hospitals (70%) and VA hospitals (81%).

Table 22-19   Expenditures of state and county mental hospitals, by size of hospitals, 1973

Size (based on number of beds)	Total expenditures (in $000's)
All hospitals—U.S.	$2,574,803
Size (based on number of beds)	
Less than 100 beds	71,080
100–199 beds	122,696
200–299 beds	110,824
300–499 beds	139,973
500–999 beds	516,109
1,000–1,499 beds	471,480
1,500–1,999 beds	354,436
2,000 beds and over	788,205

Costs per Patient Day

Total patient maintenance expenditures for state and county mental hospitals in the United States in 1974 were $2.47 billion. Daily maintenance expenditures per resident patient for inpatient services jumped from $8.84 in 1967 to $30.86 in 1974, an increase of 250%.

Table 22-20   Daily maintenance expenditures per resident patient of state and county mental hospitals, U.S.

Year	Daily expenditure per patient day
1967	$ 8.84
1973	25.20
1974	30.86

Source: DHEW, April 1975.

23

PUBLIC HEALTH

Public Health Nursing—History*

In the U.S. modern public health nursing developed in the latter part of the 19th century with the organization in many cities of voluntary agencies called "visiting nurse associations." The purpose of these agencies was to care for the sick at home on a part-time basis.

As time went on the services of nurses in public health broadened to include prevention and control of disease, health education, rehabilitation, and the promotion of healthful living, as well as care of the sick. The services of the public health nurse became an important part of official health departments. Her concern from the beginning was not only for individuals but for families, neighborhoods and communities. In the beginning, public health nursing efforts (like all public health efforts) were directed largely toward the prevention of communicable disease. However, today they are aimed more at the prevention and control of chronic illness and its effects, and at the rehabilitation of individuals and families to the fullest extent possible. The public health nurse is concerned not only with their physical health but with their social and mental health.

She also serves, along with other members of the public health team, in the scientific diagnosis and treatment of the whole community as a patient.

In recent years, with the advent of Medicare and the opportunity for more comprehensive care of the patient at home, the public health nurse has operated within a team comprised of a registered nurse, licensed practical nurse, aide, physical therapist, speech therapist and others. Hence, she has greater responsibility for developing comprehensive plans for nursing care, for team leadership and for the supervision of auxiliary personnel. With the increasing number of auxiliary nursing personnel, she has become responsible for the teaching of licensed practical nurses and aides, as well as volunteers. She also cooperates with civic groups and leaders, church groups, the community's social agencies and similar organizations.

In the public health agencies providing nursing care of the sick at home, the nurse works closely with the physician. She explains and teaches nursing care and treatments to patients and their families. Under organized home care programs, she assists in the coordination of care to the family, serving as liaison between the hospital and the home. And with the growing number of agencies serving some of her patients and their families, the public health nurse is frequently the person who helps patients to understand and integrate the services provided and aids them in taking responsibility for determining and planning their own care.

The nurse assists in the provision of services for healthy mothers and children. This includes health guidance and immunization services for the protection of health. Clinics are provided for the examination, treatment, and health supervision of the tubercular person and his family; for the diagnosis, treatment, and health supervision of persons with venereal diseases or physical handicaps such as orthopedic or cardiac conditions, and for the detection of illness or defects, such as cancer and diseases of the eye. Other specialized clinics are provided wherever they are required.

The nurse in public health helps families to better understand mental, emotional or social problems which are a handicap to the family's well-being and an obstacle to the recovery of the sick. She helps families to use other health and welfare services which the community offers through interagency referrals, conferences with other health workers and in other means.

An increasing number of agencies are providing nursing care to families where there is mental illness. The use of newer drugs and treatments has facilitated the home care of many of the mentally ill. The nurse assists in preparing the family for the return of the patient and with the care and rehabilitation of the patient in the home and the community.

In the program for the promotion of healthful living, nurses in public health assist in prenatal and maternity service and health service for infants, children in preschool years, school children, adolescents, adults and the aged. Consultation in nursing homes and working in rehabilitation programs are also part of the nurse's work as well as service in daycare centers for children and adults, and in programs for the alcoholic and the addict.

---

*Source: R. Spalding, *Professional Nursing* (Lippincott, 1970).

461

Employment

Job Types*

POSITIONS AVAILABLE
IN COMMUNITY HEALTH PROGRAMS

Positions Usually Restricted to Nurses

- Director of a nursing service in a public health agency, generalized or specialized.
- Associate or assistant director in such agency (administrative or educational).
- Supervisor
  a. General service
  b. Field service
  c. Area service
  d. Special service (see list under staff nurse)
- Assistant supervisor.
- Staff nurse rendering general service or special service, such as school nursing, camp nursing, occupational health nursing, midwifery, maternity nursing and child health, orthopedic nursing, psychiatric nursing, tuberculosis nursing, venereal disease nursing and other clinical nursing.
- Community nurse, i.e., a nurse working alone in a small town.
- Rural or urban nurse.
- Consultant in various nursing specialties to official or private agencies, such as the Public Health Service and the Children's Bureau of the U.S. Department of Health, Education, and Welfare, or other government units such as state boards of health, or a community organization such as a council of social agencies.
- Infant welfare nurse.
- Preschool nurse—day care nursery nurse.
- School nurse.
- Nurse teacher in school system.
- Health supervisor in private or public schools, camps and similar places.
- Obstetric, infant or child health nurse.
- Midwife.
- Occupational health nurse in administrative, supervisory or staff position, such as in factory, bank, theater, store, office building and many industries.
- Tuberculosis nurse.
- Nurse for cancer service.
- Cardiac nurse.

*Source: R. Spalding, *Professional Nursing* (Lippincott, 1970).

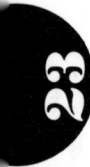

*Positions in Which Nurses Are
Sometimes Employed*

- Administrator of an organization such as a community health center or a day nursery.
- Camp counselor.
- Director of or teacher in a nursery school.
- Medical, psychiatric or family social worker.
- Mental health supervisor.
- Missionary worker, home or foreign.
- Nutritionist.
- Recreation director.
- Playground supervisor.
- Quarantine officer.
- Sanitary inspector or investigator.
- Social hygiene consultant.
- Specialist in parent education.
- Specialist in child guidance.
- Health educator, as in normal school, college or public school system.
- Prevention-of-blindness worker.

Where They Work**

In January 1972, a total of 11,455 public health/community health agencies employed 58,241 registered nurses and 3,305 licensed practical nurses for full-time and part-time public health work in the United States. These agencies also employed 36,419 other health personnel and 26,104 auxiliary personnel.

**Source: DHEW.

Figure 23-1 Public health R.N.s and L.P.N.s employed, by type of local agency

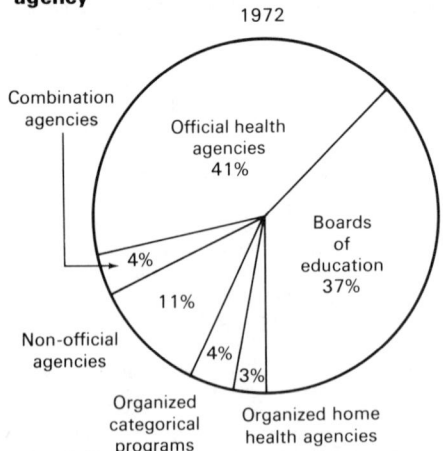

1972

Combination agencies

Official health agencies 41%

Boards of education 37%

4%

11%

Non-official agencies

4%

3%

Organized categorical programs

Organized home health agencies

Source: DHEW.

Table 23-1   Agencies and nurses employed for public health work, by type of agency (January 1972)

Type of agency	Number of agencies	Number of nurses		
		Total	Registered nurses	Licensed practical nurses
Total	11,455	61,546	58,241	3,305
National	8	886	885	1
University	270	916	916	—
State	151	2,194	2,140	54
Local	11,026	57,550	54,300	3,250
Health departments and agencies	2,950	23,854	22,436	1,418
Neighborhood and mental health centers	320	2,198	1,700	498
Combination	70	2,341	2,177	164
Visiting nurse associations and others	648	6,118	5,511	607
Hospital based home care and other organizations	337	1,614	1,361	253
Board of education	6,701	21,425	21,115	310

Table 23-2   R.N.s and L.P.N.s employed for public health work, by employment status and position level (January 1972)

Type of agency	Full-time nurses			Part-time nurses		
	Total	Admin-istrative	Staff	Total	Admin-istrative	Staff
Total	53,852	8,674	45,178	7,694	1,199	6,495
National	835	433	402	51	32	19
University	789	789	—	127	127	—
State	2,104	1,240	864	90	15	75
Local	50,124	6,212	43,912	7,426	1,025	6,401
Official	20,502	2,959	17,543	3,352	553	2,799
Organized categorical program	1,946	388	1,558	252	43	209
Combination	2,150	402	1,748	191	21	170
Non-official	4,786	1,059	3,727	1,332	174	1,158
Organized home health	1,115	393	722	499	85	414
Board of education	19,625	1,011	18,614	1,800	149	1,651

23

Trends in Employment

Despite the numerical gain of nearly 27,000 full-time registered nurses in all local agencies between 1942 and 1972, the increase in terms of nurse to population ratio was negligible.

Figure 23-2   Full-time registered nurses in public health work, by type of agency, 1938–1972[1]

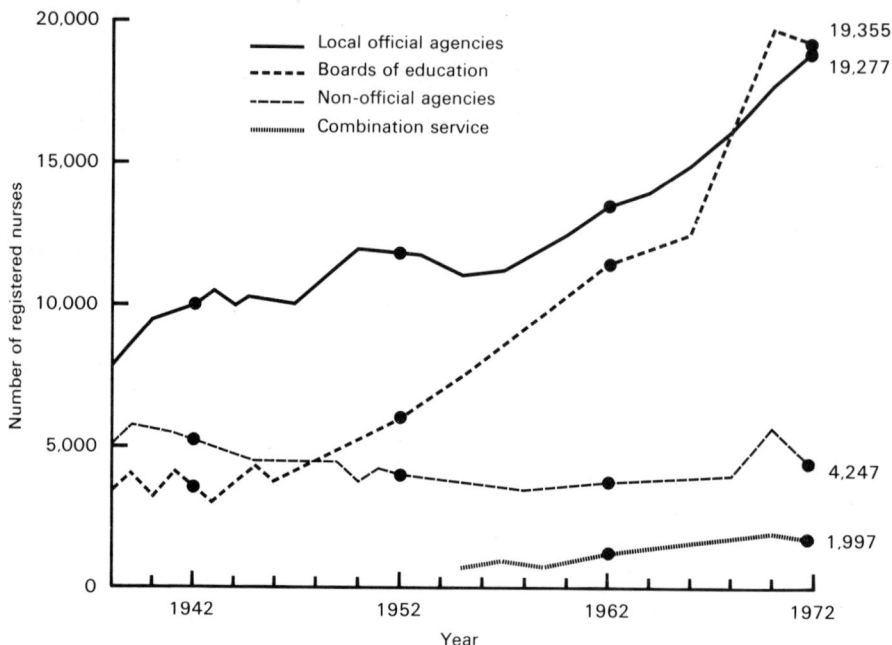

[1]Excludes organized categorical programs, hospital-based and other home health agencies which were not reported separately until 1966.

The ratio of public health nurses to the general population in 1972 was 14.5 registered nurses per 100,000, or one nurse for nearly 7,000 people in the country as a whole. Among the 50 states the ratio varied from 6 registered nurses per 100,000 in Nebraska to 33 per 100,000 in Alaska.

Public Health Nurse Characteristics

Age and Position*

Table 23-3   Full-time and part-time R.N.s employed for public health work; by age group and by position level (January 1972)

| | Position level | | | | | Position level | | | |
| | Administrative | | Staff | | | Administrative | | Staff | |
Age group	Number	Percent	Number	Percent	Age group	Number	Percent	Number	Percent
Total	8,492	100.0	47,948	100.0	40–49	2,199	25.9	14,153	29.5
					50–59	2,671	31.5	11,757	24.5
Under 30	576	6.8	7,478	15.6	60 and over	1,386	16.3	4,981	10.4
30–39	1,536	18.1	8,579	17.9	Not reported	124	1.4	1,000	2.1

*Source: DHEW.

The 8,492 nurses employed by state and local agencies at the administrative level are composed of 1,927 directors, 1,180 consultants and 5,385 nurses classified as supervisors, coordinators and other administrators. The 51,673 staff nurses are composed of 17,-588 public health nurses, 30,360 other registered nurses and 3,304 licensed practical nurses.

Salaries*

Table 23-4   Earnings of other full-time personnel usually found in larger agencies (1976)

Position[1]	Median annual salary
Registered nurse	
Assistant director	$18,900
Educational director	16,150
Other administrator	13,825
Consultant	15,660
Assistant supervisor	15,236
Licensed practical nurse	8,371
Auxiliary nursing personnel	
Public health assistant	7,615
Home health aide	6,366
Other auxiliary personnel	7,162
Nonnurse specialist	
Physical therapist[2]	13,029
Other	12,675

[1] Includes nonofficial agencies, official state and local health agencies and combination services.
[2] Some physical therapists are also R.N.s.

Public Health—State and Local Level

A local health agency may operate clinics, conduct immunization programs, inspect and license certain public facilities and monitor air pollution, among its other services. A state agency enforces state health laws and regulations and coordinates and provides overall direction for programs and services in local communities.

Most state departments of public health provide some local nursing services by assigning staff directly to areas where nursing programs or agencies have not been established, by supplementing local staff, or, by providing

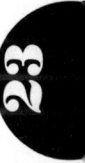

Table 23-5   Annual salaries in public health by position and by type of agency

Type of agency and position	1976 median	1975 range of middle 50%
Local official health agency		
Nurse director	$18,100	15,350–20,200
Supervising nurse	15,260	12,442–16,579
Staff nurse	12,160	9,941–13,020
P.H.N. fully qualified	12,830	
Other registered nurse	11,470	
Nonofficial agency		
Nurse director	18,007	14,014–19,200
Supervising nurse	13,463	11,271–14,709
Staff nurse	10,932	9,284–11,251
P.H.N. fully qualified	11,400	
Other registered nurse	10,543	
Board of education		
Supervising nurse	17,600	12,017–18,388
Staff nurse	12,901	9,214–14,379

service directly out of the state office. The type of health program carried on varies considerably within each state, but usually includes: the compilation of vital statistics and the development of environmental health and public health laboratory services, communicable disease control, maternal and child health, public health nursing and health education. Many health departments, however, have much more extensive programs involving activities such as mental health and retardation, chronic disease services, accident prevention, medical care for the indigent and important licensing functions.

About 84% of the 11,177 state and local agencies provide school health services; 56% engage in home visiting; and 38% offer clinic services.

Suburban health departments have grown in response to population increase, requiring services such as a potable water supply, sewage disposal, school health and mental health services. On the other hand, the large city health departments have been beset by tremendous problems resulting from the increase in children and senior citizens, which has produced a growing demand for services. Thus, city health departments have, in many cases, had to develop extensive health services, including medical care services, for increasing numbers of economically deprived persons, unable to provide these services for themselves.

D. Wilner (*Introduction to Public Health*) estimates that more than 1,500 of the approximately 3,100 counties in the nation are covered by organized local health departments, and about 700 more are covered by state health departments.

Public Health Nursing Services

Public Health Nursing Services are characterized by six major areas of services. These are home visiting, clinic services, school health, occupational/industrial health and group teaching. Other services include administration, coordination, consultation, supervision, in-service education, conferences, office or clerical work and travel.

Thirty-nine percent of the registered nurses in public health are primarily engaged in school health, and 38% listed generalized nursing as their primary area of practice. Home care was the next largest category of major responsibility, accounting for 7% of the registered nurses. The remaining 16% were spread across the categories of clinic services, child health and pediatrics, mental health, maternity, specialized nursing, administration, chronic illness and geriatrics, occupational and industrial health, education, communicable diseases, rehabilitation and physical therapy, and hospital coordination.

Obviously, registered nurses in certain areas of practice are highly concentrated in specific types of agencies. The most highly concentrated are the 22,063 registered nurses engaged principally in school health, with 91% of these being employed by boards of education.

Seventy-four percent of the nurses reporting generalized nursing as their primary area of practice are employed by local agencies; 16% of these are employed on the administrative level and 84% on the staff level.

Public Health Services Data*

Home Visiting Service

Table 23-6 Estimated home visiting services by number of persons served and types of home visits (January 1972)

Persons served and home visits per year	Type of program area								
	Maternity	Communi-cable diseases	Disease/ disability	Mental health	Infant/ family planning	Child health	School health	Promo-tion	Other
Persons served	1,396,596	1,642,170	1,669,013	286,672	234,673	782,362	119,510	3,939,107	289,637
Home visits	3,140,543	3,322,171	13,336,405	1,038,239	402,977	1,745,983	230,654	7,793,000	1,665,353
Visits per person	2.24	2.02	7.99	3.62	1.71	2.23	1.93	1.97	5.74

Clinic Services

Table 23-7 Estimated utilization of clinic services provided by local health agencies (January 1972)

Clinic sessions and persons served per year	Type of clinical services							
	Maternity	Communi-cable diseases[1]	Chronic disease/ disability	Mental health	Family planning	Infant/ child health	School health	Other
Persons served	2,191,361	13,774,343	2,854,653	267,840	2,083,911	18,044,704	751,988	5,141,675
Clinic sessions	272,850	640,753	408,547	100,521	262,499	863,728	72,634	642,199
Persons per clinic	8.03	21.49	6.98	2.66	7.93	20.89	10.35	8.00

[1]TB, VD and measles.

*Source: DHEW.

School Health Services

Table 23-8   Boards of education and local health agencies providing school health service by service and school types (January 1972)

Type of school served	Number of agencies in sample providing school health services	Type of school health service									
		Health coun- seling	Class- room instruc- tion	Home visiting	Physical exami- nation	Care of medical/ nursing emer- gency	Vision screen- ing	Audio- metric screen- ing	Tubercu- losis skin test	Other ser- vices
Public elementary	1,350	91.7%	66.5%	85.2%	57.6%	73.3%	85.7%	76.4%	72.9%	40.9%
Public secondary	1,122	92.8	73.1	86.1	54.3	74.3	83.0	75.7	72.7	43.9
Nonpublic elementary	505	85.1	50.6	78.6	56.3	62.7	80.2	63.0	71.5	46.4
Nonpublic secondary	233	90.2	60.0	77.3	51.4	61.7	74.5	70.3	71.6	48.1

Source: DHEW.

Home Care*

Overview

Home care is the provision of health care and supportive services to the sick or disabled person in his place of residence. It may be provided in a wide range of patterns of organization and service. At one end of the range is the simplest form, nursing service. At the other end is the coordinated home care program, which fulfills the concept of comprehensive patient care.

The generally accepted goal of a coordinated home care program is to provide selected patients who do not require all the facilities of a hospital, but otherwise would have to be in a hospital or other institution, with a range of medical, nursing, dietary, social and rehabilitative services in their own home, the services coordinated through one central administration. The home situation and family relationships must be capable of supporting the home care program to make it work.

Home care can work for short-term convalescent patients recovering from acute illness, the homebound chronically ill, those who usually receive treatment on an outpatient basis but are temporarily unable to do so, and certain patients with terminal illnesses. For the patient who needs a program of rehabilitation, home care may be superior to inpatient care if the home is suitable and if he does not need continuous nursing attention or use of equip-

*Source: *Role and Responsibility of Hospitals for Home Care,* 1976. Reprinted by permission of the American Hospital Association.

ment that cannot practicably be provided outside the hospital.

Although the home is not appropriate for all long-term or chronically ill patients in all stages of illness, often it can provide a desirable setting for far more patients that at present.

The Hospital's Role

Whether the hospital or another community agency provides the administrative structure, the hospital has a key role to play in stimulating development of home care, in fact-finding to determine extent of need, in identifying the desirable and appropriate scope of service, and in helping to secure stable financing.

A basic function of the hospital is to develop and maintain an effective mechanism for identification of patients potentially suitable for home care and for their prompt referral to the program. Involvement of at least the medical and nursing staff is necessary for successful performance of this function. Suitability for home care should not be related to the patient's financial condition: many patients who can pay for the service either are unaware of the service or are denied access to home care.

The hospital must also back up the home care program by ensuring that the patient will be admitted immediately or readmitted to the hospital if a change in his condition requires hospitalization.

When the hospital is the administrative agency for the home care program, its role includes direct provision of professional and related services to the patient at home. Nursing, social service, physical therapy, occupational therapy, and, in some programs, physician service are among these.

Data*

Nearly 7.8 million home visits were made to 3.9 million people for the purposes of health promotion during 1971. Some 13.3 million home visits were made to nearly 1.7 million persons with a chronic disease or disability. Clinic services were provided to more than 18.0 million infants and children in about 864,000 clinic sessions.

Home Care Survey**

In 1973 an NLN survey of home health services produced these findings:

Patient Characteristics

Home health services were utilized primarily by the older age group. The median age was 69

---

*Source: DHEW.
**Source: *Type, Length and Cost of Care for Home Health Patients,* NLN Pub. No. 21-1589, 1975.

years, and the middle 50% fell between ages 59 and 79. Sixty-three percent were female, and 24% lived alone.

Source of Referral and Medical Care

Source of referral: Sixty-eight percent of the cases were referred by hospitals and 14% by private physicians, with patient or family accounting for 13% of the referrals.

Source of physician care: Family physicians provided medical care to almost half the cases (49%). Forty-five percent of the patients received their care from clinics and 6% from health groups and other sources.

Prior hospitalization: Sixty-two percent of the cases had been discharged from hospital within the two weeks prior to admission to home health.

Costs

The average cost was $22.50 for each professional visit, $28.40 for a four-hour home health aide visit, and $228 per case through discharge.

Discharge Diagnoses

Table 23-9   Analysis of discharge summary data (exclusive of one-day cases)

Diagnosis[1]	Cases %	Visits %	Visits per case	Services	Median no. of days[2]	Median age
Infective/Parasitic	1.0	0.6	9.5	N[3]	27.0	21
Neoplasms	14.5	13.1	14.4	N,PT,OT,MS,HHA,O	35.5	66
Alergic/Endocrine/ Metabolic/Nutritional	14.0	10.2	11.7	N,PT,MS,HHA,O	26.5	64
Blood	1.4	0.7	7.7	N,PT	24.0	70
Mental/Psychoneurotic/ Personality	0.9	0.6	11.7	N,PT	48.0	38
Nervous system	7.4	9.2	19.7	N,PT,OT,MS,HHA	42.5	68
Circulatory	25.4	30.2	18.9	N,PT,OT,SP,MS,HHA,O	47.2	74
Respiratory	5.1	6.8	21.5	N,PT,MS,HHA	39.0	68
Digestive	3.9	3.0	12.0	N,PT,HHA,O	29.8	63
Genitourinary	4.0	5.9	23.3	N,PT,MS,HHA,O	19.8	76
Skin and Subcutaneous	2.4	1.8	11.5	N,PT,HHA	41.0	68
Musculoskeletal	9.1	10.7	18.6	N,PT,OT,HHA	49.1	73
Ill-defined conditions	1.1	0.6	8.5	N,MS,HHA	27.0	77
Injuries	9.8	6.6	10.6	N,PT,OT,MS,HHA,O	37.8	68
All diagnoses	100.0	100.0	15.9		36.0	69

[1] Based on the International Classification of Diseases.
[2] Number of calendar days between admission visit and final visit.
[3] Abbreviations as follows: N, nurse; PT, physical therapist; OT, occupational therapist; MS, medical social worker; SP, speech pathologist; HHA, home health aide; and O, other.

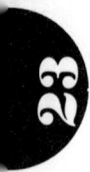

Analysis of One-Day Cases—The diagnoses of greatest concentration were circulatory (21%), neoplasms (13%) and digestive (13%). The source of referral was more frequently from self and family (30%) and from private physician (21%) and less frequently from hospital (38%) than in the larger group, where the majority (68%) of patients were referred by the hospital.

Visits per Case

Table 23-10   Average number of visits per case

Discipline	Number of visits
Nurse	10.85
Physical therapist	.61
Occupational therapist	.03
Speech pathologist	.04
Medical social worker	.02
Other	.09
Professional subtotal	11.64
Home health aide	4.25
Total, all disciplines	15.89

Medicare and Medicaid Reimbursements for Home Health Services

Medicare—Title XVIII

Medicare reimburses for home health services under both Parts A and Part B of Title XVIII. After a minimum of 3 days' stay in a hospital or after a discharge from an ECF, Part A pays for up to 100 hospital-related home health visits within a 12-month period. These visits must be ordered by a physician according to a plan established within two weeks after institutional discharge. The home health agency must be a participant in the Medicare program, and the patient must be treated for the same condition for which he was hospitalized. Part B of Medicare pays the providing home care agency for up to 100 home health care visits each year when a patient has no prior hospital stay if such services are provided according to a plan of treatment approved by a physician. Part B of Medicare also may be used if the patient's Part A visits have been exhausted.

Part A pays reasonable costs of home health services, while Part B pays 80% of the reasonable cost of services after the patient has met the overall annual $50 deductible for Part B services.

Medicare cost data for fiscal year 1971 indicate that both the number of claims and the amount paid comprise an extremely small portion of the total expenditures for the program. Home health services accounted for less than 20% of the number of claims and less than 1% of the dollars paid out under Medicare.

Medicaid—Title XIX

Medicaid statutes list services that are eligible for federal matching, including home health care services. Home health care services are defined in Medicaid regulations to include nursing and therapy services, as well as other services provided through a home health agency under direct supervision of the physician. About 80% of the individual state Medicaid programs have included home health services either for the categorically indigent or the medically indigent.

Federal Public Health Service*

Highlights of PHS Nursing History

Hospital Nursing—Professional nurses—men as well as women—were first employed in the marine hospitals in the 1890s. They were assigned to the hospital for the care of immigrants arriving at Ellis Island in New York harbor. Professionally trained women nurses began to be employed generally in marine hospitals in about 1912.

The first superintendent of nurses was Lucy Minnigerode, who was appointed to the position in 1919. She also organized a nursing service for all the marine hospitals at that time.

Public Health Nursing—Even before World War I, a few nurses had been employed for special projects which today would be considered public health work. Notable among them were the pellagra and trachoma control programs, begun in the Kentucky mountains in 1914. During the next 14 years, public health nurses assigned to these programs covered 18,000 square miles of mountainous terrain in 27 counties, traveling on horseback, muleback or on foot to visit homes, examine families and teach personal hygiene and the fundamentals of good health.

---

* Source: R. Spalding, *Professional Nursing* (Lippincott, 1970).

Consultant Services—In 1934, a public health nursing section was added to the consultant service which the PHS provided to state health departments. Following the enactment of the Social Security Act of 1935 and the authorization of grants to the states for public health programs, the nursing consultation service was greatly expanded. Among its more important accomplishments are the improvement of general qualifications for nurses in public health; the promotion, through state nursing directors in public health, of programs of in-service training; and the improvement of educational programs for the preparation of public health nurses.

In World War II, nursing consultants helped to develop civilian defense plans. By early 1945, nurses in public health, recruited by PHS, were serving state and local health departments in war impact areas in 39 states and Puerto Rico. PHS nurses served with the armed forces and, in the years after the war, with international relief agencies.

The administration of the U.S. Cadet Nurse Corps program during World War II, created by the acute need for nurses in civilian and military service, was a major wartime activity. Authorized by the Boston Act of 1943, the Cadet Nurse Corps recruited 180,000 students for preservice programs and provided instruction to 17,000 graduate nurses.

Indian Health—Although nurses had worked with Indians as early as 1890, their services were performed largely in hospitals operated under the auspices of various mission groups. It was not until 1924 that Elinor D. Gregg was appointed to the position of supervisor of field nurses and field matrons in the Bureau of Indian Affairs (BIA), under the U.S. Department of Interior. In 1926, all BIA nurses—hospital and public health—were placed under the direction of Miss Gregg.

The nursing service for the Indians was transferred to the PHS in 1955. By June 1968, the Indian health program staff included approximately 1,050 professional nurses and 1,050 auxiliary nursing personnel, employed in all types of nursing positions—public health, clinic, school and hospital.

Federal Public Health Agencies

Services

- Community Mental Health Centers.
- Alcoholism Services.
- Rat Control.
- Lead-based paint.
- Immunizations.
- Veneral disease.
- Comprehensive Health Centers.
- Family Planning.
- Maternal and Child Health.
- Emergency Medical Services.
- Migrant Health Services.
- Health Planning, Construction, and Resources Development.

Federal Agencies*

The Assistant Secretary for Health of HEW has the responsibility for supervising all the regional health administrators, who in turn function in each of ten health regions into which the country has been divided.

Reporting to the Assistant Secretary for Health are six major "health administrations."

1. *The National Institutes of Health.* This, the major health research arm of the federal government, is based in Bethesda, Maryland, just outside the nation's capital. In addition to the research carried out at the institutes, federal grant support is extended to agencies throughout the country. Studies are supported in such areas as cancer, heart disease, dental health, arthritis and metabolic diseases, neurologic diseases and blindness, child health and human development as well as environmental health. On the NIH campus there is also located the Clinical Center, a large hospital dedicated to research and treatment. Extensive intramural and extramural health training activities are centered or funded at the NIH facilities.

2. *Food and Drug Administration.* This agency is responsible for the overall surveillance of food, including safety, wholesomeness and purity. It also has responsibilities relating to the clinical investigation and licensing of drugs, and, therefore, wields great power concerning the marketing and use of any new drug which industry may wish to introduce. Radiological health activities are also now included in this administration.

3. *Center for Disease Control.* This agency is located in Atlanta, Georgia, and maintains a constant watch on the prevalence of disease in the United States. It carries out

---

*Source: M. Grant, *Handbook of Community Health* (Philadelphia: Lea & Febiger, 1975).

epidemiological investigations on request of state agencies and has a rather extensive laboratory system particularly capable of performing testing procedures which are other than routine, such as virus studies. It is also responsible for operating the National Institute for Occupational Safety and Health, and for foreign quarantine.

4. *Health Resources Administration.* This, a newly established entity, attempts to bring together many of the national health programs dealing with human health resources. Included under its umbrella are a national center for research and development, the center for health statistics, as well as health planning and evaluation. Also located here is that section dealing with construction grants to hospitals and other health facilities.

5. *Health Services Administration.* This arm of the Assistant Secretary for Health's organization is responsible for providing a variety of direct medical services. For example, it examines immigrants and is responsible for the operation of the Public Health Service hospitals which provide medical care for certain federal beneficiaries. This administration is intimately involved in the surveillance of medical care and health delivery systems. It also is the principal branch of the Department of HEW, dealing with community health services in the states including maternal and child health and family planning services as well as with local health department activities.

6. *Alcohol, Drug Abuse and Mental Health Administration.* This administration has the major federal responsibilities in the area of mental health and is charged with helping support and monitor the states' programs including the development of community mental health centers as well as those programs dealing with alcoholism and drug addiction. It also provides specialized care for drug addicts in federal hospitals in Lexington, Kentucky, and Fort Worth, Texas.

Bureau of Community Health Services*

The Bureau of Community Health Services seeks particularly to service certain groups of people:

---

* Source: *Promoting Community Health,* DHEW 1975.

- Those who live in communities where there are critical shortages of health manpower and services.
- Mothers and children who need preventive care or care for special conditions.
- Migrants and seasonal farmworkers.
- Those in need of family planning services.

Community Health Centers—There are three types of centers—neighborhood health centers, family health centers and community health networks.

Neighborhood health centers offer a broad scope of comprehensive services tailored to fit specific community needs in either rural or inner city areas where there is inadequate health manpower. The centers use hospitals or other health care institutions for services not available at the center location. Neighborhood residents help in identifying the services needed and also work at the centers. In 1975 there were 127 neighborhood health centers.

Family health centers are designed to provide a prescribed package of benefits to a specifically enrolled population residing in a defined medical scarcity area. The basic minimum service benefit package includes: emergency ambulance and other medical services; physicians' services; and other medical and health services such as outpatient services, physical therapy, and diagnostic laboratory and x-ray services. Hospital and other nonambulatory services are arranged for and coordinated by the family health centers, but grant funds cannot be used for these services.

In 1975 there were 30 operational family health centers in 26 states and the District of Columbia. These centers anticipated serving 105,000 patients in 1975.

Community health networks were developed as research and demonstration projects in the Office of Economic Opportunity. Their control was later transferred to HEW.

Community Health Centers are sponsored by many groups, such as community corporations, hospitals, medical schools, citizen's groups, medical societies and departments of health.

Usually the neighborhood residents served by the center have a substantial voice in policy-making. Most centers provide medical and dental care services, laboratory, x-ray and pharmacy services and other support services needed for providing comprehensive care.

Public Program Health Expenditures

Table 23-11 Expenditures for public health services and supplies, by program and type of expenditure (in millions)

Public program and source of funds	Total	Hospital care	Physicians' services	Dentists' services	Other professional services	Drugs and drug sundries	Eye glasses and appliances	Nursing-home care	Government public health activities	Other health services	Administration
F.Y. 1975											
Total	$45,584.7	$25,643.3	$5,855.4	$414.8	$508.7	$904.6	$102.2	$5,201.3	$3,457.0	$2,293.6	$1,203.8
Health insurance for aged and disabled	14,781.4	10,710.6	2,967.1	—	186.1	—	—	257.0	—	—	660.6
Temporary disability insurance (medical benefits)	73.3	53.6	17.0	—	1.2	0.8	0.7	—	—	—	—
Workmen's compensation (medical benefits)	1,830.0	922.6	777.7	—	56.4	36.6	36.7	—	—	349.7	—
Public assistance (vendor medical payments)	12,968.0	4,270.5	1,685.7	337.1	224.8	836.6	—	4,782.4	—	103.3	481.2
General hospital and medical care	5,491.7	5,369.7	13.9	3.2	—	1.6	—	—	—	—	—
Defense Department hospital and medical care (including military dependents)	3,011.0	1,903.8	216.8	10.8	40.2	9.7	16.1	—	—	848.3	21.6
Maternal and child health services	540.0	81.9	49.8	12.3	—	11.8	—	—	—	323.3	4.6
School health											
Other public health activities									3,457.0		
Veterans' hospital and medical care	3,242.3	2,253.6	32.4	51.4	—	7.5	30.7	161.9	—	669.0	35.8
Medical vocational rehabilitation	190.0	77.0	95.0	—	—	—	18.0	—	—	—	—
Office of Economic Opportunity	—	—	—	—	—	—	—	—	—	—	—
Federal	30,776.3	18,263.5	4,262.3	254.8	342.0	477.6	57.1	2,981.8	1,201.0	1,939.0	997.2
Health insurance for aged and disabled (Medicaid)	14,781.4	10,710.6	2,967.1	—	186.1	—	—	257.0	—	—	660.6
Workmen's compensation (medical benefits)	50.6	32.9	12.6	—	3.0	1.0	1.1	—	—	—	—
Public assistance (vendor medical payments) (Medicare)	6,966.4	2,288.6	903.4	180.7	120.5	448.3	—	2,562.9	—	187.4	274.6
General hospital and medical care	1,089.6	967.6	13.9	3.2	—	1.6	—	—	—	103.3	—
Defense Department hospital and medical care (including military dependents)[5]	3,011.0	1,903.8	216.8	10.8	32.4	9.7	10.4	—	—	848.3	21.6
Maternal and child health services	277.0	42.8	37.6	8.7	—	9.5	—	—	—	131.0	4.6
Other public health activities	1,201.0								1,201.0		
Veterans' hospital and medical care	3,242.3	2,253.6	32.4	51.4	—	7.5	30.7	161.9	—	669.0	35.8
Medical vocational rehabilitation	157.0	63.6	78.5	—	—	—	14.9	—	—	—	—
Office of Economic Opportunity	—	—	—	—	—	—	—	—	—	—	—

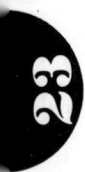

State and local	14,808.4	7,379.8	1,593.1	160.1	166.7	427.0	45.1	2,219.5	2,256.0	354.5	206.6
Temporary disability insurance (medical benefits)	73.3	53.6	17.0	—	1.2	0.8	0.7	—	—	—	—
Workmen's compensation (medical benefits)	1,779.4	889.7	765.1	—	53.4	35.6	35.6	—	—	—	—
Public assistance (vendor medical payments)	6,001.7	1,981.9	782.3	156.5	104.3	388.3	—	2,219.5	—	162.2	206.6
General hospital and medical care	4,402.1	4,402.1	—	3.6	7.8	—	5.7	—	—	192.3	—
Maternal and child health services	263.0	39.1	12.2	—	2.3	—	—	—	—	—	—
School health	—	—	—	—	—	—	—	—	—	—	—
Other public health activities	2,256.0	—	—	—	—	—	—	—	2,256.0	—	—
Medical vocational rehabilitation	33.0	13.4	16.5	—	—	—	3.1	—	—	—	—

Source: U.S. Social Security Administration, February 1976.

Public Programs— Personal Expenditures

Table 23-12 Estimated personal health care expenditures under public programs, by program and age groups (in millions)

Program	All ages			Under 19			19-64			65 and over		
	Total	Federal	State and local	Total	Federal	State and local	Total	Federal	State and local	Total	Federal	State and local
Total	$40,924	$28,578	$12,346	$3,749	$2,391	$1,358	$17,258	$9,856	$7,402	$19,917	$16,331	$3,586
Health insurance for the aged and disabled	14,121	14,121	—	—	—	—	1,355	1,355	—	12,762	12,762	—
Temporary disability insurance	73	—	73	3		3	73	—	73	—	—	—
Workmen's compensation (medical benefits)	1,830	51	1,779	—	—	—	1,773	49	1,724	57	2	55
Public assistance (vendor medical payments)	12,487	6,692	5,795	2,098	1,125	974	5,475	2,934	2,541	4,914	2,633	2,280
General hospital and medical care	5,492	1,090	4,402	518	320	198	3,638	685	2,954	1,335	85	1,250
Defense Department hospital and medical care (including military dependents)	2,989	2,989	—	726	726	—	2,173	2,173	—	90	90	—
Maternal and child health services	535	272	263	365	186	179	171	87	84	—	—	—
School health	—	—	—	—	—	—	—	—	—	—	—	—
Veterans' hospital and medical care	3,206	3,206	—	—	—	—	2,450	2,450	—	756	756	—
Medical vocational rehabilitation	190	157	33	38	31	7	148	122	26	4	3	1
Office of Economic Opportunity	—	—	—	—	—	—	—	—	—	—	—	—

Source: U.S. Social Security Administration, February 1976.

474

In 1966, community health centers were authorized by Congress to provide comprehensive health services to urban or rural areas where there are shortages of medical personnel and services.

Early in the development of the program, neighborhood health centers became the principal method used to reach these medically underserved areas. Later, in response to the President's Health Message of 1971 calling for services to the underserved in rural areas, family health centers were developed. And in July 1973, OEO introduced Community Health Networks—later transferred to HEW.

In 1975 there were 157 community health center projects funded by the Comprehensive Health Planning and Public Health Service Act and serving approximately 1,425,000 patients. Average annual cost per person was estimated to be $206.

Critics of the program have noted that even in 1971, with more centers in operation, the proportions of target and registrant population to the total poverty population in the United States was only 19.7% and 4.3%, respectively.

SERVICES OFFERED BY COMMUNITY HEALTH CENTERS

- Medical
- Laboratory
- X-ray
- Pharmacy
- Mental health
- Dental
- Home health
- Hospitalization
- Physical or speech therapy

- Optometry
- Sickle cell anemia program
- Lead poisoning program
- Social service
- Transportation
- Training
- Community organization
- Research and evaluation
- Environmental
- Family Planning
- V.D. testing
- Podiatry

Public Health Expenditures

Government spending—federal, state, and local—for health services and supplies totaled $45.6 billion in 1975. Almost $31 billion came from federal sources, the remaining $15 billion from state and local governments.

Expenditures by governments for health services and supplies rose $8.3 billion, an increase of 22.4% over 1974.

Fifty-six percent of all public spending for health care was for hospital care. Almost one-fourth of public funds went for physicians' services and nursing-home care. Seventy percent of Veterans Administration expenditures went for hospital costs. Department of Defense health expenditures were also mainly for hospital care (63%). Expenditures by state temporary disability programs and state and federal workmen's compensation programs reflected their emphasis on both hospital and medical care.

23

24

HEALTH MAINTENANCE ORGANIZATIONS (HMOs)

Background*

History

The first *prepaid* group practice plan (PGP) was developed in 1929, when Dr. Michael Shadid established the Farmer's Union-Cooperative Health Association (Elk City, Oklahoma), in the face of strenuous opposition from the medical community. Originally, supporters of the plan purchased shares at $50 each and received health care services at a discount from a closed panel of physicians. In 1931, the cooperative initiated an annual dues schedule which ranged from $12 per year for an individual to $25 for a family of four or more. The physician-owned Ross-Loos Medical Group (Los Angeles, California), which is the nation's oldest PGP model HMO that has been in continuous existence, also began offering prepaid health care to employee groups in 1929. Today, there are approximately 115,000 enrollees in the Ross-Loos plan.

Four years later, in 1933, the Kaiser-Permanente Medical Care Program (KPMCP) began to develop when the Kaiser organization contracted with Dr. Sidney Garfield to establish an industrial group practice plan for Kaiser's Southern California construction workers in areas that were remote from medical services. Kaiser then established a similar program for its employees in Washington state in 1938, extended the program to its west coast shipyard workers in 1942, and finally opened enrollment to the public on a communitywide basis in 1945. Currently, KPMCP operates in six states and serves almost three million members.

In 1937, four years after the first seeds of KPMCP were sown, the Group Health Association (GHA) was established in Washington, D.C. Membership in GHA, which was the first *urban* health cooperative, was open to federal employees and their families, and GHA's charter mandated the provision of comprehen-

sive health care services in GHA facilities, including pharmacies. In 1947, GHA added dental care. Current enrollment in GHA is in excess of 100,000 members.

The year 1947 saw the establishment of two important PGP model HMOs at opposite ends of the country—the Group Health Cooperative of Puget Sound (GHC) in Seattle, Washington, and the Health Insurance Plan of Greater New York (HIP) in New York City. The former was developed with the support of the State Grange and a number of union groups and has served as a model for other health care cooperatives. The GHC's current enrollment is over 200,000. HIP, which was established with the support of New York City as well as New York City employee unions, represented the first large-scale effort to make a PGP model HMO option available on a communitywide basis; HIP has weathered several severe financial crises, and still has almost 750,000 enrollees.

By the late 1960s, interest in developing PGP model HMOs was spreading to the private insurance industry, and in 1969, the Connecticut General Life Insurance Company (Hartford, Connecticut) financed development of the first proprietary PGP model HMO, the Columbia Medical Plan (CMP), which is based in the new city of Columbia, Maryland. The plan is operated jointly by Connecticut General and the Johns Hopkins University and Hospitals, and presently has approximately 20,000 enrollees. Blue Cross and Blue Shield followed by establishing the first Blue Cross and Blue Shield owned and operated PGP plan in Milwaukee, Wisconsin, in 1971. The plan, called Compare, has an enrollment of almost 20,000 members.

Growth of HMOs

Between 1970 and 1975 enrollments in HMOs grew from 3.6 million to 5.9 million. The number of prepaid plans grew from 33 to 167. However, only ten of these plans have met federal government requirements for approval.

---

*Source: J. A. Prussin, *Employee Health Benefits: HMOs and Mandatory Dual Choice* (Aspen Systems Corporation, 1976). (Unless otherwise noted.)

476

Sponsoring categories of the 167 projects funded under Public Law 93-222 are as follows:

Consumer groups	74
Public organizations	6
Hospitals	23
Physician organizations	48
Private organizations	9
Medical schools	5
Other	2
Total	167

Note: In most cases people are not actually using these projects since almost all are still in the developing stages and are not yet operational.

As of June 30, 1975, HEW had received 375 grant applications but had awarded only 180 grants totaling about $22.5 million to 167 projects.

Of the 108 grantees awarded feasibility studies in fiscal year 1975:

- twenty-two have decided it non-feasible,
- eleven have gone from feasibility into planning, and,
- seventy-five are still in progress to complete feasibility,

Only one of the feasibility grantees proceeded to become a qualified HMO.

Organization and Benefits

HMOs Defined

Basically, an HMO may be defined as a direct service health plan which assumes responsibility for organizing and delivering comprehensive health care services. The HMO combines prepayment, which is a financing mechanism, with group practice or individual practice, which are delivery mechanisms, in order to provide health care services to a voluntarily enrolled population on a contractual basis.

Contractual Responsibility

As direct service health plans, HMOs go beyond the obligation of Blue Cross, Blue Shield or the commercial health insurer—which is merely to pay or reimburse for covered services up to the particular policy's limits—and accept *contractual* responsibility for the actual delivery of health care services. It must hire and/or contract with appropriate personnel and make other necessary arrangements for delivering the covered services, as well as for maintaining their quality and guaranteeing their availability and accessibility to enrollees.

Enrollees

Basic to any HMO are its enrollees, or the individuals who are served by the plan. The enrollees generally pay a fixed monthly premium, regardless of utilization, in return for which the plan agrees to provide, or arrange for the provision of, comprehensive health care services. Through payment of their premiums, the enrollees in an HMO generally provide the bulk of the plan's income.

Prepayment

The member of an HMO generally pays, or has paid on his behalf by an employer or other third party, a monthly premium. While some HMOs impose moderate point-of-service copayments, such as $1.00 or $2.00 for each office visit, payment of the premium to the HMO generally represents *prepayment*, or payment in advance, for the delivery of *all* covered health care services which might be required by the individual during the contract period.

Many HMOs offer several different benefits packages, as well as certain optional benefits, such as coverage for psychiatric services, and charge different premiums for the different benefits packages and options. HMOs' benefits packages are generally somewhat broader than those offered by commercial insurance companies and Blue Cross and Blue Shield plans.

HMO premiums are sometimes substantially higher than those for commercial insurance company and Blue Cross and Blue Shield plans in the HMO's geographic area—especially in areas in which the non-HMO health insurance plans offer benefits packages that are considerably narrower, in terms of quantity and/or scope, than those offered by the HMO.

Choice of Physician or Facilities

HMOs are direct health services delivery programs and, as such, generally limit their enrollees' freedom to select physicians and facilities participating in the plan. In the case of a large HMO which has a large proportion of the physicians in a particular area under contract, freedom of choice among the physicians participating in the plan is important and meaningful. However, in the case of a smaller HMO, which may only have one or two physicians in primary care areas such as internal medicine and pediatrics—let alone some specialty areas—the theoretical freedom to choose from among the physicians participating in the plan may be rather vacuous to the HMO's enrollees.

Second, in order to prevent HMO enrollees from feeling that they are locked into the HMO system, and in order to provide an alternative for dissatisfied HMO enrollees, HMOs are generally offered in a *dual or multiple choice* setting, under which subscribers are initially and periodically permitted to choose from among two or more commercial health insurance, Blue Cross and Blue Shield, and HMO plans. This type of arrangement affords the enrollee freedom to opt out of the HMO plan and enroll in an alternative plan, if he is dissatisfied with the HMO for any reason. Thus, the HMO must satisfy its membership or lose its enrollees to the alternative plan(s).

Comprehensive Benefits

PGP and FMC model HMOs usually provide comprehensive health care benefits, including: physicians' services in the office, hospital and home; hospitalization services; diagnostic and therapeutic services in the office and hospital; and, in many cases, nursing home, drug, mental health, dental, and other such services. Generally, HMOs have found that the provision of a comprehensive range of benefits tends to contain health care costs by permitting services to be rendered in the most appropriate setting by the most appropriate provider, without regard to the source of payment for such services. Thus, for example, the HMO eliminates the practice of using unnecessarily expensive modes of treatment, such as hospitalizing patients for routine diagnostic procedures, in order that the patient's commercial insurance company or Blue Cross and Blue Shield plan can cover the costs of the procedures.

Payments and Doctors Salaries

Payment to the HMO's medical group, if it is a true medical group, is generally on a *capitation* basis, under which the medical group receives a fixed number of dollars per member per month, regardless of utilization, in exchange for which the group agrees to provide all appropriate physicians' services to the HMO's enrollees. In addition, depending upon the organization of the plan, the medical group may be responsible for the provision of allied health professionals' and ancillary services. The capitation payment system, which itself is an incentive payment system, may be coupled with *other* incentives under which the medical group may share in any excesses in revenues over expenditures that are created by efficient operation of the HMO, low hospital utilization rates and so forth.

Under all four of the basic PGP physician payment mechanisms—that is, straight salary, salary plus incentives, capitation, and capitation plus incentives—the conventional *piecework* economics of medical care are reversed, or at least neutralized. The *financial* incentives of traditional fee-for-service physicians are oriented toward providing the largest possible quantity of the most complex procedures, because the physician's income increases directly with the number and complexity of the services he provides.

The *straight salary* arrangement under the HMO neutralizes the financial incentive of physicians to provide numerous, complex procedures, because the physician's salary remains constant and is unrelated to the number and complexity of the procedures he performs. The *other* PGP physician payment mechanisms, however, go beyond merely neutralizing the financial incentives resulting from the traditional fee-for-service payment mechanism to actually reversing them by creating new incentives for the physician. These incentives, in turn, are generally based upon the financial performance of the medical group and/or the HMO, which is closely and inversely related to the utilization of services by HMO members.

HMOs in Action

HMO Performance

Several well-controlled studies have indicated that HMOs tend to reduce hospital utilization and elective surgery rates, lower health care costs, reduce infant mortality and prematurity rates, and lower mortality rates for the elderly. For example, a 1976 study compared Medicaid costs under the GHA, a Washington, D.C., based HMO, with Medicaid fee-for-service costs in Washington, D.C. The average saving under GHA for a three-year period was over 37%. An earlier study in 1965 compared the costs of health care services for KPMCP enrollees in Northern California with those for the state of California as a whole (see Table 24-1). Furthermore, the health care costs increased by 19.1% between 1960 and 1965 for KPMCP members, while the increase for the United States as a whole during the same period of time was 43.5%.

Table 24-1   Comparison of health care costs, 1965

Item	KPMCP N. California region (per capita)	State of California (per capita)	KPMCP as a percent of California
Hospital costs	$34.30	$56.06	61%
Physicians' services	44.32	67–88	66–50
Other expenses	7.69	8.76	88
Total expenses	81.83	131.82–152.82	65–54

One of the prime factors contributing to lower health care costs for HMO enrollees is the lower utilization of elective surgery and expensive hospitalization services by HMOs. For example, a 1968 study of the Federal Employees' Health Benefits Program (FEHBP) revealed age adjusted hospital utilization figures of 934 days per 1,000 enrollees under indemnity insurance plans, compared with 429 days per 1,000 enrollees under PGP model HMO plans.

Even more dramatic were the differences in the numbers of inpatient surgical procedures between individuals covered under Blue Shield's high option benefits package and those enrolled in PGP model HMOs. For example, the Blue Shield tonsillectomy rate was over 250% of that for the PGPs. In addition, Blue Shield had an annual rate of 9.2 procedures per 1,000 for female surgery, compared with a PGP rate of 4.8. Finally, the rates for all surgical procedures were: Blue Shield, 75 per 1,000, and PGP model HMOs, 34 per 1,000. Thus, the PGP surgery rate was less than half that of Blue Shield. Indeed, while an empty bed represents *lost* revenues to the traditional hospital, an empty bed in an HMO-owned hospital represents a savings to the

plan. Thus, the traditional hospital administrator is judged, at least in part, on the basis of the amount of the revenues generated by his hospital, which translates, in large part, into high utilization. The administrator of an HMO-owned hospital, on the other hand, is judged on the basis of the revenues he does *not* generate for the hospital—from the HMO.

HMO Impact on Quality of Care*

Table 24-2   Surgery performed only when medically necessary

	HMO	Other providers
1960 Data		
Hospitalized surgical cases per 1,000 persons per year	49	60
1975 Data		
Hospitalized surgical cases per 1,000 persons per year	54	90
Medicaid admissions for surgery per 1,000 persons per year	18	33

Competitiveness of HMOs

Table 24-3   Price comparisons of HMO and insurance plans

	Monthly family premium	Range of family premiums
Federally mandated HMO benefit package	$75	$57–90
Typical operating HMO	60	39–82
Typical Blue Cross/Blue Shield plan	53	45–65
Typical indemnity plan	48	21–82

Problems in Expansion of HMO Concept

Start-up Money

Appropriate implementation of the HMO act has been hampered by the lack of HMO spend-

*Source: Senate Subcommittee on Health, January 1976.

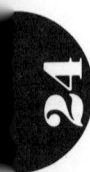

ing by HEW. Indeed, while Congress authorized a total of $80 million for HMO grants in FYs 1974 and 1975, the administration requested appropriations of $40 million for the same period and spent only $22.5 million. Furthermore, while the FY 1976 authorization level was $85 million, HEW only requested a $15 million appropriation.

Open Enrollment

The HMO act mandates that HMOs have an *open enrollment* period of not less that 30 days each year, during which the HMO must enroll individuals up to its capacity, in the order in which they apply, regardless of their health status. Many HMO proponents, however, have argued that competitive plans, such as those offered by indemnity insurance companies and Blue Cross and Blue Shield, are *not* subject to open enrollment requirements; and, therefore, HMOs might be forced to enroll disproportionate numbers of high risk members, which could cause high HMO utilization rates and result in high HMO premiums. (HMOs *cannot* charge *higher* premiums for such individuals.) Furthermore, there may be substantial differences between the utilization and cost experiences of different groups. Therefore, it is argued, indemnity insurance and Blue Cross and Blue Shield plans, which are *not* subject to community rating requirements and which generally *experience rate* their premiums, can more effectively compete for groups with low utilization and cost experiences than can HMOs. Thus, the HMO may fall into the spiral created by adverse selection—that is, a situation in which the HMO's premiums for low utilization, low cost groups are higher than those of the competing health insurance plan(s), thereby creating an environment in which the relatively high risk individuals within the particular group enroll in the HMO and, in turn, cause higher premiums and greater premium differentials.

Benefits Package

The capitalization and/or operating costs involved in offering the *mandated minimum benefits package* may also create competitive problems for HMOs. For example, commercial health insurance company and Blue Cross and Blue Shield plans are not required to, and generally do not, offer such benefits as preventive dental services and routine eye care for children, which are included under the required HMO minimum benefits package.

Nursing by Telephone*

The Harvard Community Health Plan is a health maintenance organization serving 36,-000 members in Boston. A recent survey in the health center revealed that 50% of patient care was given by telephone. The telephone saves time and money for both the patient and the health care agency. Unnecessary visits can be avoided, and necessary visits appropriately scheduled.

The telephone interview, intended to determine when a patient should be seen, reveals a vivid clinical picture: "What is your temperature?" When did your symptoms start? Are you coughing? What are you coughing up? Does your chest hurt at all?"

The guidelines in the standing orders include a list of specific symptoms to elicit from the patient in each disease category and indicate when a patient should be called in or referred to a physician.

Triage nurses staff the phones after regular working hours from 5:00 to 9:00 P.M., on Saturdays from 8:30 A.M. to 8:00 P.M., on Sundays and holidays from 8:30 A.M. to 6:00 P.M. These nurses also see and evaluate patients who come in. Their telephone role differs in that calls must necessarily be shorter and are geared toward treating immediate problems or referring the patient to the correct daytime person. Nurses who provide coverage evenings and weekends continue to manage new fevers, send patients with fractures to emergency wards and calm hysterical patients.

Triage nurses process calls to all departments and refer to the physician on call those matters that they cannot handle according to standing orders.

When patients know they will speak to a nurse, they call with questions that they might not ask otherwise—how to prevent contracting a coworker's hepatitis, what are the symptoms of syphilis, how many aspirin will control a temperature. Some patients who would be embarrassed by asking a "stupid" or personal question appreciate the anonymity of the telephone.

---

*Source: Donna Murphy and Eleanor Dineen, "Nursing by Telephone," *American Journal of Nursing*, July 1975.

HMO Personnel

Table 24-4   Clinic manpower for HMO examples

	Providers per 1,000 members							
	George-town	HIP of New York	Kaiser No. Cal.	Kaiser So. Cal.	Kaiser Oregon	GHA of D.C.	HMO Jeffrey Prussin	HMO Dallas
Physicians (MD)	1.002	.950	.950	.99	.728	.948	1.030	.969
General	.330	.370	.325	.45	.231	.362	.430	.340
Pediatric	.275	.220	.175	.16	.117	.197	.185	.157
Obstetrics-Gyn	.110	.110	.090	.10	.072	.090	.085	.116
Ophthalmology	.030	.030	.030	.02	(1)	.027	.035	.026
Psychiatry			.015			.025	(2)	(2)
Surgery	.140	.130	.210	.18	.170	.146	.110	.119
Secondary specialist	.117	.090	.090	.08	.098	.107	.185	.087
Non-care specialist								
Physicians (DO)								
Dentists						.150		
Optometrists						.084		
Podiatrists						.004		
Pharmacists						.082		
Veterinarians								
Registered nurses	.200	.200		.437		.526	.360	.211
Physician extender	.150	.150				.017		.211
Allied health manpower		1.975				4.414	1.180	.369
Administration	.350	.325		.066		.083		
Medical librarian							(4)	.263
Medical record	.350	.350		(3)		.499	.575	.158
Clinical lab	.065	.075		.684		.365		
Dietary						.013	(5)	.132
Radiologic	.065	.075		(5)		.189	(5)	.105
Therapy	.100	.125		(5)		.080		.079
General medical				.165		.053	.510	.488
Nursing care	.500	.500		.418		.760		
Vision care						.133		
Pharmacy						.053		.081
Dental care						.426		
Hosp. & clinic supp.	.500	.525		1.130		1.041	(5)	.447

The physicians service both the Clinics and Hospital Care.
[1] Included in Surgery.
[2] Included in Secondary Specialist.
[3] Included in Hospital and Clinic Support.
[4] Included in Administration.
[5] Included in Clinical Laboratory.

Source: DHEW, August 1974.

Table 24-5 HMO clinic care: physician utilization rates by specialty

| | Physicians visits per member | | |
	HIP New York	GHA Wash., D.C.	Kaiser So. Cal.
General	2.100	1.48	1.757
Pediatric	.474	.82	.728
Obstetrics-Gyn.	.279	.30	.259
Psychiatry		.02	.001
Surgery	.684	.28	.615
Other care	.659	.21	.239
Ophthalmology	.147	.10	.094
Total	4.199	3.21	3.60

Source: DHEW, August 1974.

Federal Requirements for HMOs

In order to qualify for any federal benefits, an HMO must meet all of the "Requirements for Health Maintenance Organizations" as specified in the HMO Act of 1973.

The Benefits Packages

The HMO must provide no less than the "basic health services," or minimum benefits package, to each of its enrollees. Included in the minimum benefits package are:

1. Physicians' services, including consultant and referral services.
2. Inpatient and outpatient hospital services.
3. Medically necessary emergency health services.
4. Short-term (20 visits) ambulatory evaluative and crisis intervention mental health services.
5. Medical treatment and referral services for alcohol and drug abuse and addiction.
6. Diagnostic laboratory services.
7. Diagnostic and therapeutic radiologic services.
8. Home health services.
9. Voluntary family planning and infertility services.
10. Eye examinations for children.
11. Preventive dental care for children under 12 years of age.

In addition to the minimum benefits package, HMOs are required to offer "supplemental health services" to their enrollees on an optional basis, insofar as the health manpower necessary to provide the services are available in the area served by the HMO. Included are:

- Intermediate-term and long-term care facilities' services.
- Vision care services.
- Dental services.
- Mental health services.
- Long-term physical medicine and rehabilitative services, including physical therapy.
- Prescription drugs which are prescribed in the course of rendering basic or supplemental health services.

Premiums and Other Charges

The HMO must provide "basic health services" for a "basic health services payment," which must be a fixed periodic payment calculated under a *community rating* system whereby all subscriber units of the same size and with the same coverage pay the same premium rate. Therefore, HMOs are precluded from the practice of *experience rating*—that is, basing premiums upon the past utilization and cost experiences of particular groups of enrollees and increasing premiums for groups which have high utilization and cost histories. However, the HMO may charge additional premiums, which must be fixed on a prepayment basis under a community rating system, for the "supplemental health services" which must be offered to the HMO's members on an optional basis.

Enrollment and Members

The legislation requires HMOs to enroll individuals who are "broadly representative of the various age, social and income groups within their service areas." However, it specifically precludes the enrollment of more than 75% of an HMO's members from medically underserved populations, unless the service area has been designated as a rural area by the secretary. Nonetheless, since the indemnity insurance and Blue Cross and Blue Shield plans, with which HMOs compete, are not required to enroll broadly representative populations, some HMOs may again be put at what could be a competitive disadvantage.

To exacerbate the situation, the legislation requires the HMO to have an *open enrollment* period of not less than 30 days per year, during which it accepts, up to its capacity, individuals in the order in which they apply for enrollment.

24

482

Consumer Participation

The legislation further protects the consumer by requiring that at least one-third of the HMO's board of directors be members of the HMO and that there be equitable representation on the HMO's board of directors from medically underserved populations served by the HMO.

Initial Development Costs

The federal government provides two basic types of support: grants, contracts and loan guarantees for HMO *planning;* and grants, contracts and loan guarantees for HMO *initial development costs.*

Initial Operating Losses

The legislation authorizes the secretary of HEW to make loans to public or nonprofit private HMOs in order to assist them in covering their *operating deficits,* if any, for the first three years of their operation. The secretary may also make loans to public or nonprofit private HMOs to assist them in covering any operating deficits which are attributable to significant expansion in their memberships or service areas and which are incurred during the first three years of operation after expansion.

25
NURSING ABROAD

The International Scene

World Distribution of Nurses

"A shortage of qualified nurses exists in nearly every country in the world. Moreover, the distribution of qualified nurses is very unequal: the Americas and Europe, including the USSR, between them have almost three-quarters of the total, leaving one quarter for the rest of Asia, for Africa and Oceana."*

Ratio of Nurses to Inhabitants (Range depends on the country)

Europe	1 for 330 to 1,200
Americas	1 for 230 to 6,000
Asia	1 for 430 to 8,000
Africa	1 for 800 to 12,500

Table 25-1   Number of nurses and health characteristics of selected countries[1]

Country	Nursing personnel	Physicians	Population per physician	Crude death rate (per 1,000)	Infant mortality (per 1,000 live births)	Life expectancy Male	Life expectancy Female
North America							
United States	1,349,000	338,111	622	9.1	16.6	67.4	75.2
Canada	—	36,095	613	7.5	15.6	69.3	76.3
Mexico	—	38,000	1,385	8.4	51.4	61.0	63.7
South America							
Brazil	24,315	48,726	2,025	9.5	—	57.6	61.0
Peru	16,397	8,023	1,802	11.1	65.1	52.5	55.4
Venezuela	24,205	13,017	866	7.8	53.7	63.8	63.8
Europe							
Austria	23,742	14,747	510	12.5	23.5	67.4	74.7
England & Wales	165,400	62,000	787	11.9	15.8	68.9	75.1
Italy	—	109,166	502	9.6	22.6	68.9	74.8
Sweden	55,580	12,610	645	10.6	9.6	72.1	77.6
Yugoslavia	43,761	24,247	864	8.4	40.0	65.5	70.4
Asia							
Jordan	1,659	654	—	16.0	36.3	52.6	52.0[2]
Israel	—	4,143	351	7.3	23.5	70.2	73.2
Japan	316,803	124,684	868	6.6	11.3	70.4	75.9
Pakistan	5,751	16,485	4,049	12.0	124.0	53.7	48.8
Africa							
Congo (Brazzaville)	572	162	6,173	22.8	180.0	41.0	41.0
Morocco	—	1,163	13,345	16.5	149.0	50.5	50.5
Southern Rhodesia	4,459	836	6,579	14.4	122.0	50.0	51.4
Kenya	3,711	766	16,292	17.5	55.0	46.9	51.2

[1]Mortality rates and life expectancy are mainly 1974 data; some data (South America and Africa) are from the late 1960s. Manpower statistics (physicians and nurses) are mainly 1970s data.

[2]1959–63 estimate.

Source: United Nations, 1975.

Service Abroad

Primary Health Care

Primary health care relies on active individual participation from within the community; the use of local resources to meet health and social development problems; and support from national health care systems. It also implies that health personnel must be trained on new lines, whether they be primary health care workers recruited from the community, or doctors and nurses responsible for planning, supervising and evaluating the use of such

---

*World Health Organization.

workers and for training them in the light of recognized community needs.

The way this approach is made differs of course from one country to another, but it is based on a few general principles such as:

- Primary health care should be shaped around the life patterns of the population it should serve and should meet the needs of the community.
- Primary health care should be an integral part of the national health system, and other echelons of services should be designed in *support* of the needs of the peripheral level, especially as this pertains to technical supply, supervisory and referral support.
- Primary health care activities should be fully integrated with the activities of the other sectors involved in community development (agriculture, education, public works, housing and communications).
- The local population should be actively involved in the formulation and implementation of health care activities so that health care can be brought into line with local needs and priorities. Decisions upon what are the community needs requiring solution should be based upon a continuing dialogue between the people and the services.
- Health care offered should place a maximum reliance on available community resources, especially those which have hitherto remained untapped, and should remain within the stringent cost limitations that are present in each country.
- Primary health care should use an integrated approach of preventive, promotive, curative and rehabilitative services for the individual, family and community. The balance between these services should vary according to community needs and may well change over time.
- The majority of health interventions should be undertaken at the most peripheral practical level of the health services by workers most suitably trained for performing these activities.

Serving Abroad as a Nurse

Schools of nursing, like schools of medicine, have focused on the care of the sick in hospitals, to the detriment of disease prevention, health maintenance and health promotion. Training fails to emphasize the care of the sick and disabled outside institutions, although they far outnumber hospital patients in any community. Thus the preparation of nurses to provide community health care in its full sense, or to feel responsible for meeting the health needs of communities, is often lacking.

The situation is particularly acute in underdeveloped countries and rural and peripheral areas, where the provision of care tends to be more challenging and complex and at the same time lacks administrative direction or consultation. The most dramatic change for the nurse who chooses to serve abroad as a community health nurse will be the wider range of diagnostic and therapeutic responsibilities. In addition to teaching primary health workers many of the functions traditionally performed by nurses, they will have to carry out tasks more usually assigned to general medical practitioners. These include examining the sick and disabled, determining the source of the problems presented, and treating acute conditions as well as the main prevalent diseases. The role of the community health nurse should thus be that of a generalist, able to work in a team and (if appropriate) provide leadership, to teach and encourage other health workers, to communicate with and motivate population groups and to interrelate community nursing with other systems.

World Health Organization (WHO) and Nurses

In the field of nursing WHO has been helping countries to train more nurses, to improve the quality of nursing services, to investigate problems and to exchange information. Many WHO nurses have also worked as members of international health teams collaborating with their national counterparts in fighting disease—tuberculosis, malaria, trachoma and smallpox among others.

WHO is an intergovernmental agency dedicated to raising the peoples of the world to the highest possible level of health. It has 137 member states and carries out work of global importance such as administering international health regulations, running a worldwide Telex service for information on disease outbreaks, setting up international standards for biological substances of importance in medicine and publishing the International Pharmacopoeia. It provides assistance to governments, on request, for improving health services or for attacking special health problems. It promotes medical research.

WHO's activities are financed by annual contributions from its member states (the total was about $93 million for 1973) and by voluntary contributions from governmental and private sources. In the United States its activities are combined with those of the Pan American Health Organization. WHO also works closely with a number of specialized agencies of the United Nations (for example the Food and Agriculture Organization and the International labor Organization) and maintains official relations with nongovernmental international organizations concerned with health. In the field of nursing these are the International Committee of Catholic Nurses, the International Confederation of Midwives, the International Council of Nurses and the League of Red Cross Societies, all of which have cooperated with WHO in a variety of tasks.

The WHO Nursing Program

Assistance in nursing has been requested from WHO by countries at varying stages of economic and social development. They range from those where there are long-established health services and the human and material resources to provide a high standard of medical and nursing service, to those where modern concepts of health and social well-being are in an earlier stage of development. In other words, WHO is concerned with specialized problems in technically advanced countries as well as with fundamental problems in developing countries.

In the very early days of WHO, governments asked for nurses to serve chiefly as members of specialized teams concerned with malaria, venereal diseases, tuberculosis and maternal and child health; and such requests are still being received. Gradually, however, it was realized that only by developing nursing and midwifery education programs, could sufficient numbers of nurses and midwives be made available, and governments began to be more interested in the services of nurses and nurse midwives to help in expanding and strengthening schools of nursing and mid-wifery, or in creating new ones. WHO fellowships that enable nurses to acquire new knowledge and skills abroad have also been constantly in demand over the years.

Service with WHO

Besides nurses to work in specialized fields, WHO requires experienced nurse educators to fill vacancies as they occur in various parts of the world. Their duties are to assist member governments in their efforts to strengthen health services, to develop education and training programs to meet the nursing and midwifery manpower needs, planning programs for the control of communicable diseases and other related fields. In addition to basic qualifications, successful candidates require preparation and experience appropriate to the requirements of the post to which they are assigned; for example, specialization in education, administration, a clinical specialty such as maternal and child health, psychiatric nursing or public health.

Starting salaries range between $9,274 and $13,578 a year net of national tax, plus allowances. An increase of $200 to $300 a year, depending on the level of appointment, is awarded after one year's satisfactory service. Annual leave is six weeks a year, and travel expenses for home leave are paid every two years. All appointments over one year are pensionable. The staff member contributes 7% and the organization 14% of the pensionable salary, which is slightly higher than the net salary. The organization also carries a comprehensive accident and health insurance policy for staff members and their dependents.

Application forms can be obtained from the Chief of Personnel, WHO, Avenue Appia, 1211 Geneva, Switzerland, or from the nearest regional office of WHO.

International Nurse Organization

International Conference of Nurses (ICN)

ICN has grown from a membership of three countries in 1899 to a membership of 81 associations today. In addition, ICN is in contact with 20 to 30 additional countries to help nurses prepare for membership.

During its 78 years of growth, the ICN has had 17 presidents from 12 countries and seven executive secretaries from six countries, attesting to its international focus.

ICN's *1973 National Reports of Member Associations* (International Council of Nurses, Geneva, 1973) is a basic reference on nursing

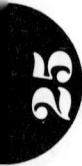

conditions abroad. This volume includes information on the professional nurses' associations in membership with the International Council of Nurses and on national nursing resources in those countries. Included are titles of different kinds of nurses, numbers of nurses, numbers employed and registration authorities.

Table 25-2 ICN member associations, year of admission to ICN and number of member nurses, 1974

1904		**1957**	
Great Britain	45,566	Barbados	140
United States	173,990	Colombia	553
Germany	6,708	Ethiopia	150
1909		Iran	400
Canada	104,124	Liberia	300
Denmark	31,766	Malaysia	726
Finland	19,847	Panama	200
Holland	6,249	Uruguay	242
1912		**1961**	
India	10,073	Guyana	140
New Zealand	8,324	Burma	520
1922		Egypt	500
Belgium	1,704	Ghana	2,316
Italy	890	Jordan	179
Norway	13,954	Kenya	903
1925		Mexico	800
France	2,299	Nigeria	2,030
Ireland	4,072	Taiwan	2,294
Poland	6,000	Singapore	1,000
1929		Thailand	1,490
Brazil	1,520	Venezuela	1,855
Greece	948	**1965**	
Philippines	5,005	Gambia	90
Sweden	40,593	Hong Kong	927
Yugoslavia	2,500	Peru	815
1933		Sierra Leone	120
Austria	3,528	Spain	12,000
Iceland	671	**1969**	
Japan	143,766	Argentina	1,000
1937		Bermuda	145
Australia	18,676	Bolivia	380
Switzerland	7,062	Costa Rica	993
1949		Ecuador	400
Haiti	193	Lebanon	300
South Korea	5,000	Morocco	150
Rhodesia	562	Nepal	233
Turkey	487	Portugal	450
1953		El Salvador	863
Sri Lanka	325	Uganda	100
Chile	2,180	**1973**	
Jamaica	750	Bahamas	188
Luxemburg	32	Botswana	200
Zambia	230	Nicaragua	350
Pakistan	615	Senegal	228
Trinidad and		Tanzania	800
Tobago	170	Zaire	500
1955		**1975**	
Israel	4,200	Fiji	700
		Swaziland	150

U.S. Nurse Volunteers

Action/Peace Corps

Peace Corps, the ACTION international program, has had volunteers from every state in the union, serving in more than a thousand different projects per year, in countries in Africa, the Near East, Asia, the Pacific, South America, Central America and the Caribbean. In 1973 there were only 130 nurses who had volunteered to work in the Peace Corps.

Experienced registered nurses are needed in most of the countries who have asked for Peace Corps help. These host countries usually ask for nurses who are experienced in one or several areas of nursing care. In addition the emphasis now is placed on teaching. The volunteer will find that her duties often include supervising, planning and teaching, as well as ward care.

Recent Projects

- Kenya—staffing 80% of faculty in School of Nursing.
- Swaziland—training physical therapists.
- Kingdom of Tonga—organizing and training hospital personnel.
- Paraguay—teaching sanitation and nutrition.
- Liberia—teaching of communicable diseases.
- Honduras—training practical nurses.
- Zaire—maintaining smallpox surveillance.

Requirements, Training and Compensation

The volunteer must be a U.S. citizen, minimum 18 years of age.

In order to better prepare volunteers an initial three-month training session is provided in the area of assignment. This includes conversational language training, technical training to suplement professional skills and cross-cultural studies.

Compensation includes a monthly allowance for food, lodging, incidentals and medical care; a readjustment allowance of $125 per month, set aside in the U.S., usually payable at completion of service; and optional life insurance at minimum rates.

Missionary Nursing

In general, missionary nurses engage in much the same kinds of work as nonmissionaries: they work in hospitals and dispensaries, visit the sick in their homes and open and conduct nursing schools, where local, qualified youth are trained so that eventually they may do all the nursing for their own people. Missionary nurses also assist in establishing and maintaining health standards and start nursing organizations when the situation warrants this progressive measure.

Public health nurses are usually involved in social action. They identify problems, provide possible solutions and present these to the appropriate local authorities for approval and initiation. They also work on social welfare committees, serve as consultants to professional nursing groups and serve as consultants to personnel in hospitals and schools of nursing.

There is a great need for nurses specially prepared in administration, teaching and consultation in both nursing service and nursing education. Maternity nurses and nurse midwives are also in demand.

Conditions of mission life vary widely with the climate, the language, the cultural differences to which one must adapt, the country, the particular part of the country, the degree of development of the people, the age of the mission, whether just beginning or long established, and the general economic, political and social condition of the immediate community.

The term of a missionary nurse can be anywhere from two to six years, depending on the policy of the mission organization, the country to which she is assigned and the type of assignment. Some mission boards have a short term plan.

In 1976, the Catholic Medical Mission Board utilized 23 nurse volunteers in eight countries and sent medical supplies to 48 countries.

Other International Volunteer Opportunities

Option

OPTION is a nonprofit organization which places health care professionals in *medical shortage areas* throughout the world. In the past decade, nearly 1,000 concerned health care professionals have accepted OPTION assignments in over 50 countries. These individuals have made invaluable contributions toward the development and expansion of preventive health care systems throughout Africa, Asia, Latin America, the West Indies, Mexico,

the Middle East, the Pacific . . . and in United States areas of medical need.

The opportunities for involvement are countless: . . . specialized training of indigenous personnel . . . supervision of vaccination programs . . . eradication of tropical diseases . . . development of family planning programs . . . organization of nutrition and health education services . . . and the ever-present problems of curative medicine.

Registration in any of the following volunteer organizations can be arranged by writing to: OPTION, 3502 Hancock Street, P.O. Box 81122, San Diego, California 92138.

Medico/Care

MEDICO was founded in 1958 by Dr. Peter D. Comanduras, now a member of its Advisory Board, and the late Dr. Thomas Dooley to act as "Physicians to the world." In 1962 it merged with the CARE organization, which carries out an integrated attack on hunger, poverty and disease in more than 30 developing countries with a wide variety of relief, nutrition, community development and health programs.

MEDICO's role in CARE's program is to recruit physicians, specialists, nurses and technicians to provide a balanced program of medical assistance at the least cost; to train host country medical personnel while giving medical care; to utilize and upgrade existing facilities as much as possible and to phase out the service when local personnel are able to carry on at an efficient level of medical care.

- Service period: two years.
- Requirements: trained in U.S./Canada and at least one year of professional experience.
- Training: appropriate language studies are provided when needed.
- Compensation: monthly living allowances plus modest salaries for nurses. First year—$2,700 to 4,200; second year: $3,000 to 4,500.
- Recent projects:

Afghanistan: expanding in-service training for nurses.
Dominican Republic: establishing in-service training for nurses.
Indonesia: training paramedical personnel to serve in outlying, rural areas.
Honduras: staffing rural health centers with auxiliary nurses.

Project Concern

An international, nonprofit, charitable health care organization serving the medically indigent. Project Concern clinics, hospitals and outreach programs are located in Tennessee, New Mexico, Arizona, Hong Kong, Ethiopia, Bali, Mexico and Guatemala. Services include curative medicine and dentistry, with emphasis on preventive medicine and health education. Minimum assignment is six months, although there are occasional short-term needs. Compensation is variable depending upon location—at least 1 year's professional experience required.

International Voluntary Services

A private, nonprofit organization providing technical assistance in many fields, including health and nutrition. IVS seeks qualified health professionals of all nationalities willing to share their expertise. Personnel are currently working in Algeria, Bangladesh, Botswana, Ecuador, Honduras, Indonesia, Mauritania, Papua New Guinea, The Sudan and The Yemen Arab Republic. There is a travel, living and housing allowance, excellent benefits and two-year contractual assignments.

Partners of the Americas

Seek primary care and allied health professionals for short-term service in Latin American countries linked with 42 states in the U.S. As well as providing care, volunteers train local paramedical personnel, help develop prevention programs, restructure health delivery systems and train workers for crisis recovery work. There are short-term assignments only. Compensation is dependent upon available funds—usually volunteer assumes expenses.

United Nations Development Program

Aids developing countries in implementing health care delivery systems, supplying necessary medical and dental professionals to structure programs and train indigenous personnel. There are two-year assignments, salary and travel, resettlement allowance, housing and comprehensive medical and dental insurance.

Miscellaneous

- World Mercy Fund—long-term assignments only.
- The Thomas A. Dooley Foundation, Inc.—long-term assignments only.
- Catholic Relief Services—long-term assignments only.
- Board of Global Ministries.
- Medical Missionaries of Mary.

Advice for the Traveler*

Medical Precautions

A prospective traveler's medical history should be reviewed and his immunization status checked. If he has an allergy, perhaps to penicillin, or a chronic condition such as diabetes, he'll need to carry a wallet card or wear a bracelet or tag that identifies his problem. A cardiac patient might carry a small photocopy of his electrocardiogram.

Any patient who requires maintenance medication should have an adequate supply. He can avoid delays or detainment by customs officials by having each bottle labeled and accompanied by a written prescription; a letter signed by the physician stating the nature of his illness and listing each medication needed will also be helpful. A blank prescription form may be included in case the supply of one of the medicines runs out, but the patient must be warned that he cannot assume the drugs he needs are available in the same form in other countries.

Patients should be cautioned about buying any drug overseas, whether prescription or over-the-counter. Drugs may be sold under names slightly or completely different from those used in the U.S., and quality and ingredients may vary. Drugs such as antibiotics that are available only by prescription in the United States are often sold over-the-counter in other countries, and the "patent medicine" the traveler buys may prove to be more potent than he expects.

Water

Only water from adequately chlorinated sources can be considered truly safe. In areas of the world where hygiene and sanitation are poor, only beverages made from boiled water, canned or bottled carbonated beverages—including bottled water and soft drinks—and beer and wine may be safe to

*Source: "Protecting Patients Going Abroad," *Nursing Update,* July 1976. Reprinted with permission from the July 1976 issue of *Nursing Update,* Intermed Communications, Inc., 132 Welsh Rd., Horsham, Pa. 19044. Further reproduction in whole or in part expressly prohibited by law.

drink. Where water is contaminated, ice must also be considered contaminated. Water of uncertain purity may be made safe for drinking by the use of either chemicals or heat.

Food

Since tapeworms are a common problem in underdeveloped areas all meat and fish should be well cooked and eaten while still hot. The same advice holds for vegetables, particularly those grown in the ground, such as carrots or radishes, which may be contaminated with bacteria and parasites; lettuce and salads are particularly risky. Milk and milk products are also suspect; use powdered milk instead. Fruits that can be peeled are usually safe.

Jet Lag—The disruption of circadian rhythm as the traveler crosses time zones is probably overemphasized as a source of disorientation. Nonetheless, to reduce fatigue and irritability, pace yourself and get ample sleep both during the time abroad and also the night before departure.

High Altitudes—Pace yourself to avoid shortness of breath in cities at high altitudes, particularly those over 8,000 feet such as La Paz, Quito, Bogota, or Addis Ababa.

Eyeglasses—Carry an extra pair of eyeglasses or contact lenses and a copy of the corrective prescription.

Finding Medical Help—If in need of a physician and not staying in a hotel where medical aid is available, call the nearest American embassy or consulate. Also, some travel agencies and local offices of U.S.-based airlines furnish lists of qualified English-speaking physicians. For a small fee, organizations such as the World Medical Association, 10 Columbus Circle, New York, NY 10019, or Intermedic, 777 Third Avenue, New York, NY 10017, will supply listings of physicians in foreign cities; Intermedic members are charged for medical services at a special low fee-schedule by some physicians abroad.

A Travel Kit

Diarrhea—("Turista" and "Montezuma's revenge"). Some authorities recommend giving diphenoxylate HCl combination (Lomotil) in tablet form for convenience in carrying; some prefer paregoric, but it has the disadvantage of potential leakage. Lomotil tablets are not recommended for children.

Constipation—Suppositories should be kept cool since they melt in warm temperatures.

Nausea and Motion Sickness—A mild gastric sedative may be included for stomach upset or vomiting.

Aches and Pain—The active tourist with limited vacation time often "over-does it," so an analgesic is often prescribed for aching muscles or painful joints. It can also be taken for relief of severe toothaches or other significant pain.

Respiratory Infection—An antihistamine is usually the prescription of choice for treating colds, sinusitis, upper respiratory congestion and allergies. Since an antihistamine may also double as a sedative, it eliminates the hazards of prescribing a narcotic. A traveler to the tropics should take along salt tablets. If he will be crossing several time zones, he may also need sleeping pills to help him adjust to his new schedule.

In addition to these medical supplies, other basic kit items include antiseptic, gauze, adhesive bandages and a Red Cross first-aid book.

Vaccinations

Certificate and Recommended Doses—For travel to countries requiring smallpox, cholera or yellow fever vaccination, a patient must carry the World Health Organization-approved International Certificate of Vaccination, available from local health departments, passport offices or travel agents. To avoid quarantine or revaccination, perhaps under less than desirable conditions during the trip, the certificate must be complete in every detail, with the traveler's name on the cover and every page, and the manufacturer and the batch number of smallpox or yellow fever vaccine used listed. It's also advisable to list all vaccinations given the patient even if some are not required. Certificates must be validated with an official stamp of the health department or other appropriate agency.

A yellow fever vaccination must be administered at one of the 250 Public Health Service-designated vaccination centers to be acceptable for international travel.

Specific Disease Requirements—The trend is clearly toward giving fewer vaccinations than in the past.

The following are the key points on necessary or advisable immunizations:

No immunization is required or even recommended for travel directly between the U.S., Canada and any country in Europe.

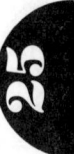

25

The U.S. now requires vaccination against *smallpox* only if the traveler within the preceding 14 days has visited a country any part of which is infected. Smallpox is currently limited to Ethiopa. However, some other countries require that all foreign visitors have this vaccination.

The U.S. no longer requires or recommends cholera vaccination even if a traveler visits an infected area. Therapy to maintain adequate fluid intake and prevent severe dehydration will effect a cure, and in so doing, will limit the spread of the infection. In any case, the vaccine is considered to be only about 50% effective.

The United States no longer requires vaccination against yellow fever, but the Public Health Service recommends it—and some other countries require it—for travel to infected areas. At present, the endemic zones are in Africa, roughly between latitudes 15 degrees N and 15 degrees S, and in South America from latitudes 15 degrees S northward including Panama.

The U.S. Public Health Service recommends, but does not require, vaccination or prophylaxis against polio, typhoid, hepatitis, and malaria for some travelers to underdeveloped areas. Vaccination against plague is not recommended for travel to most countries. It is advisable for travel to the interior regions of Viet Nam, Cambodia, and Laos. The risk of typhus for United States travelers is extremely low. Vaccination is suggested only for special risk groups.

If it has been more than 10 years since a prospective traveler last received tetanus or diphtheria toxoid, it would be reasonable to give a booster. For travel to the rural sections of tropical areas or developing countries off the usual tourist routes, a booster dose of trivalent oral polio vaccine is recommended for those having completed the primary series. If the traveler has not been previously immunized, the primary series is recommended.

PATIENT NEEDS AND SERVICES

Health Facilities

Types of Health Facilities*

Inpatient Health Facilities

Facility for alcoholics
 Home for alcoholics.
 Resident(ial) facility for alcoholics.

Facility for the blind and/or deaf
 Home for blind and/or deaf children.
 Institution for the visually handicapped.
 Resident(ial) school for the blind and/or deaf.

Facility for dependent children
 Home for dependent and neglected children.
 Resident(ial) facility for dependent children.

Facility for drug abusers
 Home for drug abusers (or, addicts).
 Hospital for treatment of drug abusers.
 Resident(ial) facility for drug abusers.

Facility for the emotionally disturbed
 Home for the emotionally disturbed.

*Source: DHEW.

Resident(ial) school for the emotionally disturbed.
School for exceptional children.
Facility for the mentally retarded
 Facility for the mentally deficient.
 Home for the mentally retarded.
 Home for retarded children.
 Hospital for the mentally retarded.
 Mental retardation facility.
 Resident(ial) school for the mentally retarded.
 School for retarded children.
Facility for the physically handicapped
 Home for crippled children.
 Home for the physically handicapped.
 Resident(ial) school for the physically handicapped.
Facility for unwed mothers
 Home for unwed mothers.
 Maternity home.
 Rescue home.
Juvenile correctional facility
 Detention home.
 Home for delinquent boys (or, girls).
 Reformatory.
 Training school for delinquents.
Orphanage

Table 26-1   Outpatient and nonpatient health services

Primary title	Alternate title	Primary title	Alternate title
Ambulance Services:		Migrant health	
Ambulance	Emergency vehicle.	program	Migrant health project.
Ambulance service	Ambulance company.		Migrant health service.
	Emergency ambulance service.	Neighborhood health center	Community health center.
	Rescue squad.		Comprehensive neighborhood health center.
Blood Banks:			Comprehensive neighborhood health service program.
Blood bank	Blood bank service.		Health care center.
	Community blood bank.		Public health center.
	Hospital blood bank.		Rural health center.
	Regional blood center.		
	Transfusion facility.	Dental Group Practices:	
	Transfusion service.	Group dental	
Clinical (Medical) Laboratories:		practice	Closed (dental) panel.
Clinical laboratory	Bacteriological laboratory.		Dental clinic.
	Hospital laboratory.		Dental dispensary.
	Independent (clinical) laboratory.		Dental group (practice).
	Medical laboratory.		General practice dental group.
	Public health laboratory.		Multispecialty dental group.
			Single-specialty dental group.
Comprehensive Health Services Programs:		Dental Laboratories:	
Community mental		Dental laboratory	Commercial dental laboratory.
health center	(Comprehensive) (community) mental health center.		Dental processing laboratory.
			Institutional dental laboratory.
			Private (practice) dental laboratory.

(continued)

Table 26-1   (continued)

Primary title	Alternate title	Primary title	Alternate title
Family Planning Facilities:			Community pharmacy.
Family planning			Drug chain.
clinic	Birth control clinic.		Hospital pharmacy.
	Family planning unit (in		Independent pharmacy.
	hospital).		Industrial pharmacy.
	Family planning service.		Noncommunity pharmacy.
	Maternal and child care clinic.		Nursing home pharmacy.
	Planned parenthood clinic.		Prescription pharmacy.
	Postpartum clinic (in		(Retail) drugstore.
	hospital).	Poison Control Centers:	
	Vasectomy clinic.	Poison control center	Poison information center.
	Well-baby clinic.		Poison treatment center.
Home Health Services:		Psychiatric Outpatient Services:	
Home health		Psychiatric clinic	(Free-standing) outpatient
agency	Community nursing service.		psychiatric clinic.
	Home care program.		Hospital-affiliated outpatient
	Home health aide service.		psychiatric service.
	Visiting nurse association.		Hospital-based outpatient
Medical Group Practices:			psychiatric service.
Medical group practice	(General practice) medical	Rehabilitation Facilities:	
	group.	Rehabilitation	
	Group clinic.	facility	(Comprehensive) rehabilita-
	Medical group clinic.		tion center.
	Medical group practice.		Free-standing rehabilitation
	Multispecialty medical group.		center.
	Single-specialty medical		Homebound program.
	group.		Rehabilitation program.
Opticianry Establishments:			(Sheltered) workshop.
Opticianry establish-			Speech and hearing center.
ment	Retail optical shop.		
	Optical department (of store).	Suicide Prevention Centers:	
Pharmacies:		Suicide prevention	
Pharmacy	Chain drugstore.	center	Crisis intervention agency.
	Chain pharmacy.		Suicide "hotline."
	Clinic pharmacy.		Suicide prevention program.

Miscellaneous Health Facilities *

Multiphasic screening centers—The examination focusing on preventive medicine and early detection of disease is called multiphasic screening. It is a multipurpose examination utilizing the latest developments in laboratory testing, x-ray technology, electrocardiograms, and a variety of other tests to determine whether any symptoms are present that might be detected so that early treatment can be given. There are a number of such screening centers located throughout the country. Some are in fixed locations, as described under the Kaiser plans. Others are located in mobile units enabling the workers to take these tests to a factory, neighborhood center, or other location, making the tests readily accessible to the population with a minimum of inconvenience.

Neighborhood Health Centers—Neighborhood health centers are found throughout the country and offer service to the residents of an immediate geographic area. Supported to a large extent by federal money, most are in low income areas in which the health center is the focus for members of the community to receive diagnosis and treatment for a wide range of health needs on an ambulatory basis. Many of these neighborhood health centers are affiliated with hospitals in order for patients who need that type of care to be admitted readily, although their emphasis is on prevention and ambulatory diagnosis and treatment.

Extended Care Facilities—Many hospitals have developed extended care facilities that serve patient needs after the acute phase of their illness. The large advantage of providing such care is an economic one in that there is

---

*Source: Sloane, Robert M., and Sloane, Beverly LeBov: *A Guide to Health Facilities,* 2nd ed., St. Louis, 1977. The C.V. Mosby Co.

no need for intensive care staffing, although adequate staffing is available for the needs of these patients while they are undergoing the recuperative phase of illness.

Industrial Medical Clinics—Many corporations have clinics for their employees, which provide preemployment examinations and routine annual examinations, and which are prepared to take care of industrial accidents as they may occur. They are staffed with phy-

sicians, nurses, x-ray and laboratory technicians and clerical supporting personnel.

Health Departments—Health departments have long been involved in preventive medicine, disseminating health information and providing sanitation standards and inspection services. Clinics are run by health departments in areas such as venereal disease, well-baby clinics, x-ray examinations and family planning.

Table 26-2   Miscellaneous inpatient health facilities, by type, 1973

U.S.	Total facilities	Mentally retarded	Dependent children	Emotionally disturbed	Unwed mothers	Drug abusers or alcoholics	Deaf and/or blind	Physically handicapped	All other facilities
Total	4,836	1,348	917	1,282	144	809	167	65	104
		Number of beds in other inpatient health facilities by type of facility							
Total	400,899	217,067	48,568	60,195	6,015	33,128	24,321	4,812	6,793

Source: DHEW, 1974.

Blood

Overview*

About 7% of a person's weight is blood. The amount of blood varies according to height and weight, but an average size man has about 12 pints of blood and an average size woman has about nine pints.

The average adult has 30 trillion red blood cells in the blood stream, or about 1 billion red cells in each two or three drops of blood. There is one white cell for every 600 red cells and one platelet for every 10 or 20 red cells.

The blood cells are made principally in the bone marrow, with the help of the spleen, lymph glands, stomach, liver and other specialized tissues. (Blood cells are constantly being produced. The red blood cell, for example, wears out after about 120 days when it is replaced by a new cell.) Plasma, the fluid part of blood, receives water, nutrients and other vital substances from the digestive tract and other organs and tissues.

What is hemoglobin?

Hemoglobin is a protein substance in the red blood cells which gives blood its red color. It is the substance that carries oxygen and carbon

dioxide to and from the cells of the body. To make hemoglobin, the body must have iron, which comes from the food we eat. People who do not have enough hemoglobin to be blood donors are frequently anemic or said to have "low hemoglobin."

Can Blood Be Preserved by Freezing?

The red cells of blood can be preserved for years if frozen within five days of donation, using very special techniques and stored at a temperature of 125 degrees below zero Fahrenheit. Since the freezing and thawing procedures are costly and involved, this method of preservation is limited at present to rare blood. Fresh plasma, however, is frequently frozen to zero degrees Fahrenheit for storage up to one year.

Blood Types

Blood type and Rh	How many have it	Frequency
O Rh positive	1 person in 3	37.4%
O Rh negative	1 person in 15	6.6%
A Rh positive	1 person in 3	35.7%
A Rh negative	1 person in 16	6.3%
B Rh positive	1 person in 12	8.5%
B Rh negative	1 person in 67	1.5%
AB Rh positive	1 person in 29	3.4%
AB Rh negative	1 person in 167	.6%

*Source: "Q & A" about Blood and Blood Banking, American Association of Blood Banks.

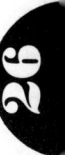

Blood Components and Derivatives

Cellular elements are 45% of blood	Red cells			Can serve for 30-50% of all blood transfusions. For treatment of anemia.
	White cells			For combating infections. Clinical use experimental at present.
	Platelets			Essential for blood clotting. For treatment of leukemia, cancer, and other diseases associated with platelet deficiency.
Plasma is 55% of blood	Plasma			Fresh frozen plasma used to control bleeding. Single-donor liquid plasma used to restore plasma volume.
	Cryoprecipitate			Prepared from fresh frozen plasma. Contains AHF (antihemophilic factor). Therapeutic for hemophiliacs.
	Plasma proteins	Serum albumin		For treatment of shock and low blood protein.
		Gamma globulin		Contains antibodies against diseases. For prevention of hepatitis and measles. For treatment of gamma globulin deficiency.
		Specific immune globulins		A special variety of gamma globulin prepared from plasmas with specific antibodies.
		Clotting factor concentrates; e.g., fibrinogen, AHF, and II, VII, IX, X		Essential for blood clotting. For controlling bleeding due to deficiencies of specific coagulation factors.

Source: "Q & A about Blood & Blood Banking," American Association of Blood Banks.

Most of the plasma is obtained by a process called plasmapheresis. "Single" plasmapheresis involves withdrawing whole blood from the donor into an anticoagulant fluid. The mixture is spun in a centrifuge so as to separate blood plasma from the red cells. The red cells are then transfused back to the donor to diminish the risk of anaemia.

Blood Properties*

Blood is a key tissue in the human body in that it serves as the body's principal transport medium, carrying oxygen, nutrients and chemicals to all body tissue and carrying waste products and synthesized metabolites away.

Blood is essentially an aqueous fluid that transports dispersed or dissolved nutrients, metabolites, electrolytes, hormones, and substances to counteract infection and hemorrhage. Blood maintains equilibria between the cells so that they sustain the narrow range of conditions of temperature, dissolved solids, and chemical reactivity necessary to their survival and proper functioning.

Various elements in the blood from different species interact unfavorably. Only properly matched human blood can be given to humans with a high probability of success. Antigen-antibody reactions from mixing human blood of different types frequently form clots that cannot pass through the circulatory system and that can cause significant problems.

In addition to the blood types routinely characterized in four types (O, A, B, AB) two additional classes, Rh(+) and Rh(−), denoting individuals who have or are missing the Rh antigen, divide each type into two more categories (O+, O−, A+, A−, B+, B−, AB+, or AB−). A host of other antigens further separate blood types of groups of individuals.

These antigens have the capacity to stimulate the formation of, and to react with, substances in the blood called "antibodies." Antibodies for A and B are routinely found in human blood. However, a person with antigen A (type A blood) will not have antibody A, but rather antibody B. If both antigen and antibody A were present or became mixed through transfusion, these would react and could cause destruction of the red cells. The case is similar for other antigens of this blood group system.

*Source: DHEW, 1972.

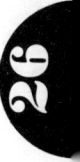

Blood type	Antigen present	Antibody present
A	A	B
B	B	A
AB	A and B	Neither A or B
O	Neither A or B	Both A and B

Cells—45% of whole blood volume

- Red blood cells (erythrocytes)
- White blood cells (leukocytes)
- Platelets

Liquid portion (plasma)—55% of whole blood volume

- Water
- Proteins, enzymes, fats
- Soluble materials such as salts, waste products and others mentioned previously

In a proper preservative medium, held at a proper temperature, red blood cells survive and remain functional for as long as 21 to 28 days. Platelets, on the other hand, are functional for shorter times (as little as 24 hours) once outside the body. Just as the body depends on blood to maintain the conditions for life, so does blood, interdependent with the rest of the organism, depend on other tissues and organs to support and maintain its vitality. Unlike the cells, most noncellular portions maintain functionality outside the body for long periods, if held under the right conditions. However, some labile materials, such as enzymes and hormones, may survive only for hours when the blood is removed from the body. Unless held under sterile conditions, blood rapidly decomposes and becomes both useless and a potential source of injury to a recipient.

Components and fractions from a single pint of blood can serve a wide variety of needs. Red blood cells can be used to treat anemia or conditions associated with poor oxygen-carrying capacity, but not heavy loss of fluids. Platelets can be used to control massive bleeding and some of the many conditions in which certain fractions are required to produce clotting.

- Fibrinogen, a protein derivative, can be used to aid clotting.
- Globulins, another protein of the noncellular portion, can be used to modify effects of disease.
- Albumin, the major protein of the noncellular portion, can be used to modify blood volume where there are fluid losses (as in shock), since this material will aid in the

26

retention of fluids within the circulatory system.

- Special materials, such as antihemophilia globulin, can be used in special disorders (hemophilia in this case) where the specific factor is missing and can only be provided from outside.

Blood Banks*

In 1972 approximately 9,350,000 units of whole blood were collected.

In 1971, of the total 5,400 blood facilities, 4.4% were licensed by the federal government, 26.7% were licensed by state governments, and only 1.2% were licensed by both. Seventy percent were unregulated by either federal or state government. Approximately 8,799,700 units of whole blood were collected by the blood-banking sector in 1971.

The subsectors in the blood-banking industry contributed to the collection of the above amount the following ratio:

Organizations	Percent of Total Supply Collected
Red Cross	39.5%
Community blood banks	29.1
Hospitals	17.9
Commercial blood banks	11.0
Military	2.5

A total of 1.7 million liters of plasma and 550,-000 units of whole blood were obtained from donors by the pharmaceutical firms surveyed. Collections by these firms contributing to the total blood resource obtained by the nation in 1971 included approximately:

- 1.5 million liters of plasma collected from donors by plasmapheresis,

- 550,000 units of whole blood drawn from donors,

- 200,000 liters of plasma recovered from 600,000 placentas.

*Source: DHEW, 1972.

Figure 26-1 Types of Blood Bank Facilities: Number, Percent and Collections

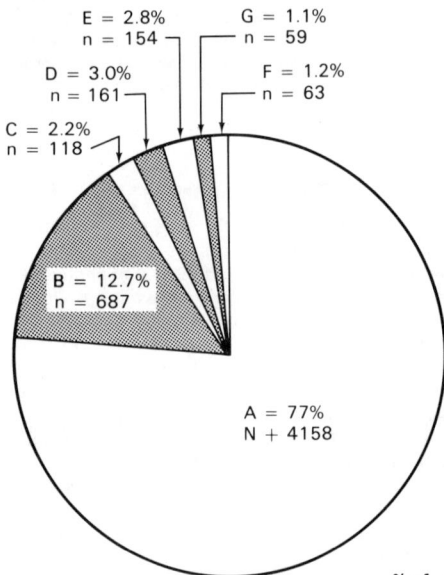

E = 2.8% n = 154
G = 1.1% n = 59
D = 3.0% n = 161
F = 1.2% n = 63
C = 2.2% n = 118
B = 12.7% n = 687
A = 77% N + 4158

	No. of facilities in %	% of whole blood collected
A. Dependent* hospital blood bank or transfusion service	77%	5%
B. Collecting hospital blood bank	13%	9
C. Collecting and supplying hospital blood bank	2	4
D. Military hospital blood bank	3	3
E. Community blood bank	3	40
F. Red cross regional blood center	1	
G. Commercial blood bank	1	39

*(Depend on outside sources for regular blood supply).

Blood Donations**

Number and Characteristics of Donors

Approximately 6½ million persons, 5.3% of persons 17–64 years of age, donated blood during a 12-month period, according to data gathered by the Health Interview Survey during 1973. Many more males than females gave

**Source: DHEW, 1976.

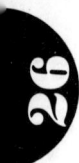

blood: 8.0% compared to 2.9% of persons of eligible age. More persons aged 25–44 years donated blood (6.7%) than persons of other ages did (4.3%). Proportionately, about twice as many white persons (5.6%) as persons of other colors (2.9%) were blood donors. A greater proportion of the population in the higher income brackets donated blood than persons with smaller family incomes did: 6.5% of persons with family income of $10,000 or more compared with 4.0% with incomes less than $10,000. Approximately two-thirds of all donors (67.1%) gave blood one time during the year, whereas only slightly more than 1 in 10 donors (13.4%) gave three or more times.

An estimated 10.2 million donations were made by the 6½ million blood donors, an average of 1.6 donations per donor.

Why People Donate Blood

The four categories used in Table 26-3 show the reasons donations are made: sold, given for replacement, given to a blood bank and "other donation." Examples of "other donations" are donations made for altruistic reasons or to receive time off from work. The proportions of donations made to blood banks and classified as other donations were similar, 35.2 and 36.5%, respectively. They are the two major categories of donations. About 20% of all donations replaced blood used by a relative or friend, while donations that were sold made up the smallest category, 8.1%. Over one-third of donations that were sold (35.0%) were given by persons donating blood five or more times during the year.

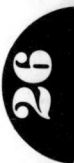

Table 26-3   Distribution of blood donations by reason for donation (1973 data)

Sex	Total donations in thousands	All reasons	Sold blood	Replaced blood	Gave to blood bank	Other donation
			Percent distribution			
All ages 17–64 years	10,215	100.0	8.1	19.8	35.2	36.5
White	9,542		7.6			
All other	673		16.3			
17–24 years						
White	2,016		14.9			
All other	165		38.2			

Table 26-4   Characteristics of blood donors (1973 data)

Color	Both sexes	Male	Female
	Percent of population		
Total	5.3	8.0	2.9
White	5.6	8.3	3.1
All other	2.9	5.0	1.2
Education			
Less than 12 years	2.7	4.2	1.2
12 years	5.6	9.0	3.1
13 years or more	8.2	11.0	4.8
Working or not			
In labor force	6.7	—	—
Not in labor force	2.0	—	—

Table 26-5   Percent of donors who sold blood; by select characteristics (1973 data)

Age and education of donor	Percent of donors who sold blood
17–24 years	
Less than 12 years	32.9%
12 years	13.8
13 years or more	15.0
25–44 years	
Less than 12 years	13.5
12 years	6.7
13 years or more	4.7
Place of Residence of Donor	
Central city	13.7
Outside central city	6.3

Table 26-6 **Number of multiple donations made during the year, according to reason for donation (1973 data)**

Reason for donation	Total donations in thousands	Number of donations made in year				
		5 or more	4 or more	3 or more	2 or more	1 or more
		Cumulative percent distribution				
All reasons	10,215	8.3	19.6	32.9	57.5	100.0
Sold blood	832	35.0	51.6	65.1	82.9	100.0

Hepatitis

The FDA estimates that the risk of acquiring post-transfusion hepatitis from commercially acquired blood is three to ten times that from donated blood. That is why one of its major concerns is to encourage efforts designed to bring into being an all-voluntary blood donation system and to eliminate commercialism in the acquisition of whole blood and blood components for transfusion purposes.

The Red Cross, which is responsible for obtaining about 40% of all whole blood collected by the blood banks in this country, rejects about 12% of all prospective donors.

Hospital Use of Blood*

The "average" nonsupplying hospital:

- Collects 11.0% of its total blood supply itself.
- Discards 6.0% of its total blood supply because of outdating, contamination, spillage, hepatitis antigen positivity, etc.
- Transfuses 56.5% of its transfusable supply.
- Performs 3.1 cross-matches for every unit of blood transfused.
- Transfuses 45.2% of its blood as packed red cells.

Transplants**

Organ Transplantation

Over the past 20 years, significant progress has been made in the field of transplantation. Laboratory research has enabled surgeons to apply experimental findings to animal models, and finally to humans. Although this transition had an initially high mortality rate, the number

---

*Source: DHEW, 1975.
**Source: House Appropriations Committee Hearings, 1977.

of long-term survivors of kidney, heart and bone marrow transplants has dramatically increased. Immunology must now solve the remaining problems, such as graft rejection, which prevent transplantation from being a routine procedure.

To achieve this goal, scientists are trying to learn how to manipulate the immune response of a recipient so that he will accept the "foreign" graft but retain his ability to fight off disease-producing organisms. This delicate balance requires a more complete understanding of the major histocompatibility complex—the group of inherited genes that regulate an individual's immune response—and of the types of cells and mechanisms involved in organ rejection.

Donor Selection

Since not enough kidneys are donated to meet today's needs, every organ must be given the best possible chance for survival, that is, it must be transplanted into the most closely matched recipient. It has been shown that more than 60% of transplanted kidneys that fail do so because of genetic differences between the donor and recipient. These genetic differences can be recognized by serologic (blood) tests which identify specific HLA antigens. These serologically-defined (SD) HLA antigens are substances which are found on the surface of certain cells, mainly white blood cells called lymphocytes.

Each individual possesses four of these antigens, two from each parent. Consequently, identical twins who have the same genetic markers are the ideal donor–recipient combination. A brother or sister offers the next best hope of genetic compatibility since there is a one in four chance that they inherited the same antigens from their parents. However, the source of most transplanted organs today are cadavers, totally unrelated to the recipient. Thus, the importance of precise typing techniques for matching donors and recipients is obvious.

Preformed Antibodies

In addition to selecting a donor who is genetically compatible, scientists have realized that they must be certain that a recipient does not have any preformed antibodies against the donor's cells. These antibodies may have been formed when the recipient was preimmunized to the histocompatibility antigens by a previous transplant, blood transfusions, pregnancies or, possibly, some types of infection. Such antibodies can destroy the transplanted cells.

Immunosuppression

Since genetically identical matches of a donor and recipient are difficult to achieve, scientists have had to rely on various techniques to manipulate the patient's immune responses. One commonly employed method is to treat the recipient with drugs, such as corticosteroids, which suppress his ability to mount an immune response not only to his graft, but unfortunately, to disease-producing organisms as well. It is the goal of scientists to understand the mechanism of action of these drugs so that eventually they can be used to block only the immune response to the graft.

Kidney Transplantation

A successful kidney transplant can "cure" chronic kidney disease. Kidney dialysis—in which a patient's blood is mechanically purified—keeps the patient with kidney failure alive, but the quality of his life is rather poor. He must spend six to eight hours a day, two to three times a week, connected to the dialysis machine. This machine dependence consumes a major part of his time, confines him to one locale, and can affect him psychologically. Furthermore, dialysis is often a downhill road since the patient continues to be ill, and it is usually only a matter of time until he has no suitable veins with which to be connected to the machine. An analysis of kidney transplant patients at the Medical College of Virginia by NIAID grantee Dr. Hyung Lee, showed that 50% of his patients who received transplants were still alive after ten years. This ten-year survival is a great deal better than for those on dialysis.

Thus, the ideal situation for a person with kidney failure is to be kept alive by dialysis until a suitable donor is found for a kidney transplant. Should the transplant fail, dialysis can again keep the patient alive until there is another opportunity for a transplant.

Most transplanted kidneys that fail do so because of genetic differences that cause rejection. HLA typing to detect these genetic differences has been recognized as very important to graft survival when the donor is a living relative of the recipient. However, the value of HLA matching in transplants involving cadaver kidneys—the most common source of today's transplants—has not been established.

Heart Transplantation

The wave of enthusiasm for heart transplantation that followed hard upon the first successful operation in 1967 diminished considerably during subsequent years. But substantial progress continues to be made in those centers with the facilities, staff, and expertise to cope with immunological and related problems that almost inevitably develop during the postoperative period.

The largest series of heart transplants, and one of the most successful, is that of Dr. Norman Shumway and colleagues at Stanford. As of August 1, 1975, this group had performed 90 heart transplants. Thirty-two recipients were still alive, the longest survivor having gone for five and two-thirds years. For the 53 patients who made it through the critical first three post-operative months, the survival rate was 76% after one year and 59% after three years. Forty-eight of these were restored to normal activity status by the procedure and many resumed their previous occupations.

The percentage of transplant recipients surviving for a year or more has continued to increase, thanks largely to improved techniques for very early detection of rejection episodes and for monitoring the effects of immunosuppressive therapy. Rejection episodes remain a recurrent problem among long-term survivors, but are no longer a major cause of death. The leading cause of death in this group is infections, resistance to which is inevitably lowered by the immunosuppressive therapy employed to prevent or control rejection episodes.

Bone Marrow Transplantation

Supported by NIAID and the National Cancer Institute, Dr. E. Donnall Thomas and other investigators at the University of Washington have become the leading transplanters of bone marrow in the world. In 1975, they performed

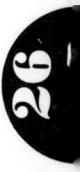

64 marrow transplants for patients with acute leukemia, or aplastic anemia—a disorder in which the bone marrow fails to produce blood cells. Thirty-five of these patients are still alive. The longest aplastic anemia survivor is now four years post transplant. The longest acute leukemia survivor who received a transplant from a twin has now been free of his disease for five years, thus demonstrating a "five-year cure" by bone marrow grafting. Another leukemia patient, who no longer responded to chemotherapy, received a bone marrow graft from his sister. His bone marrow is still female and after five years; he is still free of his disease.

These two leukemia patients with long-term cures indicate the feasibility of intensive therapy designed to destroy both normal and abnormal marrow cells followed by a marrow transplant to restore normal marrow function. There are, however, many problems to be solved before this treatment can help all who need it.

Cornea Preservation

During the past year new methods have been developed which promise to extend the benefits of corneal transplantation by improving the quality of donor tissue and reducing the risk of graft failure. Of the nearly 3,000 corneal transplants performed each year in the United States, between 75 and 85% are successful. In the remaining 15 to 25% one of the main problems associated with graft failure is loss of tissue transparency following the operation. Often this is caused by an inability to preserve the cornea's endothelial cells from the time the tissue is obtained until it is used for transplantation. This layer of cells functions as a biologic pump, removing water from the cornea and, thus, helping to maintain its transparency. Loss of these cells, not always apparent prior to transplantation, causes the grafted tissue to swell and become opaque.

Donor Selection—Because of the absence of blood vessels in the cornea, matching of antigens between donor and recipient is less crucial in corneal transplantation than in other organ or tissue transplant operations. Immune graft rejection occurs in only 5 to 10% of all corneal transplantations. However, when, in the course of certain diseases, the cornea becomes densely vascularized, the graft rejection rate increases substantially; as many as 25 to 60% of transplants involving a vascularized cornea are not successful. Furthermore, as in kidney transplants, patients receiving a donor cornea are at even greater risk of experiencing graft rejection if they have been presensitized to HLA antigens following pregnancy, blood transfusion or a previous corneal transplant.

Organ Donation*

Some 10,000–15,000 kidneys must be donated nationally each year. And there are 30,000 people waiting for sight-restoring corneal transplants.

Today, transplant techniques have developed to the point where kidney, eye-tissue and skin transplants are considered routine medical procedures. More than 30,000 kidney transplants have been performed, and many thousands of people whose vision was seriously impaired now see again. Skin grafts are routinely used in the treatment of severe burn cases.

Sight-restoring corneal transplants are 90% successful, while kidney transplants from living related donors are successful 80% of the time.** Success rates of transplants from non-related donors who leave their organs when they die are lower, around 50%. Many more parts of the body including heart, lungs, pancreas, tendons, bone marrow and cartilage have also been transplanted with varying degrees of success.

Donor Law

A model law, the Uniform Anatomical Gift Act, endorsed by legal and medical organizations, has been approved in most states. The law authorizes donations of organs by any mature person before death or by his relatives after death.

In most states, the donor's written authorization alone is sufficient. If there has been no written request when death occurs, the spouse, adult child, parent or brother or sister may still make a donation, by any recorded message or written statement. The written authorization can be by (1) will, (without the usual waiting period) or (2) any written document, including a card which may be carried by the person. (See sample on following page.)

---

*Source: N.Y.-N.J. Regional Transplant Program, 1976.
**Success rate is measured as survival of the kidney graft longer than one year.

Uniform Donor Card (Front)

> Print or type name of donor
>
> In the hope that I may help others, I hereby make this anatomical gift, if medically accept-able, to take effect upon my death. The words and marks below indicate my desires.
>
> I give: (a) _____ any needed organs or parts
> (b) _____ only the following organs or parts
>
> Specify the organ(s) or part(s)
>
> for the purpose of transplantation, therapy, medical research or education;
> (c) _____ my body for anatomical study if needed.
>
> ---
> Limitations or special wishes, if any.

Uniform Donor Card (Back)

> Signed by the donor and the following two wit-nesses in the presence of each other:
>
> | | |
> |---|---|
> | Signature of Donor | Date of Birth of Donor |
> | City and State | Date Signed |
> | Witness | Witness |
> | Name of Registry | Phone |
>
> This is a legal document under the Uniform Anatomical Gift Act or similar laws.

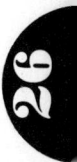

Donations can be made without naming any person or place as recipient. A donor, however, may list a qualified institution, physician or an individual needing treatment or transplanta-tion.

Some Donor Agencies

- The Eye-Bank for Sight Restoration, Inc.
- The National Kidney Foundation
- The National Association of Patients on Hemodialysis and Transplantation, Inc.
- The New York-New Jersey Regional Trans-plant Program
- The Ruth Gottscho Kidney Foundation

Nurse or Physician Procedure with Potential Donors

- Identify the potential donor
- Report the donor to the local organ recovery program
- Maintain the potential donor until the nephrectomy*

---

*The determination of death of a potential organ donor, as with any patient, traditionally remains the clinical judgment of the physician. The declaration of death must be made by a physician (two physicians in New York state and Connecticut) not affiliated with the transplant team. This provision protects the rights of the potential donor by avoiding any conflict of interest by the physicians involved.

- Obtain consent from the next-of-kin (or social worker, clergy, administrator)
- Obtain consent from the medical examiner (physician only)
- Assist with the nephrectomy (OR nurses and staff)

Number of Transplants

The current world total summary is as follows:

Table 26-7   Update on organ transplantation in the world

	Heart	Liver	Lung	Pancreas
Transplant teams	65	42	22	15
Transplants	339	299	37	52
Recipients	331	284	37	50
Alive with functioning grafts	74	39	0	0
Longest survival with function-ing graft	8.6 yr.	7.4 yr.	10 mo.	4.2 yr.
Longest current survival with functioning graft	8.6 yr.	7.4 yr.	—	—

Cases reported to the NIH Organ Transplant Registry—June 1, 1977.

Chronology of Transplants*

The following table indicates chronology of nonrenal transplantation. As of June 1977, 74 heart recipients were alive at one to 89 months; 39 liver recipients were living from one to 74 months.

Table 26-8   World totals and chronology—nonrenal organ transplantation

Year	Heart	Liver	Lung	Pancreas
1963		6	2	
1964		4	0	
1965		7	3	
1966		3	1	2
1967	2	8	6	1
1968	101	39	6	6
1969	47	46	7	7
1970	17	31	2	9
1971	18	15	4	1
1972	18	23	3	5
1973	33	25	2	5
1974	29	30	0	7
1975	32	22	1	6
1976	31	32	0	3
1977	11	8	0	0
Total transplants	339	299	37	52
Total recipients	331	284	37	50
Alive with functioning grafts	74	39	0	0

Cases reported to the Registry—June 1, 1977.

The team at Stanford University is responsible for 86 of the 155 cardiac transplants performed between 1970 and 1976. Of the 152 liver transplants performed in that time period, 87 were done in Denver under Dr. Starzl's direction, and 29 were performed by Professor Calne's group at Cambridge.

Cardiac Transplantation

As indicated in the summary, 339 cardiac transplants have been recorded by the Registry. Seventy-four patients survive currently. The longest survival with a functioning graft was 8.6 years. The principal cause of death in these patients has been chronic rejection accompanied by infection and recurrent or immunologically induced atherosclerosis.

Dr. Norman Shumway in 1975 provided the following information to the House Subcommittee on Health and Environment. As of April

*Source: *Newsletter,* Jan. 1977, American College of Surgeons, NIH Organ Transplant Registry.

1, 1975, 83 patients received transplants, with 29 currently living. One year survival has risen from 22% during the first year to 56% during the seventh (most recent) year. Of those living three months after their transplant, 36% five-year survival is currently projected. I believe this is impressive when it is considered that a transplant candidate has a less than 5% chance of one year survival untreated surgically.

Table 26-9   Stanford cardiac transplantation

	Number of patients	Number of transplants
1968	9	10
1969	9	9
1970	8	8
1971	12	12
1972	13	14
1973	15	15
1974	13	15
*1975	4	4
Total	83	87

*Through April 1.

Table 26-10   Stanford cardiac transplantation survival statistics

Overall
48% 1 Year survival
37% 2 Year survival
26% 3 Year survival
22% 4 Year survival
22% 5 Year survival

1st Program year	22% 1 Year survival
2nd Program year	44% 1 Year survival
3rd Program year	50% 1 Year survival
4th Program year	42% 1 Year survival
5th Program year	54% 1 Year survival
6th Program year	47% 1 Year survival
7th Program year	56% 1 Year survival

3 Months survivors
76% 1 Year survival
59% 2 Year survival
42% 3 Year survival
36% 4 Year survival
36% 5 Year survival

Stanford cardiac transplantation (83 patients)	
Total 1-year survivors	30
Percent rehabilitated	87
Currently living (1 month to 5 years)	29

Kidney Disorders, Transplants and Machines*

(Authorities estimate that the total number of people with kidney disease is well over 8,000,-000. Recent samplings have indicated that at least 3,300,000 Americans have unrecognized undiagnosed diseases of the kidneys.)

Kidney Failure and Treatment

The kidney is the organ most frequently transplanted with tens or thousands of kidney transplantations having been performed throughout the world. Depending on the selection of the donor organ and how close donor and recipient tissue types are matched, between 40 and 80% of kidney transplants remain functional after two years. Some recipients who have received a kidney from their identical twin are now in their second decade since receiving a kidney transplant.

However it begins, irreversible and potentially fatal kidney failure strikes more than 52,000 patients annually, of which perhaps 10,000 are suitable candidates for maintenance dialysis (or renal transplantation if a matching organ is available).

Patients who do receive dialysis treatment, which continues to be very costly, may experience a number of undesirable complications and must, of course, adjust their lives to the necessity of regular sessions on the kidney machine. Kidney transplantation is a possible alternative, but many patients (especially older ones) cannot withstand major surgery, and even those who do undergo transplantation must be sustained on dialysis until an appropriate donor organ is found. The patient may also need dialysis again if the new kidney is rejected or does not function properly at first. In fact, on the average, approximately one half of transplanted patients return to maintenance dialysis by the end of the third year, post-transplant, because of eventual failure of the grafted organ. Artificial kidneys have other important uses as well: they are used as a means of life-sustaining support in cases of acute kidney failure, and in treatment of moribund patients with accidental or suicidal drug overdosage. In such cases, use of dialysis can be decisive to the outcome.

For a decade and a half, dialysis has been used successfully to maintain life in a significant and increasing number of end-stage kidney disease patients (at present—22,000). A great deal has been achieved over these years, and clinicians now have an adequate—though not optimal—mode of dialysis based on treatment three times each week, each usually lasting six hours. Dialysis therapy, however, is only partially successful in reversing all of the lesions and dysfunctions caused by chronic kidney failure. Patients maintained on dialysis at present exhibit varying degrees of rehabilitation from poor to excellent.

Warning Signs of Kidney Disease

1. Burning or difficulty during urination
2. More frequent urination, particularly at night
3. Passage of bloody-appearing urine
4. Puffiness around eyes, swelling of hands and feet, especially in children
5. Pain in small of back just below the ribs
6. High Blood Pressure

The Artificial Kidney Machine**

The artificial kidney is a life-saving substitute for the patient's kidneys, removing from the blood waste products that would be fatal, if allowed to accumulate for more than a few days.

How Do Artificial Kidneys Work?—The artificial kidney machine provides the "blood-washing" which the human kidney usually performs. The blood slowly migrates over a cellophane membrane which together with a cleansing solution filters out body wastes but permits the flow of blood and other substances needed by the body. Cellophane, which is porous, substitutes for the kidney's glomeruli, or microscopic tufts of blood vessels, which ordinarily do the filtering.

The patient is connected to the machine by a tube inserted in an artery of his arm or leg, to conduct his blood, pumped by his heart, into the machine and over one side of the cellophane filter. When cleansed, the blood is then routed back to a vein in the body by another tube. During the entire period of treatment, the blood flows through the machine, back through the patient's body, back through the machine, making the round trip about twice an hour, filtering out some impurities each trip. Chronic

---

*Source: House Appropriations Committee Hearings, 1977.

**Source: National Kidney Foundation.

dialysis patients usually require two to three treatments a week of four to eight hours each.

The Cost of Artificial Kidney Care—Dialysis treatments are prohibitively expensive. Costs can range from $7,000 to $30,000 per year, depending on the facility which must be used by the patient. With the passage of Public Law 92-603, Amendments to the Social Security Act, in 1972, for the first time, the U.S. government recognized and financially aided persons with a catastrophic illness.

After an initial waiting period of 60–90 days, Medicare funds cover many of the costs incurred by a patient requiring dialysis and most of the cost for a kidney transplant. A number of states have passed legislation aimed at carrying the remainder of the financial burden.

At least 50,000 persons of both sexes and of all ages died each year of some form of diseases of the kidneys before the artificial kidney and transplantation became available.

Drugs

Drug Abuse

Highlights*

- Best recent estimates of the extent of drug abuse problems in the United States include the finding that there were 725,000 active narcotics users in 1974. Other user statistics include 12.4 million for marijuana, and 6.8 million and 5.3 million, respectively, using stimulants and sedatives for nonmedical purposes. The highly dangerous practice of utilizing a mixture of drugs, including alcohol, is likewise extensive and growing.

- Emergency room incidents involving heroin episodes rose 66% during the July–September 1974 period compared to the same period in 1973.

- The projected number of cases of hepatitis type A and B was 61,100 in 1974 compared to 59,200 in 1973. Primarily, this

increase can be explained by the spread of Mexican brown heroin into both larger as well as some smaller U.S. cities, and the resumption of Turkish production.

- Of Army enlisted men in Vietnam, 44% tried a narcotic at the peak of drug availability; about 20% were addicted to heroin.

- There has been a tenfold increase over eight years in the rate of drug-related hepatitis, a disease associated with the unsterile injection equipment frequently used by intravenous drug abusers.

Marijuana**

Marijuana has joined alcohol and tobacco as one of the three most commonly used drugs in America. Today almost 20% of the adults and 23% of youth ages 12 to 17 have used marijuana, and 7% of the adults and 12% of the youth are currently using it. Thus far evidence indicates that marijuana has not become popular with older groups and that its use may be diminished as adult roles are adopted.

Recent findings raise important questions concerning the possible effects of marijuana on the body's immune response system, cell metabolism, and male sex hormone levels. Accordingly, further marijuana studies are underway to clarify these issues, which take on special importance because of the millions of people, young and old alike, who are using marijuana today.

Marijuana Research

1. Reputable investigators have recently reported conflicting results with regard to possible relationships between marijuana use, chromosomal damage and birth anomalies. Some studies report no increased chromosomal damage, others a significant increase, and others mixed patterns. These differing reports require further study and clarification.

2. Completed and ongoing studies on the immediate effects of marijuana use at typical social dosage levels demonstrate various types of temporary mental impairment during periods of intoxication. Generally, there

*Source: House Appropriations Committee Hearings, 1975.

**Source: House Appropriations Committee Hearings, 1974, 1975, 1976.

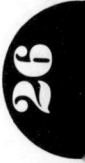

is evidence that short term memory is impaired and that impairment of other modes of intellectual and psychomotor functioning increases as task complexity increases. Recently, evidence has shown that marijuana intoxication produces impairment in driving function, which in turn may contribute to motor vehicle accidents.

3. The question of long-range effects of chronic use requires further clarification. Some studies of chronic users here and abroad seem to show little impairment after many years of use.

4. A preliminary finding that a marked reduction of sperm count (58%) occurred in five cannabis smokers following controlled conditions of smoking has been reported. While this poses the possibility of diminished fertility in chronic users, the small size of the sample and the study's preliminary nature make the work inconclusive.

Marijuana Users

The National Commission on Marijuana and Drug Abuse sponsored national household surveys of marijuana and other drug use in late 1974—early 1975.

The survey data indicate that in the 8–25 age group a majority (53%) have now tried the drug, up from 48% in 1972. Among those surveyed under 18, nearly one in four (23%) has ever tried marijuana—an increase from the one in seven (14%) who reported in the 1972 survey ever having done so.

Current use—defined as use within the past month preceding the survey—has also significantly increased among those under 18. Seven percent reported such use in 1972; 12% did so in the most recent survey. There does not appear to have been a similar increase in such use among those over 18—among whom current use has remained the same or has slightly diminished depending on age, since 1972.

Heroin

According to recent estimates based on Drug Enforcement Administration (DEA) laboratory analyses, Mexican brown heroin now accounts for about 65% of all heroin smuggled into the United States. In 1976 HEW estimated that of adult American males aged 20 to 30, 6% have *experimented* with heroin, 3% use it *occasionally*, and 1% use it on a *regular* basis.

Drug Related Deaths and Injuries

The DEA collects data in 23 major (SMSA) cities under the DAWN program—drug related deaths are reported by medical examiners; drug related injuries are reported by hospitals.

Table 26-11   Marijuana use—1974

	% Ever used	% Current use[1]
All adults		
Age:		
18–25	53	25
26–30	29	
35–49	7	1
50+	2	—
Male	24	9
Female	14	5
All youth		
Age:		
12–13	6	2
14–15	22	12
16–17	39	20
Male	24	12
Female	21	11

[1]Used during last month.
Source: DHEW, 1976.

Table 26-12   Drug related deaths

Drug	Q1 FY 74	Q2 FY 74	Q3 FY 74	Q4 FY 74	Q1 FY 75
Heroin/morphine	311	353	347	360	348
Methadone	173	251	254	232	229
Other narcotics	11	26	17	39	37
Barbiturates	322	272	302	269	296
Other depressants	116	124	134	150	139
Stimulants	36	21	22	26	36
Cannabis	4	0	2	0	1
Hallucinogens	3	1	2	5	0
Other	21	30	26	35	34
Total	997	1,078	1,106	1,116	1,120

Table 26-13   Controlled substances:

	Drugs	Sched-dule*	Often prescribed brand names	Medical uses	Dependence Physical
Narcotics	Opium	II	Dover's Powder, Paregoric	Analgesic, antidiarrheal	High
	Morphine	II	Morphine	Analgesic	High
	Codeine	II III V	Codeine	Analgesic, antitussive	Moderate
	Heroin	I	None	None	High
	Meperidine (Pethidine)	II	Demerol, Pethadol	Analgesic	High
	Methadone	II	Dolophine, Methadone, Methadose	Analgesic, heroin substitute	High
	Other Narcotics	I II III V	Dilaudid, Leritine, Numorphan, Percodan	Analgesic, antidiarrheal, antitussive	High
Depressants	Chloral Hydrate	IV	Noctec, Somnos	Hypnotic	Moderate
	Barbiturates	II III IV	Amytal, Butisol, Nembutal, Phenobarbital, Seconal, Tuinal	Anesthetic, anti-convulsant, sedation, sleep	High
	Glutethimide	III	Doriden	Sedation, sleep	High
	Methqualone	II	Optimil, Parest, Quaalude, Somnafac, Sopor	Sedation, sleep	High
	Tranquilizers	IV	Equanil, Librium, Miltown Serax, Tranxene, Valium	Anti-anxiety, muscle relaxant, sedation	Moderate
	Other Depressants	III IV	Clonopin, Dalmane, Dormate, Noludar, Placydil, Valmid	Anti-anxiety, sedation, sleep	Possible
Stimulants	Cocaine†	II	Cocaine	Local anesthetic	Possible
	Amphetamines	II III	Benzedrine, Biphetamine, Desoxyn, Dexedrine	Hyperkinesis, narco-lepsy, weight control	Possible
	Phenmetrazine	II	Preludin	Weight control	Possible
	Methylphenidate	II	Ritalin	Hyperkinesis	Possible
	Other Stimulants	III IV	Bacarate, Cylert, Didrex, Ionamin, Plegine, Pondimin, Pre-Sate, Sanorex, Voranil	Weight control	Possible
Hallucinogens	LSD	I	None	None	None
	Mescaline	I	None	None	None
	Psilocybin-Psilocyn	I	None	None	None
	MDA	I	None	None	None
	PCP‡	III	Semylan	Veterinary anesthetic	None
	Other Hallucinogens	I	None	None	None
Cannabis	Marijuana Hashish Hashish Oil	I	None	None	Degree unknown

*Scheduling classifications vary for individual drugs since controlled substances are often marketed in combination with other medicinal ingredients.

Source: *Drugs of Abuse*, U.S. Justice Dept., Drug Enforcement Administration (Booklet).

Uses and effects

potential: Psychological	Toler- ance	Duration of effects (in hours)	Usual methods of administration	Possible effects	Effects of overdose	Withdrawal syndrome
High	Yes	3 to 6	Oral, smoked			
High	Yes	3 to 6	Injected, smoked			
Moderate	Yes	3 to 6	Oral, injected	Euphoria, drows- iness, respiratory depression, con- stricted pupils, nausea	Slow and shal- low breathing, clammy skin, convulsions, coma, possible death	Watery eyes, runny nose, yawning, loss of appetite, irrita- bility, tremors, panic, chills and sweating, cramps, nausea
High	Yes	3 to 6	Injected, sniffed			
High	High	3 to 6	Oral, injected			
High	Yes	12 to 24	Oral, injected			
High	Yes	3 to 6	Oral, injected			
Moderate	Probable	5 to 8	Oral			
High	Yes	1 to 16	Oral, injected			
High	Yes	4 to 8	Oral	Slurred speech, disorientation, drunken behav- ior without odor of alcohol	Shallow respira- tion, cold and clammy skin, di- lated pupils, weak and rapid pulse, coma, possible death	Anxiety, insom- nia, tremors, de- lirium, convul- sions, possible death
High	Yes	4 to 8	Oral			
Moderate	Yes	4 to 8	Oral			
Possible	Yes	4 to 8	Oral			
High	High	2	Injected, sniffed			
High	Yes	2 to 4	Oral, injected	Increased alert- ness, excitation, euphoria, dilated pupils, increased pulse rate and blood pressure, insomnia, loss of appetite	Agitation, in- crease in body temperature, hallucinations, convulsions, possible death	Apathy, long periods of sleep, irritability, de- pression, disori- entation
High	Yes	2 to 4	Oral			
High	Yes	2 to 4	Oral			
Possible		2 to 4	Oral			
Degree unknown	Yes	Variable	Oral			
Degree unknown	Yes	Variable	Oral, injected			
Degree unknown	Yes	Variable	Oral	Illusions and hal- lucinations (with exception of MDA); poor per- ception of time and distance	Longer, more in- tense "trip" epi- sodes, psycho- sis, possible death	Withdrawal syndrome not reported
Degree unknown	Yes	Variable	Oral, injected, sniffed			
Degree unknown	Yes	Variable	Oral, injected, smoked			
Degree unknown	Yes	Variable	Oral, injected, sniffed			
Moderate	Yes	2 to 4	Oral, smoked	Euphoria, re- laxed inhibitions, increased appe- tite, disoriented behavior	Fatigue, para- noia, possible psychosis	Insomnia, hy- peractivity, and decreased ap- petite reported in a limited number of indi- viduals

† Designated a narcotic under the Controlled Substances Act.
‡ Designated a depressant under the Controlled Substances Act.

Table 26-14   Drug related injuries

Drug	Q1 FY 74	Q2 FY 74	Q3 FY 74	Q4 FY 74	Q1 FY 75	Q2 FY 75
Heroin/morphine	1,042	1,817	1,767	2,160	2,643	2,608
Methadone	271	696	746	935	801	648
Other narcotics	707	794	916	913	1,044	1,068
Barbiturates	1,910	2,820	2,733	2,436	2,343	2,410
Other depressants	6,264	7,905	8,246	8,508	8,887	9,460
Stimulants	733	884	874	951	995	994
Cannabis	358	619	560	565	630	582
Hallucinogens	506	765	705	741	758	657
Other	423	475	552	468	488	552
Total	12,214	16,775	17,100	17,677	18,589	18,979

Source: Hearings of Senate Subcommittee on Alcoholism and Narcotics, March 1975.

Drug Crimes in the Hospital Pharmacy*

Altered or Phony Prescriptions

In a survey of 168 hospitals, altered or phony prescriptions were reported by 72 hospitals; 81% of the prescriptions were reported in metropolitan hospitals of larger than 200 beds. Most of these prescription blanks were stolen from the hospital.

Internal Theft

Sixty-four percent or 106 hospitals reported internal thefts of controlled substances, and almost half of these hospitals reported an increase in thefts during the past year. However, hospitals of 200 beds and under reported little internal theft, a fact probably attributed to their having fewer employes involved in the handling or dispensing of drugs and to their smaller inventories.

The primary cause of thefts could be attributed to poor inventory records of drugs left in nursing divisions. In fact, in 73 hospitals drugs that are not used by patients are never returned to the pharmacy. Thefts also could be attributed to poor lock and key control of narcotic cabinets located on the nursing units.

Twenty-one thefts from the pharmacy itself were reported.

Burglaries and Holdups

Nineteen burglaries of hospital pharmacies were reported. Eleven hospitals reported a

total of 15 holdups during which no injuries were sustained by hospital personnel. In addition, one holdup was reported to have taken place in the emergency room and one on a nursing station.

Drug Addict Language

blast	smoke, by cupping hands and drawing deeply
busted	arrested
buzz	mood of elation, from euphoria to intoxication
caps	ampoules, capsules
connection	peddler, referred to also as "the man"
crazy	good, fine or excellent
feds	federal narcotic agents
fix	shot with a needle
goof	being knocked out with an overdosage
H	heroin; also called "horse"
high	feeling of euphoria
junkie	an addict
kick	to quit the habit
meet	place where seller is met
pot	marijuana
reefers	marijuana cigarettes
shoot	to inject with a hypodermic needle
sick	to suffer the shakes of the withdrawal syndrome; also described as "having a monkey on your back"
stash	a secret or hidden package
take it slow	to undergo withdrawal agonies without complaining
weed	marijuana plant

*Source: Robert J. Lee, "Study of Drug-Related Crimes." Excerpted with permission from *Hospital Progress,* March 1975. Copyright 1975 by The Catholic Hospital Association.

Prescription Drugs*

(In 1976 more than 75-million Americans consumed at least one drug a week, mostly every day. As a nation we spent $11 billion on prescription drugs and another $2.6 billion on over-the-counter pharmaceuticals.)

Based on 1974 data, the two most important categories of ethical drugs are products acting on the central nervous system and anti-infectives. These two categories account for 40% of domestic sales of prescription drugs.

Table 26-15   Where prescription drugs are dispensed

| | | Outpatient | | | | |
| | | | Community pharmacy | | | |
Total	Hospital inpatient	Total	Inde-pendent	Chain	Other retail	Hospital
100.0	35.0	65.0	37.9	10.5	7.8	8.8

Expenditures for Prescription Drugs

Between 1950 and 1974 per capita expenditures for "drugs and drug sundries" increased from $10.70 to $45.14. Primarily because hospital care and other components have risen more rapidly than have expenditures for drugs and drug sundries, drugs as a percentage of total health care expenditures declined from 14.6 to 9.9% between fiscal 1950 and 1974.

By comparison, the elderly, with total expenditures of $2.3 billion, accounted for 10.2% of the population but 23.3% of expenditures. Per capita drug and drug sundry expenditures by the elderly were $103.17 in fiscal 1974—more than twice the figure for those in the 19 to 64 age category.

Costs of Prescription Drugs**

In April 1976, the federal government set MAC limits for so-called multiple source drugs, which represent about one-fourth of the prescription drugs on the market today. MAC is shorthand for "maximum allowable cost"—the maximum price the government will pay for certain drugs dispensed to patients in Medicare and Medicaid programs.

Three-fourths of prescription drugs can be obtained only from a single manufacturer or source, and thus, each of these drugs is available to pharmacists and other retail dispensers at just one price. The remainder are those drugs that are available from more than one source or manufacturer, and prices for the same drug under different brand names often vary widely. The maximum cost which will be established for these drugs will be the lowest price charged by any source from which the drug is "widely and consistently" available. FDAs role in this process will be to determine whether different brands or formulations of the same generic drug are bioequivalent—that is whether they are equal in their therapeutic effect. The purpose of these regulations is to assure that prescription drugs that are intended for the same use can be used interchangeably.

Drug Effectivenesst

After the 1962 amendments concerning drugs were passed, the FDA began to review the effectiveness of the prescription drugs marketed between 1938 and 1962, a period in which only safety was considered. The results show how important the federal effectiveness requirement for drugs is.

Substantial evidence of effectiveness was lacking for 41% of the 4,300 drugs that entered the market from 1938 to 1962. Evidence in the form of controlled clinical studies could be found for only 19% of the indicated uses. The FDA asked the National Academy of Sciences/National Research Council to assist in the review.

Of the 16,573 drug claims (not over-the-counter) evaluated by the NAS/NRC, 3,493 or 21.1% were found to be lacking in substantial evidence of effectiveness or were found ineffective as a fixed combination. Another 7,145 or 43.2% were found "possibly effective" and 2,112, or 12.7%, "probably effective." Only 3,823 claim—23% of the total—were found flatly "effective."

Generic vs. Brand Drugs (Special Study Panel recommendations to FDA)

A system should be organized as rapidly as possible to generate an official list of inter-

---

*Source: DHEW, 1976.
**FDA Consumer, December 1975–January 1976.

† Source: Senate Subcommittee on Health Hearings, July 1974.

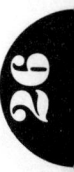

changeable drug products. In the development of the list, distinctions should be made between two classes of drugs and drug products:

1. Those for which evidence of bioequivalence is not considered essential and that could be added to the list as soon as standards of pharmaceutical equivalence have been established and satisfied.

2. Those for which evidence of bioequivalence is critical. Such products should be listed only after they have been shown to be bioequivalent or have satisfied standards of pharmaceutical equivalence that have been shown to insure bioequivalence.

RX Terminology *

Chemical name	The term by which the chemical structure of a drug is described.
Generic name	As applied to pharmaceuticals, refer to the common, established or nonproprietary name by which a drug is known as an isolated substance, or as a drug product, irrespective of its manufacturer. "Generic" denotes one drug, though not any particular formulation of it as a drug product.
Brand name	Any word, name, symbol or device or any combination adopted and used by a manufacturer or merchant to identify his goods and distinguish them from those manufactured or sold by others. It is the manufacturer's chosen name for his product.

To illustrate
each term.

Chemical name	6-chloro-7-sulfamyl-3,4-dihydro-1,2,4-benzothiadiazine-1,1-dioxide.
Generic name	hydrochlorothiazide.
Brand names	Esidrix, HydroDiuril and Oretic.
Bioavailability	A measure of the rate at which a drug dissolves and makes its active ingredient available to a part of the body to do what it's supposed to do—help the patient.
Chemical equivalence	A demonstrated comparability between two or more drug products which contain essentially identical chemically active ingredients.
Bioequivalence	A demonstrated comparability between chemically equivalent drugs showing that, when given to the same individuals in the same dosage form, similar levels of bioavailability will result. If there is a significant difference in bioavailability, the drug product is then bio*in*equivalent.
Therapeutic equivalence	A drug showing that bioequivalent products which, when given to the same individual in the same dosage form, provide essentially the same effects in patients.

The following are some of the factors that can affect the bioavailability and therapeutic effectiveness of a drug product:

Disintegration time	The time required for a tablet or capsule to break into granules or aggregates in water or body fluids.
Dissolution time	The time required for the particles in a tablet or capsule to break down into molecules or ions evenly dispersed in fluid.
Binders	Inert ingredients used to give cohesive qualities to the powdered materials used in tablets or capsules.
Fillers	Inert substances added to a drug formulation to increase the bulk, in order to make the tablet a practical size for compression. Sometimes known as *diluents* or *excipients*.
Lubricants	Inert ingredients that prevent tablets from sticking to the surface of dies (molds used to shape tablets) and to reduce interparticle friction.

*Source: Pharmaceutical Manufacturers Association, 1976.

RX Terminology **(continued)**

Disintegrators
Substances (or mixtures of substances) added to a tablet to facilitate its breakup or disintegration after administration.

Coaters
Inert ingredients that cover the surface of a tablet to protect ingredients against the atmosphere, to mask unpleasant taste and odor, to improve appearance, and to control the time and location in the body when the tablet will disintegrate.

Coloring agents
Colors help the manufacturer control the product during its preparation, serve as a means of identification to the user and the medical profession, and make the dosage more pleasing in appearance.

Drug Reactions and Interactions

(The number of Americans who died in 1976 from adverse drug reactions was estimated at 18,000 in the Journal of the American Medical Association (Feb. 28, 1977).)

Drug Allergy*

Since generalized reactions such as anaphylaxis, serum sickness and asthma are classical immunological responses to allergens, their occurrence in an adverse drug reaction indicates an allergy.

The presence of the sensitizing antibody, IgE, in someone believed to be allergic to a drug has generally been very difficult, if not impossible, to prove. Nevertheless, some experts believe that probably 25% of adverse drug reactions actually represent allergies to drugs.

Whatever the reasons for an allergic drug reaction, there are three steps in its development. First, there is at least one experience of previous exposure to the drug. This is followed by a latent period during which the antibodies or cells sensitized to the drug are formed. Usually this takes about one or two weeks. Third, the drug is administered again, and this time the sensitized cells lead to the symptoms of allergy.

Three common drugs are the most frequent causes of drug allergy—penicillin, sulfonamides and aspirin (acetysalicylic acid). These medications may be responsible for as much as 80 to 90% of all allergic drug reactions.

Drug and Diet Interactions**

The more drugs used at the same time, the greater the risk of undesirable effects. Also, certain foods and alcoholic drinks may interact with drugs to produce harmful reactions. Many cases involving suicide and deaths from accidental overdose are attributable to interaction with alcohol. Among the combinations that require extreme caution are sedatives, tranquilizers, or antidepressants plus alcohol.

Drug Administration in Relation to Meals

Take on an empty stomach (2–3 hours a.c.):
benzathine penicillin G
cloxacillin (Tegopen)
erythromycin
lincomycin (Lincocin)
methacycline (Rondomycin)
phenoxymethyl penicillin (penicillin V)
tetracyclines, except demethylchlortetracycline (Declomycin), which can easily upset the stomach

Take ½ hour before meals:
belladonna and its alkaloids,
chlordiazepoxide hydrochloride (Librax)
hyoscyamine sulfate (Donnatal)
methylphenidate (Ritalin)
phenmetrazine hydrochloride (Preludin)
phenazopyridine (Pyridium)
propantheline bromide (Pro-banthine)

Take with meals or food:
aminophylline
antidiabetics
APC (acetylsalicylic acid, phenacetin, caffeine)
chlorothiazide, (Diuril) (Hydrodiuril)
diphenylhydantoin (Dilantin)
mefenamic acid (Ponstel)
metronidazoie (Flagyl)
nitrofurantoin (Furadantin) (Macrodantin)
prednisolone
prednisone
rauwolfia and its alkaloids
reserpine (Serpasil)
triamterene (Dyrenium)

---

*Source: DHEW, 1975.
**Source: Martin A. Lambert Jr., *Drug and Diet Interactions,* ©American Journal of Nursing Co., 1976.

trihexyphenidyl hydrochloride (Artane)
trimeprazine tartrate (Temaril)

Do not take with milk:
bisacodyl (Dulcolax)
potassium chloride
potassium iodide
tetracyclines except doxycycline (Vibramycin)

Do not take with fruit juices:
ampicillin
benzathine penicillin G
cloxacillin (Tegopen)
erythromycin

Do not drink alcohol while taking:
acetohexamide (Dymelor)
antihistamines
chlorpropamide (Diabinese)
chloridazepoxide (Librium)
chloral hydrate
diphenoxylate hydrochloride (Lomotil)
MAO inhibitors
meclizine hydrochloride (Antivert)
methaqualone (Quaalude)
metronidazole (Flagyl)
narcotics
phenformin hydrochloride (DBI)
tolbutamide (Orinase)

Common Drug Reactions*

In the following list of common drug reactions and the drugs that cause them, italicized entries have the greatest potential for reaction.

Anemia

chloramphenicol
chloroquine
gold salts
hydantoins
mephenytoin
methyldopa
phenothiazines
phenylbutazone
primidone
quinacrine
sulfonamides
thiouracils
trimethadione

Asthma

antihistamines
dextran
penicillin
pollen extracts
reserpine
salicylates
serum

Bullous Eruptions

antibiotics
bromides

hydantoins
Insulin
iodides
penicillins
phenothiazines
sulfonamides

Granulocytopenia

acetazolamide
ACTH
aminopyrine
antihistamines
arsenicals
chloramphenicol
chloroquine
gold salts
hydantoins
hydralazine
novobiocin
phenacemide
phenacetin
phenothiazines
phenylbutazone
procainamide
salicylates
streptomycin
sulfonamides
sulfonylureas

tetracyclines
thiazides
thiouracils

Hepatic Damage

adrenergic hormones
anabolic agents
anesthetics
antimalarials
barbiturates
chlorothiazide
chlorpromazine
estrogens

Eczemalous Dermatitis

antibiotics
antihistamines
arsenicals
bromides
chloral hydrate
iodides
mercurials
PAS
penicillin
quinacrine
streptomycin
sulfonamides

Eosinophilia

ACTH
isoniazid
kanamycin
penicillin
phenothiazines
streptomycin

Eruptions Resembling Erythema Multiforme

antibiotics
barbiturates
bromides
gold salts
iodides
meprobamate
penicillin
gold salts
hydantoins
isoniazid
novobiocin
PAS
phenacemide
phenothiazines
phenylbutazone
probenecid

---

*Source: Warner/Chilcott.

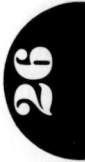

sulfonamides
sulfonylureas
thiouracils
triacetyloleanodmycin

Reactions Resembling Löffler Syndrome
mercurials
nitrofurantoins
PAS

Nephritis and/or Nephrosis
acetazolamide
amphotericin B
antibiotics
cycloserine
gold salts
iodides
mercurials
paramethadione
phenacetin
phenylbutazone
probenecid
phenacetin
phenolphthalein
salicylates
sulfonamides

Erythema Nodosum
bromides
iodides
salicylates
sulfonamides

Exanthematous Eruptions
antibiotics
barbiturates
belladonna
bromides
chloroquine
diethylstilbestrol
gold salts
hydantoins
mercurials
PAS
penicillin
phenothiazines
quinacrine
quinidine
reserpine

salicylates
serums and organ extracts
sulfonamides
thiouracils
serums
sulfonamides
sulfonylureas
thiazides
trimethadione

Periarteritis Nodosa
hydantoins
iodides
mercurials
penicillin
phenylbutazone
serums
sulfonamides
thiouracils

Photosensitivity
dimethylchlortetra-cycline
quinidine
sulfonamides
thiazides

Purpura, Nonthrombocytopenic
barbiturates
gold salts
heparin
isoniazid
penicillin
phenacetin
phenothiazines
quinidine
sulfonamides

Exfollative Dermatitis
acetazolamide
barbiturates
chloroquine
gold salts
hydantoins
iodides
mercurials
penicillin
phenothiazines

phenylbutazone
quinacrine
sulfonamides

Fever
isoniazid
mercurials
nitrofurantoins
penicillin
procainamide
quinidine
sulfonamides

Fixed Eruptions
acetophenetidin
barbiturates
gold salts
iodides
phenolphthalein
quinacrine
quinidine
sulfonamides

Purpura, Thrombocytopenic
chloramphenicol
penicillin
quinidine
quinine
sulfonamides

Reactions Resembling Serum Sickness
antibiotics
antihistamines
barbiturates
heparin
hydantoins
hydralazine
mercurials
organ extracts
penicillin
procainamide
quinidine
salicylates
serums
streptomycin
sulfonamides
thiouracils
vaccines

Shock
ACTH
anesthetics, local
antibiotics
B.S.P.
chymotrypsin
dehydrocholic acid
dextran
diphenhydramine
D-P-T
folic acid (I.V.)
gamma globulin
heparin
iodides
meperidine
meprobamate
mercurials
nicotinic acid
nitrofurantoin
organ extracts
oxytocin
penicillins
pollen extracts
salicylates
sedative-hypnotics
serums
sulfonamides
tetanus toxoid
thiamine
vaccines

S.L.E.-Like Picture
hydantoins
hydralazine
penicillin
procainamide
sulfonamides
thiazides

Urticaria
ACTH
antibiotics
insulin
liver extracts
penicillin
pollen extracts
serums
streptomycin
sulfonamides

Note: An excellent little pocket size booklet called *Drug Interactions Index* is available free of charge from Warner/Chilcott Division of Warner-Lambert Company, Morris Plains, N.J. 07950.

Lethal Drug Combinations*

Table 26-16 Some potentially lethal drug combinations

Primary Drug	Interactant	Primary drug	Interactant
ACTH	Vaccines	Anticonvulsants	Methylpenidate (Ritalin)
Alcohol	Barbiturates		Narcotics
	Carbamazepine (Tegretol)	Antidepressants, tricyclic	Alcohol
	Chloral hydrate	(Aventyl, Elavil,	Diphenylhydantoin (Dilantin)
	Disulfiram and other	Norpramine,	Guanethidine (Ismelin)
	acetaldehyde	Pertofrane,	MAO inhibitors
	Insulin dehydrogenase inhibitors	Sinequan, Tofranil,	Methyldopa (Aldomet)
	Meprobamate	Vivactil)	Reserpine
	Methotrexate		Salicylates
	Morphine and narcotic	Antidiabetics, oral	Anticoagulants (oral)
	analgesics	(Diabinese, Dymelor,	MAO inhibitors
	Muscle relaxants	Orinase, Tolinase)	
	Nitrates and nitrites	Antihistamines	CNS depressants (barbiturates,
	Sedatives and hypnotics		etc.)
	Tricyclic antidepressants	Antihypertensives	Anesthetics
Aminopyrine	Acetaminophen (long term)	Antineoplastics	Attenuated live virus vaccines
Amitriptyline (Elavil)	Chlordiazepoxide (Librium)	Appetite depressants	MAO inhibitors
Amphetamines	Cocaine	Caffeine (excessive	MAO inhibitors
	MAO inhibitors	amounts)	Propoxyphene (Darvon)
	Propoxyphene (Darvon)	Carbamazepine (Tegretol)	Alcohol
	Tyramine-Rich Foods		MAO inhibitors
Analgesics	MAO inhibitors	Carbon tetrachloride	Barbiturates
Anesthetics	Adrenergic neuron blockers	Carbrital	Alcohol
	Antibiotics (neuromuscular	Catecholamines	Anesthetics (chloroform, ether,
	blockers)		etc.)
	Antihypertensives		Guanethidine (Ismelin)
	Barbiturates	Cheese (strong, ripe)	MAO inhibitors
	Catecholamines	Chicken livers	MAO inhibitors
	Corticosteroids	Chloral hydrate	Alcohol
	Guanethidine (Ismelin)	Chloramphenicol	Anticoagulatts, oral
	Kanamycin (Kantrex)	(Chloromycetin)	Antidiabetics, oral
	MAO inhibitors	Chloroform	Catecholamines
	Mebutamate (Capla)		Propranolol (Inderal)
	Neomycin	Clofibrate (Atromid-S)	Anticoagulants, oral
	Oxytocics with vasoconstrictor	Cocaine	Sympathomimetics (amphet-
	Propranolol (Inderal)		amines, etc.)
	Rauwolfia alkaloids	Colistimethate	Antibiotics (neuromuscular
	Sedatives and hypnotics	(Coly-Mycin)	blocking)
Anorexiants	MAO inhibitors		Muscle relaxants, peripherally
Antibiotics (neuro-	Anesthetics		acting
muscular blockers)	Antibiotics (neuromuscular	Corticosteroids	Anesthetics
(Bacitrain, dihydro-	blockers)		Sympathomimetics (in asth-
streptomycin, genta-	Muscle relaxants		matics)
mycin, gramicidin,	Procainamide (Pronestyl)		Vaccines (live, attenuated)
kanamycin, neomycin,	Promethazine (Phenergan)	Curariform drugs	Antibiotics (neuromuscular
polymyxin B, strepto-	Quinidine		blocking)
mycin, viomycin, etc.)			Furosemide (Lasix)
Anticholinesterases	Fluorophosphate insecticides		Quinidine
	Muscle relaxants (depolarizing)	Cyclopropane	Epinephrine
Anticoagulants	Analgesics (aspirin, pyrazolones,		Levarterenol (Levophed)
(Coumadin, Dicu-	etc.)	Dextromethorphan	MAO inhibitors (phenelzine,
marol, (Panwarfin,	Antidiabetics, oral		etc.)
Sintrom, etc.)	Antineoplastics	Dextrothyroxine	Anticoagulants (oral)
	Carbon tetrachloride	(Choloxin)	Epinephrine (coronary insuffi-
	Clofibrate (Atromid-S)		ciency)
	Dextrothyroxine (Choloxin)	Diazoxide (Hyperstat)	Anticoagulants (oral)
	Indomethacin (Indocin)	Digitalis	Calcium salts (IV)
	Mefenamic acid (Ponstel)		Diuretics (hypokalemia)
	Oxphenbutazone (Tandearil)		Propranolol
	Phenylbutazone (Butazolidin)	Diphenylhydantoin	Analeptics (in overdosage)
	Salicylates	(Dilantin)	Disulfiram (Antabuse)
	Thyroid preparations		Folic acid antagonists (metho-
			trexate, etc.)
			Phenyramidol (Analexin)
			Sulfonamides

*Lethal with high dosage or in susceptible patients.

Table 26-16 (continued)

Primary drug	Interactant	Primary drug	Interactant
Disulfiram (Antabuse)	Alcohol		Cheese (strong, ripe)
Dopa	MAO inhibitors		CNS depressants
Echothiophate	Anticholinesterase insecticides		Dextromethorphan
(Phospholine)	Succinylcholine		Dopa
Ephedrine	Ergonovine		Ephedrine
	MAO inhibitors		Guanethidine (Ismelin)
Epinephrine	Chloroform		Isoproterenol (Isuprel)
	Cyclopropane		Levodopa (Dopar, Larodopa,
	Dextrothyroxine (Choloxin)		etc.)
	Fluroxene (Fluoromar)		Liver (beef and chicken)
	Halothane (Fluothane)		Meperidine (Demerol)
	Isoproterenol (Isuprel)		Methyldopa (Aldomet)
	Levothyroxine		Methylphenidate (Ritalin)
	Methoxyflurane (Penthrane)		Propranolol (Inderal)
	Phenylephrine (Neo-Synephrine)		Reserpine
	Sympathomimetics (status		Tyramine-rich foods
	asthmaticus)	Meperidine (Demerol)	Anesthetics
	Thyroid preparations		MAO inhibitors
Ethacrynic acid (Edecrin)	Anticoagulants (oral)	Methotrexate	Salicylates
Ether	Neomycin		Sulfonamides
	Propranolol (Inderal)	Methyldopa (Aldomet)	Antidepressants
Furosemide (Lasix)	Muscle relaxants		MAO inhibitors
Guanethidine (Ismelin)	Anesthetics	Morphine	Propranolol (Inderal)
	Antidepressants	Muscle relaxants,	Anesthetics (halogenated)
	MAO inhibitors	depolarizing	Antibiotics (neuromuscular
Indomethacin (Indocin)	Anticoagulants (oral)		blocking)
	Salicylates		Anticholinesterases
Insulin	Alcohol	Nitrates and nitrites	Alcohol
Isoproterenol (Isuprel)	Epinephrine	Oxytocics	Vasoconstrictors
	MAO inhibitors	Quinidine	Antibiotics (neuromuscular
Kanamycin (Kantrex)	Anesthetics		blocking)
	Antibiotics (neuromuscular		Muscle relaxants
	blocking)	Reserpine	Anesthetics
	Muscle relaxants		Antidepressants
	Procainamide		Digitalis
Levarterenol (Levophed)	Anesthetics (halogenated,		MAO inhibitors
	cyclopropane, etc.)	Salicylates	Anticoagulants, oral
	Antidepressants, tricyclic		Antidepressants, tricyclic
	Guanethidine (Ismelin)		Indomethacin (Indocin)
	Reserpine (in bronchial asthma)		6-Mercaptopurine (Purinethol)
	Thyroid preparations		Methotrexate
MAO inhibitors	Amphetamines	Sedatives and hypnotics	Alcohol
(Eutonyl, Furoxone,	Anesthetics		Antidepressants
Marplan, Matulane,	Anorexiants	Sulfonamides, long acting	Antidiabetics, oral
Nardil, Niamid,	Antidepressants (MAO inhibitors		Diphenylhydantoin (Dilantin)
Parnate, etc.)	and tricyclics)		Folic acid antagonists
	Antidiabetics (oral)		Methotrexate
	Caffeine (excessive amounts)	Tetracyclines	Methoxyflurane (Penthrane)
	Carbamazepine (Tegretol)		

Source: Eric Martin, *Hazards of Medication,* J. B. Lippincott, 1971.

Medical Devices

Highlights

- The value of medical device shipments increased 225% between 1958 and 1972, reaching $3.3 billion. A recent Commerce Department study projects even more rapid growth in the future, with sales reaching $12 billion by 1985.

- There are some 8,200 different medical devices involving hundreds of thousands of different items produced by some 2,000 manufacturers.

- An analysis of the medical literature undertaken in 1969 uncovered 10,000 known injuries directly related to medical devices during a single decade. Of the 10,000 injuries, 751 proved fatal. The FDA reviewed

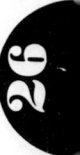

death certificates in ten states and found 858 deaths directly related to medical devices in a ten-year period. The Commission on Professional and Hospital Activities, an independent health group, estimated 36,000 complications from medical devices for a one year period.

- Since 1972, about 30,000 troublesome cardiac pacemakers have been recalled, as have hundreds of defective heart valves.
- The Downstate Medical Center, in Brooklyn New York, established a laboratory to examine medical devices to be used in their hospital. After two years of testing, they reported that 40% of the devices tested were defective.

Persons Using Special Aids

Table 26-17   Number of persons using special aids, by type of aid, 1969

Type of aid	Special shoes	Cane or walking stick	Brace Leg or foot	Brace Other	Crutches	Wheel-chair	Walker	Artificial limb Leg or foot	Artificial limb Arm or hand	Other aid for getting around
			Number in thousands							
Number of persons using aid	2,377	2,156	233	869	443	409	404	126	46	140

Source: DHEW.

Potentially Harmful Devices

In testimony before the House Subcommittee on Health and Environment in July 1975 the following types of devices were identified as potentially harmful to the consumer:

- Devices which are used in life-threatening situations and which are ineffective or fail in use—for example, heart valves, cardiac pacemakers, vascular implants. About 23,-000 individual pacemakers have been involved in recalls since 1972. FDA was involved in the "recalls" of about 256 pacemakers and 54 myocardial leads for use with pacemakers. Two children had died from problems associated with the leads.
- Devices that are hazardous to patients and/or medical personnel due to defects in design or manufacture. There have been cases of faulty monitoring devices in intensive care units that have caused fatal electric shock, and cases of defective anesthesia machines that caused explosions in operating rooms. Also in this category are EKG machines that give faulty readings and result in serious misdiagnosis.
- Devices in which the traditional risk-benefit assessment cannot now be made prior to marketing—and in which the risks outweigh the benefits—for example, certain IUDs.

FDA learned of 43 deaths and 315 septic abortions associated with IUDs. While these devices have been shown to be a relatively safe and reliable form of contraception, comparing favorably with oral contraceptives, the injury data clearly indicates the need to evaluate the potential hazards of all IUDs.

- Devices that are useless and can cause delay in diagnosis, and treatment of serious conditions, such as the old "quack" colored lights devices.
- Devices that are probably harmless but are useless and therefore economic frauds, such as "hot pants" for weight reduction.

X-Rays

In a recent report on the increasing incidence of x-ray examinations in the U.S., The New York *Times* found that surveys conducted by the U.S. Public Health Service indicate an increase in usage, from 1964 to 1970, of 12% per individual in medical x-ray examinations, and of 25% per individual for dental x-ray examinations. It was further reported that over 60% of the population is subjected annually to x-ray examinations, at the average rate of five per person. Some experts emphatically stated that both the large number of exposures and the high levels of radiation dosage involved are unnecessary.

Although usually of little diagnostic value lumbar spine films have become a routine part of many preemployment physical exams because of the fear of law suits arising from the development of lower back pain later on. One lateral lumbar spine film yields a radiation dose to the patient equivalent to 50–100 regular chest x-rays, and a dose to the gonads in the male about 500 times that received from a chest x-ray.

Clinical Labs*

The clinical laboratory represents a major and costly component of the nation's health network. In 1971, it was estimated that more than 2 billion clinical laboratory tests were conducted. In 1974, almost 3 billion tests were conducted at an average cost of $15 per test. The total cost to the nation of clinical laboratory tests that same year was estimated at more than $8 billion. By 1980, it is estimated that some 8.8 billion clinical laboratory tests will be conducted annually at a cost of about $15 billion. While general expenditures for health have been increasing at the rate of 11% per year, laboratory services (and fees) have been expanding at the rate of 15% per year.

In the United States, there are an estimated 14,000 to 15,000 clinical laboratories located in about 7,000 hospitals and other facilities. In addition, an estimated 50,000 to 80,000 physicians conduct clinical laboratory tests in their own private facilities. Of the above, the federal government regulates some 3,000 independent laboratories and 7,000 hospital laboratories. Approximately 950 are licensed by the Center for Disease Control (CDC). None of the physicians' office laboratories is covered by the existing statute.

Evidence indicates that the accuracy of performance of clinical laboratories is, at best, variable from day to day and includes a wide range of error. A National Bureau of Standards study published in 1973 (NBSIR 73-163) reveals that in microbiology 7.6% of the interstate laboratory determinations were in error, while 16.5% of the determinations by other large laboratories were incorrect. Unsatisfactory performance similarly has been demonstrated by 10 to 40% of laboratories in bacteriological testing; by 30–50% of laboratories in various simple clinical chemistry tests; by 12–18% of laboratories in blood groupings and typing; by 20–30% of laboratories in hemoglobin measurements; and by 20–25% in measurement of serum electrolytes.

Many clinical laboratories have never been inspected and for many that have, the litany of abuses is revealing: dirty and broken laboratory equipment being used by inexperienced technicians; reagents frequently unlabeled and outdated; and patient specimens often tested inappropriately with unsanitary equipment.

Under the provisions of the Clinical Laboratories Improvement Act (1976), the Secretary of HEW licenses clinical laboratories which solicit or accept diagnostic specimens for testing services. The licensure system is based upon compliance with quality assurance standards. The Secretary of HEW is authorized to set these standards and to assure that these standards provide for adequate internal quality control programs, including the maintenance of records, surveillance of equipment and facilities, establishment of personnel qualifications and the development of an objective system of proficiency testing and safeguards to assure the accuracy of the collection, processing and transmission of materials by collection stations.

(In a nationwide sampling of lab results by the National Bureau of Standards, up to 17% of bacteriological test results were found to be in error. In another study by the Center for Disease Control, nearly 15% of labs showed an unacceptable level of proficiency in the relatively simple measurement of sugar in the blood.)

Emergency Medical Services**

In 1975 alone, 70 million Americans were treated in hospital emergency departments. Statistics show that 800,000 emergencies terminated in death annually in the United States. The American College of Emergency Physicians estimates that effective EMS systems could save more than 60,000 persons who die each year from traumatic injury and heart attacks.

*Source: Senate Report, 1976.

**Source: American College of Emergency Physicians, Testimony before House Subcommittee on Health and Environment, January 1976.

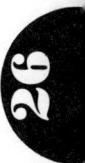

Facts, Goals and Recommendations

Facts

1. Accident	Accidents remain the leading cause of death in the age range 1 to 44.
2. Cardiovascular disease	Cardiovascular disease accounted for about 1,100,000, or 54%, of the total deaths in the United States in 1972. About 600,000 of these were sudden deaths, and more than 350,000 occurred within the community outside the hospital.
3. Total deaths from emergencies	Some 700,000 medical and surgical emergencies which terminate in death occur annually in the United States.
4. Emergency hospital visits	More than 70 million patients visited hospital emergency departments last year. In some hospitals these visits have shown an increase of 600% since World War II. Nationally the average annual increase in visits is 10%.
5. Physicians in emergency medical practice	There are approximately 15,000 physicians practicing emergency medicine in hospitals throughout the country.
6. Ambulance surveys	A survey of ambulances has shown that as few as 37% meet minimal design standards.
7. Training of ambulance personnel	In 1970, only 5% of the nation's ambulance attendants met minimum standards of training recommended by the American College of Surgeons, the Department of Transportation, the National Academy of Sciences or the Department of Health, Education, and Welfare. Five percent had no training. A standard American Red Cross first-aid course had been given to only 33%.
8. Ambulance-hospital communication	Direct communication with the hospitals served is not within the communication capability of 94% of ambulances.

Goals

1. Accident victim salvage	It has been projected that 18,000 accident victims out of the 115,000 who die annually might be saved if proper immediate care were rendered.
2. Coronary heart disease salvage	Preventable pre-hospital coronary heart disease deaths have been conservatively estimated to number 50,000/year.
3. Salvage of other emergency victims	At least 5,000 of the deaths from other causes such as poisonings, drownings, obstetrical complications, etc., are deemed preventable.

Recommendations of American College of Emergency Physicians

Nurse education	
a) Undergraduate education	
1) First aid and life support	All nursing students should be given explicit training and experience in proper methods of rendering first-aid and in basic elements of life-support procedures such as CPR.
b) Postgraduate/continuing education	

1) Comprehensive
     A) Breadth
     B) Depth
	Comprehensive training in the breadth of emergency medical problems must be made available. In-depth training aimed at appropriate clinical areas is also essential.

2) Directed to needs A) EDNA	Training programs should be related to the needs of emergency nurses as they are defined by the Emergency Department Nurses Association and should be conducted with their sponsorship.

c) Emergency nurse practitioner (R.N.)
   1) Curriculum
   2) Programs
   3) Certification
	While there is evidence to suggest the special benefits to be derived through the use of this specialized nurse practitioner, the training programs and their curricula as well as the certification mechanism and criteria must be developed.

Highlights

Ambulances and equipment (medical and communications):

- There are presently 27,500 ambulances in operation in the United States. This number is considered to approximate the number of ambulances actually needed, based upon 1 ambulance per 10,000 population.
- Fifteen percent of the ambulances do not have two-way radios, and 25% do not carry essential life support equipment.
- Only 20% of the present ambulances in operation meet federal (DOT-GSA) specifications for proper emergency care vehicles which facilitate life support equipment and procedures. The other 80% or 22,000 vehicles will be replaced over the next five years. Of the three basic ambulance types, two are modular and one is a van type. The cost of modular types is approximately $24,000 each, and the cost for the van type is approximately $12,500.

The Federal Emergency Medical Services Program (EMS)

In the first three years of its existence, EMS has had a considerable impact on the effectiveness of emergency medical services. In testimony before the House Subcommittee on Health and Environment in 1976, HEW noted the following examples: Serious spinal cord injury, which was viewed as a hopeless condition, is now being successfully treated in Illinois by rapid evacuation to a specialty care center in Chicago. Approximately 62% of the victims returned to active employment within six months. The Maryland trauma center estimated that 750 lives of accident victims were saved as a result of the use of helicopters in their program. The rural EMS program in Charlottesville, Virginia, estimated that the actual death risk from acute heart attacks has decreased some 26% for all persons under the age of 70 since the development of their prehospital care system. Arkansas reported that during the first four months of 1974, 45 life threatening poisonings were averted. The rate of infant mortality in New Jersey has decreased by 58% and in San Antonio, Texas, by 50% due to improvements in their EMS systems.

Emergency Medical Technicians & Physician Assistants*

The emergency medical technician, with a minimum 81 hours emergency medical training, has emerged as the national standard, replacing the poorly trained ambulance attendant of yesterday. The paramedic, a relatively new category of emergency care personnel, offers the ultimate in prehospital critical care by providing definitive treatment (i.e., defibrillation, intravenous medication and endotracheal intubation) at the scene of an injury or illness. They are revolutionary additions to the emergency health care team. Their widespread acceptance has opened a new era of emergency care and has provided previously unthought of care at the scene and during patient transport. Strangely enough, any resistance to paramedics defibrillating, intubating or starting IVs in the field is dissipating rapidly; and most physicians now welcome the patient care benefits paramedics can provide.

*Source: Teresa Romano, "The Future of Nursing in Emergency Care," *JEN*, January–February, 1976.

In some existing EMS programs, an even newer category of emergency personnel is in the early stages of development—the emergency department physician assistant. Much like the paramedic, emergency department physician assistants, with anywhere from three to four years training, administer definitive emergency care in the absence of a physician. Unlike paramedics, they are stationed in the emergency department.

[Teresa Romano in JEN strongly recommends that emergency department nurses also begin.] ". . . defibrillating, intubating and starting IVs in the emergency department. As a nurse, she/he should have these skills, and the knowledge and judgment to initiate them."

Poisoning**

Cases of Poisoning

During 1974, over 200,000 accidental ingestions of household substances were reported to the Food and Drug Administration's National Clearinghouse for Poison Control Centers. (Approximately 130,000 involved children under five years of age.) In 1971, 3,000 of all accidents were fatal; 250 deaths occurred in children under five years of age.

The annual report of the Clearinghouse for 1972 lists the cases reported by all poison control centers and by state health departments. Most of the victims as always, were children. And among them aspirin again was the most common substance ingested. There were 8,146 such cases.

Medicines as a group accounted for 47,625 ingestions among children under five. Other important categories, in descending number of cases, were cleaning and polishing agents, petroleum products, cosmetics, pesticides, gases and vapors, plants, and turpentine and paints. Vitamins accounted for 4,000 cases.

The single most vulnerable ages were one to two (33,476 cases) and two to three (41,227 cases). After that the totals drop off sharply.

Not all poisonings are accidental. Some 5,737 were listed as cases of intended suicide. "Kicks" was listed as the reason for 3,935 cases, which involved not only medicines but petroleum products, pesticides and paint, as well as plants. In all, 39,661 cases—nearly a quarter of the total—were considered other than accidental.

**Source: *FDA Consumer,* November 1973.

Poison Control Centers

There are presently 580 Poison Control Centers in the United States that maintain information for the physician or the public on necessary treatment for the ingestion of household products and medicines. They are familiar with the toxicity (how poisonous it is) of most substances found in the home or know how and where to find this information. For a current list of these centers write: National Clearinghouse for Poison Control Centers, DHEW, Public Health Service, FDA, 5401 Westbard Ave., Bethesda, Md. 20016.

Food Poisoning*

There are four common causes of food poisoning—Salmonella, Clostridium perfringens, Staphylococcus, and Clostridium botulinum.

Salmonella (sal' mo-nel' a) is one of the most common causes of food poisoning. While it is not often fatal, it is widespread. More than two million cases of illness from Salmonella poisoning are believed to occur in the U.S. each year.

Salmonella is most commonly found in raw meats, poultry, eggs, milk, fish and products made from them.

Symptoms of Salmonella infection are fever, headache, diarrhea, abdominal discomfort and, occasionally, vomiting. These appear in 24 hours after eating contaminated food. Most people recover in two to four days.

Clostridium perfringens (klos-trid' i-um per-fringe'-ins) is widely distributed in nature—in the soil, dust, on food, and in the intestinal tracts of man and other warm-blooded animals. It is more widespread over the earth than any other disease-causing micro-organism.

Disease outbreaks frequently occur when foods are held in large quantities at improper temperatures for several hours or overnight. Perfringens outbreaks are closely associated with restaurants or other large feeding establishments where foods are held for long periods of time on steam tables or other warming devices.

Large numbers of perfringens bacteria can cause diarrhea and abdominal pain in from four to 22 hours—usually in about 12 hours.

Staphylococcus (staf' y-lo-kok' us)—known as staph—is quite common. Staph organisms are in your respiratory passages and on your skin. They usually enter food from a human or an animal.

Staph germs grow in a wide variety of foods—all meats, poultry and egg products, egg, tuna, chicken, potato or macaroni salads, cream filled pastries, and sandwich fillings. If staph germs are allowed to multiply to high levels, they form a toxin which you cannot boil or bake away.

Symptoms of staph food poisoning are diarrhea, vomiting and abdominal cramps. They appear two to four hours after eating and may bother you for 24 to 48 hours. Staph food poisoning is rarely fatal.

Clostridium botulinum (klos-trid' i-um, bot' u-li' num), while rare, is usually fatal. A tiny amount of the toxin poison from botulism germs can kill you. Botulism spores are found throughout the environment and are harmless. However, in the proper environment, and when not destroyed by heat, the spores divide and produce poisonous toxins. When you eat food containing the toxin, you can become ill or die. High heat makes the toxin harmless.

Only five deaths from botulism in commercially canned foods have been reported since 1925. But poisoning from home-canned foods happens more often. About 700 people have died from botulism since 1925 from eating contaminated home-canned products.

Signs of botulism poisoning begin 12 to 36 hours after eating the food. They include double vision, inability to swallow, speech difficulty, and progressive paralysis of the respiratory system.

Medical help must be obtained fast. If botulism is suspected, call your doctor immediately.

Poisonous Plants

John M. Kingsbury, in his book *Poisonous Plants of the United States and Canada,* states that more than 700 species of plants are known to have caused death or illness. Included in these 700 are some of nature's most delicate creations: the oleander bush, the lily-of-the-valley, and the rhododendron. Each year

---

*Source: *Facts About Food Poisoning,* FDA Consumer Memo.*

an estimated 12,000 children ingest these plants and others like them.

Burns and Insect Bites

Burns

Each year more than 2 million Americans are burned; 75,000 of them are burned severely enough to require hospitalization, and 12,000 perish. The bleakness of the situation is emphasized by the estimate that the net effect of today's shortage of medical skills and facilities for burn treatment is that approximately 90% of all patients do not receive the quality of care they need.

One doctor testified before a House Subcommittee on health that the national survival rate of children who have suffered burns over 60% of their body is between 10 and 20%, depending on the age of the child. However, he stated that the survival rate for children with the same extent of injury who are treated in specially equipped and staffed hospitals, jumps to between 50 and 60%.

Treatment*

The management of severe burns still is a critical problem. Although there are effective means of treating the acute shock phase by judicious intravenous fluid replacement and other supportive measures, this has not been associated with a decrease in the overall mortality. Rather, there has been a shift in the time of death, so that many of those who survive the initial crisis subsequently die from overwhelming infections or from pulmonary or renal complications.

At the University of Cincinnati burn and trauma research center, Dr. William Altemeier and his associates have found that the indiscriminate use of antibiotics in burned patients has caused the normal skin bacteria to change into forms which are more resistant to most types of therapy and cause an overwhelming infection. In another study on burn patients, this same team has devised a test to determine the loss of ability of the patient's white blood cells to kill bacteria, thereby permitting the clinician to predict impending infection.

Investigators have found some of the necessary sequential steps for treatment of severe burns involving 80% of the total body surface with 70% being third-degree burns. The previous mortality rate of 100% for such extensive burns has been reduced to 64%. The technique includes skin transplantation, ummunosuppression, hyperalimentation, and a bacteria-controlled environment.

Fresh, tissue-matched skin is transplanted from parents, siblings, or other close relatives. The survival of these grafts is enhanced by the administration of immunosuppressive agents. To help combat life-threatening infections, the patient spends the most serious part of his illness (usually about three months) in a bacteria-controlled nursing environment. Increased metabolism demands an extraordinarily high calorie intake. Thus, hyperalimentation, a technique pioneered in part by these investigators, supplies the necessary amounts of calories, particularly as protein. During the four to eight week period of temporary skin grafts, autografting is being performed. When all but 20% of the burned areas have thus been covered by the patient's own skin, the immunosuppression is discontinued and grafts from cadaver skins are used to cover the remaining parts of the body. Reconstructive surgery is begun soon after removal from the bacteria-controlled unit. Usually the patient leaves the hospital six to seven months after admission. Unfortunately, considerable disfigurement still occurs.

Burn Centers**

As of now there are only 12 burn centers in the United States and of the 6,000 general hospitals in this country only 78 of them provide specialized burn care. The centers and hospitals now existing are treating only 8% of the total number of burn victims. The vast majority are being treated in regular hospitals and clinics.

The U.S. National Commission on Fire Prevention and Control in its report "America Burning" wrote, "The average hospital stay for a burn victim is over three times that of medical and surgical patients. An individual's hospital stay and later treatment can add up to $60,000 or more."

---

*NIH Hearings, House Appropriations Committee, F.Y. 1977, February 1976.

**Source: House Interstate and Foreign Commerce Committee, May 5, 1976.

26

Insect Bites*

Insect bites kill at least 100 people annually and cause thousands to become ill, some very seriously.

The victim of a poisonous sting will usually experience a severe headache and an intense throbbing in the ears.

_____
*Source: *Nursing Care,* June 1976.

Because a sting is already potentially infected, the lay practice of applying a mud pack will only increase the danger of infection. Instead, vasopressor agents are recommended.

The toxins common to bee, wasp, hornet and ant stings are similar to snake venom. They all contain a similar hemolyzing factor and similar histamines which cause some people to react more violently than others.

27

PATIENT PROBLEMS AND CONCERNS

Family Planning

Risks of Hospitalization and Death*

Serious health risks associated with the use of various methods of family planning and their result in deaths are small. An evaluation of risks associated with a particular method of contraception will need to consider not only the deaths related to the use of the method itself and, therefore, attributable to it, but also the deaths due to pregnancies which may result because of method failure.

Table 27-1   Annual number of live births, induced abortions and deaths associated with control of fertility, per 100,000 women

Regimen of control and outcome	Age group					
	15–19	20–24	25–29	30–34	35–39	40–44
No control						
Live births	48,250	59,260	54,290	49,160	37,810	18,250
Birth-associated deaths	5.3	5.0	6.6	12.3	15.5	12.6
Abortion only						
Induced abortions	96,520	128,470	121,770	108,220	85,720	37,690
Abortion-associated deaths	2.2	2.4	2.3	4.5	7.9	3.8
Oral contraception, no abortion						
Live births	1,120	1,870	1,770	1,560	1,090	380
Birth-associated deaths	0.1	0.2	0.2	0.4	0.4	0.3
Method-associated deaths	1.3	1.3	1.3	4.8	6.9	24.5
Total deaths	1.4	1.5	1.5	5.2	7.3	24.8
IUD, no abortion						
Live births	1,120	1,870	1,770	1,560	1,090	380
Birth-associated deaths	0.1	0.2	0.2	0.4	0.4	0.3
Method-associated deaths	1.0	1.0	1.0	1.0	1.0	1.0
Total deaths	1.1	1.2	1.2	1.4	1.4	1.3
Traditional contraception, no abortion						
Live births	9,950	15,490	14,520	12,890	9,190	3,430
Birth-Associated deaths	1.1	1.3	1.8	3.2	3.8	2.4
Traditional contraception and abortion						
Induced abortions	13,310	19,860	18,820	17,300	12,550	4,900
Abortion-associated deaths	0.3	0.4	0.4	0.7	1.2	0.5
Deaths due to motor vehicle accidents	23.6	19.0	13.0	12.4	11.8	12.4

Source: "Mortality Associated with the Control of Fertility," Tietze, C. *et al., Family Planning Perspectives,* January–February 1976.

It is important to note that the estimated rate of hospitalization related to intrauterine devices appears to be higher than that attributable to oral contraceptives.

The rate of hospitalization related to intrauterine devices is estimated to range from three to ten per 100,000 women years of IUD use whereas the rate of hospitalization attributable to combination oral contraceptives is

*Source: House Appropriations Committee Hearings, 1977.

estimated to be about one per 1,000 women years.

The serious risks associated with available methods of contraception are low and indeed lower, for the most part, than mortality risks associated with pregnancy and child birth.

Costs

In 1972, Professors F. S. Jaffee and Charlotte Muller of City University of New York issued a study which demonstrated the essential interrelationship between each of the health services related to childbearing and their projected costs.

Table 27-2 Average unit costs of selected fertility-related health services, 1970–71

Maternity:	
Live births[1]	$1,118.00
Fetal losses	250.00
Fertility control:	
Infertility services	500.00
Sterilizations	183.00
Contraception[2]	61.46
Termination of pregnancy	332.00
Pediatric care[3]	98.77

[1] Average cost of a live birth includes prenatal, delivery, and nursery care costs.
[2] Average cost of contraception for 1 yr.
[3] Average cost of pediatric care during the first year of life.

Source: House Ways and Means Committee Hearings, December 1975.

Table 27-3 Operating responsibility for family planning clinics

Operating responsibility	Percent of clinics
United States and territories (4,494 clinics)	100.0
Government-operated	66.0
State	17.3
County	29.1
City or metropolitan area	4.8
Health district	5.7
Indian Health Service	1.8
Other Federal Government (Department of Defense, Veterans Administration, Public Health Service, etc.	6.8
Other non-Federal government	0.6
Nongovernment-operated	34.0
Planned Parenthood affiliates	10.3
University	3.8
Church	0.1
Hospital	5.6
Corporation	13.2
Individual	0.3
Partnership	0.1
Other nongovernment	0.6

Family Planning Clinics

Operating Responsibility for the Clinic

Like the nonmedical service sites, the largest proportion of medical family clinics is government-operated, the greater number of these by state and county governments.

Parenthood Federation of America, Inc., a national nonprofit organization, in 1974 provided family planning services to more than 900,000 women of low or marginal income at some 700 clinic facilities.

Medical Services Provided

Nineteen medical services ranked as follows in terms of the percentage of clinics that performed each service. (The space between items 13 and 14 is used to separate the services commonly provided by most clinics from those less commonly or rarely performed.)

Table 27-4 Medical services performed in family planning clinic

Rank	Medical services	Percent of responding clinics that performed the service
1	Blood pressure	98.8
2	Pap smear	98.4
3	Medical history record	98.1
4	Pelvis examination	97.4
5	Reproductive history record	96.8
6	Breast examination	96.5
7	Contraceptive prescription	95.3
8	Gonorrhea testing	94.8
9	Routine lab tests	91.1
10	Insertion of IUD	87.6
11	Social history record	85.8
12	Syphilis testing	82.1
13	Pregnancy testing	80.8
14	Sickle cell screening	41.5
15	Infertility counseling	38.5
16	Other medical service	24.7
17	Infertility diagnosis	22.4
18	Female sterilization	18.9
19	Male sterilization	14.4

Source: DHEW, 1976 (1974 Survey).

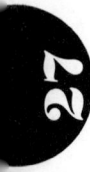

Ancillary Services Provided

From an overall perspective, the ancillary services ranked as follows in terms of percentage of clinics that provided each service.

Table 27-5 Ancillary services in clinics

Rank	Ancillary service	Percent of responding clinics that provided the service
1	Individual counseling about family planning	98.4
2	Referral to appropriate agency for social services	92.2
3	Referral to other clinic for family planning or medical services not provided at clinic site	91.6
4	Followup program (followup activities included contacting persons who had missed appointments and the scheduling of reappointments)	87.8
5	Outreach program (i.e., activities which informed prospective patients of family planning services and assisted them in availing themselves of the services)	72.9
6	Classroom or group sessions about family planning	60.7
7	Transportation to the clinic or service site (provided or subsidized)	39.7
8	Classroom or group sessions on sex education (in addition to family planning and contraceptive education)	35.4
9	Baby sitting (while patient was at clinic or service site)	29.2
10	Other ancillary service	4.6

Source: DHEW, 1976 (1974 Survey).

Contraceptive Methods Used

The use of 11 specific methods of contraception ranked as follows in terms of the percentage of clinics that employed each method.

Table 27-6 Contraceptive methods used in clinics

Rank	Contraceptive method	Percent of responding clinics using the method
1	Oral (pill)	99.6
2	IUD	94.2
3	Foam	90.1
4	Condom	75.7
5	Diaphragm jelly	64.3
6	Sterilization (female)	34.4
7	Basal temperature method	24.0
8	Sterilization (male)	23.7
9	Ovulation method	5.2
10	Morning-after pill	4.7
11	Injection	3.8

Source: DHEW, 1976 (1974 Survey).

Contraception and Conception*

Table 27-7 Percent exposure of married couples to the risk of conception, (1970)

Type of exposure	All couples (wife < 45)	White couples	Black couples
Pregnant, postpartum or trying to get pregnant	14.5	14.5	13.9
Sterile and subfecund	12.9	12.6	16.7
Other nonusers	7.5	7.2	10.2
Noncontraceptive Total	34.9	34.3	40.8
Wife sterilized[1]	5.5	4.9	11.4
Husband sterilized[1]	5.1	5.5	0.6
Pill[2]	22.3	22.4	22.1
IUD[3]	4.8	4.8	4.5
Diaphragm[4]	3.7	3.8	3.1
Condom[5]	9.2	9.7	4.0
Withdrawal	1.4	1.5	0.4
Foam	3.9	4.0	3.6
Rhythm	4.1	4.4	1.0
Douche	2.1	1.9	4.7
Other[6]	2.9	2.8	3.8
Contraceptive Total	65.0	65.7	59.2
Percent Total	100	100	100

[1-6]See footnotes accompanying Table 27-8.

*Source: Data from the 1970 National Fertility Study (NFS). "The Modernization of U.S. Contraceptive Practices." Reprinted with permission from *Family Planning Perspectives,* Vol. 4, No. 3, 1972.

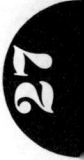

The Pill

In 1970, nearly six million married women of reproductive age were using the oral contraceptive—more than one out of every five. The Pill is by far the most popular method of contraception; it accounted for 34.2% of all current contraceptive practice in 1970, taking a commanding lead over all other methods (see Table 27-8). Its closest competitor was contraceptive sterilization (16.0%).

Table 27-8   Methods of contraception used by married couples† (1965 and 1970)

	All Couples (Wife < 45)					
Current Method	Total		White		Black	
	1965 (N = 3,032)	1970 (N = 3,810)	1965 (N = 2,441)	1970 (N = 3,273)	1965 (N = 554)	1970 (N = 462)
	Percents					
Wife sterilized[1]	7.0	8.5	6.3	7.5	14.4	19.3
Husband sterilized[1]	5.1	7.8	5.4	8.3	0.5	1.1
Pill[2]	23.9	34.2	24.0	34.0	21.7	37.4
IUD[3]	1.2	7.4	1.0	7.3	2.9	7.6
Diaphragm[4]	9.9	5.7	10.4	5.7	5.1	5.2
Condom[5]	21.9	14.2	22.4	14.8	17.0	6.7
Withdrawal	4.0	2.1	4.1	2.2	2.2	0.6
Foam	3.3	6.1	3.1	6.1	6.1	6.1
Rhythm	10.9	6.4	11.6	6.7	2.5	1.7
Douche	5.2	3.2	4.2	2.9	17.5	8.0
Other[6]	7.5	4.6	7.3	4.4	10.2	6.2
Percent Total	100	100	100	100	100	100

† Who were living together currently.
[1] Surgical procedures undertaken at least partly for contraceptive reasons.
[2] Includes combination with any other method.
[3] Includes combination with any other method except pill.
[4] Includes combination with any method except pill or IUD.
[5] Includes combination with any method except pill, IUD or diaphragm.
[6] Includes other multiple as well as single methods and a small percentage of unreported methods.

Contraceptive Failure*

Twenty-six percent of couples who use contraception report that within their first year of exposure to risk of unintended conception they fail to delay a pregnancy which they want to have at a later time; 14% of users fail to prevent a pregnancy which they do not intend to have at all, according to data from the 1970 National Fertility Study, analyzed by life table procedures. Those women who are relatively young at the beginning of exposure to risk are much more likely to fail than those who are older. Blacks are much less successful than whites both in delaying the next wanted pregnancy and in preventing the next unwanted pregnancy.

Standardized for intention and relative age, the failure proportions associated with each method are: pill, 6%; IUD, 12%; condom, 18%; diaphragm, 23%; foam, 31%; rhythm, 33%; and douche, 39%. These proportions reflect the characteristics of those who use each method, as well as of the method itself.

*Source: N. Ryder, "Contraceptive Failure in the U.S." Reprinted with permission from *Family Planning Perspectives*, Vol. 5, No. 3 1973.

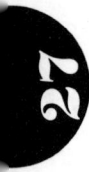

Figure 27-1 Percent of contraceptors who fail to delay a wanted pregnancy or to prevent an unwanted pregnancy in the first year of exposure to risk of unwanted conception, by selected contraceptive method.

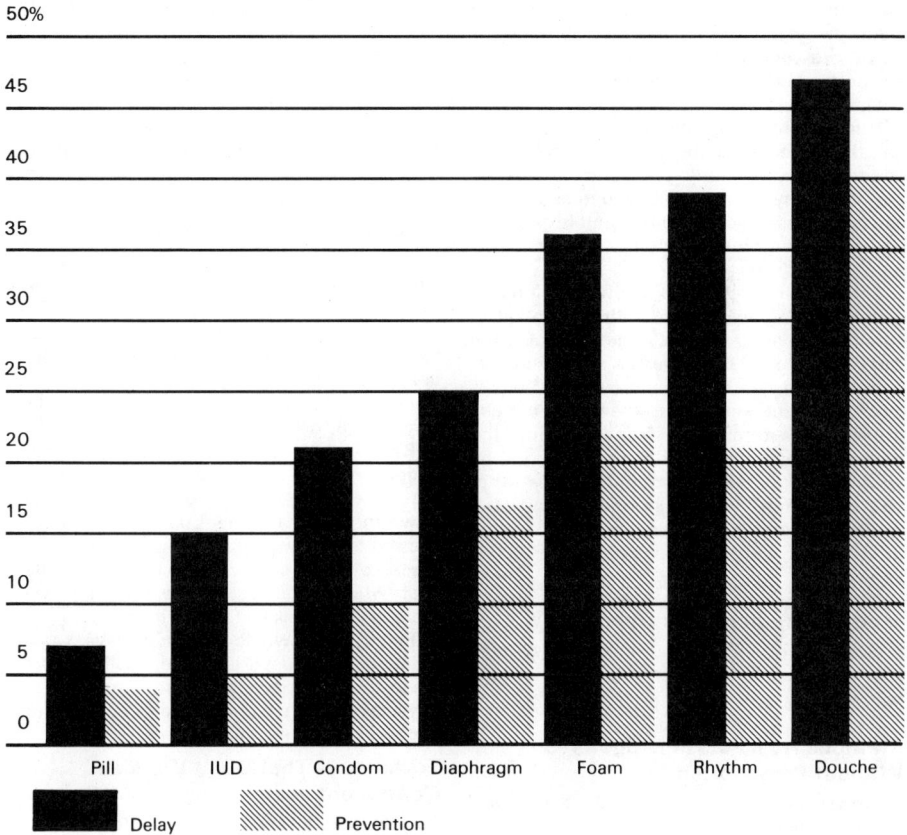

Delay Prevention

Contraceptive Methods*

Overview

There are many contraceptive methods—some are available without a doctor's prescription in drugstores; others must be either prescribed or fitted by a medically qualified person.

Methods Requiring a Fitting or Medical Prescription

Birth Control Pills—These must be prescribed by a doctor. There are many types

---

*Source: Planned Parenthood Federation, 1976.

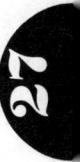

of birth control pills but basically most work by preventing an egg cell from being released by an ovary. If there is no egg, conception cannot take place. When a woman uses birth control pills, she usually takes one each day for three weeks, then either takes no pill or a substitute sugar or iron pill for one week. During the fourth week, she has her menstrual period.

After long-time use of the Pill, about 75% of women are able to become pregnant within two months after stopping. (A more detailed discussion of birth control pills can be found in a separate section below.)

27

IUD—This is also called the intrauterine device, IUD or loop. It is usually a small piece of plastic, in one of a variety of shapes, that is inserted into the uterus by a doctor or other medical practitioner to remain until a woman wants to become pregnant. Insertion and removal are very delicate procedures and must be performed only by someone medically qualified.

It is not known exactly how the IUD works but its presence in the uterus seems to be effective in preventing pregnancy. However, the IUD may be expelled spontaneously or cause cramps in some women and is generally painful during insertion and the first few months after insertion.

Diaphragm—This is a shallow cup of rubber which a woman covers with sperm-killing cream and inserts into the vagina to cover the cervix (opening of the uterus). A woman inserts it before she has sexual intercourse. It works by blocking the entrance to the uterus thereby preventing sperm cells from entering the uterus and combining with the egg cell. The sperm-killing cream immobilizes any other sperm which might swim around the diaphragm rim. The diaphragm must be fitted by a doctor because the size of the cervix varies.

Methods Requiring an Operation

Sterilization—Male and female procedures are discussed in detail in separate sections below.

Methods Available in Drugstores Without Prescription

Contraceptive Foams, Creams and Jellies—These are sperm-killing substances a woman inserts into her vagina just before sexual intercourse to block off the entrance to the uterus and kill sperm cells. Foams come in aerosol containers like shaving cream and are inserted into the vagina with a long, narrow applicator. Creams and jellies work by the same principle except that they come in tubes.

Condoms—The condom (also called a rubber or prophylactic) is shaped like the finger of a glove and is made of rubber or animal tissue. A man uses a condom by rolling it onto his erect penis before sexual intercourse. Its purpose is to catch sperm cells and semen that are ejaculated, preventing them from entering the uterus. A man should be careful to leave about ½ inch of room at the tip to catch the sperm and help prevent the condom from bursting. He should also be careful to keep the condom from slipping off his penis by holding the base as he withdraws. Rubber condoms should be discarded after each use.

Condoms are particularly effective as contraceptives if a woman at the same time also uses contraceptive foam, cream or jelly. Condoms should *not* be used with Vaseline or similar petroleum-based lubricants which may cause the rubber to disintegrate. The condom is also the only contraceptive that provides some protection against venereal disease.

Other Contraceptive Methods

Withdrawal—This is a method of withdrawing the penis from the vagina just before a man's climax to keep sperm cells away from the uterine opening. It is unreliable for most people because it requires a great deal of control from a man. Even then it's risky since some sperm are released from his penis involuntarily before climax.

Rhythm Method—With this method a couple avoids sex during the three or more days each month when the egg is traveling down the fallopian tube. Couples who want to use this method should consult a doctor or nurse to find out how to use a temperature chart which is the best way to determine when the egg is most likely to be in the tube.

Since most women do not have regular menstrual periods, it is very difficult to predict when the three days are. Also, emotional and physical changes can cause a woman to have unpredictable menstrual periods.

Techniques That Don't Work as Contraceptives

Douching: thousands of sperm enter the uterus before douching can reach them.

Plastic food wrap used like a condom: it's not made for this purpose and may break or slip off.

Having sex during menstruation: it's possible for an egg to be in the fallopian tube, even at the least likely time of the month.

New Contraceptive Methods—Research*

Drug Synthesis Program—The goals of this program are: to develop for women new and

---

* National Institutes of Health, 1977.

efficacious chemical contraceptives that will not have undesirable side effects, and, equally important, to develop safe, effective contraceptives that men will find acceptable.

A promising new drug, which is a modification of the female sex hormone (estrogen), has been shown to have high antifertility activity. This result was obtained in the rat and the drug is now being tested in other species, including the monkey.

Devices—A new type of intrauterine device under study consists of reinforced, synthetic silastic rubber in the form of a pouch which, after insertion, is expanded by fluid pressure and takes on the configuration of the uterine cavity itself. It appears to be tolerated better than the presently available IUDs and has a low expulsion rate.

An instrument to visualize the female reproductive tract now has been tested in baboons under operating room conditions. It has also been used successfully to insert plugs to close the tubes which carry eggs from the ovary to the uterus. The program calls for preliminary use of this steerable instrument in women scheduled for hysterectomy. Such an instrument, which allows the surgeon to see the inside of the uterine cavity in a safe manner, is a first step in the development of new procedures for fertility regulation.

Development and testing of devices intended for the achievement of easily reversible vasectomy have resulted in major advances. Some devices have been in laboratory animals more than 12 months and have been found to be effective. Preliminary data indicate that animals implanted with devices in the open position are fertile. The problem of the adhesion of the devices to body tissues has been resolved.

Male Reproductive Tract—Significant new knowledge of the basic physiology of the male reproductive tract is providing new ideas on possible ways of limiting male fertility without interfering with the other functions of the testis or with libido. After the sperm leave the testis and before they are ejaculated, they undergo a process of maturation, i.e., they become motile and acquire the enzymatic ability to fertilize or penetrate the egg. This occurs while the sperm are passing through the elongated ducts (epididymedes) of the male reproductive tract. We now know that there is an unusual

mechanism in the epididymis which concentrates the hormones produced by the testis so that their levels are many times higher than they are in peripheral blood. In addition, measurement of the various androgens in the epididymis has shown that testosterone, the principal testicular androgen in peripheral blood of men, is not the androgen in highest concentration in the epididymis. After castration, the epididymal function of white rats cannot be restored by hormone injection. These data suggest the possibility of male fertility regulation through drugs acting specifically on this structure.

Birth Control Pills*

Types and Trade Names

Oral contraceptives, listed in Table 27-9 are now of two basic types.

The combination oral prevents pregnancy by preventing ovulation.

The combination-type pill contains both estrogen and progestogen. The estrogen suppresses secretion of FSH by the pituitary, probably by acting directly on the pituitary as well as indirectly on the hypothalamus. It also renders the endometrium inhospitable to the implantation of a fertilized ovum. The progestogen suppresses secretion of LH and makes the cervical mucus resistant to the penetration and movement of sperm.

A tablet containing the two steroids is taken daily, beginning on the fifth day of menstruation, for 20 or 21 days. For the rest of the 28-day cycle, a placebo containing some form of iron such as ferrous fumarate may be supplied to help keep track of the days by maintaining the daily habit of taking a pill.

Progestogen-only type (the "mini-pill"): is a continuous-dosage drug that relies on adverse changes in the endometrium and cervical mucus to prevent pregnancy. It causes more breakthrough bleeding and permits more pregnancies than the combination type. Since it is not yet in widespread use, women taking it should be under direct supervision of a physician.

---

*Source: Adapted from "Oral Contraceptives" by N. Cowart and D. W. Newton, *Nursing '76,* June 1976.

Table 27-9   Trade names and ingredients of available oral contraceptives

	Ingredients	
Trade name	Estrogen (mg)	Progestogen (mg)
Combination Type		
Demulen	ethinyl estradiol 0.05	ethynodiol diacetate 1
Enovid 10 mg	mestranol 0.15	norethynodrel 10
Enovid 5 mg	mestranol 0.075	norethynodrel 5
Enovid-E	mestranol 0.10	norethynodrel 2.5
Loestrin 1/20	ethinyl estradiol 0.02	norethindrone acetate 1.0
Loestrin 1.5/30	ethinyl estradiol 0.03	norethindrone acetate 1.5
Ortho-Novum 10 mg	mestranol 0.06	norethindrone 10
Ortho-Novum 2 mg	mestranol 0.10	norethindrone 2
Ortho-Novum 1 mg	mestranol 0.05	norethindrone 1
Ortho-Novum 1/50	mestranol 0.05	norethindrone 1
Ortho-Novum 1/80	mestranol 0.08	norethindrone 1
Norinyl 10 mg	mestranol 0.06	norethindrone 10
Norinyl 2 mg	mestranol 0.10	norethindrone 2
Norinyl 1 mg	mestranol 0.05	norethindrone 1
Norinyl 1 + 50	mestranol 0.05	norethindrone 1
Norinyl 1 + 80	mestranol 0.08	norethindrone 1
Norlestrin 2.5 mg	ethinyl estradiol 0.05	norethindrone acetate 2.5
Norlestrin 1 mg	ethinyl estradiol 0.05	norethindrone acetate 1
Ovulen	mestranol 0.10	ethynodiol diacetate 1
Ovral	ethinyl estradiol 0.05	norgestrel 0.5
Zorane 1/20	ethinyl estradiol 0.02	norethindrone acetate 1.0
Zorane 1.5/30	ethinyl estradiol 0.03	norethindrone acetate 1.5
Zorane 1/50	ethinyl estradiol 0.05	norethindrone acetate 1.0
Progestogen Type		
Micronor		norethindrone 0.35
Nor-Q.D.		norethindrone 0.35
Ovrette		norgestral 0.075
Sequential (off the market)		
Norquen	mestranol 0.08	norethindrone 2
Oracon	ethinyl estradiol 0.10	dimethisterone 25
Ortho-Novum SQ	mestranol 0.08	norethindrone 2

What If A Pill Is Missed?

A woman who misses taking a Pill runs an increased risk of ovulation. Manufacturers' literature suggests that a woman who misses one or two Pills should take them as soon as she realizes the lapse, and that she should use another means of contraception until she has taken seven Pills in succession. If she misses three or more Pills, she should discard the Pills remaining in that cycle and begin a new one seven days after taking the last Pill.

Ironically, playing "catch-up" by taking missed Pills can increase the chance of pregnancy.

Annoying Side Effects

- Nausea, the most common side effect, occurs in 10 to 15% of all new patients. It is the most frequent reason for changing the type of Pill or stopping it altogether.
- About 3 to 5% of new Pill users also experience headache during the first month or so.
- Half the women taking the Pill gain weight, probably because of sodium chloride and fluid retention.
- After a woman begins to take the Pill, her first menstrual period will be delayed six to ten weeks. Then she will resume a normal or

near-normal rhythm. But the Pill will reduce the quantity and duration of her menstrual flow.

- During the initial adjustment period, and after incidents of missed Pills, many women experience "breakthrough bleeding," a light pink, serous-like spotting about three centimeters in diameter. It usually disappears after several months of adjustment to the hormonal level.
- Another frequent symptom is breast engorgement and tenderness, a pseudopregnancy effect of estrogen. In some women, the tenderness is temporary, but the breasts remain engorged.
- Some women find that the Pill's effect on the mucosa increases the incidence of vaginal discharge and infections.
- After a year or two on the Pill, some women develop brown patches on the face resembling the mask of pregnancy. This also probably stems from the high level of estrogen in the blood. The patches can be limited by avoiding exposure to direct sunlight.

Adverse Affects

Thrombosis—The most widely documented adverse effect of oral contraceptives concerns the increased risks of thrombosis (blood clot formation). It was not previously known whether brain or cerebral thrombosis (stroke) also occurred. Relationships of dose, formulation and predisposing factors also remained unknown. Current studies show that oral contraceptives do increase the risk of stroke.

The frequency of such complications can be reduced by lowering the dosage of the drugs. Hypertension, regular cigarette smoking and a history of migraine headaches increase the risk of stroke when combined with current use of oral contraceptives.

Chromosome Breakage—Analysis of the data on chromosome breakage in cultured blood cells from women taking oral contraceptives and control subjects has demonstrated a small but significant increase in breakage in cells from oral contraceptive users.

Broken chromosomes are seen in 7.1% of cells from oral contraceptive users who have never been pregnant, as compared with 5.3% of cells from women who have never used the pill or been pregnant. Women who have previously been pregnant also show more chromosome breakage than those who have not been pregnant.

Myocardial Infarction—Two recently completed projects in the United Kingdom strongly suggest an increased risk of myocardial infarction among oral contraceptive users. The risk is particularly high in the presence of other factors known to be associated with cardiovascular disease such as obesity, hypertension, diabetes and smoking. Of considerable significance was the observation of a sizable increase in the risk of myocardial infarction among women on oral contraceptive steroids who were 40 years of age and over.

Heart Attack—A recent Food and Drug Administration (FDA) bulletin states that there is an increased risk of heart attack in women over the age of 35—and especially in women aged 40 to 45—who take birth control pills. For the age group 30 to 39, the incidence of heart attacks is 5.6 per 100,000 as opposed to 2.1 per 100,000 women not using the pill. For ages 40 to 44, the incidence of heart attack is 56.1 per 100,000 as opposed to 9.9 per 100,000 not using the pill.

Birth Defects—According to an FDA announcement in early 1975, the effects of oral contraceptives on fetal development may be teratogenic, i.e., causing birth defects. So, a woman who misses two consecutive menstrual periods should find out whether she's pregnant before continuing to take the Pill.

Other Problems—Surveillance of a large population of women has revealed an increase in the prevalence of hypertension (high blood pressure) from 1.2 per 1,000 among women not using oral contraceptives to 6.8 per 1,000 women using oral contraceptives. An increase in asymptomatic urinary tract infections was also observed among oral contraceptive users. Preliminary analysis of two case-control studies shows no relationship between breast cancer and the use of oral contraceptives.

Who Should Not Take the Pill

Nursing '76 listed women with the following types of histories who should avoid the Pill:

- a family history of cancer of the genital organs
- a history of varicosities or thromboembolic conditions (because the pill may increase the clotting ability of blood)
- a history of hypertension (it may elevate blood pressure)

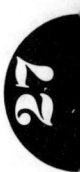

- a history of depression
- a history of severe migraine headaches, cardiovascular diseases, severe diabetes, nephritis or uterine myomas.

Sterilization

Overview

One of the most dramatic findings in the 1970 NFS is the fact that voluntary sterilization—typically, tubal ligation for women and vasectomy for men—has become the most popular method of contraception currently used by older couples (in which the wife is aged 30–44). One-quarter of all older couples who were currently practicing contraception had been surgically sterilized; the operations were almost equally divided between men and women.

Reliance on contraceptive sterilization is evidently more common among black than among white women, but much less so among black than white men. While almost one-third (32.5%) of older black women compared with 11.6% of older white women report having been sterilized, only 1.7% of older black men

compared with 12.9% of older white men were reported to have had vasectomies. This difference probably reflects a combination of differences between whites and blacks in the role of the woman in the control of fertility and in the concern for the presumed implications of vasectomies for sexual potency. Thus, the use of the male methods, condom and withdrawal, is much greater among whites than blacks. There is also a considerable difference between black and white women in their belief that a vasectomy will impair male sexual ability: 36% of black compared with 13% of white women held such beliefs in 1970. This appears to be primarily the result of educational differences.

Teenagers

The likelihood that a never-married teenage female has experienced coitus rises from 14% at age 15 years to 27% at age 17, and to 46% at age 19 years. Less than one-half of those sexually experienced used any method of contraception for the most recent exposure to the risk of conception and less than one-fifth have always utilized a means of contraception.

The Rapid Increase in Sterilization*

In 1970 alone some 320,000 vasectomies and an almost equal number of tubal ligations were performed; it is estimated that over 2.75

million married couples of reproductive age had been sterilized for contraceptive reasons as of 1970.

While vasectomies and tubal ligations were prevalent about equally in 1965, by 1970 vasectomy had become somewhat more prevalent.

* Source: Association for Voluntary Sterilization.

Table 27-10   Risk population with contraceptive sterilization, or who would "seriously consider" it (1970)*

Race	Percent sterilized				Percent who would seriously consider sterilization			Percent sterilized or who would seriously consider sterilization			
	Tubal ligation	Vasectomy	Other[1]	Total	Female operation	Male operation[2]	At least male or female	Female operation[3]	Male operation	At least male or female	Number of cases
Total	7	8	3	18	36	28	47	46	37	65	3,361
White	6	9	2	18	36	29	48	44	38	66	2,901
Black	15	1	4	21	34	9	38	54	10	59	460

* Couples who intend no more children and who are not sterile for noncontraceptive reasons.
[1] Includes hysterectomies and other sterilizing operations performed for contraceptive reasons, and couples reporting two types of contraceptive operations.
[2] Based on wife's report of husband's attitude.
[3] Includes contraceptive hysterectomies.

Source: T. Presser and W. Bumper, "The Acceptability of Contraceptive Sterilization Among U.S. Couples, 1970" Reprinted with permission from *Family Planning Perspectives*, Vol. 4, No. 4, 1972.

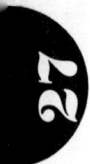

Table 27-11 Estimate of voluntary sterilizations performed

	Males	Females	Total number
1970	750,000 (80%)	192,000 (20%)	942,000
1971	825,000 (80%)	207,000 (20%)	1,032,000
1972	771,000 (70%)	331,000 (30%)	1,102,000
1973	538,000 (57%)	398,000 (43%)	936,000
1974	682,000 (51%)	652,000 (49%)	1,334,000
1975[1]	639,000 (49%)	674,000 (51%)	1,313,000

[1]Preliminary figures for 1975 indicate the total number of sterilizations in the United States is now 8,244,607. Of these, 4,635,313 are men and 3,609,294 are women.
Source: Association for Voluntary Sterilization.

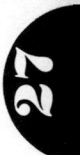

Special Consent for Voluntary Sterilizations

Only Georgia, Virginia and New Mexico have laws requiring the consent-of-spouse unless the husband has separated from or abandoned his wife. In the absence of statute a husband's consent is not required to a wife's voluntary sterilization, or vice versa. In other words, in the vast majority of states, there will be no liability on a physician or hospital who performs voluntary sterilization on a competent adult without the consent of that adult's spouse. However, if one spouse elects to be sterilized against the opposition of the other, the non-consenting spouse may have the basis for divorce or separation.

Health Insurance Coverage

Of 47 million Americans participating in group health insurance plans, 28 million are covered for voluntary sterilization, according to a report in September–October 1975 issue of *Family Planning Perspectives*.

Eighty-seven percent of the carriers offered some kind of coverage for vs., with 60% of participants in the health insurance plans actually being provided such coverage.

Questions & Answers on Sterilization*

When is sterilization indicated?

It is indicated:

- if no pregnancies are wanted in the future
- if pregnancy is likely to endanger a woman's health
- if physical, mental or emotional factors prevent fulfilling the responsibilities of parenthood

---

* Source: Association for Voluntary Sterilization.

- if there is possibility of transmitting an hereditary defect.

It is not indicated:

- if there is uncertainty about the desire to terminate fertility
- if the wish is to delay assuming the responsibilities of parenthood
- if the hope is to reverse the operation in case of remarriage, death of children, or other change of circumstances.

Is sterilization effective?

There is no guarantee that a surgical procedure of any kind will be 100% effective, or that after a sterilization the tubes will not grow back together. The risk of this is extremely small, however, and sterilization is the most reliable form of birth control available today.

Are there physical changes?

Other than the inability to reproduce, there are no known physical changes. A woman's menstrual periods and age of menopause are unaffected. A man continues to have an erection and ejaculate but his semen contains no sperm.

Are there emotional changes?

Voluntary sterilization obtained after thorough consideration, with full understanding of the nature of the operation, and without coercion, usually results in relief and peace of mind for both partners. Many patients report increased enjoyment of sex when the fear of pregnancy has been removed.

Is it permanent?

The operation is ordinarily performed as a permanent measure and should not be considered unless the individual is sure no children will be wanted in the future. Continuing research is improving the techniques for surgical restoration of fertility (reversal), but a successful reversal cannot be assured in any individual case.

Is it legal?

Yes. In all 50 states, sterilization is legal without restriction as to the reason it is performed.

Is spousal consent required by law?

Only three states require it: Georgia, Virginia, and New Mexico. Throughout the country, however, many doctors and hospitals are reluctant to perform a sterilization for the married without spousal consent.

Is it expensive?

Charges vary according to such factors as type of surgery or hospital arrangements. If other medical costs are usually paid by Medicaid, welfare or private health insurance, all or part of the costs for sterilization may be covered.

How much does the operation cost?

There is no meaningful answer on costs since physicians' fees and hospital or clinic charges vary. For the female operation, doctors' fees generally range from $150 to $350; hospital charges depend on several factors such as type of accommodation (private, semi-private, ward), length of stay required by physician (from a few hours to several days), etc. Costs for the male operation are about $150, or less if performed in a vasectomy clinic. Almost all insurance companies pay for contraceptive sterilization.

Table 27-12   Cost estimates for sterilization

	Private sector	Public sector
Tubal ligation		
Total	$586	$168
Physician	250	88
Hospital	296	80
Anesthesia	40	—
Vasectomies	$150	$ 50

Source: C. Muller, "The Cost of Contraceptive Sterilization." Reprinted with permission from *Family Planning Perspectives,* Vol. 6, No. 1, 1974. (A study conducted in Jacksonville, Florida.)

Vasectomy*

Sterilization for a man, vasectomy, is minor surgery and is usually performed in the physician's office or clinic under local anesthesia.

Vasectomy, performed on healthy, psychologically well-adjusted men, does not significantly affect male hormonal balance, sexual desire, capacity for erection, or ejaculation of semen. The operation involves the cutting or blocking of each vas deferens, the two tubes which carry sperm from the testes to the

*Source: *Population Reports,* December 1973, January and May 1975, George Washington University Medical Center. (Unless otherwise noted.)

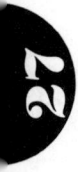

penis (see Fig. 27-2). Through a small incision in the scrotum, the surgeon cuts, ties, electrocoagulates, and/or clips the vasa. Local anesthesia is commonly used. After resting briefly from the 10 to 15 minute procedure, the patient walks out of the office, clinic or mobile unit.

For some time after the operation residual sperm are found in the semen, which is the fluid ejaculated at sexual climax, and other contraception must be used until tests show sperm are no longer present in the ejaculate. After the operation the testicles continue to produce sperm which then disintegrate and are absorbed by the body.

Although considered virtually 100% effective, vasectomy can fail because, among other reasons, the cut ends of the vas may reconnect (spontaneous reanastomosis). This occurs, however, in less than 1% of cases.

Side Effects

The most common side effects are local problems like scrotal skin discoloration, bruising, swelling and discomfort. These normally disappear a week or two after the operation. Psychological problems resulting from conscious or unconscious fears about the operation can usually be reduced by careful and sympathetic counseling.

Figure 27-2   Male reproductive system showing the area of vasectomy

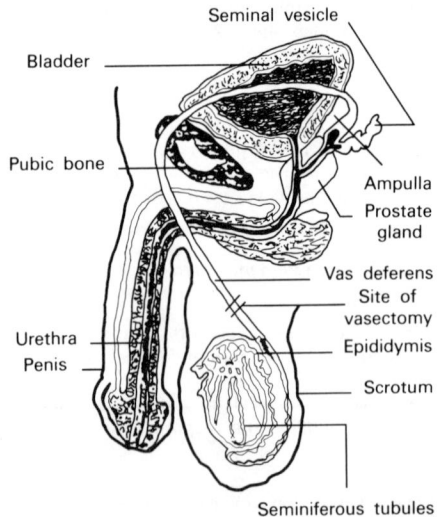

Seminal vesicle
Bladder
Pubic bone
Ampulla
Prostate gland
Vas deferens
Site of vasectomy
Urethra
Penis
Epididymis
Scrotum
Seminiferous tubules

Complications

Complications can occasionally occur after any surgery. These include hemorrhage and infection. Other possible complications following vasectomy, although less common, include epididymitis and sperm granuloma. Epididymitis is an infection of the epididymis frequently associated with a previous history of infection. Sperm granuloma is a chronic inflammatory reaction which is postulated to develop as a result of leakage of sperm from the cut ends of the vas. Occasionally the body fails to resorb the granuloma causing it to become troublesome and requiring further treatment.

The overall incidence of either hematoma, epididymitis or infection is less than 2%; for sperm granuloma, less than 1%.

Vasectomy Clinics*

Although some clinics have arbitrary requirements of age, parity and marital status, all consider younger men with fewer children. Around three-fourths will consider men who are divorced, separated or single. Nearly two-thirds will consider the young husband in a childless-by-choice couple, and slightly less than half will consider the young single man. One-fourth of the clinics do not require spousal consent for married vasectomy candidates.

In the majority of clinics the medically needy man can obtain the operation at no charge, low charge or through Medicaid. Only 10% of the clinics charge more than $150. Many charge about $75. Just under three-fourths of the clinics indicate they will consider the mentally retarded patient under given circumstances.

Reversibility

The reasons for requesting reversal cited most frequently are:

- remarriage after divorce or death of wife
- death of one or more children
- improved economic situation
- psychological desire to overcome supposed ill effects of vasectomy.

Three approaches to reversibility are:

- vas anastomosis (surgical reversal of vasectomy)
- frozen semen storage (fertility insurance without the necessity for surgical or mechanical reversal)

- vas occlusive devices (mechanical reversal of vasectomy).

Vas Anastamosis—To date, there are neither standard techniques nor criteria by which to assess the success of vas anastomosis. Success is dependent, to a large extent, on the vasectomy technique used as well as on the anastomosis technique. If the vasectomy has been done in the convoluted part of the vas and if a large segment of vas was removed, chances of successful anastomosis decrease. The experience of the surgeon performing the operation is also a factor.

There is a substantial difference between the rate of anatomical success (40–90%) as determined by reappearance of sperm and that of functional success (18–60%) as determined by pregnancy rate.

At present, vas anastomosis, the least experimental of the three approaches to reversibility, is used most widely.

Many investigators in recent years have been turning to a new technique—mucosa-to-mucosa anastomosis without a splint, performed using an operating microscope. This technique appears likely to offer potential for the greatest success. Vas anastomosis procedures require surgery and take about two hours to perform, and most procedures require general anesthesia.

Vas Occlusive Devices—Most vas occlusive devices are experimental and are not readily available. However, preliminary results with several devices appear promising. Vas occlusive devices have the potential of making a simple, reversible, safe and effective method of contraception available for men, but the development and testing of these devices are necessarily long-term processes.

Frozen Semen Storage—Frozen semen storage, a type of fertility insurance which does not involve surgery or use of mechanical devices, is another approach to reversible male sterilization. At present, it remains in the experimental stage due to its high cost, limited availability and uncertain results.

Infertility*—There has been established a cause and effect relationship between sperm antibodies and infertility. Because these antibodies have been found in nonvasectomized men with fertility problems, it is believed that sperm antibodies induce an "immunologic" infertility. This could explain why there exists a

---

*Source: Association for Voluntary Sterilization

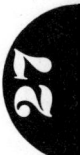

low incidence of fertility among men who have had their vasectomy reversed. Therefore, for those selecting vasectomy for contraception, the method should be considered permanent.

Sterilization for Women*

Sterilization for a woman, salpingectomy or "tubal ligation," can be achieved by a variety of surgical procedures.

These approaches permit occlusion of any part of the fallopian tube. For example, the infundibulum (distal, fimbrial end of the tube) can be excised, buried, plugged or capped; the ampulla or isthmus (middle of the tube) can be tied, cut, excised, fulgurated, clipped, banded or buried; and the interstitial portion of the tube (near the uterotubal junction) can be coagulated or blocked with chemicals or plugs.

Procedures

Laparotomy—This is the classic approach through an incision in the abdominal wall in order to cut and close the fallopian tubes. This procedure may be done at the time of delivery or other surgery, including cesarean section, making a separate hospital stay unnecessary.

Mini-Laparotomy—In the mini-laparotomy procedure—or mini-lap, as it is sometimes called—a small suprapubic incision is made and the uterus is manipulated to bring the fallopian tubes into the field of vision. Because of the small incision, local anesthesia may be substituted for general anesthesia. This simplifies the procedure and reduces recovery time, making it possible to perform mini-lap on an outpatient basis.

The mini-laparotomy approach can be adapted to various methods of tubal ligation. Mini-laparotomy is unlike laparoscopy in that it permits direct visualization of the fallopian tubes which are brought through the incision for ligation or other occluding techniques. Special endoscopic training and equipment are not necessary. With ordinary surgical skills, a physician can perform the operation in ten to thirty minutes. The patient recovers in one to four hours with a scar that eventually disappears from view.

---

*Sources: *Population Reports*, Jan., March, June 1973; March, Nov. 1974; May 1975; May 1976—George Washington University Medical Center.

Laparoscopy—This is a technique which permits a trained physician to view the abdominal cavity by means of a laparoscope, a tube containing a telescope and light. A harmless gas is used to distend the abdomen to prevent internal injuries. Through one or two small incisions below the navel, the physician inserts the laparoscope and an instrument into the cavity to seal off the fallopian tubes. After the instruments are removed and the gas is released, the incision may be covered with a band-aid and therefore the operation has become known as "band-aid" surgery.

The failure rate in surgical sterilization with a laparoscope ranges from 0.1 to 2 per 100 operations. The main reasons for failure are an undetected pregnancy already established or mistaken identification of the round ligament for the fallopian tube.

Morbidity and side effects average about five percent and are usually short-lived, but some emergencies, estimated at one percent, may require laparotomy and full hospital facilities.

Side effects of laparoscopic tubal sterilization might include some discomfort and shoulder pain from the gas introduced into the abdomen, bleeding from the incision or in the abdomen near the tubes. The electric current can cause a short, sharp pain as it seals the tubes.

Mortality in laparoscopic procedures overall has been identified as 3 per 12,000 cases, or 20–30 per 100,000. This rate, reported by some of the world's most experienced laparoscopists, should be compared with a patient mortality rate of 25 per 100,000 for nonlaparoscopic tubal ligation.

A new technique, still in experimental stages, involves the use of plastic clips which are applied with a special laparoscopic clip applicator to close the fallopian tubes.

The present operating laparoscopes depend on electrocautery, however, and therefore may cause serious burns. The use of clips instead of electrocautery might make female sterilization simpler and safer while offering an increased likelihood of reversibility, should that be desired later.

Colpotomy—This is a vaginal approach leaving no external scars. In the usual posterior approach, the cul-de-sac, or pouch of Douglas, located between the front of the rectum and the back of the uterus, is opened through the vagina to expose the fallopian tubes. In the anterior approach, which is seldom used today, the peritoneum is incised between the bladder and the uterus. The uterus is then rotated until the fallopian tubes are identified.

The two most common operative techniques on the tube itself are a fimbriectomy, in which the lateral portion of the tubes including the fimbria is removed, and the classical Pomeroy sterilization. With the Pomeroy approach, the tubes are first tied into a loop with an absorbable suture. Then the top of the loop is removed surgically, leaving two open ends which separate when the catgut suture dissolves.

Only five to fifteen minutes are normally required for the operation.

Culdoscopy—Also a vaginal approach, this technique, like laparoscopy, employs the use of a lighted instrument, a culdoscope, by which a trained physician is able to view the fallopian tubes and seal them. The physician inserts the culdoscope through a small vaginal incision to visualize the tubes while a second instrument is used to bring the tubes through the incision into direct view for ligation or other methods of tubal occlusion.

Need for Hospitalization

Laparotomy is considered major surgery under general anesthesia and usually requires several days hospitalization. For the other techniques, local or general anesthesia may be used and hospitalization ranging from a few hours to several days may be required. Not all techniques are suitable for all women, and the physician will determine which technique is advisable in consultation with the patient.

If desired, sterilization can be performed in conjunction with abortion making a separate hospitalization unnecessary.

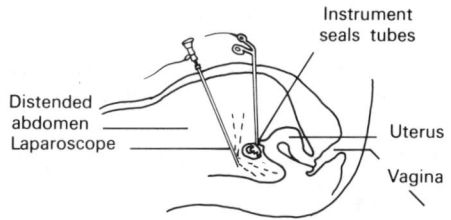

Laparoscopy

Instrument seals tubes

Distended abdomen
Laparoscope

Uterus

Vagina

Reversibility

Although some plugs offer potential for reversibility because theoretically they may be withdrawn from the tube, reversibility has not been adequately assessed by tests in humans. In animal experiments, the tubal epithelium is sometimes destroyed beyond repair when plugs are removed. Clips or bands, on the other hand, destroy a narrow segment of tube, but there is virtually no experience with reversibility. Reversal would require a second operation to cut out the crushed section of tube and anastomose (join) the two remaining ends. Ligation is the procedure most often reversed successfully, but the same operative procedure for anastomosis is required. The use of cautery makes reversibility virtually impossible to achieve because a large segment of tube is destroyed. Likewise, most chemical methods are not reversible because the epithelium is permanently damaged.

Abortion

Highlights

- Since legalization of abortion, deaths from abortion dropped from 83 in 1972 to 51 in 1973; admissions to New York City municipal hospitals for septic and incomplete abortions dropped from 6,524 in 1969 to 3,253 in 1973 (the New York law was liberalized in July of 1970). Data on maternal deaths associated with legal first trimester abortions in 1972 and 1973 show a rate of 1.7 per 100,000 abortions, compared with 14 deaths per 100,000 live deliveries in 1973. (For comparison, the surgical removal of the tonsils and adenoids had a mortality risk of 5 deaths per 100,000 operations in 1969.)

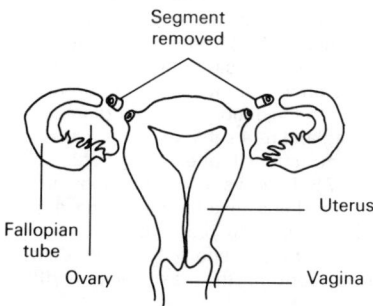

Tubal ligation

Segment removed

Uterus

Fallopian tube

Ovary

Vagina

- The abortion ratio (number of abortions per 1,000 live births) increased from 180 in 1972 to 195 in 1973.

- More than four out of five abortions were performed in the first trimester, most often by suction or D&C.

- Approximately 25% of the reported 1973 abortions were obtained outside the woman's home state.

- Approximately one-third of the women obtaining abortions were less than 20 years old, another third were between 20 and 25, and the remaining third over 25 years of age.

- In all states where data were available, about 25% of the women obtaining abortions were married.

- White women obtained 68% of all reported abortions, but nonwhite women had abortion ratios about one-third greater than white women.

The 1973 Supreme Court Decision

Nonrestrictive conditions have theoretically existed throughout all 50 states since January 22, 1973, the date of the Supreme Court decision.

However, a recent survey of abortion needs and services by the Alan Guttmacher Institute found only 15% of public hospitals across the country provide abortion services although they provide other reproductive health treatment.

- The principal impact of the decision was to permit a small number of nonhospital clinics to function and to account for more than half of all U.S. abortions.

- While abortion services, like all services, are generally more available in metropolitan areas than in rural areas, in scores of smaller and medium sized metropolitan areas not one abortion was performed in the five quarters following the Supreme Court decision.

- About a quarter of a million low income women at minimum, and 200,000 adolescents who needed abortions, could not obtain them in 1975. For many women,

this denial of treatment forces them to travel to another country or state—or to turn to an illegal abortionist. Another factor that contributes to the maldistribution of services is that Medicaid financing of abortions is often inadequate; in eleven of fourteen states reporting data to the Guttmacher Institute survey, less than 30% of the need for low income women was met.

Federal Direction

In 1977 Joseph A. Califano, Jr., secretary of Health, Education and Welfare, told Congress: I believe that federal funds should not be used for providing abortions, but if the courts decide that as a constitutional right in this country there is an entitlement to federal funds for abortion, I will enforce the law.

Congress has since passed legislation limiting the use of Federal money for abortions to cases in which the life of the mother was endangered or in which she was a victim of rape or incest.

The restriction cut deeply into the $45 million to $55 million spent each year to pay for some 250,000 to 300,000 abortions, most performed under the Medicaid program for the poor.

Numbers and Methods of Abortion

Methods most frequently used in the United States to induce abortion during the first trimester of pregnancy are suction (vacuum aspiration) or dilatation and curetage (D&C). Abortions in the second trimester are usually performed by replacing part of the amniotic fluid that surrounds the fetus with a concentrated salt solution (saline abortion), which usually induces labor 24 to 48 hours later. Other second trimester methods are hysterotomy, a surgical entry into the uterus; hysterectomy, removal of the uterus; and, recently, the injection into the uterine cavity of a prostaglandin, a substance that causes muscular contractions that expel the fetus.

In 1975 there were an estimated 1,000,000 illegal abortions in addition to the estimated 750,000 legal and reported abortions in the U.S.A. Of those reported to the Center for Disease Control, the vast majority (83% in

1973) were performed by the end of the 12th week of gestation when abortion is safest.

There were only 24 maternal deaths reported as resulting from these abortions, half of which were from the relatively rare abortions performed at 16–20 weeks of gestation.

The majority of all legal abortions (61%) were for women ages 15–24.

Over two-thirds (68%) were for women who were not married at the time either because they had never married or were separated, divorced or widowed.

Figure 27-3   Abortion Patterns: U.S. and Abroad. Legal abortions per 1,000 women aged 15–44. Selected countries, 1968–74 (Semilog scale)

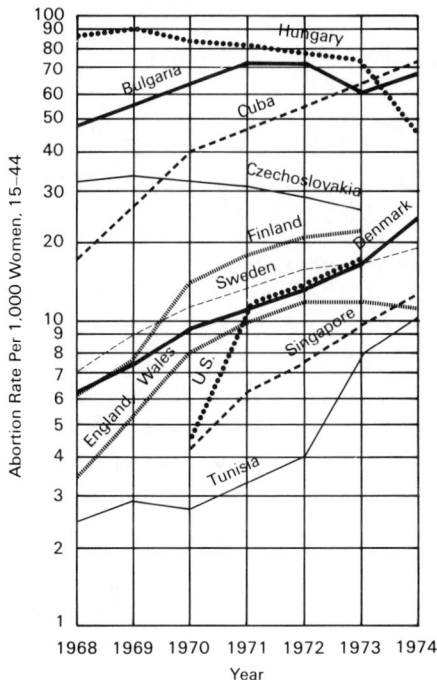

Source: House Appropriations Committee Hearings, 1977.

Table 27-13   Reported legal abortions, by age and marital status, 1973

Age and marital status	Percent distribution
Age	
Total from age-reporting states	100.0
Under 15 years	1.5
15–19 years	30.0
20–24 years	30.8
25–29 years	17.1
30–34 years	9.6
35–39 years	5.3
40 years and over	2.1
Age unknown	3.5
Marital Status	
Total from marital status-reporting states	100.0
Married	25.6
Unmarried	67.9
Marital status unknown	6.5

Source: Center for Disease Control, DHEW.

Table 27-14   Number of reported legal abortions and maternal deaths rate per 100,000 abortions (1973)

Period of gestation and method of abortion	Number of abortions	Maternal death rate per 100,000 abortions
Period of gestation		
Total	615,831	3.9
Under 8 weeks	222,100	0.0
9–10 weeks	181,326	1.7
11–12 weeks	110,178	3.6
13–15 weeks	42,604	9.4
16–20 weeks	49,193	24.4
21 weeks and over	10,430	9.6
Method of abortion		
Total	615,831	3.9
Curettage	544,402	1.1
Suction	461,369	1.3
Sharp	83,033	0.0
Amniotic fluid exchange	63,852	21.9
Hysterotomy/hysterectomy	4,117	72.9
Other	3,460	28.9

Source: Center for Disease Control, DHEW.

Abortion Patterns

Table 27-15 Reported legal abortions by age: selected status,* 1974

State	<15 No.	<15 %	15-19 No.	15-19 %	20-24 No.	20-24 %	25-29 No.	25-29 %	30-34 No.	30-34 %	35-39 No.	35-39 %	40 No.	40 %	Unknown No.	Unknown %	Total No.	Total %
Alaska	21	2.0	365	35.6	301	29.4	170	16.6	101	9.9	42	4.1	15	1.5	10	1.0	1,025	100.0
Arkansas	47	2.8	612	36.1	482	28.5	242	14.3	169	10.0	102	6.0	40	2.4	0	0.0	1,694	100.0
California	1,973	1.5	45,409	33.4	42,111	31.0	24,146	17.8	12,444	9.2	6,325	4.7	2,093	1.5	1,261	0.9	135,762	100.0
Colorado	133	1.5	2,953	32.7	3,207	35.5	1,495	16.6	694	7.7	388	4.3	139	1.5	18	0.2	9,027	100.0
Connecticut[1]	59	0.8	1,877	26.5	2,384	33.7	1,358	19.2	638	9.0	460	6.5	224	3.2	83	1.2	7,083	100.0
Dist. of Col.	369	1.6	5,999	26.4	7,775	34.3	4,236	18.7	1,848	8.1	942	4.2	387	1.7	1,132	5.0	22,688	100.0
Georgia	435	2.0	7,053	32.0	6,893	31.3	3,781	17.2	1,874	8.5	897	4.1	287	1.3	789	3.6	22,009	100.0
Hawaii	38	0.9	991	23.8	1,435	34.5	837	20.1	453	10.9	270	6.5	132	3.2	2	0.0	4,158	100.0
Illinois	270	0.8	8,614	25.8	10,765	32.3	6,290	18.8	3,750	11.2	2,116	6.3	896	2.7	669	2.0	33,370	100.0
Indiana	123	2.0	1,999	33.2	1,798	29.8	1,004	16.7	576	9.6	353	5.9	148	2.5	28	0.5	6,029	100.0
Kansas	238	2.3	4,408	43.3	2,873	28.2	1,334	13.1	698	6.9	420	4.1	194	1.9	6	0.1	10,171	100.0
Kentucky[2]	199	4.0	1,898	37.7	1,678	33.3	723	14.4	295	5.9	173	3.4	63	1.3	4	0.1	5,033	100.0
Louisiana[3]	17	1.7	331	34.0	317	32.5	157	16.1	86	8.8	33	3.4	24	2.5	9	0.9	974	100.0
Maryland	445	2.8	6,225	39.0	4,544	28.4	2,421	15.2	1,346	8.4	708	4.4	277	1.7	9	0.1	15,975	100.0
Minnesota[4]	120	1.4	2,992	34.3	3,237	37.1	1,170	13.4	609	7.0	392	4.5	212	2.4	0	0.0	8,732	100.0
Mississippi	3	2.1	40	27.9	40	28.6	23	16.4	18	12.9	11	7.9	6	4.3	0	0.0	140	100.0
Missouri[5]	174	2.2	2,369	29.7	2,599	32.6	1,390	17.4	784	9.8	465	5.8	202	2.5	2	0.0	7,983	100.0
Montana[3]	7	1.0	273	37.3	227	31.0	106	14.5	66	9.0	32	4.4	19	2.6	2	0.3	732	100.0
Nebraska	57	1.8	1,204	38.9	1,020	33.0	364	11.8	225	7.3	158	5.1	66	2.1	0	0.0	3,094	100.0
Nevada	70	4.3	457	28.3	541	33.5	273	16.9	135	8.4	87	5.4	24	1.5	27	1.7	1,614	100.0
New Hampshire	11	1.6	253	37.9	196	29.3	105	15.7	56	8.4	32	4.8	14	2.1	1	0.1	668	100.0
New York	1,715	1.1	41,202	25.5	49,887	30.9	33,188	20.5	20,026	12.4	10,806	6.7	4,147	2.6	550	0.3	161,521	100.0
(City)	(1,219)	(1.0)	(28,439)	(23.5)	(37,691)	(31.2)	(26,545)	(22.0)	(15,577)	(12.9)	(8,060)	(6.7)	(2,852)	(2.4)	(446)	(0.4)	(120,829)	(100.0)
(Upstate)	(496)	(1.2)	(12,763)	(31.4)	(12,196)	(30.0)	(6,643)	(16.3)	(4,449)	(10.9)	(2,746)	(6.7)	(1,295)	(3.2)	(104)	(0.3)	(40,692)	(100.0)
N. Carolina	388	2.4	5,791	35.2	4,805	29.2	2,708	16.4	1,597	9.7	788	4.8	341	2.1	45	0.3	16,463	100.0
Oregon	129	1.5	3,193	36.3	2,794	31.8	1,450	16.5	714	8.1	348	4.0	136	1.5	30	0.3	8,794	100.0
Pennsylvania[4]	706	1.9	12,682	33.3	12,351	32.4	5,835	15.3	3,550	9.3	2,024	5.3	829	2.2	133	0.3	38,110	100.0
Rhode Island	34	1.2	849	29.6	868	30.3	526	18.3	312	10.9	191	6.7	80	2.8	7	0.2	2,867	100.0
S. Carolina	76	2.0	1,186	31.5	1,242	33.0	592	15.7	345	9.2	156	4.1	60	1.6	103	2.7	3,760	100.0
S. Dakota	13	0.8	588	36.7	588	36.7	165	10.3	117	7.3	51	3.2	40	2.5	39	2.4	1,601	100.0
Tennessee	150	2.0	2,653	35.8	2,434	32.9	1,075	14.5	615	8.3	309	4.2	125	1.7	45	0.6	7,406	100.0
Utah[6]	10	0.8	331	27.8	419	35.2	200	16.8	97	8.2	60	5.0	23	1.9	49	4.1	1,189	100.0
Vermont	17	0.9	642	33.3	664	34.4	326	16.9	170	8.8	84	4.4	27	1.4	0	0.0	1,930	100.0
Virginia	328	2.3	5,205	36.2	4,373	30.4	2,256	15.7	1,233	8.6	677	4.7	290	2.0	10	0.1	14,372	100.0
Washington	255	1.4	6,553	36.0	5,887	32.4	2,971	16.3	1,405	7.7	789	4.3	313	1.7	12	0.1	18,185	100.0
Total	8,630	1.5	177,196	30.9	180,735	31.5	102,917	17.9	57,046	9.9	30,689	5.3	11,873	2.1	5,073	0.9	574,159	100.0

*All states with data available (33). [1]Based on distribution of data from special health department sample of total abortions reported. April–December. [2]Based on distribution of data from 1 facility reporting approximately 85% of total abortions. [3]July–December. [4]Based on distribution of data from state health department, partial year reporting. [5]Based on distribution of data from 1 facility reporting approximately 80% of total abortions. [6]April–December.

Source: Center for Disease Control. August 1976.

Attitudes Toward Abortion

Public Attitudes Toward Abortion *

Table 27-16   Making abortions up to three months' pregnancy legal

	Favor	Oppose	Not sure
1976	54%	39%	7%
1972	48	43	9

Key segment analysis on abortion issue

	%	%	%
Nationwide	54	39	7
By religion			
Catholic	41	53	6
Protestant	54	39	7
Jewish	84	9	7
By education			
8th grade or less	27	56	17
High school	49	43	8
College	68	29	3
By political philosophy			
Conservative	48	46	6
Middle of the road	52	39	9
Liberal	71	25	4
By age			
18–29	62	30	8
30–49	57	38	5
50 and over	44	47	9
By sex			
Men	55	37	8
Women	52	41	7

Nurses' Attitudes Toward Abortion * *

(Estimates are that 10–25% of American women have had abortions. A 1969 survey by *Psychology Today* found that 14% of responding women had had *illegal* abortions.)

Have you ever had an abortion?

Age is a factor: incidence of abortions among nurses over 50 years of age is highest; 17% said they'd had an abortion. Only 8% of the nurses under age 22 say they've had one. For nurses between 22 and 50, the abortion rate is 11%. Separated and divorced nurses show a higher abortion rate than single or married nurses.

* Source: Harris Survey, April 12, 1976.
* * Source: *Nursing '75,* September. (Survey of 10,000 readers.)

Religious denomination also is a factor. Only 8% of the Roman Catholic nurses report having had an abortion, as compared to 11% of the Protestants and about 15% of the Jewish, others and no denomination nurses. The more religious a nurse is, the less likely she is to have had an abortion: 5% of the very religious nurses have, 10% of the moderately religious have, 12% of the slightly religious have, and 17% of the not-at-all-religious nurses have had an abortion.

Have you ever assisted in an abortion procedure?

Eighteen percent of all respondents have, but only 11% of the nurses in the Midwest have. The highest proportion of nurses who assisted was in the West (30%).

Regardless of denomination, very religious nurses tend just as strongly to believe a fetus has rights at conception (70%) or when viable outside the womb (19%). For example, 66% of the very frequent church attenders and 60% of the frequent attenders believe a fetus has rights from the moment of conception.

Attitudes toward the rights of a fetus also are very strongly related to a nurse's self-rating of liberalism-conservatism. Very conservative nurses tend to believe that a fetus has rights at conception, whereas very liberal nurses tend to believe the fetus has rights when it is viable or at birth.

Is abortion justified when a mother's life is endangered by the pregnancy? Forty-five percent of the nurses who believe that a fetus has rights at conception nevertheless approve of abortion. There is a dramatic jump in approval (95%) with nurses who believe rights begin when the fetus can become viable and a nearly unanimous approval (98%) by nurses who believe such rights begin at birth.

In the survey, nurses between 23 and 34 years of age also were the most likely to approve of abortion for any of the discretionary reasons, but younger nurses—17 to 22 years of age—tended to be just as disapproving as older nurses over 35. Perhaps this reflects their lower likelihood of sexual involvement; women most sexually involved (and hence possibly in need of abortion) tend to be most liberal about abortion.

Disapproval of abortion for rape victims, however, is relatively high among Roman Catholic nurses (39%). But it is just as high among very religious and very frequent church-going nurses, regardless of religious denomina-

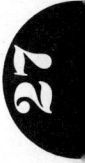

Student Attitudes Toward Abortion

Table 27-17 **"Abortion should be permitted whenever desired by the Mother"**

	Strongly agree	Percentages (rounded off)			Strongly disagree
		Agree	Undecided	Disagree	
Nursing students	21	28	17	20	15
Registered nurses	12	19	11	40	18
Medical students	44	28	7	11	11
College students	45	21	8	12	13

Source: H. Lief and T. Payne, "Sexuality—Knowledge and Attitudes," *American Journal of Nursing,* November 1975. © American Journal of Nursing Company (Survey of 1,774 nursing students and 828 R.N.s—1.4% male.)

tion. Also, 40% of the conservative nurses do not approve of abortion when a woman has been raped.

L.P.N.s are the least likely to approve of abortion (29%) when the child is not wanted, followed by diploma R.N.s (35% approve) and student nurses (35%).

Nurses who disapprove of abortion are not only the most likely to refuse to care for an abortion patient but they also are much less likely to be assigned to care for such patients.

Ob/Gyn nurses are the most likely to be assigned to abortion patient care, and 67% of Ob/Gyn nurses have never refused such assignments. But these nurses have a moral conflict on their hands; most Ob/Gyn nurses (67%) do not approve of abortion for discretionary reasons, such as the child isn't wanted or can't be afforded. Ob/Gyn nurses lead all other nursing specialties in saying fetal rights begin at conception (55% vs. 45% for all nurses), and the least likely to believe that rights begin at birth (10% of the Ob/Gyn nurses vs. 20% of all nurses).

Child Abuse*

How Many Abused?

According to Vincent De Francis, director of the Children's Division of the American Humane Association, some 10,000 children are severely battered each year; at least 50,000 to

75,000 are sexually abused; 100,000 are neglected physically, morally or educationally and 100,000 suffer emotional neglect. Abraham Levine reports that neglect is estimated to be 2½ to 20 times more prevalent than abuse, with estimates ranging between 500,000 and 2,000,000 incidents a year. David Gil and John Noble, however, place the upper limits of physical abuse at least eight times higher than De Francis' overall estimate and twice as high as Levine's maximum estimate of neglect: approximately 2,500,000 to 4,000,000 incidents of abuse annually, or about 13,000 to 21,000 incidents per million population in the United States.

A Closer Look in Connecticut

No one knows the true incidence of child molestation in the United States today. In Connecticut, for example, passage of an expanded child abuse reporting law which involves a $500 fine for mandated reporters who fail to report suspected child abuse, resulted in 1,957 reported cases in fiscal year 1974—an increase of nearly 200% over the preceding fiscal year. A breakdown of the total by reporting source is shown in Table 27-18 below.

In fiscal years 1973 and 1974 in Connecticut, the relationship of the perpetrator to the child in all cases of suspected abuse was that of a parent or a parent-substitute in 80% of the cases. The most frequently named perpetrator in cases of sexual abuse is the father or a male relative or boyfriend.

The lack of preparation and willingness of many physicians to assist patients with sexual problems in general has often been noted.

*Source: DHEW, 1975.

Table 27-18   Suspected abuse cases of children reported in Connecticut*

	Physicians	Hospitals	Police	Schools	Social workers	CCWA care-line	Others	Total
F.Y. 1973								
number	37	205	107	122	65	* *	133	669
Percent	5.5%	30.6%	16%	18.2%	9.8%	* *	19.9%	100%
F.Y. 1974								
number	98	396	456	401	327	104	175	1957
Percent	5%	20.3%	23.3%	20.5%	16.7%	5.3%	8.9%	100%

*Connecticut State Welfare Department statistics.
* *A statewide toll-free child abuse hotline has been operated by the Connecticut Child Welfare Association, a private citizen's organization, since October 1, 1973.
Source: DHEW, 1975.

Characteristics of Abused Children

Abused or neglected children are likely to share at least several of the following characteristics:

- They appear to be different from other children in physical or emotional makeup, or their parents inappropriately describe them as being "different" or "bad."
- They seem unduly afraid of their parents.
- They may often bear welts, bruises, untreated sores, or other skin injuries.
- Their injuries seem to be inadequately treated.
- They show evidence of overall poor care.
- They are given inappropriate food, drink or medication.
- They exhibit behavioral extremes, for example, crying often, or crying very little and showing no real expectation of being comforted; being excessively fearful; seeming fearless of adult authority; being unusually aggressive and destructive, or extremely passive and withdrawn.
- Some are wary of physical contact, especially when it is initiated by an adult; they become apprehensive when an adult approaches another child, particularly one who is crying. Others are inappropriately hungry for affection, yet may have difficulty relating to children and adults. Based on their past experiences, these children cannot risk getting too close to others.
- They may exhibit a sudden change in behavior, for example, displaying regressive behavior—pants wetting; thumb sucking; frequent whining; becoming disruptive; or becoming uncommonly shy and passive.
- They take over the role of the parent, being

protective or otherwise attempting to take care of the parent's needs.
- They have learning problems that cannot be diagnosed. If a child's academic, IQ and medical tests indicate no abnormalities but still the child cannot meet normal expectations, the answer may well be problems in the home—one of which might be abuse or neglect. Particular attention should be given to the child whose attention wanders and who easily becomes self-absorbed.
- They are habitually truant or late to school. Frequent or prolonged absences sometimes result when a parent keeps an injured child at home until the evidence of abuse disappears. In other cases, truancy indicates lack of parental concern or ability to regulate the child's schedule.
- In some cases, they frequently arrive at school too early and remain after classes rather than going home.
- They are always tired and often sleep in class.
- They are inappropriately dressed for the weather. Children who never have coats or shoes in cold weather are receiving subminimal care. On the other hand, those who regularly wear long sleeves or high necklines on hot days may be dressed to hide bruises, burns, or other marks of abuse.

Characteristics of Parents of Abused Children

The parents of an abused or neglected child *may* exhibit any of the following traits:

- They are isolated from family supports such as friends, relatives, neighbors, and com-

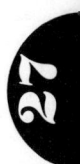

munity groups; they consistently fail to keep appointments, discourage social contact, and never participate in school activities or events.

- They seem to trust no one.
- They themselves were abused or neglected as children.
- They are reluctant to give information about the child's injuries or condition. When questioned, they are unable to explain, or they offer farfetched or contradictory explanations.
- They respond inappropriately to the seriousness of the child's condition, either by overreacting, seeming hostile or antagonistic when questioned even casually; or by underreacting, showing little concern or awareness and seeming more preoccupied with their own problems than those of the child.
- They refuse to consent to diagnostic studies.
- They fail or delay to take the child for medical care—for routine checkups, for optometric or dental care, or for treatment of injury or illness. In taking an injured child for medical care, they may choose a different hospital or doctor each time.
- They are overcritical of the child and seldom, if ever, discuss the child in positive terms.
- They have unrealistic expectations of the child, expecting or demanding behavior that is beyond the child's years or ability.
- They believe in the necessity of harsh punishment for children.
- They seldom touch or look at the child; they ignore the child's crying or react with impatience.
- They keep the child confined—perhaps in a crib or playpen—for overlong periods of time.
- They seem to lack understanding of children's physical, emotional, and psychological needs.
- They appear to be misusing alcohol or drugs.
- They cannot be located.
- They appear to lack control, or fear losing control.
- They are of borderline intelligence, psychotic, or psychopathic. While such diagnoses are the responsibility of a psy-

chiatrist, psychologist, or psychiatric social worker, even the lay observer can note whether the parent seems intellectually capable of child-rearing, exhibits generally irrational behavior, or seems excessively cruel and sadistic.

Evidence of Physical Abuse

More specifically, physically abused children will probably fit some of the following descriptions:

- They bear signs of injury—bruises, welts, contusions, cuts, burns, fractures, lacerations, strap marks, swellings, lost teeth. The list of possibilities is long and unpleasant. While internal injuries are seldom detectable without a hospital workup, anyone in close contact with children should be alert to multiple injuries, a history of repeated injury, new injuries added to old, and untreated injuries—especially in the very young child.
- The older child may attribute the injury to an improbable cause, lying for fear of parental retaliation. The younger child, on the other hand, may be unaware that severe beating is unacceptable and may admit to having been abused.
- They are behavior problems. Especially among adolescents, chronic and unexplainable misbehavior should be investigated as possible evidence of abuse. Some children come to expect abusive behavior as the only kind of attention they can receive, and so act in a way that invites abuse. Others have been known to break the law deliberately so as to come under the jurisdiction of the courts to obtain protection from their parents.
- Their parents sometimes provide such necessities for the child as adequate food and clean clothes; but they anger quickly, have unrealistic expectations of the child, use inappropriate discipline, and are overly critical and rejecting of the child.

Sexual Abuse

Sexual abuse, a form of physical abuse, ranges from exposure and fondling to intercourse, incest, and rape. Approximately 75% of the offenders, usually males, are known to the child or the child's family. Some 90% of the victims are girls, from infants through adolescents.

Since the sexually abused child lacks the telltale symptoms of battering, sexual abuse is difficult to identify and even harder to prove. Short of the child telling someone, the best indicators are a sudden change in behavior and signs of emotional disturbance. The child, for example, may unexplainably begin to cry easily and seem excessively nervous. Dr. Vincent De Francis reported in 1969 that two-thirds of the children detected in a three-year study of sexual abuse in New York City evidenced some degree of emotional disturbance.

Physical Neglect

Dr. Abraham Levine notes that, to some extent, neglect "defies exact definition, but it may be regarded as the failure to provide the essentials for normal life, such as food, clothing, shelter, care and supervision, and protection from assault." Physically neglected children tend to exhibit at least several of the characteristics below:

- They are often hungry. They may go without breakfast, and have neither food nor money for lunch. Some take the lunch money or food of other children and hoard whatever they obtain.
- They show signs of malnutrition—paleness, low weight relative to height, lack of body tone, fatigue, inability to participate in physical activities, and lack of normal strength and endurance.
- They are usually irritable.
- They show evidence of inadequate home management. They are unclean and unkempt; their clothes are torn and dirty; and they are often unbathed. As mentioned earlier, they may lack proper clothing for weather conditions, and their school attendance may be irregular. In addition, these children may frequently be ill and may exhibit a generally repressed personality, inattentiveness, and withdrawal.
- They are in obvious need of medical attention for such correctable conditions as poor eyesight, dental care, and immunizations.
- They lack parental supervision at home. The child, for example, may frequently return

from school to an empty house. While the need for adult supervision is, of course, relative to both the situation and the maturity of the child, it is generally held that a child younger than 12 should always be supervised by an adult or at least have immediate access to a concerned adult when necessary.

- Their parents are either unable or unwilling to provide appropriate care. Some neglecting parents are mentally deficient; most lack knowledge of parenting skills and tend to be discouraged, depressed, and frustrated with their role as parents.

Emotional Abuse or Neglect

Emotional abuse or neglect is far more difficult to identify than its physical counterparts. Such maltreatment includes the "parent's lack of love and proper direction, inability to accept a child with his potentialities as well as his limitations, ... (and) failure to encourage the child's normal development by assurance of love and acceptance." The parents of an emotionally abused or neglected child may be overly harsh and critical, demanding excessive academic, athletic or social performance. Conversely, they may withhold physical and verbal contact, care little about the child's successes and failures, and fail to provide necessary guidance and praise. Though emotional maltreatment may occur alone, it is almost always present in cases of physical abuse or neglect. The emotional damage to children who are physically abused or whose basic physical needs are unattended is often more serious than the bodily damage.

The indicators of emotional maltreatment are often intangible, but sooner or later the consequences become evident. The child may react either by becoming "hyperaggressive, disrupting and demanding ... shouting his cry for help," or by becoming "withdrawn ... whispering his cry for help." In a class of psychologically healthy children, the emotionally abused child often stands out unmistakably. Emotional maltreatment has a decidedly adverse effect on a child's learning ability, achievement level, and general development. The strongest indicators are unaccountable learning difficulties and changed or unusual behavior patterns.

States in which Nurses must Report Child Abuse Symptoms*

State

Alabama	Nebraska
Alaska	Nevada
† Arizona	† New Hampshire
Arkansas	† New Jersey
California	New Mexico
Colorado	New York
Connecticut	North Carolina
Delaware	North Dakota
† D. of C.	Ohio
Florida	Oklahoma
Georgia	Oregon
Hawaii	Pennsylvania
Idaho	† Rhode Island
Illinois	† South Carolina
† Indiana	† South Dakota
Iowa	† Tennessee
Kansas	† Texas
Kentucky	† Utah
Louisiana	† Vermont
† Maine	Virginia
Maryland	Washington
Massachusetts	West Virginia
Michigan	Wisconsin
Minnesota	Wyoming
Mississippi	Guam
Missouri	Virgin Islands
Montana	

Under most state laws child abuse symptoms must be reported. Only those states indicated (†) have no such provision for nurses.

*Source: DHEW data, 1974.

Adoptions**

The majority of petitions for adoption are granted to related individuals—parents, step-parents and other relatives. For both related and nonrelated petitioners, most of the adopted children for whom race/ethnic group was reported were of the white race. (Race/ethnic group was not reported for a substantial proportion). The majority of children adopted by unrelated petitioners for whom birth status was reported were born out of wedlock. Agency placements exceeded in-

**Source: National Center for Social Statistics, DHEW, April 1976.

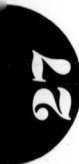

dependent placements in all but two of the states reporting type of placement; there were more placements by public agencies than by private or independent.

Age of Adopted Children

The median age for adopted children ranged from less than one month in six states to 10.3 months in Delaware.

Table 27-19   Age (at time of placement) of children adopted by unrelated petitioners by state, 1974

State	Median age in months
Alabama	4.7
Arkansas	4.3
Delaware	10.3
Florida	2.5
Georgia	3.2
Hawaii	0.5
Indiana	1.6
Iowa	0.5
Kansas	0.5
Kentucky	5.7
Louisiana	0.5
Maine	3.5
Maryland	6.3
Massachusetts	5.3
Michigan	5.4
Minnesota	5.3
Missouri	2.9
Nevada	4.0
New Hampshire	2.8
New Jersey	4.5
New Mexico	0.5
New York	5.0
North Carolina	2.8
North Dakota	2.0
Oregon	3.9
Puerto Rico	2.0
South Dakota	2.5
Tennessee	3.2
Texas	1.3
Utah	0.5
Vermont	7.2
Virginia	4.8
Washington	3.6
West Virginia	4.9

Who Adopts Children?

Table 27-20   Accepted adoption petitions by state, 1974

State	Total adopted	Unrelated petitioner (%)	Own parent stepparent (%)	Other relative (%)	Relationship not reported (%)
		Children adopted by . . .			
Alabama	2,463	18	58	20	4
Arkansas	898	34	48	18	1
California	13,559	32	68		
Connecticut	713	74	24	2	
Delaware	263	31	63	6	
District of Columbia	325	63	30	7	
Florida	6,718	26	66	8	1
Georgia	2,551	39	49	11	
Hawaii	887	20	56	24	
Indiana	4,860	31	61	8	
Iowa	2,680	33	62	4	
Kansas	889	80	2	15	3
Kentucky	1,398	36	47	14	2
Louisiana	2,796	30	60	11	
Maine	1,075	25	40	4	31
Maryland	2,332	29	63	8	
Massachusetts	1,508	78	13	8	1
Michigan	7,177	29	40	3	27
Minnesota	3,045	30	48	2	
Missouri	1,982	33	57	6	3
Nevada	315	37	61	3	
New Hampshire	716	30	65	3	2
New Jersey	2,631	37	57	6	
New Mexico	980	27	56	15	2
New York	8,054	47	48	5	
North Carolina	4,061	33	52	15	
North Dakota	552	35	63	2	1
Ohio	7,847	36			1
Oklahoma	810	85	2	13	
Oregon	2,768	28	66	5	
Pennsylvania	5,963	35	60	5	
Puerto Rico	279	40	27	32	
South Dakota	521	43	54	3	
Tennessee	1,477	34	55	10	1
Texas	3,608	31	52	13	4
Utah	385	91		8	1
Vermont	430	38	58	3	1
Virginia	3,333	34	57	7	2
Washington	3,093	29	62	5	4
West Virginia	1,352	20	73	8	
Wyoming	580	—	—	—	100

Birth Status and Placement Process of Adopted Children

Table 27-21 Children adopted by unrelated petitioners, by birth status and placement method, by state, 1974

State	Total	Birth status			Type of placement		
					By agency		Independent
		Born out of wedlock	Born in wedlock	Not reported	Public	Private	parent relative or others
Alabama	438	182	66	190	263	26	133
Arkansas	302	223	78	1	188	11	98
California	4,337	—	—	4,337	1,965	591	1,731
Connecticut	528	—	—	528	—	—	—
Delaware	82	53	29	—	24	51	7
District of Columbia	205	—	—	205	—	—	—
Florida	1,726	1,327	336	63	263	809	593
Georgia	999	701	288	10	497	96	382
Hawaii	178	136	37	5	26	52	98
Indiana	1,511	1,131	319	61	661	404	238
Iowa	889	626	202	61	147	476	257
Kansas	708	447	125	136	180	217	305
Kentucky	508	320	76	112	324	101	73
Louisiana	826	722	94	10	99	422	268
Maine	269	181	38	50	100	62	—
Maryland	678	511	148	19	328	138	149
Massachusetts	1,171	878	231	62	281	825	64
Michigan	2,080	1,306	774	—	421	1,322	—
Minnesota	1,537	1,146	189	202	294	1,164	78
Missouri	657	455	151	51	397	151	106
Nevada	115	72	43	—	90	3	21
New Hampshire	213	138	39	36	86	102	—
New Jersey	980	774	189	17	511	160	306
New Mexico	260	220	33	7	89	58	108
New York	3,825	3,064	507	254	1,419	1,410	916
North Carolina	1,342	1,098	205	39	642	356	343
North Dakota	191	163	15	13	8	179	2
Ohio	2,816	—	—	2,816	—	—	—
Oklahoma	688	—	—	688	—	—	—
Oregon	784	480	255	49	247	204	322
Pennsylvania	2,088	—	—	2,088	854	617	563
Puerto Rico	112	68	39	5	21	7	80
South Dakota	224	187	36	1	85	105	34
Tennessee	508	406	100	2	211	97	139
Texas	1,109	686	222	201	241	471	171
Utah	349	292	45	12	57	238	48
Vermont	164	79	57	28	112	49	2
Virginia	1,149	824	304	21	649	219	281
Washington	901	611	206	84	265	362	235
West Virginia	266	135	61	70	160	—	35

Sexuality

Nurses Knowledge and Attitudes Toward Sex*

Education in human sexuality has lagged in nursing schools. At the beginning of this decade, the Sex Information and Education Council of the United States (SIECUS) serveyed 176 baccalaureate schools of nursing. Only one responding school offered a course in human sexuality, and that was an elective. In five schools, such courses were available as electives outside the school of nursing.

Although all nursing schools appeared to offer some minimal content on human sexuality (as part of other programs), the emphasis was almost exclusively on reproductive biology.

The Sex Knowledge and Attitude Test (SKAT), designed by Lief and Reed and revised with the help of Ebert, was developed as a teaching and research instrument.

Among the various groups tested with SKAT, two nursing groups were compared with three other groups: 1,774 nursing students (24 or 1.6% were male), 828 registered nurses (9 or 1.4% were male), 1,104 female medical students and 1,243 female college students.

A comparison of nursing students with registered nurses indicated that nursing students were more knowledgeable and more liberal on all four attitude scales of the SKAT. This difference was most marked on attitudes toward heterosexual relations and masturbation. Both nurses' groups were significantly

* Source: Adapted from "Sexuality—Knowledge and Attitudes" by Harold I. Lief and Tyana Payne, *American Journal of Nursing,* Nov. 1975. ©American Journal of Nursing Company.

less knowledgeable than the female medical students and were more conservative on all four attitude scales. The registered nurses did not possess significantly more information than did college students.

Although age might be considered to be the most important cause of the registered nurses' conservatism, in all likelihood, social class accounted for more of the differences in liberalism and conservatism between nursing students and registered nurses. Fifty-three percent of the nursing students' fathers were either professionals or executives, in contrast to 19% of the registered nurses' fathers. Forty-one percent of the fathers of nursing students but only 9% of the fathers of registered nurses were college graduates.

Kinsey in the 1940s reported that 65% of females masturbated, so one can easily believe that the current percentage is probably 75% or higher. [Of those experiencing] "mouth-genital sex-play," Kinsey reported an incidence of two-thirds among the married couples in his study. Twenty-eight percent of the nursing students and 53% of the registered nurses [thought such practices wrong].

"Certain conditions of mental and emotional instability are demonstrably caused by masturbation." Forty-six percent of female medical students still clung to this erroneous belief. Twenty-eight percent of the nursing students and 33% of the registered nurses still hold to this false belief.

Based on self-reports by male medical students, Mudd and Siegel report there was no correlation between personal sexual experience and the degree of anxiety (or, conversely, comfort) that students exhibited in various clinical situations such as breast, pelvic, or rectal examinations, or in sexual history taking. In other words, those with many coital experiences were as nervous as the "virgins."

Table 27-22   Selected sexual behaviors

Groups	Virgins	More than 5 coital partners	Never masturbated
Nursing students	35%	13%	31%
Registered nurses	15%	17%	32%
Medical students	19%	32%	18%
College students	42%	14%	29%

Table 27-23 Responses to statement: "premarital intercourse is morally undesirable"

	Percentages (rounded off)				
	Strongly agree	Agree	Undecided	Disagree	Strongly disagree
Nursing students	5	18	9	41	28
Registered nurses	21	35	12	27	4
Medical students	5	11	6	28	51
College students	6	14	7	34	39

Sex in the Hospital*

Side by side with the increased focus on human sexuality, there has been a growing consideration of sexuality as a legitimate component of patient care. Dr. Mary Calderone, director of the Sex Information and Education Council of the United States, reported recently a listing of about 80 workshops for health professionals; the World Health Organization has issued a technical report on the training of health professionals in human sexuality.

The attitudes of health personnel toward sexuality can have a significant impact on the quality of care in two areas: patient concerns and patient behavior.

Patients are seeking more sexual counseling from medical professionals, including nurses (especially nurses in the gynecological and obstetrical areas). Nurses are in a prime position to give counsel in such areas as family planning, abortion, the effects of gynecological conditions on sexual functions. As nurses may be confronted with questions of a frankly sexual nature, these confrontations may necessitate changes in attitude and willingness to accept sexual values quite different from their own—particularly in areas of abortion counseling, management of venereal disease and contraceptive counseling for unmarried young girls.

Even in areas seemingly unrelated to sexual functions, patients may have sexual concerns: whether sexual activity will affect their health; whether a particular treatment or surgical procedure will affect their ability to perform sexually. The freedom to ask such questions and the right to receive carefully deliberated answers are crucial for patients having

*Source: Adapted from "Sexuality in a Health Care Setting," by Gregg W. Downey, *Modern Health Care,* May 1976.

prostate surgery, hysterectomies and a host of other surgical procedures.

Patients' sexual behavior within the hospital setting enters the controversial realm of "patient's rights." According to Gregg W. Downey there are five sexual issues to be considered (particularly in caring for the elderly):

● Conjugal Privacy

In nursing homes and rehabilitation centers, a patient's right to periods of privacy has been well established, although it is honored more in theory than in fact. Similarly, it is no longer considered radical to suggest that health facilities should permit conjugal encounters, unless they are medically contraindicated.

● Homosexuality

Regarding homosexuality, the experts advise tolerance. Doctors and nurses who have difficulty dealing with homosexual patients should explore their own feelings. Most professional groups now acknowledge that there is nothing innately unhealthy about homosexuality and that homosexual patients should be accorded the same rights and privileges as heterosexual patients.

● Masturbation

Because masturbation is usually practiced with discretion, it has not been encountered regularly in most facilities. It would probably be encountered even less often if health personnel merely would knock on patients' doors and wait for a response before entering.

Discreet masturbation is generally accepted and sometimes recommended. In situations where a patient has no other sexual outlet, for example, masturbation is now considered a valuable means of preventing sexual dysfunction.

- Oral-genital Sex

  Oral-genital sex—and, indeed, all alternative forms of sexual function—usually surface as specific issues in health facilities only when patients are unable to engage in ordinary sexual activities. Short of abstinence, patients with spinal cord injuries, for example, frequently have no choice but to employ alternatives. The imposition of health professionals' arbitrary biases against such practices can markedly reduce the quality of life for disabled patients, say most of the experts.

- Sexual Interaction Between Patient and Staff

  Overt sexual interaction between patients and staff members is probably rarer than might generally be supposed. A gentle rebuff usually is all that's necessary when a patient "makes a pass" at a doctor or a nurse. Frequently, the patient is trying only to reassert the sexual identity that has been threatened as the result of institutionalization. If a nurse understands the behavior, or in the case of the elderly patient, if she understands there is a need for touching, she can get this across to the family and to other staff members.

American Sexual Myths*

MYTH: The male instinctively knows what the female wants and needs.

REALITY: Men in our society are burdened with the impossible responsibility of somehow supposing to know what the female likes and dislikes. This completely neglects the teaching aspects of sex. Part of good sex comes from sharing and teaching each partner about his/her likes and dislikes.

MYTH: It takes longer for the female to get turned on than the male.

REALITY: Physiologically, it takes both males and females 3–15 seconds as measured by erection in the male and lubrication in the female. Psychologically, either partner may desire unhurried, tender foreplay for a while.

MYTH: Lovemaking should always result in intercourse.

REALITY: A common complaint of females

is that males expect that touching will lead to intercourse. This negates the touching, kissing and holding that can be rewarding without intercourse.

MYTH: Intercourse should always result in orgasm for both partners.

REALITY: The orgasmic reflex can be triggered or inhibited by many things. One or both partners may really enjoy intercourse and choose not to have an orgasm.

MYTH: Simultaneous orgasm is the goal.

REALITY: It is a neat trick if you can have that kind of timing, but it has nothing to do with satisfactory and enjoyable sex.

MYTH: The "Big O" (orgasm)—bells ring, the sky shakes, and Sherman tanks come though.

REALITY: Orgasms vary tremendously from time to time and person to person, from very slight subjective feelings to very intense subjective feelings.

MYTH: If you have a clitoral orgasm, you are immature; vaginal orgasms are the only kind to have.

REALITY: We now know that the clitoris is the transmitter of the orgasmic reflex to the brain. The vagina actually has fewer nerve endings. The physiological reaction of the body is the same regardless of where the orgasm originates. Women do report some subjective difference between clitoral and vaginal orgasms. Again, the origin of the orgasm has no bearing on any kind of maturity or immaturity.

MYTH: It's the male's duty to *give* the woman an orgasm.

REALITY: Each person is responsible for his or her own orgasm. If a woman chooses not to have an orgasm, there is little the man can do because she can psychologically cut off the orgasmic reflex.

MYTH: The male knows or must know when and if the female has an orgasm.

REALITY: Some women are experts at faking orgasm. The only way the male is really going to know is to check it out with her.

MYTH: Now that women are becoming liberated, they are supposed to be supersexy and multiorgasmic.

REALITY: Women can *choose* when and how to be sexy. The goal of good sex is enjoyment and fun, not six orgasms in a row.

*Source: Andra J. Allen, "All American Sexual Myths, *American Journal of Nursing,* October 1975. ©American Journal of Nursing Company.

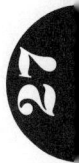

MYTH: The older you get, the more you should lose interest in sex.

REALITY: This is primarily a cultural myth. Physiologically, our body functions slow down with age, but barring debilitating illness, there is no reason why we cannot be sexually active until death.

MYTH: "Normal" sex . . .

REALITY: *Anything* is normal in sex, as long as it is consented to by the people involved.

MYTH: The evils of masturbation: you will wear out your organ, go blind, go crazy, grow hair on your palms.

REALITY: The sex organs can never be overused. Many people now consider masturbation a very beautiful, healthy way of getting in touch with their bodies and enjoying it.

MYTH: The longer the penis, the better the sex.

REALITY: Penis size has nothing to do with good sex. The vagina can expand or contract to accommodate any size penis.

Sexuality—Questions and Answers*

What are sperm?

Sperm are manufactured in the testicles located in the scrotum. During development, they pass through a complicated system of chambers and tubes and into the seminal vesicle (see drawing) where they are mixed with other fluids—which form semen—and stored until released through sexual climax.

Males produce sperm continuously from puberty to old age. Because new sperm are being manufactured each minute in the testicles, stored sperm are pushed out of the body naturally to make way for new sperm. These sperm are released by males during wet dreams, masturbation, and sexual intercourse.

Sperm cells can live in a woman's body for three to five days after they have been ejaculated. This means that it is even possible to have intercourse on Monday and become pregnant on Friday.

What is puberty and when does it happen?

Puberty is the time between childhood and physical adulthood when the body undergoes sexual and physiological changes. Most young people begin these changes at age nine or ten and continue until their mid-teens.

In the female, puberty is signaled by the onset of menstruation which means her ovaries are beginning to produce eggs. In the male, the first "wet" dream means puberty is underway and that his testicles are beginning to produce sperm.

In females, the ovaries produce eggs—usually one, approximately each month from puberty through age 45 to 55 except when a woman is pregnant.

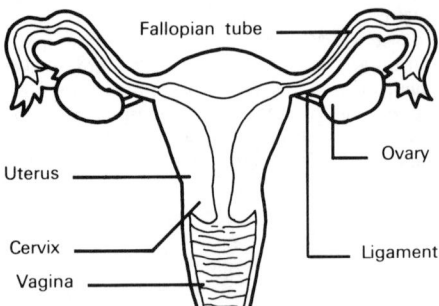

Bladder
Prostate
Penis
Seminal vesicle
Vas deferens
Testicle
Scrotum
Glans

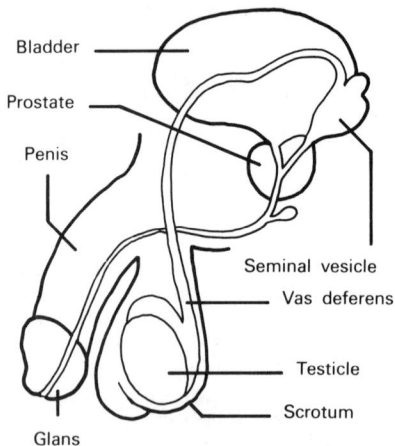

Fallopian tube
Uterus
Ovary
Cervix
Ligament
Vagina

What is menstruation?

It is the monthly shedding of the lining of the uterus after an egg cell has reached the uterus without fertilization taking place.

Because the uterus has been preparing for possible pregnancy, its lining has become spongy and full of extra blood and other tissue to nourish a developing embryo. If fertilization does not take place, the lining is not needed and is pushed out of the uterus.

"Periods" usually come monthly and last from three to seven days, although some women may be irregular. It's not unusual during adolescence for periods to happen once every three, four, five or six months.

What is a normal penis size?

There is no "normal" size. The erect penis varies from three or four to eight inches long—about six inches is average, regardless of its size when not erect. Penis size has nothing to do with sexual enjoyment for either partner.

What makes a penis erect?

When a male becomes sexually excited, the veins in his penis fill with blood causing the organ to grow larger and stiffen. After sexual climax the erection quickly subsides. Without a climax, the erection will subside gradually by itself.

Can sperm supply be used up?

No, not unless there has been an illness or an operation which interrupts sperm production. Sperm are continuously being manufactured in the testicles until old age.

Do boys need more sex than girls?

In general, boys are more easily sexually aroused than girls. But there is no evidence that boys need more sex than girls or that *not* having sexual intercourse is physically damaging to either sex. Sperm cells that are ejaculated to make room for new sperm cells will be released during a "wet" dream or by masturbation if a male does not have sexual intercourse.

How does a woman know she's pregnant?

The first sign of pregnancy is usually a missed menstrual period. If a woman has had sexual intercourse and suspects her missed menstrual period means pregnancy, she should go to her doctor, or a Planned Parenthood or other family planning clinic for a pregnancy test. This is the only sure way to tell; other symptoms of pregnancy vary for each individual. Worrying about being pregnant sometimes can delay menstruation although a woman may not be pregnant.

What is homosexuality?

Very little is known about what causes homosexuality—or for that matter, what causes heterosexuality (the preference for the opposite sex). It is known, however, that a child's sexual orientation is well established by the time he or she is an adolescent.

Sometimes during preadolescence and early adolescent years, boys and girls experiment sexually with friends of the same sex and some become concerned that they might be homosexuals. Both they and their parents should understand that for most children this is only a phase of development and that most will make primary emotional and physical relationships with the opposite sex as adults.

Sexual Dysfunction & Therapy*

The majority of sexual dysfunctions in men are secondary impotence, premature ejaculation and sometimes ejaculatory incompetence. In women the major complaint is failure to have orgasm. Another common complaint is painful coitus which tends to be associated with lack of orgasm.

Often clinic physicians are young, inexperienced residents who have little insight into the sexual complaint. The R.N., on the other hand, is likely to be a woman, older, married, with more experience than the resident and is a stable part of the clinic scene. As a result, when a patient has an apparent need for sex therapy, the R.N., oftentimes unwittingly, fills the vacuum.

Sex Therapy Clinics

Masters estimates that over 3,000 such clinics operate in the United States; many of them, however, are of questionable quality.

There is a center for marital and sex studies in Long Beach, Calif., that trains therapists. The Long Island Jewish-Hillside Medical Center, New Hyde Park, N.Y., has a training program under the direction of a physician cotherapist team trained by Masters and Johnson. (Incidentally, three of the original seven female cotherapists trained by Masters and Johnson were registered nurses.) And there are many other training centers throughout the country.

*Source: "Sexual Therapy and Nursing." Reprinted from *RN Magazine*, March 1975. Copyright ©1975 by Litton Industries, Inc. Published by Medical Economics Co., a Litton division, at Oradell, N.J. 07649. All rights reserved.

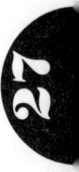

Breast Enlargement*

Some interesting insights into the importance of breast size have been a gained from the literature dealing with augmentation mammoplasty. It has been documented that small breast size has negative effects on women's sexual involvement. In a sample of 132 women having augmentation mammoplasty who were surveyed by questionnaire, 56% indicated that small breast size had adversely affected breast play; 30% indicated that it had affected their ability to have intercourse; 13% said that small breast size had interfered with their ability to have orgasm; and 10% said it had affected their decision to marry.

In all instances, the feelings of inadequacy were apparently within the patient herself, and not those of her partner. Using a means such as a padded bra was unacceptable to these women, and perhaps their responses were biased by their attitudes toward a prosthesis. After augmentation mammoplasty, 93% experienced increased self-confidence, 84% had strong feelings of self-adequacy, 74% had an increased interest in sex, 53% experienced an increased frequency in sexual intercourse, 69% perceived an improvement in the quality of their sexual intercourse, 52% reported an increased frequency of orgasm, and 78% indicated an increased desire for breast play. The investigators indicated that the implant used during the surgery should be incorporated as a part of the woman's body image. This usually required tactile and visual exploration by the woman of her own body.

Sex and the Elderly

In a 1976 workshop for nursing home operators conducted by the National Association of Social Workers and funded by the Department of Health, Education and Welfare, a proposal was entertained for providing "privacy rooms" in which aged persons could hold hands, pet or engage in sexual relations.

In defending his proposal Prof. E. Hargrove, a specialist in studies on aging, contended that segregation of the sexes and lack of privacy in institutions for older persons afford almost no opportunity for physical or emotional contact.

"I am not advocating copies of Hustler magazine and a water bed, but these people are human beings," he said." They enjoy petting, holding hands, kissing. All those things that make us feel good make them feel good, too. Age has nothing to do with the fact that you need nurture and comfort."

The professor conceded that some patients might abuse "privacy rooms," but he added, "Alcohol is abused also. Those who are capable of having sex should not be denied just because there might be a possibility of abuse."

Rape**

Caring for the Victim

Medical care should be administered to the rape victim in a most sensitive and sympathetic manner to help her begin to overcome the trauma of the experience. It must be remembered that the initial contacts the woman has with the police and health care professionals do affect the victim's ability to resolve her feelings about the attack upon her person.

The nurse must be involved in the admission of the rape victim to the hospital setting. If possible the woman is placed in a private area during the initial interview. A social worker should be called, but information already on the record should be transmitted by the nurse in order to reduce repeatedly asking the patient for the same information. The patient needs to be informed of the policies, procedures and forms that will be filed in this situation.

A general physical examination is conducted with special note of bruises, scratches, marks and wounds. The external genitalia are examined very carefully for blood, edema or trauma around the vaginal orifice. An internal gynecological examination with a non-lubricated speculum is also done so that the vaginal canal and cervix can be inspected. When pictures are to be taken, clear permission for this procedure and clear, careful identification of source must be done.

If the patient consents, specimens can be taken from the vaginal pool and cervix to

*Source: Nancy F. Woods, "Psychological Aspects of Breast Cancer," *JOGN*, September–October 1975.

**Source: "The Law, the Nurse and the Rape Victim" (Adapted from the article by Rita R. Wieczorek and Bernice H. Rosner in *Journal, NYSNA*, June 1976).

permit analysis for the presence of sperm. Three slides of material are taken in these situations: two from the vaginal pool and one from the cervix. All slides should be labeled with the patient's identification number and the anatomical location the specimens were taken from. Swabs used to obtain these specimens should also be labeled and saved in protective, sealed containers. The date and time the specimens were obtained should be clearly identified on the containers used to store these materials, along with the name of the patient and the person performing the tests.

A vaginal pool specimen should also be obtained for acid phosphatase and blood group antigen of semen determinations. These two tests, performed with the consent of the patient, are valuable in cases where the rapist has either a low sperm count or a vasectomy.

Some victims refuse to have specimens taken because at this time they feel they do not wish to press charges against the rapist. All sexually assaulted women should be encouraged to have these tests for sperm done because it is important evidence that they may want to use in the future. They may change their minds about the prosecution of the perpetrator.

A tranquilizer may be given to help the victim relax and sleep. It is natural for the assaulted woman to feel emotionally upset and nervous. This medication should be offered to the patient, when deemed necessary, because she may not feel comfortable requesting it.

It is important for the nurse in the emergency room to interview and gather data about the victim's pattern of contraception. The patient should be informed that the highest rate of pregnancy with unprotected intercourse occurs during the middle of the menstrual cycle. However, it should also be remembered that the incidence of pregnancy with rape is low.

When the sexually assaulted woman is at risk for pregnancy she should be given the following options:

1. To wait until five to six weeks have past from her last period and have a pregnancy test done. If necessary, an abortion may then be arranged.
2. To take the morning-after pill called Diethylstilbestrol (DES), 25 mg. given orally within 72 hours following unprotected in-

tercourse. DES 25 mg. is then taken for five consecutive days afterward to prevent pregnancy.

The morning-after pill may make the woman feel nauseated. An antiemetic may be given so the patient does not suffer from nausea. If the victim experiences headaches or dizziness from the medication, she should be instructed to seek medical care.

Diethylstilbestrol, although considered by authorities to be highly effective, may not work in preventing pregnancy. The drug itself may make the woman's period late. If the patient is one to two weeks late with menstruation she should have an immediate pregnancy test done.

The nurse must instruct the rape victim that the morning-after pill should not be considered an appropriate method of contraception for the rest of her cycle. Another method of contraception should be employed after the fifth day if the patient does not wish to conceive.

When the victim reports sodomy, specimens for sperm should be taken from her rectum with her consent. In cases of fellatio only, vaginal and anal specimens are not necessary. Venereal disease protection still needs to be considered.

Rape victims are potentially exposed to venereal disease, and in the emergency room they should be given penicillin or another antibiotic if they are allergic to penicillin. Women who develop itching or vaginal discharge post-penicillin therapy should be instructed by the nurse to notify a physician or seek medical care from a health source. Antibiotics are not always completely effective in preventing venereal disease, so the victim should be instructed to return to the clinic or her private physician's office for a gonorrhea test within two weeks and for a syphillis test within six weeks.

Tetanus toxoid may also be administered to the rape victim who suffers from cuts, scratches, or wounds. Where appropriate this immunization booster should be administered.

In a few cases, the rape victim may suffer from lacerations around the vaginal canal that are extensive enough to require surgical repair. If this is necessary, special notation should be made on the patient's chart in terms of the extent of the injury and the repair required.

When the rape victim has received the medical care she needs in the emergency room

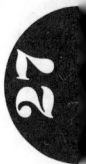

she should be escorted home and receive written instructions concerning the time and place to return for follow-up care necessary for pregnancy and venereal disease detection. Counseling services available in the community should be identified for her with names, addresses and phone numbers.

Evidence for Court

A woman who has been raped and wishes to report the crime to the police to help identify her offender and press charges against the assailant should be instructed to do the following things after the rape:

- Do not bathe or shower.
- Do not change clothes, including underwear.
- Do not attempt to alter her appearance until the rape has been reported and recorded by law enforcement officials and medical care has been obtained.
- Sign consent for medical care, including obtaining specimens and sharing medical records with law enforcement officials.
- Answer questions of law enforcement officials in regard to the identity of the rapist and the circumstances surrounding the rape itself.
- Examine her nails for particles of the rapist's hair.
- Save any item of clothing or part of clothing she may have gotten from the rapist during the attack.
- Make sure that the sperm specimens taken from her have been identified and turned over to the police.
- Discuss the rape with the District Attorney and plan to testify in court if the perpetrator is arrested.
- If witnesses were present during the rape, identify them to the police.

Questions that Will Be Asked

The following chart has been devised to list the types of information the police may need to know about the rapist and the victim. It is presented so that the nurse is made more aware of the questions asked in interviews with the assaulted female who reports the rape.

Victim

- Name
- Date of occurrence
- Time of occurrence
- Day of the week
- Crime reported within hours, days, weeks, months
- Number of times sexually attacked by the perpetrator
- Sex, race, age and marital status
- Occupation
- Residence (e.g. alone, parents, spouse)
- Treatment of victim (e.g. raped in front of children or spouse, fetish, kidnapped)
- Premises accosted were inside or outside
- Number of perpetrators
- Vehicle (if one was used and its description)

- Injury received (e.g. beaten, choked, kicked, slapped, shot, stabbed, struck with an object)
- Medical assistance (e.g. refused medical help, treated and released, private doctor, serious injury requiring hospitalization)
- Actions during attack (e.g. no resistance, physical or verbal resistance, used a weapon on the attacker)
- Resistance was overcome by threat or force
- Means employed by perpetrator (e.g. gun, knife, threat, blunt instrument)
- Modus Operandi (e.g. presented self as: delivery man, policeman, repairman or gave a con story requesting assistance or information)

Rapist

- Number of perpetrators (a separate form is generally filled out for each assailant)
- Sex of perpetrator
- Crime committed by perpetrator (e.g. rape, multiple sodomy, cunnilingus, fellatio, sexual abuse, attempted rape and robbery)
- Age of perpetrator (e.g. under 14, 15–19 years, 45 and over) If the victim cannot re-

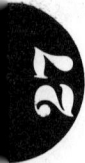

member the approximate age of the perpetrator she may be asked questions related to whether she was blindfolded or if the perpetrator wore a mask

- Race of perpetrator
- Height of perpetrator
- Weight of perpetrator
- Marks/scars (e.g. birthmarks, freckles, moles, pockmarks)
- Location of marks/scars
- Hair style (e.g. Afro long or short, curly long or short, kinky, straight)
- Hair color
- Facial Hair, (e.g. beard, mustache, long sideburns)
- Eye color
- Deformity (any unusual characteristics)
- Tattoos
- Complexion
- Teeth, (e.g. braces, missing lower or upper, buck, discolored)

- Voice and speech characteristics, (e.g. accent, stutter, lisp, harsh, effeminate)
- Clothing, (e.g. business, casual, gang jacket)
- Headgear, (e.g. fatigue cap, baseball cap)
- Jewelry, (e.g. bracelet, eyeglasses, medallion, ring)
- Perpetrator's actions, (e.g. fetish, masturbated, tied victim, verbal abuse)
- Behavior of perpetrator during the act (e.g. abusive language, apologetic, impotent, sadistic)
- Behavior of perpetrator upon termination of act (e.g. fled silently, suggested future contact, threat of retaliation)
- Relationship of perpetrator to victim (e.g. date, pick-up, total stranger)
- Additional information which may be helpful (e.g. alcohol user, drug user, gang member)

Alcoholism*

Highlights

Alcohol is the most abused drug in the United States. The extent of problems related to alcohol abuse and alcoholism is increasing and has reached major proportions.

An estimated 7% of the adult population manifest the behavior of alcohol abuse and alcoholism. Among the more than 95 million drinkers about 9 million men and women are alcohol abusers and alcoholic individuals. The National Council on Alcoholism estimates there is one alcoholic for every 12 to 14 social drinkers.

The most visible victims of alcoholism are inhabitants of skid rows. Yet most alcoholic individuals are in the working and homemaking population. As many as 5% of the nation's work force are alcoholic individuals and another 5% are serious alcohol abusers.

Alcohol-related problems are the cause of more than 85,000 deaths in the United States each year. Alcoholism shortens life expectancy 10 to 12 years. Approximately 35,000 accidental deaths at home, work, or recreation involve abuse of alcohol.

Alcohol plays a major role in half the highway fatalities in the United States, and cost 28,000 lives in one recent year. The ratio of alcohol-related traffic fatalities among youths aged 16 to 24 rises to six out of ten highway deaths.

Alcohol abuse and alcoholism drain the economy of an estimated $15 billion a year. Of this total, $10 billion is attributable to lost work time in business, industry, civilian government, and the military ... $2 billion is spent for health and welfare services provided to alcoholic persons and their families ... and property damage, medical expenses, and other overhead costs account for another $3 billion or more.

An estimated 2.5 million arrests are related to alcohol each year.

Public intoxication alone accounts for one-third of all arrests reported annually. If such alcohol related offenses as driving while under the influence of alcohol, disorderly conduct, and vagrancy are considered, the proportion would rise to between 40 and 49%.

Among American Indians, the incidence of alcoholism is at an epidemic level. The rate is estimated to be at least two times the national average. On some American Indian reservations, the rate of alcoholism is as high as 25 to 50%.

---

*Source: House Appropriations Committee Hearings, February 1976.

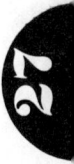

Attitudes and Myths*

Table 27-24   American attitudes toward alcohol from 1971 to 1973

	1971	Sept. 1972	March 1973	Sept. 1973
Heavy drinking is a very serious problem in the country today:	59%	64%	67%	72%
Alcohol is a drug:	61%	67%	71%	72%
No known cure for a hangover:	45%	52%	53%	50%
Drunkenness is usually like an overdose of drugs:	31%	38%	41%	43%
Host who encourages heavy drinking by guests can be described as a				
drug pusher:	19%	31%	33%	33%
bad host:	50%	58%	56%	58%

Source: Louis Harris & Associates, 1974.

Myths

- "The really serious problem in our society is drug abuse." The number one drug problem is alcoholism, with over 9,000,000 Americans having drinking problems. In a recent survey, one out of five persons claimed someone close to him was a heavy drinker and had been one for at least ten years.
- "Most alcoholics are skid row bums." Only 3 to 5% are. Most alcoholic people—about 70%—are married, employed, regular people. About one in every ten executives has a drinking problem.
- "Most alcoholic people are middle-aged or older." The highest proportion of drinking problems is among men in their early twenties. The second highest incidence occurs among men in their 40s and 50s.
- "Very few women become alcoholics." In the 1950s, there was one alcoholic female to every five or six alcoholic men. In 1974 the ratio was one to three.
- "If the parents don't drink, the children won't drink." The highest incidence of alcoholism occurs among offspring of parents who are either teetotalers or alcoholic. And drinking problems are rising among the young.

*Source: Adapted from "Drinking Myths; a Guided Tour," NIAAA, 1975.

- "Alcohol is a stimulant—makes people happier, more friendly ..." Alcohol acts as a depressant on the central nervous system. Alcohol, for example, may stimulate interest in sex but it interferes with the ability to perform. As for that "sociable" aura, half of all murders and one third of all suicides are alcohol-related.

Health and Alcohol

When taken in large doses over long periods of time, alcohol can be physically destructive, reducing a person's life span by about 10 to 12 years. The illnesses associated with alcohol abuse and alcoholism include emotional disorders and chronic progressive diseases of the central and peripheral nervous systems and of the liver, heart, muscles, gastrointestinal tract and other bodily organs and tissues.

Mortality—Within the general population heavy drinkers die younger than moderate drinkers. Among the groups with alcohol-related increased death rates, women have higher rates than men, and the youngest age classes have the highest rates of all. Abstainers have somewhat higher death rates than moderate drinkers.

Coronary Heart Disease—Drinkers have coronary heart disease less often than abstainers or ex-drinkers. Drinking apparently has no detrimental effects leading to coronary attacks, but a suspected protective effect of alcohol has not been confirmed. A less common form of heart disease, cardiomyopathy, is linked to alcoholism.

Liver Diseases—Cirrhosis of the liver is a major cause of incapacitating illness and premature death in alcohol persons. It occurs about six times more often in alcoholic people than in the general population. In large urban areas, cirrhosis represents the fourth largest cause of death between the ages of 25 and 45. Primary liver-cell cancer is also more frequent in persons with alcoholic cirrhosis. The exact relationship between alcoholism and cirrhosis has remained a mystery. In general, it is thought that the excessive intake of alcohol is not sufficient to produce cirrhosis and that dietary factors may play a key role.

Pregnancy—Heavy drinking during pregnancy can adversely affect the off-spring of alcoholic mothers, causing physical abnormalities including heart, facial and limb defects as well as overall growth deficiencies.

The Drinking Driver

Figure 27-4   Analysis of drinking driving problem

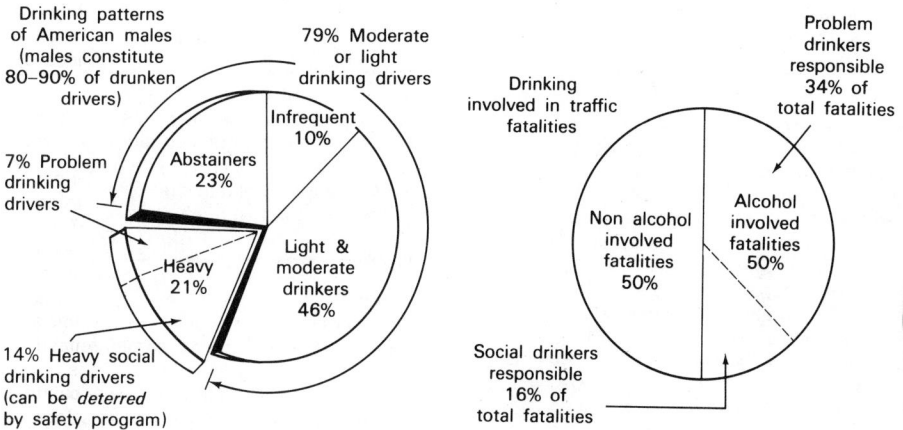

Drinking patterns
of American males
(males constitute
80–90% of drunken
drivers)

79% Moderate
or light
drinking drivers

7% Problem
drinking
drivers

Abstainers
23%

Infrequent
10%

Heavy
21%

Light &
moderate
drinkers
46%

14% Heavy social
drinking drivers
(can be *deterred*
by safety program)

Drinking
involved in traffic
fatalities

Problem
drinkers
responsible
34% of
total fatalities

Non alcohol
involved
fatalities
50%

Alcohol
involved
fatalities
50%

Social drinkers
responsible
16% of
total fatalities

*Degree of drinking was classified according to a rather complex combination of the quantity of alcohol consumed per occasion and the frequency of drinking.

Heavy drinking. Drink nearly every day with five or more per occasion at least once in a while, or about once weekly with usually five or more per occasion.

Moderate drinking. Drink at least once a month, typically several times, but usually with no more than three or four drinks per occasion.

Light drinking. Drink at least once a month, but typically only one or two drinks on a single occasion.

Infrequent drinking. Drink at least once a year, but less than once a month.

Abstainers. Drink less than once a year or not at all.

Source: DHEW, December 1971.

Services for the Alcoholic

Outpatient service—Handles the majority of those seeking treatment, as well as those discharged from inpatient and intermediate care services. Services often include: nonacute medical and psychosocial treatment, chemotherapy, counseling, and such resources as Alcoholics Anonymous.

Emergency service—Provides immediate acceptance, evaluation, and care for alcoholic persons in urgent need of medical or psychiatric care, or who require emergency assistance for social problems. Hospitals should treat the medical needs of the alcoholic client as an integral part of general emergency services.

Inpatient service—Meets subacute medical needs and provides a minimum alcohol-free period during which the cycle of dependency may be interrupted, the needs of the client may be assessed, and a followup treatment plan drafted. The inpatient service should be an integral part of the community's social and health care delivery system.

Intermediate care—Provides for persons who need a strongly supportive environment while learning to cope with alcohol and other problems. Examples include: sheltered living arrangements, such as halfway houses or foster homes; rehabilitation services, including sheltered workshops; and physical, social, and vocational services.

After-care service—Offers long-term followup care for clients whose prognosis for recovery is doubtful. For people who continue to be disabled by the taking of alcohol, residential or other facilities should be available.

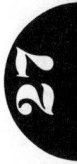

Followup service—Consists of active, periodic contact with clients for a minimum of one year after discharge or dropout from a recovery program. This service should respond to crisis situations and be linked with other crisis services in the community.

The General Hospital Role

The local general hospital occupies a strategic position because of the large number of alcoholics using its services, because it is a place where alcoholics can potentially be identified, and because it makes contact with these individuals at a time when they are more motivated for treatment.

Several surveys have shown that some 20 to 25% of male ward patients and some 6 to 7% of female ward patients of urban general hospitals can be diagnosed as suffering from alcoholism. Two-thirds of these admissions are for illnesses directly related to the patient's alcoholism. Intoxicated, injured, withdrawing and sick alcoholic patients similarly overutilize the general hospital's emergency room services, often with considerable regularity.

Considerable effort is being made on many sides to include the resources of the general hospital in the total social system of care for alcoholic people. For example, the American Hospital Association is involved in a national action to promote alcoholism programs in all general hospitals.

One approach proposes an alteration of hospital admission policies so that alcoholic patients may be admitted to general wards with the diagnosis of alcoholism. Another type of utilization allows the hospital to provide medical care while nonprofessional community workers conduct an alcoholism program in specialized wards. A third approach is the development of professionally managed alcoholism wards. Yet another tack is the development of hospital alcoholism programs managed by professional alcoholism workers but conducted throughout the general hospital.

Current models developed by the American Hospital Association focus on functional alternatives. Thus, some large urban hospitals may operate hospital-wide programs while others support specialized alcoholism units. Many smaller hospitals may form consortiums with community agencies. A general-hospital alcoholism program will usually not offer definitive alcoholism treatment. It can provide treatment for the complications of alcoholism, serve as a diagnostic center, act as a funnel into the community alcoholism care system, and be a triage agency.

Treatment*

Treatment of alcoholism has tended to be based on one of two common policies. Some treatment centers specialize in a single modality: disulfiram, conditioned reflex, behaviour modification, group therapy, psychodrama, individual counseling or diet control.

Other treatment centers use a combination of several methods and often include Alcoholics Anonymous meetings.

Methods:

- Detoxication—an effective first step in engaging alcoholics in a successful rehabilitation effort.
- Drug treatment—recent reviews of drug treatment indicate no therapeutic effectiveness; however, the image of a drug therapy program is considered supportive to the alcoholic because of the positive benefits from the transaction of drug-giving and receiving.
- Deterrent therapy—use of disulfiram (Antabuse), on the scene since 1950, sensitizes the patient to alcohol and makes consequences of even one drink agonizing. Conditioned response therapy commonly adds an emetic to patient's alcoholic beverage to produce an unfavorable experience.
- Behavior modification—based on learning and conditioning theories, treatment consists of analysis of behavior patterns, and the application of rewards, modeling and guiding experiences.
- Group therapy—increased trend towards family therapy. Transactional analysis, with its emphasis on catchy game and role playing, has become popular recently.
- Alcoholics Anonymous—considered by many therapists as the most useful adjunct to any treatment.

Recovery

A recent survey of NIAAA-supported treatment centers, which deal with severely impaired individuals drinking nine times more al-

---

*Source: Adapted from *Handbook for the Alcoholism Counselor*, Baltimore City, 2nd Edition, 1970, Dept. of Health.

cohol than the average individual, shows recovery rates of 70% for patients who had received treatment. (Consumption of one ounce or less alcohol daily was criterion for recovery.) About 54% were reported abstaining from alcohol altogether. But this figure was reduced to 10% after a time lapse of 18 months. Another result of the treatment programs was a decrease in time spent in hospitals and jails.

Table 27-25   Change in client characteristics upon exposure to NIAAA alcoholism treatment

	All clients		
	Intake	6 Mos. later	% change
Alcohol consumption (during preceding month)			
Average ounces per day[1]	6.3	1.6	75%
Average days drank	13.7	5.3	61%
% abstainers	15.4%	54.6%	355%
Behavioral pattern (during preceding month)			
Impairment index[2]	12.4	4.3	65%
% quarreled	37.2%	14.8%	60%
% drank on job	38.7%	16.1%	58%
% missed work (1 or more times)	40.1%	14.8%	63%
Employment data (during preceding month)			
Average days worked (labor force)	12.4	14.9	20%
% unemployed (labor force)	40.5%	25.4%	37%
Average earned income (all clients)	$275	$313	14%
Number of clients—range for variables shown[3]		1443–1846	

[1] Absolute alcohol calculated from all beverages.
[2] Impairment index ranges from 0 for no impairment to 33 for maximum impairment.
[3] Number of clients at intake and 6 months after intake is the same for any given variable.

Source: NIAAA.

Generally, alcoholics are considered treatable. So far, recovery rates do not seem to be correlated with any single treatment method, neither in locales such as hospitals, halfway houses, or outpatient care, nor to specific treatment techniques such as group counseling, individual therapy, anti-abuse therapy or Alcoholics Anonymous. It appears that the fact of treatment is more important than the type of treatment the individual receives; many treatments given in sufficient amounts and intensity produce positive outcomes.

Further Information—Alcoholism

- National Clearinghouse for Alcohol Information, P.O. Box 2345, Rockville, Maryland 20852, (301) 948-4450
- National Institute on Alcohol Abuse and Alcoholism, 5600 Fishers Lane, Rockville, Maryland 20852

The Institute maintains a state-by-state listing of most private and public treatment facilities currently available.

- Veterans Administration, Alcohol and Drug Dependent Service, 810 Vermont Avenue, N.W., Washington, D.C. 20420
- State Authority on Alcoholism, in your state capital.
- National Council on Alcoholism, Inc., 2 Park Avenue South, New York, New York 10016
- Alcohol and Drug Problems Association, 1130 17th Street, N.W., Washington, D.C. 20036
- Alcoholics Anonymous, P.O. Box 459, Grand Central Station, New York, N.Y. 10017
- Al-Anon Family Group, 115 East 23rd Street, New York, N.Y. 10010

Terminally Ill*

Nursing '75 surveyed 15,000 nurses in August and October of 1975 on the subject of terminal illness. Here are some of their findings.

How often has caring for an incurable, terminally ill patient made you feel discouraged, depressed, or angry?

	Discouraged	Depressed	Angry
Almost always	19%	21%	6%
Occasionally	62	58	41
Seldom	16	18	32
Never	3	3	21

Very few nurses escape being depressed and discouraged by terminal illness.

The vast majority of respondents had a high degree of confidence in their own nursing abilities in general and in their ability to provide technical care to terminally ill patients. But not so with ability to manage the psychological needs of terminally ill patients.

---

* Sources: David Popoff and *Nursing '75:* "What Are Your Feelings About Death," *Nursing '75,* August, and "Taking Life Away," *Nursing '75,* October.

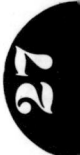

Self-confidence ratings by nurses

	Nursing abilities in general	Provide technical care to terminally ill	Manage psychological needs of terminally ill
Very confident	35%	42%	10%
Mostly confident	59	48	48
Slightly confident	5	8	35
Not at all confident	1	2	7

Should a nurse call a "code" for an unexpected cardiac arrest in a terminally ill patient when the doctor has left no instruction?

Yes	46%
No	54%

You might say that half of the nurses would take it upon themselves to let a patient die; on the other hand, you could say that half of the nurses would allow the patient the dignity of a natural death and, perhaps, death without prolongation of pain and suffering.

When should a patient with a terminal illness be told that he is dying?

As soon as possible after diagnosis	60%
Only when he asks	21
Slowly over extended period of time as illness progresses	16
Never, only that he has a serious illness	2
Only in last stages of dying when death is imminent	0.5

When a patient who has a terminal illness bluntly asks you if he is dying and his physician does not want him to know, what do you usually do?

Ask why he brought up the question, try to get him to talk about his feelings	81%
Tell him that only the physician can answer the question	14
Say you don't know	2
Reassure him that he is not dying, just ill	1
Avoid the question and try to distract him	1
Tell him the truth	1

When physicians have refused to tell your patients that they were dying, how many of these patients nevertheless clearly knew of and referred to their impending death?

Less than 10%	6%
Up to 25%	8
About half	12
Up to 75%	24
Up to 90%	23
Every one, without exception	3
Have not cared for enough dying patients to estimate	24

At least three out of four patients who were not told nevertheless knew of their impending death, according to nearly half of the respondents. The more frequently a nurse cares for dying patients, the higher is her estimate: one-third of the nurses who care for dying patients daily said that 90% of the patients knew; 61% said that at least 75% knew.

When a terminally ill patient brings up the topic of his death or dying, what is your honest, inner reaction?

	All respondents
Feel anxious and uncomfortable	15%
Feel somewhat uncomfortable	32
Feel relieved	45
Never involved in such a situation	8

Having experienced some kind of positive feedback from terminally ill patients or their families is a key element in the make-up of nurses who are able to provide care and comfort to those who are about to die.

In your own experience, how many terminally ill patients continued to deny, until the very end, that they would die?

Very few, less than 10%	46%
A small proportion, up to 25%	19
About half	7
A large proportion, up to 75%	5
Up to 90%	1
Everyone, without exception	0.05
Have not cared for enough dying patients to estimate	21

Many nurses who are also mothers of young children reported that they sometimes identify too much with young dying patients.

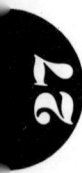

Care of dying newborns: Of all respondents, only 18% said they wouldn't mind, but 32% of pediatric nurses said they wouldn't. Some 21% of Ob/Gyn nurses said they wouldn't. Far fewer psychiatric nurses said they wouldn't.

Care of a dying young child: Again, pediatric and Ob/Gyn nurses appeared most able to cope with their own discomfort; psychiatric and emergency-room nurses, least able. But more than half of the nurses said that caring for terminally ill children, adolescents and mothers with young children would lead to very uncomfortable feelings. Caring for the elderly and middle-aged would produce the least emotional discomfort in nurses.

Care of a dying young adult: Age was a factor among young nurses, 17 to 22 years old, to the question on caring for a dying young adult: 59% of this age group would find themselves very uncomfortable or unable to cope, as compared to 48% of all older nurses.

Care of the body after death. Sociologists find that most people develop generalized anxiety, fear, and disgust when they have to handle a dead body. Nurses, it appears, are not likely to let such feelings overcome them.

What is your predominant feeling about having to care for the body of a patient after death?

Acceptance of the necessity of this task	75%
No special feeling	17
Distaste	6
Fear	2

Nurses over age 40 are the least likely to experience fear or distaste when caring for a body. They apparently have developed ways of handling their emotional reactions.

Young nurses (under age 22) are the most likely to experience distaste or fear when caring for a body. A young nurse said simply: "I don't enjoy doing it."

Death*

Overview

Until recently death was primarily due to acute communicable diseases and gastro-intestinal

---

*Source: Adapted from "Dying in the U.S.A." by Ruth Elder, *NURSING DIGEST, 1975 Review of Medicine and Surgery,* (Contemporary Publishing Co.).

upsets. Now the primary causes of death are associated with old age, heart disease, cancer, and stroke.

In earlier times, most people were nursed and died at home. Death took place with the comfort of familiar surroundings and loved faces. After death, it was generally the family who bathed and dressed the body for the last symbolic goodbyes of friends and relatives. Usually a family member sat up all night with the deceased.

Today, most deaths take place in institutions. It is estimated that about three-quarters of the deaths in America occur there despite the fact that most people say they would rather die at home. Those which do not take place in institutions are likely to be sudden. This means that the dying phase of life usually occurs in surroundings unfamiliar to the persons concerned.

The average person attends few of them apart from those of his immediate family, until he is elderly himself. [Therefore] the extent to which death interrupts the orderly structuring of everyday life [is minimized]. However, it can also have negative consequences due to the impersonality of the people and settings associated with its management.

The modern hospital is committed to the routinization of the handling of life and death crises. As a consequence many people are needlessly isolated and lonely when they become patients in hospitals during their last days.

Patient Attitudes

Most studies indicate that old people think about death, are willing to talk about it, and have made preparations for it. Few show marked fear of it, and the prevailing view is one of acceptance. Those in poor health tend to actually look forward to it.

Death is upsetting primarily when it occurs prematurely, or is accompanied by suffering or violence, for premature death and suffering are no longer accepted as natural in this society.

Physician Attitudes

The strong emphasis on preserving life in the medical culture may make health professionals unfit for dealing with the dying patient; death defeats them and makes them feel like failures.

Physicians are much less likely to want to inform patients of an unfavourable prognosis than patients would wish. One study found that 88% of the 219 physicians studied pre-

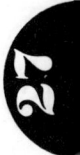

ferred not to tell cancer patients their unfavourable prognosis.

The physician's motive in curtailing information may be to maintain control over the doctor-patient relationship, as the patient who is aware of his fate may be more difficult to handle. However, it may simply be that through avoiding death talk, the physician hopes to avoid inflicting unnecessary pain. He may also wish to avoid the emotional scenes which sometimes follow informing the patient, because he does not feel equipped to deal with them. It is not an easy task to support the patient through the phases of depression and grief which often follow the disclosure that death is imminent, and most physicians, and nurses too, have had little training for it.

[In the book *Awareness and Dying,* Glazer and Strauss noted that] the management of communication and actions designed to keep the patient in ignorance of his health status were left almost entirely to the nursing staff. Physicians focused on technical aspects of care and kept their visits to a minimum, thereby escaping problematic conversations. They acted as if the patient were not dying but only ill, and they talked about the future as if it were certain that the patient would have a part in it.

Nurse Attitudes

Nurses have to carefully manage facial expressions and gestures so as not to give the show away. They have to control any sadness they feel about the patient's approaching death. Under such exhausting conditions they almost invariably reduce the amount of time they spend with the patient. If the situation goes on long enough, the [relationship] usually shifts into one of suspicion, pretense or open awareness.

Changes in priorities, policies and practices in administration as well as in clinical care also will be required.

As one authority points out, when active treatment becomes irrelevant to the patient's real needs, then care of the patient should change to focus on comfort, to making the patient's life as peaceful, contented and meaningful as possible until he dies. When comfort becomes the primary goal of care, the nursing professional could legitimately claim ascendency in its management.

An expanded role for the nurse directed at maintaining the patient's comfort and capability as he desired it could be developed. It would require additional preparation in learning how to manage medications in the control of pain, and in learning how to assess and meet the needs of dying patients and their families more adequately than is now the case.

Definition of Death

Is it the physician's and the nurse's duty to prolong life simply because it is scientifically possible to do so? How much consideration should be given to a previously expressed wish of the patient or his relatives to let nature take its course? When should one desist from trying to prolong life with heroic measures?

Dr. Wasserman (*World Medical Journal,* September-October 1967) speaks of cytological death, organ death, spiritual death, theological death, legal death, social death, physiological death and pathological death. In Wasserman's opinion, legal problems revolve around the social responsibility of man's culture to the living. According to Professor Gunner Biorck of the Karolinska Institute in Stockholm, there may be several levels of death: for example, social death may occur when freedom, mobility and contacts are exchanged for restriction, loneliness and isolation; spiritual death when intellectual activity and emotional experience give way to failure to understand or remember and to emptiness of mind; vegetative death when basic life processes no longer are maintained spontaneously; metabolic death when despite the application of life-supporting techniques, cells and tissues finally disentegrate.

A code by the Ad Hoc Committee of the Harvard Medical School to examine the definition of brain death established that irreversible coma or death occurs when these conditions are present:

1. Total lack of response to external stimuli.

2. Absence of all spontaneous muscular movements, notably breathing.

3. Absence of reflexes.

4. Flat encephalogram or absence of "brain waves."

Birth and Death Certificates

Figure 27-5   General pattern of vital registration

Responsible person or agency	Birth certificate	Death certificate	Fetal death Certificate (Stillbirth)
Physician, Other Professional Attendant, or Hospital Authority	1. Completes entire certificate in consultation with parent(s). Physician's signature required. 2. Files certificate with local office of district in which birth occurred.	1. Completes medical certification and signs certificate. 2. Returns certificate to funeral director.	1. Completes or reviews medical items on certificate. 2. Certifies to the cause of fetal death and signs certificate. 3. Returns certificate to funeral director. 4. In absence of funeral director, files certificate.
Funeral Director		1. Obtains personal facts about deceased. 2. Takes certificate to physician for medical certification. 3. Delivers completed certificate to local office of district where death occurred and obtains burial permit.	1. Obtains the facts about fetal death. 2. Takes certificate to physician for entry of causes of fetal death. 3. Delivers completed certificate to local office of district where delivery occurred and obtains burial permit.
Local Office (may be Local Registrar or City or County Health Department)	1. Verifies completeness and accuracy of certificate. 2. Makes copy, ledger entry, or index for local use. 3. Sends certificates to State Registrar.	1. Verifies completeness and accuracy of certificate. 2. Makes copy, ledger entry, or index for local use. 3. Issues burial permit to funeral director and verifies return of permit from cemetery attendant. 4. Sends certificates to State Registrar.	
	City and county health departments use certificates in allocating medical and nursing services, followups on infectious diseases, planning programs, measuring effectiveness of services, and conducting research studies.		
State Registrar, Bureau of Vital Statistics	1. Queries incomplete or inconsistent information. 2. Maintains files for permanent reference and as the source of certified copies. 3. Develops vital statistics for use in planning, evaluating, and administering State and local health activities and for research studies. 4. Compiles health related statistics for State and civil divisions of State for use of the health department and other agencies and groups interested in the fields of medical science, public health, demography, and social welfare. 5. Prepares copies of birth, death, fetal death, marriage, and divorce certificates or records for transmission to the National Center for Health Statistics.		
Public Health Service National Center for Health Statistics	1. Prepares and publishes national statistics of births, deaths, fetal deaths, marriages, and divorces; and constructs the official U.S. life tables and related actuarial tables. 2. Conducts health and social-research studies based on vital records and on sampling surveys linked to records. 3. Conducts research and methodological studies in vital statistics methods including the technical, administrative, and legal aspects of vital records registration and administration. 4. Maintains a continuing technical assistance program to improve the quality and usefulness of vital statistics.		

NOTE.—In some States there is no central file for marriage and divorce records at the State level.

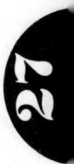

Hospices for Dying Patients*

What people need most when they are dying is relief from the distressing symptoms of their disease, the security of a caring environment, sustained expert care, and the assurance they and their families won't be abandoned.

The goal of hospice care is to help a patient continue life as usual: work, being with family, doing what is especially significant before life comes to a close, and feeling a part of ongoing life.

Hospices, expressly designed to provide such services, have come into being in the past decade. The most widely known is St. Christopher's Hospice in London, whose founder and medical director is Cicely Saunders. Hospice is a medieval term, used because it signifies that the doors are open to the traveler on a journey from one life to the next; it also emphasizes that spiritual and emotional care are as important as medical care.

The hospice movement is beginning on the American continent. New facilities are being established at Santa Barbara and in Marin County in California; in Branford, Conn., to serve the greater New Haven region; and in Paoli, Pa., to name a few.

Some hospitals are developing units within their walls to give hospice-like care. St. Luke's Hospital in New York City and the Royal Victoria Hospital in Montreal, Canada, are two examples. Facilities originally designed for care of terminally ill patients such as Calvary Hospital in New York City, the seven nursing homes of the Catholic Order of the Hawthorne Dominicans scattered throughout the country, and Youville Hospital in Cambridge, Massachusetts—all have made significant contributions to the hospice movement.

Euthanasia

Public Attitudes

A Gallup Opinion Index (Princeton, N.J., August 1975, Report #122) found that 51% of Americans believe a person does not have the moral right to end his or her life even though suffering great pain with no hope of improvement. Forty-one percent hold the opposing view.

Fifty-three percent think an individual does not have this right when he or she has an incurable disease, while 40% believe this to be morally acceptable.

However, taking one's own life to avoid being a heavy burden to one's family is thought to be morally wrong by a 72% to 20% margin.

Nurse Attitudes**

Does a dying patient have the right to refuse treatment? An overwhelming majority of nurses responding to the survey answered "yes." But when it comes to active euthanasia or mercy killing, only a minority answered yes.

How do you feel about withholding all life-sustaining treatment for dying patients who don't want it?

In favor	73%
Mixed, slightly in favor	23
Mixed, slightly against	3
Against	1

How do you feel about mercy killing or active euthanasia for dying patients who request it?

In favor	17%
Mixed, slightly in favor	31
Mixed, slightly against	16
Against	36

Are you in favor or against deliberately allowing newborns with gross abnormalities to die when there is no possibility of any meaningful existence?

In favor	42%
Mixed, slightly in favor	39
Mixed, slightly against	11
Against	8

The great majority of nurses favor letting a deformed newborn die.

Hastening death: Some 44% of the respondents said they've worked with doctors and nurses who have hastened the death of a terminally ill patient, but only 21% were willing to admit they themselves ever hastened the death of such patients.

*Source: "Hospice Care for Dying Patients," *American Journal of Nursing,* Oct. 1975, © American Journal of Nursing Company.

**Source: "Taking Life Away" by David Popoff and *Nursing '75, NURSING '75,* October 1975 (Survey of 15,000 nurses).

**Have you ever knowingly helped
to hasten the death of a terminally
ill patient?**

Yes, several times, or more	11%
Yes, once	10
No, never	79

As might be expected, intensive and coronary care unit nurses are the most likely to be involved in situations where they may hasten the death of a patient. Some 20% of such nurses said they have, several times or more, knowingly helped to hasten the death of terminally ill patients.

When it comes to *intentionally* causing the death of terminally ill patients, nine out of ten nurses say they have never observed such action by doctors or nurses they work with.

The Coroner (Medical Examiner's Office)

In the case of a murder, a suicide or other untimely death, the local government is invested with the responsibility of investigating these deaths and determining their causes.

The usual method of investigation, which the American colonies inherited from Great Britain, is the coroner system. The best coroner systems—now called medical examiner's offices—are under the direction of trained medicolegal specialists called forensic pathologists. This group is a recognized medical subspecialty of the American Board of Pathology.

In 1974 only 40% of the American people lived in jurisdictions with medicolegal death investigating systems. Only ten states have complete statewide medical examiner systems.

Suicide*

Highlights

- There appears to be a direct relationship between social status and suicide. The higher one is on the socioeconomic scale, the more susceptible he is to suicide.
- More than 65% of all suicide victims seek medical attention within three months prior

---

* Source: Adapted from *Suicides in the United States* 1950–64 DHEW (HSM) 73-1259 August 1967.

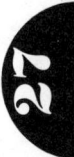

to the suicide. A careful interviewer should be able to identify the high-risk patient.
- Physicians have a much higher incidence of suicide than the lay population.
- There were 25,700 suicides in the U.S.A. in 1974.
- During the last 25 years, the rate of suicide in the U.S. has remained virtually unchanged—about 16 per 100,000 population per year. Suicide is the seventh leading cause of death for all ages, and the second leading cause, after accidents, among college students.
- Most suicides occur in April and May. The lowest suicide rate occurs in December. Suicide is most likely on Friday or Monday and Sunday is a strong third—people feel loneliest at those times and loneliness is one of the major causes of suicide.
- Three times as many women as men *attempt* suicide, but three times as many men as women complete the act.
- Men over the age of 15 are likely to commit suicide with a gun, while women usually use barbiturates and other less violent forms. Some experts feel that women use these methods because they fear disfigurement.
- While only 3% of all suicides on the national average are a result of jumping from high places, the rate goes up to 33% in New York City, where there are many very high buildings.
- Suicide occurs more frequently in the white population than in the nonwhite. In 1964 the ratio between rates for white and nonwhite persons was two to one.
- Divorced persons show the highest suicide rates—from three to five times the rates for married persons under 65. The rates for widowed persons are eight times those for married persons at ages 20–24, but this ratio gradually declines with age and the rates are almost identical after reaching age 60. Suicide rates for single persons in most age groups ranged from 1½ to 2½ times those for married persons. Married persons do indeed have the lowest suicide rate, with the single, widowed, and divorced ranking next, in that order.
- There are six metropolitan areas with rates higher than 15 suicides per 100,000 and all but one are in California and Florida. Most of the statistical areas with low suicide rates are located in the northeastern and southern sections of the country.

568

Methods Used

Firearms and explosives are more frequently used for committing suicide than any other means of injury. This category, comprised principally of deaths attributed to self-inflicted gunshot wounds, accounted for 56% of all suicides. Hanging and strangulation were the next most frequent means and accounted for about 14% of the total suicides. About 12% were from poisoning by analgesic and soporific substances (nearly three-fourths of these involved the use of barbituric acid and its derivatives.) and about 11% from "poisoning" by motor vehicle exhaust gas.

The choice of a way to commit suicide varies by sex. For instance, analgesic and soporific substances were used by only 6% of males committing suicide, compared with 30% of females. Except for suicides from poisoning by other gases (which includes motor vehicle exhaust gases), poisonous substances were used by a greater percentage of females than of males. Also, a greater percentage of females drowned themselves. Firearms and explosives accounted for 63% of all suicides for males but only 36% of those for females.

Suicide Trends, U.S.A.

Table 27-26   Suicides, by method, 1960–1974

	1960		1965		1970		1972		1973		1974	
Item	Male	Fe-male	Male	Fe-male	Male	Fe-male	Male	Fe-male	Male	Fe-male	Male	Fe-male
Suicides	14,539	4,502	15,490	6,017	16,629	6,851	17,768	7,236	18,108	7,010	18,595	7,088
Firearms	7,879	1,138	8,457	1,441	9,704	2,068	10,852	2,496	11,057	2,260	11,813	2,532
Percent of total	54.2	25.3	54.6	23.9	58.4	30.2	61.1	34.5	61.1	32.2	63.5	35.7
Poisoning	2,631	1,699	3,179	2,816	3,299	3,285	3,242	3,208	3,149	3,107	2,944	3,049
Hanging and strangulation	2,576	790	2,453	744	2,422	831	2,510	790	2,671	877	2,661	816
Other	1,453	875	1,401	1,016	1,204	667	1,164	742	1,231	766	1,177	691

Source: U.S. National Center for Health Statistics, *Vital Statistics of the United States,* annual.

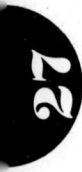

Table 27-27   Suicide mortality rates, by age groups, 1965 to 1974. (Rate per 100,000 population. Beginning 1970, excludes deaths of nonresidents of the United States)

	Male								Female							
	White				Negro and other				White				Negro and other			
Age	1965	1970	1973	1974	1965	1970	1973	1974	1965	1970	1973	1974	1965	1970	1973	1974
Total	17.4	18.0	18.8	19.2	7.7	8.5	10.0	10.2	6.6	7.1	7.0	7.1	2.5	2.9	3.0	3.0
5–14 year	0.5	0.5	0.7	0.8	0.2	0.2	0.3	0.4	0.1	0.1	0.2	0.2	0.1	0.2	0.1	0.2
15–24 year	9.6	13.9	17.4	17.8	8.5	11.3	14.0	12.9	3.0	4.2	4.3	4.8	3.1	4.1	4.1	3.9
25–34 year	17.7	19.9	21.8	23.3	14.2	19.8	22.6	22.9	7.6	9.0	8.5	8.7	6.0	5.8	5.3	6.3
35–44 year	23.4	23.3	22.8	23.8	15.0	12.6	14.3	15.6	12.0	13.0	12.2	12.1	4.2	4.3	5.4	4.5
45–54 year	30.8	29.5	28.4	28.3	13.5	14.1	13.4	11.9	13.6	13.5	13.7	14.1	4.1	4.5	3.2	4.0
55–64 year	39.7	35.0	32.4	32.1	14.2	10.5	12.1	12.5	12.3	12.3	12.0	11.0	2.8	2.2	4.4	3.4
65 year and over	43.3	41.1	40.7	38.9	15.0	10.8	11.9	15.3	9.1	8.5	8.2	7.7	3.2	3.6	3.1	2.3

Source: U.S. National Center for Health Statistics, *Vital Statistics of the United States,* annual.

Table 27-28   Suicides by race and sex, 1930 to 1974

Year	Total	White Male	White Female	Negro and other Male	Negro and other Female
Number					
1930	18,323	13,877	3,863	442	141
1935	18,214	13,465	4,094	477	178
1940	18,907	13,990	4,294	476	147
1945	14,782	10,374	3,920	380	108
1950	17,145	12,755	3,713	542	135
1955	16,760	12,430	3,662	531	137
1960	19,041	13,825	4,296	714	206
1965	21,507	14,624	5,718	866	299
1968	21,372	14,520	5,692	859	301
1969	22,364	14,886	6,152	971	355
1970	23,480	15,591	6,468	1,038	383
1971	24,092	15,802	6,775	1,058	457
1972	25,004	16,476	6,788	1,292	448
1973	25,118	16,823	6,589	1,285	421
1974	25,683	17,263	6,660	1,332	428
Rate[1]					
1930	22.1	36.4	10.4	11.3	3.6
1935	19.6	31.8	9.8	10.8	3.9
1940	19.2	31.3	9.6	10.4	3.1
1945	15.1	25.6	8.2	8.5	2.1
1950	15.6	26.0	7.4	10.4	2.4
1955	14.5	24.5	6.9	9.6	2.3
1960	15.4	25.7	7.6	11.7	3.1
1965	16.1	25.3	9.2	12.9	4.0
1968	15.2	24.2	8.8	12.1	3.8
1969	15.7	24.4	9.3	13.3	4.3
1970	16.2	25.3	9.6	13.4	4.3
1971	16.2	25.0	9.9	13.4	4.8
1972	16.5	25.6	9.7	15.9	4.8
1973	16.3	25.7	9.3	15.4	4.4
1974	16.4	26.0	9.3	15.5	4.3

[1] Per 100,000 resident population 15 years old and over.

Source: U.S. National Center for Health Statistics, *Vital Statistics of the United States,* annual.

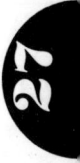

World Suicide Rates

Table 27-29   Suicide rates, selected countries, 1973. (Crude rate per 100,000 population)

Country	Suicides Male	Suicides Female	Country	Suicides Male	Suicides Female
United States	17.5	6.8	Finland	39.0	10.0
Austria	33.3	14.5	France	23.3	9.3
Australia	17.9	9.3	Germany, Fed. Rep. of	26.3	14.1
Belgium	21.5	9.6	Greece	3.9	1.5
Canada	17.4	6.9	Ireland	4.3	1.7
Denmark	30.2	17.7	Israel	8.4	6.5

(continued)

Table 27-29   (continued)

Country	Suicides	
	Male	Female
Italy	8.2	3.6
Japan	19.4	14.2
Mexico	1.1	0.3
Netherlands	10.0	6.5
Norway	13.0	5.1
Philippines	0.9	0.4
Poland	20.3	4.1
Portugal	13.4	3.6
Puerto Rico	17.0	3.7
Spain	6.7	2.3
Sweden	29.4	11.2
Switzerland	28.2	11.2
United Kingdom:		
England and Wales	9.2	6.2
Northern Ireland	4.1	2.0
Scotland	9.5	6.8

Source: United Nations World Health Organization.

Suicide Evaluation Sheet*

Every *yes* answer increases the possibility of suicide.

1. Has the patient sustained a recent loss (of job, friend, money, loved one, home, status, or part of the body by subtractive surgery)? Include miscarriage or post-partum state.   □ Yes   □ No
2. Is he isolated from others socially, without friends?   □ Yes   □ No
3. Has he ever attempted suicide?
    □ Yes   □ No
4. Has a member of his family ever attempted suicide?   □ Yes   □ No
5. Has he ever been treated for mental illness?   □ Yes   □ No
6. Is he old, bereaved or in physical pain?
    □ Yes   □ No
7. Does he view suicide as a release?
    □ Yes   □ No
8. Is he diagnosed as a psychotic?
    □ Yes   □ No
9. If so, does he hear voices telling him to kill himself?   □ Yes   □ No
10. Is he depressed?   □ Yes   □ No
11. Has he said he wished to die, or has he failed to perform life-saving acts (refused to give himself insulin, or refused to take

digitalis or other medical treatment, or said he cannot irrigate his colostomy or has "no need to learn")?   □ Yes   □ No
12. Does he have a history of self-destructive behavior (consistently reckless, accident-prone, addicted to alcohol or other drugs, given to self-mutilation)?   □ Yes   □ No
13. Does he lack a religious background that enjoins against suicide?   □ Yes   □ No

Funerals**

The average cost in the U.S. today for funeral and burial arrangements is $2,000. In 1973, the National Funeral Directors Association estimated the average adult funeral cost at $1,116. In 1974, an FTC staff report estimated it at $1,137. In addition, cemetery or grave marker costs average $800.

At The Funeral Home: Procedures

Typically, consumers use funeral homes to handle death arrangements. There are many important decisions facing consumers at the funeral home which must be made in a matter of hours after a death has occurred. One consideration is the casket; first whether or not to use a casket and if desired, which casket to select. Casket exteriors and interiors come in a variety of colors and materials. The outer materials differ and are available in fiberglass, wood and metal; interiors can be simply lined or fully padded. More expensive sealer caskets purport to be airtight or watertight and to provide "security" for the deceased, but they do not prevent decomposition of the remains. Other decisions involve whether or not embalming and restoration of the deceased are to be performed, deciding if viewing of the deceased will occur, and, if so, the number of days and whether or not to use the facilities of the funeral home for viewing. The funeral director usually does not sell cemetery property but can sell burial vaults or grave liners. These may or may not be required by cemetery rules, but the funeral buyer will often face this buying decision at the funeral home. Consumers must also decide if they want the funeral director to write an obituary and to apply for any benefits the deceased is eligible to receive. This can include benefits from the Veteran's Administra-

*Source: M. O. Diran, R.N., "You Can Prevent Suicide," *Nursing '76,* January 1976.

**Source: Adapted from *The Price of Death,* Consumer Survey Handbook 3, pub. by Seattle Regional office of FTC.

tion, Social Security, labor unions or insurance companies.

The day of the funeral ceremony must be determined and a decision is necessary as to whether to have the body present or in another room before or during the ceremony, and, if present, to have the casket open or closed. The family must decide if the funeral director, the clergy or a friend of the deceased will officiate at the ceremony.

Although the standard adult funeral is sold often as a "package," the consumer may not have to buy the whole package. If a buyer wishes to decline some of the "included" services or merchandise, such as embalming, viewing, etc., some funeral directors will reduce their total charge.

The purchase of a casket for cremation is usually not required by law. However, some container may be required by the funeral home, cemetery or crematory. A fiberboard or plain wooden box may be adequate.

Cremation after viewing does not always require the purchase of a casket. Sometimes the deceased may be placed on a day bed or couch, or a casket may be loaned for viewing purposes. While some states do not allow the reuse of a casket, some do. Check this in your state.

After cremation, the deceased's remains may be scattered or placed in an urn or other container for burial or housing in a columbarium. Urn prices vary substantially, just like caskets.

The purpose of embalming is to make the corpse presentable for viewing during a funeral. If viewing is not desired or if a corpse is to be viewed only during the period immediately after death, embalming may not be necessary. Embalming fluid preserves the body for only a few days. It is a mistake to think that the fluid retards deterioration for any significant amount of time.

Making Funeral Arrangements

Funeral arrangements sold by funeral homes generally include the following services and merchandise: in a single "package" price.

Cost of casket
Removal of remains to funeral home
Embalming
Use of chapel and funeral home facilities
Arranging for obituary notices
Use of viewing room
Church services

Burial permits
Transcript of death certificates
Arranging and care of flowers
Providing guestbook and acknowledgment cards
Use of hearse
Arranging for veterans', social security, fraternal, labor union or life insurance benefits
Use of one limousine for family
Providing prayer cards
Arranging for pallbearers
Services of professional staff
Extension of credit

Additional charges are made for the following:

Grave liner
Vault or interment receptacle
Burial clothing
Extra limousine
Flower car
Newspaper death notices
Clergyman's honorarium
Organist
Soloist
Flowers
Additional certified copies of death certificates

The price of a funeral varies according to the casket chosen. Casket prices range from $100 to $2,000. A higher priced casket will increase the total price of a standard adult funeral. Thus, a $900 funeral and a $400 funeral may differ only in the choice of casket.

Caskets are usually displayed in a room within the funeral home or at the casket manufacturer's display room or by means of photographs. Sometimes the lowest priced caskets are not on display in the display room, or low priced caskets which are on display are shown in colors or materials which are less desirable than others. However, other low priced or more suitably colored caskets are often available and must be specifically requested. It is important that consumers be fully informed of all caskets available, because the price range is great and the price of the casket is the largest cost factor of the standard adult funeral.

Burial Charges

Often the burial charges in cemeteries owned by nonprofit groups or municipalities are less expensive than privately owned cemeteries. There are also 103 national cemeteries, about half of which have openings for additional

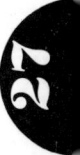

burial of eligible veterans and their eligible family members.

The cost of a grave space may include a charge for the care of the cemetery property. Some cemeteries have established what is called an endowment care fund. This means that a portion of the purchase price of the cemetery property is placed in a trust fund, the proceeds or earnings of which are used for maintaining the grounds long after the people who supply the funds are gone.

If a cemetery is not an endowment care cemetery, the property may or may not be maintained; but, if it is, the owner may have to pay some additional cost for care.

Most cemeteries require the purchase of a grave liner, a concrete container into which a casket is placed, to prevent the earth from caving in. Vaults are more elaborately designed and more expensive than grave liners but are used basically for the same purpose.

The purchase price of cemetery property (the grave space, crypt or niche) is only one of many cemetery charges. Other items include: grave opening and closing, grave liner, grave marker and its installation, and perpetual care. Some even choose above ground entombment in a mausoleum.

Disposition of cremated remains in a cemetery may be ground burial, in what the industry calls an "urn garden," or above-ground inurnment in a columbarium.

Grave Markers

Consumers generally buy grave markers from the cemetery where the burial is to take place. However, grave markers are also available from independent monument dealers, and in some cases these firms offer lower prices than cemeteries.

There is a wide variety of choices to consider. First, the kind of material for the grave marker must be selected. Monuments and memorials in cemeteries are fashioned from many kinds of materials, but the most common are granite and bronze. Granite is the least expensive. The size and type of the marker also affect the total price. Markers can be elaborately designed from large pieces of stone and placed upright at the grave site, or they can be simple and flush to the ground.

Often cemeteries have grave marker requirements as to material, size, style, etc., which may severely limit a consumer's choices.

Consumers may find some cemeteries which will not permit installation of a monument purchased from an independent monument dealer. Buyers may find some cemeteries charge a higher installation fee if a monument is purchased from an independent monument dealer.

A standard single grave marker usually includes a two-line inscription of the person's name and the years of birth and death. A longer inscription is more expensive. Special border carvings will also increase the price. Most cemeteries also charge a fee for installation (setting the marker in a concrete foundation).

The endowment care fund for cemetery property maintenance may not include care of the marker. Independent monument dealers may also charge for delivery of the marker to the cemetery.

Eligible veterans can receive a head stone or grave marker through the Veterans Administration at no charge, whether burial is in a national or a private cemetery. A private cemetery usually charges an installation fee.

Cutting Costs

If cost is a primary concern, the overall lowest priced alternative in making death arrangements is to donate the body to medical research. The next lowest priced choice is immediate cremation; that is, within 24 hours after death. This choice eliminates embalming, viewing and other funeral home services and merchandise, often including the casket. Having the ashes scattered (this can be arranged through a funeral home but does not need to be) will eliminate the purchase of a container or an urn. Finally, if a ceremony is desired, a memorial service can be held in a private home. Through these choices, the services and merchandise needed from a funeral home, cemetery and monument dealer can be minimized.

The Veterans Administration offers death benefits for eligible veterans and their families which include $250 toward funeral costs, free burial in a national cemetery, $150 toward cemetery costs if in a nongovernment cemetery, and a head stone or monument supplied at no charge.

Social Security benefits, currently $255 may also be available.

28

DISEASES, DISABILITIES AND ACCIDENTS

Overview

Acute Conditions

Table 28-1   Acute conditions summary

	Incidence of acute conditions in thousands	Percent distribution	Number of acute conditions per 100 persons per year
All acute conditions	364,278	100.0	175.7
Infective and parasitic diseases	40,465	11.1	19.5
Common childhood diseases	3,996	1.1	1.9
Virus, N.O.S.	15,332	4.2	7.4
Other infective and parasitic diseases	21,137	5.8	10.2
Respiratory conditions	195,741	53.7	94.4
Upper respiratory conditions	94,868	26.0	45.8
Common cold	70,311	19.3	33.9
Other upper respiratory conditions	24,557	6.7	11.8
Influenza	92,809	25.5	44.8
Influenza with digestive manifestations	15,012	4.1	7.2
Other influenza	77,796	21.4	37.5
Other respiratory conditions	8,065	2.2	3.9
Pneumonia	1,851	0.5	0.9
Bronchitis	3,266	0.9	1.6
Other respiratory conditions	2,947	0.8	1.4
Digestive system conditions	16,193	4.4	7.8
Dental conditions	3,511	1.0	1.7
Functional and symptomatic upper gastrointestinal disorders, N.E.C.	7,436	2.0	3.6
Other digestive system conditions	5,246	1.4	2.5
Injuries	63,085	17.3	30.4
Fractures, dislocations, sprains, and strains	18,310	5.0	8.8
Fractures and dislocations	5,884	1.6	2.8
Sprains and strains	12,426	3.4	6.0
Open wounds and lacerations	17,448	4.8	8.4
Contusions and superficial injuries	13,226	3.6	6.4
Other current injuries	14,101	3.9	6.8
All other acute conditions	48,794	13.4	23.5
Diseases of the ear	11,573	3.2	5.6
Headaches	3,145	0.9	1.5
Genitourinary disorders	8,537	2.3	4.1
Deliveries and disorders of pregnancy and the puerperium	2,760	0.8	1.3
Diseases of the skin	2,310	0.6	1.1
Diseases of the musculoskeletal system	4,673	1.3	2.3
All other acute conditions	15,796	4.3	7.6

Note: Excluded from these statistics are all conditions involving neither restricted activity nor medical attention.

N.O.S.—not otherwise specified; N.E.C.—not elsewhere classified.

Source: DHEW, 1976 (1974 Survey).

Table 28-2 Acute conditions by age and sex

Sex and condition group	All ages	Under 6 years	6–16 years	17–44 years	45 years & over	All ages	Under 6 years	6–16 years	17–44 years	45 years & over
	Incidence of acute conditions in thousands					Number of acute conditions per 100 persons per year				
Both sexes										
All acute conditions	364,278	61,121	102,172	141,483	59,503	175.7	309.0	236.7	175.1	93.5
Infective and parasitic diseases	40,465	9,371	13,062	12,958	5,074	19.5	47.4	30.3	16.0	8.0
Respiratory conditions	195,741	34,149	55,671	74,696	30,225	94.4	172.6	131.3	92.5	47.5
Upper respiratory conditions	94,868	20,233	27,982	33,134	13,520	45.8	102.3	64.8	41.0	21.3
Influenza	92,809	11,928	27,228	38,685	14,968	44.8	60.3	63.1	47.9	23.5
Other respiratory conditions	8,065	1,987	1,462	2,878	1,738	3.9	10.0	3.4	3.6	2.7
Digestive system conditions	16,193	1,449	4,598	7,076	3,070	7.8	7.3	10.6	8.8	4.3
Injuries	63,085	6,697	16,429	27,277	12,682	30.4	33.9	38.1	33.8	19.9
All other acute conditions	48,794	9,455	11,412	19,476	8,452	23.5	47.8	26.4	24.1	13.3
Male										
All acute conditions	171,661	31,560	52,269	63,560	24,272	171.6	312.2	237.9	163.2	83.7
Infective and parasitic diseases	18,086	4,246	6,979	5,007	1,853	18.1	42.0	31.8	12.9	6.4
Respiratory conditions	92,228	17,135	28,023	33,793	13,277	92.2	169.5	127.6	86.8	45.8
Upper respiratory conditions	44,249	10,178	12,849	15,690	5,531	44.2	100.7	58.5	40.3	19.1
Influenza	43,753	5,843	14,403	16,493	7,014	43.7	57.8	65.6	42.3	24.2
Other respiratory conditions	4,227	1,114	771	1,609	733	4.2	11.0	3.5	4.1	2.5
Digestive system conditions	6,043	803	1,940	2,483	817	6.0	7.9	8.8	6.4	2.8
Injuries	36,059	3,939	9,835	16,541	5,693	36.0	39.0	45.0	42.5	19.5
All other acute conditions	19,245	5,436	5,442	5,736	2,631	19.2	53.8	24.8	14.7	9.1
Female										
All acute conditions	192,617	29,561	49,903	77,922	35,231	179.5	305.6	235.3	186.3	101.8
Infective and parasitic diseases	22,379	5,125	6,083	7,950	3,221	20.9	53.0	28.7	19.0	9.3
Respiratory conditions	103,513	17,014	28,648	40,904	16,947	96.5	175.9	135.1	97.8	49.0
Upper respiratory conditions	50,619	10,055	15,133	17,443	7,989	47.2	103.9	71.4	41.7	23.1
Influenza	49,056	6,085	12,825	22,192	7,954	45.7	62.9	60.5	53.1	23.0
Other respiratory conditions	3,838	874	691	1,268	1,005	3.6	9.0	3.3	3.0	2.9
Digestive system conditions	10,150	646	2,658	4,594	2,253	9.5	6.7	12.5	11.0	6.5
Injuries	27,026	2,758	6,543	10,735	6,989	25.2	28.5	30.9	25.7	20.2
All other acute conditions	29,549	4,019	5,970	13,740	5,820	27.5	41.5	28.2	32.8	16.8

Note: Excluded from these statistics are all conditions involving neither restricted activity nor medical attention.

Source: DHEW, 1976 (1974 Survey).

Table 28-3   Acute conditions: comparative data

Characteristic	July 1973– June 1974 per 100 persons	Characteristic	July 1973– June 1974 per 100 persons
All acute conditions	172.0	Geographic region	
Sex		Northeast	152.8
Male	169.7	North Central	179.5
Female	174.1	South	167.0
		West	195.1
Age			
Under 6 years	303.4		
6–16 years	232.2		
17–44 years	170.2	Type of disability day	
45–64 years	98.3	Days of restricted activity	922.2
65 years and over	75.7	Days of bed disability	400.4
		Days lost from work among cur-	
Place of residence		rently employed persons	355.8
All SMSA	177.1	Days lost from school among	
Outside SMSA:		children aged 6–16 years	493.2
Nonfarm	162.8		
Farm	142.8		

Source: U.S. Bureau of Labor Statistics.

Hospital Illnesses

Table 28-4   Discharges by condition and by age, race, and sex—1974

Condition	Total	<15	15–44	45–64	65+	White	Non-white	Male	Female
Total, all conditions	153,040	18,188	65,141	36,268	33,443	132,933	20,107	61,363	91,677
	(100.0%)	(11.9%)	(42.6%)	(23.7%)	(21.9%)	(86.9%)	(13.1%)	(40.1%)	(59.9%)
Infective and parasitic	1,729	437	759	306	227	1,414	315	882	847
diseases	(1.1%)	(0.3%)	(0.5%)	(0.2%)	(0.1%)	(0.9%)	(0.2%)	(0.6%)	(0.6%)
Neoplasms	10,437	300	3,371	3,712	3,054	9,190	1,247	3,602	6,835
	(6.8%)	(0.2%)	(2.2%)	(2.4%)	(2.0%)	(6.0%)	(0.8%)	(2.4%)	(4.5%)
A. Malignant	5,644	75	853	2,306	2,410	5,068	576	2,560	3,084
	(3.7%)	r[1]	(0.6%)	(1.5%)	(1.6%)	(3.3%)	(0.4%)	(1.7%)	(2.0%)
1. Sex-specific	999	—	251	307	441	818	181	315	684
	(0.7%)		(0.2%)	(0.2%)	(0.3%)	(0.5%)	(0.1%)	(0.2%)	(0.4%)
a. Male	315	—	—	49	266	267	48	315	—
	(0.2%)			r	(0.2%)	(0.2%)	r	(0.2%)	
b. Female	684	—	251	258	175	551	133	—	684
	(0.4%)		(0.2%)	(0.2%)	(0.1%)	(0.4%)	(0.1%)		(0.4%)
2. Not sex-specific	4,645	75	602	1,999	1,969	4,250	395	2,245	2,400
	(3.0%)	r	(0.4%)	(1.3%)	(1.3%)	(2.8%)	(0.3%)	(1.5%)	(1.6%)
B. Benign	4,793	227	2,558	1,550	458	4,122	671	1,042	3,751
	(3.1%)	(0.1%)	(1.7%)	(1.0%)	(0.3%)	(2.7%)	(0.4%)	(0.7%)	(1.7%)
1. Sex-specific	2,148	9	1,279	787	73	1,802	346	—	2,148
	(1.4%)	r	(0.8%)	(0.5%)	r	(1.2%)	(0.2%)		(1.4%)
a. Male	—	—	—	—	—	—	—	—	—
b. Female	2,148	9	1,279	787	73	1,802	346	—	2,148
	(1.4%)	r	(0.8%)	(0.5%)	r	(1.2%)	(0.2%)		(1.4%)
2. Not sex-specific	2,645	218	1,279	763	385	2,320	325	1,042	1,603
	(1.7%)	(0.1%)	(0.8%)	(0.5%)	(0.3%)	(1.5%)	(0.2%)	(0.7%)	(1.0%)
Allergic, endocrine,	4,248	312	1,175	1,451	1,310	3,539	709	1,535	2,713
metabolic, & nutri-	(2.8%)	(0.2%)	(0.8%)	(0.9%)	(0.9%)	(2.3%)	(0.5%)	(1.0%)	(1.8%)
tional conditions									

(continued)

Table 28-4 (continued)

Condition	Total	<15	15–44	45–64	65+	White	Non-white	Male	Female
A. Hay fever, asthma	726	147	203	211	165	547	179	305	421
	(0.5%)	(0.1%)	(0.1%)	(0.1%)	(0.1%)	(0.4%)	(0.1%)	(0.2%)	(0.3%)
B. Diabetes mellitus	2,086	67	394	737	888	1,755	331	796	1,290
	(1.4%)	r	(0.3%)	(0.5%)	(0.6%)	(1.1%)	(0.2%)	(0.5%)	(0.8%)
C. Other	1,436	98	578	503	257	1,237	199	434	1,002
	(0.9%)	(0.1%)	(0.4%)	(0.3%)	(0.2%)	(0.8%)	(0.1%)	(0.3%)	(0.7%)
Conditions of blood and	953	138	210	223	382	797	156	433	520
blood-forming organs	(0.6%)	(0.1%)	(0.1%)	(0.1%)	(0.2%)	(0.5%)	(0.1%)	(0.3%)	(0.3%)
Mental, psychoneurotic,	4,328	131	2,309	1,335	553	3,765	563	1,932	2,396
and personality disorders	(2.8%)	(0.1%)	(1.5%)	(0.9%)	(0.4%)	(2.5%)	(0.4%)	(1.3%)	(1.6%)
Conditions of the	8,352	1,054	1,372	2,075	3,851	7,495	857	3,982	4,370
nervous system &	(5.5%)	(0.7%)	(0.9%)	(1.4%)	(2.5%)	(4.9%)	(0.6%)	(2.6%)	(2.9%)
sense organs	1,220	441	329	303	147	1,153	67	596	624
A. Conditions of ear and mastoid process	(0.8%)	(0.3%)	(0.2%)	(0.2%)	(0.1%)	(0.8%)	r	(0.4%)	(0.4%)
B. Cataract and other	2,352	372	265	534	1,181	2,142	210	1,111	1,241
conditions of eye	(1.5%)	(0.2%)	(0.2%)	(0.3%)	(0.8%)	(1.4%)	(0.1%)	(0.1%)	(0.8%)
C. Other	4,780	241	778	1,238	2,523	4,200	580	2,275	2,505
	(3.1%)	(0.2%)	(0.5%)	(0.8%)	(1.6%)	(2.7%)	(0.4%)	(1.5%)	(1.6%)
Conditions of the	14,448	274	2,206	5,075	6,893	12,032	1,516	7,283	7,165
circulatory system	(9.4%)	(0.2%)	(1.4%)	(3.3%)	(4.5%)	(8.5%)	(1.0%)	(4.8%)	(4.7%)
A. Congestive heart	983	5	23	194	761	837	146	466	517
failure	(0.6%)		r	(0.1%)	(0.5%)	(0.5%)	(0.1%)	(0.3%)	(0.3%)
B. Arteriosclerosis	385	—	12	85	288	352	33	194	191
	(0.3%)	—	r	(0.1%)	(0.2%)	(0.2%)	r	(0.1%)	(0.1%)
C. Other	13,080	269	2,171	4,796	5,844	11,743	1,337	6,623	6,457
	(8.5%)	(0.2%)	(1.4%)	(3.1%)	(3.8%)	(7.8%)	(0.9%)	(4.3%)	(4.2%)
Conditions of the	17,737	7,492	4,028	2,930	3,287	15,821	1,916	9,172	8,565
respiratory system	(11.6%)	(4.9%)	(2.6%)	(1.9%)	(2.1%)	(10.3%)	(1.3%)	(6.0%)	(5.6%)
A. Upper respiratory	2,090	1,084	497	249	260	1,857	233	1,056	1,034
infection, acute	(1.4%)	(0.7%)	(0.3%)	(0.2%)	(0.2%)	(1.2%)	(0.2%)	(0.7%)	(0.7%)
B. Pneumonia	3,828	1,358	563	752	1,155	3,241	587	2,037	1,791
	(2.5%)	(0.9%)	(0.4%)	(0.5%)	(0.8%)	(2.1%)	(0.4%)	(1.3%)	(1.2%)
C. Bronchitis, acute	999	333	182	259	225	908	91	509	490
	(0.7%)	(0.2%)	(0.1%)	(0.2%)	(0.1%)	(0.6%)	(0.1%)	(0.3%)	(0.3%)
D. Other	10,820	4,717	2,786	1,670	1,647	9,815	1,005	5,570	5,250
	(7.1%)	(3.1%)	(1.8%)	(1.1%)	(1.1%)	(6.4%)	(0.7%)	(3.6%)	(3.4%)
Conditions of the	21,544	2,434	7,329	6,814	4,967	19,456	2,088	10,686	10,858
digestive system	(14.1%)	(1.6%)	(4.8%)	(4.5%)	(3.2%)	(12.7%)	(1.4%)	(7.0%)	(7.1%)
A. Ulcers of stomach,	2,413	26	819	964	604	2,158	255	1,493	920
duodenum, jejunum	(1.6%)	r	(0.5%)	(0.6%)	(0.4%)	(1.4%)	(0.2%)	(1.0%)	(0.6%)
B. Appendicitis	1,814	560	1,001	169	84	1,632	182	1,009	805
	(1.2%)	(0.4%)	(0.7%)	(0.1%)	(0.1%)	(1.1%)	(0.1%)	(0.7%)	(0.5%)
C. Inguinal hernia	2,689	552	654	952	531	2,443	246	2,402	287
	(1.8%)	(0.4%)	(0.4%)	(0.6%)	(0.3%)	(1.6%)	(0.2%)	(1.6%)	(0.2%)
D. Cholelithiasis and	2,613	5	799	1,020	789	2,467	146	648	1,965
cholecystitis	(1.7%)	r	(0.5%)	(0.7%)	(0.5%)	(1.6%)	(0.1%)	(0.4%)	(1.3%)
E. Other	12,015	1,291	4,056	3,709	2,959	10,756	1,259	5,134	6,881
	(7.9%)	(0.8%)	(2.7%)	(2.4%)	(1.9%)	(7.0%)	(0.8%)	(3.4%)	(4.5%)
Conditions of genito-	14,642	1,086	7,064	3,928	2,564	12,734	1,908	4,906	9,736
urinary system	(9.6%)	(0.7%)	(4.6%)	(2.6%)	(1.7%)	(8.3%)	(1.2%)	(3.2%)	(6.4%)
A. Cystitis	963	107	363	253	240	871	92	225	738
	(0.6%)	(0.1%)	(0.2%)	(0.2%)	(0.2%)	(0.6%)	(0.1%)	(0.1%)	(0.5%)
B. Sex-specific	8,176	373	4,364	2,072	1,367	6,969	1,207	2,254	5,922
	(5.3%)	(0.2%)	(2.9%)	(1.4%)	(0.9%)	(4.6%)	(0.8%)	(1.5%)	(3.9%)
1. Male	2,254	317	368	587	982	1,931	323	2,254	—
	(1.5%)	(0.2%)	(0.2%)	(0.4%)	(0.6%)	(1.3%)	(0.2%)	(1.5%)	—
2. Female	5,922	56	3,996	1,485	385	5,038	884	—	5,922
	(3.9%)	r	(2.6%)	(1.0%)	(0.3%)	(3.3%)	(0.6%)	—	(3.9%)
C. Other	5,503	606	2,337	1,603	957	4,894	609	2,427	3,076
	(3.6%)	(0.4%)	(1.5%)	(1.0%)	(0.6%)	(3.2%)	(0.4%)	(1.6%)	(2.0%)

28

Table 28-4 (continued)

Condition	Total	<15	15–44	45–64	65+	White	Non-white	Male	Female
Deliveries and compli-	23,175	84	23,041	50	—	18,335	4,840	—	23,175
cations of pregnancy, childbirth, and puerperium	(15.1%)	(0.1%)	(15.1%)	r	—	(12.0%)	(3.2%)	—	(15.1%)
A. Abortion	1,756	5	1,739	12	—	1,369	387	—	1,756
	(1.1%)	r	(1.1%)	r	—	(0.9%)	(0.3%)	—	(1.1%)
B. Normal delivery	14,938	38	14,869	31	—	12,120	2,818	—	14,938
	(9.8%)	r	(9.7%)	r	—	(7.9%)	(1.8%)	—	(9.8%)
C. Delivery with	3,606	25	3,574	7	—	2,635	971	—	3,606
complications	(2.4%)	r	(2.3%)	r	—	(1.7%)	(0.6%)	—	(2.4%)
D. Other	2,875	16	2,859	—	—	2,211	664	—	2,875
	(1.9%)	r	(1.9%)	—	—	(1.4%)	(0.4%)	—	(1.9%)
Conditions of skin and	2,145	309	886	574	376	1,818	327	1,031	1,114
cellular tissues	(1.4%)	(0.2%)	(0.6%)	(0.4%)	(0.2%)	(1.2%)	(0.2%)	(0.7%)	(0.7%)
Diseases of bones and	5,476	359	2,036	1,971	1,110	4,979	497	2,527	2,949
organs of movement	(3.6%)	(0.2%)	(1.3%)	(1.3%)	(0.7%)	(3.3%)	(0.3%)	(1.7%)	(1.9%)
A. Osteoarthritis	697	—	76	284	337	651	46	286	411
	(0.5%)	—	r	(0.2%)	(0.2%)	(0.4%)	r	(0.2%)	(0.3%)
B. Other	4,779	359	1,960	1,687	773	4,328	451	2,241	2,538
	(3.1%)	(0.2%)	(1.3%)	(1.1%)	(0.5%)	(2.8%)	(0.3%)	(1.5%)	(1.7%)
Congenital malforma-	1,259	682	363	154	60	1,136	123	694	565
tions	(0.8%)	(0.4%)	(0.2%)	(0.1%)	r	(0.7%)	(0.1%)	(0.5%)	(0.4%)
Certain conditions of	279	279	—	—	—	202	77	157	122
early infancy	(0.2%)	(0.2%)	—	—	—	(0.1%)	(0.1%)	(0.1%)	(0.1%)
Miscellaneous or ill-	6,279	874	2,372	1,700	1,333	5,503	776	3,034	3,245
defined symptoms or conditions	(4.1%)	(0.6%)	(1.5%)	(1.1%)	(0.9%)	(3.6%)	(0.5%)	(2.0%)	(2.1%)
Injuries and adverse	16,009	2,551	7,291	3,435	2,732	13,777	2,232	9,320	6,689
external effects	(10.5%)	(1.7%)	(4.8%)	(2.2%)	(1.8%)	(9.0%)	(1.5%)	(6.1%)	(4.4%)
A. Fractures	5,735	914	1,841	1,304	1,676	5,113	622	3,024	2,711
	(3.7%)	(0.6%)	(1.2%)	(0.9%)	(1.1%)	(3.3%)	(0.4%)	(2.0%)	(1.8%)
B. Sprains, strains of	1,523	23	911	467	122	1,385	138	779	744
back and neck	(1.0%)	r	(0.6%)	(0.3%)	(0.1%)	(0.9%)	(0.1%)	(0.5%)	(0.5%)
C. Lacerations	1,928	290	1,199	338	101	1,465	463	1,397	531
	(1.3%)	(0.2%)	(0.8%)	(0.2%)	(0.1%)	(1.0%)	(0.3%)	(0.9%)	(0.3%)
D. Other	6,823	1,324	3,340	1,326	833	5,814	1,009	4,120	2,703
	(4.5%)	(0.9%)	(0.2%)	(0.9%)	(0.5%)	(3.8%)	(0.7%)	(2.7%)	(1.8%)

[1]r = percent less than 0.1%.

Sources: Vital and Health Statistics, DHEW, 1973; and House Report, "Issues in the National Financing of Health Care," November 1976.

Stress and Illness*

We rarely think of a car accident or a suicide attempt as an illness. Surgical operations are not illnesses. But all of them involve a certain disruption of the state of health and functioning. (That's why the word "illness" is really too limited and the term "health change" is used here.)

The sophisticated instruments and laboratory tests we use to diagnose ailments still do not tell us what accounts for individual susceptibility to illness.

We say that we get sick when our resistance is down. But resistance is hard to define. Is it related to fitness? Is resistance related to mental attitude? Is resistance related to exposure to illness producing agents?

Psychiatric disorders such as depression and schizophrenia involve more than emotional imbalance. Depressed people, for example, almost always experience marked decreases in appetite and sex drive, along with weight loss, insomnia, fatigue and constipation.

Whatever the contributing factors, when our resistance goes down our risk goes up. One approach to the problem of what determines the behavior we call sick is to find a measure of risk, or susceptibility, to health change.

*Source: Adapted from "Stress," published by the Blue Cross Association.

Adolf Meyer, professor of psychiatry at Johns Hopkins, around the turn of the century began keeping "life charts" on his patients. They were abbreviated biographies that showed time and again that people tended to get sick around the time when clusters of major events took place in their lives.

In 1949, Dr. Thomas H. Holmes began to apply Dr. Meyer's life chart idea systematically to the case histories of more than 5,000 patients.

Over a 15-year period, between 1949 and 1964, Dr. Thomas Holmes and Dr. Richard Rahe studied the correlation between the number and types of changes in people's lives and incidences of illness.

A number of life-change items were found to occur over and over and tended to cluster in the brief time period just prior to the onset of major illnesses. The items are listed in the chart shown here. The "Social Readjustment Rating Scale" is an instrument intended to help predict general illness or disability by the use of scoring values assigned to 43 common life occurrences.

Some of the changes in life situation and life style are socially desirable and some are undesirable. We are all aware of the drain on energy and resources associated with such "stressful"

Table 28-5   Holmes-Rahe social readjustment rating scale

Rank	Event	Value	Rank	Event	Value
1	Death of spouse	100	23	Son or daughter leaving home	29
2	Divorce	73	24	Trouble with in-laws	29
3	Marital separation	65	25	Outstanding personal achieve-	
4	Jail term	63		ment	28
5	Death of close family member	63			
6	Personal injury or illness	53	26	Spouse begins or stops work	26
7	Marriage	50	27	Starting or finishing school	26
8	Fired from work	47	28	Change in living conditions	25
9	Marital reconciliation	45	29	Revision of personal habits	24
10	Retirement	45	30	Trouble with boss	23
11	Changes in family member's		31	Change in work hours, condi-	
	health	44		tions	20
12	Pregnancy	40			
13	Sex difficulties	39	32	Change in residence	20
14	Addition to family	39	33	Change in schools	20
15	Business readjustment	39	34	Change in recreational habits	19
16	Change in financial status	38	35	Change in church activities	19
17	Death of close friend	37	36	Change in social activities	18
18	Change to different line of		37	Mortgage or loan under	
	work	36		$10,000	17
19	Change in number of marital				
	arguments	35	38	Change in sleeping habits	16
20	Mortgage or loan over		39	Change in number of family	
	$10,000	31		gatherings	15
21	Foreclosure of mortgage		40	Change in eating habits	15
	or loan	30	41	Vacation	13
22	Change in work responsi-		42	Christmas season	12
	bilities	29	43	Minor violation of the law	11

Note: The probability of illness increases with the frequency and severity of life change events. An individual's score is figured by adding the values of all occurrences on the list experienced during the past year. If you scored below 150 points, you are on pretty safe ground—about a one in three chance of serious health change in the next two years. Remember, you already have a 10% chance of winding up in the hospital some time during the year. If you scored between 150 and 300 points, your chances rise to about 50-50. The odds on Russian roulette are better than that. If you scored over 300 points, be sure your health insurance is paid up—your chances are almost 90%.

Source: *Journal of Psychosomatic Research*, 11:213–218, 1967 (Pergamon Press, Ltd.)

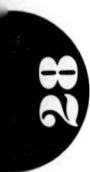

events as divorce, troubles with the boss and death of a spouse.

But not all life changes are stressful in the usual negative sense. What could be more gratifying to a singer than finally to hit the big time? Concert tours, recording dates, parties, money and meeting famous people may represent all his dreams come true. But the way he lives his life will be radically changed. Think of the many changes brought about by the happiest marriage. Even a long awaited vacation requires certain change if only for a relatively short time—eating in restaurants instead of at home, sleeping in a sleeping bag instead of a bed, snorkeling or playing tennis for the first time. Whether "positive" or "negative" to our way of thinking, all such events require us to cope, adapt or change to some degree.

The numbers in the right-hand column of the chart represent the amount, duration and severity of change required to cope with each item, averaged from the responses of hundreds of people. Marriage was arbitrarily assigned the magnitude of 50 points, and the subjects then rated the other items by number as to how much more or how much less change each requires in comparison with marriage. For instance, the scale implies that losing a spouse by death (100) requires, in the long run, twice as much readjustment as getting married (50), four times as much as a change in living conditions (25), and nearly 10 times as much as minor violations of the law (11).

The more changes you undergo in a given period of time, the more points you accumulate. The higher the score, the more likely you are to have a health change. All the kinds of health changes previously discussed—serious illnesses, injuries, surgical operations, psychiatric disorders, even pregnancy—have been found to follow high life change scores. And the higher your score, the more serious the health change will likely be.

What's your own risk? Take a moment and add up the score for all the items that applied to you in the last year.

Leading Causes of Death

The excess of male death rates over female death rates has increased for most causes of death during recent decades. Of the 15 leading causes of death 14 show an advantage for females. The only exception is diabetes mellitus, and even this cause of death has shown a steady decline in the male advantage. Only for suicide and peptic ulcers has there been a dis-

tinct erosion of the female mortality advantage. Several other conditions, such as homicide, congenital anomalies, cirrhosis of the liver, and arteriosclerosis reveal no definite trend in the sex ratio of mortality, although women are still less likely to die from these causes than men.

Causes of Death: Male vs. Female

Table 28-6   Ratio of female to male death rates and age-adjusted female death rate by cause of death. (Based on age-specific death rates per 100,000 population in specified group)

Causes of death	1973	1952
All causes		
Female age-adjusted rate	513.1	658.9
Age-adjusted sex ratio[1]	0.56	0.67
Diseases of the heart	167.4	225.6
Sex ratio	0.49	0.60
Malignant neoplasms	108.7	118.8
Sex ratio	0.68	0.89
Cerebrovascular diseases	58.5	84.6
Sex ratio	0.83	0.93
Accidents	27.4	32.0
Sex ratio	0.35	0.37
Influenza and pneumonia	15.2	19.7
Sex ratio	0.57	0.69
Certain causes of mortality in early infancy	11.8	33.5
Sex ratio	0.68	0.69
Diabetes mellitus	13.3	16.4
Sex ratio	1.03	1.43
Arteriosclerosis	7.3	13.9
Sex ratio	0.82	0.82
Bronchitis, emphysema, and asthma	4.5	3.2
Sex ratio	0.25	0.48
Cirrhosis of the liver	9.9	6.2
Sex ratio	0.47	0.48
Suicide	6.6	4.3
Sex ratio	0.37	0.28
Congenital anomalies	6.0	11.4
Sex ratio	0.81	0.81
Homicide	4.5	2.4
Sex ratio	0.27	0.28
Nephritis and nephrosis	2.5	11.8
Sex ratio	0.68	0.77
Peptic ulcer	1.6	1.8
Sex ratio	0.39	0.22

[1]Ratio of female rate to male rate.

Source: National Center for Health Statistics.

Causes of Death by Age

Table 28-7 Leading causes of death—by age

Expected number of deaths per 100,000 from ages 15 through 24

Cause of death	White males	Nonwhite males
Motor accidents	807	661
Other accidents	310	545
Suicide	113	82
Neoplasms	103	82
Homicide	75	771
Influenza and pneumonia	29	58
Heart diseases	28	69
All causes	1,690	2,777

Expected number of deaths per 100,000 from ages 35 through 44

Cause of death	White males	Nonwhite males
Heart diseases	999	1,831
Neoplasms	507	803
(lung cancer)	(146)	(285)
Motor accidents	351	596
Other accidents	321	787
Suicide	232	126
Cirrhosis of liver	188	557
Homicide	98	1,146
Influenza and pneumonia	79	422
All causes	3,458	9,203

Expected number of deaths per 100,000 from ages 55 through 64

Cause of death	White males	Nonwhite males
Heart diseases	9,940	11,679
Neoplasms	4,697	6,484
(lung cancer)	(1,848)	(2,148)
Cerebrovascular disease	1,196	3,519
Cirrhosis of liver	645	677
Other accidents	508	945
Influenza and pneumonia	505	1,210
Motor accidents	383	628
Suicide	348	120
Homicide	62	508
All causes	21,902	32,607

Source: House Report, *Issues in Nat'l. Financing of Health Care,* November 1976.

Medic Alert Name Tags

The Medic Alert Foundation International (Turlock, California 95380. Tel. (209) 632-2371) is a nonprofit, charitable and tax-exempt organization. The Foundation provides the very best emergency medical identification system available in the world, serving persons with hidden or special medical problems that cannot be easily seen or recognized. Diabetes, special allergies, heart conditions, and epilepsy are among more than 200 common reasons persons join Medic Alert.

Medic Alert's lifesaving system of protection is available for a one-time lifetime basic membership fee of $7.00.

A. The first of the three-part system is the metallic alerting device or emblem in the form of a bracelet or necklace. It bears the insignia of the medical profession and the words "Medic Alert" in red. On the reverse side is engraved the medical problem or problems of the wearer, such as "Taking Anticoagulants" or "Wearing Contact Lenses." The member's unique membership number and the telephone number of the Emergency Answering Service are also engraved.

B. The system of protection also includes a wallet card which is issued annually and contains additional personal and medical information to that on the emblem.

C. The third part of Medic Alert's system is the Emergency Answering Service which is available to all emergency personnel around the clock via a collect telephone call from any world location. The telephone number is engraved on the emblem and printed on the wallet card. Within seconds of receiving a call, emergency operators can relay emergency information from the computerized data base that might save a life.

The top ten medical problems of Medic Alert members, in descending order are: allergy to penicillin, diabetes, heart condition, taking anticoagulants, wearing contact lenses, allergy to sulfa, epilepsy, allergy to insect stings, allergy to bee stings and allergy to codeine.

Among many organizations endorsing Medic Alert are: American Hospital Association, American Nurses' Association, American College of Physicians.

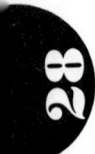

Accidents and Injuries

During 1971 and 1972 an average of about 63.4 million persons per year were injured, an incidence of 311.9 persons injured per 1,000 persons per year.

Table 28-8   Number injured per 1,000 persons, by type of accident, U.S.A., 1971–2

Type of accident	No. of persons injured per 1000 persons/ year	Type of accident	No. of persons injured per 1000 persons/ year
Total persons injured	311.9	Struck by moving object	20.2
Moving motor vehicles	23.2	Twisted or stumbled	14.2
Injured person inside vehicle or getting in or out	20.2	Injury caused by animal or insect	13.2
Collision between 2 or more vehicles on road	11.6	Complication of medical or surgical procedure	12.1
Ran off road	2.8	One-time lifting or exertion	11.6
Accident not on road	2.3	Handled or stepped on rough object	11.4
Other and unknown	4.0		
Injured person outside vehicle	2.2	Foreign body in eye, windpipe or other orifice	7.2
All other accidents	288.7	Machinery in operation	6.2
Falls	67.0	Nonmotor vehicle in motion	5.9
On stairs, steps or from a height	(21.7)	Discharge of firearm	.8
All other falls	(45.3)	Uncontrolled fire or explosion	.5
Bumped into object or person	27.8	Other	16.8
Cutting or piercing instrument	20.6	Unknown	42.4

Source: National Center for Health Statistics.

Accidental Deaths

Table 28-9   Accidental deaths by type of accident

Type of accident or manner of injury	1974[1]	1973	1972	1971
All accidental deaths	104,622	115,821	115,448	113,439
Transport accidents	50,659	59,986	60,480	58,529
Railway accidents	716	789	692	750
Motor vehicle	46,402	55,511	56,278	54,381
Traffic	45,314	54,347	55,214	53,366
Nontraffic	1,088	1,164	1,064	1,015
Other road vehicle	275	293	306	263
Water transport	1,579	1,725	1,568	1,531
Drowning (excluded from drownings below)	1,413	1,573	1,390	1,375
Other water transport	166	152	178	156
Air and space transport	1,687	1,668	1,636	1,604
Poisoning by solids and liquids	4,016	3,683	3,728	3,710
Poisoning by drugs and medicaments	2,742	2,444	2,516	2,528
Poisoning by other solid and liquid substances	1,274	1,239	1,212	1,182
Poisoning by gases and vapors	1,518	1,652	1,690	1,646

(continued)

Table 28-9   (continued)

Type of accident or manner of injury	1974[1]	1973	1972	1971
Falls	16,339	16,506	16,744	16,755
Fires and flames	6,236	6,503	6,714	6,776
Conflagration in private dwellings	4,369	4,362	4,654	4,401
Conflagration in other buildings or structures	224	280	268	265
Conflagration not in buildings or structures	75	87	92	123
Ignition of clothing	445	517	542	655
Ignition of highly inflammable materials	185	254	224	223
Other and unspecified fires and flames	938	1,003	934	1,109
Natural and environmental factors	1,427	1,348	1,800	1,366
Excessive heat	140	181	234	112
Excessive cold	348	381	490	361
Hunger, thirst, exposure and neglect	201	240	268	283
Bites and stings of venomous animals and insects	53	49	42	48
Other accidents caused by animals	139	164	146	163
Lightning	112	124	94	122
Cataclysm	384	193	500	248
Other natural and environmental factors	50	16	26	29
Other accidents	20,711	21,936	20,320	20,241
Drowning, submersion (excl. water trans. drownings above)	6,463	7,152	6,196	6,021
Inhalation and ingestion of food	2,181	2,210	2,088	2,227
Inhalation and ingestion of other object	810	803	742	650
Mechanical suffocation	1,083	1,109	1,104	1,176
In bed or cradle	234	287	322	435
Other and unspecified mechanical suffocation	849	822	782	741
Struck accidentally by falling object	1,143	1,196	1,218	1,168
Striking against or struck accidentally by objects	927	882	846	836
Caught accidentally in or between objects	521	598	536	548
Cutting or piercing instruments	112	133	126	147
Explosion of pressure vessel	57	73	60	72
Firearms	2,513	2,618	2,442	2,360
Self-inflicted	512	516	538	524
Other and unspecified firearms	2,001	2,102	1,904	1,836
Explosive material	459	512	518	544
Fireworks	3	5	10	3
Blasting materials	24	21	24	24
Explosive gases	230	234	242	228
Other and unspecified explosive material	202	252	242	289
Hot substance, corrosive liquid, and steam	216	279	282	248
Electric current	1,157	1,149	1,088	1,065
Home wiring and appliances	203	232	206	216
Industrial wiring and appliances	163	181	142	155
Other electric current	636	564	604	534
Unspecified electric current	155	172	136	160
Radiation	1	0	0	0
Machinery accidents not elsewhere classified	783	884	896	874
Other and unspecified	2,285	2,338	2,178	2,305

Table 28-9   (continued)

Type of accident or manner of injury	1974[1]	1973	1972	1971
Surgical and medical complications and misadventures	3,021	3,525	3,324	3,740
Operative therapeutic procedures	2,151	2,612	2,504	2,736
Other and unspecified therapeutic procedures	638	646	628	787
Other and unspecified nontherapeutic procedures	232	267	192	217
Late effects (death more than a year after accident)	695	682	648	676
Motor vehicle	166	152	132	137
Falls	172	190	156	181
Other and unspecified late effects	357	340	360	358

[1] Latest official figures.

Source: National Center for Health Statistics.

Home Accidents

Table 28-10   Home accident deaths by type of accident, 1950–1975

Year	Total home	Falls	Fires, burns[2]	Suffo.- ing. obj.	Suffo.- mech.	Poison (solid, liquid)	Poison by gas	Fire- arms	Other
1950	29,000	14,800	5,000	(3)	1,600	1,300	1,250	950	4,100
1955	28,500	14,100	5,400	(3)	1,250	1,150	900	1,100	4,600
1956	28,000	13,700[1]	5,500	(3)	1,300	1,150	900	1,150	4,300
1957	28,000	13,500	5,200	(3)	1,300	1,150	850	1,200	4,800
1958	26,500	11,900	6,000[1]	(3)	1,400	1,150	900	1,100	4,050[1]
1959	27,000	12,100	5,700	1,700	1,700	1,350	800	1,150	2,500
1960	28,000	12,300	6,350	1,850	1,500	1,350	900	1,200	2,550
1961	27,000	12,000	5,850	1,950	1,400	1,400	800	1,100	2,500
1962	28,500	12,600	6,200	1,400[1]	1,400	1,400	1,000	1,000	3,500[1]
1963	28,500	11,900	6,700	1,500	1,300	1,600	1,000	1,100	3,400
1964	28,000	11,400	6,200	1,400	1,300	1,700	900	1,200	3,900
1965	28,500	11,700	6,100	1,300	1,200	1,700	1,100	1,300	4,100
1966	29,500	11,900	6,800	1,300	1,100	1,800	1,200	1,400	4,000
1967	29,000	12,000	6,200	1,300	900	2,000	1,100	1,600	3,900
1968	28,000	10,800	6,100	2,000[1]	1,200[1]	2,100	1,100	1,300[1]	3,400[1]
1969	27,500	10,300	6,000	2,400	1,100	2,400	1,100	1,300	2,900
1970	27,000	9,700	5,600	1,800	1,100	3,000	1,100	1,400	3,300
1971	26,500	9,300	5,600	1,900	1,000	3,000	1,000	1,300	3,400
1972	26,500	9,300	5,500	1,800	900	3,000	1,000	1,400	3,600
1973	26,500	9,200	5,300	1,900	1,100	3,000	1,000	1,500	3,500
1974	26,000	9,000	5,100	1,800	900	3,200	900	1,400	3,700
1975	25,500	8,400	5,100	1,900	800	3,300	1,000	1,400	3,600

[1] Data for this year and subsequent years not comparable with previous years due to classification changes.
[2] Includes deaths resulting from conflagration, regardless of nature of injury.
[3] Included in Other.

Source: NSC estimates based on data from National Center for Health Statistics and state health departments.

Figure 28-1   How people died in home accidents, 1975

	Death total	Change from 1974	Death rate ‡

Type of accident and age of victim

All home — 25,500   -2%   12.0

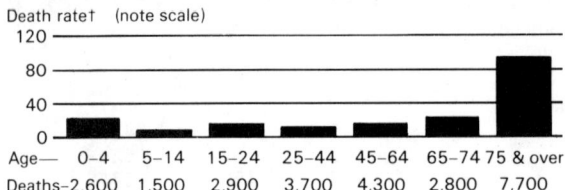

Death rate† (note scale)

Age—	0–4	5–14	15–24	25–44	45–64	65–74	75 & over
Deaths–	2,600	1,500	2,900	3,700	4,300	2,800	7,700

Includes deaths in the home and on home premises to occupants, guests and trespassers. Also includes domestic servants but excludes other persons working on home premises.

Falls — 8,400   -7%   3.9

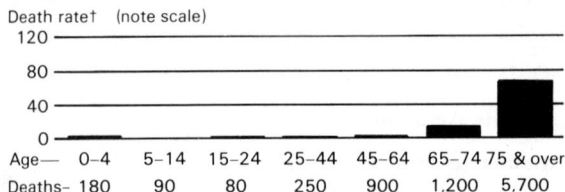

Death rate† (note scale)

Age—	0–4	5–14	15–24	25–44	45–64	65–74	75 & over
Deaths–	180	90	80	250	900	1,200	5,700

Includes deaths from falls from one level to another (stairs, ladder, roof, etc.); and on the same level (floor ground, sidewalk, etc.).

Fires, burns, and deaths associated with fires — 5,100   0%   2.4

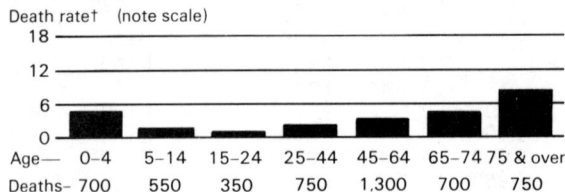

Death rate† (note scale)

Age—	0–4	5–14	15–24	25–44	45–64	65–74	75 & over
Deaths–	700	550	350	750	1,300	700	750

Includes deaths from fires, burns, and injuries in conflagrations in the home—such as asphyxiation, falls and struck by falling objects. Excludes burns from hot objects or liquids.

Poisoning by solids and liquids — 3,300   +3%   1.5

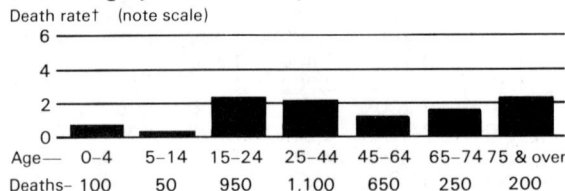

Death rate† (note scale)

Age—	0–4	5–14	15–24	25–44	45–64	65–74	75 & over
Deaths–	100	50	950	1,100	650	250	200

Includes deaths from drugs, medicines, mushrooms and shellfish, as well as commonly recognized poisons. Excludes poisonings from spoiled foods, salmonella, etc.— which are classified as disease deaths.

Poisoning by gases and vapors — 1,000   +11%   0.5

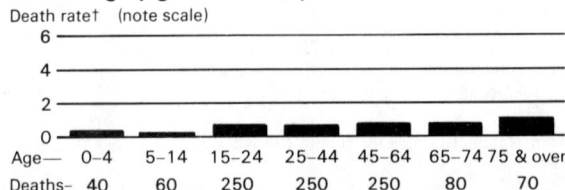

Death rate† (note scale)

Age—	0–4	5–14	15–24	25–44	45–64	65–74	75 & over
Deaths–	40	60	250	250	250	80	70

Principally carbon monoxide due to incomplete combustion, involving cooking stoves, heating equipment and standing motor vehicles. Gas poisonings in conflagrations are classified as fire deaths.

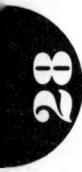

Figure 28-1 (continued)

	Death total	Change from 1974	Death rate‡

Suffocation-ingested object
1,900 +6% 0.9

Death rate† (note scale)

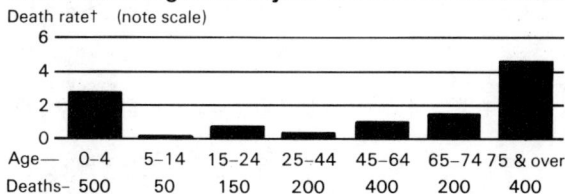

Age—	0–4	5–14	15–24	25–44	45–64	65–74	75 & over
Deaths–	500	50	150	200	400	200	400

Includes deaths from accidental ingestion or inhalation of objects or food resulting in the obstruction of respiratory passages.

Suffocation-mechanical
800 -11% 0.4

Death rate† (note scale)

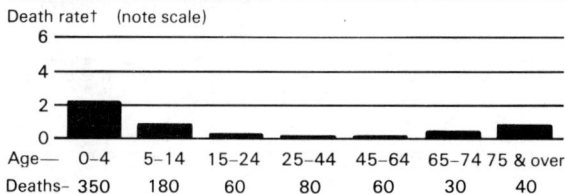

Age—	0–4	5–14	15–24	25–44	45–64	65–74	75 & over
Deaths–	350	180	60	80	60	30	40

Includes deaths from smothering by bed clothes, thin plastic materials, etc., suffocation by cave-ins or confinement in closed spaces, and mechanical strangulation.

Firearms
1,400 0% 0.7

Death rate† (note scale)

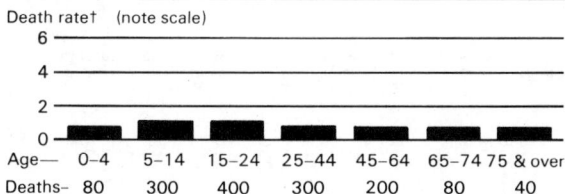

Age—	0–4	5–14	15–24	25–44	45–64	65–74	75 & over
Deaths–	80	300	400	300	200	80	40

Includes firearm accidents in or on home premises. Many occur while cleaning or playing with guns. Excludes deaths from explosive materials.

All other home
3,600 -3% 1.7

Death rate† (note scale)

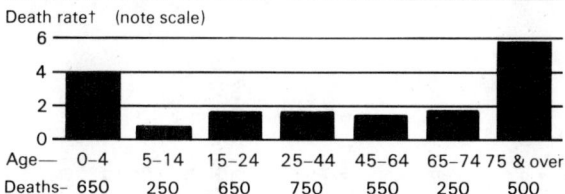

Age—	0–4	5–14	15–24	25–44	45–64	65–74	75 & over
Deaths–	650	250	650	750	550	250	500

Most important types included are: drowning, electric current, explosive materials and blow by falling object.

Principal type in each age group:

		Population death rate†
Under 1 year	Suffocation—ingested object	11.4
1 to 4 years	Fires, burns	4.5
5 to 14 years	Fires, burns	1.5
15 to 24 years	Poisoning by solids and liquids	2.4
25 to 44 years	Poisoning by solids and liquids	2.1
45 to 64 years	Fires, burns	3.0
65 to 74 years	Falls	8.6
75 years and over	Falls	66.8

† Deaths per 100,000 population in each age group, 1975.
‡ Deaths per 100,000 population.

Source: National Safety Council, *Accident Facts, 1976 Edition.*

28

Consumer Product Injuries

Table 28-11 Injuries associated with consumer products—treated at hospitals

| Product descriptions | Number of cases fiscal year 1976 | Percent of victims for report year | | | | | | | Rate per 100,000 pop. report year | Mean severity |
| | | By ages | | | | | By sex | | | |
		00–04	05–14	15–24	25–64	65 +	Male	Female		
General household appliances										
Washing machines with wringers	349	27.2	32.1	8.6	13.2	18.9	37.5	62.5	5.14	118
Water heaters	134	15.7	9.7	18.7	49.3	6.7	67.9	32.1	0.96	95
Kitchen appliances										
Blenders, mixers, choppers, & grinders (elec.)	241	3.7	12.4	21.6	57.7	4.6	33.2	66.8	2.91	37
Cooking stoves/ranges/ovens, electric	70	32.9	11.4	17.1	34.3	2.9	48.6	51.4	1.06	109
Cooking stoves/ranges/ovens, gas	296	5.7	12.2	38.2	39.5	4.4	32.8	67.2	3.65	200
Cooking stoves/ranges/ovens, not otherwise specified	878	29.8	12.8	19.2	33.4	4.7	44.8	55.2	8.72	89
Counter-top appliances	228	23.7	13.6	18.0	40.4	4.4	39.0	60.5	2.26	87
Irons	107	51.4	10.3	16.8	16.8	4.7	45.8	54.2	0.81	122
Refrigerators & freezers	75	10.7	8.0	25.3	53.3	2.7	57.3	42.7	1.28	104
Space heating, cooling & ventilating appliances										
Furnaces & floor furnaces	330	25.2	10.3	15.5	44.2	4.8	67.0	32.7	4.73	151
Space heaters & heating stoves	487	43.3	15.8	11.7	22.6	6.2	56.3	43.7	5.63	126
Housewares										
Coffeemakers & teapots, unpowered	24	16.7	12.5	12.5	54.2	4.2	45.8	54.2	0.21	76
Cutlery, unpowered, 'kitchen knives'	2,923	4.2	16.5	30.2	46.5	2.5	50.5	49.4	37.53	13
Drinking glasses, glass	2,761	5.4	12.1	38.8	41.4	2.1	30.6	69.4	37.36	14
Pots & pans (inc. lids)	494	14.4	10.5	23.1	46.0	6.1	34.6	64.8	4.88	62
Tableware & accessories	2,086	7.9	12.5	32.2	44.9	2.4	29.6	70.4	23.13	17
Home communication, entertainment & hobby equip.										
Sound recording & reproducing equipment (elec.)	879	27.4	20.0	20.9	29.5	2.2	53.0	46.9	9.46	35
Television sets	836	45.1	19.7	9.1	21.7	4.4	56.0	43.9	8.73	31
Home furnishings and fixtures										
Appliance & extension cords	108	29.6	17.6	6.5	32.4	13.9	43.5	56.5	1.24	70
Bathtub & shower structures	2,344	21.5	14.2	12.7	37.8	13.7	48.0	52.0	22.27	57
Beds (including springs & frames)	7,003	41.8	22.1	9.4	16.7	9.9	51.6	48.3	65.47	35
Carpets & rugs	795	6.8	7.5	13.0	44.4	28.3	27.8	72.2	7.52	45
Electrical fixtures (outlets, circuit breakers)	225	29.8	19.6	16.9	29.8	3.6	64.4	35.6	2.47	134
Ladders & step stools	3,540	4.2	6.8	11.9	63.4	13.5	70.1	29.8	39.66	41
Lamps, light fixtures, & chandeliers (electric)	830	18.4	19.9	28.4	29.9	2.9	63.5	36.5	9.18	35

Non-upholstered chairs	5,311	28.1	17.3	11.3	32.3	10.9	42.6	57.4	52.88	31
Plumbing fixtures	684	28.4	16.7	15.1	28.2	11.5	55.1	44.9	7.20	34
Storage furniture	3,799	24.1	28.2	16.0	26.8	4.9	49.7	50.3	40.09	26
Tables, non-glass	8,080	53.0	18.3	8.3	17.3	3.1	56.8	43.1	81.47	29
Upholstered furniture	1,532	38.3	15.1	15.5	27.3	3.8	49.2	50.8	15.04	29
Home alarm, escape, and protection devices										
All products except 0705	166	14.5	29.5	31.3	22.3	2.4	66.3	33.7	1.92	38
Home workshop apparatus, tools, and attachments										
Batteries, all kinds	508	2.3	3.6	41.3	50.8	1.8	89.8	10.0	5.88	173
Hammers	1,507	5.3	17.5	21.4	53.2	2.6	83.6	16.3	17.83	20
Home workshop saws (electric)	1,498	0.7	7.6	20.2	60.0	11.5	94.5	5.5	19.27	83
Home and family maintenance products										
Cleaning agents, caustic compounds	2,034	51.2	8.6	11.3	26.5	2.4	48.6	51.3	20.56	98
Household chemical products, other	914	37.1	14.6	21.9	29.8	1.5	64.2	35.6	10.86	98
Liquid fuels, kindling & illuminating	1,082	30.9	19.8	23.7	23.6	1.9	77.2	22.6	13.51	189
Paints & solvents	784	45.9	10.1	16.2	25.1	2.5	60.2	39.7	7.37	77
Waxes & polishes	141	80.9	6.4	2.1	8.5	2.1	56.0	43.3	1.48	56
Farm supplies and equipment										
Combine, threshing machine, harvesting equip.	40	—	20.0	27.5	52.5	—	92.5	7.5	1.17	285
Farm elevator, conveyor	34	20.6	35.3	8.8	26.5	8.8	76.5	23.5	1.44	46
Farm tractor	242	6.6	21.5	20.7	45.5	5.8	85.1	14.5	5.21	119
Picker or picker/sheller	23	8.7	26.1	13.0	43.5	8.7	87.0	13.0	0.46	177
Power take-off	13	—	23.1	38.5	38.5	—	92.3	7.7	0.56	26
Packaging and containers for household products										
Cans (inc. self-openers & resealable closures)	3,277	14.4	24.9	22.7	34.8	3.2	47.5	52.4	36.44	16
Glass bottles & jars	3,322	10.1	27.1	27.3	33.1	2.3	57.5	42.4	32.33	18
Glass containers (malt beverages)	479	5.6	16.3	42.4	34.2	1.5	75.4	25.6	5.72	20
Glass soft drink bottles (carbonated beverages)	1,292	16.4	31.7	24.5	25.6	1.7	52.7	47.2	16.38	18
Paper & cardboard objects, wrapping products	701	17.8	21.0	17.0	40.2	4.0	48.5	51.4	6.98	37
Pressurized containers, aerosol containers	247	23.3	24.7	16.2	31.6	4.0	59.9	40.1	2.73	67
Sports and recreational equipment										
Baseball, activity, related equip. & apparel	15,094	1.6	33.0	37.9	27.3	0.1	76.0	24.0	171.84	11
Basketball, activity, & related equipment	15,466	0.1	22.8	60.3	16.7	—	85.6	14.3	161.19	16
Bicycles & bicycle equipment	21,105	10.2	64.1	17.3	7.9	0.5	66.8	33.2	229.24	34
Fishing equipment	1,792	4.9	44.9	16.5	30.8	2.8	77.0	22.8	29.74	25
Football, activity, related equip. & apparel	18,041	0.2	38.3	53.2	8.2	—	95.4	4.5	189.89	23
Golf equipment (inc. golf carts)	838	8.1	37.9	14.4	36.0	3.5	73.0	27.0	10.47	30
Guns, gas, air & spring-operated, inc. BB guns	542	5.2	63.5	22.9	8.3	0.2	79.3	20.7	6.48	41
Gymnastics, activity, & related equipment	3,219	2.2	59.1	34.9	3.7	0.1	47.1	52.8	35.61	21
Hockey equipment & apparel	2,907	0.5	31.5	52.8	15.1	—	91.5	8.4	23.11	26

(continued)

Table 28-11 (continued)

Product descriptions	Number of cases fiscal year 1976	Percent of victims for report year							Rate per 100,000 pop. report year	Mean severity
		By ages					By sex			
		00–04	05–14	15–24	25–64	65+	Male	Female		
Ice skates	1,767	1.1	39.5	35.3	23.9	0.2	54.8	45.2	19.99	24
Motor scooters, mini bikes, & other such vehic.	733	1.5	61.7	25.1	11.3	0.4	81.4	18.6	9.85	47
Snow skiing & related equipment	2,423	0.2	21.9	49.8	28.0	—	61.7	38.2	42.23	22
Soccer	2,411	0.2	41.8	46.4	11.4	0.1	82.2	17.7	22.18	18
Swimming pool diving boards	356	0.8	42.7	41.3	15.2	—	73.9	26.1	4.21	24
Swimming pool water slides	36	5.6	66.7	22.2	5.6	—	50.0	50.0	0.56	109
Swimming pool, not otherwise specified	1,430	7.4	46.4	26.2	19.5	0.6	63.0	36.7	16.20	79
Swimming pools & associated equip.	773	6.0	46.6	27.2	19.9	0.3	67.9	32.1	8.70	67
Swimming pools, above ground	130	9.2	46.9	18.5	25.4	—	59.2	40.8	2.26	40
Swings, slides, seesaws, & climbing apparatus	6,058	31.1	63.4	3.2	2.0	0.2	52.9	47.1	70.82	29
Toboggans, sleds, snow discs, & snow tubing	1,604	3.6	52.7	30.3	13.1	0.3	65.1	34.8	21.00	35
Wading pools	17	47.1	29.4	17.6	5.9	—	52.9	47.1	0.15	167
Toys										
Cars, trucks, non-flying airplanes, & boats	347	53.9	34.9	4.9	6.1	0.3	75.5	24.5	4.84	27
Fireworks	271	5.5	49.8	29.2	13.7	1.8	76.0	24.0	2.94	90
Skates, scooters, & skateboards	5,703	1.4	59.7	25.8	12.9	—	55.5	44.4	63.54	22
Tricycles	494	70.0	25.5	0.4	2.8	1.2	64.6	35.2	6.05	37
Wagons & other ride-on toys	665	55.2	39.2	2.4	3.0	0.2	69.2	30.8	8.09	29
Yard and garden equipment										
Hand garden tools	918	12.0	38.8	18.5	28.1	2.6	64.7	35.2	11.91	18
Power lawnmowers	2,167	4.0	13.4	17.7	54.5	10.3	79.6	20.3	27.88	73
Child nursery equipment and supplies										
Baby carriages, walkers, & strollers	476	87.8	9.2	1.1	1.5	0.4	57.1	42.6	4.50	31
Baby cribs, gates, & playpens	486	85.2	5.3	3.9	5.3	0.2	49.4	50.6	4.65	39
High chairs & youth chairs	430	75.8	6.3	4.4	9.8	3.7	51.2	48.8	4.43	34
Personal use items										
Cigarette/pipe/cigar lighters	122	21.3	19.7	26.2	29.5	3.3	55.7	44.3	1.00	187
Clothing (inc. day & night wear)	323	10.5	26.9	18.9	34.7	9.0	59.1	40.9	2.80	241
Desk supplies, other	440	17.3	41.4	18.2	21.4	1.6	55.7	44.3	4.37	33
Jewelry, watches, keys, & key rings	796	22.6	31.2	24.0	20.2	2.0	32.7	67.2	7.64	45

28

Money, paper & coins, inc. toy money	630	61.7	36.2	1.3	0.6	—	53.2	46.7	5.19	114
Outerwear, footwear, & clothing accessories	1,187	6.7	22.7	28.4	38.8	3.5	37.7	62.3	10.85	22
Pencils	1,305	8.6	69.1	14.6	7.2	0.2	59.9	40.1	12.18	24
Pens & marking pens	189	37.0	32.3	20.6	9.0	1.1	62.4	37.6	1.64	31
Pins & needles	2,267	8.9	30.3	26.3	31.7	2.6	32.1	67.9	21.86	21
Razors, shavers, & razor blades	2,074	7.9	14.8	34.9	39.6	2.8	61.6	38.3	19.18	15
Sun lamps & heat lamps	497	0.6	4.6	64.0	30.4	0.4	31.4	68.4	5.40	116
Miscellaneous products										
Matches	417	7.0	14.1	36.2	41.7	1.0	53.5	46.5	4.22	182
Pocket knives	490	1.6	30.4	27.1	39.4	1.4	87.3	12.7	10.04	14
Home structures and construction materials										
Architectural glass	8,673	8.7	23.8	35.1	30.4	1.9	63.3	36.6	90.91	21
Bricks, concrete blocks, not part of structure	1,420	20.3	40.4	15.1	22.1	2.0	69.2	30.8	15.83	28
Doors, other than glass doors	11,534	21.9	26.2	20.6	27.6	3.8	51.8	48.1	111.13	28
Doors, with glass panels, not storm doors	247	7.3	38.5	28.3	24.3	1.6	56.3	43.7	3.13	20
Fences, not electric, all types	3,773	8.7	52.0	21.6	16.3	1.3	72.1	27.8	37.53	22
Floors & flooring materials	5,494	21.8	18.7	13.3	30.1	16.1	43.8	56.1	49.34	38
Nails, carpet tacks, screws, & thumbtacks	12,778	6.1	37.8	23.0	31.1	1.9	65.4	34.5	152.19	14
Outside structures, inc. retaining & ext. walls	768	15.0	36.5	22.0	23.0	3.5	63.5	38.5	8.93	33
Porches, balconies, etc.	2,014	23.8	23.3	14.1	32.4	6.3	52.8	47.2	22.94	40
Roofs & roofing materials	553	1.8	30.9	23.3	40.5	3.4	90.6	9.4	6.59	51
Stairs, ramps, & landings	27,740	13.4	12.5	20.6	44.1	9.4	40.9	59.0	264.91	31
Storm doors, not otherwise specified	245	17.1	38.0	18.4	22.9	3.7	46.5	53.1	3.33	17
Window & door sills, door & window frames	1,174	27.3	24.3	16.4	26.7	5.0	52.6	47.4	14.21	29
Wire, not electric	701	4.0	41.1	23.8	28.4	2.3	69.0	30.8	12.72	19
Products covered by existing federal regulations										
Cosmetics	1,228	41.8	6.9	19.4	30.3	1.5	39.2	60.7	12.13	34
Drugs, non-prescription	2,092	73.4	11.1	7.6	7.2	0.7	48.8	51.0	21.27	53
Drugs, prescription	2,972	40.0	14.3	17.1	25.9	2.6	42.4	57.4	27.09	68
Pesticides	567	76.5	7.9	5.5	9.2	0.9	54.0	45.9	6.59	63

Source: U.S. Consumer Product Safety Commission/Bureau of Epidemiology, 1976.

28

590

Communicable Diseases

Number of Cases per Disease

Table 28-12   Reported cases of specified notifiable diseases, U.S.

Disease	1975	1970	1966	Disease	1975	1970	1966
U.S. total resident population, July 1 estimate (in thousands)	213,121	203,805	195,923	Rubella congenital syndrome	30	77	11
Amebiasis	2,775	2,888	2,921	Salmonellosis, excluding typhoid fever	22,612	22,096	16,841
Anthrax	2	2	5	Shigellosis	16,584	13,845	11,888
Aseptic meningitis	4,475	6,480	3,058	Tetanus	102	148	235
Botulism	17	12	9	Trichinosis	201	109	115
Brucellosis (undulant fever)	310	213	262	Tuberculosis (newly reported active cases)[2]	33,554	37,137	47,767
Chickenpox	154,248	—	—	Tularemia	129	172	208
Diphtheria	307	435	209	Typhoid fever	375	346	378
Encephalitis, primary	3,837	1,580	2,121	Typhus fever, flea-borne (endemic, murine)	44	27	33
Encephalitis, post-infectious	400	370	964	Typhus fever, tick-borne (Rocky Mountain spotted)	844	380	268
Hepatitis A	35,855	56,797	32,859	Venereal diseases (newly reported civilian cases)			
Hepatitis B	13,121	8,310	1,497	Syphilis	80,356	91,382	105,159
Hepatitis, unspecified	7,158	—	—	Gonorrhea	999,937	600,072	351,738
Leprosy	162	129	109	Other specified venereal diseases:			
Leptospirosis	93	47	72	chancroid, granuloma inguinale,			
Malaria	373	3,051	565	and lymphogranuloma			
Measles (rubeola)	24,374	47,351	204,136	venereum	1,113	2,152	1,294
Meningococcal infections	1,478	2,505	3,381	Rabies in animals[2]	2,625	3,224	4,178
Mumps	59,647	104,953	—				
Pertussis (whooping cough)	1,738	4,249	7,717				
Poliomyelitis, total	8	33	113				
Paralytic	8	31	106				
Psittacosis	49	35	50				
Rabies in man	2	2	1				
Rheumatic fever, acute[1]	2,854	3,227	4,472				
Rubella (German measles)	16,652	56,552	46,975				

[1] Reports of cases of acute rheumatic fever were received from 36 states.
[2] Provisional figure for 1975.

Source: National Center for Health Statistics, August 1976.

Number of Deaths per Disease

Table 28-13   Deaths from specified notifiable diseases, U.S.

Cause of death	1974	1970	1965	Cause of death	1974	1970	1965
Amebiasis	25	59	66	Rabies	—	2	2
Anthrax	—	—	—	Rheumatic fever, acute	175	256	483
Botulism	6	7	8	Rubella (German measles)	15	31	16
Brucellosis	—	2	6	Salmonellosis, including paratyphoid fever	59	81	87
Chickenpox	106	93	143	Shigellosis	86	30	99
Diphtheria	5	30	18	Streptococcal sore throat and scarlet fever	22	29	63
Encephalitis, acute infectious	276	327	500				
Hepatitis, infectious	630	1,014	707	Tetanus	44	79	181
Leprosy	2	5	3	Trichinosis	—	1	3
Leptospirosis	5	4	11	Tuberculosis (all forms)	3,513	5,217	7,934
Malaria	4	5	8	Tularemia	2	2	2
Measles (rubeola)	20	89	276	Typhoid fever	3	6	6
Meningococcal infections	305	550	890	Typhus fever, flea-borne (murine)	—	—	—
Mumps	6	16	31	Typhus fever, tick-borne (Rocky Mountain spotted)	49	29	16
Pertussis (whooping cough)	14	12	55	Venereal diseases and sequelae			
Plague	1	1	1	Syphilis	300	461	2,434
Poliomyelitis	3	7	16	Gonorrhea	1	9	9
Bulbar or polioencephalitis	—	2	6	Other	4	6	11
With other paralysis	—	1	3				
Unspecified	3	4	7				
Psittacosis	—	1	—				

Source: National Center for Health Statistics, 1976.

Table 28-14 Deaths from selected non-notifiable acute diseases

Cause of death	1974	1970	1965	Cause of death	1974	1970	1965
Abscess of lung	828	893	601	Mononucleosis, infectious	24	19	28
Empyema and pleurisy	725	730	450				
Fungal infections				Respiratory infections			
Actinomycosis	9	18	26	Bronchitis, acute	750	1,310	1,004
Aspergillosis	50	38	NA	Influenza	2,201	3,707	2,295
Blastomycosis	1	3	29	Pneumonia (primary cause			
Coccidioidomycosis	61	42	52	of death)	52,576	59,032	59,608
Cryptococcosis	122	112	62	Upper respiratory infections,			
Histoplasmosis	58	56	74	acute	377	574	745
Moniliasis	190	153	93				
Nocardiosis	37	27	26	Sepsis of			
Unspecified	61	35	NA	Abortion	14	94	158
Herpes zoster	112	79	78	Childbirth	17	18	53
Hydatid disease	5	3	7	Septicemia and pyemia	5,243	3,535	3,224
Meningitis, excluding							
meningococcal and tuber-				Worm infestation	11	9	68
culous	1,539	1,701	2,363				

Source: National Center for Health Statistics, 1976.

Figure 28-2 Communicable diseases

	Incubation period	Communi- cability period	Symptoms	Treatment
Amebiasis— *Entamoeba histolytica*	Three days to several months	During infection	Vary with severity—diarrhea (some- times intermittent), blood and mucus in feces, abdominal dis- comfort	Chemothera- peutics or antibiotics
Ascariasis— *Ascaris lumbricoides hominis*	Two months	Until fertilized female worms are killed	Vague unless heavily infected; then may exhibit digestive disturbance, abdominal pain, restlessness, exaggerated nervous reflexes	Anthelmintic
Brucellosis (Undulant Fever)— *Brucella melitensis, abortus,* or *suis*	One week to several months	Not usually communicable from man to man	Irregular fever, profuse sweating, chills, pain in joints and muscles	Antibiotics
Chancroid (Soft Chancre)— *Hemophilus ducreyi*	One to twelve days	Until etiologic organisms are destroyed	Necrotizing ulcerations at site of inoculation; usually venereal	Sulfadiazine
Chickenpox (Varicella)— Virus	Two to three weeks	One day before to six days after first appearance of vesicles	Chills, slight fever, headache, malaise, successive crops of macules, papules, vesicles, crusts	Symptomatic
¹Diphtheria— *Coryne- bacterium diphtheriae*	Two to five days, some- times longer	Several hours before onset and for about two weeks dur- ing infection	Sore throat, fever, coryza, malaise, grayish patches (pseudomembranes) on tonsils and mucosa of throat and nose	Antitoxin, antibiotics

¹Disease best controlled by prophylactic use of vaccine.

(*continued*)

Figure 28-2   (continued)

	Incubation period	Communi- cability period	Symptoms	Treatment
Dysentery, Bacillary— Species of *Shigella* bacillus	One to seven days	During infection	Acute onset, diarrhea, sometimes fever, tenesmus, and frequent defecation, often with blood and mucus; symptoms variable in mild cases	Sulfonamides, antibiotics
Enterobiasis (Pinworm or Threadworm Infection)— *Enteroblus vermicularis*	Fourteen to twenty-one days	During infection	Variable, frequently absent; anorexia, restlessness, insomnia, and pruritus ani	Anthelmintic. All members of family should be considered infected.
Ersipelas— Hemolytic streptococci, Group A strains	One to two days	Until clinical recovery	Acute febrile infection of skin, characterized by red, tender, edematous, spreading skin lesion which is sharply delineated; fever, malaise	Antibiotics
Gonorrhea— *Neisseria gonorrhoeae*	Two to nine days or longer	During infection	In the male, acute anterior urethritis with burning on urination; serous discharge, becoming profuse, greenish-yellow, and often blood-tinged. In the female, often asymptomatic.	Antibiotics
Hepatitis, Infectious— Virus	Ten to forty days	From two to three weeks before until about one month after clinical onset	Acute infection, fever, anorexia, nausea, vomiting, fatigue, lassitude, headache, abdominal discomfort, sometimes followed by jaundice	Symptomatic
Hepatitis, Serum—Virus	Forty to one hundred sixty days	Unknown	Slow onset and little fever except in fatal cases; other symptoms similar to those in infectious hepatitis	Symptomatic
[1]Influenza— Virus Type A, Type B, sub-types	Twenty-four to seventy-two hours	Unknown, probably during early and febrile stage	Sudden onset, chills and fever, prostration, aches and pains in back and limbs, coryza, sore throat, bronchitis	Symptomatic; antibiotics for secondary infection
[1]Measles (Rubeola)— Virus	Seven to fourteen days	Two to four days before appearance of rash until two to five days thereafter	Mild fever, malaise, conjunctivitis, coryza, cough, photophobia, Koplik's spots, small reddish-brown or pink macules changing to papules. Rash fades on pressure, begins behind ears (and/or on forehead and cheeks), progresses to extremities in three days, lasts about five days.	Symptomatic; gamma globulin

[1]Disease best controlled by prophylactic use of vaccine.

Figure 28-2   (continued)

	Incubation period	Communi-cability period	Symptoms	Treatment
[1]Measles, German (Rubella)— Virus	Fourteen to twenty-one days	From as long as thirteen days before onset of rash until six days after rash disappears. In the case of newborns in-fected *in utero*, virus may be re-covered from the throat, urine, and/or stool for several months after birth.	Malaise, fever, headache, rhinitis, postauricular and postoccipital lymphadenopathy with tender nodes, small pink to pale-red macules fused or closely grouped to give scarlet blush which fades on pressure, disappears within three days	Symptomatic
Meningococcus Meningitis (Cerebrospinal Fever)— Meningo-coccus or *Neisseria meningitidis*	Two to ten days	Indefinite, until meningococci are absent from nose and mouth discharges	Sudden onset, fever, intense head-ache, stiff neck, nausea, vomiting; frequently petechial rash; delirium and coma	Antibiotics, sulfonamides
Mononucleosis, Infectious (Glandular Fever)—Cause unknown	Four to fourteen days	Unknown	Acute febrile infection, sore throat, malaise, fatigue, headache, often enlargement of cervical and other lymphatic glands	Symptomatic
[1]Mumps (Infectious Parotitis)— Virus	Twelve to twenty-six days	From about seven days be-fore first symp-toms appear until swelling subsides	Slight fever, malaise, nausea, irritability; swelling, inflammation, and tenderness of salivary glands	Symptomatic
[1]Pertussis (Whooping Cough)— *Bordetella pertussis*	One to three weeks, al-most uni-formly within ten days	Greatest in catarrhal stage before onset of paroxysms; or-ganism rarely recovered after fourth week of disease	Coryza, dry tracheal cough which is worse at night; paroxysms of several staccato coughs in one ex-piration, followed by sudden, rapid, deep inspiration and whoop	Hyperimmune serum; symptomatic; antibiotics may be of value
Pneumonias (Acute Lobar)— Pneumococci	One to three days	Unknown during infec-tious discharge)	Acute infection, sudden onset with chills and fever, often pain in chest, usually cough and dyspnea	Antibiotics

[1]Disease best controlled by prophylactic use of vaccine.   (*continued*)

Figure 28-2   (continued)

	Incubation period	Communi-cability period	Symptoms	Treatment
Pneumonia, Mycoplasma (Eaton Agent)	Seven to twenty-one days	Unknown	Insidious and variable onset; frequent absence of respiratory symptoms; fatigue, muscle pains, chilliness, feverishness, sometimes cough	Symptomatic; antibiotics
¹Poliomyelitis (Infantile Paralysis)— Virus	One to five weeks	Greatest during late incubation and early days of infection; virus remains in feces for weeks	Acute illness, fever, malaise; variable, but usually include headache and stiffness of neck and spine	Symptomatic
Rabies (Hydrophobia)— Virus	From ten days to two years; average fifty to sixty days	In dogs and other animals, for three to five days before onset of symptoms through clinical course of disease; rarely from man to man	Fulminating encephalitis, almost inevitably fatal; depression, fever, headache, anorexia, nausea, sore throat, malaise, restlessness, hyperesthesia of skin, hypersensitivity to light and sound; convulsions, paralysis	Rabies vaccine and/or rabies immune globulin when bitten by rabid animal; symptomatic once symptoms occur
Ringworm of the Body— Several species of fungi	Unknown	During presence of infection	Circinate scaly patches with miliary vesicles in the active border	Fungicides
Ringworm of Scalp (Tinea Capitis)— *Microsporum audouini, M. canis,* other fungi	Unknown	During presence of infection	Vary from noninflammatory patches with short, brittle, lusterless, broken hairs to deep dusky-red, baggy, swollen areas of infection	Fungicides or x-ray depilation
Rocky Mountain Spotted Fever— *Rickettsia rickettsil*	Three to ten days	Not communicable from man to man	Sudden onset with fever, headache, photophobia, muscle and joint pains, and chills; characteristic maculopapular rash, usually first on extremities, rapidly spreads over body	Antibiotics
Scabies— *Sarcoptes scabiei*	Variable	Until itch mites and ova are destroyed	Characteristic burrows of itch mite, not inflammatory unless scratched; severe itching, especially when warm	Miticides
Scarlet Fever (Scarlatina) —Hemolytic streptococci, Group A strains	Three to five days	From onset until recovery	Sudden onset, sore throat, fever, headache, nausea, vomiting, rapid pulse. Bright-red uniform rash begins on upper chest one to three days after onset, spreads rapidly over neck, arms, trunk, and legs, velvety skin.	Antibiotics

¹Disease best controlled by prophylactic use of vaccine.

Figure 28-2 (continued)

	Incubation period	Communicability period	Symptoms	Treatment
¹Smallpox (Variola)—Virus	Seven to sixteen days	From one to two days before first symptoms until crusts drop off. Crusts are infectious.	Abrupt onset, with fever, prostration, chills, headache, myalgia, nausea, vomiting; eruption on thighs and lower abdomen on second or third day followed by true exanthema beginning on face and involving head and extremities more than trunk; duration three to six weeks	Thiosemicarbazone derivatives shorten clinical course of disease; antibiotics for secondary infections
Syphilis— Treponema pailidum (Spirochaeta paillda)	Ten to ninety days	During primary and secondary stages and during mucocutaneous relapses	In acquired infection (usually venereal), ulcer occurs at site of inoculation. Constitutional symptoms and generalized lesions of skin and mucous membranes follow. May recur over several years. Late manifestations (tertiary stage) involve circulatory and central nervous systems.	Antibiotics
¹Tetanus— Clostridium tetani	Two to fifty days; usually between five and ten days	Not communicable from man to man	Acute infectious disease characterized by stiffness of jaw and fever followed by restlessness, irritability, stiff neck, and difficulty in swallowing; rigidity and convulsions as disease progresses.	Antitoxin, sedatives, antibiotics
Trichinosis— Trichinella spiralis	One to twenty-eight days	Not communicable from man to man	Variable. Many infections asymptomatic. About twenty-four hours after infection, nausea, vomiting, abdominal pain, fever, and severe dysentery sometimes develop. Later, during migration of larvae, malaise, weakness, remittent or intermittent fever, myalgia, sweating, periorbital and facial edema, laryngitis, painful swallowing, striate hemorrhages beneath fingernails, and sometimes cardiac and respiratory difficulty occur in varying severity.	Symptomatic and supportive
Tularemia— Pasteurella tularensis	One to ten days	Not communicable from man to man	Sudden onset, chills, fever, prostration, headache, severe malaise. Ulceroglandular type is characterized by pustuloulcerative lesion with regional lymphadenopathy. Typhoidal form has no external lesion but may cause local lesions of mouth or pharynx. Fever, vomiting, severe abdominal pain, and diarrhea.	Antibiotics

¹Disease best controlled by prophylactic use of vaccine.

(continued)

Figure 28-2   (continued)

	Incubation period	Communi- cability period	Symptoms	Treatment
[1]Typhoid Fever —*Salmonella typhosa*	One to three weeks	Indefinite, as long as typhoid bacilli occur in feces or urine	Chills, fever, headache, backache, anorexia, diarrhea or constipa- tion, epistaxis, generalized aching, frequently bronchitis. Rose-colored elevated rash which appears in crops about the seventh day is most abundant on abdomen but also on chest and back. Crops last two to three days, leaving brownish stains. Delirium, listlessness, photophobia, muscle twitching, and somnolence usually indicate severe infection.	Antibiotics

[1]Disease best controlled by prophylactic use of vaccine.

Vaccination and Immunization

The Immune System

The immune system consists of the bone marrow, the thymus, the spleen and the lymph nodes, as well as the white blood cells, as shown in the attached figure.

As shown in Figure 28-3, white cells originate in the bone marrow. Some migrate first to the thymus where they mature and acquire special characteristics. These are called T lymphocytes. Another type of cell, also originating in the bone marrow, is known as the B lymphocyte. A third important white blood cell is the phagocyte, or "scavenger" cell. There is good evidence that all three cell types must interact for protection against disease.

When working properly, the immune system is the major defense against disease-causing microbes and other aliens, including malignant cells. It produces antibodies—protective blood proteins—to these aliens. Antibodies, plus phagocytes, lead to the destruction of agents causing disease. The immune system can be stimulated to do a better job. Vaccines are often used for this purpose.

NIH estimates that one out of every six Americans has a serious allergy. In these people, the immune system reacts abnormally

Figure 28-3   The immune system—a simplified view

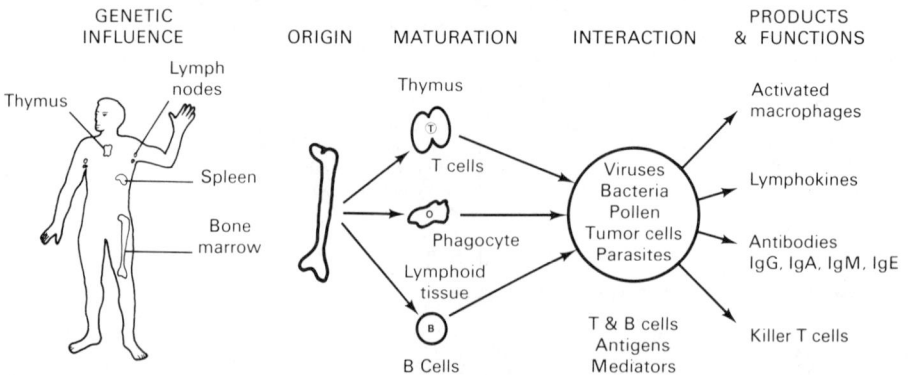

Source: National Institutes of Health, 1977.

to certain substances and produces an unusual kind of antibody. This antibody, termed IgE, triggers the release of harmful chemicals into the tissues or bloodstream. This series of events leads to asthma, hay fever, and other allergic conditions.

Disorders of the immune system are widespread and are responsible for various diseases, including kidney disease and arthritis.

Malfunction of the immune system is also frequently caused by potent drugs used to treat diseases such as rheumatoid arthritis and cancer. Patients given these drugs are very vul-

nerable to infections. Many cancer patients succumb not to cancer but to an overwhelming infection brought about by the drug-induced derangement of the immune system.

The immune system is immature at birth and not primed to perform its protective role. Soon after birth, the nasal and upper respiratory passages and the intestinal tract become the home of millions of usually harmless microbes—bacteria and viruses—which stimulate the immune system to mature so it can protect us against the microbes which cause disease.

How Many Have Been Vaccinated

Table 28-15   Children: vaccinations—United States, 1975

	Measles, mumps vaccine and chickenpox		
	Percent of population with		
Age group	History of immunizing infection and/or vaccine	History of mumps vaccine	History of chickenpox in past 12 months
1–4	67.7	44.4	7.2
5–9	80.4	47.5	9.5
10–13	80.5	30.2	4.5

DTP		Polio	
Percent of population with no history of diphtheria-tetanus-pertussis vaccine		Percent of population with specified doses of oral polio vaccine	
Age group	No doses	Age group	No doses
1–4	4.5	1–4	10.3
5–9	2.2	5–9	6.3
10–13	3.4	10–14	9.2
		15–19	13.5

Rubella		Smallpox	
Percent of population with history of rubella infection and/or vaccine		Percent of population with smallpox vaccination during past 12 months	
Age group	History of immunizing infection and/or vaccine	Age group	Percent
<1	8.3	<1	7.5
1–4	69.9	1–4	13.9
5–9	82.6	5–19	5.6
10–12	82.0		

Source: U.S. Center for Disease Control, 1976.

Table 28-16　Adults: influenza vaccine

**Percent of total persons
receiving influenza vaccine
during past 12 months—1975**

Age group	With vaccine
20–29	10.5
30–39	12.1
40–49	15.0
50–64	20.0
65 +	29.2

Source: U.S. Center for Disease Control, 1976.

Table 28-17　All ages: vaccinations

**Percentages of the population
with complete immunization
against various diseases**

Year	Polio	Diphtheria, pertussis and tetanus	Measles	Rubella
1969	67.7	77.4	61.4	—
1970	65.9	76.1	57.2	37.2
1971	67.3	78.7	61.0	51.2
1972	62.9	75.6	62.2	56.9
1973	60.4	72.6	61.2	55.6
1974	63.1	73.9	64.5	59.8

Source: U.S. Center for Disease Control, 1976.

Vaccination Schedules for Children

Since 1963, the Center for Disease Control has provided project grant and technical assistance to state and local health agencies for childhood immunization programs. With this assistance these health agencies have conducted intensive immunization programs against poliomyelitis, measles and rubella, and have carried out routine immunization programs against diphtheria, pertussis and tetanus.

These efforts have had a dramatic impact on children's health. Reported measles cases have declined from 261,904 in calendar year 1965 to 22,094 in 1974, and reported rubella cases fell from 57,686 in 1965, to 11,917 in 1974. However, both measles and rubella were up in 1975 compared to 1974 (10% and 37%, respectively).

While overall disease morbidity for childhood vaccine preventable diseases has been declining, concentrated immunization efforts will be continued. It is estimated that because of inadequate protection more than 18 million children are susceptible to poliomyelitis, 22 million to diphtheria, pertussis and tetanus, 11 million to measles, 31 million to mumps and 16 million to rubella. Recent data suggests that measles may once again be increasing.

Approximately one-fourth of preschool children have received less than the recommended three doses of DTP vaccine, and these diseases continue to occur in the United States. During 1974, there were 257 reported cases of diphtheria, 94 cases of tetanus and 1,758 cases of pertussis.[*]

This schedule for first vaccinations is based on recommendations of the American Medical Association and the American Academy of Pediatrics. A first test for TB (tuberculosis) may be recommended at one year. Your physician may suggest a slightly different schedule suitable for your individual child. And recommendations change from time to time as science gains new knowledge.

Rubella

Table 28-18　Reported new cases of rubella and congenital rubella and percent of children immunized, U.S. 1966–1974

Year	Rubella	Congenital rubella	Percent of children immunized by natural infection or vaccination	
			1–4	5–9
Prevaccine average				
1966–1968	47,562	N.A.	N.A.	N.A.
1969	57,686	77	N.A.	N.A.
1970	56,552	89	47.3	67.3
1971	45,086	52	59.4	77.8
1972	25,507	39	63.3	79.5
1973	27,804	32	62.4	77.9
1974	11,917	21	66.0	79.8

The table above shows the most up-to-date statistical information regarding reported rubella, the number of infants born with congenital rubella syndrome, and the estimated number of children immunized by natural infection or vaccination. Source: National Registry for Congenital Rubella Syndrome.

Source: U.S. Center for Disease Control.

---

[*] Source: National Institutes of Health.

Figure 28-4   Vaccination schedule

Disease	No. of doses	Age for first series	Booster
Diphtheria Tetanus Whooping Cough	4 doses	2 months 4 months 6 months 18 months	At 4 to 6 years— before entering school. As recom- mended by physician.
Polio (Oral vaccine)	4 doses	2 months 4 months 6 months 18 months	At 4 to 6 years— before entering school. As recom- mended by physician.
Rubella (German measles)	1 vaccination	about 15 months	None
Measles	1 vaccination	about 15 months	None
Mumps	1 vaccination	about 15 months	None

Source: "Memo to Parents about Immunization" (1976 pamphlet) Metropolitan Life Insurance Company.

Smallpox

In 1519 a Negro slave is believed to have brought smallpox to Mexico, where it was communicated to the Aztec population. During the Spanish conquest of Mexico it was esti- mated that one half of the Aztec population died from smallpox.

Smallpox was the first disease to be made preventable by a modern method of immuniza- tion.

In 1975 smallpox was expected to disap- pear from the earth as the World Health Orga- nization finished its mopping-up operation in the eradication program begun in 1967.

Poliomyelitis

Although we have had no major epidemics of poliomyelitis in the United States during the last decade, the proportion of adequately protected children has declined steadily from 1965 to 1974. Following the mass oral vacci- nation programs of the early 1960s, almost 90% of children aged one to four years had received three or more doses of poliomyelitis vaccine. This proportion had declined to only slightly more than 63% in 1974. In some areas, even fewer children are adequately protected. If immunization levels remain this low, the threat of localized epidemics of polio is very real.

Interestingly, the occurrence of paralytic poliomyelitis reached an all time low in 1974, with only five reported cases.

Cancer*

Trends

The overall incidence of cancer has decreased slightly in the past 25 years. Incidence decreased substantially for cancers of the stomach, uterus, rectum and eosphagus. In general, cancer between the ages of 20 and 40 is three times as common in women as men, but between the ages of 60 and 80, men ac- count for more cancer cases.

For men, there has been a much higher inci- dence of lung cancer, amounting to an increase of over 125% in 25 years; slight increases oc- curred for cancers of the colon, prostate, pancreas and bladder. Decrease for stomach cancer.

For women, decrease in incidence has been noted for cancers of the uterus (both cervical and endometrial), bladder and stomach. Inci- dence of breast and colon cancers remain un- changed, but lung cancer has steadily increased.

Overall since 1949, more men than women have been dying of cancer each year; in 1976 about 55% to 45%. But cancer is the leading cause of death among women ages 30–54.

For men, the cancer death rate per 100,000

---

*Source: '77 Cancer Facts and Figures, American Cancer Society. (Unless otherwise noted.)

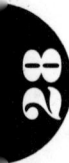

population has increased by over 50% since 1950 for blacks, and by 20% for whites. The increased death rate is mainly the result of lung cancer which rose from 18 deaths per 100,-000 in 1950 to 52 deaths per 100,000 in 1974.

For women, since 1950 the death rate has declined by 5% for blacks and 10% for whites. This is due mainly to a sharp reduction in deaths caused by cancer of the uterine cervix which is attributed to increased use of Pap tests and regular checkups. There was also a decline in stomach cancer. However, the lung cancer rate has tripled from 4.0 per 100,000 in 1950 to 12.3 in 1974.

For children, cancer is responsible for more deaths in the 3 to 14-year-old group than any other disease. In 1977, cancer will account for the deaths of about 3,000 children, about half of them from acute lymphocytic leukemia, a cancer of blood-forming tissues.

Overall five-year survival rates have increased for some cancers, and leveled off for most cancers in the past 25 years.

Table 28-19   Estimated new cancer cases and deaths by sex for all sites—1977[1]

Site	Estimated new cases			Estimated deaths		
	Total	Male	Female	Total	Male	Female
All sites	690,000[1]	347,000[1]	343,000[1]	385,000	210,500	174,500
Buccal cavity & pharynx (oral)	23,900	17,000	6,900	8,450	6,000	2,450
Lip	4,100	3,800	300	225	200	25
Tongue	4,500	6,100	1,400	2,000	1,400	600
Salivary gland				650	400	250
Floor of mouth	8,700	5,200	3,500	525	400	125
Other & unspecified mouth				1,250	800	450
Pharynx	6,600	4,900	1,700	3,800	2,800	1,000
Digestive organs	171,400	89,300	82,100	104,700	55,200	49,500
Esophagus	7,600	5,600	2,000	6,900	5,000	1,900
Stomach	23,000	14,000	9,000	14,600	8,600	6,000
Small intestine	2,200	1,200	1,000	700	350	350
Large intestine (colon-	70,000	32,000	38,000	41,200	19,200	22,000
rectum)	31,000	17,000	14,000	10,100	5,600	4,500
Liver & biliary passages	11,800	5,800	6,000	9,800	4,800	5,000
Pancreas	21,800	12,000	9,800	19,800	10,900	8,900
Other & unspecified digestive	4,000	1,700	2,300	1,600	750	850
Respiratory system	109,700	85,700	24,000	93,750	72,100	21,650
Larynx	9,200	8,100	1,100	3,350	2,900	450
Lung	98,000	76,000	22,000	89,000	68,300	20,700
Other & unspecified respiratory	2,500	1,600	900	1,400	900	500
Bone tissue and skin	15,900	8,000	7,900	8,850	5,050	3,800
Bone	1,900	1,100	800	1,900	1,100	800
Connective tissue	4,500	2,400	2,100	1,650	850	800
Skin	9,500[2]	4,500[2]	5,000[2]	5,300[4]	3,100	2,200
Breast	89,700	700	89,000	34,000	300	33,700
Genital organs	129,900	61,700	68,200	43,900	21,200	22,700
Cervix, invasive ⎫ Uterus	20,000[3]	—	20,000[3]	7,600	—	7,600
Corpus uteri ⎭	27,000	—	27,000	3,300	—	3,300
Ovary	17,000	—	17,000	10,800	—	10,800
Other female genital	4,200	—	4,200	1,000	—	1,000
Prostate	57,000	57,000	—	20,100	20,100	—
Other male genital	4,700	4,700	—	1,100	1,100	—
Urinary organs	44,900	31,300	13,600	17,100	11,400	5,700
Bladder	29,900	22,000	7,900	9,800	6,800	3,000
Kidney & other urinary	15,000	9,300	5,700	7,300	4,600	2,700
Eye	1,700	800	900	400	200	200
Brain & central nervous system	10,900	5,900	5,000	8,800	4,900	3,900

(*continued*)

Table 28-19   (continued)

Site	Estimated new cases			Estimated deaths		
	Total	Male	Female	Total	Male	Female
Endocrine glands	9,200	2,700	6,500	1,650	650	1,000
Thyroid	8,200	2,200	6,000	1,150	350	800
Other endocrine	1,000	500	500	500	300	200
Leukemia	21,300	12,000	9,300	15,000	8,400	6,600
Multiple myeloma	8,200	4,200	4,000	5,600	2,900	2,700
Lymphomas	21,900	12,100	9,800	15,700	8,600	7,100
Lymphosarcoma & reticulosarcoma	10,600	5,700	4,900	7,200	3,800	3,400
Hodgkin's disease	7,400	4,300	3,100	2,900	1,700	1,200
Other lymphomas	3,900	2,100	1,800	5,600	3,100	2,500
All other & unspecified sites	31,400	15,600	15,800	27,100	13,600	13,500

Note: The estimates of new cancer cases are offered as a rough guide and should not be regarded as definitive. Especially note that year-to-year changes may only represent improvements in the basic data.

[1] Carcinoma in situ of the uterine cervix (over 40,000 new cases) and non-melanoma skin cancers (300,000 new cases) not included in totals.

[2] Melanoma only.

[3] Invasive cancer only.

[4] Melanoma 3700, other skin 1600.

Incidence estimates are based on rates from NCI third national cancer survey, 1969–71.

Table 28-20   Estimated new cases and deaths for major sites of cancer—1977[1]

Site	No. of cases	Deaths
Lung	98,000	89,000
Colon-rectum	101,000	51,000
Breast	90,000	34,000
Uterus	47,000[2]	11,000
Oral	24,000	8,000
Skin	10,000[3]	5,000
Leukemia	21,000	15,000

[1] Figures rounded to the nearest 1,000.

[2] If carcinoma in situ included, cases total over 87,000.

[3] Estimate new cases of non-melanoma about 300,000.

Incidence estimates are based on rates from NCI third national cancer survey 1969–71.

Figure 28-5   Five-year cancer survival rates*

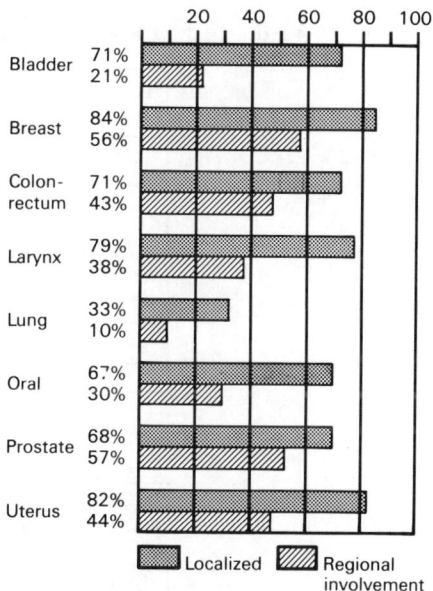

	Localized	Regional involvement
Bladder	71%	21%
Breast	84%	56%
Colon-rectum	71%	43%
Larynx	79%	38%
Lung	33%	10%
Oral	67%	30%
Prostate	68%	57%
Uterus	82%	44%

*Adjusted for normal life expectancy.
Source: end results group, National Cancer Institute 1965–69.

Figure 28-6   Cancer incidence by site and sex*—1977 estimate

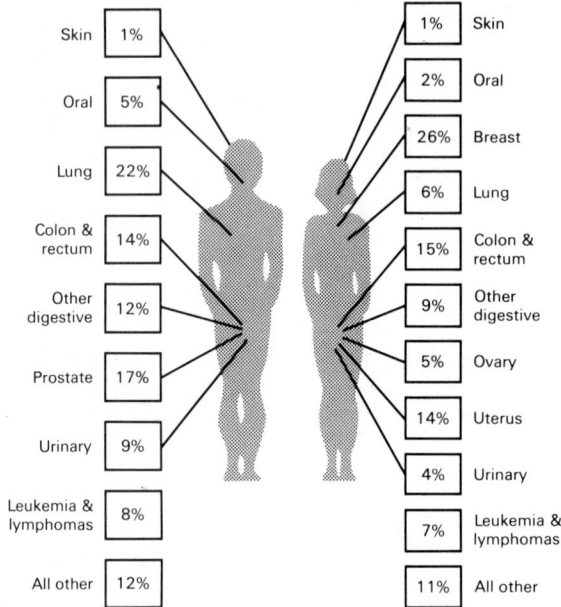

	Male		Female	
Skin	1%		1%	Skin
Oral	5%		2%	Oral
			26%	Breast
Lung	22%		6%	Lung
Colon & rectum	14%		15%	Colon & rectum
Other digestive	12%		9%	Other digestive
			5%	Ovary
Prostate	17%		14%	Uterus
Urinary	9%		4%	Urinary
Leukemia & lymphomas	8%		7%	Leukemia & lymphomas
All other	12%		11%	All other

* Excluding nonmelanoma skin cancer and carcinoma in situ of uterine cervix.

Figure 28-7   Cancer deaths by site and sex—1977 estimate

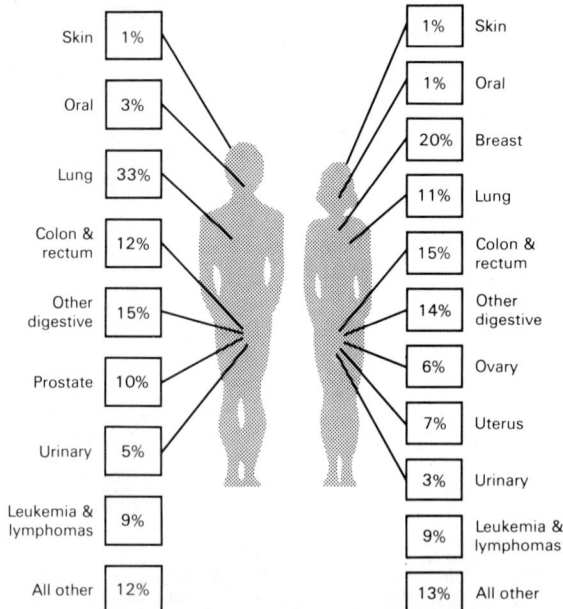

	Male		Female	
Skin	1%		1%	Skin
Oral	3%		1%	Oral
			20%	Breast
Lung	33%		11%	Lung
Colon & rectum	12%		15%	Colon & rectum
Other digestive	15%		14%	Other digestive
			6%	Ovary
Prostate	10%		7%	Uterus
Urinary	5%		3%	Urinary
Leukemia & lymphomas	9%		9%	Leukemia & lymphomas
All other	12%		13%	All other

Leading Cancer Sites

Figure 28-8   Reference chart of leading cancer sites, 1977[1]

Site	Estimated new cases 1977	Estimated deaths 1977	Warning signal if you have one see your doctor	Safeguards	Comment
Breast	90,000	34,000	Lump or thickening in the breast, or unusual discharge from nipple.	Regular checkup. Monthly breast self-exam.	The leading cause of cancer death in women.
Colon and Rectum	101,000	51,000	Change in bowel habits; bleeding.	Regular checkup, including proctoscopic examinations are included in routine checkups.	Considered a highly curable disease when digital and proctoscopic examinations are included in routine checkups.
Lung	98,000	89,000	Persistent cough, or lingering respiratory ailment.	80% of lung cancer would be prevented if no one smoked cigarettes.	The leading cause of cancer death among men and rising mortality among women.
Oral (including Pharynx)	24,000	8,000	Sore that does not heal. difficulty in swallowing.	Regular checkup.	Many more lives should be saved because the mouth is easily accessible to visual examination by physicians and dentists.
Skin	10,000[2]	5,000	Sore that does not heal, or change in wart or mole.	Regular checkup, avoidance of overexposure to sun.	Skin cancer is readily detected by observation, and diagnosed by simple biopsy.
Uterus	47,000[3]	11,000	Unusual bleeding or discharge.	Regular checkup, including pelvic examination with PAP test.	Uterine cancer mortality has declined 65% during the last 40 years with wider application of the PAP test. Postmenopausal women with abnormal bleeding should be checked.
Kidney and Bladder	45,000	17,000	Urinary difficulty, bleeding—in which case consult doctor at once.	Regular checkup with urinalysis.	Protective measures for workers in high-risk industries are helping to eliminate one of the important causes of these cancers.
Larynx	9,000	3,000	Hoarseness—difficulty in swallowing.	Regular checkup, including laryngoscopy.	Readily curable if caught early.
Prostate	57,000	20,000	Urinary difficulty	Regular checkup, including palpation.	Occurs mainly in men over 60, the disease can be detected by palpation at regular checkup.
Stomach	23,000	14,000	Indigestion.	Regular checkup.	A 40% decline in mortality in 25 years, for reasons yet unknown.
Leukemia	21,000	15,000	Leukemia is a cancer of blood-forming tissues and is characterized by the abnormal production of immature white blood cells. Acute lymphocytic leukemia strikes mainly children and is treated by drugs which have extended life from a few months to as much as ten years. Chronic leukemia strikes usually after age 25 and progresses less rapidly.		
Lymphomas	22,000	16,000	These cancers arise in the lymph system and include Hodgkin's disease and lymphosarcoma. Some patients with lymphatic cancers can lead normal lives for many years. Five-year survival rate for Hodgkin's disease increased from 25% to 54% in 20 years.		

[1] All figures rounded to nearest 1,000.   [2] Estimate new cases of non-melanoma skin cancer about 300,000.   [3] If carcinoma *in situ* is included, cases total over 87,000.   Incidence estimates are based on rates from N.C.I. Third National Cancer Survey 1969–71.

28

Breast Cancer

Review

About 90,000 new cases of breast cancer and 33,000 deaths from the disease are expected in 1977. Breast cancer remains the foremost site of cancer incidence and death in American women.

The disease is found most often among women over 35 and is the leading cause of death of women from 40 to 44 years of age. Risk is higher for women who have never had a child or who bore the first child after age 25, women whose mothers or sisters have had breast cancer, and women who experienced early menarche and/or late menopause. Cancer in one breast increases risk for the other breast.

At present rates, one out of every thirteen American women will develop breast cancer. The incidence of breast cancer has remained about the same since 1940. Early detection, through breast self-examination (BSE) and regular checkups, is of primary importance in the control of breast cancer.

Since 1950, besides surgery, therapy has included some radiation, chemotherapy and/or hormones.

However, despite a number of improvements in surgery and cancer therapy generally, there has been no significant change in the breast cancer mortality rate in 30 to 40 years, with only 62% surviving five years and 37% living ten years after diagnosis and treatment.

Current therapy is most effective when breast cancer is discovered in a localized stage—the five-year survival rate is 84%. About 95% of women discover breast cancers themselves through BSE, but too often the cancer has already spread to the axillary lymph nodes, reducing the five-year survival rate to 56%. More localized breast cancer is being found today as a result of public education and an alert medical profession. For the very earliest cancers—called minimal tumors—which cannot be felt and are only detectable through mammography, five-year survival rates of up to 95% have been reported.

Most lumps in the breast are not malignant—eight out of ten are benign, but only a physician can make the diagnosis and recommend appropriate treatment based on individual needs.

NIH reported in 1976 that the proportion of women reporting ever having had a breast examination was 76% versus 43% in 1963. An earlier Gallup survey had shown an increased awareness and practice of self examination—23% were following a monthly program of breast self-examination.

New Treatment*

A new treatment strategy of giving anticancer drugs postoperatively to women with breast cancer and a high risk of recurrence has significantly lowered the recurrence rate among such patients. One breast cancer study used the drug, L–PAM, as a postoperative treatment; another used a three-drug combination called CMF. The second study led to an even more dramatic drop (5 times better than that prior to 1971) in the recurrence rate than did L–PAM. There is great and justifiable cause for optimism in these results, because experience has shown that prolonged tumor-free survival leads to increased survival rates.

A study of the treatment of breast cancer with less radical surgery has shown to date that it may be as effective as radical surgery. If the trend continues, the results will lead to treatment tailored to the individual patient and in many cases significantly different from the traditional radical surgery.

Radiation and Mammography

In July 1976 a committee of scientific consultants to the National Cancer Institute recommended that routine mammographic screening of women aged 35 to 50 be stopped, unless the women have symptoms of possible breast disease that should be checked by x-ray.

Of course, any woman with breast symptoms—such as pain, discharge or lump—which a physician regards as suspicious should have a mammogram promptly. Some doctors say that anxiety about breast cancer is also justification for mammography, especially since more than 99.9% of those examined are reassured because they are found not to have cancer.

But while the risk of a single mammogram is extremely small, so is the chance that it would pick up an otherwise hidden cancer in a woman 35 to 50, because breast cancer is less common in these young women. The average lifetime risk of breast cancer is 7%, but before

---

* Source: National Institutes of Health.

age 35 it is near zero and then increases with increasing age.

The most significant study found that women who received considerably higher doses of radiation to the breast (some received a cumulative dose of more than 1,000 rads—the measurement of radiation absorbed by the tissue) experienced a 100% increase in breast cancer risk, or twice the normal number of breast cancers, for each 120-rad exposure.

Women's Attitudes toward Mastectomy

A 1973 Gallup survey found that 51% of all women felt that loss of a breast would result in a woman losing her sense of feminity. The attitude was especially strong among single women 18 to 34 years of age.

The loss of a breast held a social as well as sexual significance. Fifty-six percent felt they could lead their lives as they had before surgery. Eighteen percent felt that it would be harder to adjust to breast loss than to the loss of an arm or a leg, and 4% said they would rather die than have a mastectomy.

Most women felt a happy marriage would not be endangered, but 51% of the sample believed a single woman's chances of being happily married were decreased after mastectomy.

Uterine Cancer

The combined figure for the two forms of uterine cancer, cervical (neck of the uterus) and endometrial (body of the uterus), is estimated at 47,000 new cases, excluding carcinoma *in situ* of the cervix, and 11,000 deaths. There has been a 65% decrease in deaths from uterine cancer during the last 40 years. Including both forms, uterine cancer ranks fourth highest among the major cancers in women, after breast cancer first, colon-rectum second and lung cancer third.

Cervical Cancer

Cervical cancer occurs most often in ages 45–69. Data indicate a causal relationship between cervical cancer and early sexual activity. New cases of cervical cancer are estimated at 20,000 for 1977; deaths are estimated at 7,600.

The incidence of cervical cancer is higher in low-income groups. Puerto Rican immigrant women have about four times as much cervical cancer as mainland U.S. women. There is also more cervical cancer among black women than white women with a rate for blacks of 34 per 100,000 compared to 15 for whites.

Pap Test

In cervical cancer detection, the Pap test is simple and effective. When cell samples are studied by qualified laboratory cytotechnicians, the results are 95% accurate (confirmed by tissue diagnosis). This test has made it possible to detect precancerous conditions and carcinoma-in-situ sufficiently early to make treatment almost 100% successful; it also permits diagnosis at this site before symptoms appear.

A Gallup study in 1973 found that almost nine out of ten women in the United States were aware of the Pap Test and that 78% had had a Pap test at least once. However, that still left one out of five American women who had never had a Pap test.

Endometrial Cancer

Endometrial cancer is primarily a disease of mature women. According to the 1970 census, there are about 45 million women 35 years or older. Of these, an estimated 700,000 will eventually develop this type of cancer. This year there will be about 27,000 new cases and about 3,300 deaths. Most cases of endometrial cancer are diagnosed in the 50–64 year age group. Many older women have not had a checkup since childbearing years, especially women living in rural areas. The need is to persuade older women to have regular checkups and see a physician for abnormal bleeding.

There is higher risk for women with late menopause, a tendency noted in association with obesity, diabetes and high blood pressure. It is usually not connected with family history.

Lung Cancer

In 1977 over 100,000 American men and women had lung cancer. In 1977, another 98,-000 were stricken with this disease. During the same year, 89,000 died of lung cancer—or approximately 244 a day.

This is largely a preventable disease, since most lung cancer is caused by cigarette smoking. Unfortunately, it is difficult to diagnose in time for cure. Only about 10% of all cases are being saved.

Though the general trend of smoking has been upward in the past 25 years, there were a number of years during which there was a sharp decline—1965-71—due to the impact of educational antismoking campaigns. In 1965, nearly 43% of the total adult population was smoking; by 1971, this had dropped to 36%, or about one in every three adult Americans was a smoker, with 30 million exsmokers.

While no national survey results have been published since 1971, there are indications that the total percentage of smokers in the adult population has risen slightly since then.

Recently, some vital information has been disclosed concerning women and smoking. There is evidence of a link between smoking by pregnant women and (1) stillbirths, (2) increased mortality among newborns, and (3) low birth weight of babies. Lower-than-normal birth weight is associated with a child's poor physical and emotional development.

Cigarette Smoking

Cigarette smoking causes at least 80% of lung cancer: (1) Risk increases if a close relative has had lung cancer; and (2) also there is a significantly higher risk of smokers getting cancer of the larynx, oral cavity and bladder. *For men,* most lung cancers occur in ages 60-69, and in men who have smoked two or more packs of cigarettes a day for 20 years and who started smoking before age 15; the risk is 15 to 20 times greater of dying from lung cancer for these smokers than for men who have never smoked. *For women,* most lung cancers occur in ages 55-64, and also in women who have smoked up to one or more packs of cigarettes a day for at least 20 years and began smoking before age 20; a woman in this group has a risk of dying of lung cancer five times that of a woman who never smoked.

Mortality

This is the number one site of cancer deaths among men. The death rate for men has increased more than 25 times in 45 years. It is going up steadily for women. Incidence has more than doubled in both men and women, black and white. Third in incidence overall, only skin and colon-rectum cancers have higher incidence—first after skin cancers in incidence

for men. The five-year survival rate for all stages is low: 8% for men, 12% for women. This is a very slight increase since the 1940s.

Cancer in Children

Cancer is second only to accidents as the cause of death for children under 15 years of age. Childhood cancer accounts for one out of twenty-eight deaths compared to adult figures of one out of six. The most common forms of childhood cancer are leukemia, brain and central nervous system, lymphomas, kidney and bone. Cancer kills more children between the ages of 3 and 14 than any other disease. Leukemia accounts for about one-half of these deaths.

For all forms of cancer occurring in children under 15, the five-year survival rate, age-adjusted for normal life expectancy, is 30%. For the 10 most frequent forms the range is as low as 3% for some leukemias to a high of 98% for thyroid and 85% for eye tumors. In Comprehensive Cancer Centers the five-year survival rate rises to 50% for children with acute lymphocytic leukemia; these results reflect aggressive treatment. More than 60% of leukemia cases in children are acute lymphocytic.

Skin Cancer

More than 300,000 new cases of skin cancer are reported in the United States each year. Of these cases about 9,000 are melanoma and the balance, nonmelanoma. Most nonmelanoma skin cancers are preventable through avoidance of overexposure to the sun. Early detection can be achieved through regular health checkups and seeing a physician promptly for changes in a wart, a mole or a sore that does not heal. The American Cancer Society (ACS) estimates that about 95% of skin cancer could be cured if such warning signals were heeded. Deaths run about 5,000 a year and are caused mainly by melanoma.

Risk is highest for farmers, sailors, and those with outdoor occupations requiring frequent sun exposure, also workers who deal with coal, tar, pitch or creosote. Excessive sunning is a high risk for those with fair complexions, particularly Northern Europeans; some families appear to be prone to skin cancer.

28

Colon-Rectum Cancer

Cancer of the colon and rectum will strike 101,000 Americans in 1977, more than any other cancer except nonmelanoma skin cancers. It occurs about equally in men and women. Over 51,000 die of it annually—though almost three out of four patients might be saved by early diagnosis and prompt treatment. The key to early diagnosis is the proctosigmoidoscopy as part of the health checkup. This is an examination with a lighted tube passed into the rectum and lower colon by which the physician can inspect the wall visually. Colonoscopy, a more elaborate technique for direct examination of the entire large bowel, is usually performed in the hospital.

Colon cancer occurs more frequently in urban and developed countries; the risk may be as high as 50% if close relatives have such genetic conditions as familial polyposis, or the patient has suffered more than ten years of ulcerative colitis. Possible dietary influence is being studied, especially highly processed foods in relation to slower transit time and increased exposure of the intestinal tract to carcinogens.

New Treatment

The first successful combination drug treatments of advanced cancers of the colon-rectum and stomach have been reported. Trials of these drug combinations immediately after surgery to increase the cure rates after the primary treatment are now in progress. If this therapy is as successful as it appears, it could significantly reduce the 49,000 annual deaths due to cancer of the large intestine.

Oral Cancer

Cancers of the mouth afflict some 24,000 Americans annually and kill about 8,000. So many deaths arising from a site so easily observable underline the need for a more intensive program of education. By the time of diagnosis, 50% of oral cancers have already metastasized to the lymph nodes. The five-year survival rate for localized lesions of the oral cavity is 67%; the rate drops to 30% when the cancer has metastasized.

Since oral cancer in its earliest stages may be painless or even asymptomatic, regular and complete examination of the oral cavity is essential, especially for high risk groups.

Environmental factors are an important cause of oral cancers including the tongue, especially habits of cigarette smoking, chewing tobacco and alcohol. Risk increases with poor oral hygiene and lack of dental care. Excessive sunlight is a factor in lip cancer; blacks, other dark-skinned people and Orientals have less risk.

Leukemia

Leukemia is a disease of the blood-forming organs.

The normal white blood cells are concerned with fighting infection. In the leukemic patient the overproduction of abnormal (or immature) white cells disrupts the production of red blood cells and interferes with clotting. In addition, these abnormal white cells are unable to fight infection. Infection and hemorrhage account for some 80% of the serious manifestations of leukemia and are immediate causes of death in leukemic patients. The uncontrolled increase in the number of white cells also results in fever, pain in the joints and bones and swelling of the lymph nodes, the spleen and liver.

HEW predicted that leukemia and related diseases would strike approximately 50,000 Americans in 1977 while an additional 33,800 would die of them.

Generally considered a disease primarily of children, leukemia actually strikes many more adults and at a rapidly increasing rate. There is no prevention or cure as yet, but some cancer experts believe the latter may be imminent. The first temporary remissions in acute lymphatic leukemia were achieved by chemotherapy in 1947. Today, with adequate treatment, survival times are improving dramatically and patients have longer symptom-free periods with near-normal blood pictures. Some drugs, in combinations, have prolonged the life of leukemia patients for well over ten years. In some medical centers, remissions are being achieved in up to 90% of so-called childhood or acute lymphocytic leukemia.

In 1960, only a few patients could be expected to live five years, while under today's optimum treatment regimen, almost 50% are expected to live that long.

In 1977 there will be 21,000 new cases of leukemia and 15,000 deaths. It strikes both sexes as well as all ages.

If leukemia strikes, families in need are directed to consult the nearest ACS Unit to

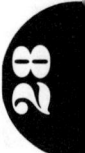

find out what help is available from the society and other local agencies.

Causes

The causes of the different types of leukemia are still unknown. For acute leukemia the participation of a virus in the causation is widely suspected, in part because in virtually every species of animals (other than man) in which similar leukemias have been observed, viruses have been found to play a causative role. For chronic myelogenous, as well as acute leukemia, ionizing radiation has been proved to be an important causative factor. Thus the incidence of leukemia of these types increased sharply in the Japanese population exposed to the atom bomb in 1945. Leukemia was also a hazard for physicians working with x-rays, until proper protective measures were adopted, and in patients formerly treated with x-rays for certain conditions. For chronic lymphatic leukemia, radiation does not seem to be a factor. Finally, certain birth defects have been found to be associated with increased risk of acute leukemia. It is widely believed that all these mechanisms—viruses, radiation and abnormal genes—alter the genetic constitution of the leukemic cells, resulting in a "somatic mutation" that endows them with new and undesirable properties and allows them to escape from the normal regulatory mechanisms of the body.

Acute Leukemia

In acute leukemia the bone marrow is replaced by the abnormal cells, so that it cannot produce either normally functioning white cells or red cells or so-called platelets, a third kind of formed element of the blood that plays a vital role in preventing bleeding from capillaries. As a result, the patient becomes (1) susceptible to infection, (2) anemic, and (3) prone to hemorrhage. These are the principal hazards of acute leukemia. Because the leukemic cells are carried to every tissue through the blood stream and may proliferate like cancer cells at remote sites, tumor-like effects may occur, notably in the central nervous system, even if the blood and bone marrow manifestations are under control as the result of treatment.

Children

Leukemia is a comparatively rare disease, but is the principal killer of children (other than accidents) beyond infancy in the U.S. It occurs at all ages, but the chronic forms predominate in older people. It is not contagious, and not heritable.

More than 50% of children with acute childhood leukemia treated at various centers in the nation now survive more than five years without disease. In 1972, in the best of institutions and under the best of circumstances over 90% of children with this disease could be put into remission and that about 50% were alive a full five years after diagnosis. In 1972, only about 25% of American children had access to this kind of treatment. Now (1977) at least 75% of our children are getting this kind of diagnosis, referral and treatment. Even this accessibility will be improved, not only for acute lymphocytic leukemia, but for other childhood cancers as well. *

At the present time, there are a number of drugs that can be used, either one at a time or in combination, for the control of acute leukemia in children. The mode of action of the various drugs differs, but in general they aim at interfering with or killing off the leukemic cell population, thus allowing the normal blood-forming cells to repopulate the bone marrow and produce normal blood cells. When this is achieved, a remission occurs. Now the average survival following diagnosis is measured in years, in contrast to the weeks expected prior to the use of drugs. Survival beyond five years is no longer exceptional. Even ten and twenty years of survival, free of disease, are being observed, giving hope for a cure. In adults, acute leukemia is more resistant to treatment, but improved modes of treatment are being developed and the outlook for adults has been improved.

Chronic Lymphocytic Leukemia

This disease is usually a very chronic condition of older people which may be manifest only by an increase in the number of circulating white blood cells of the lymphocyte type in the blood and in the bone marrow. Often the lymph glands are also infiltrated; many patients develop multiple tumors of these glands and other symptoms. The treatment is entirely different from that of acute leukemias.

Chronic Myelogenous Leukemia (CML)

This condition is the result of an overgrowth and overproduction of normally functioning

---

*National Institutes of Health, House Hearings, 1977.

elements of the bone marrow with increased numbers of white cells, and often platelets as well, in the blood stream. The leukemic cells in this condition are derived from the cell population that carries an abnormal marker chromosome. CML is usually readily controlled for years, but most often converts into acute leukemia.

Hodgkin's Disease

Hodgkin's disease is a rather rare disease which yearly strikes about 5,000 Americans. It is a disorder of the lymphatic system where the body manufactures plasma cells and white blood cells (lymphocytes)—major links in its chain of defense against infection. As the disease runs an unchecked course, lymphocytes proliferate in a variety of abnormal forms, depleting the body of normal cells to fight infection. Because it attacks white blood cell-producing organs, Hodgkin's disease is akin to leukemia.

The most frequent first symptom of Hodgkin's disease is a swollen lymph gland, usually in the neck, but also in the armpits or groin. Sometimes pain may occur in the abdomen, back or legs along with persistent fever, sweating, itching, appetite loss, nausea and vomiting.

Biopsy, a microscopic study by a doctor of tissue removed by surgery from an affected lymph node, is the major method of diagnosis.

With the treatments now available at certain centers, more than 90% of patients with early Hodgkin's disease, and about 70% with advanced disease, are surviving five years. Many of these are free of disease and are expected to live normal lifetimes. Recent update of these data show that those achieving a complete remission with drugs have a 66% chance of remaining free of disease up to ten years.

Some patients with various types of advanced non-Hodgkin's lymphomas can be cured (have up to nine years without evidence of disease) by use of drug combinations.*

Other Cancers

Ovary

Death rates increased slightly in last 25 years. Five-year survival rate shows slight gain from 25% in 1940s to 32% in 1960s. *Kidney*—sur-

vival rates for both men and women have continued to increase from 1940s to 1960s. *Brain, oral cavity, thyroid*—all showed improvement in survival rates from 1940s to 1950s; rates have leveled in 1960s.

Incidence is infrequent under age 35, most frequent in ages 65–69. Risk is higher if close relatives have had cancer of this site.

Prostate

Rare in men under age 50, familial risk. Uncommon in Orientals, Indians, Mexicans and Filipinos.

Has increased in incidence by more than 20% in past 25 years. Five-year survival rate has continued to show steady improvement from 1940s up to the present.

Stomach

Steady decrease in incidence, more than 50% in 25 years, both men and women; about one-third the death rate of 30 years ago. No known reason.

Gastric cancer

Risk is about three times higher if close relatives have had it, high incidence in Japan, declining in U.S. Data show higher incidence continues for Japanese who migrate to Hawaii but does not persist among their offspring. There is some association with blood group A. Another factor is diet with higher incidence for frequent consumers of smoked fish or meats, pickled vegetables, dried salted fish.

Pancreas

Highly fatal; five-year survival rate is still only 1%. Incidence increasing, more than 20% for men and women. No known reason.

Larynx

Strikes few women; survival rate for men has continued to improve through the 1960s.

Bladder

Slight decline in death rate for women in 25 years, with 26% decline in incidence; an increase of 21% for incidence in men. Five-year survival rates show improvement for men from 41% to 61% and from 44% to 60% for women.

Occupational Cancers

There is evidence of occupational risks for workers in certain industries: fibers and dust associated with asbestos, glass fiber products, sawdust; chemical fumes from manufacturing

---

*Source: National Institutes of Heatlh.

28

processes and arsenic compounds used in paints, sprays; contact with inks and dyes.

Carcinogens*

The following list indicates the year each substance was "reported" or "recognized" as being carcinogenic to man.

Substance	First reported as human carcinogen
Beta-naphthylamine	1954 (case reports since early 1900s).
Benzidine	1954 (case reports since 1930s).
4-aminobiphenyl	1955 (case reports since 1930s).
4-nitrobiphenyl	(Known to be metabolically converted to 4-amino-biphenyl).
Chlornaphazine	1964.
Mustard gas	1957.
Diethylstilbestrol	1971.
Bis (chloromethyl) ether	1973.
Vinyl chloride	1974.
Aflatoxin	1975.
Asbestos	1955 (case reports since 1930s).
Arsenicals	1947–57.
Chromates	1951.
Conjugated estrogens	1975.
Tobacco (chewing)	1933.
Tobacco smoke	1950.
Soots	1775.
Tars	1892.
Pitches	1892.
Asphalts	1947.
Cutting oils	1950.
Shale oils	1876.
Creosote oils	1924.
High boiling petroleum oils	1953.
Coke oven effluents	1974.
Various combustion products	1947.
Betel nut (chewing)	1959.
Radium[1]	1940s.
Thorotrast[1]	1940s.
Uranium ores[1] (radon and radon daughters)	1940s.
Other radioactive materials[1]	1940s.

[1] Carcinogenicity due to radiation.

* Source: House Appropriations Committee Hearings, 1977.

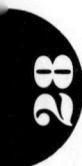

In addition, certain manufacturing exposures have been clearly identified as showing evidence of carcinogenic effects in exposed people:

Substance	Reported as human carcinogen
Auramine	1954.
Magenta	1954.
Isopropyl oil	1959.
Wood dust	1975.
Nickel refining	1958.

Cancer Centers

Currently, 17 Comprehensive Cancer Centers funded by the National Cancer Institute are carrying out high priority research and providing expert treatment for cancer.

1. Memorial Sloan-Kettering Cancer Center, New York, N.Y.
2. University of Texas System Cancer Center, M.D. Anderson Hospital and Tumor Institute, Houston, Tex.
3. University of Wisconsin, Wisconsin Clinical Cancer Center, Madison, Wis.
4. Roswell Park Memorial Institute, Buffalo, N.Y.
5. Fred Hutchinson Cancer Research Center (affiliated with the University of Washington), Seattle, Wash.
6. Sidney Farber Cancer Center, Boston, Mass.
7. University of Alabama, Cancer Research and Training Center, University of Alabama, Birmingham, Ala.
8. Johns Hopkins University Comprehensive Cancer Center, Baltimore, Md.
9. Duke University, Duke University Medical Center, Durham, N.C.
10. University of Southern California, LAC–USC Cancer Center, Los Angeles, Calif.
11. Comprehensive Cancer Center of Greater Miami, Miami, Fla.
12. Mayo Comprehensive Cancer Center, Mayo Clinic, Rochester, Minn.
13. Yale University Cancer Research Center, Yale University School of Medicine, New Haven, Conn.

14. Colorado Regional Cancer Center, Inc., Denver, Colo.
15. Illinois Cancer Council which includes: Rush-Presbyterian-St. Lukes Hospital, Chicago, Ill., University of Chicago Cancer Center, University of Chicago, Chicago, Ill. and Northwestern University Cancer Center, Northwestern University School of Medicine, Chicago, Ill., Illinois Department of Public Health.
16. Georgetown University Hospital, Vincent T. Lombardi Cancer Research Center, Washington, D.C., and Howard University Cancer Research Center, College of Medicine, Washington, D.C.
17. Fox Chase Cancer Center, Philadelphia, Pa., and University of Pennsylvania Cancer Center, School of Medicine, Philadelphia, Pa.

Cancer—Quackery

An unapproved drug called Laetrile, derived from apricot kernels, has long been promoted and sold to the public for the prevention or cure of cancer.

Recently, promoters have claimed it safe for oral consumption. Capsules of ground, defatted apricot kernels and concentrates of apricot and peach pits have been marketed as a source of Laetrile. FDA has seized such products and has charged that they are adulterated and misbranded.

On April 18, 1975, Judge Malcom Lucas of the U.S. District Court for the Central District of California granted the government's request for a permanent injunction which prohibits further marketing of these products because they were misbranded and adulterated. The Judge found capsules of defatted apricot kernels are adulterated because they are unfit for food due to their hydrogen cyanide content.

In Glenn D. Kittler's book, *Laetrile—Control for Cancer,* Laetrile was hailed as a miracle product "which will be to cancer what insulin is to diabetes."

After five years of testing, Sloan-Kettering Cancer Institute announced in June 1977 that Laetrile was totally ineffective in the cure or remission of cancer. Nevertheless, a number of states have passed special legislation to permit its sale.

Other Illnesses and Diseases

Allergies*

Allergy is a reaction to substances ordinarily harmless. These may be taken into the body by being inhaled, by being swallowed, or through contact with the skin. Sensitizing substances are called *allergens.*

Some of the common allergens are pollens, molds, house dust; animal danders (skin shed by dogs, cats, horses, rabbits): feathers (as in feather pillows); dyes, kapok, wool, chemicals used in industry; foods and medicines; insect stings. There are many possible allergens.

Approximately 17 out of every 100 Americans—or 35,277,000—suffered from one or more major allergies in 1973, according to the National Institute of Allergy and Infectious Diseases (NIAID), National Institutes of Health. Forty-four percent suffered from hay fever, 25% from asthma and 33% from other allergies. Included among "other allergies" are conditions such as *atopic* (allergic) *eczema, angioedema* (a swelling of body tissue), *urticaria* (hives on the surface of the skin), food allergy, drug allergy, and bee sting allergy. Individuals with contact dermatitis—such as poison ivy, oak, or sumac—and those who in recent years have reported allergic reactions to detergents containing enzyme additives are not included in this figure.

Numerous surveys have provided evidence of a familial incidence of allergic diseases. As many as 70% of adult asthmatics, and up to 80% of patients with hay fever, give family histories of allergic diseases.

It is true that emotions—anxiety, fear, anger, strong excitement—may precipitate allergic attacks or make an existing condition suddenly worse. However, this does not deny the physical basis of the allergy which is primary and very real.

What does an allergen do in the body?—The response to allergens results in production of blood proteins, or antibodies, which sensitize the individual to the allergic substance. With each succeeding exposure to the allergen, more sensitizing antibodies, known as immunoglobulin E (IgE), are produced until eventually the symptoms of allergy develop whenever the allergen is encountered.

---

*Sources: National Institutes of Health and The Allergy Foundation of America.

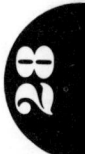

Scientists do not understand completely how antibodies cause allergic symptoms. They do know, however, that IgE causes certain sensitized cells, called mast cells, to release chemical mediators. These mediators, in turn, lead to the varied symptoms of allergy, such as nasal swelling and congestion, or bronchial constriction.

Further information: contact The Allergy Foundation of America, 801 Second Ave., N.Y. City.

Arthritis and Rheumatic Diseases*

Arthritis, rheumatic diseases, and related disorders represent a grave public health problem, afflicting more than 18 million people in the United States with pain and severe crippling. The most severely crippling form of these disorders, rheumatoid arthritis, afflicts about 5 million Americans. The most prevalent form of arthritis, known as osteoarthritis, affects more than half of all people between the ages of 55 and 64, who show evidence of this degenerative joint disease.

Arthritis, including numerous disorders of the joints characterized by inflammation and eventual degenerative changes, is man's oldest known chronic illness. Arthritis refers to the diseases which attack the joints. Other types, such as those that involve the muscles, tendons, ligaments or bursae are referred to as rheumatism. The effects of rheumatic disease may vary from a slight pain, stiffness or swelling to crippling and total disability.

The terms "arthritis" and "rheumatism" encompass about 100 different disorders, of which more than a dozen represent serious public health problems. These include rheumatoid arthritis, degenerative joint disease, also called osteoarthritis, connective tissue disorders such as systemic lupus erythematosus, and arthritis associated with metabolic abnormalities such as gout.

Common Forms of Arthritis

Rheumatoid Arthritis—This is the most serious, because it can lead to crippling. It is inflammatory and often chronic. Although it attacks the joints primarily, it can also cause

disease in the lungs, skin, blood vessels, muscles, spleen and heart. It tends to subside and flare up unpredictably, often causing progressive damage to tissues. Women are affected three times more often than men.

In children it occurs in a form known as *juvenile rheumatoid arthritis* and sometimes can be quite serious. It may involve many organs, including the spleen, liver and heart. Chiefly it attacks the joints. One or more joints may be affected, including those of the fingers, wrists, elbows, hips, knees and feet. There is inflammation, swelling, pain and resulting disabilities.

Research scientists are continuing their efforts to discover the cause(s) of rheumatoid arthritis. This disease often leads to severe disability and no permanent cure has yet been found. Researchers have sometimes found certain infectious agents in close association with tissues inflamed by rheumatoid arthritis, but none of these organisms has been found to be a cause of the disease. Many investigators believe that the mechanism which causes the widespread chronic inflammation affecting various systems of the body is an abnormal reaction of the body's immune system. Such a reaction may be stimulated by infection and may result in a misdirected attack by the body's defense systems on its own tissue (an autoimmune reaction).

Chief symptoms: Rheumatoid arthritis usually begins with general fatigue, soreness, stiffness and aching followed by the gradual appearance of localized symptoms in a joint or in several joints consisting of pain, swelling, warmth and tenderness. Sometimes there is a sudden onset of these joint symptoms. In most cases several joints become involved, particularly those of the hands and feet.

Usually there is weakness and fatigue, loss of appetite and loss of weight. Frequently patients have cold, sweaty hands and feet.

The symptoms may leave or return with flare-ups and periods of improvement.

Gradually, joint motion can be lost, and in time deformities of the joints may occur.

In addition to joint symptoms patients may have other changes such as lumps or nodules under the skin, inflammation of the eyes, pleurisy and anemia.

Osteoarthritis—Also called degenerative joint disease, this is principally a wear-and-tear disease of the joints which comes with getting older. It is usually mild and is not generally

---

*Source: The Arthritis Foundation and National Institutes of Health.

inflammatory. It does not cause general illness or affect parts of the body other than the joints. Sometimes there can be considerable pain. Mild to severe disability may develop gradually.

Symptoms: Many people with osteoarthritis are not bothered by it, even though x-ray pictures show they have it.

For those who do have trouble, pain in and around joints is the major symptom. It may be mild aching and soreness, particularly when joints are moved, or it may be a nagging, constant pain.

The pain is caused by pressure on nerve endings and by tense muscles and muscle fatigue. Occasionally pain is felt at a distance from the joint where the trouble is.

The second most common symptom is loss of ability to move a joint easily and comfortably. Muscle weakness in the area of the joint is part of the problem.

In advanced cases, when bone changes have taken place on the inside, joints take on an outwardly knobby look.

Ankylosing Spondylitis—This is chronic, inflammatory arthritis of the spine. It usually begins in the teens or early twenties.

Systemic Lupus Erythematosus—Called "SLE," or "lupus," or "lupus arthritis" for short, this is an acute systemic disease, a cousin of rheumatoid arthritis. It can inflame and damage joints and organs throughout the body, including the kidneys, heart, lungs, brain and blood vessels. A skin rash on the face is common. It strikes women more often than men. A mild form of the disease, which affects the skin only, is called discoid lupus erythematosus.

Gout—Gout, also called gouty arthritis, is an acutely painful form of arthritis and far more prevalent than is generally supposed. There are at least 1,000,000 victims in the United States

The disease often results from an inherited defect in body chemistry, but may occur after the use of diuretic pills, given to get rid of excess body fluid or to lower blood pressure. Uric acid, a normal body substance, is either overproduced or produced faster than the kidneys can get rid of it. In about one out of ten people who have too much uric acid in their blood, the excess uric acid forms needle-like crystals in joints. This leads to severe inflammation. The affected joints become hot, swollen and extremely tender.

In three out of four cases, the large joint of the big toe is attacked first, but gouty arthritis can settle in almost any part of the body. Most victims are men.

Rheumatic Fever—Rheumatic fever, caused by a streptococcus infection and chiefly damaging the heart, is considered an arthritic disease because it inflames joints. The arthritis, though painful, does not cripple and usually clears up completely with proper treatment.

Quackery in Arthritis

Arthritis sufferers are the most exploited of all victims of disease in the country today. More than $403 million a year is spent by arthritics on worthless or harmful treatments, cures and devices, according to a recent Arthritis Foundation survey. These include such nostrums as filtered sea water, so-called "immune" milk, honey and apple vinegar combinations, alfalfa tablets, glorified aspirin and all manner of treatments and devices offering "miracle" cures. These are generally worthless, almost all are expensive, and some are in fact harmful.

To help you recognize the species Common Quack, we offer some simple clues to how he operates—clues to help you be wary and think twice before you buy.

1. He may offer a "special" or "secret" formula or device for "curing" arthritis.
2. He advertises. He uses "case histories" and testimonials from satisfied "patients."
3. He may promise (or imply) a quick or easy cure.
4. He may claim to know the cause of arthritis and talk about "cleansing" your body of "poisons" and "pepping up" your health. He may say surgery, x-rays and drugs prescribed by a physician are unnecessary.
5. He may accuse the "medical establishment" of deliberately thwarting progress, or of persecuting him . . . but he doesn't let his method be tested in tried and proved ways.

Bursitis

A bursa is a small sac containing slippery fluid, a cushioning device located at potential friction points between adjoining tissues within a joint structure. Irritation from pressure or injury can trigger inflammation of a bursa, causing extreme tenderness and pain. The whole joint may become red and swollen. Bursitis most often affects a shoulder but may occur in other joints such as hips or elbows.

Blindness*

It is estimated that there are about 6.4 million persons in the United States with some kind of visual impairment, that is, persons who have trouble seeing even with corrective lenses. Of these, 1.7 million are severely impaired. This means that they cannot read a newspaper with either eye, even with glasses. Only about 400,-000 of the severely visually impaired, however, have no usable vision at all.

Over one million persons—or about 65% of the severely visually impaired—are 65 years old or older.

A person is said to be "legally blind" if his central visual acuity does not exceed 20:200 in the better eye with correcting lenses or his visual field is less than an angle of 20 degrees. In simpler terms, a person is considered "legally blind" if he can see no more at a distance of 20 feet than someone with normal sight can see at a distance of 200 feet.

Table 28-21   Incidence and prevalence of vision disorders

	Number of people afflicted	Number of blind persons	Number of newly blind each year	Percent of all blindness
Retinal and choroidal diseases	1,177,000	151,000	15,000	32%
Corneal diseases	311,000	22,000	N/A[1]	6%
Cataract	3,013,000	64,000	4,400	14%
Glaucoma	1,016,000	56,000	3,100	12%
Sensory-motor disorders of vision	890,000[2]	36,000	3,000	9%
Other causes	4,708,000	138,000	N/A[1]	27%

[1] Not available.
[2] Nerve atrophy and myopia only.

Source: National Institutes of Health, 1977.

Vision Disorders**

Retinal and Choroidal Diseases—Diabetic retinopathy, the leading cause of blindness in the United States, is the result of tiny blood vessels in the retina breaking and causing little hemorrhages on or in the retina.

Diabetic retinopathy, macular degeneration, retinitis pigmentosa, and other retinal degenerative diseases are primary causes of more than one-third of all blindness in this country. These diseases which can neither be prevented nor cured, are considered by ophthalmologists to be the most difficult to treat and most in need of further research.

An estimated 15,000 people become blind each year from retinal and choroidal diseases, which already accounts for 32% of all blindness in the United States.

Corneal Diseases—Corneal diseases are a leading cause of blindness worldwide and are the most painful of eye disorders. There are an estimated 22,000 Americans blind from corneal disease, accounting for about 6% of all blindness in the country. Many more individuals, though not legally blind, have varying degrees of visual impairment because of corneal diseases. These disorders have great impact, not only in reducing visual acuity but also in causing suffering, for they are the most painful eye disorders.

Transplantation of the cornea may soon become more successful and its benefits extended to more people because of a new method for preserving the life of fresh donor tissue. During the past year, NEI-supported investigators developed an improved method for storing donor corneas that reduces the risk of graft failure and extends the survival period of healthy donor tissue from the traditional 48 hours to one week.

The method is now being used by eye banks across the country to preserve donor corneas for transplantation.

Cataract—Any cloudiness or opacity in the normally transparent lens is called a cataract. The more serious types of cataract will

---

*Source: American Foundation for the Blind.
**Source: National Institutes of Health, 1977.

obstruct the passage of light to the retina and impair vision. Although there are different types of cataract, the most common are those associated with old age, the so-called senile cataract.

Nearly 3,013,000 Americans have cataracts, 64,000 of whom are legally blind. Therefore, ways are being sought to prevent cataracts or medically retard their progression. Although surgery is 95% successful, social, psychological and economic factors contribute to cataracts being responsible for 14% of all blindness in this country. With a cataract operation costing about $2,500, the 400,000 procedures performed annually cost about $1 billion.

Glaucoma—Glaucoma is one of the leading causes of visual disability in the nation. It is responsible for 12% of all blindness in the U.S. and 14% of all new cases of blindness.

Glaucoma results when an obstruction in the outflow of a fluid, aqueous humor leads to increased pressure within the eye with subsequent damage to the optic nerve and loss of vision.

Sensory-Motor Disorders and Rehabilitation—Sensory and motor disorders of vision may be either congenital or acquired and account for 16% of all blindness. Research into the visual system in health and disease is hoped to improve the diagnosis and treatment of strabismus (crosseye), amblyopia (decreased vision without apparent organic cause) and other sensory and motor problems. A total of 37,000 Americans are blind from optic nerve atrophy and myopia alone (9.2% of all legal blindness) and each year 3,000 more people are blinded by this disorder.

Seeking Help

The *Directory of Low Vision Aids Facilities in the U.S.A. (AFB)* lists available facilities and their services throughout the country. These include:

Services	Referrals
Complete ophthalmological examination	Ophthalmologist (staff)
Refractive	Ophthalmologist (private)
Optician	Other M.D.
Prescribing optical aids	Optometrist
Instruction in use of aids	Agency for the blind
Loan of optical aids	Vocational rehabilitation
Social services	School for the blind
Follow-up	Department of education
Large print materials	Nursing home
Electric visual aids	Self-referral
Referral for complete ophthalmological examination	Service organization
Referrals to other agencies	Social welfare agency
Consultation	Public health department
Psychological counseling	Mobile eye clinic
Rehabilitation	Braille institute
	Veterans Administration

Note: There are both ophthalmologists and optometrists who, in their private practices, do low vision work but are not included because of the purpose of this list.

Information on these could probably also be obtained through local or state medical, ophthalmological or optometric societies.

Further information: For more information write:

● American Foundation for the Blind, Inc.
  15 West 16th Street
  New York, N.Y. 10011

● The National Society for the Prevention of Blindness, Inc.
  79 Madison Avenue
  New York, N.Y. 10016

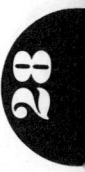

616

- The Library of Congress receives federal funds to maintain libraries for the blind. Some of the services available are large-print literature, a music library and books in the form of braille, talking discs and tape. Nearly 50 libraries throughout the country serve as regional distributing centers for these materials which can be mailed free of charge. Address inquiries to Division for the Blind and Physically Handicapped, Library of Congress, Washington, D.C. 20542.
- The National Center for Deaf-Blind Youths and Adults
  105 Fifth Avenue
  New Hyde Park, N.Y. 11040
- Recording for the Blind, Inc. lends taped educational materials free of charge to visually and physically handicapped students and others who require such materials in their professions. Recording is done by trained volunteers at the specific request of the borrower. Address inquiries to:
  Recording for the Blind Inc.
  215 East 58 Street
  New York, N.Y. 10022

- Bureau of Education for the Handicapped
  Office of Education
  7th and D Streets, S.W.
  Washington, D.C. 20202
- Office for the Blind and Visually Handicapped
  Department of Health, Education, and Welfare
  330 C Street, S.W.
  Washington, D.C. 20201
- The Seeing Eye
  P.O. Box 375
  Morristown, N.J. 07960
- American Printing House for the Blind
  1839 Frankfort Avenue
  Louisville, Ky. 40206
- The R. R. Bowker Company lists more than 1,200 titles in *Large Type Books in Print.* Today a number of newspapers and magazines regularly issue large-print editions. One magazine, the *Enlarged Type Reader's Digest,* reported that 93% of its subscribers were over 65; the oldest claimed to be 102.

Cerebral Palsy*

Cerebral palsy is a condition caused by damage to the human brain, usually at birth. "Cerebral" refers to the brain and "palsy" to lack of control over the muscles. At least 40% of all persons with cerebral palsy have a history of having been born prematurely.

In addition to lack of motor control, there may be seizures, spasms, mental retardation, abnormal sensation and perception, or impairment of sight, hearing or speech, all in varying degrees.

There is no single effective preventive measure and no cure. However, careful medical care and good nutrition throughout pregnancy can prevent some cerebral palsy. Also, as a result of the development and use of the rubella vaccine and of the Rh immuno-globulin serum, fewer babies may be born today with cerebral palsy than five years ago.

The United Cerebral Palsy Associations, Inc., estimates that there are 750,000 persons in the United States with cerebral palsy. Each year, 15,000 babies are born with brain damage that causes cerebral palsy.

Kinds and Degrees of Cerebral Palsy

There are six clinical types of cerebral palsy: cases exhibiting *spasticity,* in which the muscles are under a continuous state of tension, with increased reflex activity; *athetosis,* characterized by disorganized, spontaneous muscular movements; *ataxia,* manifested as a disturbance in balance while walking or standing; *tremor,* similar to the fine tremulousness seen in adults who have Parkinsonism; those with *rigidity,* a slow, sustained contraction of the muscles, leading to clumsiness; and *mixed,* a combination of two or more of the above types.

The degree of disability is dependent upon the site and amount of damage in the brain. Sometimes damage is so slight that the victim may have only a mild clumsiness or incoordination of the hands, a slight loss of balance in walking or a minor speech impediment. In very severe cases, he may be confined to wheelchair or bed and be totally dependent upon others. At times, speech may be so involved that verbal communication is impossible. In some patients, only the right or left half of the body is affected. In others, both legs may be involved so that walking is associated with awkward or involuntary movements and irregular

---

*Source: National Institutes of Health.

gait. Complete loss of hand function may make it impossible for the cerebral palsied victim to provide himself any degree of self care.

Because the brain controls so many functions other than purely motor acts, other defects are also associated with cerebral palsy. Thus defective vision or hearing, convulsive tendencies, intellectual impairment and personality change may occur in cerebral palsy. These associated defects in some instances may be more disabling than the motor disability itself.

Symptoms

The child may be tense or irritable, may feed poorly or have difficulty in sucking. Often, abnormally slow development of the infant's muscular control and coordination may be the first sign of trouble.

Causes of Cerebral Palsy

Cerebral palsy is caused by damage to the part of the brain which controls and coordinates muscular action.

It is known that anoxia—lack or reduction of oxygen—can harm the developing brain, though it is not yet clear whether the lack of oxygen or its secondary effects are directly responsible for the damage. Maternal infection during pregnancy, blood type incompatibility and metabolic disturbances in the newborn are also factors.

Maternal infection is considered an especially serious threat to the fetal brain, either by interfering with its normal development, as in rubella (German measles) or cytomegalovirus (CMV) infection, or by damaging it later, as in toxoplasmosis, a lesser known parasitic infection.

Brain damage may occur in the newborn period to infants seemingly predisposed to it by such factors as low birth weight or difficulty in adapting to life immediately after birth. Disordered brain function in the premature or low birth weight infant may also be of genetic or embryonic origin, or it may be a consequence of severe nutritional lack during pregnancy.

In later infancy and early childhood, such infectious diseases as meningitis and encephalitis, as well as other neurological disorders, account for an appreciable percentage of cerebral palsy cases. Direct trauma from accidents, especially traffic accidents, is an increasingly alarming cause of this condition. Battering (nonaccidental injury) is also a factor in a significant proportion of cases.

Management and Treatment of Cerebral Palsy

Attention is directed at assisting the child to achieve his maximum intellectual and physical potential, using specialized techniques for specific defects. Physical therapy, bracing and, at times, orthopedic surgery are indicated if the potential for functioning warrants it. Drugs may be effective in reducing tension and in limiting other problems connected with nerve damage. Physical, speech and hearing therapy by skilled professionals are important features of any program to prepare the cerebral palsied child to succeed in school and in life.

A child with cerebral palsy or any other physical disability is often handicapped as much as a consequence of having a disability as by the degree and type of the disorder itself. Personality, emotional development and educational achievement are all affected by the motor disorder, associated sensory, intellectual and other disabilities. As a result of this combination of disadvantages, progressive social deprivation and isolation often occur, and in time become the greatest handicap.

Further Information

For additional information contact:

- The American Academy for Cerebral Palsy
  1255 New Hampshire Ave., N.W.
  Washington, D.C.
- United Cerebral Palsy Associations, Inc.
  66 East 34th St.
  New York, N.Y.
- The National Easter Seal Society for Crippled Children and Adults
  2026 Ogden Ave.
  Chicago, Ill.

Cystic Fibrosis*

Striking one in every 1,500 infants, cystic fibrosis (CF) is characterized by malfunctioning exocrine glands that secrete abnormal fluid to internal and external body surfaces, particularly to the gastrointestinal and respiratory mucosal linings and the skin.

Cystic fibrosis, an inherited metabolic disorder, results in three principal clinical problems. The first is the production of sweat with a high salt content. Because of this defect,

---

*Source: National Institutes of Health.

patients are unable to conserve salt and are therefore at risk of developing profound dehydration or heat exhaustion in the summer, either of which may be fatal.

The second is that in CF, the mucus-secreting glands of the body fail to secrete normal, clear, free-flowing fluid. Instead, they produce abnormally thick, viscous mucus which tends to obstruct the ducts or openings of these glands. When the mucus accumulates in the ducts of the pancreas, it interferes with the ability of this gland to supply digestive enzymes to the intestinal tract, thus leading to poor digestion of food and to malabsorption of a number of essential nutrients. Depending on the severity of this complication, the patient may suffer from general underdevelopment, poor musculature and retarded bone growth.

The third and most serious complication is the development of progressive, chronic lung disease. Thick mucus obstructs the smaller air passages in the lung, causing labored breathing and chronic cough. In time, bacteria multiply in the accumulated secretions, predisposing the child to chronic bronchitis or pneumonia—the leading cause of death in these patients. The lung changes may also restrict pulmonary blood flow, leading to increased blood pressure in the lung, consequent chronic heart strain and eventual heart failure.

The key to prolonged survival for most cystic fibrosis patients is control of respiratory complications. Chronic pulmonary disease is responsible for death in 90% of the cases.

Although much has been accomplished toward alleviating the symptoms of cystic fibrosis, its basic defect and means of permanent control still elude investigators. Malnutrition due to pancreatic insufficiency, formerly a serious complication of the disease, can now be readily managed in most cases by administration of supplementary pancreatic enzymes of animal origin. Through improved antibiotic therapy the consequences of chronic pulmonary disease can now be forestalled in many patients. These measures and others have prolonged the life of the cystic fibrosis patient, and have also enhanced the quality of that still unduly short life.

Deaf and Mute*

There are 1.8 million deaf people in the United States. Many of them are without useful speech despite years of training. Many have limited language skills. They receive messages principally through their eyes. They send messages by combinations of signs, gestures, speech and writing. Most of them have normal strength, mobility and intelligence.

There are currently 203 deaf persons for every 100,000. In all there are between 13 and 14 million people in this country with sufficient hearing loss to significantly affect their ability to function effectively in everyday activities.

Americans with communication disorders exceed 20,000,000. Some have disorders of the ears, the normal channels for receiving verbal messages. Some have defects in the vocal mechanisms, the main means for sending verbal messages. Some have disorders of the central nervous system which interfere with receiving and sending even though the ears and vocal apparatus are whole. Some have peripheral involvements that curb free verbalization. Some have combinations of causes.

Diabetes*

Authorities now estimate that the number of reported diabetic patients is more than 4,250,000 in the United States alone. It is further estimated that another six million Americans are potential diabetics, persons who at present have no symptoms of the disease, but who may develop diabetes sometime during their lives.

A complicated disease, for which there is no known cure, diabetes has been known for some time to have a strong hereditary component. As a result of the body's inability to metabolize carbohydrates normally (which results from impaired production or activity of the hormone insulin, normally secreted by the beta cells of the pancreas, and from excessive secretion of the insulin antagonist glucagon), the diabetic patient is unable to convert dietary carbohydrates properly into the stored form, glycogen, or to utilize them normally to produce the energy required for body functions. Thus, carbohydrates, in the form of glucose, accumulate in the blood and, because of their high concentration, overflow into the urine. It appears that as the disease progresses, derangement in the metabolism of fats and proteins also results.

*Source: National Institutes of Health.

Juvenile diabetes is the severe form of the disease which is generally characterized by onset early in life. This classic type of severe, "brittle" or "unstable" diabetes primarily occurs in children or young adults with a history of diabetes in their families; it is now recognized that it occasionally emerges in adults. If untreated, juvenile diabetes rapidly progresses to a state of grave metabolic imbalance, believed to be caused mainly by a relatively severe deficiency in insulin output or severe impairment in insulin activity. One result may be the excessive breakdown of fat with the production of ketoacids (diabetic ketoacidosis) which may lead to coma and death unless controlled by insulin and other supportive therapy. Patients with juvenile diabetes require lifelong maintenance therapy based on daily insulin injections, which control the more obvious clinical symptoms and permit the patient to engage in near-normal activities. Nevertheless, patients with juvenile diabetes have a decreased life expectancy and are subject to a gradual onset of progressive changes in various organ systems, leading to the long-term complications of diabetes. These complications involve an abnormality characteristic of diabetes in the small blood vessels of the body; an accelerated, degenerative process in the large blood vessels akin to atherosclerosis; and a characteristic, irregular degeneration in the nervous system. With the passage of time, these underlying pathologic processes may result in one or more of the following:

1. premature heart attacks, strokes or impairment of the blood supply to the extremities
2. kidney failure
3. progressive deterioration of vision and eventual blindness
4. disabling disorders of the nervous system including impotence.

The majority of patients with diabetes are afflicted with the more common, less severe type termed "Maturity-Onset Diabetes." This form of the disease, as its name implies, usually has a gradual onset in the 50s and 60s and in most cases does not require insulin. Many overweight patients benefit from reducing body weight and all patients must adhere to a proper diet. Some patients with maturity-onset diabetes may, like those with juvenile diabetes, gradually develop serious long-term complications.

The theory that diabetes may be triggered by an infectious process in persons who are genetically predisposed to the disease has gained more and more advocates in recent years.

Digestive Diseases*

The diversity and magnitude of the category of digestive disorders is evident in that it includes diseases of the esophagus, stomach, intestine, colon, liver, gallbladder and pancreas. Among the well-known disorders in this category are peptic ulcer, hepatitis, cirrhosis of the liver, gallstones, Crohn's disease and ulcerative colitis. Some of the causes are infections, cancer, alcoholism, genetic defects and reactions to stress.

The economic and social costs of digestive diseases are high. Chronic digestive disease affects at least 18 million Americans and is of enormous economic cost in direct medical expenditures and indirect hours lost from work. In a recent year the cost was estimated at $16.5 billion or some $80 for every man, woman and child. More than 10% of the cost of the nation's medical care is for digestive diseases. One-ninth of hospital admissions and almost one-third of all surgery are for digestive diseases. One-quarter of cancer deaths are due to malignancies in the digestive system. Cirrhosis of the liver has become the fifth most common cause of death in men in the United States. Peptic ulcer strikes one of every ten men at some time during their lives.

Gallstones*

Little is known about how gallstones are formed, yet gallstone disease ranks fifth among causes of hospitalization. Some 15 million Americans have gallstones; in many cases they cause no symptoms while in others they result in debilitating disease. Surgery is the standard form of treatment and some 375,000 gallbladder operations are performed each year at an average cost of $2000 each. Many gallstone patients are poor surgical risks and an estimated 6,000 patients die each year after surgery.

Drs. Johnson L. Thistle and Alan F. Hofman and associates at the Mayo Foundation,

---

* Source: National Institutes of Health.

28

Rochester, Minnesota, first reported three years ago that long-term oral administration of a primary bile acid, chenodeoxycholic acid, can result in dissolution of long-standing cholesterol gallstones.

One of the causes of gallstone formation is cholesterol oversaturation of the bile in the human body. Cholesterol, a natural component of bile, is kept in solution by two other components of the bile, lecithin and bile acids. When the ratio of cholesterol to lecithin and bile acids is too great, gallstones form. If the concentration of bile acids can be increased, the cholesterol will again become soluble in bile and there will be no reason for cholesterol precipitation and consequent cholesterol stone formation, or, in the case of existing cholesterol stones, there will be a tendency for their dissolution in the acid-rich bile fluid.

Obese individuals who are subject to gallstones are even more susceptible during a period of active weight reduction and should, therefore, avoid the see-saw of alternately losing and regaining weight, according to studies by NIAMDD scientists at the Institute's Clinical Research Section in Phoenix, Arizona.

It is well-known that the obese tend to have gallstones more frequently than lean persons and that permanent weight reduction and maintenance of normal weight diminish the risk of developing such accretions.

Emphysema and Chronic Bronchitis*

Emphysema and chronic bronchitis are separate diseases. However, they usually occur together and involve many of the same physical and biochemical components within the lung. They also trigger many of the same physiological mechanisms.

Chronic obstructive pulmonary disease (COPD) is a serious health problem in this country. In 1973 it killed 39,000 Americans. Of the 1.3 million people with emphysema, it is estimated that 700,000 are under age 65.

Chronic bronchitis afflicts 6.5 million Americans. One hundred eighty thousand citizens are limited in activity as a consequence of this disease.

Chronic Bronchitis

Chronic bronchitis is characterized by a persistent inflammation and swelling of the lin-

---
* Source: National Institutes of Health.

ings of the bronchial airways, excessive production of mucus (phlegm) and other fluids that tend to block the airways and that lead to coughing, spitting and shortness of breath. The onset of chronic bronchitis may be slow, and usually follows episodes of acute bronchitis. Early symptoms are often shrugged off as "smokers cough" and "winter colds." By the time the condition is diagnosed, the delicate lung tissue may be irreversibly damaged and the patient well on the way to respiratory disability. The principal, known factors contributing to the prolonged bronchial irritation of chronic bronchitis are smoking, air pollution and recurrent respiratory infections. These same irritants can promote the development of the companion disorder, emphysema.

Emphysema

The exact cause of emphysema is not known, but the initial event appears to be a breakdown in the thin coating of mucus and the many hair-like cilia that line all air passageways throughout the respiratory system. This lining normally protects lung tissues against inhaled dust, bacteria and other harmful materials. The constant waving motion of the cilia acts to propel these particles on a mucus-lubricated path toward the throat where they can be eliminated from the body.

With the breakdown of this protective lining, the noxious materials begin to destroy the normal physical properties and architecture of the lung, producing large, inefficient air spaces. As a result, resistance to air flow increases and breathing becomes progressively more difficult.

Late in the disease, blood oxygen levels decrease, and the toxic gaseous waste product, carbon dioxide, accumulates. Death usually results from heart failure (the heart is overworked in a vain attempt to meet body oxygen needs by more vigorous pumping of oxygen-poor blood), or from suffocation during a respiratory crisis precipitated by a cold or other respiratory infection.

Diagnostic Techniques

Emphysema and chronic bronchitis develop so insidiously that many victims are unaware that anything is seriously wrong until 50% or more of their lung function has been destroyed. At this late stage, the damage cannot be undone.

Although the causes of COPD are still poorly defined, two factors—cigarette smoking and air pollution—are strongly suspected of contributing importantly to the development of emphysema and chronic bronchitis in both their "pure" and combined forms and of aggravating their clinical course. Emphysema, for example, is 13 times more prevalent among cigarette smokers than among nonsmokers.

Epidemics and Famine

The devastating epidemics of antiquity and medieval times—and even later—resulted in a great mortality toll. Speculations as to the rapid spread of disease then suggest several causes: ignorance of the laws of health, dense overcrowding within circumscribed walled towns, total lack of drainage with filthy streets poisoning water well supplies and insufficient care for the sick and diseased. Reasons for famine conditions include widespread failure of crops through lack of water and destruction by diseases and pests.

B.C. 436: Famine at Rome; thousands threw themselves into the Tiber
767: First recorded plague; affected all parts of the world

A.D. 80: Plague in Italy; ten thousand destroyed daily
1193: Dreadful famine in England and France, followed by pestilential fever
1348: The great epidemic of Black Death (bubonic plague) over most of world; estimated death toll—25 million in Europe, 25 million in Asia
1466: Famine accompanied by plague wastes great numbers in Ireland
1510: Worldwide epidemic of influenza
1529: Sweating sickness sweeps through England and north Germany
1583: Diphtheria epidemic rages in Spain
1611: Pestilence slaughters 200,000 at Constantinople
1630: Plague spreads through major Italian centers
1664: Great plague of London

A.D. 1769: Great famine in Bengal; a third of population, 10 million, starves to death
1792: Devastating plague in Egypt; 800,000 perish
1831: Asiatic cholera first appears in England; continues on to rage in Scotland, Ireland and United States
1865: Cholera spreads in Turkey, France and Italy
1876: Vast famine in Bombay, Madras and Mysore; five million perish
1877: Severe famine in China; nine million said to have perished
1910: Pneumonic plague epidemic in North Manchuria
1918: Worldwide epidemic of Spanish influenza
1921: Famine in U.S.S.R.; again in 1931
1960: Famine conditions averted in Congo by United Nations action

Epilepsy*

Our brains are constantly working, receiving information from inside and outside our bodies by way of our sense organs and their nerve networks. The brain sorts that information, evaluates it, stores some of it for future reference and acts on the rest through a network of motor nerves to our muscles.

To keep this intricate mechanism working, brain cells (neurons) generate electrochemical energy impulses which sweep rhythmically along the neuronal networks. When there is a job to be done, neurons which control the brain or body part to be activated send impulses until the work is finished, then "turn off." Sometimes, in some brains, some neurons or groups of them do not shut off when a job is done, but keep sending action messages. When these excessive impulses continue, the body or brain parts on the receiving end operate erratically and the brain may even shut down conscious operation although in some cases, normal movements can continue without apparent purpose. Sometimes, adjacent neurons get excited and send additional, unnecessary impulses involving the whole

*Source: National Institutes of Health.

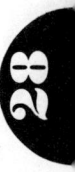

body in erratic movements. These fitful physical and mental activities are seizures. When they happen repeatedly, the brain parts where they originate are termed "epileptic" and the person is said to have epilepsy.

Seizures are classified as *simple partial, complex partial, generalized* and *partial, secondarily generalized. Simple partial* seizures are usually without loss of consciousness and consist of flickers, shakes, jerks of body parts, dizziness or unpleasant sight, sound, taste or stomach sensations. *Complex partial* seizures are usually with loss of consciousness where the individual appears to be in a dreamy state, at rest or moving automatically and purposelessly. He or she may also show outward signs of fear, anger, elation or irritability although there is usually no memory of such feelings later.

In *generalized* seizures, most of the brain becomes involved, unconsciousness occurs and both sides of the body react. Such seizures are classified as *absence, tonic-clonic, tonic, clonic, myoclonic* or *akinetic.*

Sometimes *partial* seizures progress to *generalized* seizures, as nearby cells join the malfunctioning cells in the uncontrolled discharges until the whole brain and then the entire body are involved.

Seizure frequency varies from seldom to often. Seizures may last from a split second to several minutes. In "status epilepticus," they follow one another so closely that they appear continuous and can be fatal unless stopped by therapy. Seizures may be preceded by "auras" and are often followed by periods of exhausted confusion.

Causes

It appears that brain damage is basic to epilepsy. Difficult births, high fever, some infectious diseases, head injuries and chronic drug or alcohol addiction are often followed by seizures. Accidental or surgically associated brain injuries can cause seizures in man. In animals, they can be caused by various experimental chemical or electrical stimulations. They often accompany brain tumors, abscesses or inborn brain malfunctions. Where no brain injury possibility can be cited, the epilepsy is termed *idiopathic* (cause unknown).

The Victims

The Epilepsy Foundation of America estimates the number of epileptics in the United States as four million. Other medical groups estimate one to two million cases.

Some 60% of epileptic patients can live relatively "normal" lives because their seizures are controlled by drugs or surgical removal of damaged brain tissue. The other 40% go partially controlled or without any control. Even those who have only a few brief attacks a year find it difficult, often impossible, to get jobs or drivers' licenses. Those who have frequent seizures have trouble existing without help.

Persons who have epilepsy but no other brain damage are as intelligent as the general population and have similar abilities for learning and working. Epileptics are not insane nor is epilepsy contagious. Susceptibility to epilepsy may be hereditary in some cases. More than half of the epilepsy cases are in people under 20. Yet, through brain injury, anyone can become epileptic at any age.

Therapy—Drugs and Surgery

Phenobarbital, first used for epilepsy in 1912 and diphenylhydantoin (Dilantin), developed in 1938, are still the most effective and safest drugs for controlling seizures.

Headaches*

Brain tissue does not feel pain on direct stimulation, nor does the bone of the skull. But other structures of the head are extremely sensitive to pain, including the scalp, blood vessels and certain of the brain coverings. Here are some ways of classifying head pains:

1. Swelling (dilation) of arteries of the head. Just as your ankle hurts when it is swollen, so the pain-sensitive blood vessels hurt (ache) when they swell inside or outside of the head. Headaches of migraine, fever, carbon monoxide poisoning and other toxic states, hangovers, and hunger are some which relate to pain in the cranial arteries.
2. Pulling (traction) on pain-sensitive structures within the head. A brain tumor, abscess or hemorrhage does not cause pain because of direct pressure on brain tissue, but because it pulls on the arteries or other pain-sensitive structures.
3. Inflammation or irritation of pain-sensitive structures. Like an infected finger, an

---

* Source: National Institutes of Health.

inflamed brain artery produces pain; an inflamed brain covering is accompanied by severe headache.

4. Prolonged contraction of neck muscles. Holding your head stiffly with tense neck muscles may be an instinctive reaction to events which anger or worry you, or simply a poor posture habit. This produces one of the commonest of headaches—the muscle-contraction (tension) headache. Because a head already aching from swollen arteries or inflammation probably will be held stiffly, muscle-contraction headache often complicates and confuses the diagnosis of headaches from other sources.

5. Spreading pain. Pain may spread into a general headache from local pain in the eye, ear, nose, sinuses or infected teeth.

   These physical sources of headache may be duplicated by research experiment. When no physical mechanism to explain headache can be discovered, the source may be considered.

6. Psychogenic. An emotional conflict or anxiety is "converted" ("conversion reaction") into a body symptom—a "real" not an "imaginary" headache.

Research has proven that a temporary narrowing (vasoconstriction) of the blood vessels in the head marks the early painless stage of migraine. Perhaps eight to ten percent of migraine patients experience a warning of the impending headache, such as jagged streaks of light or other "fireworks" of vision, numbness, tingling and perhaps nausea. Some feel weak, tired or overexcited.

This warning "aura" allows the individual to lie down in a dark, quiet room or to take immediately the medicine his doctor has prescribed. These means may ward off the threatening head pain.

Heart Disease*
Arteriosclerosis

For some reason still not clearly understood, fatlike substances build up on the inside walls of the arteries. Gradually they accumulate and form thick deposits called "plaques." These deposits both roughen the artery's normally smooth inner lining and narrow the channel for

---

* Source: National Institutes of Health,

blood flow, making it more difficult for enough blood to get through. Making matters worse, the artery also loses elasticity with age and loses its flexibility.

It is believed that some, but probably not all, of the fatty substances that build up on the artery wall come from the blood fats. People with high concentrations of fat in their blood develop hardening of the arteries earlier and are more likely to suffer serious consequences in later years.

More than half of all deaths from the various kinds of heart disease are the consequence of hardening of the arteries.

For instance, hardening of the arteries sets the stage for many "strokes" by clogging arteries carrying blood to the brain. The damaged artery or arteries may be located either inside the brain itself or in the neck.

When kidney arteries harden, one type of hypertension—or "high blood pressure"—may develop.

Another site of hardening, and by far the most frequent troublespot, is the "coronary arteries," the network of vessels that bring the heart muscle its own blood supply. Gradual reduction in blood flow in a coronary artery due to hardening may cause heart pain, known as "angina pectoris." When more drastic or sudden restriction in the flow of food- and oxygen-laden blood occurs anywhere in the coronary artery network, starving a part of the heart muscle, a "heart attack" may result. Often this is precipitated by formation of a clot at an area affected by hardening.

Angina Pectoris

Even when fatty deposits have narrowed one or more of the coronary arteries, the blood supply reaching the heart muscle may still be adequate to fill the need for food and oxygen which this steady workload imposes.

These same arteries, however, may not be capable of furnishing the extra blood the heart demands when a person exerts himself more than usual, such as in dashing to catch a bus, or when he becomes overexcited by some especially good or bad news.

At such times "angina"—as angina pectoris is often called—may be felt in the chest.

Heart Attack

Blood fighting its way through a narrowed and roughened coronary artery may form a clot that seals off the channel, halting further blood flow through that vessel and all of its "downstream" branches. With its source of life cut off, that segment of heart muscle normally fed by the blocked artery will die. Doctors call a heart attack occurring in this way a "coronary thrombosis." The most common type of attack, coronary thrombosis, can happen during sleep as well as during normal daily activity or in the midst of a stressful or exciting situation.

In the second type of heart attack, the fatty deposits themselves plug the vessel, without the help of a clot. The deposits simply become so greatly enlarged that they merge and shut off the flow of blood.

An attack occurring in either way may be so mild that the victim doesn't notice it (although this is most uncommon), or it could be so severe as to bring sudden death. How serious it is depends on the size of the blocked vessel, and the extent of the heart muscle area damaged by blood starvation. This damaged or killed region of heart muscle is called a "myocardial infarct."

Each year in this country over 300,000 deaths occur from what is called sudden cardiac death, that is, death within six hours from onset of acute symptoms. The majority of these deaths occur before the individual reaches the hospital or other medical attention.

Checklist of Heart Attack Early Warnings—None of the symptoms below is conclusive proof of a heart attack. But the more of them present, the more likely it is that the patient *is* undergoing a heart attack.

- difficulty breathing
- palpitations
- nausea
- vomiting
- cold sweat
- paleness
- weakness
- anxiety

New Developments

The extent of damage to the heart muscle can now be determined by measuring certain enzymes in the blood by a special kind of electrocardiogram, and by using certain radioactive isotopes that are selectively attracted to either the damaged or the normal part of the heart muscle.

There has been progress in the development of noninvasive diagnostic techniques like echocardiography—ultrasound—and computer-based x-ray image intensification to harmlessly and noninvasively measure the extent of cardiac and blood vessel disease both before and after clinical symptoms appear. Such new techniques are now being used selectively in several hospitals and clinics across the United States.

Figure 28-9   The heart

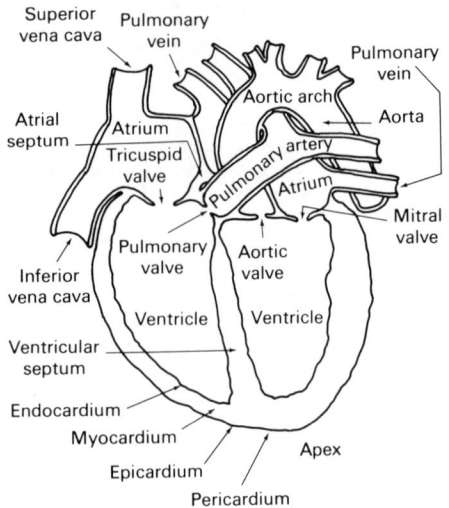

RIGHT SIDE OF HEART   LEFT SIDE OF HEART

Source: *A Handbook for Heart Terms,* DHEW, 1976.

Hemophilia*

Hemophilia is a disorder of the blood's clotting mechanism affecting males primarily and being transmitted through the unaffected female.

An estimated 20,000 Americans suffer from severe hemophilia. About 15,000 of these

_____

*Source: National Institutes of Health.

have hemophilia A, some 5,000 hemophilia B, and an undetermined number have von Willebrand's disease, which is a relatively mild bleeding disorder in most.

Both hemophilia A and hemophilia B affect males almost exclusively, but are nearly always transmitted by female carriers. In these sex-linked forms of hemophilia, if a male hemophiliac has children, his sons will be normal, but his daughters will be carriers. But if the daughters bear children, their sons have a 50–50 chance of being hemophiliac and their daughters a 50–50 chance of being carriers. Hemophilia can occur in women, but this is rare because it requires a union between a hemophilic male and a female carrier. Daughters born of this union have a 50–50 chance of being hemophiliacs and those who escape the disease will be carriers. Sons born of this marriage have a 50–50 chance of being hemophiliacs.

About 30% of all cases of hemophilia apparently occur de novo, with no previous family history of the disease. Some of these cases probably represent errors or omissions in reconstructing the victim's family tree, but others may represent recent genetic mutations. At present, it is impossible to determine which of these possibilities obtains in most instances of "unexplainable" hemophilia.

In victims of hemophilia, the chief threat to health or life is not excessive blood loss from surface cuts, abrasions or related injuries. Bleeding from such causes can usually be staunched even if the coagulation defect of hemophilia remains uncorrected. The real threat is internal bleeding into organs, soft tissues and joints, which may occur with no apparent reason in severe hemophilia and is very likely to follow even seemingly minor trauma. The only effective means of controlling such bleeding episodes is to supply the specific clotting factor needed to correct (temporarily) the victim's coagulation abnormality.

The major causes of death among hemophiliacs are thought to be cerebral hemorrhage and severe internal bleeding due to trauma, but there are no reliable data on this. The major causes of permanent disability in these patients are orthopedic problems resulting from repeated hemorrhages into the joints. These may result in progressive muscular atrophy, unstable joints and related conditions that may eventually prove crippling.

In addition to all the other miseries that hemophilia visits on its victims and their families are the heavy financial burdens imposed by the disease. For the threatment of severe hemophilia, the cost of blood products alone may exceed $6,000 a year. Physicians' fees and hospital expenses average about $2,000 a year.

The prevention and treatment of serious bleeding episodes in hemophiliacs improved dramatically during the sixties with the introduction of clotting factor concentrates which, administered by intravenous infusion, could temporarily restore normal coagulability to blood deficient in AHF or AHF activity.

For further information contact: National Hemophilia Foundation, 25 West 39 St., N.Y., N.Y. 10018.

Hypertension

Review

High blood pressure (hypertension) affects an estimated 23 million American adults. Of these, about 14 million have hypertensive heart disease (chiefly heart enlargement) resulting from the elevated blood pressure. The prevalence rate of high blood pressure among U.S. Blacks is about twice as high as that among whites, and the prevalence rate of hypertensive heart disease among Black males is nearly three times that of white males. Nearly 15 million Americans with high blood pressure are under age 65 and more than 4 million are under 45.

Probably, at least in part, due to the availability and widespread use of effective drugs for blood pressure control, the United States death rate from high blood pressure has declined more than 65% since 1950. But the disease still claims over 20,000 deaths a year directly and contributes to hundreds of thousands of deaths from heart attacks and strokes, because it increases susceptibility to these events, the number one and number three causes of death. In addition, high blood pressure places an added burden on the heart that may ultimately drive it into failure and may stress or damage arteries and the organs they

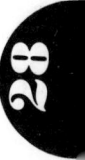

supply throughout the body. The kidneys are highly vulnerable to such damage, and kidney failure is a common complication of severe hypertension.

High blood pressure alone roughly doubles the risk of heart attacks and other manifestations of coronary heart disease. The threat is amplified by the presence of other risk factors. For example, if the person with high blood pressure is a cigarette smoker, the risk from coronary heart disease is increased by a factor of 3.4. If, in addition, blood fats are elevated, the risk is more than 10 times that of persons with none of these risk factors.*

What is Normal—The upper level of normal systolic pressure in adults is considered to be around 140, the upper level of normal diastolic pressure around 90; this would be recorded as 140/90.

Diastolic pressures between 90 and 95 are called "borderline" by some investigators, and a diastolic pressure that persistently exceeds 95 is hypertension as defined by the World Health Organization.

Measurement Errors—The measuring instrument, the sphygmomanometer, has been in relatively unchanged use for 70 years. It has a small inaccuracy for both diastolic and systolic pressures in normal individuals even under ideal conditions. Potential measurement errors can be introduced by arm size, arm and subject's position, emotional state of the subject, observer digit selection, cuff position, arrhythmia, respiration, recent eating and individual discomfort. Some part is also played in measurement considerations by the well-known lability in blood pressure.

Effectiveness of Drugs

Although drugs capable of lowering elevated blood pressures have been available for more than 20 years, it has only been objectively demonstrated relatively recently (1970) that lowering the blood pressure can lower the morbidity and mortality associated with moderate hypertension (diastolic pressures

equal to or greater than 105 mm Hg) and its complications. This demonstration markedly altered the public health status of hypertension. Whereas hypertension had previously been recognized as one of the major causes of illness and death in this country, it has now become the major disease for which simple and effective treatment is available but largely unused. Of the estimated 23 million Americans that have hypertension, about a third of them have hypertension in the range where drug therapy has been demonstrated to be beneficial. At present, however, most of the 8 million Americans with treatable hypertension do not have effectively controlled blood pressures.

Side-Effects—These agents are not without side effects, especially in higher doses. With some drugs, the side effects are relatively mild and work no hardship, neither impeding the patient's job nor other pursuits. However, all of the most effective antihypertensive drugs may cause undesirable side effects, including blurred vision, bladder dysfunction, constipation, anemias, liver disease, abnormal heart rhythms and sexual impotence in males. Fortunately, side effects can usually be minimized by using several agents in combination, each in relatively low doses.

Blood Pressure

Table 28-22   Mean systolic and diastolic blood pressures for adults by age and sex, U.S. 1971–2

Blood pressure and age in years	Men		Women	
	White	Negro	White	Negro
Mean blood pressure in mm. Hg				
Systolic				
18–44 years	124.9	129.2	117.2	121.0
45–59 years	136.2	141.0	133.0	149.4
60–74 years	144.6	151.7	149.6	165.8
Diastolic				
18–44 years	80.4	83.7	74.6	78.4
45–59 years	87.3	91.5	82.9	92.6
60–74 years	85.0	90.9	85.1	92.4

Source: Blood Pressure of Persons 18–74 years. U.S.A. 1971–72 DHEW Pub No. (HRA) 75-16.

*Source: National Institutes of Health.

Systolic Blood Pressure

Figure 28-10   Percent distribution of systolic blood pressure of the population 18–74 years by age and sex: United States, 1971–72

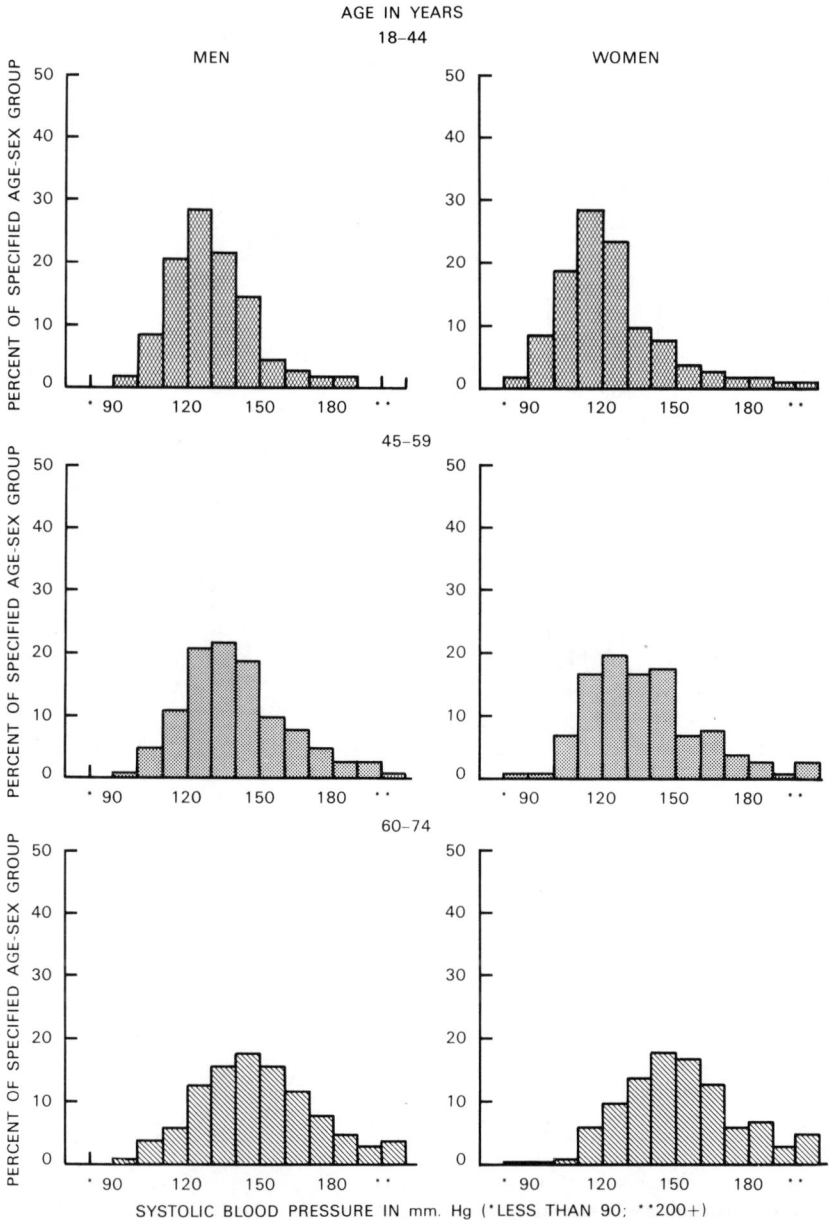

AGE IN YEARS
18–44

MEN   WOMEN

45–59

60–74

SYSTOLIC BLOOD PRESSURE IN mm. Hg (*LESS THAN 90; **200+)

*Source: Blood Pressure of Persons 18–74 years. U.S.A. 1971–72 DHEW Pub No (HRA) 75-16.

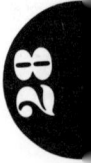

Diastolic Blood Pressure

Figure 28-11   Percent distribution of diastolic blood pressure of the population 18–74 years by age and sex: United States, 1971–72

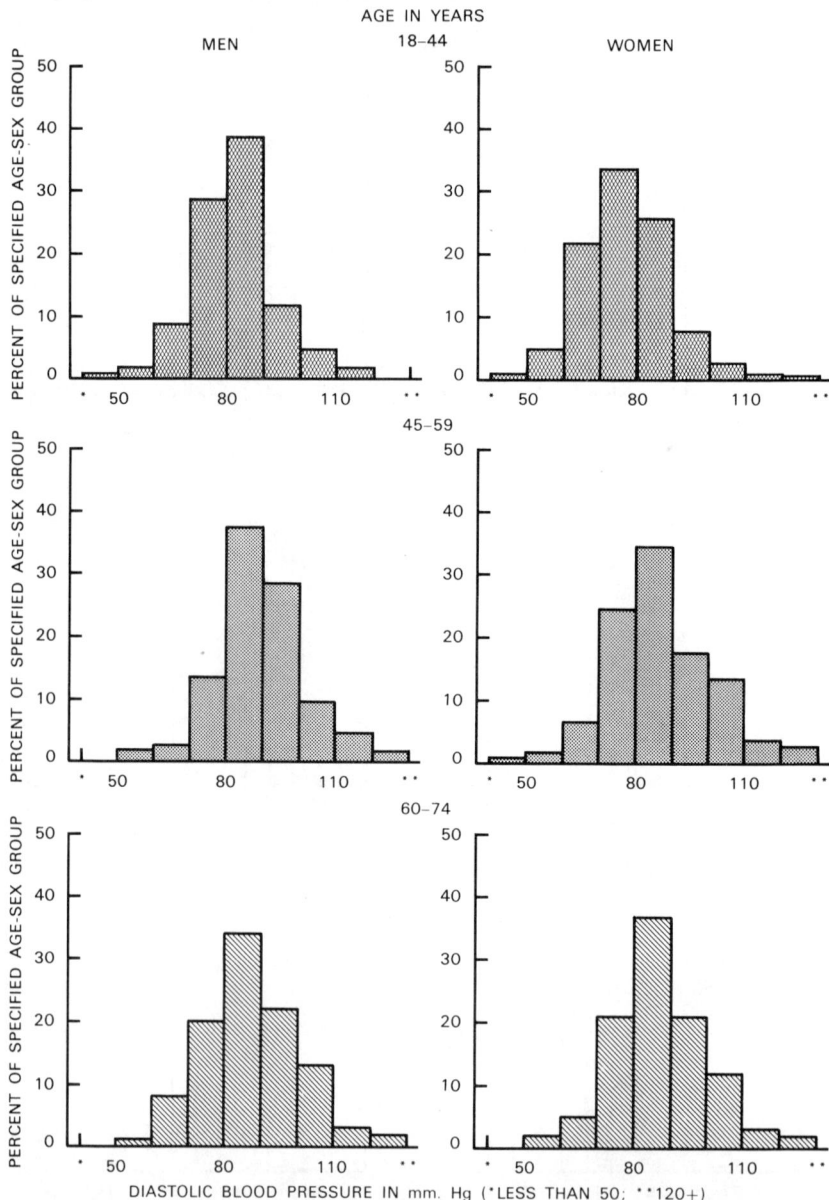

AGE IN YEARS

DIASTOLIC BLOOD PRESSURE IN mm. Hg (*LESS THAN 50; **120+)

*Source: Blood Pressure of Persons 18–74 years. U.S.A. 1971–72 DHEW Pub No (HRA) 75-16.

Sudden Infant Death Syndrome*

In the United States, the sudden infant death syndrome (SIDS), also known as crib death, is the leading cause of death among infants between the first and the twelfth months of life. It is estimated that each year approximately 7,500 to 10,000 infants, about 2 to 3 infants per 1,000 live births, succumb to this syndrome. Most victims are between the ages of one and six months. The incidence is highest between the second and fourth months of life.

The sudden infant death syndrome is defined as the sudden death of any infant or young child which is unexpected by history and in which a thorough post-mortem examination fails to demonstrate an adequate cause of death. Other terms frequently used to describe the syndrome include crib death or cot death.

The peak incidence is consistently found worldwide to be between the second and fourth months of life. SIDS occurs more frequently in males than in females in a ratio of 3:2. The incidence is higher in non-white than in white babies, in one of twins as compared to single born babies, in families of lower socioeconomic status, in low birth weight infants and particularly in premature infants who had gestational ages between 34 and 35 weeks, and in babies who had recent upper respiratory infections.

SIDS strikes without warning, usually during a sleep period. The SIDS victim has usually been well cared for and considered to have been in good general health and eating well before death. A number of infants have been seen by a physician for a routine checkup within 24 to 48 hours before death, during which no major health problems were found. The infant is placed in his crib for a nap or for the night and several hours later is found dead.

Following autopsy, no cause of death can be identified. In about one-half of the cases there is a history of a slight upper respiratory infection which is usually of such a minor degree that medical advice was not sought. In a large proportion of the victims, however, minute hemorrhages have been found within the chest; the babies are otherwise free of abnormal tissue changes.

Influenza and Pneumonia*

The earliest recorded evidence of influenza appeared when Hippocrates described its symptoms. The armies of Marcus Claudius Marcellus, a Roman general, suffered an outbreak of influenza in A.D. 212. Symptoms of the disease were described as a sudden onset of chills, cough, sweating, and a dry throat and mouth, accompanied by difficulty in swallowing and expectoration and wasting.

A disease known as "sweating sickness" appeared in England in 1485, lasting about five weeks. The disease attacked all economic levels, causing a very high mortality. From England the disease spread to other countries where it became generally known as the "English sweat."

The Virus

Over the years scientists have explored the genetic makeup of more than 100 respiratory viruses. They have found that, in general, these agents consist of a continuous strand of nucleic acid (RNA or DNA) which are the genes that carry instructions for viral self-duplication.

But the influenza virus is different. Its nucleic acid—RNA—consists of seven to ten discrete pieces, each of which controls a specific viral function. The fragmented nature of this genetic material is believed to be the key to the influenza agent's unique and puzzling ability to undergo periodic changes in its hemagglutinin and neuraminidase. Indeed, in the laboratory, "recombination" or reassortment of genes during simultaneous infection of the same cell with different influenza A viruses yields new viruses that differ from both parents.

This explains why human beings have never developed a complete immunity to influenza because the virus is capable of shuffling its eight genes through either mutation or recombination, and is therefore continually producing variations of the basic types that are strange to the body's immunological or defense mechanism.

Scientists know that the influenza virus occurs in three immunologically distinct types—A, B, and C. Local outbreaks and epidemics are caused more frequently by type A

* Source: National Institutes of Health.

than by B, while type C rarely causes detectable disease.

Investigators have concentrated, therefore, on the influenza A virus and few microorganisms have been more intensively studied. These studies have shown that each year the flu virus changes slightly and that every 10–12 years a major modification takes place, rendering whole populations susceptible to the new strain.

The shifty nature of the influenza virus is related to changes in two chemical substances found on the outer surface of the virus.

The last major shift in the influenza A virus—and the last world-wide epidemic—took place in 1968. This was the Hong Kong flu. The next such pandemic is predicted for the late 1970s.

Vaccine Research and Development

Influenza vaccines presently approved for use are inactivated (killed) preparations made from strains causing disease in humans. Each year, due to genetic drift (as explained earlier) the vaccine must be changed and during an epidemic year, the necessary change may be so drastic that manufacturers find it difficult to get an effective product on the market quickly enough to reduce the number of illnesses and excess deaths.

Mycoplasma Pneumoniae

Although mycoplasmas—the smallest of free-living organisms—are found in many species of plant and animal life, only one—*M. pneumoniae*—is known to cause disease in man. Frequently isolated from the nose and throat of children, *M. pneumoniae* causes disease most often in teen-agers and young adults—particularly those housed in close quarters, such as military recruits.

More than fifteen years ago, it was established that *M. pneumoniae* was susceptible to treatment with antibiotics. It was soon discovered, however, that while this treatment shortened the duration of fever and the acute phase of the pneumonia, symptoms such as cough and malaise often continued for weeks. Even more important, antibiotic therapy failed, in most instances, to eradicate *M. pneumoniae* from the respiratory tract, and shedding of the organism often continued for a prolonged period.

Streptococcus pneumoniae

Pneumococcal pneumonia, caused by *Streptococcus pneumoniae* (formerly called *Diplococcus pneumoniae*) remains a serious disease. In spite of the availability and use of effective antibiotics, a 20–30% fatality rate of patients hospitalized with pneumococcal pneumonia has remained unchanged over the past decade.

Table 28-23   Deaths due to pneumonia and influenza, 1957–1975

Period of excess mortality	Population (1,000's)	Estimated number of excess deaths due to pneumonia and influenza	Rate of excess per 100,000	Type of influenza
Oct. 1957–Mar. 1958	173,232	18,500	10.7	A(Asian)
Mar.–Apr. 1959	176,420	1,400	0.8	A(Asian)
Jan.–Mar. 1960	179,323	12,700	7.1	A(Asian)
Jan.–Mar. 1962	185,890	3,500	1.9	B
Feb.–Mar. 1963	188,658	11,500	6.1	A(Asian)
Feb.–Mar. 1965	193,818	2,900	1.5	A(Asian)
Feb.–Apr. 1966	195,875	3,700	1.9	A(Asian)
Jan.–Feb. 1968	199,846	9,000	4.5	A(Asian)
Dec. 1968–Jan. 1969	201,921	12,700	6.3	A(HK)
Jan.–Feb. 1970	203,736	3,500	1.7	A(HK)
Jan.–Feb. 1972	208,232	5,600	2.7	A(HK)
Jan.–Feb. 1973*	209,851	6,700	3.2	A(HK-Eng)
Jan.–Feb. 1975*	211,390	4,800	2.3	A(HK-PC)

*Estimates based on pneumonia and influenza mortality data collected from 121 U.S. cities by CDC. Mortality data in earlier years based on data obtained from the National Center for Health Statistics.

Source: U.S. Center for Disease Control, February 1976.

Kidney Diseases*

The most important function of the kidney is to maintain a stable chemical state within the body by regulating the quality and quantity of urine. Two important kidney diseases are pyelonephritis and glomerulonephritis (Bright's Disease and Nephritis). Both of these diseases have acute and chronic stages. Adequate treatment in the acute stage prevents the chronic stage. The chronic stage causes progressive destruction of the kidney, resulting in decreased function, uremia and ultimately death. Other renal diseases are nephrotic syndrome, nephrosclerosis and kidney stones.

Estimates indicate at least 100,000 deaths occur each year in the United States as a result of various diseases of the kidneys. Mortality from this disease through age 34 exceeds that due to many other chronic diseases including diabetes, neurological conditions, stroke, rheumatic heart disease and hypertension.

It is estimated that more than 3.3 million Americans have an unrecognized and undiagnosed infection of the kidneys. Chronic pyelonephritis is more common in women up to middle age, and chronic glomerulonephritis is most frequent in the early periods of life and is more common in men than in women.

Cause

Pyelonephritis is an infection of the kidneys by a microorganism. The organism enters the kidney by way of the blood stream or ascends through the urinary tract.

Glomerulonephritis in most cases is not an actual infection of the kidneys. This disease damages the kidneys because of an allergic response to an upper respiratory infection which creates a hypersensitivity in the kidneys.

Other kidney diseases may be caused by hypertension, tumors, clots, stones, congenital defects and toxic elements.

Symptoms

Lassitude, mental depression, diminution of vigor and mental acuity which lead in time to torpor, confusion and psychosis. There may be loss of appetite, morning sickness, tendency to bleed, hypertension and heart failure.

*Source: DHEW, 1973.

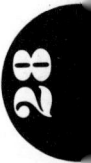

Treatment and Subtitutes for the Sick Kidney

Antibiotics have contributed to the treatment of pyelonephritis. Prolonged steroid therapy produces remission in nephrosis in many cases. Renal hypertension due to the narrowing of one or both of the renal arteries is amenable to surgical treatment. Certain tumors also are treated surgically.

Recent medical efforts have been directed toward developing substitutes for sick kidneys. One approach has been the transplantation of kidneys obtained from normal donors. This procedure has been most successful in transplantation between identical twins. However, most transplants from other persons have not been successful, since the patient's immunization mechanisms reject the donor kidney. Destruction of the donor kidney by the patient's antibody response occurs even when the donor is a close relative.

Another approach to the control of uremia has been the use of artificial kidneys. The artificial kidney, like the natural kidney, can remove wastes from the body, regulate the internal chemistry of the body and control the amount of water in the body. The patient is "hooked up" to the kidney by means of tubes in his arm which permit his blood to pass through a cellophane compartment surrounded by a cleansing fluid. Wastes and other chemical substances can pass back and forth between compartments through microscopic holes in the cellophane. This process is known as renal or kidney dialysis, or hemodialysis.

The carefully selected patient checks into the hospital one or two nights a week and spends ten or more hours "hooked up" to the artificial kidney. Recent technological advances have reduced the size and complexity of the equipment to permit dialysis in the patient's home.

There are only a few Artificial Kidney Centers in the United States and each center can handle only a small number of patients. The cost of taking care of one patient for a year is over $10,000. There are approximately 3,000 to 5,000 "ideal candidates" for renal dialysis who die each year of renal failure. Because of their nature, hemodialysis programs for chronic kidney conditions become deeply involved with medical, moral, ethical and socioeconomic problems.

Figure 28-12   The kidneys

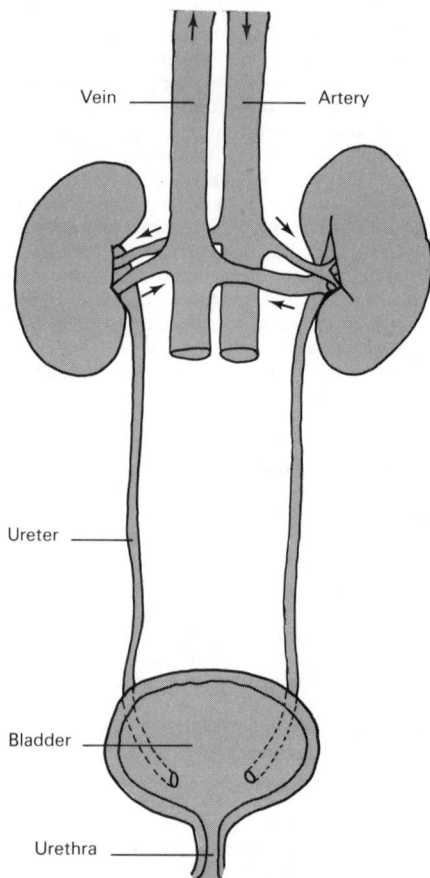

Source: National Kidney Foundation.

Lead-Based Paint Poisoning*

It has been estimated that 600,000 children each year suffer from undue lead absorption. Of these, 6,000 may suffer permanent neurologic damage and 200 deaths may result. In addition, recent studies indicate that levels of lead absorption previously thought tolerable can result in metabolic disorder, mild neurological disability and hyperactivity.

The potential for lead poisoning exists wherever lead-based paint is accessible to children, especially in deteriorating housing where peeling paint and paint chips are found. There are an estimated 2.5 million children in the United States between the ages of one and six years who are living in dilapidated housing with interior surfaces containing lead paint.

In a special series of screening projects in 40 communities 275,000 children were tested. It was found that 10% had more than acceptable levels of lead in their blood. Of these 4,600 required actual treatment.

During 1975 a total of 77 local communities were federally funded to provide detection, treatment and hazard control services, and through these programs only 440,650 children were tested.

The number of children receiving chelation treatment has remained relatively constant over the past three years, while the number of children found with undue lead absorption has increased by 76% in 1975 alone.

Early identification of children with undue lead absorptions, followed by appropriate pediatric management and environmental intervention, can result in a significant reduction in the later sequelae of lead poisoning, including mental retardation, neurologic impairment, hyperactivity and death.

Local Childhood Lead Poisoning Prevention activities are coordinated with and are often an integral part of the Maternal and Child Health Services provided by the health department, Neighborhood Health Centers and Early Periodic Screening, Diagnosis and Treatment (EPSDT) programs in a community.

Leprosy**

In the United States, the disease is known to affect only about 2,000 persons. Since leprosy takes a long time to develop, it has been suggested that many U.S. patients actually contract their disease outside this country. For example, in a survey of 320 leprosy patients seen at the Public Health Service Hospital in San Francisco from 1960–1970, 90 were of Mexican birth or descent, 66 were Filipinos, 26 were Samoans, 21 were Chinese, 11 were Hawaiians, 7 were Indians, and 68 were Cau-

* Source: National Institutes of Health.

** Source: U.S. Center for Disease Control, 1972.

casians. Of the Caucasians, only 16 had never lived outside the United States.

The skin on the forehead and face thickens, the natural lines become exaggerated and, in extreme instances, a so-called "lion face" develops. Spread of the disease around the hair follicles results in loss of hair, especially noticeable on the outer sides of the eyebrows. In advanced cases, the mucous membranes of the nose may be involved and as ulcers develop, the nose itself may be destroyed.

Leprosy is only mildly contagious. The incubation period of the disease ranges from six months to eight years or longer, with an average of three to five years. Although leprosy itself is not inherited from one's parents, susceptibility may be. The mode of transmission is not definitely known but many experts believe the disease is transmitted to a susceptible individual by direct skin-to-skin contact with a person who has an untreated case.

DDS (4,4-diaminodiphenyl sulfone, Dapsone) is now the treatment of choice. Daily doses of the drug may be needed for very long periods in cases of generalized lepromatous leprosy. In milder forms, more susceptible to treatment, one or two years may be sufficient.

Today, leprosy patients are usually hospitalized only for a relatively short while until it can be determined that their disease is responding satisfactorily to treatment and can no longer be transmitted.

Menopause*

Literally, the word menopause means an end (pause) to the menses, or monthly bleeding. When used precisely this term refers only to the permanent ending of menstruation which occurs because the ovaries become depleted of eggs and hormone-producing cells. In a normal woman of reproductive age the ovaries produce the hormone estrogen in fluctuating amounts as part of the monthly cycle. A gradual decline in this periodic release of estrogen normally takes place in women between the ages of 48 and 52. As a result, menstruation becomes irregular, occurs less often and eventually stops. Unlike menstruation which begins abruptly, menopause usually occurs so gradually that there are no clear markers for its beginning and end. A woman

may begin producing less estrogen before there is any irregularity in her periods. Likewise, the general rule of thumb for marking the completion of the menopause is the absence of a menstrual period for one full year. However, the menopause may occur abruptly, this is unusual, but not abnormal. The menopause may also occur prematurely as a result of certain ovarian disorders or surgical removal of the ovaries.

The climacteric is more commonly referred to as a woman's change of life. When used precisely, the climateric means a group of hormonal, physical and psychic changes that a woman may undergo in the years just before, during and after the menopause. The menopause, that is, the permanent ending of menstruation, is only one event among many that occurs during this stage in a woman's life. Some of these changes may result from the decreased amounts of estrogen a woman is producing, some from the natural aging process, and some from a combination of the two. The *only* signs and symptoms which are uniquely characteristic of the menopausal period are hot flashes and genital atrophy.

Hot flashes, or sudden waves of heat, are generally felt on the upper chest and arms, neck and head. Frequently this sensation is accompanied by reddening of the skin, or hot flushes, and is followed by profuse sweating. In most instances these symptoms are not severe or especially troublesome. Occasionally, they can become severe and frequent enough to interfere with a woman's sleep or routine.

Genital atrophy refers to the degenerative changes that can occur in the vagina and external sex organs. The vagina gradually shortens and becomes narrower and less elastic. Its lining undergoes cellular changes and loses its thickness, while vaginal secretions lose their normal acidity, increasing susceptibility to vaginal infections. The tissues and structures of the external sex organs shrink and lose some of their fat.

Mononucleosis**

Infections with the clinical symptoms of mononucleosis are more numerous in countries with a high standard of living than in other parts of the world.

---

*Source: National Institutes of Health, 1975.

**Source: National Institutes of Health, 1976.

Infectious mononucleosis—known popularly as "the kissing disease," "glandular fever," or just "mono"—has been recognized for more than a century but remains largely a scientific mystery. Experts believe it is caused by a "herpes-like" virus, known as the Epstein-Barr or EB virus.

In many countries, the symptoms of mononucleosis are rare. Where living conditions are crowded and methods of sanitation primitive, children are exposed to EB virus infection at a young age, develop a usually symptomless infection and have immunity for many years after. Only in the more industrialized countries, especially the United States, Canada, Great Britain, Denmark, Norway and Sweden, is significant exposure to the virus often delayed until young adulthood—the second and third decades of life. Then infection is accompanied by the familiar symptoms of mononucleosis—sore throat, swollen lymph glands and fever.

Seventy to eighty per cent of all documented cases have occurred in persons between the ages of 15 and 30. There is evidence suggesting that the disease is spread through close personal contact—probably the oropharyngeal (mouth and throat) route in children and young adults and possibly the fecal-oral route in children. The oropharyngeal route has earned mono its name—"the kissing disease." Prolonged kissing probably allows exchange in the saliva of virus-infected cells from the mouth. What now seems clear is that mono with symptoms is not a highly contagious disease and patients with it need not be isolated.

The illness develops slowly and early symptoms are usually vague. They may include a general complaint of "not feeling good," headache, fatigue, chilliness, puffy eyelids and loss of appetite. Later, the familiar triad of symptoms appears: fever, sore throat, and swollen lymph glands in the upper part of the body, especially at the side and back of the neck. A fever of 101° to 105°F lasts for approximately five days and sometimes continues intermittently for another week. The swollen lymph glands, varying in size from a bean to a small egg, are tender and firm and disappear over a few days or weeks. The spleen is enlarged in 50% of mono cases. Tonsillitis, difficulty in swallowing, bleeding gums, and, rarely, jaundice or rash may also accompany these symptoms.

Multiple Sclerosis*

Multiple sclerosis is one of the most common chronic diseases affecting the human brain and spinal cord. It is characterized by a loss of the fatty sheaths or myelin that surround the nerve fiber and derives its name from the plaques or patches of scarred (sclerosed) nervous fibers that dot the central nervous system (CNS). It is estimated that between 100,000 and 250,000 Americans suffer from multiple sclerosis and perhaps an additional 250,000 may be affected by other demyelinating disorders.

Multiple sclerosis proceeds in a series of unpredictable attacks in most patients. In earlier stages, attacks are more often followed by periods of improvement known as remissions. With successive episodes, resulting scars in the central nervous system (CNS) become more numerous, more dense and more destructive, causing progressively severe disability. It should be noted, however, that multiple sclerosis symptoms are not always progressive. Some patients experience one or two episodes and are never bothered again. Autopsies sometimes show evidence of multiple sclerosis on bodies of persons who were never aware of an attack when alive.

The onset of symptoms is rare before age 15 or after 55. The disease most commonly strikes between 20 and 40 years of age, with the peak of onset at age 30; it affects women more often than men.

The cause of multiple sclerosis remains unknown despite the compiling of enormous amounts of information from basic research, clinical studies and epidemiologic investigations.

The course of multiple sclerosis is totally unpredictable and different for each patient, which generally includes extensive and sometimes disabling muscular weakness, dizziness and blurred vision. Symptoms appear episodically, in a varying rhythm of periods of exacerbations (recurrence and usually worsening of symptoms) and remissions (cessation of symptoms). While a majority of patients can expect to live up to 75% of their normal lifespan, those years can often be marred by frustrating incapacitation and dependency on their families, placing an enormous psychological and economic burden on all in-

---

* Source: National Institutes of Health.

volved. And, in their later years, multiple sclerosis patients may experience other resultant distressing symptoms including partial or near-total blindness, kidney disease, and bladder incontinence. Although multiple sclerosis is rarely regarded as the direct cause of death, accompanying lung or bladder infections can be fatal.

For more information contact: National Multiple Sclerosis Society, 205 East 42nd Street, New York, N.Y. 10017, Tel. (212) 532-3060.

Muscular Dystrophy and the Neuromuscular Disorders*

The neuromuscular disorders characterized generally by weakness, wasting, and fatigue of the muscles, generally claim children and young adults as their victims. Some of the neuromuscular diseases cause rapid death and some cause chronic paralysis and invalidism. The two most common disorders in this group, the muscular dystrophies and myasthenia gravis, afflict some 200,000 and 100,000 patients respectively. When other less prevalent neuromuscular disorders are included, estimates of the number of patients with these conditions range from 300,000 to as many as one million.

The muscular dystrophies are a group of chronic, inherited disorders characterized by progressive weakening and wasting of the skeletal or voluntary muscles. Most types of muscular dystrophy are inherited, but any may occur spontaneously in a family as the result of a mutation or a new genetic change.

As the disease progresses, a patient may become confined to a wheelchair or have difficulty performing the ordinary activities of living. A common cause of death in these patients is respiratory failure which results from infection. Heart failure also is found in some patients.

Accurate diagnosis of the specific type of muscular dystrophy is vital since patients with other closely related neuromuscular diseases that simulate muscular dystrophy can be treated successfully, even though there is no treatment yet for any type of muscular dys-

*Source: National Institutes of Health.

trophy. In addition, accurate diagnosis facilitates evaluation of any treatment and aids the physician in his efforts to counsel the patient and his family.

The Muscular Dystrophy Association, Inc., through a nationwide network of 155 clinics, offers differential diagnosis free to anyone suspected by his physician to be suffering from muscular dystrophy or related neuromuscular disorders.

For further information contact: Muscular Dystrophy Association, Inc., 810 Seventh Avenue, New York, N.Y. 10019, Tel. (212) 586-0808.

Occupational Illnesses and Injuries

Table 28-24   Distribution of occupational injury and illness fatalities, by industry division, U.S. 1975

	Fatalities	
Industry	Number (in thousands)	Percent
Private sector	5.3	100.0
Agriculture, forestry, and fisheries	.3	5.7
Mining	.4	7.5
Contract construction	1.0	18.9
Manufacturing	1.2	22.6
Transportation and public utilities	1.0	18.9
Wholesale and retail trade	.9	17.0
Finance, insurance and real estate	.1	1.9
Services	.4	7.5

Source: Bureau of Labor Statistics, U.S. Department of Labor.

The incidence rate indicates that, on the average, 1 out of every 11 workers experienced a job-related injury or illness. About 163,300 recognized occupational illnesses were estimated for 1975 and skin diseases accounted for 40% of these.

Total occupational injuries in 1975 were 4.8 million, or 8.8 injuries per 100 full-time workers. The number of work-related fatalities in 1975 was 5,300.

Table 28-25 Distribution of occupational illnesses by category: private sector, U.S. 1974

Category of illness	Total illnesses		Category of illness	Total illnesses	
	Number (in thousands)	Percent		Number (in thousands)	Percent
Total	200.4	100.0	Disorders due to physical agents	27.1	13.5
Occupational skin diseases or disorders	89.4	44.6	Disorders due to repeated trauma	24.6	12.3
Dust diseases of the lungs	1.7	.8	All other occupational illnesses	37.4	18.7
Respiratory conditions due to toxic agents	12.7	6.3			
Poisoning	7.4	3.7			

Source: U.S. Bureau of Labor Statistics.

Chemicals Causing Occupational Diseases

Table 28-26 Chemical agents producing occupational disease

Agent	System(s) affected	Principal manifestation(s)	Representative occupations in which exposure occurs
Metals			
Lead	Gastrointestinal	Abdominal pain (colic)	Battery makers
	Neuromuscular	Palsy (wrist drop)	Enamelers
	Blood forming	Anemia	Painters
	Central nervous system	Encephalopathy	Welders
Mercury	Central nervous system	Tremor	Dentists
	Oral mucous membranes	Inflammation of mouth and gums	Fluorescent lamp makers
	Renal	Erethism	Thermometer makers
Cadmium	Pulmonary	Pulmonary edema (acute)	Cadmium smelters
	Renal	Emphysema (chronic)	Engravers
		Nephritis	Solderers
Chromium	Respiratory	Dermatitis	Dye makers
	Cutaneous	Skin ulcers	Leather tanners
		Nasal septal perforation	Printers
		Lung cancer	
Beryllium	Pulmonary	Pulmonary inflammation and scarring	Ceramic makers
			Neon tube workers
			Nuclear physicists
Solvents			
Benzene (benzol)	Hematopoietic	Aplastic anemia	Organic chemists
	Central nervous system	Leukemia	Furniture strippers
		Narcosis	Rubber makers
Carbon tetrachloride	Hepatic	Toxic hepatitis	Dry cleaners
	Renal	Kidney shutdown	Ink makers
			Wax makers
Carbon disulfide	Central nervous system	Mania	Glassmakers
	Renal	Acceleration of atherogenesis	Rayon makers
		Chronic renal disease	Rubber makers
		Parkinsonian syndrome	
Methyl alcohol	Ocular	Blindness	Rubber workers
Gases			
1. Irritants			
Amonia	Upper respiratory	Irritation	Refrigerator maker
Sulfur dioxide	Middle respiratory	Bronchospasm	Smelter workers
Ozone	Lower respiratory	Delayed pulmonary edema	Welders

Table 28-26   **(continued)**

Agent	System(s) affected	Principal manifestation(s)	Representative occupations in which exposure occurs
Gases (continued)			
2. Asphyxiants			
Carbon monoxide	Blood oxygen transport	Headache	Auto mechanics
		Dizziness	Policemen
Hydrogen sulfide	Respiratory center paralysis	Decreased ventilation	Miners
		Irritation of respiratory tract	Sewer workers
Cyanide	Cellular enzymes	Deficient oxygen in tissues	Nylon makers
			Plastic workers
Dusts			
1. Inorganic			
Silica	Pulmonary	Nodular fibrosis or scarring (silicosis)	
		Chronic obstructive lung disease	
Asbestos	Pulmonary	Diffuse fibrosis or scarring (asbestosis)	Pipe insulators
			Textile workers
	Peritoneum	Lung cancer	Floor tile sanders
		Mesothelioma (rare malignant tumor)	Brake liners
Talc	Pulmonary	Fibrosis or scarring	Talc miners
		Pleural thickening	Rubber workers
Coal	Pulmonary	Chronic obstructive lung disease	Coal miners
		Coal worker's pneumoconiosis (black lung)	
2. Organic			
Cotton	Pulmonary	Chronic obstructive lung disease (byssinosis—brown lung)	Textile workers Weavers
Detergent enzymes	Pulmonary	Bronchitis	Housewives
		Pneumonitis	Detergent packers
		Asthma	
Hay	Pulmonary	Granulomatous reaction (farmer's lung)	Farmers
Sugar Cane	Pulmonary	Granulomatous reaction (bagassosis)	Bagasse processors

Source: Health, Jean Mayer, copyright 1974 by D. Van Nostrand Company. Reprinted by permission.

Parkinson's Disease*

Parkinson's disease is one of the most severely crippling chronic disorders of the nervous system. Estimates of prevalence range from one case per 1,000 to one case per 200 population. The disease most frequently attacks people in their 50s and 60s. Parkinson's disease is rarely a primary cause of death but it often weakens the victim so that he falls prey to other diseases.

First described in 1817 by James Parkinson, a London physician, Parkinson's disease affects the brain centers involved in the control and regulation of movement. Due to disordered control of movement, rigidity of the muscles develops, accompanied by uncontrollable trembling of the extremities, stooped posture, loss of facial expression, and difficulty in walking, talking, writing, or any action requiring a high degree of muscular coordination.

The cause or causes of Parkinson's disease are still unknown. Certain forms may result from a still undetected virus and a few metallic poisons have been suspected.

Advances in the treatment of parkinsonism have comprised one of the major neurological research success stories of the decade.

However, in spite of exciting progress in alleviation of symptoms, the disease progresses, and many patients continue to have severe problems.

*Source: National Institutes of Health.

The Plague (Black Death)

From the thirteenth to the seventeenth centuries plague was epidemic over all of Asia, Europe, the islands of the Mediterranean and the British Isles. The exact number of persons who succumbed to the disease is unknown, since accurate mortality records were not maintained. It is believed that deaths far exceeded those indicated in the records. Various estimates placed the number of deaths from one-fourth to three-fourths of the entire population. It has been reported that some towns had a 90% mortality rate and that some small villages were completely wiped out. Defoe reports that during the 1665 epidemic in London there may have been as many as 10,000 deaths a week. In 1711 two thirds of the population of Italy, Spain and Constantinople had died.

Today plague occurs in a common cyclical pattern in squirrels and other rodents in the western third of the United States. It is transmitted to humans through fleas from infected animals.

The most common rodent carrier is the rock squirrel, a large gray-brown ground squirrel with a bushy tail whose favorite habitat is New Mexico, Arizona and Colorado.

The symptoms of plague in humans include fever, headache and often swollen lymph nodes near the site of the flea bite.

In 1975 there were 20 reported human cases, four of them fatal.

Bubonic plague is treatable with antibiotics if identified quickly. The most serious aspect of the disease is that a sick person can develop secondary plague pneumonia, a highly contagious disease transmitted to other humans by droplets, like the common cold.

The area most susceptible to plague has been northern New Mexico from Albuquerque and Gallup to the Colorado border. Fourteen human cases were reported in that state.

Rabies*

Rabies—an acute, severe viral infection of the central nervous system—is one of the most terrifying diseases known to man. Although each year there are now only one or two human deaths from rabies in the United States, as many as 30,000 Americans undergo the prolonged and discomforting series of inoculations used to furnish protection after known or suspected exposure to the disease.

No treatment has proved dependably effective once symptoms appear.

Rabies is caused by a virus which is present in the saliva of infected (rabid) animals and is commonly transmitted by bites. All warm-blooded animals are susceptible, and some serve as natural reservoirs of the disease. When a bitten individual does contract the illness, symptoms usually develop in 31 to 60 days. In dogs, the usual incubation period is 21 to 60 days, but it may, at times, be much longer.

Rabies in man is suspected if weeks or months after exposure, the individual experiences headache, fever, malaise, nausea, sore throat or loss of appetitie. Abnormal sensations around the site of infection are of particular diagnostic significance. Other early symptoms include unusual sensitivity to sound, light, and changes of temperature, muscle stiffness, dilation of pupils and increased salivation.

Sickle-Cell Anemia**

Sickle-cell anemia is a hereditary blood disease found preponderantly, but not exclusively, in Black people. It afflicts an estimated 50,-000–60,000 Americans. These persons suffer from chronic blood deficiency and are subject to painful, frequently disabling episodes called sickle-cell crises. The disease may also result in jaundice, increased susceptibility to infections, retarded growth and shortened life expectancy.

Sickle-cell anemia occurs only when the child inherits from each parent a gene for producing an abnormal form of hemoglobin, the oxygen-carrying pigment of red blood cells. Under certain conditions, such as reduced blood oxygen levels or increased blood acidity, the abnormal pigment, called sickle hemoglobin, may aggregate to form long rods that force the red blood cells into rigid crescent or sickle shapes whence the disease derives its name. Sickled cells do not flow readily through the smaller blood vessels and may plug them, impeding bloodflow to various organs and

---

* Source: U.S. Center for Disease Control, 1975.

** Source: National Institutes of Health.

tissues and thereby causing many of the complications of the disease.

An additional two million Americans have the sickle-cell trait. They carry one gene for sickle hemoglobin, but also one for normal hemoglobin, which predominates in their red blood cells. The sickle-cell trait rarely causes health problems, but carriers can transmit the gene to their children. If two carriers of the trait marry, the odds are two in four that a child born of this marriage will have sickle-cell trait, one in four that the child will have completely normal hemoglobin, and one in four that the child will have sickle-cell anemia.

There is presently no cure for sickle-cell anemia, although supportive treatment continues to improve and measures to reduce the threat of sickle-cell crises and other complications of the disease are being more widely applied.

In 1977 there were 24 sickle-cell clinics scattered across the country funded by HEW's Bureau of Community Health Services.

Strep Infections*

Streptococcal diseases are the most common bacterial infections in man, yet huge gaps remain in our knowledge of them. Diagnostic tests are not completely reliable and frequently can only indicate the presence of a previous infection. Treatment, in most cases, consists of penicillin, but the increasing number of patients with penicillin allergy necessitates the search for new drugs. Although there were over 400,000 cases of strep throat and scarlet fever reported in the United States in 1972, no vaccine is commercially available.

The primary focus of Group A streptococci, or strep, is the respiratory tract, where they cause sore throat or scarlet fever, and the skin, where impetigo is the common infection. Invasion of the bloodstream, usually by streptococci other than Group A, results in bacteremia and subacute bacterial endocarditis. Urinary tract infections can be caused by two groups of strep, one of which also affects the central nervous system in babies born of infected mothers. Permanent damage to the heart and kidney can result from rheumatic fever (RF) and acute glomerulonephritis (AGN)—aftereffects, or sequelae, of strep infections.

Stroke**

A stroke is a sudden loss of brain function resulting from interference with the blood supply to the brain. It is often the culmination of progressive cerebrovascular disease, which may extend over many years, and which is usually not detectable in the course of a normal physical examination. Some strokes are minor episodes, while others may cause death in a few minutes. Usually they are brought on by one of four events: thrombosis—a clot within a blood vessel of the brain or neck; cerebral embolism—the blocking of a blood vessel in the brain by a piece of clot or other material carried through the circulation from some other part of the body; narrowing (stenosis) of an artery supplying blood to the brain; or cerebral hemorrhage—the rupture of a cerebral blood vessel with bleeding into the brain tissue.

An important underlying cause of cerebrovascular disease is atherosclerosis. In atherosclerosis, fatty deposits form within the inner lining of an artery wall and decrease the size of the channel carrying blood to the brain. Also, material from the deposits may break off and cause blocking of one of the cerebral arteries. High blood pressure (hypertension) has been associated with a considerable increase in the frequency and severity of vascular diseases of the brain, especially cerebral hemorrhage. Among other causes of stroke are aneurysms and abnormalities in the clotting process. Aneurysms are sac-like swellings which may rupture, and are usually caused by congenital weaknesses in the artery walls. Abnormalities in the blood clotting mechanism may result in spontaneous hemorrhage.

Whatever the specific process involved, interference with the blood supply to the brain for more than about five minutes invariably leads to death of some brain cells and impairment of function. Temporary or permanent loss of movement, thought, memory, speech or sensation is the result.

Stroke (cerebrovascular disease) ranks third among causes of death in the United States, exceeded only by heart disease and cancer. Each year about 500,000 Americans are stricken, and about 200,000 die. Strokes incapacitate far more people than they kill and are

---

*Source: U.S. Center for Disease Control, 1975.

**Source: National Institutes of Health.

640

probably the leading cause of long-term disability in the United States. There are about 2.5 million stroke survivors in the country, 30% of whom have gone back to work or to their normal activity, with 55% disabled but capable of carrying on the activities of daily living, often with help. Fifteen percent are so helpless that total nursing care is required for the rest of their lives.

The following table, based on figures collected by the National Center for Health Statistics, shows the principal categories used by physicians in certifying stroke deaths.

Table 28-27   Stroke mortality, U.S. 1973

Acute but ill-defined cerebro-vascular disease	67,730
Generalized ischemic cerebro-vascular disease	39,261
Subarachnoid hemorrhage	9,191
Cerebral hemorrhage	33,909
Occlusion of precerebral arteries	3,177
Cerebral thrombosis	56,648
Cerebral embolism	967
Transient cerebral ischemia (minor strokes)	61
Other and ill-defined cerebro-vascular diseases	3,369
Total	214,313

Tuberculosis

(Note: Hawaii, Alaska, South Carolina and Alabama had the highest rate of incidence of tuberculosis in 1974.)

Table 28-28   New active tuberculosis cases and deaths, U.S. 1953–1974

	New active cases				Tuberculosis deaths			
			% Change				% Change	
Year	Number	Rate	Number	Rate	Number	Rate	Number	Rate
1953	84,304	53.0	—	—	19,707	12.4	—	—
1954	79,775	49.3	− 5.4	− 7.0	16,527	10.2	− 16.1	− 17.7
1955	77,368	46.9	− 3.0	− 4.9	15,016	9.1	− 9.1	− 10.8
1956	69,895	41.6	− 9.7	− 11.3	14,137	8.4	− 5.9	− 7.7
1957	67,149	39.2	− 3.9	− 5.8	13,390	7.8	− 5.3	− 7.1
1958	63,534	36.5	− 5.4	− 6.9	12,417	7.1	− 7.3	− 9.0
1959	57,535	32.5	− 9.4	− 11.0	11,474	6.5	− 7.6	− 8.5
1960	55,494	30.8	− 3.5	− 5.2	10,866	6.0	− 5.3	− 7.7
1961	53,726	29.4	− 3.2	− 4.5	9,938	5.4	− 8.5	− 10.0
1962	53,315	28.7	− 0.8	− 2.4	9,506	5.1	− 4.3	− 5.6
1963	54,042	28.7	+ 1.4	0.0	9,311	4.9	− 2.1	− 3.9
1964	50,874	26.6	− 5.9	− 7.3	8,303	4.3	− 10.8	− 12.2
1965	49,016	25.3	− 3.7	− 4.9	7,934	4.1	− 4.4	− 4.7
1966	47,767	24.4	− 2.5	− 3.6	7,625	3.9	− 3.9	− 4.9
1967	45,647	23.1	− 4.4	− 5.3	6,901	3.5	− 9.5	− 10.3
1968	42,623	21.3	− 6.6	− 7.8	6,292	3.1	− 8.8	− 11.4
1969	39,120	19.4	− 8.2	− 8.9	5,567	2.8	− 11.5	− 9.7
1970	37,137	18.3	− 5.1	− 5.7	5,217	2.6	− 6.3	− 7.1
1971	35,217	17.1	− 5.2	− 6.6	4,501	2.2	− 13.7	− 15.4
1972	32,882	15.8	− 6.6	− 7.6	4,376	2.1	− 2.8	− 4.5
1973	30,998	14.8	− 5.7	− 6.3	3,875	1.8	− 11.4	− 14.3
1974	30,122	14.2	− 2.8	− 4.1	3,770[1]	1.8	− 2.7	0.0

[1]Provisional, Deaths for 1974 are based on the NCHS ten percent sample.

Source: U.S. Center for Disease Control, July 1975.

Venereal Disease

"Venereal" comes from "Venus," the Roman goddess of love. Thus venereal disease, or VD, is associated with lovemaking.

In the last two decades, syphilis and gonorrhea have reemerged as significant health threats to the United States. In recent years, other sexually transmitted diseases have also increased—disease such as genital herpes virus, nonspecific urethritis and trichomoniasis. The federal government's Center for Disease Control estimates that in a year, eight to ten million Americans have gonorrhea, syphilis, genital herpes, trichomoniasis or nongonococcal urethritis. These diseases all have in common the fact that they are spread through very intimate—usually sexual—contact. Accordingly, persons most affected by venereal diseases are those in the most sexually active group—15 to 30 years of age.

While there are over 80,000 new cases of syphilis each year, there are almost 430,000 cases in the country at this time. While there are nearly a million new cases of gonorrhea each year, there are estimated to be 2.6 million people who need treatment for gonorrhea.

The age distributions for both syphilis and gonorrhea are similar and show the 20–24-year-old age group to be at the greatest risk of acquiring infection. Among gonorrhea patients, the second highest risk group is teenagers (15–19 years of age), and for syphilis patients it is the 25–29-year-old age group.

Table 28-29   Extent of veneral disease, U.S. 1971–1975

	Reported veneral disease (new cases)				
	Syphilis		Gonorrhea		
Year	Total syphilis	Primary and secondary	Total gonorrhea	Males	Females
1971	94,333	23,336	624,371	448,731	175,640
1972	95,076	24,000	718,401	494,652	223,749
1973	90,609	25,080	809,681	504,706	304,875
1974	84,164	24,728	874,161	523,298	350,863
1975	82,397	25,746	¹938,778	557,058	381,720

¹All time high.

Syphilis and Gonorrhea Questions

Questions your Patients may ask About[*]

Syphilis

Q. *Can a person get syphilis from kissing? From a toilet seat?*

A. The most common way to get syphilis is through sexual intercourse. But if the person you kiss happens to have the infection in his mouth, you can get it that way, too. No, you can't get syphilis from a toilet seat, nor from using someone's comb, or from holding hands.

Q. *Will a condom keep me from contracting syphilis?*

A. You're safer than if you don't use one, because you avoid contact of penis and vagina. But it is no sure guarantee against infection.

Q. *What can I do to protect myself?*

A. Wash your genital area with soap and water before and after intercourse. That goes for your partner, too. This will reduce the chance of infection.

Q. *How would I know if I had syphilis?*

A. In the first stage, a woman may have a painless sore in or near the vagina. A male may have a hard, painless sore on the penis. Or the sore can sometimes appear on the lips or in the mouth or around the rectum.

Q. *What are the signs of the second stage of syphilis?*

A. A common sign is a rash all over the body, which may appear in a few weeks. There may also be lesions in the mouth or a rash on the hands and feet rather than the whole body.

[*]Source: Syphilis and Gonorrhea," *Nursing '76,* January.

Q. *What can syphilis do to me if it is not treated?*

A. It can destroy the cells in your brain or spinal cord, or damage your heart and blood vessels. In fact, it can drive you insane, paralyze you or cripple you.

Q. *I wouldn't die from syphilis, would I?*

A. Fifteen to twenty-five percent of victims of untreated syphilis die prematurely.

Q. *If a pregnant woman has syphilis, will her baby be born with the disease?*

A. If she doesn't get treated, syphilis may cause a stillbirth. If she does have the baby, it will probably be deformed or have later medical problems.

Q. *Is syphilis easily cured?*

A. Yes—especially in the early stage. A series of penicillin shots is all it takes, provided you take the required number. The trouble is, many people don't bother to get the shots because they don't realize they have syphilis. Or, if they do start the shots, they don't finish the series.

Q. *Once I'm cured, will I be immune to the disease?*

A. No. Having syphilis once is no guarantee that you won't get it again.

Gonorrhea

Q. *How does a person get gonorrhea?*

A. The same way you get syphilis ... through sexual contact with someone with the disease.

Q. *What are the signs in a male?*

A. He usually gets a painful, burning sensation when he urinates and a yellow-white discharge from his penis.

Q. *What are the signs in a female?*

A. Four out of five women who have gonorrhea show no immediate signs at all.

Q. *What can gonorrhea do to me?*

A. If you don't get treatment, it can damage you in a lot of different ways. If you're a male, it can injure your sperm ducts. If you're a female, it can injure your fallopian tubes. In both cases, it can cause sterility. If you have the germs on your hands and accidentally rub your eyes, you could get a bad eye infection. Gonorrhea can also lead to a crippling form of arthritis or heart disease.

Q. *How long after contact does gonorrhea appear?*

A. Three to five days after contact.

Q. *If I am cured of gonorrhea, can I contract it again?*

A. You can get it again and again. There is no immunity against gonorrhea.

Q. *If I have a venereal disease what should I do about others who may be infected?*

A. If you have been diagnosed and are undergoing treatment for gonorrhea or syphilis, do not conceal the names of your sex partners—you are not doing them any favor. Early diagnosis and treatment are important. You and your sex partners who have the disease will be given confidential treatment.

Gonorrhea

Gonorrhea accounted for approximately 1 million reported infections in this country in 1975 but the actual figure is probably many times higher—perhaps 2.7 million. Most people are treated by private physicians who often do not report their cases to public health authorities.

Gonorrhea can almost always be traced to sexual exposure to an infected individual. Rarely, if ever, does gonorrhea result from contact with inanimate objects such as toilet seats. This is because the gonococcus is extremely delicate and survives very poorly outside the human body in open air or under significant changes in temperature.

Gonorrhea does not confine itself to the genital and urinary tracts, however. Physicians are finding evidence of gonococcal infection in places like the rectum and throat. This may be related to changing sexual preferences and practices.

Treatment—Treatment for gonorrhea consists of two injections of penicillin, given at the same time, with a tablet of a medication (probenecid) used to increase the efficacy of penicillin. An oral medication related to penicillin (ampicillin) may also be used. People allergic to these drugs may be given either of two other antibiotics, tetracycline or spectinomycin hydrochloride.

Once treatment is begun, symptoms begin to clear quickly, and the person may no longer be contagious within 24 hours.

Cause—Gonorrhea is caused by a bacterium known as the gonococcus. Its scientific name is *Neisseria gonorrhoeae*.

Typically, the gonococcus infects the mucous lining of the genitourinary tract. In males, this involves an acute, purulent (with pus) infection of the urethra (the canal carrying urine from the bladder to the outside of the body). In females, infection of the urethra and the cervix (opening of the womb) is usual. Newborn children may acquire a purulent infection of the eyes after passing through an infected birth canal in the mother. To prevent this and other eye infections, physicians place silver nitrate solution in the eyes of all infants immediately after birth. Complications of gonococcal infection often include sterility and arthritis, but rarely may also result in infection of the brain (meningitis) or heart (endocarditis), or the widespread presence of gonococci in the blood (gonococcemia).

Symptoms—The early symptoms of gonorrhea usually begin within two to eight days after exposure by sexual contact. However, many people—especially females—may have no apparent symptoms of the disease until much later. Such early symptom-free infections may be one reason for the current uncontrolled spread of this disease.

Complications for Women—As indicated by recent studies, the complications of gonorrhea in women are serious and costly. In one study, area pelvic inflammatory disease (PID) occurred in 17% of all women known to have gonorrhea, and 4.5% of women with PID were surgically sterilized. If these percentages are applied nationally, some 220,000 cases of PID occur yearly, resulting in the surgical sterilization of 9,900 women during their childbearing years. Additional data from Sweden suggest that sterility occurs in 15–40% of women after one episode of PID. Such results indicate that from 33,000 to 80,000 women become sterile annually in the United States from PID.

Syphilis*

It was long believed that syphilis was a New World infection first brought to Europe by the crews of Columbus' ships. New evidence now contradicts this explanation for the great epidemic which swept Europe in the late fifteenth century.

Whatever its origin, syphilis is now not as widespread as gonorrhea. Syphilis was reported in more than 80,000 Americans in 1975. Not all cases are reported by physicians,

*Source: National Institutes of Health.

however, and the actual number might be as high as 500,000.

Syphilis, like gonorrhea, is spread by direct intimate contact with the lesions of someone in the infectious stages of the disease. Also like the gonococcus, the syphilis bacterium is fragile and, thus, unlikely to be contracted from inanimate objects.

Symptoms—Symptoms begin 10 to 90 days after exposure to syphilis with the appearance of the characteristic, although sometimes unnoticed, chancre. This is a small, firm sore which develops at the site of infection, usually the tip of the penis in men and in the cervix or vagina in women. Without treatment, this symptom of *primary syphilis* disappears in three to five weeks.

If early syphilis is not diagnosed and treated, the disease may progress through three other stages. After the second stage, *secondary syphilis*, some untreated people (perhaps one out of four) experience a spontaneous cure. About the same number, although not cured, never have further evidence of disease. But the rest eventually develop the complications of *late syphilis*.

Secondary syphilis is heralded by a rash which appears anywhere from 2 to 12 weeks after the chancre disappears. The rash may cover the body or appear only on the hands or feet. It may be accompanied by tiredness, fever, loss of hair and lesions in the mouth. These symptoms, too, disappear without treatment, but meanwhile, the bacteria have probably begun to invade other organs in the body.

Only during these first two stages, which last for up to two years, is an individual infectious to others. An exception is a pregnant woman who, for a much longer period, may transmit her disease to her unborn child.

If untreated, secondary syphilis is followed by *latent syphilis*—a stage of undetermined length. After a long period of dormancy, the bacteria may begin their damage in the heart, brain or spinal cord. Thus, *late syphilis*—the final stage—may involve mental illness, blindness, heart disease or even death.

Treatment—Treatment of primary and secondary syphilis usually consists of injections of penicillin given in a single visit. Tetracycline, erythromycin or cephaloridine are the antibiotics given to people allergic to penicillin. Dosages will vary for the later stages of the disease.

A patient is usually no longer infectious 24 hours after therapy, and with early treatment, a positive blood test becomes negative within six months to two years.

Genital Herpes*

The herpes simplex virus is best known as the cause of fever blisters or cold sores which affect many persons from time to time. This, however is only one form of herpes simplex—type 1—which produces its familiar lesions generally anywhere above the waist, but most commonly near the mouth.

Another herpes simplex form—type 2—is commonly found in lesions below the waist, especially in the genital area. Although usually not as serious as gonorrhea or syphilis, genital herpes infections may be quite painful and temporarily disabling. Like fever blisters, these infections tend to recur.

In addition, herpes virus infection of the female genital region may cause disseminated herpes virus infection of the newborn—frequently a fatal or crippling disease. Obstetricians, when they diagnose genital herpes in an expectant mother, often make plans for delivering the baby by caesarean section to avoid its exposure to the virus.

Genital herpes is not a disease which physicians are asked to report, but recent esti-

_____

* Source: National Institutes of Health.

mates of this infection in this country are as high as 300,000 cases each year.

The herpes virus is present in the fluid of the skin lesions, as well as in some bodily secretions such as saliva and urine, and is believed to be transmitted by close human contact.

Treatment for genital herpes infections, as with most viral infections, is not specific. Antibiotics, which are useful against bacteria, are of little help in fighting a virus.

Therefore, treatment is directed toward relieving the symptoms until the body itself fights off the infection.

Other Sexually Transmitted Diseases

Sexually transmitted diseases, other than the traditional "venereal" diseases, continue to be increasingly recognized as major public health problems because they produce severe morbidity, cause patient loss of productivity and impose enormous demands on medical care facilities. Among the most important STDs are nongonococcal urethritis, with an estimated incidence of more than 2.5 million cases annually; trichomoniasis, with an estimated incidence of more than 3 million cases annually; and genital herpes, with some 300,000 cases annually. Data obtained from a national survey of private physicians found that for every 100 cases of gonorrhea treated by private physicians, approximately 57 cases of nongonococcal urethritis, 204 cases of trichomoniasis, 11 cases of genital herpes, 10 cases of pediculosis pubis and 27 cases of venereal warts were treated.

29
PATIENT RIGHTS

The HEW Secretary's Commission on Medical Malpractice recommended:

- that hospitals and other health care facilities adopt and distribute statements of patients' rights in a manner which most effectively communicates these rights to all incoming patients;
- that the functions of teaching hospitals be explained to all patients entering such hospitals, and that those functions be emphasized in other forms of consumer education;
- that distinctions in the treatment of patients in teaching hospitals based on the patient's race or socioeconomic status be eliminated.

Differing Versions of Patient Rights

American Hospital Association's "A Patient's Bill of Rights"*

(Many state nurses' associations have endorsed the AHA statement and have passed resolutions on patients' rights.)

1. The patient has the right to considerate and respectful care.
2. The patient has the right to obtain from his physician complete, current information concerning his diagnosis, treatment and prognosis in terms the patient can be reasonably expected to understand. When it is not medically advisable to give such information to the patient, the information should be made available to an appropriate person in his behalf. He has the right to know, by name, the physician responsible for coordinating his care.
3. The patient has the right to receive from his physician information necessary to give informed consent prior to the start of any procedure and/or treatment. Except in emergencies, such information for informed consent should include but not necessarily be limited to the specific procedure and/or treatment, the medically significant risks involved and the probable duration of incapacitation. Where medically significant alternatives for care

or treatment exist, or when the patient requests information concerning medical alternatives, the patient has the right to such information. The patient also has the right to know the name of the person responsible for the procedures and/or treatment.
4. The patient has the right to refuse treatment to the extent permitted by law and to be informed of the medical consequences of his action.
5. The patient has the right to every consideration of his privacy concerning his own medical care program. Case discussion, consultation, examination and treatment are confidential and should be conducted discreetly. Those not directly involved in his care must have the permission of the patient to be present.
6. The patient has the right to expect that all communications and records pertaining to his care should be treated as confidential.
7. The patient has the right to expect that within its capacity a hospital must make reasonable response to the request of a patient for services. The hospital must provide evaluation, service and/or referral as indicated by the urgency of the case. When medically permissible, a patient may be transferred to another facility only after he has received complete information and explanation concerning the needs for and alternatives to such a transfer. The institution to which the patient is to be transferred must first have accepted the patient for transfer.
8. The patient has the right to obtain information as to any relationship of his hospital to other health care and educational institutions insofar as his care is concerned. The patient has the right to obtain information as to the existence of any professional relationships among individuals, by name, who are treating him.
9. The patient has the right to be advised if the hospital proposes to engage in or perform human experimentation affecting his care or treatment. The patient has the right to refuse to participate in such research projects.
10. The patient has the right to expect reasonable continuity of care. He has the right to know in advance what appointment times and physicians are available

---

*Reprinted by permission of the American Hospital Association.

and where. The patient has the right to expect that the hospital will provide a mechanism whereby he is informed by his physician or a delegate of the physician of the patient's continuing health care requirements following discharge.

11. The patient has the right to examine and receive an explanation of his bill regardless of source of payment.

12. The patient has the right to know what hospital rules and regulations apply to his conduct as a patient.

Note: * The AHA itself warned hospitals not to reproduce and distribute copies of the Bill of Rights until the document had been carefully scrutinized and approved by both the hospital attorney and the board of trustees. The association particularly stressed that a hospital should modify the PBR to accommodate any local law or custom and that it should avoid the specification of any rights that it was not prepared to fulfill.

"Citizen's Bill of Hospital Rights"**

We believe that you have rights regarding hospitals whether you're a patient or not. Every member of the public pays for hospitals through his health insurance, his Blue Cross and Blue Shield premiums, and his tax dollars. So the bill of rights should apply to all citizens—to all members of the public—not just patients.

We think a bill of rights should be more than words and rhetoric, and so we have formulated rights which are based on law or are otherwise enforceable through procedures which the public has access to. If these rights are not already recognized, there are private and public agencies that can demand their recognition.

The patient (and/or the public) has a right—

- to good quality care and high professional standards that are continuously monitored and reviewed. This includes frank disclosure to the patient when it is discovered that poor quality care has been delivered or when there has been medical or hospital malpractice.

* Source: *Nursing Outlook,* April 1974. ©American Journal of Nursing Company.
** By Herbert S. Denenberg, Pennsylvania Insurance Department, April 1973.

- to economical care and to hospital management that operates efficiently and eliminates waste, such as unnecessary services and duplicative and unsafe facilities.

- to have its voice heard in the management, control and planning of hospitals, and in the case of community hospitals it should be assured of a board of directors that represents a broad cross-section of the community.

- to full information on his diagnosis, treatment, and prognosis in terms he can understand. This should include information about alternative treatments and possible complications. The patient is entitled to have his questions answered on any phase of his hospital and medical care.

- to personal dignity at all times. Among others, this includes the right to be treated without discrimination based on race, color, religion, national origin, ability to pay or source of payment; the right to considerate and respectful care; and the right to privacy and confidentiality of personal records. Those not directly involved in the treatment should affirmatively disclose their purposes and obtain permission of the patient to be present.

- to control his body and life. This includes the patient's right to refuse treatment to the extent permitted by law, to be informed of the medical consequences of his action, and to leave the hospital when he desires to do so.

- to redress of grievances in a reasonably efficient and timely fashion. This means the hospital should establish formal grievance procedures and appoint ombudsmen or patient advocates to be certain that problems are identified and remedied. Hospitals should let patients know about how to assert complaints. Forms for doing so should be readily available.

- to full information about the finances and activities of the hospital. This should include general information about assets, expenses, costs, profits, charges, occupancy and the like.

- to full disclosure of any hospital relationships that pose an immediate or potential conflict of interest.

- to full information about his stay, including information about his bill and access to his hospital records. This includes detailed information about his hospital bill, including

The U.N.'s Patient Bill of Rights

Declaration on the Rights of Disabled Persons*

1. The term "disabled person" means any person unable to ensure by himself or herself wholly or partly the necessities of a normal individual and/or social life, as a result of a deficiency, either congenital or not, in his or her physical or mental capabilities.

2. Disabled persons shall enjoy all the rights set forth in this Declaration. These rights shall be granted to all disabled persons without any exception whatsoever and without distinction or discrimination on the basis of race, colour, sex, language, religion, political or other opinions, national or social origin, state of wealth, birth or any other situation applying either to the disabled person himself or herself or to his or her family.

3. Disabled persons have the inherent right to respect for their human dignity. Disabled persons, whatever the origin, nature and seriousness of their handicaps and disabilities, have the same fundamental rights as their fellow-citizens of the same age, which implies first and foremost the right to enjoy a decent life, as normal and full as possible.

4. Disabled persons have the same civil and political rights as other human beings; article 7 of the Declaration of the Rights of Mentally Retarded Persons applies to any possible limitation or suppression of those rights for mentally disabled persons.

5. Disabled persons are entitled to the measures designed to enable them to become as self-reliant as possible.

6. Disabled persons have the right to medical, psychological and functional treatment, including prosthetic and orthetic appliances, to medical and social rehabilitation, education, vocational education, training and rehabilitation, aid, counselling, placement services and other services which will enable them to develop their capabilities and skills to the maximum and will hasten the process of their social integration or reintegration.

7. Disabled persons have the right to economic and social security and to a decent level of living. They have the right, according to their capabilities, to secure and retain employment or to engage in a useful, productive and remunerative occupation and to join trade unions.

8. Disabled persons are entitled to have their special needs taken into consideration at all stages of economic and social planning.

9. Disabled persons have the right to live with their families or with foster parents and to participate in all social, creative or recreational activities. No disabled person shall be subjected, as far as his or her residence is concerned, to differential treatment other than that required by his or her condition or by the improvement which he or she may derive therefrom. If the stay of a disabled person in a specialized establishment is indispensable, the environment and living conditions therein shall be as close as possible to those of the normal life of a person of his or her age.

10. Disabled persons shall be protected against all exploitation, all regulations and all treatment of a discriminatory, abusive or degrading nature.

11. Disabled persons shall be able to avail themselves of qualified legal aid when such aid proves indispensable for the protection of their persons and property. If judicial proceedings are instituted against them, the legal procedure applied shall take their physical and mental condition fully into account.

12. Organizations of disabled persons may be usefully consulted in all matters regarding the rights of disabled persons.

13. Disabled persons, their families and communities shall be fully informed, by all appropriate means, of the rights contained in this Declaration.

*Adopted by the General Assembly of the United Nations, December 9, 1975.

itemized charges. This information should be readily available regardless of the patient's source of payment.

- to continuity of care. This includes timely response to his needs and appropriate transfer to other facilities.
- to expect a hospital to behave as a consumer advocate rather than as a business headquarters for doctors and hospital.

Approaches to Patients' Rights

Patients' Rights and the Federal Government*

Promulgation of patients' rights is a burgeoning field within the health bureaucracy. Following are five different examples of patients' rights.

1. Protection of human research subjects—the focus of considerable effort especially by the FDA, the National Institutes of Health, ADAMHA and the Center for Disease Control in their various biomedical research activities.

2. Procedural rights—for example, within the Bureau of Health Insurance, beneficiaries have access to a process for review of grievances arising out of payment of claims in the Medicare program.

3. Protection of patients' civil rights—particularly for mental patients. Efforts are being focused specifically on that problem in the Mental Health Care Financing and Services Branch of the National Institute of Mental Health.

4. Confidentiality of medical records, especially with regard to records of drug abuse and alcoholism given attention by ADAMHA as demonstrated in recently published federal regulations assuring safeguards.

5. More informed consent of patients, other than in the context of biomedical experi-

mentation—the goal of at least two agencies. The Center for Disease Control has a new, more aggressive informed consent program seeking to supply more information to patients participating in public health immunization programs across the nation for which CDC gives technical and financial assistance. The FDA has taken a new approach to informed consent by consumers of prescription drugs through FDA requirements that patient-directed inserts be included with certain prescription drugs informing consumers of the drug's proper use and potential side effects. The most prominent example to date has been the requirement of patient inserts with oral contraceptives.

The Hospital Ombudsman (The Patient Representative)**

The patient representative or hospital ombudsman, little known as recently as five years ago, is a rapidly expanding profession. Among a patient representative's functions in various institutions are patient and health education, liaison with the hospital community to open access to health services, conducting tours of facilities, providing information about resources outside the institution, providing language banks for non-English-speaking patients, and linking elderly patients who are being discharged from the hospital with telephone reassurance programs.

The President's Commission on Medical Malpractice recommended that all hospitals establish effective patient grievance mechanisms, and urged the secretary of HEW to make such programs a prerequisite of Medicare and Medicaid payments. In many hospitals, this recommendation could lead to appointment of a patient representative who can function as an advocate for the patients without being an adversary to the system.

The AHA Society of Patient Representatives, which was organized in 1972, has 350 members from hospitals in 41 states.

---

*Source: Health Services Administration, DHEW.

**Source: "Patient Relations," by Ruth Ravich, *Hospitals, JAHA,* April 1975. Reprinted by permission of the American Hospital Association.

Research and Patients' Rights

The American Nurses' Association's guidelines for the nurse researcher in clinical research stress the protection of human rights in research: (1) the right to privacy; (2) the right to self-determination; (3) the right to conservation of personal resources; (4) the right to freedom from arbitrary hurt; and (5) the right to freedom from intrinsic risk of injury.

The Tuskegee (Alabama) Syphilis Experiment

In this experiment, begun 40 years ago, 399 victims of the disease were left untreated and uninformed of the nature of their illness even after penicillin therapy became generally available. The victims, all black and all men, were told they were joining a health program. The purpose of the study was to determine the long-term effects of syphilis on untreated victims. All of the participants, 85% of whom had less than a sixth grade education, were persuaded to join a social club named after the public health nurse who supervised the study in the field.

This case brought into sharp focus the whole question of protecting patients' rights while conducting meaningful research projects.

The media have also reported instances of sterilization among mentally defective women where the irreversibility of the procedure had not been fully explained.

Medical Records*

Medical records are generally exempt from inspection except for the individual involved, but the bureaucratic barriers make it difficult for that person to see his own records. However the time in which there is a choice in the matter of sharing the record may be ending. While it is legally recognized that the patient's record is the property of the hospital or physician (in his office), the information that the record contains is not similarly protected. Currently, only nine states allow patients access to their records, either through the patient's attorney (California, Illinois, and Utah) or directly (Massachusetts, Wisconsin, New Jersey, Louisiana, Mississippi and Connecticut). The one sure way in which the patient has access to that information, however, is through a malpractice suit in which the record is subpoenaed—a costly process for both provider and consumer.

The Commission on Medical Malpractice in 1975 suggested making records available to the patient's attorney when a patient demands access.

Nurses' Response to Patient's Right to Know**

The physician and hospital administrator often think in clinical terms: the efficiency of diagnosis and the availability of clinically effective treatment modalities—surgery, drugs and the like. The patient, on the other hand, generally defines quality from a more humanistic point of view. He usually agrees that quality starts with scientific medicine, but he wants it to be delivered in a respectful and dignified manner at a price he can afford. Increasingly, he wants to know what is going on and why.

How are nurses, who probably spend more time with the patient than any of the other health professionals, going to react to this new type of consumer-patient? Tell him they "don't know," he'll have to ask the doctor? Imply that he shouldn't take up their time with all these questions? Submerge his individual needs to the hospital routine and to their own and the physician's convenience?

To what extent should a nurse explain when asked by a patient?[1]

As much as possible	76%
Only in a general way	13%
Only with doctor's permission	8%
Should not attempt	3%

[1]Source: "Nursing Ethics," *Nursing '74,* Oct. (Survey of 11,000 nurses).

---

*Source: Lucie Y. Kelly, "The Patient's Right to Know," *Nursing Outlook,* Jan. 1976. ©American Journal of Nursing Company.

**Source: Nancy Quinn and Anne R. Somers, "The Patient's Bill of Rights," *Nursing Outlook,* April 1974.

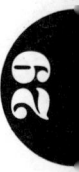

Psychiatric Patient Attitudes Toward Nursing Interventions[1]

Table 29-1

Statement	Rank order of mean	Statement	Rank order of mean
I feel good about myself:		6. When staff encourages me to participate in activities	10
1. When a certain staff member will take time to really sit and talk with me	7	7. When I am given something worthwhile to do	4
2. When staff will pay special attention to one person if they need it	3	8. When staff won't put up with any nonsense from me	9
3. When staff approaches me to ask how I am feeling	6	9. When I have something to keep me busy for awhile	5
4. When I can do something for staff or other patients	2	10. When staff will talk to me about their own feelings	1
5. When I can express my feelings about certain staff members or patients	8	11. When staff encourages me to improve my appearance	11

Source: Calista V. Leonard, "Patient Attitudes Towards Nursing Intervention," *Nursing Research*, September–October 1975. ©American Journal of Nursing Company.

[1] A study of 103 psychiatric hospital inpatients.

30

NUTRITION, OBESITY AND EXERCISE

Nutrition

The Balanced Diet*

The guarantee of a balanced diet is the Basic Four, with everyday foods from the grocery store.

1. **Milk Group**—Everyday everyone should have some milk, or its equivalent, for calcium, protein and vitamins. Recommended daily amounts are: one to two glasses for adults, two to four glasses for children and teenagers and one quart for nursing mothers. This can be whole milk or skim milk, evaporated or dry milk, or buttermilk. One ounce of cheese or one serving of ice cream may be substituted for one glass of milk.

2. **Vegetable-Fruit Group**—Everyday everyone should have four or more servings of vegetables and fruits to supply vitamins, minerals and fiber. One serving should be citrus or tomato (for vitamin C). At least four times a week the intake should include a dark green or deep yellow vegetable or fruit for vitamin A.

3. **Meat Group**—Twice a day everyone should have beef or veal or pork or lamb or liver or poultry or fish or eggs. These supply protein, iron, vitamins and also fat. One serving should be dinner size (two or three ounces without bone or fat). One serving should be lunch size—for instance, one egg or an ounce of cheese or meat or canned fish. Two eggs or one cup of dried peas, beans or lentils are equivalent to a medium serving of meat. Other sources of protein include nuts or cereal with milk.

4. **Bread-Cereal Group**—Four servings daily of enriched or whole-grain breads and cereals provide carbohydrates, minerals and vitamins. A serving is a slice of bread, three-quarters of a cup of ready-to-eat cereal, or about one-half a cup of cooked cereal, cornmeal, grits, macaroni, noodles, rice or spaghetti.

Food Labeling

All fortified foods and all foods for which a nutrition claim is made must display a "nutrition information" panel on the product label.

All nutrient information listed on the panel is calculated on the basis of a serving. The label tells the size of a serving and number of servings in the container. Immediately below are listed the number of calories and the amounts of protein, carbohydrates and fat in a serving.

The lower part of the nutrition label must give the percentages of the U.S. RDA of protein and seven vitamins and minerals in a serving of the product. A label may say, for example:

Percentage of U.S. Recommended Daily Allowances (U.S. RDA)

Protein	30%	Riboflavin	15
Vitamin A	35	Niacin	25
Vitamin C	10	Calcium	2
Thiamine	15	Iron	25

This means that one serving of that food contains 30% of the U.S. RDA for protein, 35% of the U.S. RDA for vitamin A, 10% of the U.S. RDA for vitamin C and so on.

The label below is an example of what to look for.**

NUTRITION INFORMATION
(Per serving)
Serving size = 8 oz.
Servings per container = 1

Calories	560	Fat (percent of	
Protein	23 g	calories	
Carbohydrate	43 g	53%)	33 g
		Polyunsat-	
		urated	2 g
		Saturated	9 g
		Cholesterol[1]	
		(20 mg/	
		100 g)	40 mg
		Sodium	
		(365 mg/	
		100 g)	830 mg

Percentage of U.S.
Recommended Daily Allowances
(U.S. RDA)

Protein	35	Riboflavin	15
Vitamin A	35	Niacin	25
Vitamin C		Calcium	2
(Ascorbic		Iron	25
acid)	10		
Thiamine			
(vitamin B₁)	15		

---

[1]Information on fat and cholesterol content is provided for individuals who, on the advice of a physician, are modifying their total dietary intake of fat and cholesterol.

---

*Source: "Your Diet: Health is in the Balance," Nutrition Foundation, Inc.

**A label may include optional listings for cholesterol, fats and sodium.

Food Values

Recommended Daily Food Allowances

The U.S. RDAs were developed by the Food and Drug Administration for use in nutrition labeling and for labeling of dietary supplements and special dietary foods.

Table 30-1 Recommended daily allowances (U.S. RDA)

Vitamins, minerals and protein	Unit of measurement	Infants	Adults and children 4 or more years of age	Children under 4 years of age	Pregnant or lactating women
Vitamin A	International units	1,500	5,000	2,500	8,000
Vitamin D	International units	400	400[1]	400	400
Vitamin E	International units	5.0	30	10	30
Vitamin C	Milligrams	35	60	40	60
Folic acid	Milligrams	0.1	0.4	0.2	0.8
Thiamine	Milligrams	0.5	1.5	0.7	1.7
Riboflavin	Milligrams	0.6	1.7	0.8	2.0
Niacin	Milligrams	8.0	20	9.0	20
Vitamin B_6	Milligrams	0.4	2.0	0.7	2.5
Vitamin B_{12}	Micrograms	2.0	6.0	3.0	8.0
Biotin	Milligrams	0.5	0.3	0.15	0.3
Pantothenic acid	Milligrams	3.0	10	5.0	10
Calcium	Grams	0.6	1.0	0.8	1.3
Phosphorus	Grams	0.5	1.0	0.8	1.3
Iodine	Micrograms	45	150	70	150
Iron	Milligrams	15	18	10	18
Magnesium	Milligrams	70	400	200	450
Copper	Milligrams	0.6	2.0	1.0	2.0
Zinc	Milligrams	5.0	15	8.0	15
Protein	Grams	18[2]	45[2]	20[2]	

[1] Presence optional for adults and children 4 or more years of age in vitamin and mineral supplements.

[2] If protein efficiency ratio of protein is equal to or better than that of casein, U.S. RDA is 45 g. for adults, 18 g. for infants, and 20 g. for children under 4.

Source: U.S. Food and Drug Administration, 1976.

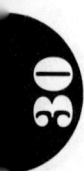

Nutrient Deficiencies

Table 30-2   Nutrients and clinical signs of deficiency

Nutrient	Clinical sign of deficiency	Severity of deficiency[1]
Protein	Dry, starving hair	L—if single
	Dyspigmented hair	M—if two or more signs present
	Easily pluckable hair	L; M—if two or more signs present
	Abnormal texture or loss of curl of hair	M
	Visible or enlarged parotids	M
	Hepatomegaly	M
	Potbelly	M
	Apathy	M
	Marked hyperirritability	M
Vitamin B complex: Riboflavin	Circumcorneal injection	L
	Conjunctival injection	L
	Angular blepharitis	M
	Angular lesions of lips ⎫ bilateral	H
	Angular scars of lips ⎭	H
	Cheilosis	M
	Magenta tongue	H
	Nasolabial seborrhea	M
Vitamin B complex other than riboflavin: Niacin	Filiform papillary atrophy of tongue	H
	Fungiform papillary hypertrophy of tongue	M
	Fissures of tongue	M
	Serrations or swelling of tongue	L
	Hyperpigmentation, hands and face	M
	Pellagrous dermatitis	H
	Scarlet beefy tongue	H
Thiamine	Absent knee jerks	M
	Absent ankle jerks	M
Vitamin D	Bossing of skull	M
	Beading of ribs	H
	Bowed legs	M
	Knock knees	M
	Epiphyseal enlargement, wrists	H
Vitamin A	Bitot's spots	H
	Keratomalacia	H
	Xerophthalmia	H
	Xerosis of the conjunctiva	H
Vitamin A and/or essential fatty acids	Follicular hyperkeratosis of upper back	L
	Follicular hyperkeratosis, arms	M ⎫ if both occur = M
	Dry or scaling skin (xerosis)	L ⎭
	Mosaic skin	L

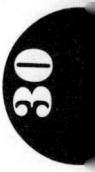

(*continued*)

Table 30-2 (continued)

Nutrient	Clinical sign of deficiency	Severity of deficiency[1]	
Vitamin C	Perifolliculosis	M	if two or more occur = H
	Petechiae	M	
	Ecchymosis	M	
	Bleeding and swollen gums	M	
	Swollen red papillae of gingivae	L	
	Diffuse marginal inflammation	L	
Iodine	Enlarged thyroid gland, Group I	M	
	Enlarged thyroid gland, Group II	H	
Calcium	Positive Chvostek's sign	M	

[1] L = low, M = moderate, H = high-risk indicator of possible deficiency.
Source: DHEW, 1975.

Table 30-3 Comparison of persons with nutrient value intake less than the standard: U.S. 1971–72 (HANES Preliminary)

Age, sex and nutrient	Percent of persons with intakes less than standard		Age, sex and nutrient	Percent of persons with intakes less than standard	
	White	Negro		White	Negro
Income below poverty level[1]			**Income above poverty level[1]**		
1–5 years, both sexes			1–5 years, both sexes		
Calcium	14.42	35.26	Calcium	12.14	24.96
Iron	94.46	93.61	Iron	94.88	95.29
Vitamin A	51.51	46.07	Vitamin A	36.91	51.01
Vitamin C	58.23	48.54	Vitamin C	42.82	52.91
18–44 years, female			18–44 years, female		
Calcium	56.39	74.50	Calcium	55.59	71.69
Iron	94.24	94.66	Iron	92.13	94.70
Vitamin A	73.54	64.42	Vitamin A	64.90	67.36
Vitamin C	72.26	59.37	Vitamin C	49.04	56.81
60 years and over, both sexes			60 years and over, both sexes		
Calcium	40.43	44.67	Calcium	34.41	47.71
Iron	62.66	67.31	Iron	46.97	64.57
Vitamin A	61.45	62.40	Vitamin A	55.56	52.24
Vitamin C	59.16	54.65	Vitamin C	38.96	43.78

Source: DHEW, 1976. [1] Excludes persons with unknown income.

Food Myths and Fallacies

Fallacies and Facts*

Fallacy: Oysters, raw eggs and rare or raw meat increase sexual potency.

Fact: These foods, as well as all others, contribute toward health and well-being, but have no special properties to increase sexual potency.

Fallacy: Vegetables should be purchased fresh because canned and frozen vegetables have been robbed of their nutrients.

Fact: Commercially processed vegetables are as nutritious as fresh vegetables cooked at home. Food containing Vitamin C will always lose some of this nutrient when exposed to heat, whether commercially processed or home cooked. To minimize loss of Vitamin C (or other heat or water sensitive nutrients), use short cooking times and minimum amounts of water. Ideally, the cooking liquid should be saved for soups and stews. Vitamin A, the major nutrient supplied by vegetables, is not destroyed by heat.

Fallacy: Foods raised on soils organically fertilized are more nutritious than food raised on chemically fertilized soil.

Fact: There is no difference in the nutritional quality of organically fertilized and chemically fertilized crops. The soil and growing plant reduce *all* fertilizers to inorganic chemical components before using the nutrients. There is no difference between a "chemically derived" chemical and a "naturally derived" chemical. Actually most nutrients, except minerals, are synthesized by the plant, not absorbed from the soil.

Fallacy: Frozen orange juice has less nutritive value than fresh.

Fact: The major contribution of orange juice to the diet is Vitamin C. Fresh and frozen products are remarkably similar in Vitamin C content.

Fallacy: Beets are high in iron.

Fact: Beets have very little iron. The fallacy probably stems from the fact that beets are red. Redness of foods is *not* related to the iron content of those foods. Beet *greens* are a good source of iron.

Fallacy: It is dangerous to leave food in a can that has been opened.

Fact: It is safe to keep the food in the original can after it has been opened. It is important to cover the can and to keep the food cool. A few acid foods may dissolve a little iron from the can, but this is not harmful or dangerous to health. It may cause discoloration of the food product.

*Source: *Food Facts Talk Back,* The American Dietetic Association.

Fallacy: White bread and white flour have no nutritional value; only whole grain products should be purchased.

Fact: White bread is white because the bran and germ (which contain many nutrients) have been removed in milling. When white flour products are enriched, thiamin, riboflavin, niacin and iron are added to equal or better the levels of the nutrients in the whole grain. Not all nutrients are returned to the flour, but these usually can be obtained in adequate amounts from a well-balanced diet. White flour, enriched or unenriched, also contributes some protein.

Fallacy: Blackstrap molasses is good for anemia and rheumatism.

Fact: Blackstrap molasses does contain calcium, iron and most of the B vitamins. The iron content of one tablespoon of blackstrap molasses is approximately 3.2 mg; this is within the range of iron content of $\frac{2}{3}$ cup dried beans or peas. A 3-oz. cooked serving of beef has 3.0 to 3.5 mg of iron; 3 ounces of beef liver has 7.3 mg iron. While not a wonder food, blackstrap molasses along with other good sources of iron can help alleviate and prevent iron-deficiency anemia. There is no scientific evidence indicating any benefit from blackstrap molasses in the treatment of rheumatism.

Fallacy: Vinegar and honey can help cure rheumatism and arthritis.

Fact: As explained, honey is a sugar comparable to table sugar in composition. Honey, alone or with vinegar, adds only calories to the diet. Neither item has an effect on rheumatism or arthritis. In fact, too many calories will add weight, which indirectly can create greater pain.

Fallacy: Athletes need more protein than the average person.

Fact: The belief held by many athletes and other active persons that hard exercise increases the need for protein has no scientific support. Carbohydrate and calorie needs are increased, however.

Fallacy: Rare roast beef or steak is more nutritious than meat cooked longer.

Fact: Medium-done meat cooked at moderate temperature is about the same in nutritive value as rare meat. Overcooked meat has greater loss of some vitamins. The degree of doneness does not affect the protein or iron content.

Fallacy: White eggs are more nutritious than brown.

Fact: The nutritive value of an egg is not related to the color of the shell. Color is determined by the breed of hen.

Fallacy: Gelatin is an excellent source of protein and will strengthen the fingernails.

Fact: Unlike eggs, milk or meat, gelatin is an incomplete protein and does not contain all of the amino acids needed for growth, repair and maintenance of the body—despite its animal origin. There are differences of scientific opinion as to whether protein in any form improves fingernails.

30

Fallacy: Fish is a brain food.

Fact: Possibly this belief arose from the fact that nerve tissue, which comprises a part of our brains, is rich in phosphorus, and fish provides phosphorus-containing compounds. But meat, poultry, eggs and milk are also rich in phosphorus, as well as good-quality protein.

Fallacy: If small amounts of a vitamin are necessary to maintain the body, then larger amounts are even better for your health.

Fact: The accepted guide for vitamin intake is the Recommended Dietary Allowances. These allowances are based on the amounts your body can use, and taking more does you no good; it can even be harmful. When you consume more of the water soluble vitamins (B complex and C) than your body needs, the vitamins are excreted. This can cause undue strain on the kidneys. However, it has been proven that fat soluble vitamins, such as A and D, are stored in the body and are toxic when taken in excessive doses on a regular basis. (Therapeutic doses of a particular vitamin may be given under a doctor's strict supervision in specific cases.)

Fallacy: Lecithin is a valuable antidote for many diseases such as heart disease, dry skin, nervous disorders and arthritis.

Fact: Lecithin is a phospholipid which contains choline (a B vitamin); it is found in egg yolks, soybeans, meats (especially liver and whole grains). Phospholipids help transport fats in the blood stream. Despite claims from health food enthusiasts, there is no proof that lecithin can reduce elevated blood cholesterol associated with heart disease risk. Large doses of lecithin have not been proven to have any curative effect.

Fallacy: Non-dairy creamers are better for your health than cream.

Fact: Non-dairy creamers are usually made from plant oils. They do not contain cholesterol, as does cream. However, the plant oil most commonly used is coconut, and this is a saturated fat. If the reduction of saturated fats in the diet is the goal, nonfat dry or liquid skim milk would be a better substitute for cream. The non-dairy creamers contain about 11 calories per teaspoon. Cream contains about 14 calories per teaspoon.

30

Health Food Myths*

In general, the term "organic food" is assumed to mean that the product has been produced under conditions where pesticides and herbicides have not been used, where the fertilization of the soil has been done with natural composting rather than with so-called manufactured fertilizers, and where the handling of the product following its production has been without the use of any type of food additive.

The fraud aspect is a very important one relative to incorrect labeling of products as "organic" because they are usually sold for more.

For example, dried apricots labeled as organic were being sold for $1.24 for ten ounces, while eight ounces of the regular dried apricots were priced at 59 cents. Spinach sold as or-

*Source: *FDA Consumer,* DHEW, 1974.

30

Table 30-4   Vitamin chart

Vitamins

Vitamin	Function	Deficiency results	Sources	History
A	Healthy skin and mucous membranes, new cell growth, adaption of eye to dim light, and color vision	Night blindness, skin lesions, changes in eye, mucous, and gland tissues after long deficiency	Carotene, found in carrots, yams, leafy green vegetables, and cereal grains are converted by body into vitamins; also found in cod and other fish liver oils, butter, egg yolks, and cheese	1913—Diet deficiency in animals corrected by butter and milk 1917—Xerophthalmia (dry, lusterless eyes) traced to lack of Vitamin A 1920—Carotene related to Vitamin A 1930—Proved body converted carotene to Vitamin A 1937—Pure Vitamin A isolated from fish liver oils
B₁ Thiamine	Normal function of all body organs and tissues with greater need during pregnancy and lactation	Beriberi—often fatal disease of the Orient characterized by nerve degeneration leading to paralysis, convulsions, and psychological disturbances often with related heart, lung, and digestive symptoms	Cereal grains, pork, liver, kidney, milk, eggs, bread, and enriched flour	1882—Diet change used to reduce beriberi in Japan 1897—Beriberi cured by adding rice polishings to diet 1913—Funk isolated Vitamin B₁ from rice polishings and coined the term "vitamine" 1936—Vitamin B₁ made synthetically (by chemical means rather than taken from food)
B₂ Riboflavin— also known as Vitamin G	Vital to proper metabolism, utilizes energy derived from carbohydrate foods, proper function of eyes, and keeps body tissues healthy	Faulty vision, skin lesions of mouth and face, nervousness, and poor blood	Most meat and vegetables, although best sources are Brewer's yeast, cheese, milk, eggs, leafy green vegetables, peas, lima beans, liver, and kidney	1920—Multiple nature established 1926—Vitamin B₂ found different from Vitamin B₁ 1933—Riboflavin isolated 1935—Riboflavin synthesized
Niacin Nicotinic acid part of Vitamin B complex	Maintains healthy body by occurring in all body tissues as an enzyme to aid in protein and carbohydrate metabolism	Pellagra (common in southern United States) characterized by diarrhea, dermatitis, dementia, and death	Yeast, wheat germ, liver, and lean meats are best sources, although also found in peanuts, potatoes, and vegetables	1913—Isolated by Funk from rice polishings with Vitamin B₁ 1926—Antipellagra factor known to exist in foods 1935—Found in many foods 1936—Liver extract cures pellagra 1937—Proved niacin in liver cured pellagra
Niacinamide Nicotinamide synthetic most often used		Less advanced stages result in digestive, skin, and psychological disturbances	Precursor is amino acid tryptophan	
B₆ Pyridoxine	Involved in protein metabolism, utilizes essential fatty acids, and helps body convert tryptophan to niacin	Dermatitis around eyes and mouth, nervousness, insomnia, abdominal pain, weakness, and partial responsibility for dental cavities and cleft palate	Liver, wheat germ, milk, yeast, peas, lima beans, meat, and vegetable fats	1934—Properties described 1938—Isolated 1939—Synthesized 1950—Deficiency artificially produced 1953—Demonstrated to be necessary in nutrition

Vitamin	Function	Deficiency	Sources	History
B_{12} Group of mixed vitamins —the cobalamins	Essential in protein metabolism, helps transform carbohydrates to fat, essential for normal development of red blood cells, growth factor in children, and antianemia factor	Growth retardation and anemia. Severe deficiency usually due to lack of "intrinsic factor" in gastric juices resulting in pernicious anemia for which Vitamin B_{12} is only cure	Meat—especially liver and kidney—and milk products	1926—Liver cured pernicious anemia 1929—Castle's famous theory—"intrinsic factor" versus "extrinsic factor" of red blood cell development; "extrinsic factor," later identified as Vitamin B_{12}, needed to build red blood cells, but cannot work unless "intrinsic factor," made in normal stomachs, is present; pernicious anemia patients do not make "intrinsic factor" in stomach 1948—Isolated and named
Folic acid Formerly known as Vitamin M and also part of Vitamin B complex	Important in protein metabolism, used with Vitamin B_{12} to combat anemia, and helps in normal function of blood cells	Lack of bone marrow growth which leads to anemia	Liver, kidney, leafy green vegetables and yeast	1948—Used against pernicious anemia 1934—Yeast used to combat anemia in pregnancy 1935 to 1938—Response to yeast by diet deficient animal studies 1941—Isolated 1946—Synthesized
C Ascorbic acid	Wound healing, prevention of scurvy and important in infant feeding	Scurvy—characterized by weakness, loose teeth, spongy gums, swollen and tender joints and hemorrhage Acute scurvy—blindness, bone decay and brain damage	Citrus fruits—oranges, lemons, limes, grapefruits—are best sources, although also found in tomatoes, cabbage, broccoli, spinach, raspberries and strawberries	1906—Diet deficiency found to cause scurvy 1907—Existence of antiscurvy factor 1932—Identified as antiscurvy factor 1933—Synthesized
D	Normal bone structure, healthy teeth and muscle tone	Weak muscles, tooth decay, rickets in children and osteomalacia (disease by which bones become soft and then deformed) in adults	Fish liver oils, butter and eggs yolks Also produced in body by exposure to sunlight. Dark skin is a barrier to sun, so rickets often seen in Negroes and Latins	1807—Cod liver oil used in osteomalacia 1890—Action of sunlight against rickets demonstrated 1919—Cod liver oil used to combat rickets 1931—Isolated
K (K_1, K_2, K_3) Synthetic K_3—menadione—used often	Manufacture of prothrombin (protein in blood enabling blood to clot), useful in surgery to aid blood clotting. Vitamin K_1 only used to counteract overdose of anticoagulants	Bleeding in many tissues and organs	K_1—Alfalfa and other green plants K_2—Spoiled fish meal	1929—Danish scientist Damm reported bleeding in chicken due to diet deficiency 1935—Damm named Vitamin K for Danish word "koagulation" 1939—Vitamin K_1 synthesized 1940—Vitamin K_3 synthesized—menadione

30

ganic cost the consumer 75 cents for ten ounces, but the regular price for spinach was 39 cents for ten ounces.

The manufacturer or producer of organic foods does have some higher costs. He may lose more of his crop to pests because he doesn't use pesticides. But the opportunity for economic fraud is considerable.

The evidence today suggests that for the nutritional qualities that we expect to find in foods, there simply is no difference between those produced under "organic" conditions and those produced under normal conditions.

FDA's general position on vitamins and minerals is that people get enough from the food they eat, and therefore supplements are not necessary, although FDA has no objection to people taking reasonable supplements. It is a type of insurance that might provide some consumers with a psychological, if not a physiological, lift.

Vitamin Myths *

Vitamin C

According to all studies documented at the present time, the body uses only the amount of ascorbic acid it needs, and eliminates the rest through the kidneys.

Nobel Prizewinner Linus Pauling, Ph.D., from his studies of existing literature, is convinced that "ascorbic acid, taken in the proper amount, has much value in decreasing the incidence, severity, and integrated morbidity of the common cold and related infections." In his writing, he indicates the "proper amount," to him, means a minimum daily intake of 200 to 400 mg for "optimal health."

A more recent study has been reported in January 1974, in *The New England Journal of Medicine* by Coulehan, Reisinger, Rogers and Bradley covering 641 children at a Navajo boarding school over a 14-week period. Although there was no difference between the two groups in the number of respiratory illnesses, the children receiving vitamin C had fewer days of illness than those receiving the placebo. Among the younger children, there were 26% fewer days of illness in the vitamin C group, and 33% fewer in the older girls. No such difference was seen in the older boys.

---

* Source: *FDA Consumer.*

These and other studies indicate that vitamin C may be beneficial in reducing the severity of colds or reducing the length of time symptoms persist.

However, questions about the safety of high doses of ascorbic acid have been raised by other nutritionists and physicians. There is some indication high intake may have an effect on the menstrual cycle and even terminate pregnancy; it may interfere with treatments of patients whose urine must be kept alkaline; or it may cause problems in treating certain people with anticoagulant drugs.

Vitamin E

It will help you grow hair. Cure your skin problems. Ease your arthritis pain. Prevent ulcers. Make you sexually young.

These are just a smattering of the claims being made for vitamin E, whose sales in recent years have soared. But there is no scientific evidence that vitamin E will do any of the dramatic things that are being claimed for it, or that large supplements are needed for the treatment of disease.

Vitamin E is a chemical in the alcohol family that is soluble in fat. Its chief function is as an antioxidant. An antioxidant inhibits the combination of a substance with oxygen, and thus acts as a preservative.

What about the cosmetic usefulness of vitamin E?

In this area the claims have reached new heights. Cosmetics containing vitamin E have been promoted for healing skin blemishes, for softening dry skin, for erasing wrinkles and for giving new life to aging skin. There is no evidence from controlled studies to substantiate such benefits.

For example, no evidence has been presented to FDA, and no documentation has appeared in medical literature, to support the claim that vitamin E is effective for use as or in a deodorant.

In summary, vitamin E has not been proved scientifically to have any of the "miraculous" effects being claimed for it. And FDA sees no reason for persons in good health and eating a well-balanced diet to use a dietary supplement.

Vitamins A and D

Many people assume that the more vitamins they take, the healthier they will be. Large doses of vitamin A and/or D over a long period of time not only cease to be beneficial but also can cause adverse effects, some of them serious.

Some of the effects from high doses of vitamin A are relatively minor, such as nausea, drying and cracking of skin, irritability and headache. Others are more serious, including growth retardation in children, enlargement of the liver and spleen, loss of hair, rheumatic pain, bone pain and disturbance of the menstrual cycle.

Perhaps most dangerous, excessive use of vitamin A can cause intracranial pressure that mimics a brain tumor, sometimes resulting in unnecessary (and inherently dangerous) exploratory brain surgery. This effect has been observed in children and young people who have been given large doses of vitamin A for the treatment of acne.

Excessive intake of vitamin D can result in nausea, weakness, weight loss, excessive urination, constipation, stiffness, premature calcification of the bones, hypertension and irreversible failure of kidney function.

Calories

Calories and Dieting *

The food calories you eat must be just enough to offset your requirement for energy calories. If you eat too few calories, body fat will be burned as fuel. If you eat more than you need, the surplus will be turned into body fat and pounds will pile up. Extra calories invariably end up as extra fat. This is *always* true, whether the extras come from carbohydrate, protein or fat, or from beef or bread or bourbon or blueberries.

In other words, balancing calories is exactly like balancing your income and expenses. If you do not have an excess or a deficit, you cannot gain and you cannot lose.

How the extras add up

Extras	Approximate calorie content
Celery, 1 stalk	5
Carrot, 1 medium	20
Pretzels, 5 small sticks	20

Cottage cheese, 2 tablespoons	30
Crackers, 2 Ritz	34
Peach, fresh, medium	35
Cookie, small	50
Popped corn, 1 cup (with 1 tsp. oil)	65
Orange, medium	70
Apple, medium	70
Soft drink, 6 ounces	72
Milk, skim, 1 cup (8 ounces)	90
Pear, medium	100
Cheese, average, 1 ounce	100
Hard candy, (3¾" balls, or 20 small gum drops)	100
Whisky, 1½ ounce jigger	105
Peanuts, 20	114
Potato chips, 10 about 2" size	115
Yoghurt, 1 cup	120
Ice milk, ½ cup	121
Ice cream, standard, ½ cup	145
Cupcake, unfrosted	145
Beer, 12 ounces	150
Candy bar, small size	160
Milk, whole, 1 cup (8 ounces)	160
Pizza, ⅛ large	185
Doughnut, jelly	226
Ice cream soda	255
Hamburger on a bun	305
Peanut butter sandwich	340
Sundae with nuts	345
Pie, fruit, 4" sector	350
Milk shake with ice cream	420
Cake with icing (2" sector)	445

An average-sized person, as described below, requires about the number of calories shown:

	Calories
Teenagers:	
Girls	2,000–2,400
Boys	2,700–3,000
Housewife, normally active:	
Age 22 up to 35	2,000
Age 35 up to 55	1,850
Man, normally active:	
Age 22 up to 35	2,800
Age 35 up to 55	2,600

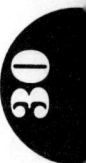

Losing Weight—For every 3,500 extra calories you get and do not use, you gain about one pound of weight. This pound represents stored food energy in the form of fat. To lose excess fat you have to somehow use up stored energy. You can—

- Eat less food (fewer calories), to force your body to draw energy from its stored fat.
- Increase your activity, to use up more energy.

30

Figure 30-1   Estimating the calories your patient needs

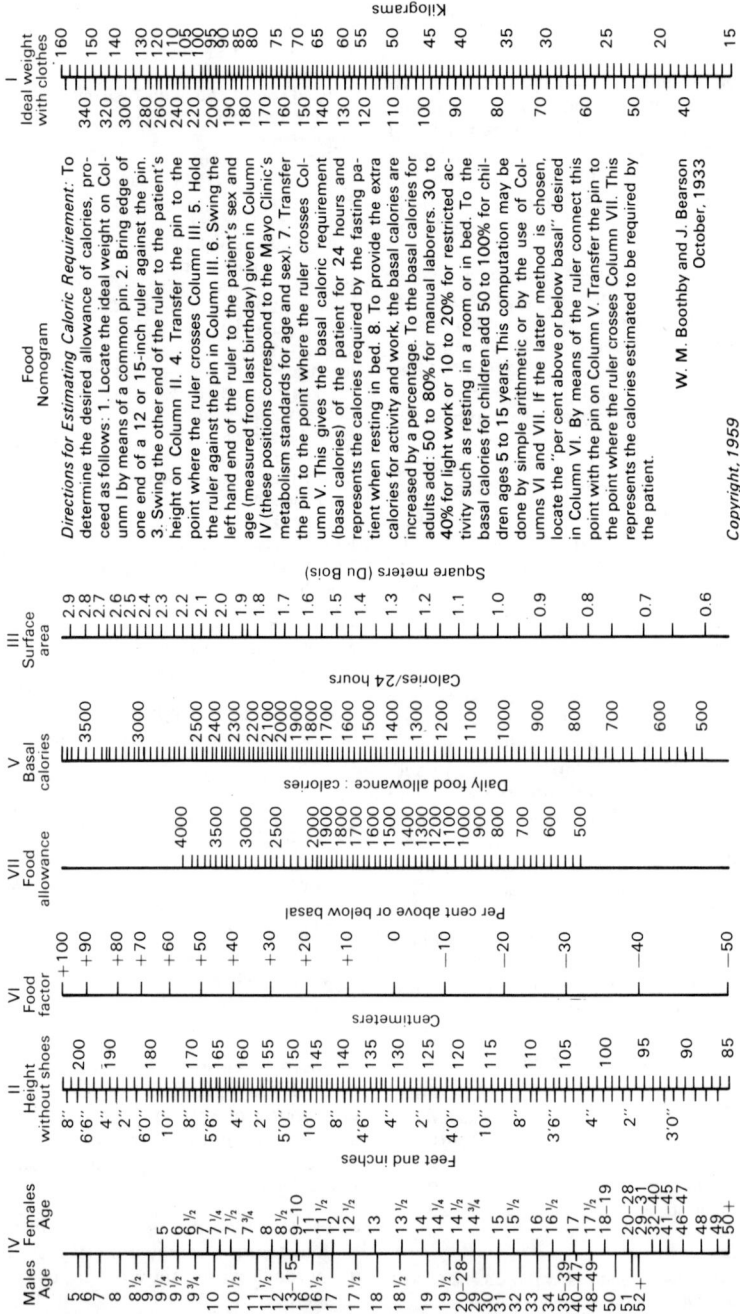

Food Nomogram

Directions for Estimating Caloric Requirement: To determine the desired allowance of calories, proceed as follows: 1. Locate the ideal weight on Column I by means of a common pin. 2. Bring edge of one end of a 12 or 15-inch ruler against the pin. 3. Swing the other end of the ruler to the patient's height on Column II. 4. Transfer the pin to the point where the ruler crosses Column III. 5. Hold the ruler against the pin in Column III. 6. Swing the left hand end of the ruler to the patient's sex and age (measured from last birthday) given in Column IV (these positions correspond to the Mayo Clinic's metabolism standards for age and sex). 7. Transfer the pin to the point where the ruler crosses Column V. This gives the basal caloric requirement (basal calories) of the patient for 24 hours and represents the calories required by the fasting patient when resting in bed. 8. To provide the extra calories for activity and work, the basal calories are increased by a percentage. To the basal calories for adults add: 50 to 80% for manual laborers. 30 to 40% for light work or 10 to 20% for restricted activity such as resting in a room or in bed. To the basal calories for children add 50 to 100% for children ages 5 to 15 years. This computation may be done by simple arithmetic or by the use of Columns VI and VII. If the latter method is chosen, locate the "per cent above or below basal" desired in Column VI. By means of the ruler connect this point with the pin on Column V. Transfer the pin to the point where the ruler crosses Column VII. This represents the calories estimated to be required by the patient.

W. M. Boothby and J. Bearson
October, 1933

*Copyright, 1959
Mayo Association*

Column labels: I Ideal weight with clothes (Kilograms); II Height without shoes (Centimeters / Feet and inches); III Surface area (Square meters [Du Bois]); IV Males Age / Females Age; V Basal calories (Calories/24 hours); VI Food factor (Per cent above or below basal); VII Food allowance (Daily food allowance: calories)

- Do both. Many dieters find a combination of eating less food and getting more exercise the best way to lose weight.

Allow yourself 500 to 1,000 fewer calories a day than you are now getting, to lose weight at the recommended rate of one to two pounds a week. You will need to cut down more than this on calories, however, if you are gaining weight on the amount of food you now eat. But *don't cut calories to fewer than 1,200 a day unless you are under a doctor's supervision.* *

Cholesterol

Cholesterol is a normal constituent of blood and tissues and is found in every animal cell. Some of the cholesterol in human blood and tissues is synthesized by the body and some is supplied by diet. The amount supplied by diet varies greatly depending on the kinds and amounts of foods included.

The amount of cholesterol in the diet is positively related to the amount of cholesterol in the blood. Ordinary diets are likely to supply 600 to 900 milligrams of cholesterol daily. A "low-cholesterol" diet usually provides about 300 milligrams of cholesterol daily.

The director of the Heart and Lung Institute of NIH testified in 1976:

> We now understand how cholesterol and other blood fats circulate in the plasma. We know there are specific proteins that can carry cholesterol and how the basic amino acid structure of these proteins makes them a vehicle for the transport of the fat—we can now synthesize proteins building on the same kind of protein structures and ultimately infuse synthetic proteins that may act eventually as chemical roto-rooters that might remove lipid from already existing deposits. . . .
>
> We now have conclusive evidence from four different groups of investigators that in nonhuman primates, monkeys, not only can one prevent progression of arteriosclerosis produced by diet, high cholesterol, or other factors, but one can actually demonstrate regression with intervention, with changing of diets and drugs—that is the arteriosclerosis disappears.

* Source: U.S. Department of Agriculture.

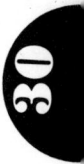

Exercise and Calorie Expenditures

Table 30-5   Energy expenditure in specified activities[1]

	Calories per minute	
	Men	Women
In bed asleep or resting	1.08	0.90
Sitting quietly	1.39	1.15
Standing quietly	1.75	1.37
Walking 3 miles/hour (4.9 km/hour)	3.7	3.0
Walking 3 miles/hour (4.9 km/hour) with a 10-kg load	4.0	3.4
Office work (sedentary)	1.8	1.6
Domestic work		
Cooking	2.1	1.7
Light cleaning	3.1	2.5
Moderate cleaning (polishing, window cleaning, chopping firewood, etc.)	4.3	3.5
Light industry		
Printing	2.3	
Tailoring	2.9	
Shoemaking	3.0	
Bakery work		2.3
Brewery work		2.7
Chemical industry		2.7
Electrical industry		1.9
Furnishing industry		3.1
Laundry work		3.2
Machine tool industry		2.5
Recreations		
Sedentary	2.5	2.0
Light (bowling, golf, sailing, etc.)	2.5–5.0	2.0–4.0
Moderate (canoeing, dancing, horseback riding, swimming, tennis, etc.)	5.0–7.5	4.0–6.0
Heavy (athletics, football, rowing, etc.)	7.5 +	6.0 +

[1] Based on weight of man 143 pounds and of woman 121 pounds.

Source: FAO, World Health Organization Techn. Rep. Ser. 1973.

Fat or Fatty Acids

Fatty acids are the building blocks of fat. Three molecules of fatty acid combined with one molecule of glycerol constitute a molecule of fat. This is called a triglyceride, the form in which fat is stored in adipose tissue.

Fats are classified as saturated or unsaturated depending on the kind of fatty acids present. Most food fats are a combination of the different saturated and unsaturated fatty acids.

A chemist describes a fatty acid as saturated if its chain of carbon atoms contains all the hydrogen it can hold (or if there are no double bonds between carbon atoms). The most common saturated fatty acids are myristic acid and palmitic acid. Saturated fats are usually hard at room temperature. They occur in both animal and vegetable fats, but chiefly in animal fats.

A chemist describes a fatty acid as unsaturated if its chain of carbon atoms has one or more double bonds where hydrogen could be added. The process of adding hydrogen to a double bond in an unsaturated fatty acid to make it more saturated is referred to as hydrogenation.

Monounsaturated fatty acids have only one double bond where hydrogen could be added. Oleic acid is the most common monounsaturated fatty acid.

Polyunsaturated fatty acids have two or more double bonds where hydrogen could be added.

Polyunsaturated fats are usually oils and are most abundant in plant seeds and fish oils. Nearly all fats from plant sources are unsaturated; the only major exception is coconut oil, which is highly saturated.

Cholesterol Content of Common Foods

Table 30-6   Cholesterol content of measures of selected foods (in ascending order)

Food	Amount	Cholesterol milligrams
Milk, skim, fluid or reconstituted dry	1 cup	5
Cottage cheese, uncreamed	½ cup	7
Lard	1 tablespoon	12
Cream, light table	1 fluid ounce	20
Cottage cheese, creamed	½ cup	24
Cream, half and half	¼ cup	26
Ice cream, regular, approximately 10% fat	½ cup	27
Cheese, cheddar	1 ounce	28
Milk, whole	1 cup	34
Butter	1 tablespoon	35
Oysters, salmon	3 ounces, cooked	40
Clams, halibut, tuna	3 ounces, cooked	55
Chicken, turkey, light meat	3 ounces, cooked	67
Beef, pork, lobster, chicken, turkey, dark meat	3 ounces, cooked	75
Lamb, veal, crab	3 ounces, cooked	85
Shrimp	3 ounces, cooked	130
Heart, beef	3 ounces, cooked	230
Egg	1 yolk or 1 egg	250
Liver, beef, calf, hog, lamb	3 ounces, cooked	370
Kidney	3 ounces, cooked	680
Brains	3 ounces, raw	more than 1700

Source: R. M. Feeley, P. E. Criner, and B. K. Watt, "Cholesterol Content of Foods," *Journal of American Diet Association,* 1972.

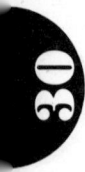

Obesity

How To Reduce*

Weight reduction should begin in the doctor's office. Apart from ruling out medical and serious psychological causes of obesity and those diseases that obesity makes more common (such as diabetes), your doctor may want to determine the amount of cholesterol in your blood.

If you are obese, and if your cholesterol level is in the high ranges, your doctor will probably want to put you on a calorie-restricted, cholesterol-lowering diet. This diet will probably contain fish at least four or five times a week, will substitute special margarines for butter and it will avoid products rich in saturated fats such as cream, hard cheeses and ice cream. The complication of high blood levels of cholesterol in obesity is infrequent in women under 45; it is more common in men 35 and over.

Although crash diets offer the promise of rapid weight loss, unbalanced diets may be hazardous by producing anemias and by creating protein, mineral and vitamin deficiencies. They induce temporary weight loss—if they cause weight loss at all. But they do not alter the basic eating habits *necessary for life-long weight control.*

The diet we propose includes a start at changing life-long eating habits. The proper choice of foods is the major secret of this diet. It is designed to provide all the essential nutrients. Its principles have been used in clinics in New York City for 15 years and it has been followed successfully by tens of thousands of people, many of whom said later that they had never eaten so well as they did during their period of weight reduction.

Motivation

Motivation is the trick in getting started. A husband's promise of a gift or a trip may suddenly stir motivation but this is not likely to last. True motivation must come from a real desire to change body image. The dieter has to say to himself "this is not the way I want to look—this is not the way I want the world to see me." In place of a sudden spurt of interest

*Source: George Christakis, M.D. and Robert K. Plumb, "Obesity" (pamphlet), The Nutrition Foundation, Inc.

in dieting, recognition is needed that being overweight presents a serious hazard to health and that a sustained program of educated eating is essential.

The recipe for successful weight reduction is simple:

- Take motivation—strong reasons for losing weight;
- Add knowledge—about good nutrition;
- Mix with self-discipline—will power;
- Dash of extra physical activity.

Knowledge

Although obesity is a complex subject, one rule stands: calories taken in must equal calories expended or overweight will result.

A calorie is a measure of energy, and it may be expressed in heat. For example, a person eating a level teaspoonful of butter consumes enough calories to bring two-and-one-half pints of room-temperature water to a boil.

Not only do all foods contain calories, but many foods are also a concentrated form of energy. This is important in impoverished areas and the world's hungry benefit from the concentration of energy in food. But this may work against people where an excess of food is available and the temptation is to eat too much. This country is a good example.

Nearly all foods are a mixture of carbohydrates, proteins, fats, minerals, vitamins, water and undigestible roughage. If taken in pure form, the components would have different caloric contents. Fats are the high calorie foods. Proteins and carbohydrates have less than one-half the caloric value of fats.

There is no one miracle food. We need about 50 food elements called nutrients. No one food contains all the nutrients in the required amounts. To get the nutrients you need in a reducing diet, you must eat a wide variety of foods. The reducing diet must, therefore, reduce the number of calories taken in while maintaining an intake of the essential nutrients and it must provide a new nutritional way of life that corrects the previous faulty diet and gives a new life pattern of eating.

The diet the New York City Health Department recommends fulfills these objectives. Its content of lean meat, fish, poultry, dairy products and legumes provides the protein that is especially needed during weight reduction—and proper quantities of minerals and vitamins as well. If these protein-rich foods are not included in a reducing diet in appropriate amounts, the body has to burn its own muscle tissue for its protein needs. This is the hazard in many crash diets.

Cereals, bread and potatoes are rich sources of the B vitamins and they provide adequate carbohydrate vital to a reducing diet. Our body has a limited ability to store carbohydrate. A carbohydrate reserve is always required by the liver to meet the body's energy needs.

Fish is a rich source of protein, unsaturated fats, vitamins and minerals that the body cannot manufacture and must derive from the diet. Fats from fish have the remarkable ability of lowering blood cholesterol in ways not yet clearly understood.

General Weight Reduction Diet

This pattern of eating is designed to help you reduce, stay reduced and form habits of eating that promote the best possible health throughout life.

1. Use the following as desired.

bouillon	horseradish	seltzer
clear soup	lemon and lime	spices
(fat-free)	paprika	tea
club soda	pepper	vinegar
coffee	salt	water
herbs		

2. Eat all you want of the following cooked or raw vegetables. Those in large print are rich in vitamin A.

artichokes	mushrooms
asparagus	MUSTARD GREENS
beans, green, snap	okra
or waxy	onions
bean sprouts	parsley
BEET GREENS	parsnips
Brussels sprouts	peppers
CARROTS	pickles
cabbage	pimentos
cauliflower	PUMPKIN
celery	radishes
CHICORY	rutabaga
Chinese cabbage	sauerkraut
COLLARDS	scallions
cucumber	SPINACH
DANDELION	squash, summer
GREENS	SQUASH, WINTER
endive	SWISS CHARD
ESCAROLE	tomato
KALE	turnips
kohlrabi	TURNIP GREENS
leeks	WATERCRESS
lettuce	

3. The following vegetables and cereals should be used more sparingly than those listed under 2.

corn (fresh or canned)	cornmeal
dried beans or peas	grits
green limas	macaroni
green peas	noodles
lentils (fresh or canned)	rice
plantain	spaghetti
potatoes	

SWEET POTATOES or YAMS

4. You may eat three servings daily of any unsweetened fruit, fresh, canned or frozen. Choose at least one vitamin C fruit daily. Those in large print are especially rich in vitamin C.

apples	LIME
apricots, fresh	ORANGE
blackberries	ORANGE JUICE
blueberries	PAPAYA
CANTALOUPE	peach
cranberries	pineapple
GRAPEFRUIT	plums
GRAPEFRUIT JUICE	raspberries
honeydew melon	STRAWBERRIES
LEMON	TANGERINES

Use more sparingly

apricots, dried	nectarine
bananas	pear
cherries	persimmon
dates	pomegranate
grapes	prunes, dried
GUAVA	raisins
MANGO	watermelon

Most canned and frozen foods are sweetened; drain syrup.

5. Eat enriched or whole-grain bread or cereal.

6. Limit eggs to four to seven a week. Cook in shell, poach or scramble without fat.

7. Include two cups of skim milk daily. Fat-free buttermilk or evaporated skim milk may be substituted.

8. Broil, pan broil, simmer, bake or roast meat, fish or poultry. Do not fry. Remove all visible fat before eating. Do not eat gravies or sauces. Eat at least five seafood meals weekly. Limit fat group to three times weekly.

Lean Group		Fat Group
Fish, Lean Meat, Poultry		*No more than 3 servings each week*
bass	mussels	beef, lean
bluefish	oysters	bologna
bonito*	pike	frankfurter
butterfish	salmon*	ham, lean
carp	sardines*	lamb, lean
chicken	scallops	liverwurst
clams	shad	pork, lean
cod	shad roe	
crabmeat	shrimp	
finnan haddie	sturgeon, fresh	
flounder	swordfish	
haddock	tongue	
halibut	trout	
herring*	tuna fish*	
kidney	turkey	
liver	veal	
lobster	weakfish	
mackerel	whitefish	

*Canned fish with added oil should be drained well.

9. Avoid excessive amounts of alcohol, rich gravies, cream dressings, fat spreads, candy, pastries and carbonated beverages.

10. Exercise contributes to the success of your diet program in several important ways. It helps tone muscles and increases the blood supply to many vital organs and tissues.

	Activity				
Food	Walking min.	Riding bicycle min.	Swimming min.	Running min.	Reclining min.
Apple, large	19	12	9	5	78
Beer, 1 glass	22	14	10	6	88
Cake, 1/12, 2-layer	68	43	32	18	274
Carbonated beverage, 1 glass	20	13	9	5	82
Carrot, raw	8	5	4	2	32
Cookie, chocolate chip	10	6	5	3	39
Egg, boiled	15	9	7	4	59
Halibut steak, ¼ lb.	39	25	18	11	158
Malted milk shake	97	61	45	26	386
Pie, apple, 1/6	73	46	34	19	290
Pizza, cheese, 1/8	35	22	16	9	138
Sandwich, tuna fish salad	53	34	25	14	214
Steak, T-bone	45	29	21	12	181
Strawberry short-cake	77	49	36	21	308

*From Dr. Frank Konishi, Southern Illinois University.
**Source: Metropolitan Life Insurance Co., "Four Steps to Weight Control."

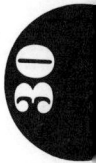

Exercise burns up calories that might otherwise be stored as fat in the body. The amount of time in minutes required at various physical activities* in order to burn up the calories in the food portions listed is given below:

Daily Low-Calorie Diets**

The foods in the following suggested daily diets may be eaten any time during the day, in varied combinations. For example, you may find it more satisfying to divide this three-meal plan into four or five smaller meals. And perhaps you prefer to take part—or all—of your milk at breakfast on your cereal or in your coffee. If you wish, have your vegetables in a tossed salad with lemon juice dressing. The only rule to remember is this: Count everything you eat and keep your *total* daily food intake within the bounds of this diet plan.

1,000-CALORIE DAILY DIET

Breakfast

Fresh fruit or juice	1 serving—½ cup
Egg—cooked without fat	1
or	
Cereal	1 small serving
Bread	1 slice
Butter or margarine	1 level teaspoon
Skim milk or buttermilk	1 glass—6 ounces
Clear coffee or tea	

Dinner

Lean meat, fish, or poultry	3 ounces (cooked)
Vegetables (raw or cooked)	½ cup cooked raw, freely
Skim milk or buttermilk	1 glass—6 ounces
Fruit (raw, cooked or canned without sugar)	1 serving—½ cup

Lunch or Supper

Cottage cheese or lean meat	½ cup of cheese 2 ounces of meat
Vegetables (raw or cooked)	½ cup cooked raw, freely
Skim milk or buttermilk	1 glass—6 ounces
Fruit (raw, cooked or canned without sugar)	1 serving—½ cup

30

Recommended Weights for Men and Women

Table 30-7   Desirable weights. Weight in pounds according to frame (in indoor clothing)

Height (with shoes on) 1-inch heels		Small frame	Medium frame	Large frame
Feet	Inches			
Men of ages 25 and over				
5	2	112–120	118–129	126–141
5	3	115–123	121–133	129–144
5	4	118–126	124–136	132–148
5	5	121–129	127–139	135–152
5	6	124–133	130–143	138–156
5	7	128–137	134–147	142–161
5	8	132–141	138–152	147–166
5	9	136–145	142–156	151–170
5	10	140–150	146–160	155–174
5	11	144–154	150–165	159–179
6	0	148–158	154–170	164–184
6	1	152–162	158–175	168–189
6	2	156–167	162–180	173–194
6	3	160–171	167–185	178–199
6	4	164–175	172–190	182–204
Women of ages 25 and over				
4	10	92– 98	96–107	104–119
4	11	94–101	98–110	106–122
5	0	96–104	101–113	109–125
5	1	99–107	104–116	112–128
5	2	102–110	107–119	115–131
5	3	105–113	110–122	118–134
5	4	108–116	113–126	121–138
5	5	111–119	116–130	125–142
5	6	114–123	120–135	129–146
5	7	118–127	124–139	133–150
5	8	122–131	128–143	137–154
5	9	126–135	132–147	141–158
5	10	130–140	136–151	145–163
5	11	134–144	140–155	149–168
6	0	138–148	144–159	153–173

For girls between 18 and 25, subtract 1 pound for each year under 25.

Source: Metropolitan Life Insurance Company.

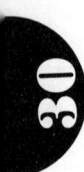

1,200-CALORIE DAILY DIET

Breakfast

Fresh fruit or juice	1 serving—½ cup
Egg—cooked without fat or	1
Cereal	1 small serving
Bread	1 slice
Butter or margarine	1 level teaspoon
Skim milk	1 glass—6 ounces
Clear coffee or tea	

Dinner

Lean meat, fish, or poultry	4 ounces (cooked)
Vegetables (raw or cooked)	½ cup cooked raw, freely
Potato or bread	1 small potato or 1 slice of bread
Butter or margarine	1 level teaspoon
Skim milk	1 glass—6 ounces
Fruit (raw, cooked or canned without sugar)	1 serving—½ cup

Lunch or Supper

Cottage cheese or lean meat	½ cup of cheese or 2 ounces of meat
Vegetables (raw or cooked)	½ cup cooked raw, freely
Skim milk	1 glass—6 ounces
Fruit (raw, cooked or canned without sugar)	1 serving—½ cup

1,500-CALORIE DAILY DIET

Breakfast

Fresh fruit or juice	1 serving—½ cup
Egg—cooked without fat or	1
Cereal	1 serving of cereal (1 cup, prepared, or ½ cup, cooked)
Bread	1 slice
Butter or margarine	1 level teaspoon
Skim milk	1 cup—8 ounces
Coffee or tea	
Cream	1 tablespoon

Dinner

Lean meat, fish, or poultry	4 ounces (cooked)
Vegetables (raw or cooked)	½ cup cooked raw, freely
Potato	1 small
Butter or margarine	1 level teaspoon
Skim milk	1 cup—8 ounces
Fruit (raw, cooked or canned without sugar)	1 serving—½ cup

(continued)

Lunch or Supper

Cottage cheese or lean meat	½ cup of cheese or 2 ounces of meat
Vegetables (raw or cooked)	½ cup cooked raw, freely
Bread	1 slice
Butter or margarine	1 level teaspoon
Skim milk	1 cup—8 ounces
Fruit, plain custard, or plain cookies	½ cup of fruit or custard, or 2 cookies

Exercise

Exercise for the Senior Citizen*

In this "reasonable" exercise program planned for senior citizens there are three series of exercises, graded according to their difficulty or the amount of stress involved. They are identified as the *Red*, the *White*, and the *Blue* programs, with Red the easiest, White next, and Blue the most difficult and sustained. They let you start where you should, and they provide for an easy progression as you improve your physical condition.

Each of these three exercise programs is designed to give you a balanced workout, utilizing all major muscle groups. Performing the program regularly will lead to improvement in the various components of physical fitness, especially in functioning of the heart and lungs.

As you grow proficient at the exercises in your program, you should increase the number of repetitions of certain exercises, and increase the duration and speed of walking and jogging.

As you become able to increase the number of repetitions and handle more complicated and demanding exercises, you can move up to the next level.

Physical fitness can be improved by gradually increasing the amount of work performed, but it is necessary to progress in easy stages. The enthusiast who tackles a keep-fit program too fast and too strenuously soon gives up in discomfort, if not in injury.

Preexercise Tests

The test on the following pages will help you select your appropriate exercise level and pace.

Activity and Calorie Consumption**

Category 0 (Less than 1 calorie per minute)

Sleeping
Lying down

Category 1 (1–2 calories per minute)

Sitting—reading
Sitting—eating
Sitting—knitting, crafts
Sitting—listening to music, talking on telephone
Passenger in a car

Category 2 (2–3 calories per minute)

Standing up
Washing face
Sweeping
Driving a car
Bathing, showering
Deskwork
Painting at an easel
Playing musical instruments
Simple calisthenics—balancing, abdominal exercises

Category 3 (3–5 calories per minute)

Walking
Scrubbing floors
Washing windows
Making beds
Vacuuming
Ironing
Washing clothes by hand
Bowling
Shopping
Polishing floors

Category 4 (More than 5 calories per minute)

Walking up and down stairs
Carpentry
Mowing the lawn
Golf
Swimming
Skiing
Ballroom dancing
Tennis
Bicycling
Outdoor gardening
Active calisthenics—hopping, arm swinging
Jogging and running

---

*Source: President's Council on Physical Fitness, 1975.
**Source: DHEW, 1975.

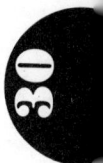

30

EXERCISE
670

Walk Test

The idea behind this walk test is to determine how many minutes, up to 10, you can walk briskly, without undue difficulty or discomfort, on a level surface. Test yourself outdoors preferably, but walking around the room indoors will do if necessary.

If you can finish three minutes, but no more, you should begin your daily exercise program with the RED level.

If you can go beyond three minutes, but not quite to ten minutes, you can *warm up* at the RED level for a week or two, and then move up to the WHITE level.

If you can breeze through the whole ten minutes, you are ready for the WHITE level.

The exercises in this program are not graded separately for men and women. More than likely, however, a man who has been active can start at a higher level or progress faster than most of the women who undertake the program.

Begin *very easily* and increase the tempo and number of repetitions *very gradually*. This will keep stiffness and soreness to a minimum. If you do get a little stiff during the first few days, don't let it slow you down; the stiffness will soon be overcome and it is an indication that you *needed* the activity.

Follow the directions for your exercise exactly. If, for example, you are at the RED level and a particular exercise should be performed only twice as a starter, stop after two repetitions—even though you may feel you can do many more. A warm-up is built into each exercise series.

RED Program

- Try to complete the entire sequence without undue rest periods between exercises, but of course, rest awhile if you feel overtaxed.

- For the first week at least, perform only the smallest number of repetitions or shortest duration of time shown for each exercise under its illustration (pages 10–18). If you find even this amount to be strenuous, or if you feel fatigued at the end of the week, do not increase the repetitions or duration but continue at the same pace for another week.

- After the first week—or as you are ready—in each exercise where a range of repetitions is shown, increase the minimum by *one*. Do this number, but no more, the second week. (If you need to stay at the lowest count, as explained above, don't increase the count at all.) In the following weeks, gradually increase the number of repetitions as you feel you can. Most people should take three to four weeks to reach the highest counts in the RED program.

- After you reach the point where you can do the higher number of repetitions shown for each exercise, continue on the RED level until you can complete the whole series without resting between exercises.

- When you can do this for three days in a row, move on to the WHITE level.

WHITE and BLUE Programs

For the WHITE and BLUE programs (as in the RED program) start at the lowest frequency of repetitions and gradually work up.

- Most people should remain at the WHITE level for three to five weeks before moving to the BLUE.

- When you reach the upper limits of the BLUE exercises and can go through the workout without stopping on three straight days, you are ready to: (1) continue with the exercises in this book, gradually increasing the number and speed of repetitions, the distances walked and jogged, and also engage in more sports and recreational activities; or (2) go on to more difficult exercises.

Note: For those ready for more difficult exercises, send for: *Adult Physical Fitness—A Program for Men and Women,* a President's Council on Physical Fitness publication, available from the Superintendent of Documents, U.S. Government Printing Office, Washington, D.C. 20402, 35 cents.

Order of exercises*

RED program sequence	WHITE program sequence	BLUE program sequence
	Exercises** to be performed in the following order.	
Walk 2 minutes	Walk 3 minutes	Alternate Walk (50 steps)/Jog (50)
Bend and Stretch (2–10 times)	Bend and Stretch (10 times)	3 minutes
Rotate Head (2–10 times each way)	Rotate Head (10 times each way)	Bend and Stretch (10 times)
Body Bender (2–5 times)	Body Bender (5–10 times)	Rotate Head (10 times each way)
Wall Press (2–5 times)	Wall Press (5 times)	Body Bender (10 times)
Arm Circles (5 each way)	Arm Circles (5–10 each way)	Wall Press (5 times)
Wing Stretcher (2–5 times)	Half-Knee Bend (5–10 times)	Arm Circles (10–15 each way)
Walk 2–5 minutes	Wing Stretcher (5–10 times)	Half-Knee Bend (10–15 times)
Lying Leg Bend (2–5 times each leg)	Wall Push-Away (10 times)	Wing Stretcher (10–20 times)
Angel Stretch (2–5 times)	Walk 5 minutes	Alternate Walk (50 steps)/Jog (50)
Walk-a-Straight-Line (walk 10 feet)	Lying Leg Bend (5–10 times each leg)	3 minutes
Half-Knee Bend (2–5 times)	Angel Stretch (5 times)	Leg Raise and Bend (2–5 times each leg)
Wall Push-Away (2–10 times)	Walk-the-Beam (walk 10 feet)	Angel Stretch (5 times)
Side Leg Raise (2–5 times each leg)	(2-inch by 6-inch beam)	Walk-the-Beam (walk 10 feet)
Head and Shoulder Curl (2–5 times, hold 4 seconds)	Knee Push Up (1–3 times)	(2-inch by 4-inch beam)
Alternate Walk (50 steps)/Jog (10)	Side Leg Raise (5–10 times each leg)	Hop (5 times on each foot)
1–3 minutes	Head and Shoulder Curl (5 times, hold 6 seconds)	Knee Push Up (3–6 times)
Walk 1–3 minutes	(arms crossed on chest)	Side Leg Raise (10 times)
	Diver's Stance (hold for 10 seconds)	Head and Shoulder Curl (5 times, hold 10 seconds)
	Alternate Walk (50 steps)/Jog (25)	(hands clasped behind neck)
	3–6 minutes	Stork Stand (10 seconds on each leg)
	Walk 1–3 minutes	Alternate Walk (50 steps)/Jog (50)
		5 minutes, gradually increasing to
		walk 100 steps/jog 100
		Walk 3 minutes

*Note: Some of the exercises illustrated are not included in the RED or WHITE exercise programs and should not be performed by those following either of these programs.
**Illustrations of each exercise and figures for number of repetitions or length of time to perform it, appear on the following pages. Where two figures are given, start at the lower figure: gradually increase the repetitions or duration over a period of days or weeks until you can perform the higher number.

30

Exercises

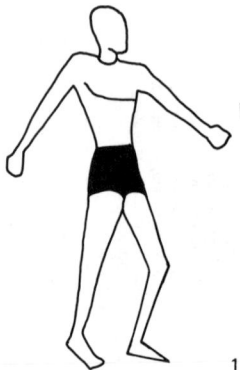

1

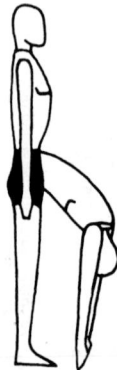

3

1. Walk

Starting position: Stand erect, balanced on balls of feet.

Action: Simply begin walking briskly on a level space, preferably outdoors, but walking around the room will do if necessary.

Value: A good warm-up exercise, loosening muscles, and preparing you for your full exercise schedule.

After vigorous exercise:

Value: Tapering off, as heart rate, breathing, body heat and other functions return to normal.

3. Bend and Stretch

Starting position: Stand erect, feet shoulder-width apart.

Action: Count 1. Bend trunk forward and down, flexing knees. Stretch gently in attempt to touch fingers to toes or floor. Count 2. Return to starting position.

Note: Do slowly, stretch and relax at intervals rather than in rhythm.

Value: Helps loosen and stretch most muscles of body; helps relaxation; aids in "warm-up" for more vigorous exercise.

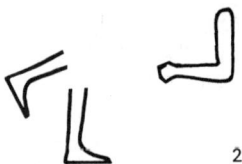

2

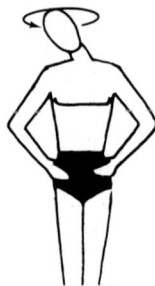

4

2. Alternate Walk-Jog

Starting position: As for walking, arms held flexed, forearms generally parallel to the ground.

Action: Jogging is a form of slow running. Begin walking for 50 steps, then shift to a slow run with easy strides, landing lightly each time on the heel of the foot and transfer weight to the whole foot in flatfooted style. (Heel-toe running in contrast to the sprint in which the runner stays on balls of his feet.) Arms should move loosely and freely from the shoulders in opposition to legs. Breathing should be deep but not labored to point of gasping.

Value: Good warm-up for more advanced exercises. Good for legs and circulation.

4. Rotate Head

Starting position: Stand erect, feet shoulder-width apart; hands on hips.

Action: Count 1. Slowly rotate the head in a full circle from left to right. Count 2. Slowly rotate head in the opposite direction.

Note: Use slow, smooth motion; close eyes to help avoid losing balance or getting dizzy.

Value: Helps loosen and relax muscles of the neck, and firm up throat and chin line.

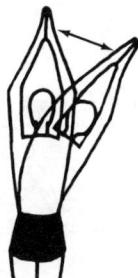

5

5. Body Bender

Starting position: Stand with feet shoulder-width apart, hands extended overhead, fingertips touching.

Action: Count 1. Bend trunk slowly sideward to left as far as possible, keeping hands together and arms straight (don't bend elbows). Count 2. Return to starting position. Counts 3 and 4. Repeat to the right.

Value: Stretches arm, trunk and leg muscles.

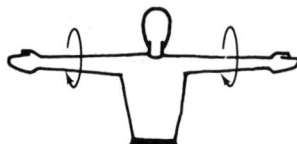

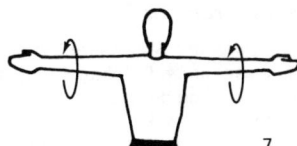

7

7. Arm Circles

Starting position: Stand erect, arms extended sideward at shoulder height, palms up.

Action: Describe small circles backward with hands. Keep head erect. Reverse, turn palms down and do circles forward.

Value: Helps keep shoulder joint flexible; strengthens muscles of shoulders.

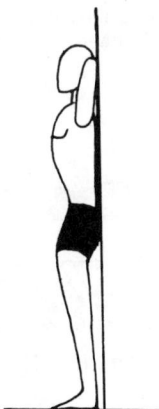

6

6. Wall Press

Starting position: Stand erect, head not bent forward or backward, back against wall, heels about 3 inches away from wall.

Action: Count 1. Pull in the abdominal muscles and press the small of the back tight against the wall. Hold for six seconds. Count 2. Relax and return to starting position.

Note: Keep entire back in contact with wall on Count 1 and do not tilt the head backward.

Value: Promotes good body alignment and posture. Strengthens abdominal muscles.

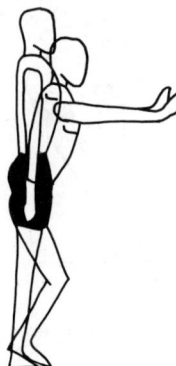

8

8. Half-Knee Bend

Starting position: Stand erect, hands on hips.

Action: Count 1. Bend knees halfway while extending arms forward, palms down. Keep heels on floor. Count 2. Return to starting position.

Value: Firms up leg muscles and stretches muscles in front of legs. Helps improve balance.

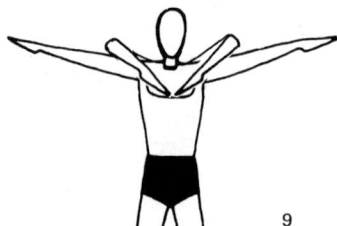

9

9. Wing Stretcher

Starting position: Stand erect, bend arms in front of chest, extended finger tips touching and elbows at shoulder height. Counts 1, 2, 3. Pull elbows back as far as possible, keeping arms at shoulder height and returning to starting position each time. Count 4. Swing arms outward and sideward, shoulder height, palms up and return to starting position.

Note: This is a bouncy, rhythmic action, counting "one-and-two-and-three-and-four."

Value: Strengthens muscles of upper back and shoulders; stretches chest muscles. Helps promote good posture and prevent "dowager hump."

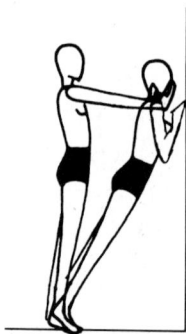

10

10. Wall Push-Away

Starting position: Stand erect, feet about six inches apart, facing a wall and arms straight in front, palms on wall, bearing weight slightly. Count 1. Bend elbows and lower body slowly toward wall, meanwhile turning head to the side, until cheek almost touches the wall. Count 2. Push against wall with the arms and return to the starting position.

Note: Keep heels on floor throughout the exercise.

Value: Increases strength of arm, shoulder and upper-back muscles. Stretches muscles in chest and back of legs.

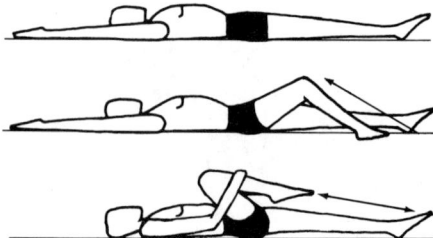

11

11. Lying Leg Bend

Starting position: Lie on back, legs extended, feet together, arms at sides.

Action: Count 1. Bend left knee and move left foot toward buttocks, keeping foot in light contact with floor. Count 2. Move knee toward chest as far as possible, using abdominal, hip, and leg muscles; *then* clasp knee with both hands and pull slowly toward chest. Count 3. Return to position at end of count 1. Count 4. Return to starting position.

Note: After completing desired number of repetitions with left leg, repeat the exercise using right leg.

Value: Improves flexibility of knee and hip joints; and strengthens abdominal and hip muscles.

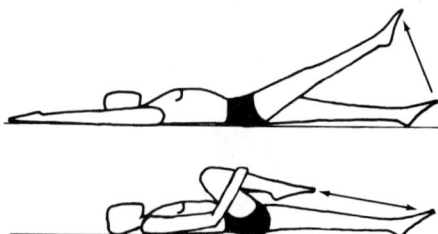

12

12. Leg Raise and Bend

(After completing desired number with left leg, do exercise with right leg.)

Starting position: Lie on back, legs extended, feet together, arms at sides.

Action: Count 1. Raise extended left leg about 12 inches off the floor. Count 2. Bend knee and move knee toward chest as far as possible, using abdominal, hip, and leg muscles; *then* clasp knee with both hands and pull slowly toward chest. Count 3. Return to position at end of count 1. Count 4. Return to starting position.

Value: Improves flexibility of knee and hip joints; strengthens abdominal muscles.

30

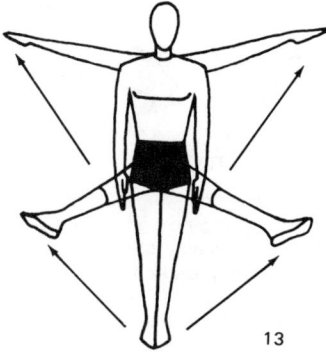

13. Angel Stretch

Starting position: Lie on back, legs straight, feet together; arms extended at sides.

Action: Count 1. Move arms and legs outward along the floor to a "spread-eagle" position. Slide—do not raise—arms and legs. Count 2. Return to starting position.

Note: Throughout the exercise try to compress the lower back against the floor by tightening the abdominal muscles. Do not "arch" the lower back.

Value: Stretches muscles of arms, legs, trunk; aids posture; improves strength of abdominal muscles.

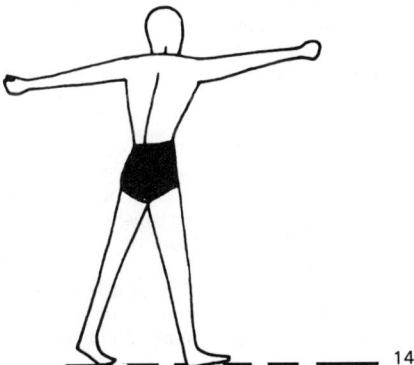

14. Walk a Straight Line

(Walk for 10 feet.)

Starting position: Stand erect with left foot along a straight line. Arms held away from body to aid balance.

Action: Count 1. Walk the length of the straight line by putting the right foot in front of the left foot with right heel touching left toe, and then placing the feet alternately one in front of the other, heel-to-toe. Count 2. Return to the starting point by walking backward along the line, alternately placing one foot behind the other, toe-to-heel.

Value: Improves balance; helps posture.

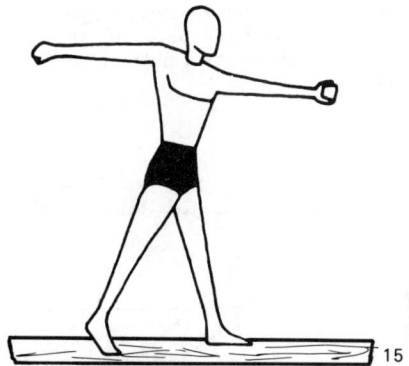

15. Walk the Beam

Starting position: Stand erect with left foot on board, long axis of foot in line with board.

Action: Count 1. Walk the length of the board by putting the right foot in front of the left foot with right heel touching left toe, and then placing the feet alternately one in front of the other, heel-to-toe. Count 2. Return to the starting point by walking backward along the length of the board, alternately placing one foot behind the other, toe-to-heel.

Note: The board is placed flat on the floor, not on the 2" edge.

Value: Improves balance; helps posture.

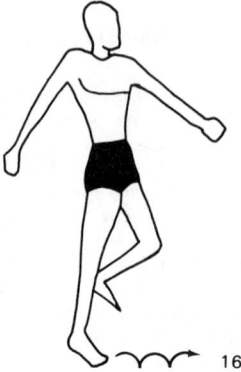

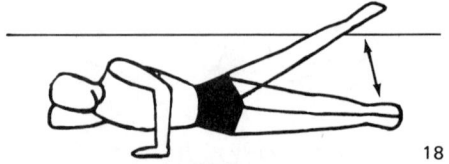

18. Side Leg Raise

Starting position: Right side of body on floor, head resting on right arm. Count 1. Lift left leg sidewards about 30" off floor. Count 2. Return to starting position.

Note: Do the desired number of repetitions with the left leg and then turn over, lie on left side and exercise the right leg.

Value: Helps improve flexibility of the hip joint and strengthens lateral muscles of trunk and hip.

16. Hop

Starting position: Stand erect, weight on right foot, left leg bent slightly at the knee, and left foot held a few inches off the floor; arms held sidewards slightly away from the body to aid balance.

Action: Count 1. Hop on right foot, moving few inches forward each hop.

Note: Perform the desired number of hops on right leg, then change to left leg and hop.

Value: Improves balance, strengthens extensor muscles of leg and foot; increases circulation.

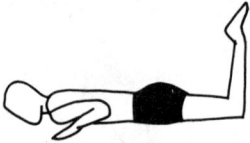

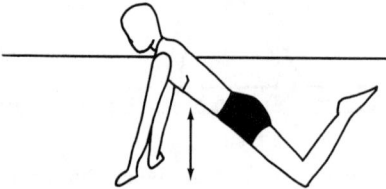

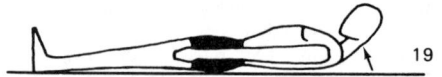

19. Head and Shoulder Curl

Starting position: Lie on back, legs straight, feet together, arms extended along the front of the legs with palms resting lightly on the thighs.

Action: Count 1. Tighten abdominal muscles and lift head and shoulders so that shoulders are about 10 inches off the floor. Meanwhile slide arms along the legs, keeping them extended. Then hold the position for 4 seconds. Count 2. Return slowly to starting position, keeping abdominal muscles tight until shoulders and head rest on floor. Relax.

Note: The head should lead in a "curling" motion, chin tucked to chest, back rounded, not arched.

Value: Excellent for improving abdominal strength and stretching back muscles.

BLUE: Same as RED except hold each for 6 seconds and on starting position arms are crossed over chest (kept in that position throughout).

WHITE: Same as RED except hold each for 10 seconds and on starting position, hands are clasped behind the neck (held that way throughout).

17. Knee Push Up

Starting position: Lie on floor, face down, legs together, knees bent with feet raised off floor, hands on floor under shoulders, palms down.

Action: Count 1. Push upper body off floor until arms are fully extended and body is in straight line from head to knees. Count 2. Return to starting position.

Value: Strengthens muscles of arms, shoulders and trunk.

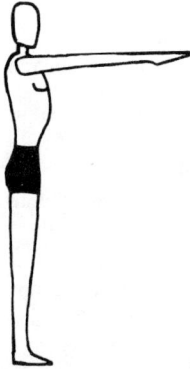

20

21

20. Diver's Stance

Starting position: Stand erect, feet slightly apart, arms at sides.

Action: Rise on toes and bring arms upward and forward so that they extend parallel with the floor, palms down. When this position is attained, close eyes and hold balance for 10 seconds.

Note: Head should be straight and body should be held firmly throughout.

Value: Improves balance; strengthens extensor muscles of feet and legs; helps maintain good posture.

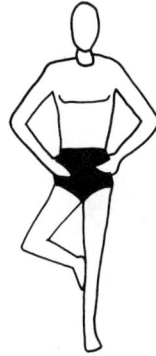

21. Stork Stand

(BLUE only—hold position 10 seconds on each leg.)

Starting position: Stand erect, feet slightly apart, hands on hips, head straight.

Action: Transfer weight to the left foot and bend right knee, bringing the sole of the right foot to the inner side of the left knee. When this position is reached, close eyes and hold for 10 seconds.

Note: After holding on left leg, change to the right leg and repeat.

Value: Improves balance.

Which Sports Provide the Best Exercise*

Seven prominent doctors were asked to rate 14 particular sports. Following are selected comments.

Walking

Excellent for reconditioning, but not a great added stimulus for those in "good" condition. Great for fitness if done at a brisk, steady pace.

Jogging

The most efficient and inexpensive approach to enhancing endurance capacity. Must be approached with warm-up preliminaries and a "starter" program of walk-jog alternations.

Excellent for cardiovascular fitness; unfit

people should start with a calisthenics program to first attain minimum muscular fitness, otherwise muscle strain, back pain, etc., often result.

Calisthenics

Value rests entirely on the vigor of the exercise program; properly prescribed exercises are particularly valuable for muscle and joint flexibility.

A good calisthenics program should contain relaxation and limbering exercises, should build up slowly from relaxation to warm-up to workout and then return to cool-off and finally relaxation.

Swimming

Good for people recovering from hip, knee and ankle problems. Magnificent exercise, but it neglects the weight bearing, antigravity musculature of the body. It should be balanced by something like jogging for all-round muscular development.

*Source: "What Sport Is Best for the Body," *Esquire,* October 1974 Quotes from: Interviews of President's Council on Physical Fitness and Sports. Reprinted by permission of Esquire Magazine © 1974 by Esquire Magazine Inc.

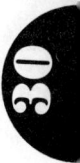

30

Bicycling

Good fitness-building activity, primarily cardio-vascular. Calorie consuming, thus weight reducing.

Golf

A very fine recreational pastime but as played today, utilizing a caddy and/or a golf cart, it provides so little exercise that it is practically useless from the physical-fitness standpoint.

Tennis

Splendid exercise for almost all purposes except bilateral symmetrical upper-body development; has value for the development of cardio-vascular fitness—depends on the manner in which one plays.

Bowling

Not enough exercise to have a pronounced effect on physical fitness, but it's better than nothing.

Touch Football

Does little for fitness, a lot for injuries; keeps the orthopedists busy.

Handball/Squash

Excellent endurance stimulation. Should warm up prior to play. Demands on ligaments and joints may cause problems in middle to later years.

Basketball

A sport for the already fit. You don't play to get fit; you must be fit to play it.

Softball

No good to create fitness; not too valuable for fitness maintenance either.

Alpine/Nordic Skiing

Alpine: can maintain and improve fitness. It is especially important to have good basic muscular tone; otherwise, there is great exposure to injury.

Nordic: excellent for fitness; need to be pre-conditioned to gain maximum muscular fitness.

Ice/Roller Skating

Good for fitness building and maintenance for people who have the necessary muscular fitness.

31

MATERNAL, INFANT AND CHILD HEALTH

Overview

Facts and Figures*

Health problems of mothers and children are best described by the following statistics, reported by the National Institutes of Health:

- Although the national infant mortality rate has fallen from 22.4 to 17.6 deaths per 1000 live births over the last six years, the United States has dropped from fourteenth to fifteenth position among developed countries.
- Approximately 7.6%, or 238,000, of the infants born in the United States in 1973 were born either too soon or too small, weighing less than 5.5 pounds. One out of every four of these babies had a teenage mother. Approximately 42,000 of these babies died within their first month of life.
- Of the low birth weight babies born each year, about 60,000 will have life-long disabilities, including mental retardation.
- Approximately 7,500 infants succumb to the sudden infant death syndrome each year.
- Of all babies born in this country, 3.5% show evidence of a birth defect during the first month of life; 7% have developed identifiable defects by the end of the first year.
- Each year an estimated 200,000 children are struck by handicaps which could have been prevented if their mothers had received early health care.

- Forty percent of the young children of this country are not fully immunized against childhood diseases.
- Approximately seven million children between the ages of 10 and 18 in the United States suffer some major impairment including communicative disorders, learning disabilities and aberrant functional and skeletal development.

Hospital Births**

(The National Hospital Panel Survey (AHA) in 1976 reported. . . .)

For the second consecutive year, the number of births in U.S. community hospitals has increased. This increase in births reflects a population increase rather than a change in the birthrate, which remains at the 13-year low point recorded in the past three years by the National Hospital Panel Survey. Nevertheless, the upswing in newborn statistics may have an important impact on the utilization of newborn and obstetrical units.

Community hospital newborn statistics, presented (below) exhibit the changes in newborn utilization that have occurred during the years ending September 30, 1971 through 1975. The number of births increased by nearly 60,000 in 1975 to a four-year high of three million births. This change was somewhat less than the 82,000 birth increase experienced in 1974.

*Source: House Appropriations Committee Hearings, 1977.

**Source: "Newborn Statistics," *Hospitals, J.A.H.A.*, March 1976. Reprinted by permission of the American Hospital Association.

Table 31-1   Newborn statistics for community hospitals

Statistics	1971	1972	1973	1974	1975
Bassinets[1]	90,547	87,840	84,699	86,209	84,783
Births	3,274,452	2,955,741	2,859,170	2,941,173	3,000,699
Newborn days	13,654,188	12,253,776	11,727,228	11,951,884	12,075,286
Newborn daily census	37,409	33,480	32,129	32,745	33,083
Newborn occupancy	41.30	38.10	37.90	38.00	39.00
Newborn length of stay	4.2	4.1	4.1	4.1	4.0

[1]12-month average.

Source: National Hospital Panel Survey.

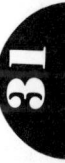

Mortality

Infant and Maternal Mortality—Summary

Table 31-2   Infant, and maternal mortality rate per live births, United States 1949–73

Year	Infant rate per 1,000			Maternal rate per 100,000		
	Total	White	All other	Total	White	All other
1973	17.6	15.2	28.8	—	—	—
1972	18.5	16.4	27.7	18.8	14.3	38.5
1971	19.1	17.1	28.5	18.8	13.0	45.3
1970	20.0	17.8	30.9	21.5	14.4	55.9
1969	20.9	18.4	32.9	22.2	15.5	55.7
1968	21.8	19.2	34.5	24.5	16.6	63.6
1967	22.4	19.7	35.9	28.0	19.5	69.5
1966	23.7	20.6	38.8	29.1	20.2	72.4
1965	24.7	21.5	40.3	31.6	21.0	83.7
1964	24.8	21.6	41.1	33.3	22.3	89.9
1963	25.2	22.2	41.5	35.8	24.0	96.9
1962	25.3	22.3	41.4	35.2	23.8	95.9
1961	25.3	22.4	40.7	36.9	24.9	101.3
1960	26.0	22.9	43.2	37.1	26.0	97.9
1959	26.4	23.2	44.0	37.4	25.8	102.1
1958	27.1	23.8	45.7	37.6	26.3	101.8
1957	26.3	23.3	43.7	41.0	27.5	118.3
1956	26.0	23.2	42.1	40.9	28.7	110.7
1955	26.4	23.6	42.8	47.0	32.8	130.3
1954	26.6	23.9	42.9	52.4	37.2	143.8
1953	27.8	25.0	44.7	61.1	44.1	166.1
1952	28.4	25.5	47.0	67.8	48.9	188.1
1951	28.4	25.8	44.8	75.0	54.9	201.3
1950	29.2	26.8	44.5	83.3	61.1	221.6
1949	31.3	28.9	47.3	90.3	68.1	234.8

Source: Vital Statistics of the United States.

Infant Mortality*

Recent Trends

Since the mid-1950s there has been serious concern about the slackening decline in the infant mortality rate which the United States has been experiencing since the early part of the century.

Despite medical advances, expansion and improvement of health facilities, greater availability of medical and other health personnel, and increased activity within public and private health and welfare agencies, there had been no sizable decrease in infant mortality during the 1950s and relatively small decreases thereafter.

*Source: DHEW, 1975.

Race—The infant mortality rate for other than white infants in 1974 was 28.8 per thousand live births, nearly twice as much as for white infants (15.2 per thousand live births).

Region—There is wide disparity in infant mortality among the states. The most favorable infant mortality is 15.95 deaths per 1,000 live births in North Dakota. The most disturbing is in Mississippi where the infant mortality rate is 31.9 per thousand live births. Infant mortality rates by age, by death and color, are consistently higher in the lowest income states than in the United States as a whole.

Urban Areas—Infant mortality rates in large urban areas tend to be higher than the national average. The infant mortality rate in the 26 U.S. cities with 500,000 or more population in 1970 was 15% higher than the national average. However, they ranged from 17.7 per 1,000 live births in San Francisco to 29.6 in Pittsburgh.

The high infant mortality rates in urban areas are generally attributed to rapid population growth, shortages of professional personnel, and inadequate expansion of facilities, as well as deterioration of some existing facilities.

Cause of Death

Seventy-five percent of infant deaths occur in the neonatal period when many deaths are ascribed on death certificates to nonspecific categories such as "immaturity unqualified" and "asphyxia of the newborn." These "catchall" categories reflect a lack of knowledge about and incomplete recording of the causes of death.

However, an analysis of causes of death from 1965–73, when total infant mortality declined from 24.7 per 1,000 live births to 17.6 per 1,000 live births, shows that while mortality decreased in all categories, there were variations. Mortality from influenza and pneumonia (65% reduction), certain gastrointestinal diseases (50% reduction), immaturity unqualified (48% reduction), and asphyxia of the newborn (47% reduction), declined by amounts greater than the decline in overall infant mortality.

Congenital anomalies decreased 24%, about the same as the decline in total infant mortality. Birth injuries showed a 14% reduction.

Underlying Causes

Causative factors underlying and leading to infant deaths include environmental or socioeconomic factors and biological or developmental factors. It is belived that biological factors are more important in the neonatal period while environmental factors play a more prominent role in the postneonatal period.

There has been an increased interest in public health with newer types of health services made available to large groups of people, especially those at high risk, primarily through federal funds. There has been growing use of family planning, changes in abortion laws and views on family size, as reflected in decreasing birth rates.

There is strong evidence of a positive correlation between the receipt of maternal health care services and the reduction of infant mortality. There is further indication that health services play a particularly important role in infant mortality reduction in the neonatal period (0–28 days) when three-fourths of all infant deaths occur. The nonmedical factors appear to have an effect more on post-neonatal period (29 days to one year).

World Rates of Infant Mortality

In 1950 a comparison of infant mortality in 18 countries with a population of 1 million or more, where virtually all vital events are registered, showed the United States ranking 6th. In 1960 the United States ranked 10th, and by 1973 had fallen to 18th.

Table 31-3 Infant mortality rates for selected countries

Country	Rates per 1,000 births	% Decrease since 1961
Sweden	9.6	39.2
Iceland	9.6	50.8
Finland	10.1	51.4
Japan	11.3	60.5
Netherlands	11.5	32.4
Norway	11.8	34.1
Denmark (1972)	12.2	44.0
Switzerland	13.2	37.1
Luxemburg	14.3	45.0
Spain	15.1	67.3
France	15.5	39.5
East Germany	16.0	52.5
New Zealand	16.2	28.9
Australia	16.5	15.4
Canada	16.8	38.2
Belgium	17.0	39.5
United Kingdom	17.2	22.2
United States of America	17.6	30.4

Source: Statistical Office of the United Nations, 1975.

Maternal Mortality

Trends

Between 1916 and 1929 the maternal mortality rate was relatively static. Toward the end of the 1920s a downward trend appeared. About 1936, however, the rate of decline in maternal mortality became precipitous. A combination of factors played a role in the decline: formation of hospital and community committees to investigate the cause and circumstances of each maternal death and assign

682

responsibility for it; increased hospitalization for delivery; availability of sulfa drugs for the control of infections; and availability of blood and blood substitutes for treatment of hemorrhage. As a result, the maternal mortality rate was cut by almost two-thirds within nine years (1936–1945).

After World War II the rate of decline accelerated and by 1949 the maternal mortality rate had dropped to 90.3 per 100,000 live births. Increased use of hospitals for delivery and the general availability of antibiotics after World War II contributed to this situation. The rate continued downward and by 1956 stood at 40.9 per 100,000. This downward trend slowed markedly, however, and in the eight years between 1957 and 1964, there were only minor decreases. The downward trend then resumed, resulting in a maternal mortality rate of 18.8 per 100,000 in 1972 reflecting the decrease in maternal deaths resulting from abortion, as state laws were reformed.

However, there continue to be marked differences between white and nonwhite maternal mortality rates. In 1950 the nonwhite maternal mortality rate of 221.6 per 100,000 live births was 260% higher than the white maternal mortality rate of 61.1 per 100,000 live births. In 1972 the data show a nonwhite maternal mortality rate of 38.5 per 100,000 live births, 170% higher than the corresponding white maternal mortality rate of 14.3. Despite a narrowing of the gap, mothers of other races are still nearly a full generation behind white mothers in mortality due to conditions arising in pregnancy and childbirth.

Causes and Related Factors

The three major causes of maternal mortality in 1972 were sepsis, toxemia, and hemorrhage. This was true for white women, but the third major cause for other than white women was abortion, rather than hemorrhage.

Though the maternal mortality rate for all women declined by 13% over the three-year period 1970 to 1972, the maternal mortality rate for two causes declined by a greater amount. Mortality from abortion declined by 38% and from toxemia by 26%. Many of the important factors in the reduction of maternal mortality are related to medical advances and changing concepts of obstetrics and public health. The expansion of maternal health programs, increased availability of prenatal care, and liberalization of state abortion laws have been major influences in reducing maternal

mortality. The fact that most deliveries now occur in hospitals where increased supervision and specialized obstetric care are available is also an important consideration, as is the improved obstetrical training of physicians and nurses.

There are several remaining problems. Many women still do not receive adequate prenatal care and many high-risk women are not being given needed, specialized care. More extensive distribution of resources and current knowledge could effect further reductions in maternal mortality.

Birth Defects*

Overview

Every year, more than 200,000 American children are born with birth defects. They may be crippled, mentally retarded, blind, deaf, anemic, diabetic or handicapped in hundreds of other ways.

About 20% of birth defects are inherited. The remaining 80% are thought to result from environmental influences or a combination of environment and heredity. When defects commonly occur together, they are termed a syndrome.

The Victims

- Birth defects strike 7% of American babies born each year, or about one in 14. Every hour, 25 children are born with defects.
- Many of these children die in infancy. The others, with medical help and special training, may overcome their defects to lead useful, though often limited lives.
- Birth defects kill more than 60,000 persons of all ages every year. Another half-million potential lives are wiped out by miscarriages and stillbirths, largely owing to faulty fetal development.
- *Marital status:* unmarried mothers are at a higher risk of perinatal complications, in particular, premature delivery. For example, one report indicated that complications of pregnancy occurred 1⅓ times as frequently for the unmarried mother as for the married mother. Complications may result more from the inadequate prenatal care than the unmarried status itself.
- *Race:* evidence indicates that women from

---

*Source: The National Foundation March of Dimes—unless otherwise indicated.

nonwhite groups have a higher degree of obstetrical risk than do Caucasian women. However, race is not considered a pure factor; social class and degree of obstetrical care are confounded with it. Race is associated as a predictive factor as it correlates with other variables, degrees of prenatal care, diet adequacy and general health.

- *Social class:* class is significant also because causal variables are correlated with it. Among the poor there is a higher rate of unmarried pregnancies, poor diet, infectious environments, and inadequate antenatal and postnatal care. Each of these characteristics can be shown to be independently related to suboptimal outcomes of pregnancy.
- *Age:* A higher proportion of defects occurs when mothers are under 17 or over 37 years of age.

The Problems

There are now 15 million Americans whose daily lives are affected in some way by birth defects. Each year, some 1.2 million infants, children and adults are hospitalized for treatment.

The National Foundation-March of Dimes estimates that birth defects are responsible for:
- 2.9 million mentally retarded
- 4 million with diabetes
- 1 million with congenital bone, muscle or joint disease
- 500,000 born completely or partially blind
- 750,000 with congenital hearing impairment
- 350,000 with heart or circulatory defects
- 100,000 with severe speech problems
- millions of others with defects of the nervous, digestive, endocrine, urinary and other body systems.

Incidence and Death Toll

Table 31-4 Estimated incidence and prevalence of selected birth defects, U.S.A., 1975

Condition	Newly affected	Under age 20 with condition currently
Anencephaly	3,100	
Spina bifida and/or hydrocephalus	6,200	53,000
Cleft lip and/or cleft palate	4,300	71,000
Congenital heart disease	24,800	248,000
Clubfoot	9,300	149,000
Congenital dislocation of hip	3,100	50,000
Polydactyly	9,300	184,000
Syndactyly	1,000	21,000
Cystic fibrosis	2,000	10,000
Hemophilia	1,200	12,400
Phenylketonuria	310	3,100
Sickle-cell anemia	1,200	16,000
Tay-Sachs disease	30	100
Thalassemia (Cooley's anemia)	70	1,000
Diabetes	+	90,000
Down's syndrome	5,100	44,000
Other mental retardation of prenatal origin	44,000	800,000

+ Late-appearing birth defect. *Fatal soon after birth.

Note: Some children have more than one kind of birth defect; hence the total number with one or more of the specific defects cited is smaller than the sum of the numbers for each condition.

Table 31-5 Birth defects annual death toll

Cause of death		Number of deaths
Diabetes mellitus		38,208
Cystic fibrosis		519
Other hereditary metabolic diseases		1,067
Structural defects:		
Heart and other circulatory defects	6,964	
Genitourinary defects	877	
Anencephalus	795	
Hydrocephalus	706	
Spina bifida	592	
Other nervous system defects	670	
Digestive system defects	693	
Respiratory system defects	658	
Musculoskeletal defects	401	
Multiple structural defects	1,428	
Other structural defects	280	
Total structural defects		14,064
Hereditary diseases of blood		2,420
Hereditary neuromuscular diseases		1,316
Certain abdominal hernias		859
Hemorrhagic disease of newborn		454
Hemolytic disease of newborn (including Rh disease)		378
Gout		297
Diseases of newborn due to maternal infections		175
Hemangioma and lymphangioma		73
Total		59,830

Source: Vital Statistics of the United States, 1973.

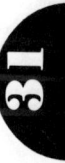

Table 31-6 Selected birth defects, U.S.A.

Birth defect	Type	Annual Incidence*	Prevalence**
Down's syndrome (mongolism)	functional/structural: retardation often associated with physical defects	5,100	44,000
Low birthweight (weighing 4 lbs. 6 oz. or less)/ prematurity	structural/functional; organs often immature	50,000	NA
Muscular dystrophy	functional: impaired voluntary muscular function	unknown (late-appearing)	200,000
Congenital heart malformations	structural	24,800	248,000
Clubfoot	structural: misshapen foot	9,300	149,000
Polydactyly	structural: multiple fingers or toes	9,300	184,000
Spina bifida and/or hydrocephalus	structural/functional: incompletely formed spinal canal; "water on the brain"	6,200	53,000
Cleft lip and/or cleft palate	structural	4,300	71,000
Diabetes mellitus	metabolic: inability to metabolize carbohydrates	unknown (late-appearing)	90,000
Cystic fibrosis	functional: respiratory and digestive system malfunction	2,000	10,000
Sickle cell anemia	blood disease: malformed red blood cells	1,200	16,000
Hemophilia (classic)	blood disease: poor clotting ability	1,200	12,400
Congenital syphilis	structural: multiple abnormalities	(newborn only) 180	NA
Phenylketonuria (PKU)	metabolic: inability to metabolize a specific amino acid	310	3,100
Tay-Sachs disease	metabolic: inability to metabolize fats in nervous system	30	100
Thalassemia	blood disease: anemia	70	1,000
Galactosemia	metabolic: inability to metabolize milk sugar galactose	70	500
Erythroblastosis (Rh disease)	blood disease: destruction of red blood cells	7,000	NA
Turner syndrome	structural/functional	575	3,100
Congenital rubella syndrome	structural/functional multiple defects	varies with occurrence of disease; less than 50	NA

*Incidence: the number of new cases diagnosed within a specific time period.

**Prevalence: total number living who have been diagnosed as having defect. Above statistics based on number less than 20 years of age.

Cause	Detection***	Treatment***	Prevention***
chromosomal abnormality	amniocentesis, chromosome analysis	corrective surgery, special physical training and schooling	genetics services
hereditary and/or environmental: maternal disorder or malnutrition	prenatal monitoring, visual inspection at birth	intensive care of newborn, high nutrient diet	proper prenatal care, genetics services, maternal nutrition
hereditary: often recessive inheritance	apparent at onset	physical therapy	genetics services
hereditary and/or environmental	examination at birth and later	corrective surgery, medication	genetics services
hereditary and/or environmental	examination at birth	corrective surgery, corrective splints, physical training	genetics services
hereditary: dominant inheritance	visual inspection of birth	corrective surgery, physical training	genetics services
hereditary and environmental	amniocentesis, prenatal X-ray, ultrasound, maternal blood test, examination at birth	corrective surgery, prostheses, physical training, special schooling for any mental impairment	genetics services
hereditary and/or environmental	visual inspection at birth	corrective surgery	genetics services
hereditary and/or environmental	appears in childhood or later; blood and urine tests	oral medication, special diet, insulin injections	genetics services
hereditary: recessive inheritance	sweat and blood tests	treat respiratory and digestive complications	genetics services
hereditary: incomplete recessive—most frequent among Blacks	blood test	transfusions	genetics services
hereditary: sex-linked recessive inheritance	blood test	clotting factor	genetics services
environmental: acquired from infected mother	blood test, examination or birth	medication	proper prenatal care
hereditary: recessive inheritance	blood test at birth	special diet	carrier identification, genetics services
hereditary: recessive inheritance—most frequent among Ashkenazi Jews	blood and tear tests, amniocentesis	none	carrier identification, genetics services
hereditary: incomplete recessive inheritance	blood test	transfusions	carrier identification, genetics services
hereditary: recessive inheritance	blood and urine tests, amniocentesis	special diet	carrier identification, genetics services
hereditary and environmental: Rh− mother has Rh+ child	blood tests	transfusion: intrauterine or postnatal	Rh vaccine, blood tests to identify women at risk, genetics services
chromosomal abnormality	amniocentesis chromosome analysis	corrective surgery, medication	genetics services
environmental: maternal infection	antibody tests and viral culture	corrective surgery, prostheses, physical therapy and training	rubella vaccine

***Last three columns list possible means now known for detection, treatment, and prevention. The techniques may not necessarily be applicable or successful in every case.

Source: The National Foundation-March of Dimes.

Inherited vs. Environmentally Caused Birth Defects

Inherited Birth Defects

Genetic Disorders—Originate by mutation—a change in a gene's molecular structure. Possible causes include natural or man-made radiation, foreign chemicals and drugs and failure of a cell's internal machinery to repair a damaged gene or duplicate a normal one during cell division. Mutation is very rare and most mutations now recognized occurred many generations ago.

A more common way in which genetic disease appears in families is recessive inheritance. A recessive disorder surfaces when both parents carry a defective gene whose effect in "single dose" is negligible or nil but which, when inherited in double dose from both parents, affects their offspring.

Dominantly inherited disorders, in which a single dose of a harmful gene is enough to cause disease, may also appear without family history. New mutation aside, the reason is that many dominant defects are highly variable in the extent to which they affect different individuals. Alerted by the birth of an affected child, physicians may detect minor signs of the disorder in a parent.

Some inherited traits are sex-linked. Hemophilia and certain severe disorders of body chemistry, for example, occur almost exclusively in sons of women who carry the abnormal genes.

Other traits occur mostly in particular ethnic groups, such as sickle-cell anemia in blacks, cystic fibrosis in whites, Tay-Sachs disease in Jews of eastern European ancestry and thalassemia in Italians or others of Mediterranean origin. (Other examples of inheritable birth defects include Huntington's disease, diabetes and cystic fibrosis.)

Damage to single genes can cause any of about 2,000 known, heritable disorders which affect physical structure, organic function or body chemistry mildly, severely or fatally.

Chromosomal Causes—A larger scale of damage to genetic material appears in chromosome defects. Because each of a cell's 46 paired chromosomes contains thousands of genes, the lack or excess of even a small piece of one chromosome can be disastrous. Down's syndrome is the most common serious chromosome defect. Another is Turner's syndrome in which the child is born with only one X chromosome, missing either another X chromosome or a Y chromosome needed to fully define sex. The result is a sexually underdeveloped, stunted female who is often mentally defective.

Congenital Malformations In Infants

A considerable body of knowledge is now being accumulated on the teratogenic effects of radiation, the virus of rubella, the protozoan of toxoplasmosis, folic-acid antagonists, synthetic progestins and other drugs. There is also increased understanding of the interplay between genetic and environmental factors. All of this new knowledge is markedly improving the ability to predict the possibilities of congenital anomaly in future offspring.

Diagnostic significance can be attached to detecting a single, minor anomaly. However, in studying minor defects in children with selected major defects (i.e. cleft lip and palate, ventricular septal defect, mental retardation) and in a control group, one major study found that the presence of two minor anomalies in an otherwise normal child is somewhat unusual, and three or more minor anomalies may suggest the possible presence of a major defect.

To indicate the broad range of anomalies which may be encountered by the nurse, some of the major and minor anomalies are listed in Table 31-7.

Environmentally Influenced Birth Defects

A variety of environmental influences can act on the fetus, altering the normal growth and development. The most crucial period is the embryo's first six weeks, when basic body parts are forming. Later interferences also can affect body growth, organ function, mental development or all of these.

The Mother

The mother's age and general physical and mental health are important. Women over 35 more often experience fetal loss. (In Down's syndrome for example, studies have shown that mothers between ages 20 and 30 have a risk of 1 in 1,500 for having a child with this problem. By age 45, the risk is 1 in 40.) Teenagers frequently have low weight babies. Chronic maternal illnesses such as diabetes and thyroid disorders also may affect the fetus.

Table 31-7 Major and minor anomalies in infants

Major anomalies*	Minor anomalies**
Central nervous System Hypotonicity Hydrocephalus Anencephaly Microcephaly, severe Marked hypertonicity Meningocele	**Craniofacial** Borderline small mandible Prominent occiput Flat occiput Large posterior fontanel Small nares
Craniofacial Micrognathia, severe Defect bony orbits Choanal atresia Scaphocephaly, severe Hypertelorism, severe Protruding forehead Beaklike nose Absent ramus of mandible Defect of malar bone	**Eyes** Bilateral inner epicanthal folds Upward lateral slant of palpebral fissures Short palpebral fissures Short inner canthal distance Downward lateral slant of palpebral fissures Sparse eyebrows Web of connective tissue across eyelids
Eye Cataract or corneal opacity Coloboma of iris Microphthalmos, severe	**Auricle** Lack of usual fold of helix Preauricular and/or auricular skin tags Severe slant away from eye Asymmetrical size Small Absent tragus Separate lobule
Auricle Low-set, severe Severely malformed Rudimentary Low ear canal	**Skin** Capillary hemangioma elsewhere than face or posterior of neck Low hairline posteriorly Alopecia of scalp, spotty High placed nipples
Oral and Gastrointestinal Tract Cleft lip and cleft palate Cleft palate alone Cleft lip alone Imperforate anus Intestinal atresia	
Skin Webbed neck (posterior) Multiple hemangiomas	
Hand Severe flexion of fingers Short hands Polydactyly Complete cutaneous syndactyly Absence of thumbs Index finger overlapping 3rd Absence of all metacarpals Absence of distal phalanx Ulnar deviation of hand Broad fingers Streeter's bands and deformity	**Hand** Simian crease Other unusual crease pattern Clinodactyly of 5th finger Clinodactyly of other fingers Narrow hyperconvex fingernails Long narrow fingers Single crease on fingers Rudimentary polydactyly
Foot Calcaneovalgus, severe Equinovarus Syndactyly, cutaneous Absence of nails Rudimentary distal phalanx Streeter's bands of ankle and toes Dislocation at ankle Metatarsus adductus, severe	**Foot** Prominent calcaneous Dorsal flexion of hallus
Other Skeletal Congenital dislocated hip Short neck, severe Absence of radius Absence of fibula Short thoracic cage Malleable bones	**Other Skeletal** Cubitus valgus
Genitourinary Severe hypospadias Common cloaca	**Miscellaneous** Diastasis recti
Miscellaneous Sacral teratoma Gastroschisis Absence of sternocleidomastoid muscle	

* Defined as one which has adverse effect either on function or social acceptance. Detected by surface examination of 4,412 newborns.
** Defined as one with no adverse medical or cosmetic consequence. Detected by surface examination of 90 babies having one or more major anomalies.
Source: P. N. Marden, D. W. Smith, and M. J. McDonald, "Congenital Anomalies of the Newborn," Journal of Pediatrics 64:363, 1964.

31

Another factor is how well the mother takes care of herself, both before and during pregnancy.

Among the adverse influences are:

Viral Disease and Infections—German measles (rubella) is perhaps the best known. Depending on when during pregnancy the infection occurs, the virus can cause deafness, heart defects, cataracts, gloucoma and central nervous system damage in babies. Other infectious agents damaging to the child's central nervous system include cytomegalovirus (CMV) and toxoplasmosis.

Venereal Diseases—Can cause defects, too. In the case of syphilis, the child may be born with bone malformations and infection of many body organs. Gonorrhea can cause eye infection which may lead to blindness if the baby is not promptly treated.

Drug Use—Practically any kind of drug can potentially affect the development of the fetus. In Europe, thalidomide caused numerous limb deformities in newborns during the 1960s. Evidence is accumulating against such everyday drugs as aspirin, alcohol and nicotine. They too may affect the outcome of pregnancy.

The mother's use of narcotics definitely affects her baby's health.

Radiation—X-rays and other kinds of radiation have been linked with deformities, to varying degrees.

Smoking—Stillbirths, early infant mortality and low birthweight occur more frequently among the babies of women who smoke during pregnancy. The degree of the effect appears to depend on how much the mother smokes. A recent study indicates that the risk may be lessened if smoking is stopped by the fifth month of pregnancy.

Diet—Maintaining a balanced diet plays a large role in having a healthy baby. Stillbirths and premature and underweight babies are associated with poor nutrition in the mother.

Pollutants—A recent case was the poisoning of offshore waters at Minamata, Japan, by an industrial waste, methyl mercury. Neurological defects were more frequent among children born to women who had eaten contaminated fish.

Environment and Heredity as Causes of Birth Defects

Most birth defects, however, are probably not caused by either heredity or environment exclusively. The two factors may interact to heighten each other's effects.

For example, malformations of the skull, brain, vertebrae and spinal cord, which are among the most common severe birth defects in the United States, tend to recur in some families. Their frequency also varies with a puzzling array of environmental conditions such as geography and socioeconomic status. This suggests interaction of as yet unidentified genetic and environmental factors.

Low Birth Weight

- Is associated with almost half of all infant deaths.
- Substantially increases the likelihood of birth defects.
- Is three times as likely when mothers have no prenatal care.
- Is proportionally highest among children whose mothers are under 15.

Babies weighing less than 5½ pounds are less likely to survive and develop normally. They often have problems with breathing, heart action, and control of temperature and blood sugar—difficulties which can lead to brain damage or death.

Most of these babies are born prematurely, but some are small, not because of prematurity, but because of abnormalities of the pregnancy including maternal malnutrition.

About 248,000 babies are born each year weighing less than 5½ pounds. They are 17 times more likely to die in infancy than the normal weight child. Some 45,000 have defects other than low weight.

Why Birthweight Is Important—The rate of defects increases significantly as birthweight decreases. Defects occur in about 6% of babies over 5½ pounds; in 9% of those between 4½ pounds and 5½ pounds; and in more than 30% of those less than 4½ pounds. Babies in the last group, numbering about 85,-000 annually, are at grave risk of early death or long-term physical or mental impairment.

Prenatal care remains the most important protection against the risks that accompany low birthweight. Numerous studies have shown that mothers who go to the doctor early and often during pregnancy have healthy babies more often than women who don't. Good nutrition and personal hygiene also are im-

31

portant influences in a healthy outcome of pregnancy.

Identifying Birth Defects

If a serious defect is suspected, the doctor can insert a thin, hollow needle through the pregnant woman's abdomen into the amniotic sac, or bag of waters, to withdraw a little of the fluid that surounds the fetus. This is called amniocentesis. It does not hurt the mother or harm the fetus. The amniotic fluid contains cells shed by the growing baby. The cells and fluid are carefully studied and certain fetal chromosome defects or chemical abnormalities can be detected. Prenatal diagnosis and early treatment following birth can mini-

mize the effects of some inborn errors of metabolism such as phenylketonuria (PKU).

The National Foundation-March of Dimes has helped set up screening programs for Tay-Sachs disease, sickle-cell disease, and thalassemia (Cooley anemia). Genetic counseling is another important means of prevention.

The genetic counselor helps a couple interpret the data gained from family health histories and the latest diagnostic techniques. If, for example, a husband and wife learn that they are both carriers of a genetic disorder, they may proceed to take the calculated risk in having a child, they may decide not to have any more children or they can choose adoption.

Another agency concerned with the problem is The National Genetics Foundation, 250 West 57th Street, New York, N.Y. 10019.

Figure 31-1   Birth defects that become evident long after birth of child

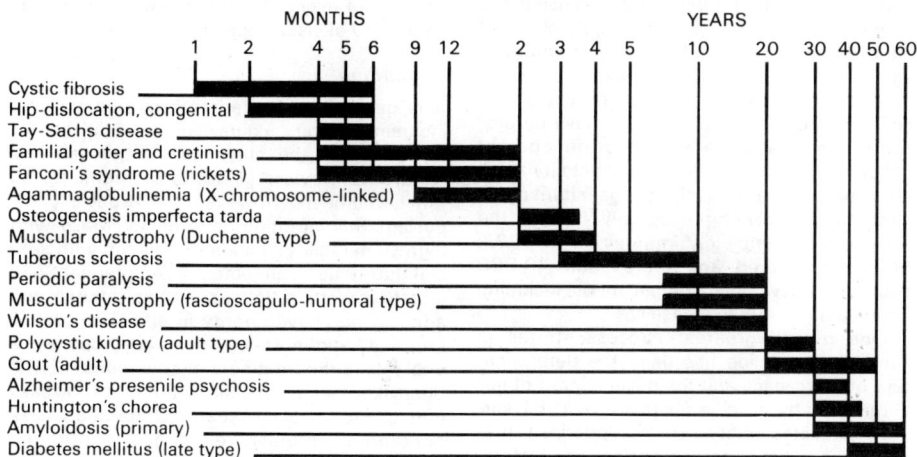

Source: The National Foundation-March of Dimes.

Child Health

Current Problems of Special Concern*

● *Genetic Disease and Development Impairment*

There are currently 15 million Americans who

have a birth defect serious enough to drastically affect their lives. Genetic defects account for developmental disabilities in up to 5% of all live births. But they account for approximately one fourth of all hospital admissions, a major portion of infant and childhood mortality, and an enormous financial burden in terms of medical care, provision of special social services and institutionalization.

Investigation sponsored by the National Institute of Child Health and Human Development has made significant progress in the

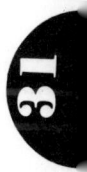

---

*Source: Subcommittee on Oversight and Investigation Hearings, October 1975.

diagnosis of phenylketonuria and other diseases. Recent work in hearing, speech and language disorders using audiometry has improved the assessment of very young children who may have an organic basis for future learning problems. The Institute intends, in the near future, to initiate new research efforts in dyslexia to assist the 15% of children who experience difficulty in learning to read.

● *Childhood Infectious Diseases and Immunization.*

In spite of the success in recent years in the control and prevention of measles, poliomyelitis and rubella, one area of concern requires special attention: the immunization of preschoolers from low-income families. Federal immunization programs will focus on Head Start, EPSDT, Day Care and Neighborhood Health Center populations because of the recent, alarming increase in the numbers of children who are inadequately immunized against childhood infectious diseases.

It is known that two out of every five children one to four years of age have no protection or inadequate protection against poliomyelitis and measles. In central city areas containing poverty pockets, the situation is even more alarming—scarcely half of the children are completely immunized. In 1973, 50 children died and more than 40,000 youngsters developed complications, including brain damage, due to measles.

One of the greatest success stories in American medicine has been the determination of the causes and the development of immunization by vaccine for polio. In 1964 surveys indicated that 88% of American preschoolers were protected against polio. However, by 1973, that figure dropped to 63%. The figure was even lower—approximately 51% —for nonwhite preschool children living in the central cities of major metropolitan areas.

In 1974 the incidence of these diseases was as follows: 22,374 measle cases in 1974, down 70.7% since 1971; 11,917 rubella cases, down 73.6% since 1971; 7 polio cases, down 66.7% since 1971; 2,402 cases of whooping cough, down 20.9% since 1971; and 272 cases of diphtheria, up 26.5% since 1971, with most cases occurring among adults.

The National Communicable Disease Center, for a five-year period, estimated that immunization efforts averted 10 million cases of measles and 3,200 cases of mental retardation. It also estimated that immunization saved 973 lives, 555,000 hospital days, 291,000 years of life, 1.6 million work days, 32 million school days and $423 million.

● *Communication and Visual Disorders*

One out of every ten children in the United States suffers from some form of communication disorder. Of these, over half have some type of speech pathology; a third have severe hearing impairment; and the remainder are totally deaf. Untreated communication disorders literally isolate a child from his environment and render him unable to carry out the myriad learning tasks of childhood.

The prevalence of vision deficits is relatively low among preschool-age children, affecting approximately 5% of this population. However, one out of every four school-age children has some kind of visual handicapping condition.

● *Nutrition*

It is generally accepted that nutritional care, including dietary counseling, should be integrated into the preventive, diagnostic and restorative services of health programs for all family members. However, it is especially important that nutrition services for those with high vulnerability to malnutrition and with special nutritional requirements, i.e., pregnant and lactating women, infants, young children and adolescents, have priority in efforts to reduce morbidity and mortality rates. Nutrition plays a vital role in the treatment of conditions such as phenylketonuria, maple syrup urine disease and cardiovascular disease. Untreated, these conditions seriously endanger health and increase stress for individuals and families as well as increase costs for long term care.

Health Care Expenditures for Children

Children under the age of 19 represented 34.1 of the population in 1974 but accounted for only 14.9% of all personal health expenditures. As might be expected, persons age 65 and over were only 10.2% of the population but accounted for 29.5% of all health expenditures.

Per capita expenditures for all personal health expenditures varied widely with age. For children under age 19, per capita expenditures in 1974 were $183, compared to $420 for persons 19–64 and $1,218 for persons age 65 and over.

On the basis of these figures there have been suggestions that the government could develop a comprehensive health care program for all children in the immediate years ahead at probably around $300 a year per child or about $1.8 billion for all children up to the age of six, plus the cost of prenatal and postnatal care for approximately 3.2 million births per year, probably at a cost of around $2 billion a year.

Table 31-8 Estimated personal health services for children under age 19, fiscal year 1974 (in millions of dollars)

	Total	%
Total	$13,416	100
Hospital care	4,477	33.4
Physicians' services	4,141	30.9
Dentists' services	1,389	10.4
Other professions' services	438	3.2
Drugs and drug sundries	1,883	14.0
Eyeglasses and appliances	354	2.6
Nursing home care	186	1.4
Other health service	548	4.1

Source: House Hearings, Subcommittee on Health and Environment, 1976.

Deaths and Accidents

Trends in Mortality Rate

Childhood mortality rates have declined steadily during the twentieth century.

The mortality rate in children aged one to four years declined from 150.2 per 100,000 population in 1949 to 84.5 in 1970.

The mortality rate in children aged five to fourteen years declined from 66.1 per 100,-000 population in 1949 to 41.3 in 1970.

Accidents as the cause of death ranked first among all children from one to fourteen years of age.

Ages 1–4 Years

In rank order, leading causes of death in children ages one to four years (excluding accidents) were:

- *Congenital anomalies:* death rates due to this category declined 16% since 1949.

- *Influenza and pneumonia:* declined from a rate of 19.4 per 100,000 in 1949 to 5.5 in 1970.
- *Malignant diseases:* within this category, leukemia accounts for almost half of the rate due to all malignant diseases.
- *Homicide:* the death rate due to homicide increased from 0.6 in 1949–51 to 1.6 in 1968–70. This finding is pertinent because of the current interest and concern about child abuse in the United States.
- *Infections:* in this age group the death rate due to infections such as enteritis and tuberculosis declined markedly from 1949–70.

Ages 5–14 Years

For the age group of children from five to fourteen years, leading causes of death after accidents were malignant diseases and congenital anomalies, both of which show very little decline in rates since 1949. However, a death rate decline is reflected in the rates for cardiovascular causes, due to a decline in rheumatic fever and heart disease.

Table 31-9 Childhood cause of death (rates per 100,000)

	1–4 years 1968–70	5–14 years 1968–70
All causes	85.3	42.0
Accidents	31.5	20.1
Motor vehicle	11.5	10.0
Other	20.0	10.1
Congenital anomalies	9.7	2.4
Malignant neoplasms	7.6	6.1
Leukemia	3.6	2.8
Other	4.0	3.3
Influeneza and pneumonia	8.5	1.7
Homicide	1.6	0.8
Major cardiovascular diseases	2.6	1.8
Rheumatic fever and chronic rheumatic heart disease	0.1	0.3
Other	2.5	1.5
Enteritis and other diarrheal diseases	1.5	0.2
Tuberculosis	0.3	0.0
Other infective and parasitic diseases	5.8	1.4
Nephritis and nephrosis	0.3	0.4
All other causes	15.9	7.1

Sources: Vital Statistics of the United States.

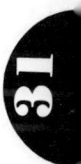

Table 31-10   Communicable

	Chickenpox	Diphtheria
Cause	A virus: Present in secretions from nose, throat and mouth of infected people.	Diphtheria bacillus: Present in secretions from nose and of infected people and carriers.
How spread	Contact with infected people or articles used by them. Very contagious.	Contact with infected people or articles used by them.
Incubation period (from date of exposure to first signs)	13 to 17 days. Sometimes 3 weeks.	2 to 5 days. Sometimes longer.
Period of communicability (time when disease is contagious)	From 5 days before, to 6 days after first appearance of skin blisters.	From about 2 to 4 weeks after onset of disease.
Most susceptible ages	Under 15 years.	Under 15 years.
Seasons of prevalence	Winter.	Fall, winter and spring.
Prevention	No prevention.	Vaccination with diphtheria toxoid (in triple vaccine for for babies).
Control	Exclusion from school for 1 week after eruption appears. Avoid contact with susceptibles. Immune globulin may lessen severity. (Cut child's fingernails.) Immunity usual after one attack.	Booster doses. Antitoxin and antibiotics used in treatment and for protection after exposure. One attack does not necessarily give immunity.

	Rheumatic Fever	Rubella (German Measles)
Cause	Direct cause unknown. Precipitated by a strep infection.	A virus: Present in secretions from nose and mouth of infected people.
How spread	Unknown. But the preceding strep infection is contagious.	Contact with infected people or articles used by them. Very contagious.
Incubation period (from date of exposure to first signs)	Symptoms appear about 2 to 3 weeks after a strep infection.	14 to 21 (usually 18) days.
Period of communicability (time when disease is contagious)	Not communicable. Preceding strep infection is communicable.	From 7 days before to 5 days after onset of rash.
Most susceptible ages	All ages; most common from 6 to 12 years.	Young children, but also common in young adults.
Seasons of prevalence	Mainly winter and spring.	Winter and spring.

Diseases

Diseases of Childhood*

Measles	Mumps	Polio
A virus: Present in secretions from nose and throat of infected people.	A virus: Present in saliva of infected people.	3 strains of polio virus have been identified. Present in charges from nose, throat, bowels of infected people.
Contact with infected people or articles used by them. Very contagious.	Contact with infected people or articles used by them.	Primarily, contact with infected people.
About 10 to 12 days.	12 to 26 (commonly 18) days.	Usually 7 to 12 days.
From 4 days before until about 5 days after rash appears.	From about 6 days before symptoms to 9 days after. Principally at about time swelling starts.	Apparently greatest in late days of illness.
Common at any age during childhood.	Children and young people.	Most common in children 1 to 16 years.
Mainly spring. Also fall and winter.	Winter and spring.	June through September.
Measles vaccine.	Mumps vaccine.	Polio vaccine.
Isolation until 7 days after appearance of rash. Immune globulin between 3 and 6 days after exposure can lighten attack. Antibiotics for complications. Immunity after one attack.	Isolation for 9 days from onset of swelling. Immunity usual after one attack but second attacks can occur.	Booster doses (see page 5). Isolation for about one week from onset. Immunity to infecting strain of virus usual after one attack.

Smallpox	Strep Infections	Tetanus	Whooping Cough
A virus: Present in skin pocks and discharges from mouth, nose and of infected people. Rare in United States.	Streptococci of several strains cause scarlet fever and strep sore throats. Present in secretions from mouth, nose and ears of infected people.	Tetanus bacillus: Present in a wound so infected.	Pertussis bacillus: Present in secretions from mouth and nose of infected people.
Contact with infected people or articles used by them.	Contact with infected people; rarely from contaminated articles.	Through soil, contact with horses, street dust, or articles contaminated with the bacillus.	Contact with infected people and articles used by them.
From 8 to 17 (usually 12) days.	1 to 3 days.	4 days to 3 weeks. Sometimes longer. Average about 10 days.	From 7 to 10 days.
From 2 to 3 days before rash, until disappearance of all pock crusts.	Greatest during acute illness (about 10 days).	Not communicable from person to person.	From onset of first symptoms to about 3rd week of the disease.
All ages.	All ages.	All ages.	Under 7 years.
Usually winter, but anytime.	Late winter and spring.	All seasons, but more common in warm weater.	Late winter and early spring.

(continued on next 2 pages)

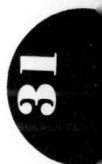

Table 31-10

| Prevention | No prevention, except proper treatment of strep infections. (See Strep infections.) | Rubella (German measles) vaccine. |
| Control | Use of antibiotics. One attack does not give immunity. | Isolation when necessary, for 5 days after onset, Immunity usual after one attack. |

Source: "memo to Parents about Immunization," Metropolitan Life Insurance Co., 1975.

Accidents

Fatal Accidents

In the age group one to four years, fatal accidents account for over one-third of all deaths. The mortality rate due to accidents was 31.5 per 100,000 out of a total mortality rate of 85.3 in 1968–70. Motor vehicle accidents account for 11.5 out of the total accident rate in this age group. The death rate due to overall accidents declined from 1949–51 but the death rate due to motor vehicle accidents did not.

Those in the age group five to fourteen years, account for almost one-half of all accidental deaths (20.1 out of a total of 42.0 in 1968–70). Motor vehicle accidents account for half of the death rate due to accidents. The death rate due to accidents declined from 1949–51 while the death rate due to motor vehicle accidents increased.

Nonfatal Accidents

Other leading causes of accidents to children fall into the following five groupings:

1. Severe Falls, Blows, Cuts, and Animal Bites
2. Suffocation and Strangulation
3. Poisoning
4. Drowning
5. Fires, Burns, and Electric Shock

The Accident-Prone

The theory of accident-proneness indicates that predictive behaviors can be identified in early childhood. The child who is, for example,

daring, excessively curious, happy-go-lucky, unable to delay gratification and easily over-stimulated is more apt to be exposed to hazards. Aggressiveness, lack of self-control, poor attention, stubbornness and "hotheaded-ness" are some characteristics associated with reduced ability to cope with hazards.

Table 31-11 Type of accident resulting in medically attended injuries

| | Annual rates per 1,000 children | |
Type of accident	All injuries	Severe injuries
Fall	56.8	11.9
Contact with sharp or rough object	20.2	2.6
Collision with person or object except vehicle in motion	22.7	3.6
Dog bite	13.4	.6
Struck by falling, flying, or thrown object	10.2	2.1
Bicycle or other pedal vehicle	9.5	2.7
Caught in, pinched, crushed	8.2	1.3
Contact with hot object or substance	6.7	2.0
Motor vehicle	6.2	1.2
Occupant	4.4	.7
Pedestrian	1.8	.5
Ingestion of poison	6.2	.5
Suffocation	5.8	.4
All injuries	246.1	37.4

Source: National Center for Health Statistics.

(continued)

Smallpox	Strep Infections	Tetanus	Whooping Cough
Vaccination (no longer given routinely in United States.	No prevention. Antibiotic treatment for those who have had rheumatic fever.	Immunization with tetanus toxoid (in triple vaccine for babies).	Immunization with whooping cough vaccine (in triple vaccine for babies).
Vaccinia immune globulin may prevent or modify smallpox if given within 24 hours after exposure. Isolation until all pock crusts are gone. Immunity usual after one attack.	Isolation for about 1 day after start of treatment with antibiotics—used for 10 days. One attack does not necessarily give immunity.	Booster dose of tetanus toxoid for protection given on day of injury. Antitoxin used in treatment and for temporary protection for child not immunized. One attack does not give give immunity.	Booster doses. Special antibiotics may help to lighten attack for child not immunized. Isolation from susceptible infants for about 3 weeks from onset or until cough stops. Immunity usual after one attack.

Health Status of Children*

The Health Examination Survey, from which the data below were obtained, is one of the major programs of the National Center for Health Statistics to determine the health status of the population.

Issued in 1974, the report contains information on health status and health history in relation to the significant examination findings among children 6–11 years and youths 12–17 years in the United States, as estimated from surveys of 1963–65 and 1966–70, respectively.

Health Picture

On direct examination, the survey pediatricians found one child in eight or an estimated 3.1 million in the population 6–11 years of age to have some significant physical abnormality—11% with some cardiovascular, neurological musculoskeletal or other condition (not including serious ear infections) and an additional 2% with an acute condition classed as severe otitis media.

Within this group, the condition showing the highest representation was neuromuscular joint abnormalities (31.8%) followed by cardiovascular abnormalities (22.9%).

Infectious Diseases

The most prevalent of the childhood infectious diseases was measles. While the disease was

reported to have occurred at any age from under one year to eleven years, about half the examinees were reported to have had measles between four and six years of age.

Children with a history of mumps most frequently had it at five or six years of age, with two-thirds having the disease between four and seven years. Serious complications were reported less frequently for mumps than for measles.

Hospitalizations and Operations

More than one child in four of those 6–11 years of age had been hospitalized for surgery other than tonsillectomy or for some other sickness or trouble. Boys of 6–11 years were significantly more likely than girls to have been hospitalized (30% compared with 24%).

Fifty percent of youths were reported to have been hospitalized over-night or longer. Over three-fourths of these youths (78%) were in the hospital for one week or less, while 1% had been confined for over six months.

The proportion of children and youths who had had at least one operation generally increased steadily with age from 24% among the 6-year-olds to 43% among the 16- and 17-year-olds.

The majority of these operations were tonsillectomies and adenoidectomies. Two-thirds of the children and three-fourths of the youths with a history of surgery had had one or both of these operations. In order of frequency the other major operations included surgery for ruptured hernia, appendectomy and circumcision. One percent of the children and 5% of the youths had had more than one type of these operations.

---

*Source: "Examination and Health History Findings among Children and Youth," *Vital and Health Statistics, Series 11, No. 129*, NCHS.

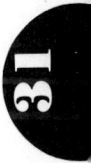

Figure 31-2   Prevalence rates for history of major types of serious accidental injuries among U.S. children (1963–65) and youths (1966–70)

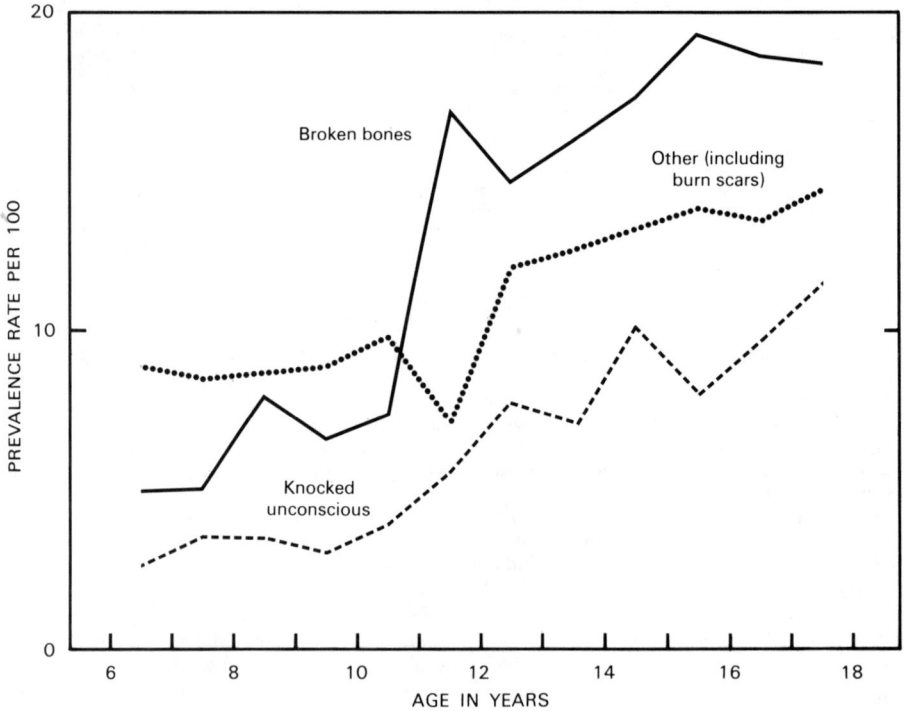

Incidence of Illness

Table 31-12   Children and youths with a medical history of selected illnesses or other physical conditions, operations, hospitalization or exercise restriction, U.S.

Medical history item	1963–65 6–11 years	1966–70 12-17 years	Medical history item	1963–65 6–11 years	1966–70 12-17 years
Infective diseases			Allergies and related conditions		
Chickenpox	—	84.1	Asthma	5.3	6.0
Measles	85.8	92.5	Hay fever	4.6	9.2
Mumps	48.8	64.6	Other allergies	11.4	13.6
Scarlet fever	3.8	5.0	Kidney condition	3.9	4.6
Whooping cough	9.4	14.5	Heart condition	3.7	4.9
			Respiratory conditions		
Accidents			Sore throat	11.7	—
			Colds	21.0	—
Broken bones	7.8	17.3	Coughs	10.7	—
Knocked unconscious	3.4	8.9	Bronchitis	15.7	—
Scars from burns	4.5	—	Chest colds	6.2	—
Other accidents	4.2	12.3	Pneumonia	—	11.2

Source: National Center for Health Statistics.

Figure 31-3   Prevalence rates for history of hay fever, asthma, or other allergies among U.S. children (1963–65) and youths (1966–70)

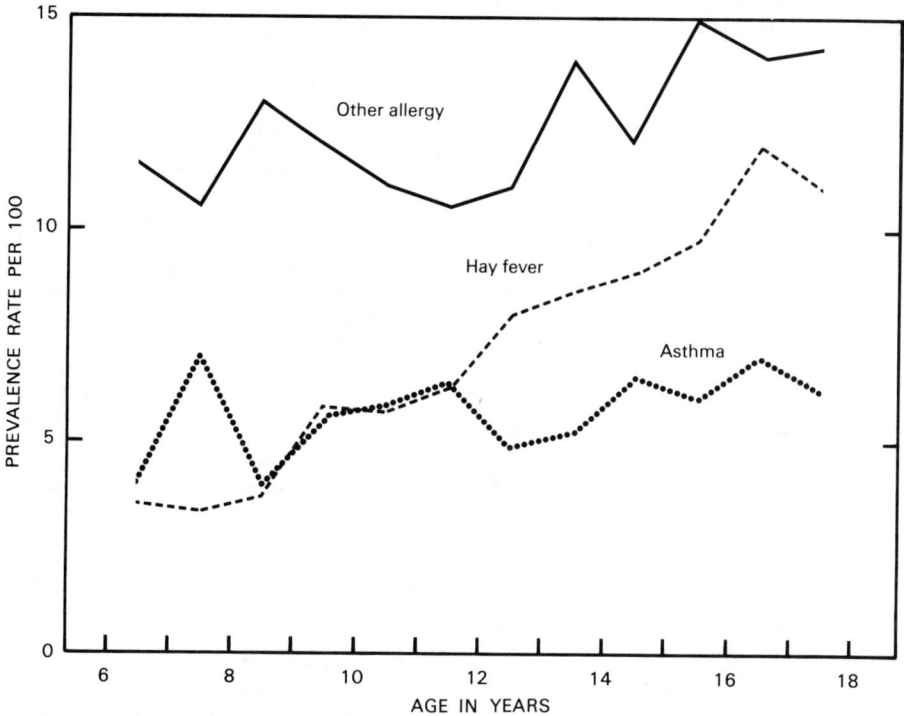

Table 31-12   (continued)

Medical history item	1963–65 6–11 years	1966–70 12-17 years
Sensory-neurological conditions		
Convulsions or fits	3.3	3.1
Eye trouble	14.0	6.8
Trouble hearing	4.3	3.7
Earaches	26.8	15.1
Running ears	11.9	9.4
Problem talking	8.4	4.3
Trouble walking	2.3	2.0
Arm or leg limitation	1.3	1.7
Operations	30.8	39.2
Hospitalized more than 1 day	26.8	50.4
Exercise restricted:		
Ever	5.4	11.1
Now	1.5	4.6
Taking medicine regularly	4.1	6.5

Factors In Growth And Development*

The types of variables which are believed to interact over time to influence child outcomes are (1) the perinatal factors, those physical characteristics of the infant that are present at birth, or those health status events that are present during pregnancy or result from the birth process, which provide a background for the infant's extrauterine growth and development; (2) the characteristics of the parents and child which help to constitute the environment and its stimuli within which the child develops; and (3) the parent-child personal interaction, the reciprocal behavior which stimulates development and promotes health.

*Source: *Child Health Assessment; A Literature Review* ed. K. Barnard and H. B. Douglas, Division of Nursing, DHEW, 1975.

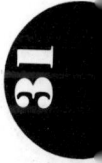

The available evidence suggests that the following environmental variables are probably of major importance for the child's healthy growth and development:

1. The amount of inanimate stimulation available to the child, e.g., the number and variety of toys or the variety of experiences provided.
2. The amount of animate stimulation, e.g., the amount of time the child is talked to, held, cuddled, etc.
3. The manner in which the animate stimulation is provided, whether "contingent," i.e., depending on something the child does or "noncontingent," i.e., given irrespective of what the child does.
4. The style of teaching used by the significant adults in the child's life. Some teaching styles, for example, seem well designed not only to teach a child new skills but also to teach him how to learn on his own. Other styles do not encompass this characteristic.
5. The mother's (or other adult's) perception of the child, e.g., whether she sees him/her as normal, supernormal, subnormal; whether she likes the child, and how she performs her role as mother.
6. The amount of stress in the family situation.
7. The general emotional stability of the mother and family members.
8. The presence of a father or some other male figure in the home. This seems to be particularly important for boys, especially in their early years.

Developmental Screening*

The management of children with developmental problems, including mental retardation, is more effective when begun early in life. Systematic developmental assessment of infants, toddlers, and preschoolers is one approach to detecting developmental delay, which allows an early referral to be made so appropriate therapy can be initiated.

Several devices for developmental screening are now available for use in daily child health practice.

The Washington Guide to Promoting Development in the Young Child was spe-

cifically designed to assist the nurse in observing, assessing, casefinding and planning developmental intervention for the child from birth to five years. It is presented in its entirety in the publication, "Teaching the Mentally Retarded Child—A Family Care Approach," by Kathryn E. Barnard and Marcene L. Powell. Organized sequentially, the developmental items are arranged progressively from simple to more complex tasks that are expected of a child at different age periods. This allows the nurse to determine where the child is functioning developmentally, to provide parental counseling, to offer anticipatory guidance and to give suggestions in promoting the child's development. Appropriate referrals can be made on the basis of the data obtained.

The Denver Developmental Screening Test was devised to provide a simple method of assessing the development of infants and preschool children from birth to six years. This screening tool enables the examiner to note whether the development of a child is within the normal range. It is not an intelligence test and does not enable one to make a diagnosis. The developers stress that it is intended only to alert the examiner to the presence of a developmental problem that needs further study.

The Developmental Screening Inventory, developed by Knoblock and Pasamanick, screens children from one month to eighteen months. It is of value for serial observations in well baby supervision and for diagnostic problems. It includes a wheel device designed to remind the nurse of basic steps in development, to be used as a quick reference for developmental milestones and to more precisely describe a child's physical limitations. This device allows both the reflexes and the milestones to be assessed at the same time.

The Developmental Profile, published in 1972, is an inventory of skills which has been designed to assess a child's development from birth to preadolescence. The inventory provides a reliable screening of five areas and a developmental age level for each.

This profile does not stress direct observation of the child; items may be passed or failed on the basis of an interview with the parent or person knowledgeable about the child.

The profile has been utilized extensively by nurses for the school age population. Until the profile was published, nurses met with some

---

*Source: DHEW, 1975.

difficulty in developmental screening of school age children by any standardized measure.

The Rapid Developmental Screening Check List is a compilation of developmental accomplishments matched against the age of the child. It was developed by the Committee on Children with Handicaps, American Academy of Pediatrics, New York. Substantial deviation from the expected age values makes further developmental evaluation mandatory.

The one-page Rapid Developmental Screening Check List can be used, filed away in the child's health record, retrieved and used over and over again.

Average Heights and Weights for Boys and Girls

Table 31-13   Weight-height-age table for girls (in schoolroom clothing, without shoes)

Height in inches	Average weight in pounds for each specified age											
	6–7 years	7–8 years	8–9 years	9–10 years	10–11 years	11–12 years	12–13 years	13–14 years	14–15 years	15–16 years	16–17 years	17-18 years
38												
39												
40	36											
41	37											
42	39											
43	41	41										
44	42	42										
45	45	45	45									
46	47	48	48									
47	50	50	50	50								
48	52	52	52	53	53							
49	54	55	55	56	56							
50	56	57	58	59	61	62						
51	59	60	61	61	63	65						
52	63	64	64	64	65	67						
53	66	67	67	68	68	69	71					
54	—	69	70	70	71	71	73					
55	—	72	74	74	74	75	77	78				
56	—	—	76	78	78	79	81	83				
57	—	—	80	82	82	82	84	88	92			
58	—	—	—	84	86	86	88	93	96	101		
59	—	—	—	87	90	90	92	96	100	103	104	
60	—	—	—	91	95	95	97	101	105	108	109	111
61	—	—	—	—	99	100	101	105	108	112	113	116
62	—	—	—	—	104	105	106	109	113	115	117	118
63	—	—	—	—	—	110	110	112	116	117	119	120
64	—	—	—	—	—	114	115	117	119	120	122	123
65	—	—	—	—	—	118	120	121	122	123	125	126
66	—	—	—	—	—	—	124	124	125	128	129	130
67	—	—	—	—	—	—	128	130	131	133	133	135
68	—	—	—	—	—	—	131	133	135	136	138	138
69	—	—	—	—	—	—	—	135	137	138	140	142
70	—	—	—	—	—	—	—	136	138	140	142	144
71	—	—	—	—	—	—	—	138	140	142	144	145

Source: Bureau of Education, United States Department of the Interior.

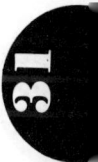

Table 31-14   Weight-height-age table for boys (in schoolroom clothing, without shoes)

Height in inches	Average weight in pounds for each specified age											
	6–7 years	7–8 years	8–9 years	9–10 years	10–11 years	11–12 years	12–13 years	13–14 years	14–15 years	15–16 years	16–17 years	17–18 years
41	38											
42	39	39										
43	41	41										
44	44	44										
45	46	46	46									
46	48	48	48									
47	50	50	50	50								
48	53	53	53	53								
49	55	55	55	55	55							
50	58	58	58	58	58	58						
51	61	61	61	61	61	61						
52	63	64	64	64	64	64	64					
53	66	67	67	67	67	68	68					
54	—	70	70	70	70	71	71	72				
55	—	72	72	73	73	74	74	74				
56	—	75	76	77	77	77	78	78	80			
57	—	—	79	80	81	81	82	83	83			
58	—	—	83	84	84	85	85	86	87			
59	—	—	—	87	88	89	89	90	90	90		
60	—	—	—	91	92	92	93	94	95	96		
61	—	—	—	—	95	96	97	99	100	103	106	
62	—	—	—	—	100	101	102	103	104	107	111	116
63	—	—	—	—	105	106	107	108	110	113	118	123
64	—	—	—	—	—	109	111	113	115	117	121	126
65	—	—	—	—	—	114	117	118	120	122	127	131
66	—	—	—	—	—	—	119	122	125	128	132	136
67	—	—	—	—	—	—	124	128	130	134	136	139
68	—	—	—	—	—	—	—	134	134	137	141	143
69	—	—	—	—	—	—	—	137	139	143	146	149
70	—	—	—	—	—	—	—	143	144	145	148	151
71	—	—	—	—	—	—	—	148	150	151	152	154
72	—	—	—	—	—	—	—	—	153	155	156	158
73	—	—	—	—	—	—	—	—	157	160	162	164
74	—	—	—	—	—	—	—	—	160	164	168	170

Source: Bureau of Education, United States Department of the Interior.

Poverty and Child Health*

Overview

The most recent estimates of poverty in the United States by the Census Bureau show that for 1974 of the 24.3 million persons with incomes below the poverty line, some 10.2 million were children under age 18. In other words, 15% of all children were living below the poverty line.

There is a very high incidence of poverty among children in families when the head of a family is a woman (51.5%) and an even higher percent when the head of the family is a black women (65.7%).

The poverty rates for black children were about four times those of white children.

It is estimated that 20 to 40% of all children in low-income families suffer from one or more chronic conditions and that only four out of every ten children are under treatment.

In certain areas, a child in a poor family has only half the chance of those with higher incomes to live to his or her first birthday. Half of

*Source: House Committee Hearings, 1976, on Maternal and Child Health Care Act.

all poor children are not immunized against polio. About two-thirds have never been to a dentist. And poor children have three times more heart disease, seven times more visual impairment, six times more hearing defects and five times more mental illnesses than the more affluent.

In spite of this need, only about half of the nation's 25 million low-income—that is, poor and working poor—children are eligible for medicaid and EPSDT services. The remainder are ineligible; yet many are too poor to pay for preventive care.

Diagnostic Services for Disadvantaged Children

In 1969 Congress passed legislation whose clear intent was to insure basic health protection for the nation's needy children. The Early Periodic Screening, Diagnosis and Treatment program (EPSDT) provides for the identification and prevention of correctable physical deficits through the provision of early health services.

However, it wasn't until 1975 that most states had initiated EPSDT programs to serve children under six years of age. And most of these programs concentrated only on the screening phase.

Guidelines issued by HEW recommend that each state actively seek eligible children by:

- informing parents that these services are available and when and where they can be obtained;
- helping parents understand the nature and purpose of the screening program;
- enlisting community agencies to locate children eligible for EPSDT services;
- providing the necessary transportation to the services.

Table 31-15   Children aged 5 through 17 in poverty families by state, 1970 census

State	State average (percent)	Low and high county percents		State	State average (percent)	Low and high county percents	
		Low	High			Low	High
50 States and District of Columbia	14.8	1.6	93.1	Missouri	14.8	4.5	52.2
				Montana	12.9	5.6	35.6
Alabama	29.5	15.7	71.4	Nebraska	12.0	2.2	44.6
Alaska	14.6	1.8	93.1	Nevada	8.8	5.8	17.9
Arizona	17.5	10.7	57.2	New Hampshire	7.7	6.3	11.4
Arkansas	31.6	12.6	59.2	New Jersey	8.7	3.1	16.7
California	12.1	5.7	26.0	New Mexico	26.3	1.6	65.0
Colorado	12.3	3.8	44.0	New York	12.2	3.9	27.9
Connecticut	7.2	4.9	10.5	North Carolina	24.0	9.0	57.1
Delaware	12.0	9.7	17.9	North Dakota	15.7	9.4	45.8
Florida	18.9	10.4	48.3	Ohio	9.8	4.1	33.0
Georgia	24.4	6.7	74.6	Oklahoma	19.5	8.9	53.1
Hawaii	9.7	8.8	12.2	Oregon	10.3	4.8	21.7
Idaho	12.0	4.0	27.2	Pennsylvania	10.6	3.8	22.3
Illinois	10.7	2.3	53.6	Rhode Island	11.0	6.1	14.8
Indiana	9.0	4.0	19.5	South Carolina	29.1	39.1	59.9
Iowa	9.8	5.4	24.6	South Dakota	18.3	7.4	50.5
Kansas	11.5	2.2	26.2	Tennessee	24.8	14.3	70.7
Kentucky	25.1	9.2	71.0	Texas	21.5	3.0	70.4
Louisiana	30.1	10.7	68.2	Utah	10.0	2.6	43.4
Maine	14.2	9.3	23.7	Vermont	11.4	7.5	21.0
Maryland	11.5	3.9	29.4	Virginia	18.2	3.3	51.4
Massachusetts	8.4	4.0	18.5	Washington	9.3	6.4	24.6
Michigan	9.1	4.2	31.1	West Virginia	24.3	6.7	48.4
Minnesota	9.5	3.8	30.9	Wisconsin	8.7	3.2	43.6
Mississippi	41.5	14.9	75.9	Wyoming	11.2	4.5	18.4
				District of Columbia	23.2	—	—

Source: U.S. Bureau of the Census.

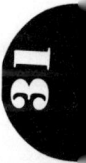

702

Considering only those who qualify for medicaid, there are approximately 13 million children eiigible for EPSDT services. Of those, only 15% (1.9 million) had been screened by the end of 1974. Of the small percentage of children who were screened, nearly one-half were found to need additional diagnostic and treatment services.

In Alabama's EPSDT program—the most successful that the General Accounting Office studied—among 39,000 children screened, more than 40,000 incidences of illness or of impairment were diagnosed. That is, an average of more than one physical problem was identified for each and every child tested.

Screening Services

The following screening services were outlined: taking a medical history and performing a physical examination; assessing immunization status; screening for dental, hearing and vision problems; screening for anemia, lead poisoning, sickle-cell disease and trait, bacteriuria, and tuberculosis.

A screening manual developed by the American Academy of Pediatrics specifically for EPSDT recommends that for preventive health care to be truly effective, seven complete physical examinations are necessary in the first 25 months alone of a child's life. This same manual recommends that additional, complete examinations be provided approximately once every two years thereafter.

Head Start—Health Services for Preschool Children

The health services component of Head Start (medical, dental, nutrition and mental health) provides that for each child enrolled in the Head Start program, a complete medical, dental and developmental history will be obtained and recorded, a thorough health screening will be given, and medical and dental examinations will be performed. These services were provided to approximately 350,000 preschool children in Head Start in 1974.

Social Services for Children

Table 31-16   Children receiving social services: state and local public welfare agencies*

Reporting states (31)	Total				Reporting states (31)	Total			
	Number	Rate per 10,000 child population[1]	In home of parent or relative	In institutions		Number	Rate per 10,000 child population[1]	In home of parent or relative	In institutions
Alabama	142,872	1,034	137,530	665	North Carolina	81,886	404	72,183	1,126
Connecticut	74,300	675	69,201[2]	1,142	Ohio	238,809	588	215,340	4,164
Florida	98,659	358	85,839	1,558	Oklahoma	33,913	346	30,569	1,802
Georgia	32,495	168	23,516	735	Oregon	36,364	443	29,919	1,200
Iowa	10,955	104	6,945	547	Puerto Rico	83,939	558	79,110	2,289
Kansas	20,377	250	16,070	1,271	South Carolina	29,806	268	27,365	365
Louisiana	7,373	48	2,461	740	South Dakota	6,779	257	5,411	147
Maine	4,200	107	2,046	224	Tennessee	37,321	245	32,380[2]	302
Maryland	47,383	308	34,772	712	Texas	18,619	39	13,491	835
Minnesota	58,534	386	46,582	2,957	Utah	6,741	127	4,978	52
Mississippi	23,460	244	21,110	107	Virgin Islands	3,925	935	3,502	53
Missouri	30,531	176	25,926	300	Washington	38,635	304	30,326	1,163
Nebraska	10,067	175	8,612	196	West Virginia	27,786	432	24,291	386
Nevada	10,942	495	10,119	89	Wisconsin	54,815	313	43,355	1,856
New Hampshire	3,618	119	2,149	207	Wyoming	1,461	104	895	135
New Mexico	6,769	141	3,623	728					

*Foster homes and group homes.
[1]Based on child population under 21 years of age, January 1, 1975.
[2]Estimated.

Source: DHEW, 1976.

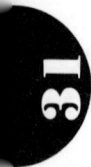

Figure 31-4   Preliminary results of a questionnaire sent to state medicaid agencies concerning early and periodic screening, diagnosis, and treatment (EPSDT)

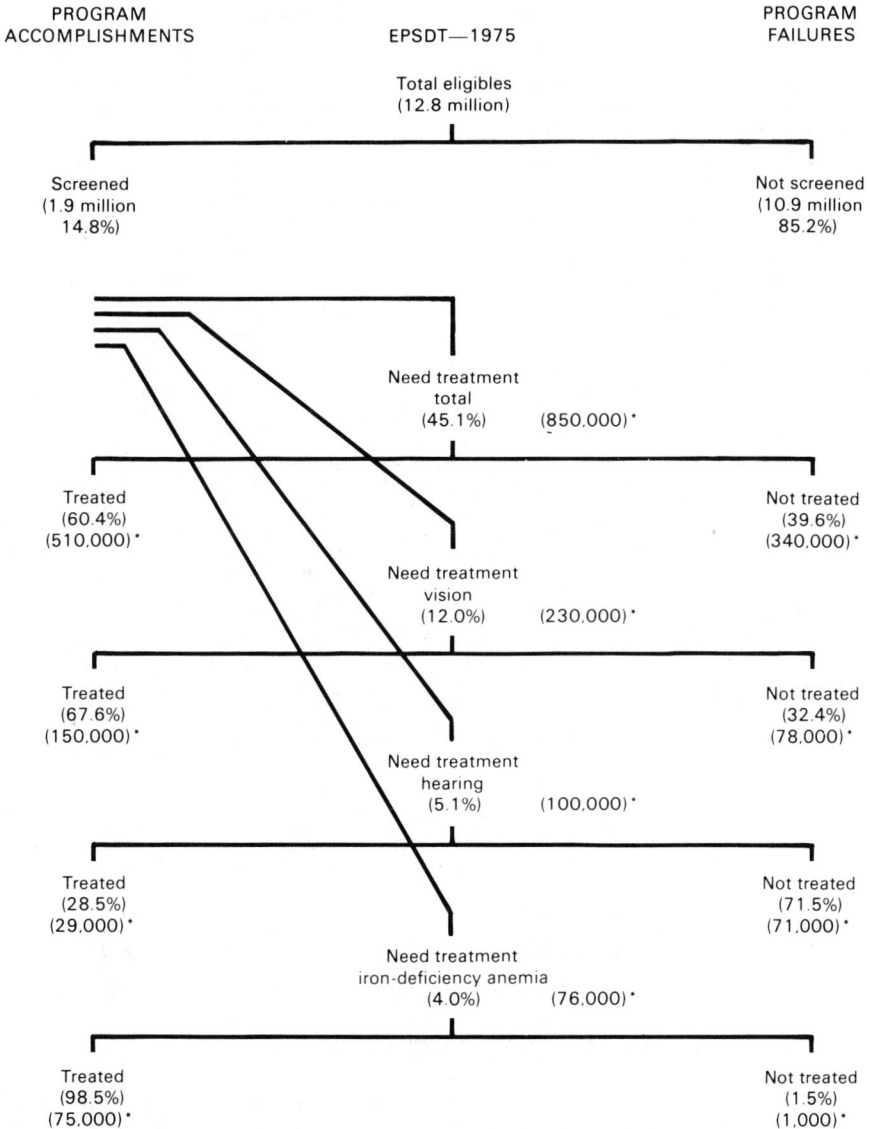

PROGRAM
ACCOMPLISHMENTS

EPSDT—1975

PROGRAM
FAILURES

Total eligibles
(12.8 million)

Screened
(1.9 million
14.8%)

Not screened
(10.9 million
85.2%)

Need treatment
total
(45.1%)   (850,000) *

Treated
(60.4%)
(510,000) *

Not treated
(39.6%)
(340,000) *

Need treatment
vision
(12.0%)   (230,000) *

Treated
(67.6%)
(150,000) *

Not treated
(32.4%)
(78,000) *

Need treatment
hearing
(5.1%)   (100,000) *

Treated
(28.5%)
(29,000) *

Not treated
(71.5%)
(71,000) *

Need treatment
iron-deficiency anemia
(4.0%)   (76,000) *

Treated
(98.5%)
(75,000) *

Not treated
(1.5%)
(1,000) *

* Staff estimates

Source: House Subcommittee on Oversight and Investigations, 1975.

Table 31-17 Licensed approved foster family homes and group homes March 31, 1975

Reporting states (35)	Foster family homes Total Number	Capacity	Group homes Total Number	Capacity
Alabama	2,184	8,337	12	112
Connecticut	2,703	4,703	22	252
Florida	2,569	13,655	83	750
Georgia	2,070	3,665	6	63
Hawaii	350	837	3	21
Illinois	10,884	18,969	64	462
Indiana	6,080	7,885	299	331
Iowa	3,100	5,518	—	—
Kansas	1,593	3,186	14	116
Louisiana	1,807	3,975	9	108
Maine	889	1,880	13	102
Maryland	4,353	10,155	39	247
Minnesota	4,643	8,793	84	736
Mississippi	1,128	3,057	—	—
Missouri	2,368	5,670	—	—
Nebraska	552	1,352	8	61
Nevada	376	841	2	21
New Hampshire	708	2,124	11	99
New Jersey	6,500	9,000	13	104
New Mexico	598	1,359	4	25
North Carolina[1]	2,783	15,915	55	363
Ohio	7,269	14,379	102	742
Oklahoma	1,858	3,504	—	—
Oregon	2,801	5,476	42	277
Puerto Rico	16	831	—	—
South Carolina	680	1,956	9	96
South Dakota	720	1,545	13	133
Tennessee	1,745	3,230	10	94
Texas	3,258	7,659	65	621
Utah	975	1,878	22	271
Virgin Islands	95	224	2	48
Washington	7,191	13,441	29	350
West Virginia	—	—	6	45
Wisconsin	5,679	10,861	70	480
Wyoming	191	393	—	—

[1]Data incomplete.

Source: DHEW.

Social Services for Unmarried Mothers

Table 31-18 Child welfare institutions and maternity homes for unmarried mothers, March 31, 1975

Reporting states (35)	Child welfare institutions Number	Capacity	Maternity homes Number	Capacity
Alabama	22	1,021	2	70
Connecticut	14	719	1	20
Florida	111	1,576	7	144
Georgia	37	2,049	2	82
Hawaii	2	72	1	10
Illinois	100	4,999	3	68
Indiana	1,302	1,746	57	68
Iowa	62	1,270	—	—
Kansas	48	721	2	66
Louisiana	39	1,494	9	197
Maine	14	378	4	34
Maryland	105	876	3	98
Minnesota	25	946	1	10
Mississippi	13	732	2	38
Missouri[1]	33	1,263	6	120
Nebraska	23	1,429	—	—
Nevada	3	202	—	—
New Hampshire	11	313	—	—
New Jersey	51	7,900	5	170
New Mexico	23	575	1	16
North Carolina[1]	31	2,357	2	76
Ohio	85	4,376	7	318
Oklahoma	35	1,606	3	120
Oregon	14	507	2	72
Puerto Rico	35	2,356	—	—
South Carolina	20	1,708	1	42
South Dakota	10	196	—	—
Tennessee	66	3,300	5	121
Texas	148	8,923	11	437
Utah	—	—	—	—
Virgin Islands	2	57	—	—
Washington	40	959	5	56
West Virginia	15	494	2	45
Wisconsin	43	1,868	4	83
Wyoming	4	215	1	9

[1]Data incomplete.

Source: DHEW, March 1976.

Federal Assistance in Child Health—Summary of Miscellaneous Programs and Services

Bureau of Community Health Services

The Bureau of Community Health Services conducts various programs concerned with the health of children.

• *Maternal and child health services*—The Maternal and Child Health program is responsible for extending and improving health services for mothers and children, especially in rural areas. These programs are designed to reduce infant mortality and also to provide maternal and child health care.

The most commonly provided direct services for women are the maternity medical clinic services, maternity nursing services and family planning services. Nationwide, about 600,000 mothers receive prenatal and postpartum care in these maternity clinics. Maternity nursing services were provided to about 2,000,000 new mothers in FY 1975. It is estimated that over one million women in 1975 received family planning services through the state maternal and child health services program.

The Maternal and Child Health program has taken on an increased emphasis in recent years. Maternal and child health programs were originally involved primarily in providing preventive health services. Currently the programs are focusing treatment services to assist states in the delivery of curative and clinical services and have expanded their provision of health care services for high risk mothers and their children, much the same as the Crippled Children's program.

- *Community health programs*—focuses support on ambulatory comprehensive health care in medically underserved communities. Centers now include a wide range of primary and preventive health services. In 1975, it was estimated that nearly a half million children received services out of the 1.7 million children estimated to reside in the 157 medically underserved areas.
- *Family planning program*—provides a high level of diagnostic health care to patients. Data suggests that the program has become a major source of preventive health care among young, low-income and fairly healthy women of childbearing age. In 1974, approximately 29% of the estimated 2.2 million served in family planning programs were 19 years of age or under.
- *Special services*—maternal and child care are included in the health services for special groups as provided by the Indian Health Service, Migrant Health Centers and National Health Service Corps.

Crippled Children's Programs*

(DHEW estimated in 1975 that 65% of all handicapped preschool children were not receiving special services.)

---

*Source: DHEW, 1975.

Every state has a crippled children's agency. Usually the agency is located in the state capital. Its job is to diagnose and then see that each child gets the medical and other health-related care, hospitalization and continuing followup that he needs. After a child is examined and the doctors, nurses and others have learned what they can about his condition and his family situation, they advise the parents about the treatment that will benefit the child and help them find the kind of treatment and care the child needs.

Usually the initial examination is given in a clinic by a team of physicians and other health workers backed up by laboratory and X-ray services.

To find out when and where a clinic will be held, parents are advised to ask the state crippled children's agency or their local health department.

The goal of well-rounded state crippled children's programs is to meet, with the cooperation of professional people and community agencies, the needs of each child for whom the state agency assumes responsibility in all stages of treatment and recovery—in the clinic, the hospital, the home, the school, and the community.

All states include children under 21 years of age who have some kind of handicap that needs orthopedic or plastic treatment. This means children with cleft lip, cleft palate, club foot, chronic conditions affecting bones and joints, paralyzed muscles and cerebral palsy.

Nearly all the states include in their crippled children's programs children with rheumatic and congenital heart disease, epilepsy, cystic fibrosis, vision problems requiring surgery and hearing problems. The states have increasingly broadened their programs to include children with many kinds of handicapping conditions or long-term illnesses, including crippled children who are mentally retarded or have multiple handicaps.

Among children currently being served, three classes of disease are predominant: diseases of the bones and organs of movement, diseases of the nervous system and sense organs, and congenital malformations.

In many states, three levels of care are provided by the crippled children's agency. Field clinics provide initial screening examinations and followup care. Children with special problems who need further diagnostic work or treatment may be referred to district centers

706

where a variety of specialists and more extensive laboratory services are available. The university medical centers, with the most advanced and specialized services, give care to children with conditions requiring the most complex treatment.

A public health nurse may visit the handicapped child's home to give health guidance and help the family carry out the doctor's instructions. A medical social worker may help a family with its emotional, social and financial problems and put the parents in touch with community agencies that can help meet their child's needs. A physical therapist may give followup therapy in the clinic or home according to the physician's recommendations. An occupational therapist may assist the mother with changes in the house to increase the child's ability to take care of himself. A nutritionist may give advice about diet for the child and food for the family.

National Institutes of Health*

National Institute of Child Health and Human Development

The National Institute of Child Health and Human Development (NICHD) serves as the focal point for DHEW biomedical and behavioral research relating to the health of mothers, children and families.

In recent research:

- NICHD scientists have developed a vaccine which has the potential to prevent a type of meningitis which is the leading cause of acquired mental retardation.

- A number of maternal diseases, complications and environmental factors that can increase infant morbidity and mortality have been identified.

National Institute of Mental Health

During FY 1975, the total amount of money spent on child mental health related activities approximated $105 million. Of this amount, $19,405,000 was spent on research grants and $2,045,000 on intramural research. Training grants and fellowships accounted for $20,285,000.

---

*Source: House Hearings, 1975.

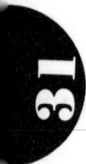

In 1975 the bulk of NIMH funds, went to fund Child and Youth Services in certain Community Mental Health Centers. These centers provided basic services to over 132,000 children under the age of 18 in 1975.

National Institute on Alcohol Abuse and Alcoholism

The National Institute on Alcohol Abuse and Alcoholism (NIAAA) in 1975 supported directly or indirectly, nearly $4.5 million of activities and programs which benefited children.

National Institute on Drug Abuse

In 1975, the National Institute on Drug Abuse (NIDA) expended approximately $39 million on programs and activities supportive of youth. Nearly $21 million augmented programs which provided services, and $11 million was employed for public information activities and consumer education.

Center for Disease Control

Among the current functions of the center are:

- Monitoring the incidence of birth defects aimed at preventing epidemics caused by new environmental agents.
- Analytical investigations seeking to discover the etiology of birth defects which are not now epidemic.
- A population-based study to demonstrate that technical assistance to state and local health departments can greatly increase the number of women who have laboratory testing to determine if a fetus has a chromosomal disorder like Down's syndrome (mongolism).

Alcohol, Drug Abuse and Mental Health Administration (ADAMHA)

ADAMHA has committed substantial Federal funds for juvenile programs in connection with intramural research, training grants, hospital improvement grants, fellowships, consultation and education, staffing grants to community mental health centers and innumerable other activities. In 1975 the budget level for ADAMHA programs identified as including activities affecting children approximated $148.5 million.

Office of Education (DHEW)

Charted below are the estimated number of students served and the federally appropriated dollars expended in the category of health services conveyed through school health programs.

Table 31-19 Federal funds for health services through school health programs (FY 1973)

	Total	Migrant	Low income	Title III	Title VII	Title VIII	Follow through	Education of the handicapped	Emergency school aid
Federal expenditures ($)	27,891,000	2,189,000	22,764,000	225,000	25,000	148,000	2,400,000	110,000	30,000
Students served	2,064,900	162,000	1,686,000	16,000	1,800	10,900	178,000	8,000	2,200

31

32
ADOLESCENTS AND HEALTH

Overview*

Population

Estimates by the U.S. Bureau of the Census for 1972 show that 45% of the 209 million people in the United States were less than 25 years of age. Within this category there were 42 million between the ages of 10 and 19 who could be labeled adolescents. Projections of present trends indicate that the number of adolescents in the United States may reach 54 million by the year 2000.

Adolescent Morbidity and Mortality

Adolescents are considered to be a healthy population group. By this age congenital anomalies have been detected and treated. Immunity—passive or acquired—has been developed against infectious diseases.

---

*Sources: Bureau of Community Services, DHEW and National Center for Health Statistics.

Degenerative processes have not begun to show their effects. Nevertheless, adolescents do die.

The number of deaths among teenagers is small and the death rate from all causes combined is low.

However, from 1960 to 1969 the mortality rate for teenagers 15–19 years of age increased 25%, from 92 to 115 per 100,000 population. The rise in teenage mortality during the sixties was due primarily to deaths from violent causes—accidents, homicide and suicide. Death rates for the major nonviolent causes declined.

For an older grouping, age 15–24 years, in 1972 the death rate from all causes was 127.7 per 100,000. Accidents are the leading cause of death. In 1972, the fatality rate for all accidents was 68.1 per 100,000 population in this group, or 53% of all deaths. Other major causes of death and the corresponding rates per 100,000 in the 15- to 24-year-old group include homicide—13.5; suicide—10.2; malignancies—7.7; and cardiovascular diseases—4.6.

Figure 32-1   Leading causes of death as percentages of all deaths, ages 12–19

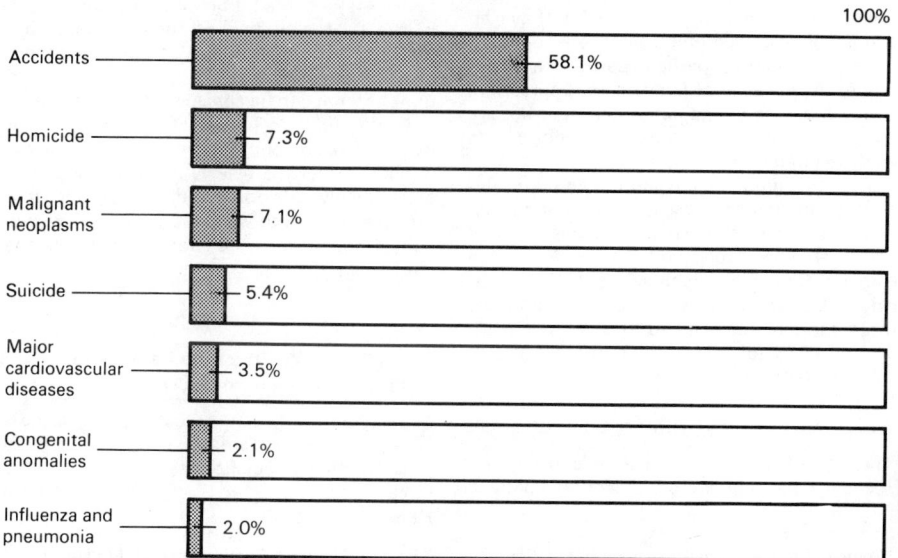

Source: National Center for Health Statistics.

Typical Health Problems

Table 32-1   Health problems identified among adolescent patients in a major hospital

Primary problems of adolescence	Problems made worse by adolescence	Problems with origin during adolescence
Scoliosis	Tuberculosis	Obesity
Slipped epiphysis	Automotive injuries	Alcoholism
Acne	Unwed pregnancy	Duodenal ulcer
Sports injuries	Suicide	Hypercholesterolemia
Mononucleosis	Diabetes	Labile hypertension
Body image	Inflammatory bowel disease	Irritable colon syndrome
Drug abuse	Menstrual dysfunction	Migraine
Venereal disease	Dental caries	Marital conflicts
Goiter	Abortion	
Sexual dysfunction	Gynecomastia	
Delinquency	Mental retardation	
Tumors	Dying	
Anorexia nervosa		
Hepatitis		
Primary amenorrhea		
School-learning problems		

Source: DHEW, 1975.

Special Health Problems of Adolescents

Mental Health*

Disorders of mental health appear to be increasing among young people. A diagnostic analysis of patients attending adolescent clinics shows that many complaints have an emotional base. Mental hospitals are admitting more young people, perhaps partly as a reflection of the absence of family care. Depression, impulse disorders, and acting-out behavior are the predominant characteristics of adolescents who are emotionally disturbed.

The most dramatic indicator of emotional instability and unhappiness is the mounting incidence of suicide. *It is the third leading cause of death for older adolescents.* According to the National Center for Health Statistics, the suicide rate for adolescent white males from 15 to 24 years of age climbed from 4.0 per 100,000 in 1955 to 9.0 per 100,000 in 1969 to 11.4 per 100,000 in 1973.

Alcohol**

The use of alcohol by children and youth is recognized as a growing problem. In a national probability study on the use of alcohol by U.S. teenagers who were in junior and senior high school during the spring of 1974, preliminary results estimated that over 15 million teenagers in school drank alcoholic beverages in the past year and of those at least 3½ million drink on a weekly or more frequent basis. This translates to 17% of school youth drink at what can be considered a heavy rate.

Furthermore, over 5% of the students, or over one million pupils, claim that they become drunk on at least a weekly basis. These figures are probably conservative due to the fact that grade school youth, sixth grade and below, and school dropouts were not included in the study.

Drugs†

Table 32-2   Youths who have used drugs: 12–17 years old, (1972)

Marijuana	23.6%
Glue and other inhalants	6.4%
LSD and other hallucinogens	4.8%
Cocaine	1.5%
Heroin	.6%

*Source: *Approaches to Adolescent Health Care.*
**Source: House Hearings, 1975.

† Source: National Commission on Marijuana and Drug Abuse.

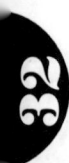

32

Venereal Disease

The alleged vices of the teenage population have attracted much publicity—sexual activity in particular.

The central health issue is not necessarily the incidence of sexual activity among teenagers, but its consequences—rising numbers of teenage pregnancies, VD and abortions performed on very young girls.

The marked increase in venereal disease clearly indicates that the freedom from preg-nancy provided by the Pill is not accompanied by freedom from infection.

The incidence of gonorrhea has reached epidemic proportions among teenagers. This condition is usually reported by the male who is experiencing painful symptoms. However, "silent" gonorrhea in males has increased to more than 10% of reported cases.

The frequent absence of primary symptoms in females allows the disease to go unnoticed until serious complications arise. The absence

Figure 32-2   Reported venereal diseases among 15–19 year olds: 1956–74

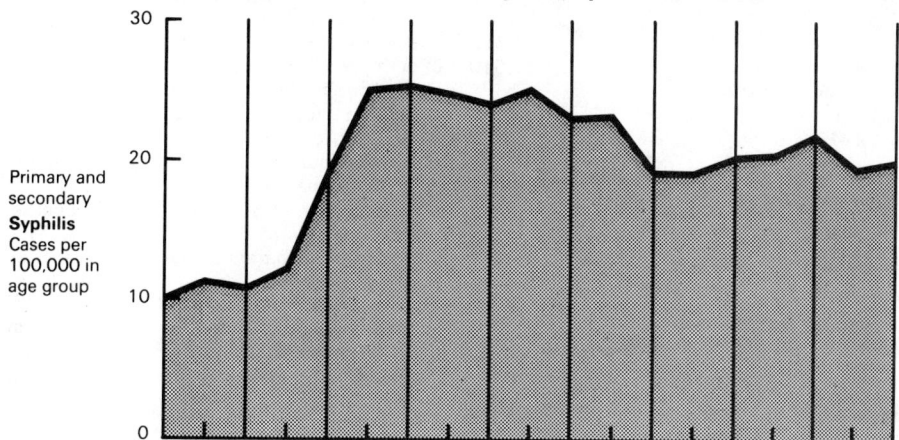

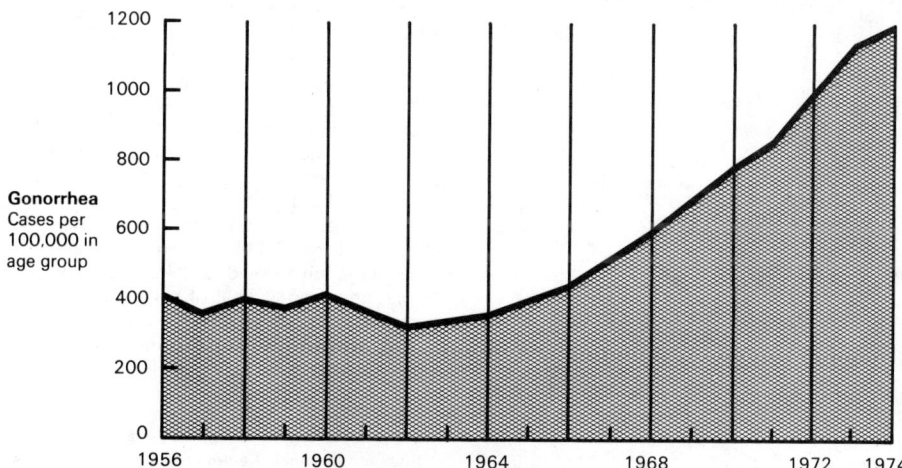

Source: U.S. Center for Disease Control, 1975.

of a serological test for gonorrhea makes diagnosis in women impossible without a cervical smear and culture.

Although the incidence of syphilis appears to have stabilized for the population at large, the incidence for adolescents continues to increase.

Note: These diseases are vastly under-reported.

Table 32-3   Gonorrhea among children 0–14 years of age

Reported cases:	
1965	4,525
1974	11,510
Rates per 100,000:	
1965	7.6
1974	21.1

Source: House Appropriations Committee Hearings, September 1976.

Smoking*

In 1972, 22.8% of youths age 12–19 years, were reported to be users of tobacco.

Figure 32-3   U.S. youths reporting themselves as regular smokers, by age and sex

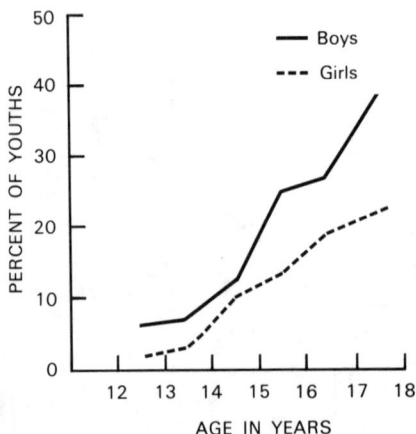

AGE IN YEARS

From an earlier collection of data from the National Health Survey which dealt with a nationally representative sample of 7,514 youths, the following details are available: the percentage of youths who reported regular smoking increased from about 4% among 12-year-olds to about 31% among 17-year-olds. Of those who reported smoking regularly, about 61% smoked less than half a pack of cigarettes per day, 25% smoked between half and one pack a day, and about 14% smoked one or more packs a day.

Nutrition

Obesity is a common problem in teenagers of both sexes. Although no significant mortality or medical morbidity is attributable to obesity during the adolescent years, there are reasons for concern about overweight teenagers. The obesity acquired in youth is particularly resistant to treatment.

In a survey of teenagers, NCHS reported that about 55% of the boys and 41% of the girls wanted to be about the same weight as they were. Satisfaction with present weight decreased as youths grew older. At age 17, about one-half of the boys but only one-third of the girls expressed satisfaction with their present weight.

Acne**

The National Health Survey (NCHS) on youths confirmed that acne, at least in mild degrees, is a fairly common condition among adolescents. About half of the youths reported that they had acne, pimples or blackheads. Girls reported an earlier onset of acne than boys did.

Of the youths who reported that they had acne, 58% indicated they were using some treatment for it. At every age girls were more likely than boys to be using some treatment. Furthermore, of the youths with acne, 11% stated that they had seen a doctor about it, a percentage which tended to increase with age. Apparently a good deal of self-medication for acne exists among youths.

Only about 14% of the youths reporting acne indicated that their acne worried them *quite a lot.*

---

*Source: *Vital and Health Statistics,* 1975.

**Source: National Center for Health Statistics, 1975.

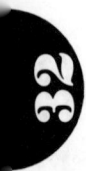

Figure 32-4   Self-perceptions and preferences of physical appearance by youths, age 12–17

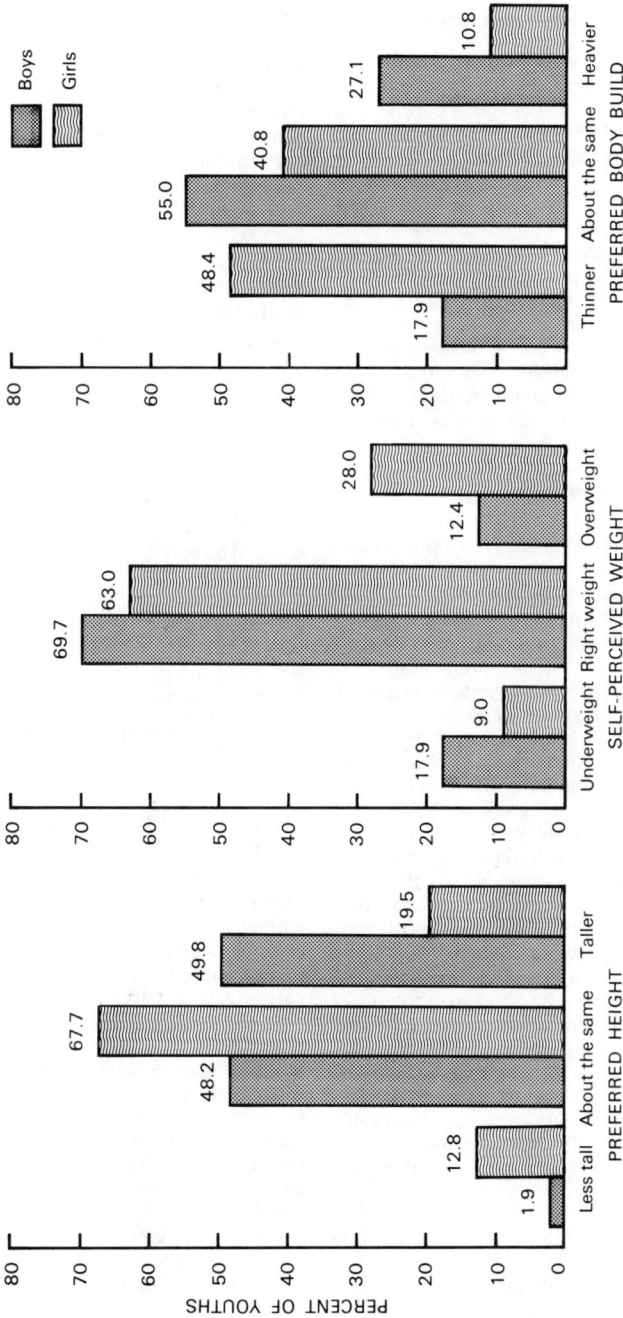

Boys

Girls

PREFERRED HEIGHT

Less tall   About the same   Taller

SELF-PERCEIVED WEIGHT

Underweight   Right weight   Overweight

PREFERRED BODY BUILD

Thinner   About the same   Heavier

PERCENT OF YOUTHS

Source: *Vital and Health Statistics*, 1975.

32

Teenage Pregnancies*

While unplanned and unwanted pregnancies have declined in the population above 20, they have increased in the teenage group. During the period from 1965–70, over two and one-half million "unwanted" babies were born, a significant proportion of which were to teenage mothers. The proportion of all births that are illegitimate doubled between 1963 and 1973 rising from 6.3 to 13.0%. Among teenage girls, the proportion of illegitimate births rose from 18 to 35% in the same period.

Studies show that pregnant adolescents have higher rates for toxemia, prolonged labor, premature delivery, pelvic disproportion and cesarean section than more mature women, and therefore require more intensive maternity care.

Illegitimacy and Premarital Pregnancy**

Data available from studies on illegitimacy and premarital pregnancy indicate that illegitimacy is a major social problem, and premarital conceptions, whether aborted or leading to forced marriage, create additional problems. The problems of illegitimacy and premarital pregnancy are greatest for teenagers, especially if they are Black. One study has shown that 30% of women age 15–19 have had intercourse, with the Black percentage about twice that of whites, and that sexual activity among unmarried teenagers is increasing. Moreover, teenagers are relatively poor contraceptors. About 30% of the sexually active teenagers become pregnant while unmarried, with the likelihood of pregnancy being four times as great for Blacks as for whites. Two-thirds of the premarital pregnancies were unwanted and were followed by marriage in 44% of the cases, by illegitimate births in 42%, and by abortion in 14%. Ninety-five percent of all live births to Black teenagers were conceived before marriage, and more than 90% of these births were illegitimate. Seventy-five percent of all live births to white teenagers were conceived prior to marriage, and 35% of these were illegitimate. Both maternal and infant mortality are

higher for teenagers. In addition, teenagers constitute the largest group of late aborters, with the concomitant high risk. Consequences of these facts include disruption of education, forced marriage with the high probability of subsequent divorce, psychological and social consequences of illegitimacy, and adverse long-term effects of early parenthood on the mother, father, child and society.

Table 32-4   Estimated illegitimate births, United States, 1968 (estimated rounded to the nearest hundred)

Age	Number Total	Ratio per 1,000 live births White	All other
Total	339,200	53.3	312.0
Under 15 years	7,700	610.1	907.7
15–19 years	158,000	158.0	549.7
20–24 years	107,900	51.0	264.0
25–29 years	35,200	20.4	168.0
30–34 years	17,200	20.5	155.3
35–39 years	9,700	24.5	157.2
40 years and over	3,300	28.4	156.5

Source: National Center for Health Statistics, 1974.

Infant Mortality Among Teenage Mothers

Infants born to teenage mothers face greater risks of death or deformity than infants born to women at older ages. Risk of death is greatest for infants physically underdeveloped at time of birth and the percentage of births in this category is greatest for births to very young mothers.

In the United States, the risk of death in the first year of life among infants who weighed 2,-500 grams or less at birth was found to be 17 times the risk among infants weighing more. In addition to the greater risk of death, there was greater prevalence among infants with low birth weight of such conditions as cerebral palsy, epilepsy, mental retardation, congenital anomalies, deafness and blindness. Infants born to teenage mothers are more likely to be of low birth weight than infants born to older mothers.

*Sources: House Hearings, 1975 and "Teenagers Marriages, Divorces. . ." NCHS (HRA, 15–1901).
**Source: House Appropriations Committee Hearings, February 1976.

Services for Teenage Pregnant Girls*

Of the 130 respondent cities, 111 (85.4%) reported that they provided a special program of some type for teenage pregnant girls. In general, the larger the city, the more the likelihood of programs. The caseloads were relatively small. For example, 48 cities reported caring for less than 100 girls a year. Only nine cities reported caring for 500 or more girls a year.

Thirty-seven cities reported a budget of less than $100,000 for the special programs. Investigators noted that almost half of the cities with programs were unable to provide information regarding cost.

In the 130 respondent cities, the most frequent services provided to teenage pregnant girls in the special programs were counseling (101), social service (100), special education (98), special health class (90), and instruction in family life education (89). The services provided least frequently were abortions (23), day care for infants (33), special services for fathers (37), maternity home care (42) and pregnancy testing (43).

Contraception—A total of 77 cities reported that contraception was available for teenagers. Forty-nine cities reported that it was not available.

Abortion—Only 22 cities reported that abortion services were available to teenagers. Restrictions on abortion services were legal (73 cities), length of gestation (28 cities), limited to inpatient service (15 cities) and religious (7 cities).

Medical Care—Sixty-eight cities provided a special program of medical care for pregnant teenage girls and 58 large cities did not. Private physicians and hospitals were the most frequent sources of medical care, followed by health departments and maternity and infant care projects. Nurse midwives were available only in two cities.

---

*Source: A study of services and needs of teenage pregnant girls in the large cities of the United States. Helen M. Wallace, Edwin G. Gold, Hyman Goldstein, and Allan C. Oglesby, University of California, Berkeley, 1973—as reported in Bureau of Community Health Service, DHEW, 1975.

Teenage Marriages**

Early marriage is more common now than it was at the turn of the century but slightly less common than it was 20 years ago. A gradual upward trend from 1890 to 1930 and a decline in the 1930s preceded an upsurge in the married teenage population right after World War II.

Teenage Marriages During the 1960s

About one-third of the women and 14% of the men who married during 1969 were teenagers. An estimated 717,000 women and 311,000 men married at ages under 20 years.

In 1969 the teenage marriage rate was 88 per 1,000 for women and 35 per 1,000 for men. This was 12% below the rate of 100 per 1,000 observed for women in 1960 and 13% above the rate of 31 per 1,000 for men.

Table 32-5   Percent of teenage population ever married, by sex and age U.S. 1890–1970

	Female			Male		
Year	15–19 years	15–17 years	18–19 years	15–19 years	15–17 years	18–19 years
1970	11.9	4.7	23.4	4.1	1.4	8.7
1960	16.1	6.8	32.1	3.9	1.2	8.9
1950	17.1	7.2	31.1	3.3	1.1	6.6
1940	11.9	4.6	22.2	1.7	0.4	3.7
1930	13.1	5.4	24.6	1.8	0.3	4.1
1920	12.9	5.2	24.6	2.1	0.5	4.7
1910	11.7	—	—	1.2	—	—
1900	11.2	—	—	1.0	—	—
1890	9.7	—	—	0.5	—	—

Teenage Divorces**

Concern over teenage marriage focuses on the stability of these unions and whether they are more likely to end in divorce than marriages contracted at older ages. In 1969 an estimated 28,000 teenage women and 6,000 teenage men were granted divorces. More significant is the large proportion of divorces granted to persons who married in their teens (46% for women and 19% for men).

**Source: National Center for Health Statistics.

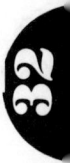

32

Table 32-6 Divorced husbands and wives who were teenagers at time of decree and married when teenagers–1969 (28 reporting states)

Divorced husbands who were teenagers at time of:		Divorced wives who were teenagers at time of:	
Decree	Marriage	Decree	Marriage
0.9%	19.2%	4.4%	45.8%

Sports Injuries and Accidents*

Recently sports medicine has begun to emerge as a specialty devoted to keeping professional and amateur athletes fit and to the application of injury prevention and of treatment to everyone.

Head Injuries

Although accidents in sports involve many parts of the body, injuries to the brain assume special importance because they are sometimes followed by incapacitating neurological damage or death.

Brain injuries occur as a result of blows to the head, sliding collisions or bodily contact. Regardless of the type of injury, the effects may be similar: loss of consciousness or balance; dizziness, vertigo, bradycardia, respiratory changes and hemiparesis or hemiplegia.

Spine and Spinal Cord Injuries

Cervical spine injuries. The most common injuries to the spine are related to hyperflexion, hyperextension or flexion compression of the vertebral column. In the upper spine, the junction between the rigid thoracic spine and the three lower cervical vertebrae is the most vulnerable.

Hyperflexion of the neck is the usual cause of injury, which may or may not result in spinal cord compression.

Dorsal and lumbar spine injuries. Dorsal or lumbar spine injuries are generally due to hyperflexion from a fall in a sitting position or

---

*Source: "Sports Injuries . . ." *American Journal of Nursing,* October 1975. © American Journal of Nursing Company.

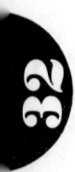

from being hit with an object while in a crouching position. The force of the blow is transmitted from the pelvis upward through the spine, and almost always results in compression of a vertebra.

School Activities

School nurses can do much in conjunction with physical education departments to evaluate health and exercise programs for children of all ages, and institute changes needed to encompass and emphasize prevention of injury.

The Athlete Profile Examination, or use of standardized evaluation methods, can be of help in evaluating each youngster's capacity and potential for athletics. Then a computerized file card containing this information can become part of the student's permanent school record from grade school to college.

Adolescent Health Care Services

Patient Care

Preventive health care is the goal toward which all health programs should strive. Preventive care for teenagers includes regular physical examinations, maintenance of immunizations and counseling on nutrition, sexuality, contraception, drug abuse and other concerns. The encounter during a health breakdown or other contact should be used as an opportunity to make a complete health evaluation of the teenager. Then the process of educating the young person to become interested in the body and its functions should begin, as the adolescent is given information about his or her own health.

The *initial medical history* probably remains the most important phase of the entire health process. Regardless of the nature of the presenting symptom, the practitioner has a responsibility to determine whether the adolescent is at ease with himself, whether his life is going smoothly, or whether he is confused and troubled. Developing a therapeutic relationship with the physician, nurse or other health worker may be of great value to the teenager. If the history is taken in an insensitive or mechanical way, the adolescent may be turned off to such an extent that he will not return.

Screening for certain prevalent conditions through specific tests that determine the presence or absence of pathology in healthy individuals may be a part of a preventive adolescent health program. For adolescents, screening should include tests for hypertension, kidney disease, sickle cell and other hemoglobinopathies, scoliosis, tuberculosis, visual defects, hearing loss, venereal disease and abnormal cervical cytology. Such tests are given at ages where the yield of positive cases will be most productive and cost-effective.

The reason for screening should always be explained so that young people understand the importance of preventive health services.

Delivery of Health Services

Although general concepts of health delivery and quality of care have been formulated to suggest the vital elements of successful health care delivery to adolescents, no coordinated approach for widespread implementation has been developed.

A 1972 survey of 43 clinics that treat adolescent patients pinpoints the dilemma. Though operated under varying auspices, private organizations, government agencies, medical schools and teaching hospitals, none of them was able or willing to identify the single most effective method for delivery of health services to adolescents.

In "Approaches to Adolescent Health Care in the 1970's," (HSA75-5014, DHEW, 1975) the following needs and requirements were discussed:

The clinical environment—The teenager requires easy access to facilities where primary health care is available. In the past, services for teenagers were available only in traditional hospital settings. These have not been generally acceptable to an essentially healthy group seeking preventive or primary care.

Neighborhood clinics, set up in many cities as satellites to a hospital, have eliminated some transportation difficulties, and brought services closer to where people live.

Services for teenagers should be provided on an age-specific basis, in areas specially designated for them and not used by young children and adults.

Practical considerations such as scheduling clinic hours after school, in the evening, or on weekends may influence the adolescent's willingness to utilize services.

Staffing—Staffing patterns in units caring for adolescents have undergone considerable changes in recent years. The advantages of multidisciplinary teams have been demonstrated. They have included a physician assisted by a nurse, a social worker and a nutritionist. Staff should have definite policies to follow concerning privacy and confidentiality, within the limits of existing state laws and regulations.

Adolescent Use of Doctors and Hospitals

Incidence: On a national scale, figures in 1972 show that the percentage of 12–19 year olds making visits to physicians was 72%, to dentists 60%. The chart below is based upon youths 12 through 17 years of age, selected and examined in the National Health Examination Survey of 1966–70.

Table 32-7   Doctor visits and hospital visits by youths, age 12–17 years: 1966–70

Selected variables	Checkup by doctor within 2 years	Hospital stay		
		Once	More than once	Never
	Percent distribution			
Total	63.0	32.6	17.1	49.4
Race				
White	65.1	34.3	18.2	46.6
Negro	49.1	21.3	10.2	66.8
Income				
Less than $3,000	45.4	23.3	12.8	62.3
$3,000–$5,000	51.2	27.1	13.4	58.2
$5,000–$7,000	58.5	30.3	17.1	51.8
$7,000–$10,000	66.8	36.2	17.0	46.1
$10,000–$15,000	71.2	36.3	19.1	43.7
$15,000 or more	79.9	38.0	19.8	41.7
Region				
Northeast	72.9	34.2	18.1	46.8
Midwest	63.4	33.3	17.9	47.4
South	54.0	28.2	15.2	55.8
West	62.2	34.5	17.0	47.9
Type of community				
Urban	66.0	32.1	17.6	49.2
Rural	57.7	33.4	16.1	49.6
Parents' education				
Elementary	49.5	26.1	13.2	59.2
High school	65.1	34.8	18.2	46.1
Beyond high school	77.6	36.6	19.4	43.4

Source: National Center for Health Statistics.

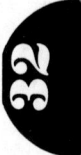

718

Views on Adolescent Health Care*

Background

The provision of health care for the adolescent sector of the U.S. population has received only minimal attention for several reasons. Teenagers have generally been viewed as an essentially healthy group whose members make few demands on the medical profession. Apart from emergency situations, they usually do not seek care between the time of the last visit to the pediatrician—traditionally made at 12 years of age—and adulthood. Many health professionals have not established rapport with the adolescent patient because they have not been adequately prepared to deal with the problems and complications stemming from unconventional life styles. Financial barriers, requirements of parental consent and other restrictive red tape often discourage teenagers from going to a clinic or hospital.

Historically, teenagers received care in pediatric settings where they often felt too big or out of place among much younger patients. The alternative was the adult clinic or ward, where teenagers were often exposed to sights and sounds associated with serious illness and the process of dying. A teenager developed an even greater sense of isolation in such an environment.

Initially, intense interest in the adolescent and his health was limited to academic settings where departments of pediatrics were enlarged to include special facilities for adolescents. Hospital services also became more responsive to the medical needs of teenagers.

Still, from 1965 to 1975, the health needs of adolescents outstripped existing capabilities both in volume and scope. There is still no satisfactory health care system available for this group in the United States and few adolescents are receiving appropriate or adequate health care.

Even within a single clinic, school or health department, services tend to be highly fragmented. Many teenage patients drift through an organization's resources, leaving a trail of uninterpreted tests and procedures. It is rare for all patient information to be coordinated into the individual health profile that could serve as the basis for a comprehensive health care plan.

Failure to recognize the patient as a human being is particularly offensive to those in their teens, who are almost by definition highly sensitive to real or implied infringement of their rights to individual respect and consideration. A related barrier to quality medical care is the reluctance of many adolescents to bring health problems to a practitioner or facility associated with their parents, which might check the independence most are striving for.

Adolescent Perception of the Need for Medical Care**

In the National Health Examination Survey of 1966–70 a number of the self-report questionnaire items required teenagers to rate selected medical conditions or symptoms according to each youth's self-perceived need for consulting a doctor. Blood in urine or bowel movement ranked as the most serious symptom, with three in four youths responding that they would definitely want to see a doctor if they had that condition.

A lump in the stomach or abdomen was considered next most serious by boys, 68%. Girls viewed this symptom with slightly more concern: about three out of four girls would definitely want to see a doctor.

The next most serious symptom for all youths was pain in chest, a symptom for which about half of the youths would definitely want to consult a doctor. The remaining conditions were ranked in the following order of seriousness: hurt all over (45%), stiff neck or back (24%), loss of appetite (19%), overtiredness (15%), nervousness (14%), vomiting (12%), sore throat (8%), stomachache (4%), and headache (3%).

Conditions which were perceived as less serious by older than younger youths were hurt all over, stiff neck or back, and stomach ache. Older boys viewed the symptoms sore throat and vomiting as less serious than younger boys did, and older girls regarded loss of appetite as less serious than younger girls did.

Legal Health Rights of Teenagers†

The factors which are the greatest deterrents to an adolescent seeking health care are: re-

---

*Source: DHEW, 1975.

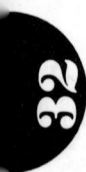

** Source: National Center for Health Statistics, 1975.

† Source: DHEW, 1975.

quirements relating to ability to pay, parental consent and other administrative red tape. Many young people complain about the health care system being immobilized by its own bureaucracy. The frustrations of endless waiting for decisions about eligibility or a referral appointment do not encourage teenagers to seek care within the system.

Yet there has been vigorous action to afford minors adult rights in matters of medical care. Since 1967 almost every state has enacted legislation enabling specific groups of minors to consent to some or all of their own health care. The trend to expand the scope of such statutes seems to be accelerating. These laws, which have arisen in part out of the recognition that many adolescents have the capacity for making a valid informed consent, are comparable to the common law exception for emancipated minors.

However, state laws governing the rights of minors are far from consistent. Several states had considered modification of their discriminatory laws by the mid-1970s.

A "Model Bill for Minors' Consent to Health Services" was published in the correspondence section of *Pediatrics* in November 1973. It states that parents should participate in all health care decisions about their minor children whenever feasible, but no legal barrier should prevent minors from receiving needed health care. "Minor," "emancipated minor," "parent" and "health services" are defined. Conditions for consent, financial responsibility and the health professionals' liability are described.

By 1975 there were efforts to make sure that all eligible older children have personal Medicaid cards. At that time such cards were available for teenagers only in California and New York State.

32

33
THE AGED

Population Growth*

The average lifespan at the height of the Roman Empire was 23 years. At the turn of the century in the United States, it reached 47 years. Today, life expectancy at birth is 70 years for the average American child. Those who reach their 65th birthday can expect, on the average, 15 additional years of life.

The older ("gerontic") population of the United States is large and continues to grow rapidly. There were in 1975, 22 million over 65, 8.5 million over 75, and 1.9 million over 85.

The population 65 and over numbered 3.1 million in 1900. By 1940 the group had nearly tripled in size to 9.0 million. It more than doubled again to 20.1 million by 1970. In the year 2000, the number of persons 65 and over is expected to be about 31 million.

The past general decline in death rates has contributed to the rapid increase in the number of aged persons, but its effect has been much less than the rise in the number of births.

The proportion of the population 65 years and over has been increasing even more rapidly (Table 33-1). It grew two and one-half times between 1900 and 1975, from 4.1% in 1900 to 10.5% in 1975.

Table 33-1   Percent increase of population by age groups: 1950 to 1990

Age	1950 to 1960	1960 to 1970	1970 to 1980	1980 to 1990
15 to 24 years	9.9	48.5	13.7	−16.6
25 to 44 years	3.2	2.7	27.7	25.5
45 to 54 years	17.9	13.3	−2.9	11.4
55 to 64 years	16.6	19.4	12.8	−2.7
65 to 74 years	30.1	13.0	23.4	13.8
75 to 84 years	41.2	31.7	14.2	26.6
85 years and over	59.3	52.3	44.6	20.1

Source: *Current Population Reports*, Series P-25, Nos. 311, 519, and 601.

Characteristics of the Aged

Sex Composition

A large majority of older persons in the United States are women, whereas at the younger ages there is an excess of males or a small excess of females. The characteristic pattern of sex ratios by age is a generally progressive decline throughout the age span, from a small

*Source: U.S. Bureau of the Census, May 1976.

excess of boys among young children to a massive deficit of men in extreme old age. At the present time there are only 69 males for every 100 females 65 and over in the United States. Only 40 years ago just as many males as females were reported at ages 65 and over, but there has been a steady decline in the proportion of men and an increasing excess of women since that time. It is now anticipated that the sex ratio of the population 65 and over will continue to fall, reaching 65 males per 100 females in the year 2000. This would represent an excess of 6.5 million women in the elderly population.

Race and Ethnic Composition

A much smaller proportion of the black population is 65 and over (7.4% in 1975) than for the white population (11.0% in 1975). This difference results principally from the higher fertility of the black population and secondarily from the relatively greater concentration of declines in mortality at the younger ages among blacks.

The population of Spanish origin currently has a very low proportion of persons 65 and over (3.6% in 1975) and a very high sex ratio at these ages (87 males per 100 females in 1975), in comparison with the white population as a whole, and even the black population.

Where They Live

Elderly persons tend to be most numerous in the largest states, of course. New York and California have the largest number of people over 65, with nearly 2 million each in 1975. They are followed by Pennsylvania, Florida, Illinois, Texas and Ohio. Each of these five states has over a million people over age 65, and together the seven states account for about 45% of the population in this age range.

Rapid growth of the number of elderly persons also occurred between 1970 and 1975 in Arizona, Florida, Nevada and Hawaii; each of these states experienced a gain of over 30% of its 1970 population, as compared with 12% for the entire country. Florida added 362,-000, Texas 170,000 and California 265,000. Other states with high growth rates (over 15%) in the 1970–75 period are South Carolina, New Mexico and Alaska. Slow growth (under 5%) was experienced by New York, Iowa and the District of Columbia.

In 1975 the proportion of elderly persons in the states varied from 2.4% (Alaska) to 16.1%

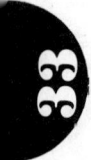

Figure 33-1 Distribution of the male and female population 65 years old and over by marital status: 1975

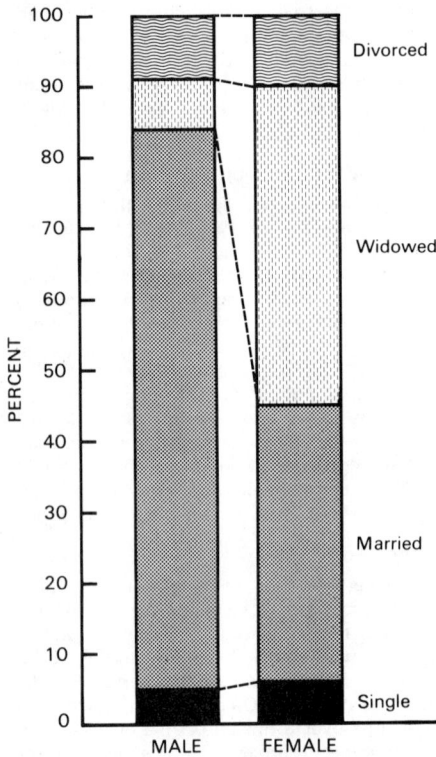

Figure 33-2 Distribution of the male and female population 65 years old and over by living arrangements: 1975

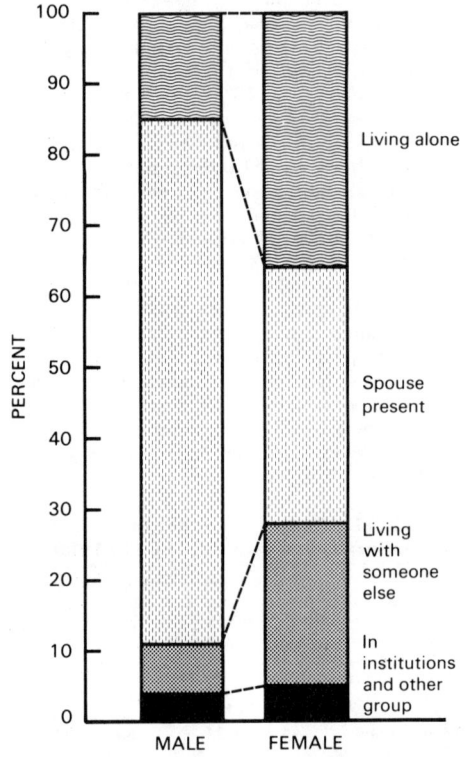

	Male	Female
Percent, total	100.0	100.0
Single	4.7	5.8
Married	79.3	39.1
Spouse present	77.3	37.6
Spouse absent	2.0	1.5
Widowed	13.6	52.5
Divorced	2.5	2.6

Source: U.S. Bureau of the Census.

Living arrangements	Male	Female
	Percents	
In households	95.6	94.4
Living alone	14.2	36.0
Spouse present	74.0	35.6
Living with someone else	7.4	22.8
Not in households	4.4	5.6

Source: U.S. Bureau of the Census.

(Florida), as compared with 10.5% for the United States as a whole. Such midwestern states as Iowa, Kansas, Missouri, Nebraska and South Dakota (that is, much of the midwestern farm belt), as well as Oklahoma, Arkansas and Rhode Island, showed high proportions (i.e., 12.0% or more) of elderly persons in 1975.

Estimates of net migration reflect a considerable movement of elderly persons out of the Middle Atlantic states and the East North Central states, and a considerable movement of elderly persons into the South Atlantic states, the West South Central states, and Pacific states, during the 1960–70 decade. New York, Pennsylvania, Ohio, Illinois and Michigan were big losers; and Florida, Texas and California were big gainers. In relative terms the District of Columbia, Alaska and Hawaii were the largest losers, and Florida and Arizona were the largest gainers.

Of the 20.1 million persons 65 and over in April 1970, over half (55%) lived in urbanized areas, (of the latter group about three-fifths lived in central cities and the remainder in the urban fringe), 27% in rural areas and the remainder in small towns and cities.

Of the 1.6 million blacks 65 and over in 1970, 61% lived in urbanized areas (of the latter group 86% lived in central cities, and 14% lived in the urban fringe), 24% in rural areas (mostly on farms) and the remainder in small towns and cities.

The population of Spanish heritage 65 and over is very largely an urban population (86% in 1970).

Marital Status

Figure 33-1 displays the statistics on the marital status of the elderly.

Living Arrangements

Contrary to the popular view, only a small proportion of the elderly population lives in institutions. Slightly less than 5% of the population 65 and over resided in institutions in 1975. See also Figure 33-2.

Income*

Only about one out of five men 65 and over (22%) works today; only one out of 12 women (8.3%) 65 and over works.

*Source: U.S. Bureau of the Census, November 1975.

Families with heads 65 and over have relatively low incomes as compared with all families. Their median income in 1974 ($7,298) was less than three-fifths (.57) the median income for all families ($12,836). The per-person income of the families with heads 65 and over was only about 18% below the corresponding figure for all families.

Table 33-2   Total money income of persons 65 years old and over, 1973

(Persons as of March, 1974)

Income and sex	White	Negro
Male		
Number of persons (thousands)	7,727	716
Number of persons with income (thousands)	7,682	705
Income Recipients Percent	100.0	100.0
$1 to $2,499 or loss	20.9	57.2
$2,500 to $3,999	25.1	20.2
$4,000 to $5,999	22.4	14.2
$6,000 to $9,999	17.2	5.4
$10,000 and over	14.5	3.0
Median income (dollars)	4,317	2,281
Female		
Number of persons (thousands)	11,027	957
Number of persons with income (thousands)	9,598	887
Income Recipients Percent	100.0	100.0
$1 to $1,499 or loss	29.3	49.2
$1,500 to $2,499	29.5	32.4
$2,500 to $3,999	22.0	13.1
$4,000 to $9,999	15.9	5.2
$10,000 and over	3.2	0.1
Median income (dollars)	2,192	1,519

Source: U.S. Department of Commerce, Bureau of the Census.

Table 33-3   Low-income status of elderly by metropolitan-nonmetropolitan residence and by race and sex (Numbers in thousands)

Metropolitan-nonmetropolitan residence and sex	White			Negro		
		Below low-income level			Below low-income level	
	Total	Number	Percent of total	Total	Number	Percent of total
Total—65 years and over	18,754	2,698	14.4	1,672	620	37.1
Metropolitan areas	11,850	1,314	11.1	1,101	320	29.1
Inside central cities	5,721	711	12.4	850	241	28.4
Outside central cities	6,129	603	9.8	251	79	31.5
Nonmetropolitan areas	6,904	1,384	20.0	571	300	52.5
Male	7,727	801	10.4	716	232	32.4
Female	11,027	1,896	17.2	957	388	40.5

Source: U.S. Bureau of the Census.

Health

Three-fourths of the non-institutional population aged 65 or older have one or more chronic conditions. Almost two out of five have a chronic condition that puts some limit on activity.

The most prevalent diseases of the aged are cardiac, cerebral and arterial disease, mental and nervous disorders, cancer, and diseases of the joints. Where these are accompanied by disability or invalidism, they may take a heavy toll of the resources of the patient, the family and the community.

Ailments

Table 33-4   Prevalence of chronic conditions by demographic characteristics: persons 65 years and over

Demographic characteristic	Arthritis (1969)	Asthma (1970)	Chronic bronchitis (1970)	Diabetes (1973)	Heart conditions (1972)	Hernia of abdominal cavity (1968)	Hypertension (without heart involvement (1972)	Ulcer of stomach or duodenum (1968)	Impairment of back or spine (except paralysis) (1971)	Hearing impairments (1971)	Vision impairments (1971)
	Number per 1,000 persons 65 years and over										
Total[1]	380.3	35.8	41.2	78.5	198.7	58.8	199.4	29.0	67.1	294.3	204.6
Sex											
Male	287.0	42.3	47.3	60.3	199.3	80.9	141.2	38.4	54.6	338.2	183.1
Female	450.1	31.1	36.6	91.3	198.3	42.2	240.9	22.0	76.3	262.1	220.4
Color											
White	376.3	35.2	42.5	75.9	200.0	61.0	194.6	29.8	65.8	299.4	200.9
All other	424.8	42.9	26.0	104.5	185.2	33.9	248.7		81.9	237.5	245.7

Table 33-4 (continued)

Demographic characteristic	Arthritis (1969)	Asthma (1970)	Chronic bronchitis (1970)	Diabetes (1973)	Heart conditions (1972)	Hernia of abdominal cavity (1968)	Hypertension (without heart involvement) (1972)	Ulcer of stomach or duodenum (1968)	Impairment of back or spine (except paralysis) (1971)	Hearing impairments (1971)	Vision impairments (1971)
Region											
Northeast	351.2	26.5	39.6	74.9	192.9	48.4	186.0	27.3	59.2	244.0	182.8
North Central	371.4	34.3	37.8	79.9	187.6	68.8	192.8	22.3	59.2	293.5	187.5
South	414.4	43.8	45.5	83.5	212.6	61.2	226.8	29.8	75.4	327.5	249.5
West	381.5	39.1	41.2	71.8	200.6	51.6	179.0	46.0	77.9	312.8	181.4
Residence											
Metropolitan	364.4	30.3	42.0	79.3	192.3	55.4	196.2	27.3	62.0	265.6	193.0
Nonmetropolitan	405.0	44.8	39.8	76.9	208.9	64.1	204.4	31.6	74.7	337.3	221.9
Family income											
Under $5,000	411.7	41.4	45.4	82.0	219.0	65.6	216.1	27.4	78.7	323.0	232.0
$5,000–$9,999	353.3	32.6	37.2	76.1	190.0	51.4	179.5	34.7	57.3	271.6	163.2
$10,000–$14,999	310.9		27.4	81.1	158.9	} 43.8	192.6	} 30.6	39.3	247.3	181.3
$15,000 and over	300.8		40.7	62.7	174.8		161.4		48.5	259.2	169.2

[1] Includes unknown income.

Source: National Center for Health Statistics, 1976.

Health Indicators

Table 33-5 Selected health indicators for elderly population by sex: 1972

Indicator	Male 65 years and over	Female 65 years and over
Total population (thousands)	8,301	11,623
Percent with activity limitation	47.0	40.5
In major activity	43.3	34.1
Persons injured per 100 persons per year	22.3	20.6
Days of restricted activity per 100 persons per year	439.9	633.2
Days of bed disability associated with injury per 100 persons per year	171.8	211.8

Source: National Center for Health Statistics.

Table 33-6 Annual physician visits per person for elderly persons—1972

Type of visit and sex	Total persons 65 years and over (thousands)	Visits per person per year
Physician Visit		
Both sexes	19,924	14.5
Male	8,301	15.8
Female	11,623	13.7

Source: National Center for Health Statistics.

Life Expectancy

Life expectancy has shown a tremendous increase since the beginning of this century, having risen from 49 years in 1900–02 to 69.5 years in 1955, 71.3 years in 1973 and 71.9 years in 1974.

At ages 65–74 in 1974 the recorded death rate for blacks and other races was a third greater than the death rate for whites, but at ages 75–84 the recorded death rate for blacks and other races was 10% below the death rate for whites.

Table 33-7 Death rates for the ten leading causes of death for the elderly—1973

Rank	Cause of death	65 years and over
	All causes	5,874.4
1	Diseases of heart	2,643.2
2	Malignant neoplasms	946.7
3	Cerebrovascular diseases	839.3
4	Influenza and pneumonia	210.3
5	Arteriosclerosis	146.0
6	Accidents	127.7
	Motor vehicle	33.2
	All other	94.5
7	Diabetes mellitus	126.3
8	Bronchitis, emphysema, and asthma	97.7
9	Cirrhosis of liver	37.9
10	Infections of kidney	22.9
	All other causes	676.4

Source: National Center for Health Statistics.

Table 33-8 Male to female ratio for the ten leading causes of death, for ages 65 and over—1973

Cause of death	65 years and over
All causes	1.455
Diseases of heart	1.434
Malignant neoplasms	1.779
Cerebrovascular diseases	1.028
Influenza and pneumonia	1.555
Arteriosclerosis	0.952
Accidents	1.516
Motor vehicle	2.295
All other	1.313
Diabetes mellitus	0.860
Bronchitis, emphysema, and asthma	5.422
Cirrhosis of liver	2.662
Infections of kidney	1.063
All other causes	1.734

Source: National Center for Health Statistics.

Health Expenditures

Table 33-9 Estimated personal health care expenditures for the aged, by type of expenditure and source of funds, fiscal years 1973–75

Type of expenditure	Amount (in millions)					Percentage distribution				
				Public					Public	
	Total	Private	Total	Medicare	Other	Total	Private	Total	Medicare	Other
Total 1975	$30,383	$10,466	$19,917	$12,762	$7,155	100.0	34.4	65.6	42.0	23.5
Hospital care	13,467	1,379	12,088	9,725	2,363	100.0	10.2	89.8	72.2	17.5
Physicians' services	4,862	1,987	2,875	2,629	246	100.0	40.9	59.1	54.1	5.1
Dentists' services	540	502	38	—	38	100.0	92.9	7.1	—	7.1
Other professional services	441	220	221	167	54	100.0	49.8	50.2	38.0	12.2
Drugs and drug sundries	2,629	2,285	344	—	344	100.0	86.9	13.1	—	13.1
Eyeglasses and appliances	506	498	8	—	8	100.0	98.4	1.6	—	1.6
Nursing-home care	7,650	3,571	4,079	241	3,838	100.0	46.7	53.3	3.1	50.2
Other health services	288	24	264	—	264	100.0	8.2	91.8	—	91.8

Source: DHEW.

The Process of Aging*

Senescence refers to degenerative changes that occur *after maturity has been reached,* which ultimately culminate in death.

Mobility Limitations

Of the total population, fewer than one out of 100 of those under 45 are affected in this way, compared to one out of 20 of those 45–64, and almost one out of five of those 65 and older.

Perception

In most sensory systems, acuity declines with advancing age. Reduction can be a consequence of age-related diseases and occupational injuries, as well as changes in the receptors that may be due to primary aging.

From age 20 to age 60, the rate of hearing impairments rises from about 10 to about 75

*Source: *Working with Older People,* Vol. I, DHEW, 1974.

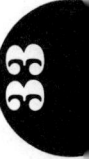

per 1,000 population. However, between ages 60 and 80, the rate accelerates to 250. Thus, one out of four very aged persons has a significant hearing impairment. In the same age group, about 80 individuals per 1,000 population are blind.

With age, most sensory receptors require more energy to reach a threshhold level of stimulation.

In general, the sensory changes associated with advancing age effectively reduce alertness. Compensations for sensory losses are achieved in part through closer monitoring, increased intensity of stimuli and slowness and cautiousness.

Aged Mental Changes *

Mental Ability—Some evidence suggests that the thought processes of older adults tend toward simple associations rather than toward analysis. The weakness in solving abstract problems seems to be a reduction in the tendency to generate hypotheses about the nature of the problem and an orderly checking out of facts.

Verbal Ability—Loss of verbal ability seemed particularly good as a clue to incipient disease.

Verbal ability improved with age, contrary to the misconception that aging must signify decline in every function. In one survey, old men did better on verbal tests than young men. However, this was a departure from the general psychological decline that comes with age. Decline in verbal ability when the men were re-tested seemed an index to a group of changes, including decline in cerebral metabolic oxygen utilization and 23 cognitive and psychomotor measures.

Senile Dementia—Senile dementia can be expected in about 4% of the population. Senile dementia seems to occur independently of, or in combination with, preexisting disease such as psychoneurosis, schizophrenia or manic depressive reactions.

Mental illness in older persons can occur commonly as a side effect of somatic illnesses. Infectious diseases and undernutrition may help produce mental symptoms, and these may not disappear until some time after the original conditions are controlled.

---

*Source: *Working with Older People . . .*, Volume I, DHEW, 1974.

As a result, geriatric psychiatry is placing more emphasis on seeking mixed causes of mental illness in older persons, taking into consideration possible interactions among physical illness, mental illness and social illness. Problems of health, finances and loss of spouse often arise in retirement when the individual has fewer resources with which to solve them. He or she begins to lose hope. As problems are solved less and less adequately, anxiety not only emerges but grows, becomes itself a barrier to successful problem solving and spreads to the family.

Vascular and senile changes are distinct, though often concomitant. Advancing age does not lead characteristically to a reduction in blood flow to the brain. Individuals with functional emotional disorders have a favorable prognosis and are likely to be discharged from specialized facilities within one year. But patients diagnosed with senile brain disease or "organic brain syndrome" have only a 50% probability of surviving the year.

In patients with organic brain disease, cognitive functioning degenerates. However, there is the possibility of a social-psychological cushioning of the consequences of senile brain disorder. An individual with an affective interpersonal relationship with another person, e.g., a "confidant," is less likely to be precipitated into a mental crisis requiring hospitalization than is the isolate.

Personality Types

One extensive study of personality showed at least three clear-cut types associated with high life satisfaction:

1. The "mature" type includes individuals who accept the facts of aging, adjust well to losses, are realistic about their past and present lives and face death with relative equanimity.
2. The "armored" type includes persons who cling to middle-aged behavior patterns, deny aging, keep as busy as ever and manage to get along very well.
3. The "rocking chair" type, which is growing as society becomes more leisure oriented, includes persons who accept passivity, sit and rock without feeling guilty about it.

The American Health Care Association in a 1975 survey of nursing home administrators asked: "About what percentage of your current patients present behavior problems or are mentally confused? Include senile patients."

CARING FOR THE AGED PATIENT

728

33

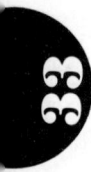

Percent of respondents according to
percentage of confused patients reported

% confused patients	% respondents
1–24%	19%
25–49%	22%
50–74%	26%
75–89%	20%
90–99%	13%

The distribution of patients reported confused ranged from 1% to 99%. Approximately 41% reported that less than half of their patients were confused, and 59% of the respondents indicated that over half of their patients were confused or had behavior problems.

Brain Damage*

Symptoms—

1. Decreases or deficits in orientation.
2. Memory loss.
3. Decreases in patient's fund of general information.
4. Decreases in patient's ability to do simple calculations.

Normal Changes in Brain—Changes take place in the *neurons* in the *cortex* of the brain. The cortex is a relatively thin, but very important, layer covering the entire brain. It is like corrugated material, so that its area, if spread out flat, is much larger than the brain area it covers.

There are billions of neurons—or cells—in the cortex, and each day we live, for a variety of reasons, we lose some of them. This continuous process over the life-time of the individual can take place without impairing the individual's ability to live in his normal environment and to deal effectively with it.

Excessive Chances—However, in addition to these gradual, not necessarily dysfunctional, losses, there are aspects of the individual's genetic inheritance or events in his life which may act as causal agents for excessive loss, which leads to brain dysfunction and perhaps to brain damage. Serious impairment or loss of a large number of brain cells is usually the result of an unfortunate combination of causal factors. Seldom is the magnitude of malfunction that brain syndrome reflects the consequence of only one cause.

Causal Agents—

1. Accidents in which there is serious injury affecting a substantial area of the brain.
2. Infectious diseases, particularly when accompanied by high fever. It seems probable that high fever does kill brain cells. Encephalitis, meningitis, scarlet fever, and whooping cough are examples of infectious diseases likely to be linked to brain damage. These may cause decrements in cellular quantity which, late in life, may render the individual more vulnerable to losses from other causes.
3. Stresses and deficiencies of early life may act as causal agents. For example, poor health and habitual malnutrition, long hours spent in unhealthy surroundings—polluted air, for example—may result in early losses far in excess of the gradual losses which normally occur. The individual is then left with insufficient resources when the losses associated with old age occur.
4. Aspects of the individual's genetic inheritance appear to predispose him to brain dysfunction or damage—for example, the condition called *senile deterioration*. Something causes a rapid loss of a substantial number of brain cells, which is reflected by the impairment in function.

Caring for the Aged Patient

The Aged Patient's Psychological Needs**

The goal of the physician—and this can be taken as a key to the goals of other practitioners—is to maintain structure without major loss, to try to promote ability to handle stress, and to help the patient attain and maintain the maximum physical and mental efficiency of which he is capable.

Practitioners should be aware:

- of the impact of retirement, loss of income and prestige and dependency;
- that the elderly man keenly feels the waning of strength, lack of usefulness in society's eyes;
- that the elderly woman, perhaps widowed, may be overwhelmed by her loss, conscious

*Source: DHEW, 1975.

**Source: *Working With Older People . . .*, Volumes I and II, DHEW, 1974.

of a fading place in her children's lives and worried about diminished income and health;

- of the impact of these anxieties on physical condition and of physical condition on these anxieties;
- that health has a greater influence on a persons's concept of himself than does age;
- that personality changes and the psychological effects attributed to aging are in large measure reactions to health states rather than to chronologically determined processes alone;
- that factors of class, culture and economics inhibit the patient's obtaining or using proper medical care, and that these factors and the patient's attitudes toward health and aging must be understood by both practitioner and patient;
- that attitudes and definitions of health vary by social class, finances, country, culture, age, sex and occupation, and that many of these outlooks lead elderly people to accept certain symptoms and disabilities as natural or inevitable;
- that the elderly patient needs assistance in sustaining a sense of his worth and dignity;
- that we must treat the person, not the symptom.

Much of the emotional disturbance in old age is the result of the loss of certain social roles and the search for new ones. The aging not only face retirement but also face further changes, particularly in health. Anxiety about the present and future may result in physical and mental health problems. These anxieties must be considered by those who have the responsibility for caring for older people.

Two of the most common mechanisms of adjusting to problems of aging are hypochondriasis and denial. In hypochondriasis, the aging person becomes excessively concerned with declining health. He complains, makes frequent visits to physicians, and busies himself in self-doctoring with patent medicines. Denial means the refusal to recognize declining health and the resistance to receiving medical care and advice.

The desire for good health may be so much a personal need that decline comes as a trauma, leading to depression and disorganization of self and role behavior. For most of the elderly, the realization is unpleasant but not shocking. Adjustment with a minimum of

social and emotional disturbance requires much effort and often much assistance.

Social isolation apparently predisposes certain types of personality toward mental illness. Loss of social role by retirement or widowhood may result in mental illness. Perhaps the quality of social contact and participation means more than the quantity in preserving mental health.

It is true that the adult can, after leaving school, lose the attitude of seeking to learn. As the years go by he tends to solve problems on the basis of what he already knows and is not inclined to change his approach—even in the face of information suggesting that he should. This "rigidity" or refusal to change was at one time thought to be related to aging. Current evidence, however, suggests that the level of rigidity in an individual is associated with the extent of schooling and the number of years that have passed since school was attended. Furthermore, the greater the person's intelligence, the less likely he is to be "rigid." There is some evidence that the thought processes of older adults tend toward simple associations rather than toward analysis, and the weakness in solving abstract problems seems to be related to a reduction in the tendency to generate hypotheses about the nature of a problem and an orderly checking out of facts.

Home Care for the Aged*

There is no firm national policy with respect to alternatives to institutionalization. Home health care receives a very low priority in the United States. While home health is authorized under both Medicare and Medicaid, expenditures for home health care constitutes less than 1% of either program.

The services which should be provided include those which are necessary to the rehabilitation and recovery of the patient, those which are necessary to prevent deterioration, and those which sustain the patient's current capacity even when full recovery or medical improvement is not expected.

Agnes Brewster, consultant for the Senate Committee on Aging, estimates that 2.6 million individuals over 65 need in-home

---

* Source: Senate Special Subcommittee on Aging, November 1975.

services: 300,000 in institutions and another 2.3 million in the community. In 1970 there were 2,800 home care programs in the United States. Almost 85% of these had been approved for Medicare.

Of the 2,250 home health agencies participating in Medicare in 1972, about 57% were official health agencies, 24% were visiting nurse associations, 3% were combined government and voluntary agencies, and 9% were hospital based. The remainder were based in rehabilitation facilities extended care facilities, retirement villages and in other types of agencies. In fiscal year 1973, Medicare paid out $75 million in home health benefits, accounting for less than 1% of the total Medicare expenditures of $12.1 billion.

A General Accounting Office survey of 11 states revealed that from 1968 to 1971:

- the number of home visits to Medicare patients decreased 42%;

- the number of nurses in home health programs and home health aides decreased by 41% and 49%.

As a consequence, few states have developed significant home health programs. In 1972 Medicaid home health expenditures totaled $24 million or less than 1% of the Medicaid $5 billion total. Some 113,372 recipients were served nationwide.

Day Care—An Alternative

The recent surge in interest in lowering health care costs and enabling long-term disabled persons to live in their homes rather than becoming institutionalized has resulted in intensive efforts to develop a program of day care for aged and long-term disabled persons. A viable day care program for the aged and long-term disabled has economic as well as social, rehabilitative and preventive advantages.

34

THE HANDICAPPED AND THE DISABLED

The Disabled: Rates and Characteristics*

Overview

The 1970 Bureau of the Census survey estimated that 11 million Americans between 16 and 64 were disabled—suffering from spinal cord injuries, cerebral palsy, multiple sclerosis, muscular dystrophy, mental retardation, blindness and other handicaps. This number was 9% of the total adult population, or one out of every 11 Americans. As expected, the national disability rate increases by age. However, the disability rate for women is lower than for men, in all age brackets—from one to three percent.

Table 34-1 United States disability rate by sex and age (percent disabled six months or more)

United States summary	Sex		
	Total	Male	Female
Total	9.3%	10.1%	8.5%
Age			
16–24	4.5	5.9	3.1
25–34	5.0	5.7	4.4
35–44	7.6	8.1	7.2
45–54	12.7	13.4	12.0
55–64	21.0	22.1	20.0

Highlights of the national 1970 Census—

- *Education*—The median educational level for the total American population was four years of high school. The average handicapped person only attended one to three years of high school.
- *Income*—The average handicapped person's income was approximately $1,000 below the average for the total American population.
- *Poverty status*—Thirty-six percent of the handicapped are in the poverty category, compared with 20% of the general population.
- *Labor force status*—Among the handicapped, 42% are employed; among the general population, 59% are employed.
- *Age*—Two-thirds of the total population between 16 and 64 are less than 45 years

*Source: President's Committee on Unemployment of Handicapped, 1976.

old; yet nearly two-thirds of the handicapped population are more than 45 years old.

Metropolitan Concentration

Table 34-2 Disability rate: 1970 noninstitutionalized disabled population 16 to 64 years old, with work disability of six months or more

In standard metropolitan statistical areas with one million or more total population	Total no. of disabled	Disability rate
Anaheim–Santa Ana–Garden Grove, California	68,767	8.1%
Atlanta, Georgia	83,640	9.7
Baltimore, Maryland	116,368	9.2
Boston, Massachusetts	129,538	7.8
Buffalo, New York	65,101	8.1
Chicago, Illinois	343,216	8.2
Cincinnati, Ohio–Kentucky–Indiana	76,752	9.5
Cleveland, Ohio	107,481	8.6
Dallas, Texas	82,360	8.7
Denver, Colorado	62,027	8.3
Detroit, Michigan	234,485	9.4
Houston, Texas	104,445	8.7
Indianapolis, Indiana	58,192	8.9
Kansas City, Missouri-Kansas	65,741	8.8
Los Angeles-Long Beach, California	435,892	10.0
Miami, Florida	79,119	10.4
Milwaukee, Wisconsin	63,164	7.7
Minneapolis-St. Paul, Minnesota	80,867	7.6
New Orleans, Louisiana	64,903	10.5
New York, New York	569,507	8.0
Newark, New Jersey	89,007	7.9
Paterson-Clifton-Passaic, New Jersey	56,493	6.7
Philadelphia, Pennsylvania	246,316	8.5
Pittsburgh, Pennsylvania	121,200	8.3
Portland, Oregon-Washington	61,630	10.2
St. Louis, Missouri-Illinois	126,333	9.1
San Bernardino-Riverside-Ontario, California	71,832	10.9
San Diego, California	74,855	8.7
San Francisco-Oakland, California	175,655	8.9
San Jose, California	54,854	8.4
Seattle-Everett, Washington	75,754	8.7
Tampa-St. Petersburg, Florida	67,339	12.2
Washington, D.C.–Maryland–Virginia	130,810	7.3

Source: President's Commission on Employment of Handicapped, 1976.

Work Performance of the Handicapped Employee

DuPont's eight-month study gathered data on 1,452 employees with physical handicaps. The key findings of the duPont study:

1. Insurance: No increases in compensation costs nor lost-time injuries.
2. Physical Adjustments: Most handicapped require no special work arrangement.

3. Safety: 96% of handicapped workers rated average or better both on and off the job; more than one-half were above average.
4. Special Privileges: A handicapped worker wants to be treated as a regular employee.
5. Job Performance: 91% rated average or better.
6. Attendance: 79% rated average or better.

The duPont study also shows there is very little difference between handicapped and nonhandicapped workers as to their ability to work in harmony with supervisors and fellow employees.

The Mentally Retarded

Where They Work

Over the years qualified mentally retarded persons have been successfully employed in the following jobs (as well as hundreds of others): general office clerks, messengers, office persons, mail carriers, stock clerks, salesclerks, domestics, dayworkers, housekeepers, nursemaids, nurses' aides, attendants, ward helpers, busboys, kitchen helpers, dishwashers, bootblacks, manicurists, ushers, personal service workers, porters, janitors, sextons, recreation and amusement workers, farmhands, landscape laborers, groundsmen, bakers, upholsterers, construction workers, unskilled laborers, textile machine tenders, welders, routemen, packers, assemblers, inspectors, laundry sorters, filling station attendants, carpenters' helpers, metal workers, warehousemen. And the list grows and grows.

A vital reason for successful placements has been preparation and training provided by the more than 300 vocational rehabilitation agencies and sheltered workshops which serve mentally retarded adults. Many are sponsored by, or have some relationship with, the National Association for Retarded Citizens. In addition, many Goodwill Industries of America workshops and Jewish Vocational Service workshops can assist mentally retarded persons.

In a typical sheltered workshop, the retarded person is given a comprehensive vocational rehabilitation program of evaluation and training, which takes about a year. He is exposed to a simulated work atmosphere and is evaluated and trained by a professional staff in a wide variety of work situations. Individual vocational

analysis is made, and suitable preparation is given for competitive employment. The trainee learns the basic skills essential to work and is given every opportunity to demonstrate his ability to use hand and machine tools. Eventually, he is ready for full-time employment.

Table 34-3   Major occupational groupings for rehabilitated mentally retarded persons. (Based on 26,762 retarded persons vocationally rehabilitated through federal-state programs, fiscal year 1969—11% of all rehabilitations that year.)

Type of occupation	Percentage
Service	36.7
Industrial	36.4
Sheltered workshops	6.1
Clerical	5.8
Homemaker	5.1
Agriculture	3.8
Unpaid family work	3.5
Sales	1.6
Professional	1.0

Source: President's Committee on Employment of Handicapped, 1976.

Advice and Assistance

Handicapped Children: Where to Get Advice

Parents should seek the best possible medical advice available to them. A diagnostic and evaluation clinic, for example, or a hearing and speech center or other special clinics may be available in their town or city. A public health nurse may be able to visit in their home from time to time. Information about assistance and guidance is usually available through the local department of welfare or department of public health.

In addition to the advice of their own pediatrician and the local services described above, there are also many national organizations concerned with helping the handicapped. Already these include associations for muscular dystrophy, cerebral palsy, birth defects, mental retardation, epilepsy, diabetes, to name only a few. These organizations are an excellent source of information and guidance, news of research and treatment possibilities, good suggestions for physical therapy, recreation, education and even the legal rights of the handicapped.

The Bureau of Education for the Handicapped has compiled a list of every educational project in the United States which offers programs for handicapped children. Requests for information can be sent to "Closer Look," Box 1492, Washington, D.C. 20013.

A complete list and description of 107 organizations directly concerned with the handicapped—*Directory of Organizations Interested in the Handicapped, 1976*—is available from the Committee for the Handicapped, Suite 610, La Salle Building, Connecticut Ave. and L St., Washington, D.C. 20036.

Employment Assistance

1. *Vocational Rehabilitation—Rehabilitation Services:* Provides funds to states to meet the costs of vocational rehabilitation services for physically or mentally handicapped persons. Special funds available for projects involving new or special services. For information, contact:

Vocational Rehabilitation Administration,
U.S. Department of Health, Education and Welfare,
Washington, D.C. 20201

2. *Aid to the Permanently and Totally Disabled:* Provides grants to states for financial assistance, medical care and social services for the permanently and totally disabled. For information, contact:

Bureau of Family Services,
Welfare Administration,
U.S. Department of Health, Education and Welfare,
Washington, D.C. 20201

3. *Youth Opportunity Centers:* Provides individual counseling, testing, placement and related services to all youths between the ages of 16 and 21. For information, contact:

U.S. Employment Service,
Bureau of Employment Security,
Manpower Administration,
U.S. Department of Labor,
Washington, D.C. 20210

4. *Bureau of Work Programs:* Provides funds and technical assistance for establishment of work-training programs for unemployed youths 16 through 21 years of age. Among eligible institutional sponsors are nonprofit hospitals. For information, contact:

Bureau of Work Programs,
U.S. Department of Labor,
Washington, D.C. 20210

5. *Job Corps Training Centers:* Offers a residential program of vocational training, remedial education and work experience for qualified youths between ages 16 to 21. Youths with limited medical conditions and disabilities are considered eligible. For information, contact:

Job Corps,
Washington, D.C. 20506

6. *Health Referral Services for Armed Forces Medical Rejectees:* Provides funds to states to establish and operate referral/counseling programs for those rejected for military service for medical reasons. For information, contact:

Bureau of Health Services,
Public Health Service,
U.S. Department of Health, Education and Welfare,
Washington, D.C. 20201

7. *Vocational Rehabilitation of Service-Disabled Veterans:* Provides vocational rehabilitation training for service-disabled veterans at appropriate training facilities and supplies all training costs plus a subsistence allowance. For information, contact: Veteran Administration Regional Office.

8. *Veteran's Restoration Program:* Assists in the return of disabled veterans to regular community life. The medical staff member responsible for his treatment and care determines the candidate's eligibility. For information, contact:

Director, Extended Care Service
Department of Medicine and Surgery
Attention: Chief, Domiciliary and Restoration Center Division
Veterans Administration,
Washington, D.C. 20420

9. *Adult Basic Education:* Enables state educational agencies to instruct illiterate persons in reading/writing English and to improve their participation in occupational training programs. For information, contact:

Adult Education Branch,
Office of Education,
U.S. Department of Health, Education and Welfare,
Washington, D.C. 20202

34

10. *Work Experience Program:* Grants made to state public welfare agency for projects at the community level which raise the employability of needy adults and provide work experience and training. On-the-job training may include work as nurse's aides, hospital orderlies or laboratory aides. For information, contact:

Office of Special Services,
Bureau of Family Services,
Welfare Administration,
U.S. Department of Health, Education and Welfare,
Washington, D.C. 20201

11. *Occupational Training in Redevelopment Areas:* Provides training for persons residing in designated redevelopment areas to qualify for existing job opportunities. For information, contact:

Office of Manpower Policy, Evaluation and Research,
Manpower Administration,
U.S. Department of Labor,
Washington, D.C. 20210

12. *Manpower Development and Training:* Provides occupational training and subsistence allowances for unemployed and underemployed persons who cannot obtain appropriate full-time employment without training. For information, contact:

Office of Manpower Policy, Evaluation and Research,
Manpower Administration,
U.S. Department of Labor,
Washington, D.C. 20210

13. *Apprenticeship and Training:* Develops training programs in skilled and semi-skilled crafts/trades by working directly with management. Sponsors may be an industry, association or organization that has access to training facilities. For information, contact:

Bureau of Apprenticeship and Training,
U.S. Department of Labor,
Washington, D.C. 20210

14. *Physically and Mentally Handicapped—Employment Service:* Provides direct employment and counseling services to the physically and mentally handicapped. For information, contact:

U.S. Employment Service,
Bureau of Employment Security,
Manpower Administration,
U.S. Department of Labor,
Washington, D.C. 20210

15. *Books for the Blind and Physically Handicapped:* Provides library service, free of charge, to blind and physically handicapped. Catalogs of books available from 32 regional libraries. Certification of eligibility may be made by a competent authority, including registered nurses. For information, contact:

Division for the Blind and Physically Handicapped,
Library of Congress,
Washington, D.C. 20540

16. *Teaching Materials for the Blind:* Provides free instruction materials for blind pupils in elementary and secondary schools, including state commissions and adult rehabilitation centers for the blind. For information, contact:

Vice President and General Manager,
American Printing House for the Blind,
1839 Frankfort Avenue,
Louisville, Ky. 40206

17. *Aid to the Blind:* Provides grants to states for the financial assistance and medical care of needy blind persons. For information, contact:

Bureau of Family Services,
Welfare Administration,
U.S. Department of Health, Education and Welfare,
Washington, D.C. 20201

18. *Captioned Film for the Deaf:* Maintains a lending library of captioned films for eligible groups, including clubs and organizations. For information, contact:

Captioned Films Branch,
Bureau of Research,
Office of Education,
U.S. Department of Health, Education and Welfare,
Washington, D.C. 20202

35
WOMEN TODAY*

Overview

Highlights**

- In July 1976 the female population of the United States was about 110.2 million, outnumbering males by 5.3 million. With increases in the total population, by the end of the century women are projected to outnumber men by 6.9 to 7.9 million.

- The changing social and economic role of women is most evident in the increase in their labor force participation. Between 1950 and 1974 the number of working women nearly doubled, while the number of working men increased by about one-fourth.

- The dramatic change in the female work force is reflected in the change in the ratio of women to men who were year-round full-time workers, from 29 women per 100 men in 1950 to 47 women per 100 men in 1974.

- The historical relationship between labor force participation and such variables as marital status and the presence and age of children has been changing. Among married women with preschool age children the participation rate has risen substantially, from 12% in 1950 to 37% in 1975.

- Although employment of women increased in the 1960s, women workers remained concentrated in a few major occupation groups in both 1960 and 1970, with over half of them working in clerical, operative and service positions.

- Income differentials of women and men workers remained substantial in 1974; the median income for women who had worked year round full-time was 57% of the median income for men who had worked year round full-time.

- Families headed by women were 13% of all families in 1975. The proportion of families below the poverty level that are headed by women has increased, accounting for 46% of all families in poverty in 1974.

- College enrollment rates of women have risen far more rapidly than those for men since 1950, but women were still only 44% of college students in 1974.

- Although younger women are approaching educational equality with men, they have not yet closed the gap; among persons 25 to 29 years old in 1975, 77% as many women as men had completed four years of college; in 1950 the comparable figure was 66%. During the period the proportion of women 25 to 29 years old who completed four years of college rose from 6% to 19%.

- Life expectancy at birth, a measure of longevity, has improved more for women than for men, advancing for women from 48.3 years in 1900 to 75.3 years in 1973, and advancing for men from 46.3 years to 67.6 years in the same period. Life expectancy of women now exceeds that of men by almost eight years.

- Of the 15 leading causes of death, women experience lower death rates than men for all causes except one (diabetes). The dramatic decrease in the maternal mortality rate in the last 50 years has eliminated this as a major cause of death among women.

- The recent trends in marriage and divorce have resulted in an increasing proportion of young women who are single or divorced. Between 1950 and 1975 the proportion of women 20 to 24 years old who were single increased from 28 to 40%; during the same period the proportion of women 25 to 34 years old who were divorced and not remarried increased from 2.5 to 6.8%.

- The fertility rates of American women have shown wide fluctuations in the past quarter century from near record highs for the century in the late 1950s to record lows in the past few years. If the current level of fertility were to continue, a natural decrease (an excess of deaths over births) would result eventually.

---

*Source: Material is adapted from literature of the Women's Bureau, U.S. Department of Labor, except where otherwise noted.
**Source: *Statistical Portrait of Women in the United States,* U.S. Bureau of the Census, April 1976.

Attitudes Toward a New Role for Women
The Public's Attitude

Table 35-1   New public attitudes toward women's roles

	Women		Men	
	1975 %	1970 %	1975 %	1970 %
Taking care of a home and raising children is more rewarding for a woman than having a job.				
Agree	51	71	52	68
Disagree	34	16	25	13
Not sure	15	13	23	19
The country would be better off if women had more to say about politics.				
Agree	57	39	39	35
Disagree	29	46	42	51
Not sure	14	15	19	14
There won't be a woman president of the U.S. for a long time, and that's probably just as well.				
Agree	41	67	51	65
Disagree	47	23	36	25
Not sure	12	10	13	10
For a woman to be truly happy she needs to have a man around.				
Agree	42	67	54	68
Disagree	52	27	33	22
Not sure	6	6	13	10
Women will always be more emotional and less logical than men.				
Agree	39	58	54	68
Disagree	53	35	35	24
Not sure	8	7	11	8
Attitude toward the efforts to strengthen and change women's role in society.				
Favor	65	40	59	44
Oppose	25	42	25	39
Not sure	10	18	16	17

Source: Harris Survey, Dec. 11, 1975.

The Nurse's Attitude

Nursing '74 (Oct. 1974), in a survey of 11,000 nurses asked:

What effect has the women's lib movement had on nursing?

Entirely positive	11%
Mostly positive, some negative	25%
Little or no effect	52%
Entirely negative	3%
Mostly negative, some positive	9%

Student nurses and nurses with bachelor's and master's degrees tend to hold a more favorable view of women's liberation; about half thought it had a positive effect.

Health and Longevity**

During the 20th century, great progress has been made in increased longevity though the discrepancy between male and female life ex-

** Source: *Statistical Portrait of Women in the United States,* U.S. Bureau of the Census.

pectancy continues to widen. Over the 75-year period 1900 to 1975, the average length of life of females increased from 48.3 years in 1900 to 76.4 years in 1975, i.e., by 28.1 years. For men, life expectancy increased only 22.2 years over the same period, advancing from 46.3 years to 68.5 years.

In 1930 women could expect to live 3.5 years longer than men; by 1970 women had a life expectancy nearly eight years longer.

The main reasons for the increasing female advantage in longevity have been the decrease in deaths due to pregnancy and childbirth and the shift from infective and parasitic diseases to chronic degenerative diseases as the major causes of death.

Pregnancy and Childbirth

The reduction in death rates of women from the complications of pregnancy and childbirth has removed one of the major causes of death among women. In the United States, the maternal mortality rate has shown a dramatic improvement in the last five decades, dropping sharply from 690 deaths related to pregnancy and childbirth per 100,000 live births in 1920–24, to 376 in 1940, 37 in 1960, and 15 in 1973. This dramatic drop may be attributed to a combination of factors, including the decline in the birth rate (specifically in the number of children born to women, particularly to older women). The expanded programs of prenatal and postnatal care, which have contributed to reductions in infant mortality, have also benefited the mother, as has the decline in the practice of employing a midwife at home as a substitute for an attending physician in a hospital. Among other factors which have resulted in the reduction of maternal mortality are the use of antibiotics to control infections and the availability of blood and blood substitutes for the treatment of hemorrhage.

Degenerative Diseases

In the past 40 years, degenerative diseases such as heart disease and malignant neoplasms have become increasingly prevalent as causes of death due to the relatively successful eradication of infective and parasitic disease. For reasons that are not entirely clear, women succumb to degenerative diseases less than men. Furthermore, medical technology has developed in such a way that some of the more serious types of cancer among women, such as breast and uterine cancer, are more easily de-tected and treated than the main types of cancer among men (e.g., cancer of the lungs and digestive system).

Male/Female Population Ratio*

Since 1910 the female population has grown faster in each decade than the male population. The sex ratio (number of males per 100 females) has declined steadily from 106.2 in 1910 to 94.9 in 1975. At the turn of the century, men constituted 51.1% of the total U.S. population; in 1950, for the first time in any decennial census, women outnumbered men.

Although the sex ratio (number of males per 100 females) at birth is a little above 105, this small preponderance of males at the start of life is reduced, first, by the higher infant mortality of males and, then, by the higher death rates of males at other ages.

The excess of women over men is projected to range between 6.2 million and 6.5 million by 1985; between 6.9 million and 7.9 million by 2000.

Select Hospitals for Women**

In an evaluation of hospitals which are superior in the treatment of women's special health problems, The Ladies Home Journal (January 1976) submitted a questionnaire to a panel of 18 top medical professionals and representatives of consumer health organizations who came up with the recommendations below.

Though chosen for a variety of reasons, all the selected hospitals are large metropolitan institutions affiliated with universities or medical schools, engaged in both treatment and research, staffed by highly qualified physicians and surgeons using the most advanced equipment to deal routinely with both esoteric and emergency conditions. They are superspecialized, with a full range of both inpatient and outpatient services; and they are primarily referral institutions, meaning that they get tough cases others cannot handle.

Besides general excellence as a basis for selection, specific reasons were also given for hospital recommendation:

---

*Source: U.S. Bureau of the Census.

**Source: Edwin Kester, "America's Ten Best Hospitals for Women," The Ladies Home Journal January 1976. © 1975 Downe Publishing, Inc. Reprinted with permission of The Ladies Home Journal.

- Boston Hospital for Women, including Boston Lying-In Hospital: stresses painless childbirth.
- Harbor General Hospital, UCLA, Torrance, Calif.: emphasis on patient's rights.
- Hartford, Connecticut Hospital: program of personal care.
- Hospital of the University of Pennsylvania, Philadelphia: treatment of female endocrine disorders/infertility.
- Los Angeles County-University of Southern California Medical Center, Women's Hospital, Los Angeles: ranks number one in Ob/Gyn care.
- McDonald House, University Hospital, Case Western Reserve University, Cleveland: research and treatment of perinatology.
- Parkland Hospital, University of Texas Health Sciences Center, Dallas: no specifics indicated.
- Sloane Hospital for Women, Columbia-Presbyterian Medical Center, New York: program of personal care.
- University of Colorado Hospitals, Denver: innovative clinic care.
- Women's Pavilion, University of Michigan Hospitals, Ann Arbor: innovative clinic care.

Education*

None of the indicators of educational achievement—attainment, enrollment, field of study or degrees awarded—shows that women have reached the same levels as men. But in most areas the educational gap between the sexes has narrowed since 1950.

The proportion of college-age women (18 to 24) enrolled in school was significantly higher in 1974 than in 1960. In 1960, 30% of the females 18 to 19 years old were enrolled in school; the enrollment ratio increased to 42% in 1970 and has since remained at approximately that level. However, while the enrollment rates of women have risen more rapidly than those of men since 1950, there were still fewer women than men attending college in 1974: 3,898,000 as opposed to 4,924,000.

As an indicator of trends among persons 25 to 29 years of age in 1950, there were only 66

*Source: U.S. Bureau of the Census, 1976.

women who had completed at least four years of college for every 100 men who had done so. The corresponding ratio in 1975 was 77 female college graduates for every 100 comparable males.

However, those women who were attending college have been moving into traditionally "male" majors in increasing numbers. For example, the percentage of engineering majors who were women rose from 2% in 1966 to 7% in 1974. The comparable figures for agriculture and forestry were 3% in 1966 and 14% in 1974.

Generally increases in college attendance by women are being reflected in the proportion of bachelor's and higher degrees awarded to women. In the academic year 1949–50, about one-fourth of all bachelor's and higher degrees were awarded to women, but only 10% of all doctorates given in that year went to females. By 1972 women earned 41% of all degrees at or above the B.A. level and 16% of all doctorates.

What College Women Major In

Table 35-2 Major fields of study for female college students

	1974		1966
Major field of study	Number	% female	% female
Total enrollment			
Female	3,898,000	44.2%	38.2%
Male & female	3,822,000	100.0	100.0
Agriculture/forestry		13.5	2.6
Biological sciences		41.0	(1)
Business or commerce		31.7	23.0
Education		72.6	67.9
Engineering		6.8	1.9
English or journalism		59.1	50.9
Other humanities		48.0	
Health or medical profession		64.2	2 44.5
Law		23.2	(NA)
Mathematics or statistics		44.6	36.5
Physical sciences		26.9	11.1
Social sciences		44.4	37.6
Vocational-technical studies		25.4	(NA)
Computer science		20.0	(NA)
Other		41.0	27.4
None and not reported		44.7	41.9

NA Not available.
[1] Included in health or medical profession.
[2] Includes biological sciences.

Source: U.S. Bureau of the Census.

Educational Levels and the Working Woman

Nearly three-fourths of all women workers were high school graduates. More than one out of four of all women in the labor force had completed one or more years of college, and one out of eight was a college graduate. Generally the more education a woman has, the more likely she is to be in the labor force.

Education level	% women in work force
Elementary	
Less than eight years	22%
Eight years	26%
High school	
Four years	51%
College	
Four years	61%
Five years or more	70%

There has been an unprecedented rise in the number of women in professional training, both absolutely and relative to men, after half a century of "little or no change." One of the primary factors in this development is the changing attitudes of women: more women are applying to professional schools. For example, women represented approximately 4 to 5% of practicing physicians to medical school prior to 1940. The percentage of women applicants rose very slowly for nearly two and a half decades. After 1965 women began applying in greater numbers, relative to men, and this has continued to the present. In 1973–74, nearly 18% of applicants to medical schools were women. Enrollment data indicate that the number of women entering professional training relative to men is likely to rise.

Table 35-3   Enrollment in professional schools

Field	1960 Women as percent of total enrollment	1973 Women as percent of total enrollment	1974 Women as percent of total enrollment
Architecture	5	8.3	9.0
Dentistry	1	4.3	6.8
Engineering	1	3.3	5.7
Law	4	14.5	19.4
Medicine	6	15.4	18.0
Optometry	1	7.7	10.2
Pharmacy	12	27.4	31.7
Veterinary medicine	4	18.2	21.1

Source: "Monthly Labor Review," November 1975.

Marriage/Divorce

Trends*

Trends in the rates of first marriage, divorce and remarriage of women since the early 20th century reflect patterns of change in the economic and social conditions in the United States. Each of the rates was at a relatively low point during the depression years of the 1930s, gradually climbing to a peak in the immediate post-World War II period, and then declining throughout the 1950s. While the rate of first marriages continued to drop during the 1960s and into the 1970s, the rates of divorce and remarriage began an upturn around 1960 and increased dramatically from 1960 to 1970.

Since 1970 the divorce rate has continued to climb, but the rate of remarriage has leveled off. Reasons suggested for these recent trends include liberalization of divorce laws, growing acceptance of divorce and of remaining single, and, implicitly, a reduction in the economic cost of divorce. Also, the broadening educational and work experience of women has contributed to increased economic and social independence, which, in the short run at least, may contribute to divorce.

Current Highlights

- There is a general movement among young people away from early marriage. From 1960–1976, the average age at which both men and women first married increased by a full year, to 23.8 and 21.3, respectively.
- Young adults are remaining single for longer periods within the 20–24 year age bracket, 62% of the males and 48% of the females were single in 1976 as opposed to 53% and 28% for the same groups in 1960.
- A parallel trend is the increase of "shared households" (shared by "unrelated" occupants of opposite sex): 327,000 in 1970; 660,000 in 1976. An estimated 1.3 million people live in these arrangements.
- In 1975 the annual total number of divorces exceeded one million for the first time.
- The dramatic escalation of divorce is reported to have doubled in the last dozen years; the increase has been greater in the

*Source: U.S. Bureau of the Census, 1976.

last six years than the entire decade of 1960–70.

- Most typical ages at divorce after first marriage are 25 to 29 for men and 20 to 24 for women. The most typical interval is two or three years from first marriage to divorce.
- Seven years is the median interval between marriage and divorce. Of women—now in their late thirties 75% had been married once and never been divorced or widowed; 22% had been divorced; and the remaining 3% had been widowed.

- Three years is the median interval between divorce and remarriage. Divorced men are five to ten percentage points more likely then divorced women eventually to remarry. For the older age range, four out of every five divorced persons eventually remarry. Among persons who had reached 50 to 75 years in 1975, five of every six men and three of every four women whose first marriage ended in divorce had remarried. Close to nine-tenths of the reported divorces occurred after the first marriage.

Male and Female Marital Status by Age

Table 35-4   Marital status by age and sex: 1950 and 1975, United States (numbers in thousands)

Year and age	Women					Men				
	Total	Never married	Married, husband present	Widowed	Di-vorced	Total	Never married	Married, wife present	Widowed	Di-vorced
1975										
Total, 14 years and over	100.0	22.8	56.9	12.1	4.8	100.0	29.5	62.3	2.4	3.3
14 to 24 years	100.0	68.9	26.6	0.1	1.6	100.0	81.6	16.7	0.0	0.6
25 to 34 years	100.0	10.9	76.2	0.7	6.8	100.0	17.2	74.7	0.1	4.6
35 to 64 years	100.0	4.8	74.5	10.1	6.6	100.0	6.9	83.1	1.9	4.8
65 years and over	100.0	5.8	37.6	52.5	2.6	100.0	4.7	77.3	13.6	2.5
1950										
Total, 14 years and over	100.0	19.6	63.4	12.2	2.2	100.0	26.2	65.9	4.2	1.7
14 to 24 years	100.0	59.2	37.4	0.3	1.0	100.0	78.4	20.5	0.0	0.3
25 to 34 years	100.0	10.8	82.0	1.2	2.5	100.0	18.5	77.8	0.3	1.4
35 to 64 years	100.0	7.9	73.9	12.4	2.9	100.0	10.3	81.5	3.4	2.3
65 years and over	100.0	8.0	34.3	55.3	0.7	100.0	8.1	62.8	23.9	2.2

Source: U.S. Bureau of the Census.

Marriage and Divorce Laws

Marriage Laws

Although the procedural requirements for marriage do vary from state to state with respect to scope of premarital physical examinations and waiting periods for issuance of marriage license, in most states the laws which apply to marriage have made few distinctions based on sex except for establishing lower minimum marriageable ages for women than for men. In recent years, the trend toward uniform treatment of the sexes has been evidenced by the movement to equalize age requirements for marriage without parental consent—as a rule

by lowering the age for males to 18 years. Undoubtedly, the major impetus for such action by the states was adoption in July 1971 of the 26th Amendment to the Constitution guaranteeing the right to vote to citizens who are 18 years or older.

At least 45 states now set a uniform age for marriage without parental consent at 18 years for both males and females, 36 of the states having done so since 1971.

Alaska, Nebraska and Wyoming have revised their marriage laws to permit both males and females to marry at 19 without parental consent. Mississippi and the Commonwealth of Puerto Rico have a uniform marriageable

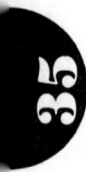

age of 21 (their legal age of majority) without parental consent.

Alabama and the District of Columbia still set an age of 21 for males and 18 for females.

Divorce Laws

In recent years reform of divorce laws has occurred in a number of states. Since January 1970, when California became the first jurisdiction to adopt the irreconcilable differences approach to marriage dissolution, both the grounds and the procedural requirements for divorce have been increasingly eased throughout the states, with the result that the majority of the states have now adopted the concept of "no-fault" divorce. This holds neither partner in a marriage responsible for commission of a specific marital offense or for the breakdown of the marriage relationship. Rather, the fact that the marriage has been a failure is sufficient grounds for divorce. The "guilt principle" and adversary system that heretofore traditionally characterized divorce proceedings are eliminated.

"No fault" divorce includes divorce based on irretrievable breakdown of the marriage relationship as the sole ground for marriage dissolution; irretrievable breakdown added to existing grounds; incompatibility added to existing grounds; separation or absence for a specified period of time; and conversion to absolute divorce after prior decree of limited divorce.

Among the strongest objections to the no-fault ground have been those voiced by women's groups. Their objections relate to the need for guidelines to insure that the terms of divorce or dissolution of marriage granted on that basis provide for fair and equitable treatment of both spouses and their minor children in determining child custody and support arrangements, visitation, alimony and property division. (See Table 35-6.)

Marriage/Divorce Records

An official record of every marriage should be available in the place where the event occurred. These records may be filed permanently either in a state vital statistics office or in a city, county or other local office. To write for a record include the following information:

1. Full names of bride and groom (including nicknames).
2. Residence addresses at time of marriage; for divorce, address on court records.
3. Ages at time of marriage or divorce (or dates of birth).
4. Date and place of marriage; or divorce.
5. Purpose for which copy is needed.
6. Relationship to person whose record is on file.
7. In addition, for divorce records, type of final decree and present residence.

To obtain addresses of the appropriate state office, send for: *Where to Write for Birth and Death Records* (HRA) 76-1142 and *Where to Write for Marriage Records* (HRA) 76-1144, available from the Superintendent of Documents, U.S. Government Printing Office, Washington, D.C. 20402.

Table 35-5 Number of divorced persons per 1,000 married persons, United States

Sex and year	Total	Under 45 years	45 years and over
Both sexes			
1976	75	82	68
1970	47	44	51
1965	41	36	48
1960	35	30	42
Male			
1976	58	63	53
1970	35	31	38
1965	34	28	40
1960	28	22	35
Female			
1976	92	98	85
1970	60	55	67
1965	49	44	57
1960	42	37	51

Source: U.S. Bureau of the Census.

Families*

Fertility

After falling during the 1920s and the Depression years of the 1930s, the U.S. birthrate started to rise, especially during the

*Source: U.S. Bureau of the Census, 1976.

Table 35-6 Divorce laws (1973)

State or other jurisdiction	Residence required before filing suit for divorce	Grounds for absolute divorce														
		No fault (see note)	Adultery	Mental and/or physical cruelty	Desertion	Alcoholism	Impotency	Non-support by husband	Insanity	Pregnancy at marriage	Bigamy	Separation or absence	Felony conviction or imprisonment	Drug addiction	Fraud, force, or duress	Prior decree of limited divorce
Alabama	6 mos.(2)	•	•	•	1 yr.	•	•	•	5 yrs.	•		2 yrs.(2)	•	•		(2)
Alaska	1 yr.		•	•	1 yr.	•	•	•	18 mos.				•	•		
Arizona	90 days	•														
Arkansas	60 days		•	•	1 yr.	•	•	•(2)	3 yrs.			3 yrs.	•	•		
California	—(2)	•							(2)							(2)
Colorado	90 days	•										7 yrs.				
Connecticut	2 yrs.1	•	•	•	1 yr.	•	•	•	5 yrs.			18 mos.	•			
Delaware	6 mos.	•	•	•	1 yr.	•	•	•	5 yrs.							
Florida	6 mos.	•	•													
Georgia	6 mos.	•	•	•	1 yr.	•	•	•	2 yrs.	•		2 yrs.(2)	•	•		(2)
Hawaii	6 wks.		•	•	6 mos.	•	•	•	3 yrs.			2 yrs.(2)	•	•		
Idaho	1 yr.1	•	•	•	1 yr.	•	•	•	3 yrs.			5 yrs.	•			
Illinois	1 yr.		•	•	1 yr.	•	•						•			
Indiana	6 mos.	•	•	•		•	•	•	2 yrs.				•	•		
Iowa	1 yr.	•														
Kansas	6 mos.	•	•	•	1 yr.	•	•	•	3 yrs.			2 yrs.	•	•	•	(2)
Kentucky	—	•														
Louisiana	—	•	•					•				2 yrs.	•			
Maine	6 mos.(1)		•	•	3 yrs.	•	•	•	3 yrs.			(2)	•			
Maryland	(x)		•	•	1 yr.				3 yrs.			(2)	•			
Massachusetts	(aa)		•	•	2 yrs.	•	•	•					•			
Michigan	1 yr.(1)	•														
Minnesota	1 yr.(1)		•	•	1 yr.	•	•	•	3 yrs.			2 yrs.(2)	•			(2)
Mississippi	1 yr.		•	•	1 yr.	•	•	•	3 yrs.	•	•		•	•		
Missouri	1 yr.(1)		•	•	1 yr.	•	•	•				1 yr.	•			
Montana	1 yr.		•	•	1 yr.	•	•	•	5 yrs.				•			
Nebraska	1 yr.	•														
Nevada	6 wks.(1)	•							2 yrs.			1 yr.				
New Hampshire	1 yr.(1)	•	•	•	2 yrs.	•	•		2 yrs.			2 yrs.	•			
New Jersey	1 yr.		•	•	1 yr.	•						18 mos.	•	•		
New Mexico	6 mos.	•	•	•	•				2 yrs.							
New York	1 yr.(1)		•	•	1 yr.							1 yr.(2)	•			
North Carolina	6 mos.		•		1 yr.		•		5 yrs.			1 yr.		•		
North Dakota	1 yr.		•	•	1 yr.	•	•	•	5 yrs.			1 yr.(2)	•	•		
Ohio	1 yr.		•	•	1 yr.	•	•	•	5 yrs.		•	1 yr.	•		•	
Oklahoma	6 mos.(2)		•	•	1 yr.	•	•	•	5 yrs.	•			•	•	•	
Oregon	6 mos.	•													•	
Pennsylvania	1 yr.		•	•	2 yrs.		•						•		•	

baby boom following World War II. It reached 26.6 births per thousand population in 1947 and 25.3 per thousand in 1954 and 1957. The birthrate then declined steeply and steadily to 15.0 per thousand in 1973.

This precipitous rise and fall in the relatively short time is unparalleled. In fact, fertility rates have recently been at levels which, if maintained, would eventually result in an excess of deaths over births. Data on children born illustrate these trends. Women 20 to 24 years old in 1960 had already had an average of one child each, but women 20 to 24 years old in 1974 had an average of about 0.6 children per woman. The average for women 25 to 29 years old in 1960 was two children; by 1974 the average was about 1.4 for women 25 to 29.

Historically, certain socioeconomic characteristics of women have been associated with varying rates of children born. For example, women in metropolitan areas, especially in the suburban sectors, bear fewer children than women in nonmetropolitan areas. High educational attainment, high labor force participation rates, and above-average age at first marriage are all associated with relatively low fertility. The long trend toward early marriage and early childbearing was reversed about 15 years ago. Only 17% of the women born between 1950 and 1955 had married by age 18, in contrast to approximately 30% of the women born between 1935 and 1939. This decrease in early marriage has been paralleled by a drop in fertility levels for women 18 years old or younger.

These and other facts show that recent trends toward higher levels of education, increased labor force activity, and the postponement of marriage have been accompanied by decreases in the average number of children born to married women.

Changes in the level of illegitimacy are noteworthy. Birth registration data on illegitimate births suggest that sizable increases in illegitimacy occurred between 1940 and 1970, but that the increases have been tapering off in more recent years. In 1940 there were only about 7.1 births per 1,000 unmarried women. In 1970 this figure was 26.4, and in 1973 it was 24.5. In 1940, 4% of all births were illegitimate; in 1970, 11% were illegitimate; and in 1973, 13%.

State	Residence required							
Rhode Island	2 yrs.(2)	•	•	•	•			5 yrs.(2)	5 yrs.
South Carolina	1 yr.	•						1 yr.	3 yrs.
South Dakota	1 yr.(1)	•	•					1 yr.	
Tennessee	6 mos.	•		•	•	•	5 yrs.	1 yr.	2 yrs.(2)
Texas	1 yr.	•			•			1 yr.	3 yrs.
Utah	3 mos.	•					3 yrs.	1 yr.	3 yrs.(2)
Vermont	6 mos.(2)	•		•	•		5 yrs.	*(2)	6 mos.
Virginia	1 yr.	•		•		•		1 yr.	2 yrs.
Washington	—	—	—	—	—	—	—	—	—
West Virginia	1 yr.(1)	•	—				3 yrs.	1 yr.	2 yrs.
Wisconsin	6 mos.	•			•			1 yr.	1 yr.
Wyoming	60 days(1)	•		•	•	•	2 yrs.	1 yr.	2 yrs.
District of Columbia	1 yr.	—						1 yr.	1 yr.

*Indicates grounds for absolute divorce.
(1)Under certain circumstances, a lessened period may be required. Note: 'No fault' is expressed variously in state laws, as irremediable breakdown of marriage relationship, irreconcilable differences.
(2)Special qualifying conditions.

Source: Women's Bureau, U.S. Department of Labor.

Family Composition

The makeup of the traditional family is being altered by the effect of recent trends in marriage and divorce: a growing proportion of women are single or divorced and have not remarried. In 1975 the percentage of women divorced and not remarried among those 25 to 34 years (prime family time) was 6.8%.

As the number of divorced women has increased, the number of female-headed families has also risen. Such families numbered over 7.2 million in 1975—13% of all families and approximately a 73% increase since 1960. Correspondingly, the number of children in female-headed families grew from 4.2 million in 1960 to 6.9 million in 1970 and to 10.5 million in 1975. More women are required and/or desire to be more economically independent, and there are associated changes in fertility, labor force participation, poverty, etc.

Women As Heads of Families

- Thirteen percent of all families were headed by females in 1975. Among all families, one out of eight was headed by a woman; in black families, one out of three.
- Around 54% of the females who headed families were in the work force. Among all women workers, one out of ten was a family head; among minority women workers, one out of five.
- Income and poverty: the number of families with female heads has grown substantially over the past quarter-century but the income of female-headed families has not increased as greatly as the income of male-headed families. In 1950 families with female heads had a median income which equaled about 56% of the median for male-headed families; in 1974 this had dropped to about 47%. Although the percent of all families with female heads below the poverty level declined from about 42% in 1960 to about 33% in both 1970 and 1974, the number of female-headed families in poverty increased between 1970 and 1974. In 1960 there were about 31 female-headed families for every 100 male-headed families below the poverty level, while in 1974 there were 85 female-headed families for every 100 male-headed families.
- Among the 3.7 million families headed by women workers, 20% had 1973 incomes below the poverty level; for the two million women workers of minority races who headed families, the corresponding figure was 33%.

Table 35-7   Households and families, by type of head, United States, 1975 (in thousands)

Type of head	Number	Percent
Households, total	71,120	
White	62,945	100.0
Husband-wife	42,951	68.2
Other male head	6,295	10.0
Female head	13,700	21.8
Negro and other	8,175	100.0
Husband-wife	4,000	48.9
Other male head	1,103	13.5
Female head	3,073	37.6
Families, total	55,712	
White	49,451	100.0
Husband-wife	42,969	86.9
Other male head	1,270	2.5
Female head	5,212	10.5
Negro and other	6,262	100.0
Husband-wife	4,002	63.9
Other male head	230	3.7
Female head	2,030	32.4

Source: U.S. Bureau of the Census.

Table 35-8   Families with female heads by number of own children under 18 years old (numbers in thousands)

Number of own children under 18 years of age	1975	1970	1960
Families with female heads	7,242	5,580	4,196
Percent of all families	13.0	10.9	10.5
With no own children under 18	2,319	2,655	2,305
With own children under 18	4,924	2,925	1,891
1 own child under 18	1,994	1,051	785
2 own children under 18	1,376	826	510
3 own children under 18	761	497	286
4 or more own children under 18	793	552	311
Total own children under 18	10,474	6,895	4,198
Mean number	1.45	1.24	1.00

Source: U.S. Bureau of the Census.

Law, Politics and Women

Overview

Women in both the Democratic and Republican parties in 1976 were working for full participation in the elective process. They were involved in developing overall and women's issues for the party platform, caucuses and delegations to conventions, and running as candidates for office.

The National Women's Political Caucus formed Women's Task Forces for the Democratic and Republican Parties to assure participation of women at all levels of organization. The Democratic Women's Agenda was articulated by a broad spectrum of women in the party to press for cooperation in addressing women's issues. The Federation of Republican Women, under the direction of newly elected Patricia Hutar, did the same in the Republican Party.

The National Women's Educational Fund sponsored regional "how-to" workshops to prepare potential women candidates for campaigning and office holding. (To obtain their curriculum package for women seeking elective office write National Women's Educational Fund, 1532 16th St. N.W., Washington, D.C. for more information.)

Their political activity was reflected in an increase of the number of women candidates for public office, the number who were elected and the growing trend of selecting females for appointive positions.

Women elected	1972	1974	1975–6
Federal congress	16	18	23
State legislature	441	596	610
State government	—	1	1

On county and municipal levels, the National Women's Political Caucus reports the following figures for 1975–6:

County commissioners	456
Mayors	578
City & township council members	5,369
School board members	11,000

As for voting, in general, a smaller proportion of women than men register and vote in both congressional and presidential elections. This difference is especially true for the oldest age groups. However, since women outnumber men at the voting ages, slightly more votes are usually cast by women than by men.

The Equal Rights Amendment (ERA)

A proposal to amend the United States Constitution to prohibit governmental denial or abridgment of equal rights on account of sex has been approved overwhelmingly by Congress, after almost 50 years of attempts to secure its passage. By 1976, 34 states had ratified the amendment; four more must do so by March 22, 1979, in order for it to become part of the Constitution.

Fifteen states have equal rights provisions in their own constitutions, and legislatures in other states have taken preliminary steps toward submitting equal rights proposals to their electorates.

Effect ERA Would Have on Laws Differentiating on the Basis of Sex*

The probable meaning and effect of the equal rights amendment was outlined in a 1975 Senate Judiciary Committee report:

1. In employment, the amendment would restrict only governmental action and would not apply to purely private action. It would prohibit discrimination and require equal pay for equal work, wherever the government is an employer—on federal, state, county and city levels.
2. Special restrictions on property rights of married women would be unconstitutional; married women could engage in business as freely as a member of the male sex; inheritance rights of widows would be same as for widowers.
3. Women would be equally subject to jury service and to military service, but women would not be required to serve (in the Armed Forces) where they are not fitted any more than men are required to so serve.
4. Restrictive work laws for women only would be unconstitutional (e.g., maximum hours, night work and weight-lifting restrictions on women).
5. Alimony laws would not favor women solely because of their sex, but a divorce decree could award support to a mother if she was granted custody of the children. Matters concerning custody and support of

---

*Source: U.S. Citizen's Advisory Council on the Status of Women, March 1976.

children would be determined in accordance with the welfare of the children and without favoring either parent because of sex.

6. Laws granting maternity benefits to mothers would not be affected by the amendment, nor would criminal laws governing sexual offenses become unconstitutional (e.g., rape, prostitution).

Attitudes Toward ERA

Table 35-9 Attitudes toward efforts to strengthen women's status in society

	1975 %	1972 %	1971 %
Favor	59	48	42
Oppose	28	36	41
Not sure	13	16	17

Source: Harris Survey, May 19, 1975.

Nationwide support for the women's movement has risen 17 points in the past four years, but ironically, more of that support comes from men. Men back the movement by 63–24%, compared to the 55–32% majority of women who support equal rights. And consistently, men have been more supportive of the women's cause than most women have.

Table 35-10 Attitudes toward equal rights amendment: 1975

	Favor %	Oppose %	Not sure %
Nationwide	51	36	13
By sex			
Men	56	31	12
Women	48	40	12
By region			
East	62	26	12
Midwest	49	39	12
South	41	44	15
West	55	34	11
By age			
18–29	66	25	9
30–49	50	37	13
50 and over	41	43	16
By race			
Black	65	22	13
White	50	38	12

Source: Harris Survey, May 19, 1975.

A 45–40% plurality does not believe that ERA "would wipe out many of the laws which have benefited women with special protection for many years," the main argument used by critics of the proposed amendment.

Other Legislation Affecting Women

In recent years extensive legislative activity, particularly in the area of employment, has sought to improve the life and opportunities of women.

Sex Discrimination in Employment— Forty states, the District of Columbia and Puerto Rico have laws prohibiting sex discrimination in private employment; this represents a dramatic increase over the last decade.

The basic federal fair employment practices law, Title VII of the 1964 Civil Rights Act, was amended in 1972 to lower the employee exemption, extend coverage to state and local government workers, and give a statutory basis to equal opportunity provisions for federal employees. The amendments also strengthened enforcement procedures and provided for coordination of federal equal employment opportunity agencies. Title VII prohibits employers, labor organizations and employment agencies from discriminating on the basis of race, color, religion and national origin, as well as sex.

Executive Order 11246, as amended by Executive Order 11375, not only prohibits discrimination by federal contractors on the same bases stated in Title VII but also requires employers to commit themselves to affirmative action programs to assure equal opportunity.

Title IX of the 1972 Education Amendments prohibits sex discrimination under educational programs or activities receiving federal assistance. It affects most admissions, financial aid, etc., as well as employment.

Equal Pay—Thirty-seven states have laws specifically prohibiting pay differentials between the sexes for equal or substantially equal work in private employment. Only five states do not have either an equal pay law or a prohibition of pay discrimination based on sex in a broader fair employment practices law.

The federal Equal Pay Act was extended effective July 1, 1972, to executive, administrative and professional employees and to outside sales personnel.

Age Discrimination in Employment—Thirty-four states, the District of Columbia and Puerto Rico have laws prohibiting age discrimination in private employment.

The federal age discrimination in Employment Act, which prohibits discrimination against persons 40 to 65 years old, was amended in 1974 to lower the employee exemption and to extend coverage to government workers.

Minimum Wage—Forty states, the District of Columbia and Puerto Rico have minimum wage laws with minimum rates currently in effect. Since the enactment of Title VII, there has been a marked increase in the proportion of state minimum wage laws that cover men as well as women—from 17 out of 32 to 39 out of 42.

The federal "wage and hour law," the Fair Labor Standards Act, was amended in 1974 to raise minimum rates and establish timetables for future raises, extend coverage to some groups immediately and provide for phasing out additional categorical exemptions, and establish special overtime provisions for certain public employees. In 1975 most covered nonagricultural workers must be paid at least $2.10 for the first 40 hours of work per week and one and one-half times their regular rates for additional hours. By January 1, 1978, all covered workers must be paid at least $2.30 an hour.

Restrictive Labor Laws for Women—State laws setting maximum daily or weekly hours for women, prohibiting or regulating nightwork by women, and limiting women's occupations have virtually disappeared because of their conflict with Title VII of the 1964 Federal Civil Rights Act, although a few are enforced with respect to workers not protected by Title VII.

Jury Duty—Women are eligible to serve on juries in all states, the District of Columbia and Puerto Rico. Some jurisdictions still permit women to be excused from jury service solely on the basis of sex or permit only women to be excused because of child care or family responsibilities.

Abortion Laws—U.S. Supreme Court rulings in January 1973 that states have no right to interfere in an abortion decision during the first trimester of pregnancy have caused a great deal of controversy. Most states have enacted new abortion laws, and many of these in turn have been found unconstitutional. Some members of Congress have proposed amending the Constitution to give the states unrestricted right to regulate or prohibit abortion.

Sex Discrimination in Credit—At least 40 states and the District of Columbia have laws or regulations on some aspect of discrimination in credit based on sex and/or marital status. Local jurisdictions also are attempting to resolve economic problems of women caused by discrimination in the granting of credit.

A federal law that became effective October 28, 1975, prohibits discrimination against any credit applicant on the basis of sex or marital status. Other federal legislation prohibits sex discrimination in housing programs.

International Women's Year*

International Women's Year in 1975 was a time during which American women, along with women from many countries, analyzed progress being made toward full partnership. Celebrations included local, national and international observances.

The year was highlighted by a world conference held in Mexico City June 19 to July 2, 1975. More than 1,000 official delegates and advisors, representing 123 nations and 21 liberation movements, 1,300 journalists and 4,500 participants gathered in a worldwide pioneering effort for women. The official United Nations Conference was held at the initial request of the United States and resulted in notable "firsts" for the women's movement and for the United States: the first meeting of worldwide governments to consider women's issues; the first U.S. delegation headed by a woman, Honorable Patricia Hutar; and the first time the majority of delegates to a conference were women.

The delegates adopted a World Plan of Action. The World Plan of Action calls for extensive social, legal and economic changes and lists specific goals to be met within the ten-year women's decade. A follow-up world conference has been scheduled by the U.N. for 1980.

---

*Source: U.S. Citizen's Advisory Council on the Status of Women, March 1976.

748

Women in the Labor Force

Characteristics of the Working Woman

Profile*

A profile of working women reveals that they are more apt to be young, city dwellers, better educated, from homes with a professional or white collar person in the family and in the higher income brackets. Those women who are less likely to be working are rural dwellers, over 50 years of age, in homes with a business executive or skilled worker in them and in upper middle income families.

These patterns make it clear that the economic status of the family is not the main reason why some women work and others do not. For example, relatively affluent women with a professional in the family are far more likely to work than are the wives and daughters of business executives in much the same income bracket. By the same token, women in blue collar families are less likely to be employed than are women in white collar families with the same income. Among young women, it is much more probable that those from more affluent families will be in the job market than will those from the less affluent sector.

Table 35-11   Reasons given why women work

	1975 %	1970 %
Total working women:		
To support self	37	23
To support family	17	18
To bring in extra money	39	48
To keep busy	7	9
Not sure	—	2

That more women now say they are working to support themselves means they are far more likely to want to be financially independent of the rest of their family and not just a source of supplemental income. This drive toward financial independence implies that women want to be less dependent on men than before.

Attitudes toward Day Care—Despite the sharp increase in the number of women who are working, another 11% of all women could

* Source: Harris Survey, December 8, 1975.

come into the work force if more child day-care centers were set up, where mothers can leave their young children during the day while they work. Public support for the day-care center has risen from 56 to 67% of the entire adult public since 1970. Significantly, the number of men who would back an expansion of day-care centers has risen from 49 to 61% in the past five years. The percentage of women who support day-care centers has risen from 63 to 72% over the same period.

If a day-care center were available, 30% of all women with children 12 years of age or under say they would then look for work. The potential work force would be augmented more heavily by young mothers in the west, those who are black and those in the $5,000 to $10,000 income brackets.

Number of Female Workers

● Women have steadily increased their representation as workers. In 1974, women accounted for 39% of the civilian labor force.

● Nearly 37 million women were in the labor force in 1975, representing 46% of all women 16 years of age and over. More than half of all women had some work experience in 1973.

● Of the 43 million women who were not in the labor force, 35 million were keeping house, nearly 4 million were students and 4 million were out of the labor force because of ill health, disability or other reasons.

Table 35-12   Number and percent in labor force by sex and marital status: 1950 and 1975 (numbers in thousands)

Sex and marital status	1975		1950	
	% labor force participation	Number in labor force	% labor force participation	Number in labor force
Single:				
Women	56.7	8,464	50.5	5,621
Men	67.1	12,233	62.6	8,898
Married, spouse present:				
Women	44.4	21,111	23.8	8,550
Men	83.1	39,576	91.6	32,912
Other ever married:[1]				
Women	40.7	6,932	37.8	3,624
Men	65.2	4,091	63.0	2,616

[1] Includes widowed, divorced and married, spouse absent.

Source: U.S. Bureau of Labor Statistics.

Age and Marital Factors

- Fifty-three percent of the women 18 to 64 years of age were in the labor force in 1974.
- The highest labor force participation rate was for women 20 to 24–63%.
- Married women (husband present) accounted for nearly 58% of all women workers; single women 23%; widowed or divorced 19%.
- Of all married women (husband present), 43% were in the labor force; of all single women, 57%; of all divorced or separated, 65%.
- In 47% of husband-wife families both were earners; in 31% of the husband-wife families the husband was the only earner in 1973. Twenty-two percent had no earners or were supported by others.

Table 35-13   Marital status of women in the labor force: 1940 to 1975 (persons 14 years old and over through 1965; 16 years old and over thereafter.)

| | Female labor force as percent of female population | | | |
| | | | | |
Year	Total	Single	Married	Widowed or divorced
1940	27.4	48.1	16.7	32.0
1960	34.8	44.1	31.7	37.1
1975	45.9	56.7	45.0	37.8

Source: U.S. Bureau of the Census.

Table 35-14   Occupations of employed married women (husband present in household)

Occupation	1975
Total, all groups (millions)	19.3
Percent distribution	100.0
Professional, technical, and kindred workers	17.6
Farmers and farm managers	0.3
Managers and administrators[1]	5.6
Clerical and kindred workers	35.0
Salesworkers	6.8
Craft and kindred workers	1.6
Operatives and kindred workers	12.5
Private household workers	2.3
Service workers, except priv. hshld.	16.6
Farm laborers and supervisors	0.9
Laborers, exc. farm and mine	0.8

[1] Excludes farm.

Source: U.S. Bureau of Labor Statistics.

Working Mothers and Children (1975 data)

- The number of working mothers (with children under 18) has increased ninefold since 1940.
- About 13.6 million mothers with children under 18 years of age are in the labor force, of whom 5.1 million have children under 6 years.
- Thirty-seven percent of women with children under 6 years are in the working force; 54% of women with children ages 6 to 17 years; and 44% of women with no children under 18 years. In 1950, only 12% of women with children under 6 years worked.
- Children of working mothers number 26.8 million. Of these children, 20.7 million are 6 to 17 years of age, and 6.1 million are under the age of 6. Among the children of working mothers, 4.6 million have mothers who are heads of families; 913,000 of these children are under the age of 6.
- The number of children in female-headed families below the poverty level increased by approximately one-third between 1960 and 1974, and in 1974 the majority of children in poverty were in families headed by women.

Table 35-15   Employed married women (husband present) by age and presence of children: 1950 to 1975

Item	1950	1960	1970	1975
Percent labor force participation[1]				
Married women, husband present	23.8	30.5	40.8	44.4
With no children under 18 yr. old	30.3	34.7	42.2	43.9
With children 6–17 yr. old only	28.3	39.0	49.2	52.4
With children under 6 yr. old	11.9	18.6	30.3	36.6
Also with children 6–17 yr. old	12.6	18.9	30.5	34.3

[1] Married women in the labor force as percent of married women in the population.

Source: U.S. Bureau of the Census.

Employment Patterns

- *Number who work:* Nine out of ten girls today will work at some time in their lives.

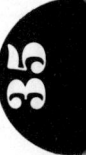

- *Annual work experience:* * Over half of the women 16 years old and over worked at some time during 1974. This represented an 84% increase over the number of women with work experience in 1950. The number of women working 50 to 52 weeks at full-time jobs grew even more dramatically during the period; in 1950 there were only about 29 women for every 100 men working year round full-time, but in 1974 this ratio had risen to 47 women per 100 men.

- *Variations in the lifetime work experience of women according to educational attainment:* 30-to-44-year-old women college graduates had worked, on the average, for two-thirds of the years since completing school, but women high school graduates of the same age worked for only about half the years since completing their education.

- *Worklife patterns:* Typically a woman enters the labor force after schooling and works a few years before marriage or her first child. A very small proportion of women leave the labor force permanently at this time. Most women who marry experience some breaks in employment during their child-bearing and child-rearing years. However, an increasing proportion of young married women with and without children are remaining in the labor force.

- *Job tenure:* Women had 2.8 median years on the job and men had a median of 4.6 years in 1973. Women with ten years or more on the job comprised 18% of female workers, while men with ten or more years on the job comprised 30% of male workers.

- *Peak work years:* The labor force participation of men peaks in their middle years with 94% of men in the labor force in the ages of 35–44. Women in 1974 peaked in their earlier years (20–24) with 62% of women working—they decrease and climb again in participation in later years. Despite this fluctuation more than half of all women in most age groups work.

- *Time pattern:* Women comprised 34% of all full-time employees and 64% of all part-time employees in 1974.

Occupations of Women Workers

Figure 35-1   Current status

WOMEN

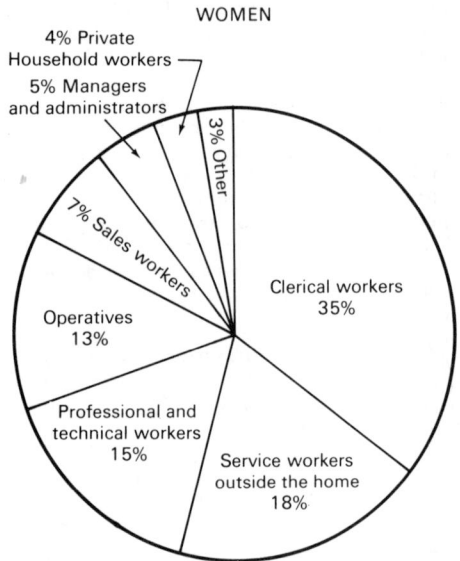

4% Private Household workers
5% Managers and administrators
3% Other
7% Sales workers
Clerical workers 35%
Operatives 13%
Professional and technical workers 15%
Service workers outside the home 18%

MEN

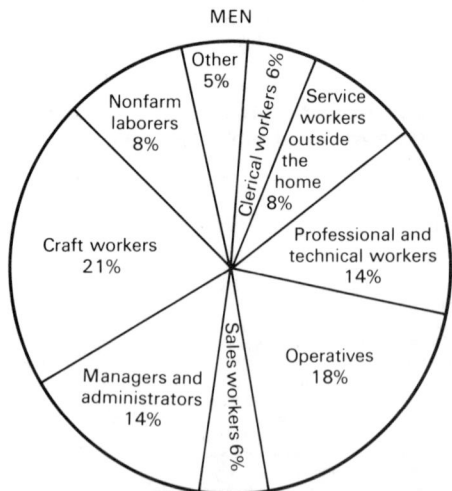

Other 5%
Nonfarm laborers 8%
Clerical workers 6%
Service workers outside the home 8%
Craft workers 21%
Professional and technical workers 14%
Managers and administrators 14%
Sales workers 6%
Operatives 18%

As White Collar Workers—Women are more apt than men to be white-collar workers, but the jobs they hold are usually less skilled and pay less than those of men. Women professional workers are most likely to be teachers, nurses and other health workers, while men are most frequently employed in professions other than teaching and health. Women are less likely than men to be managers and officials and more likely to be clerical workers.

As Blue Collar Workers—About one out of six women workers is employed in a blue collar job, but almost half the men are in such jobs. Women are almost as likely as men to be operatives but are very seldom employed as skilled craft workers—the occupation group for one out of five men workers.

As Service Workers—More than one out of five women but only one out of 12 employed men are service workers. Eight out of ten women and virtually all the men service workers are employed in occupations other than private household work.

The Trend Toward Non-Traditional Occupations for Women*—Despite the continued concentration of women in a relatively small number of traditionally women's fields, women workers entered predominantly male fields in large numbers during the 1960s. Data for 1973 from the Current Population Survey indicate that the movement of women into nontraditional jobs is continuing.

The most dramatic shift that occurred between 1960 and 1970 was the large influx of women into the skilled trades. In 1970 almost half a million women (495,000) were working in the skilled occupations—up from 277,000 in 1960. The rate of increase (nearly 80%) was twice that for women in all occupations. It was eight times the rate of increase for men in the skilled trades.

Penetration of Traditionally Male Fields

Skilled trades registering significant gains in employment of women were: electricians from 2,500 to 8,700 (0.7 to 1.8%); plumbers from about 1,000 to 4,000 (0.3 to 1.1%); auto mechanics from about 2,300 to about 11,000 (0.4 to 1.4%); painters from about 6,400 to 13,400 (1.9 to 4.1%); tool and die makers from about 1,100 to 4,200 (0.6 to 2.1%); and machinists from about 6,700 to about 11,800 (1.3 to 3.1%). In one skilled occupation, that of compositor and typesetter, the number of

*Source: *1975 Handbook on Women Workers,* Women's Bureau, U.S. Department of Labor.

Table 35-16   Employed persons, by major occupation group and sex (in thousands of persons 16 years old and over)

Occupation group and sex	1976, Apr.	Occupation group and sex	1976, Apr.
Total	86,584	Farmworkers	2,397
Male	51,812	Female	34,772
White-collar workers	21,350	White-collar workers	22,010
Percent of total	41.2	Percent of total	63.3
Professional and technical	7,612	Professional and technical	5,522
Managers and administrators[1]	7,342	Managers and administrators[1]	1,895
Salesworkers	3,165	Salesworkers	2,317
Clerical workers	3,231	Clerical workers	12,276
Blue-collar workers	23,401	Blue-collar workers	5,069
Craft and kindred workers	10,455	Craft and kindred workers	527
Operatives	9,124	Operatives	4,141
Transport equipment	3,057	Nonfarm laborers	401
Nonfarm laborers	3,822	Service workers	7,260
Service workers	4,663	Farmworkers	433

[1] Excludes farm.

Source: U.S. Bureau of Labor Statistics.

women increased from 15,500 to nearly 24,000, whereas the number of men employed in the occupation declined.

Women also made significant employment gains in some predominantly male professions. Employment of women lawyers grew from less than 5,000 to more than 12,000 between 1960 and 1970, and women nearly doubled their proportion of all employed lawyers (2.4 to 4.7%). Similar gains in employment were made in the medical professions. The number of women physicians increased from about 16,000 to nearly 26,000, and the proportion of doctors who were women rose from 7 to 9%. The number of women dentists increased from about 1,900 to more than 3,100 (from 2.3 to 3.4% of all dentists).

Enrollment data indicate that the number and percent of women in law and medicine can be expected to grow sharply. For example, the number of women enrolled in law schools in 1973 (16,760) was three and a half times the number in 1969 (4,715); the proportion women were of all law students increased from 7 to 16%. Similarly, the number of women enrolled in U.S. medical schools increased from 3,392 in the 1969–70 school year to 7,824 in the 1973–74 school year. The proportion women were of all medical school students increased from 9 to more than 15% in this four-year period.

Women appear to have made substantial inroads into some other predominantly male professional occupations. Women in engineering increased from about 7,000 to about 19,-600 between 1960 and 1970, growing by more than four and a half times the rate for men. Employment of women accountants grew from 80,400 to 183,000, also more than quadrupling the growth rate for men.

Women also have made noticeable inroads into several traditionally male sales occupations. Employment of women insurance agents and brokers increased from about 35,300 to nearly 56,600 and from 9.6 to 12.4% of all employees in this occupational field. Similarly, women real estate sales agents increased in number from about 46,100 to 83,600 and women stock and bond sales agents from 2,100 to 8,900.

Among the managerial occupations, the number of women bank officers and financial managers grew rapidly from 2,100 to 54,500; in sales management from 100 to 8,700.

Other occupational areas were penetrated effectively by female workers: as postal clerks, protective guards, bus drivers and bartenders.

In a reverse trend, it is significant that men were making inroads into traditionally female-dominated fields: as librarians, elementary school teachers, typists and telephone operators.

Earnings of Women Workers

Women's median earnings are significantly lower than men's in all occupational categories . . . and the gap continues to widen.

Table 35-17   Median earnings of year-round full-time civilian workers by sex: 1960 to 1974 (median earnings in current dollars)

Year	Women	Men	Ratio: women/men
1974	$6,772	$11,835	0.57
1973	6,335	11,186	0.57
1972	5,903	10,202	0.58
1971	5,593	9,399	0.60
1970	5,323	8,966	0.59
1969	4,977	8,455	0.59
1968	4,457	7,664	0.58
1967	4,134	7,174	0.58
1966	3,946	6,856	0.58
1965	3,828	6,388	0.60
1964	3,669	6,203	0.59
1963	3,525	5,980	0.59
1962	3,412	5,754	0.59
1961	3,315	5,595	0.59
1960	3,257	5,368	0.61

Source: U.S. Bureau of the Census.

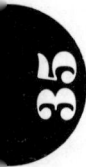

Table 35-18   Median income of year-round full-time civilian workers by age and sex: 1975 (In dollars. Age as of March of following year)

Age	Women	Men
Total with income	7,719	13,144
14–19 years	4,568	5,657
20–24 years	6,598	8,521
25–34 years	8,401	12,777
35–44 years	8,084	14,730
45–54 years	7,980	14,808
55–64 years	7,785	13,518
65 years and over	7,273	11,485

Source: U.S. Bureau of the Census.

Comparison of Earnings of Men and Women *

Despite gains toward equality in education and range of employment, differences between the income of women and men workers remain substantial. In 1974 the median income of women year-round full-time workers was about 57% of the median for comparable men. The number of women income recipients working year-round full-time increased relative to men between 1960 and 1974, from a ratio of 32 women per 100 men in 1960 to 46 women per 100 men in 1974. However, during this period the female/male income ratio for year-round full-time workers did not improve.

Part of this differential between women and men is attributable to differences in such factors as educational attainment, occupational distribution, industry of employment, and work experience. In both 1970 and 1974, however, the median income of women college graduates aged 25 and over who worked year-round full-time was only about 60% of the comparable male median income. In fact, women college graduates had incomes that were, on the average, lower than men with only a high school education.

Fully employed women high school graduates (with no college) have less income on the average than fully employed men who have not completed elementary school. However, as the level of education increased to five or more years of college the difference in the "pay-off" for education narrowed considerably.

There is some variation in female/male earnings ratios for different major occupation groups, but for most groups women year-round full-time workers earned only about 55 to 60% as much as men in 1974. The only occupation group with a relatively large number of women workers and an earnings ratio above 0.60 was professional, technical and kindred workers.

Personal services, the industry with the largest proportion of workers who were women, had one of the lowest female/male earnings ratios in 1974 (0.49); but professional and related services, in which the majority of workers are women, had a fe-

male/male earnings ratio of 0.60. Both in transportation, communication and other public utilities and in business and repair services, industries with relatively small numbers of women workers, women's median earnings were approximately two-thirds as high as men's.

The above comparisons have been restricted to persons who worked at full-time jobs for the entire year (50 to 52 weeks). However, over half of the women and over one-fourth of the men with earnings in 1974 worked at part-time jobs or worked fewer than 40 weeks at full-time jobs. The earnings for women working at part-time jobs were much closer to their male counterparts (ratio of 0.90) than was true for year-round full-time workers. Also, women working at full-time jobs for less than 40 weeks during the year had earnings equal or nearly equal with those of comparable men. Thus, the relative returns for working year-round full-time do not seem to be as great for women as for men.

Table 35-19   Median income for full-time workers 25 years old and over by educational attainment and sex: 1975

Educational attainment	Women	Men
Total	$8,117	$13,821
Elementary:		
Less than 8 years	5,109	8,647
8 years	5,691	10,600
High school:		
1 to 3 years	6,355	11,511
4 years	7,777	13,542
College:		
1 to 3 years	9,126	14,989
4 years or more	11,359	18,450

Source: U.S. Bureau of the Census.

Wives' Contribution to Family Income

- Among all working-wife families, the contribution of wives' earnings was slightly above one-fourth of family income in 1974. When the wife was a year-round full-time worker, her contribution was nearly two-fifths—38%.
- Frequently the wife's earnings raise a family out of poverty. In husband-wife families, 15% have incomes below $5,000 if the wife does not work; 4%, when she does work.

---

* Source: U.S. Bureau of the Census, 1976.

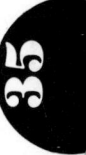

Table 35-20 Wife's contribution to family income—families with husband and wife working, by race of husband

Race, region, and wife's current occupation group	Husband-wife families, both working (1,000)	Average (mean) family income	Average (mean)	Percent of family income
		1974		
All white workers	20,101	$17,983	$4,483	24.9
North and West	13,733	18,599	4,575	24.6
South	6,367	16,654	4,286	25.7
White collar workers	10,813	20,207	5,735	28.4
North and West	7,369	20,738	5,805	28.0
South	3,444	19,073	5,585	29.3
All black workers	1,821	14,317	4,645	32.4
North and West	815	16,801	5,525	32.9
South	1,006	12,305	3,932	32.0
White collar workers	658	18,246	6,876	37.7
North and West	366	19,114	7,261	38.0
South	292	17,162	6,394	37.3

Source: U.S. Bureau of the Census.

Unemployment & Women

- The unemployment rate for adult women (20 years old and over) has historically been higher than that for adult men. Women normally have more frequent periods of withdrawal from the labor force and subsequent reentry, which contributes to higher unemployment. Also, tenure or years of experience are usually lower for women than for men, and this increases the likelihood of layoff or job loss.
- Unemployed women numbered 2.4 million and accounted for 47% of all unemployed persons in 1974. The unemployment rate for women was 6.7%, compared with 4.8% for men.
- In March 1974 nearly one-fourth of a million unemployed women were family heads. Their rate of unemployment was 6.4%, compared with 2.7% for men family heads in husband-wife families.
- Of unemployed women in 1974, 36% were re-entrants into the labor force; 16% were new entrants. Of men, 22% were re-entrants; only 11% are new entrants.

Labor Union Participation*

Between 1962 and 1972, the proportion of all union members that were women rose from 18.6% to 21.7%. In absolute terms, the number of women union members increased from 3.3 million to 4.5 million, a gain of 37%. The growing proportion of total union membership accounted for by women reflects the considerable increase of women in the labor force.

The relatively low proportion of women who are union members reflects to some extent the nature of women's employment and the industries in which they work. The types of occupations women have entered most frequently have been among the traditionally less organized. Unions have organized less than 25% of the workers in five of the nine industries in which women constitute more than 40% of total employment: textiles, finance, service, and state and local governments. In none of the industries with over 40% women were as many as 75% of the workers unionized. In addition the 7.6 million women who were part-time employees in 1972 probably felt less incentive to participate in the union movement due to their frequent entry into and exit from the labor market, as well as the traditionally low level of unionization in the two industries in which over 64% of all voluntarily part-time employees work—wholesale and retail trade and finance and service.

Although women accounted for at least half of the membership in 25 unions, more than one out of five unions—39 in all—reported there was not a single woman member. These included unions in predominantly "male" industries such as construction, maritime, coal mining and air transportation pilots.

The unions with the largest numbers of women members were the International Ladies' Garment Workers, where 80% of all members were women, and the Retail Clerks, with about 50%. Together, these two unions had a membership of 659,000 women. Other unions reporting large numbers of women workers were, in ranking order, the Electrical Workers (IBEW); Amalgamated Clothing Workers; Communications Workers; State, County and Municipal Employees; and Automobile Workers.

---

*Source: *1975 Handbook on Women Workers,* U.S. Department of Labor.

Women in Health Jobs

Figure 35-2   Percent of females in selected health occupation: United States, 1970

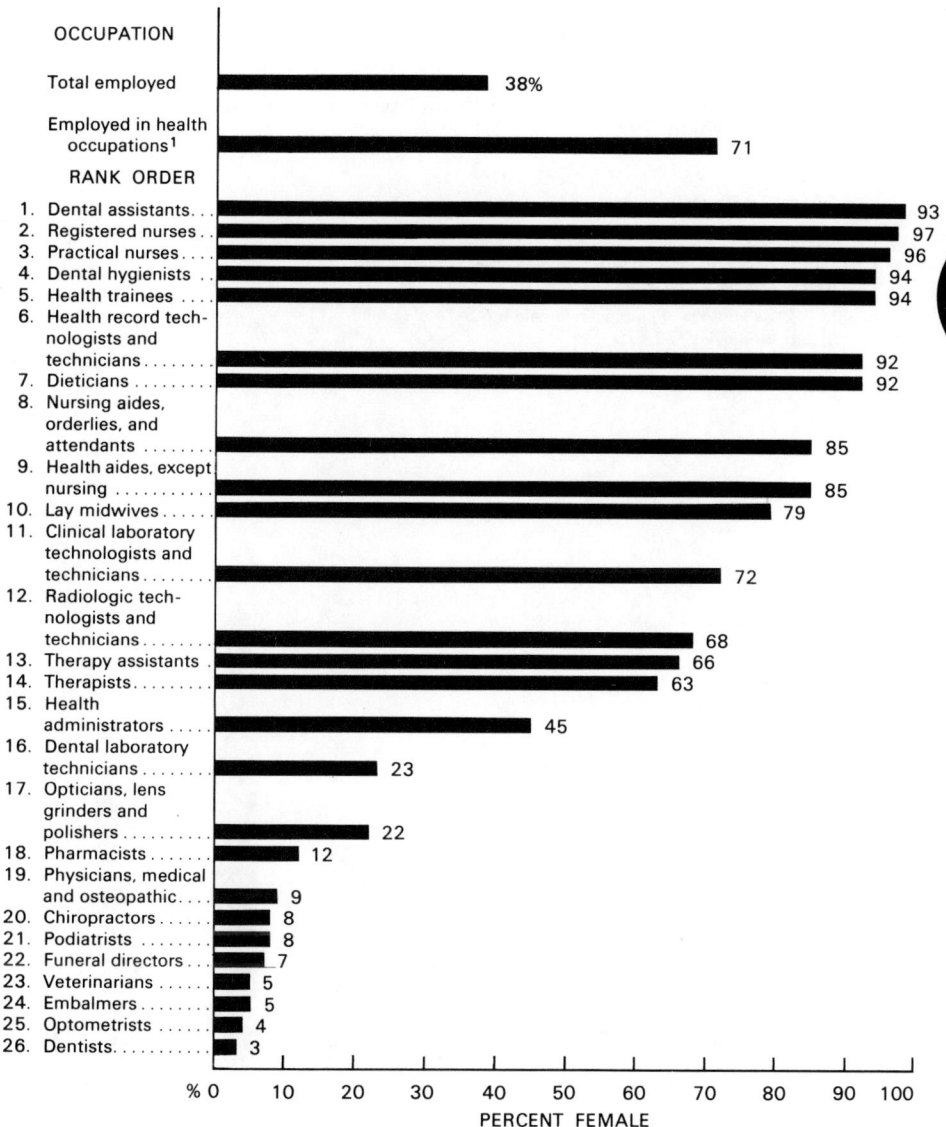

OCCUPATION

Total employed	38%
Employed in health occupations[1]	71

RANK ORDER

1. Dental assistants... — 93
2. Registered nurses.. — 97
3. Practical nurses.... — 96
4. Dental hygienists .. — 94
5. Health trainees .... — 94
6. Health record tech-
   nologists and
   technicians....... — 92
7. Dieticians......... — 92
8. Nursing aides,
   orderlies, and
   attendants .... — 85
9. Health aides, except
   nursing .... — 85
10. Lay midwives...... — 79
11. Clinical laboratory
    technologists and
    technicians....... — 72
12. Radiologic tech-
    nologists and
    technicians....... — 68
13. Therapy assistants . — 66
14. Therapists........ — 63
15. Health
    administrators .... — 45
16. Dental laboratory
    technicians....... — 23
17. Opticians, lens
    grinders and
    polishers......... — 22
18. Pharmacists...... — 12
19. Physicians, medical
    and osteopathic.... — 9
20. Chiropractors..... — 8
21. Podiatrists .... — 8
22. Funeral directors... — 7
23. Veterinarians ..... — 5
24. Embalmers....... — 5
25. Optometrists ..... — 4
26. Dentists.......... — 3

% 0   10   20   30   40   50   60   70   80   90   100

PERCENT FEMALE

[1] Includes health practitioners, n.e.c., and health technologists and technicians, n.e.c., not shown separately.
Source: U.S. Bureau of Labor Statistics, September 1975.

Positions Held by Male and Female Nurses

Numerically, female R.N.s in high level positions far outweighs those of male R.N.s. However within each group a much larger percentage of male nurses have reached administrative/supervisor positions (24%) than female nurses (14.2%).

Figure 35-3   Comparison of employed male registered nurses and female registered nurses by type of position, 1972

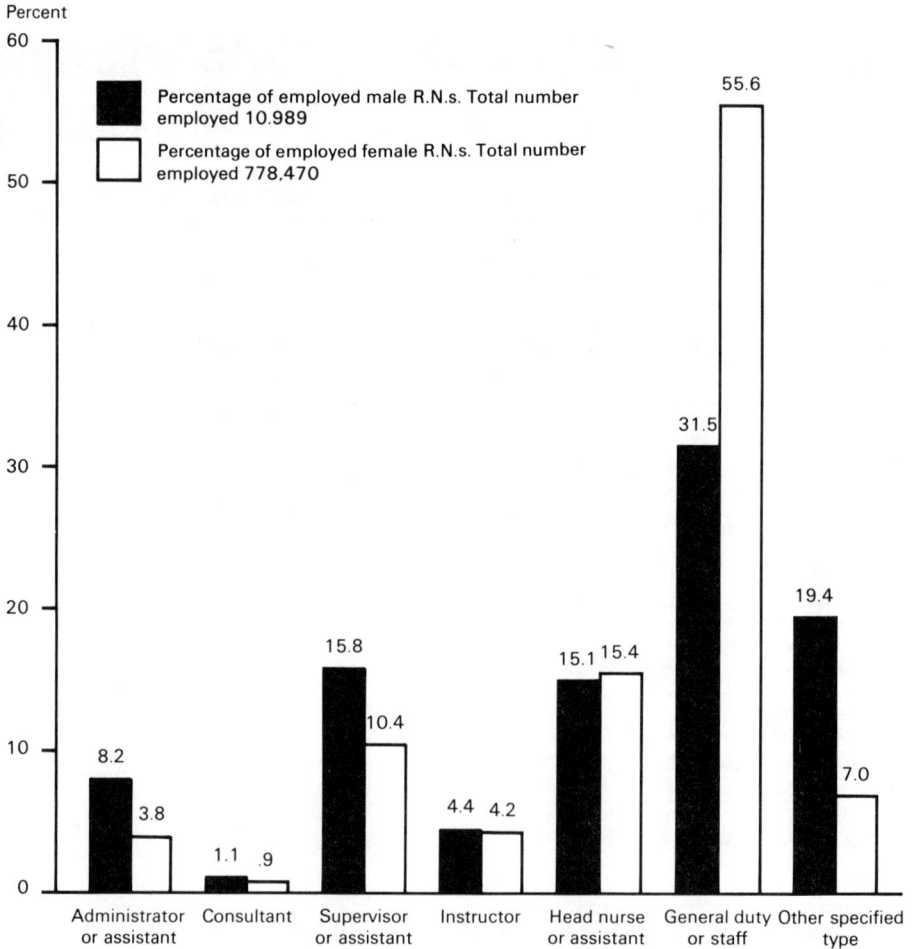

Percent

- ■ Percentage of employed male R.N.s. Total number employed 10.989
- □ Percentage of employed female R.N.s. Total number employed 778,470

Position	Male	Female
Administrator or assistant	8.2	3.8
Consultant	1.1	.9
Supervisor or assistant	15.8	10.4
Instructor	4.4	4.2
Head nurse or assistant	15.1	15.4
General duty or staff	31.5	55.6
Other specified type	19.4	7.0

Source: *The Nation's Nurses, 1972 Inventory,* American Nurses' Association, 1974.

Student Enrollments

Aside from nursing, the highest proportion of females enrolled in health professions schools was 30.4% in schools of pharmacy. In schools of medicine the proportion of females was 18.0%, and in schools of veterinary medicine, 13.6%.

Table 35-21   Total student enrollments in selected health professions schools in the United States, by sex

Profession and academic year	Both sexes	Students				
		Male		Female		
		Number	%	Number	%	
Medicine 1974–75	53,554	43,893	82.0	9,661	18.0	
Osteopathic medicine 1974–75	3,139	2,872	91.5	267	8.5	
Dentistry 1974–75	20,146	18,785	93.2	1,361	6.8	
Optometry 1972–73	3,328	3,158	94.9	170	5.1	
Pharmacy 1974–75	23,235	16,168	69.6	7,067	30.4	
Podiatry 1972–73	1,401	1,380	98.5	21	1.5	
Veterinary medicine 1972–73	5,439	4,698	86.4	741	13.6	
Nursing 1972–73	198,848[2]	9,513	4.8	189,335	95.2	
Diploma	66,949	2,533	3.8	64,416	95.2	
Associate degree	61,674	4,177	6.8	57,497	93.2	
Baccalaureate	70,225	2,803	4.0	67,422	96.0	

Source: Health Resources Administration, DHEW, 1976.

Crime

Women as Victims*

Women were the victims of about two-fifths of all crimes against persons in 1973. Personal larceny (theft of property or cash) accounted for about four-fifths of all crimes against women. Among women 12 years old and over the personal larceny victimization rate was 82 per 1,000 women; for crimes of violence as measured in the National Crime Panel (rape, robbery and assault) the rate was 23 per 1,000. Higher proportions of men than women tend to be victimized, as emphasized by the higher rates for violent crimes, where twice the proportion of men were victims. For personal larceny the ratio was four women to every five men.

Age appears to have been an important determinant in assessing the likelihood of women being victimized by personal crimes. The highest rates of victimization were for 12- to 19-year-olds, with each successive age group reporting lower rates. For incidences of violent crimes, the dividing line appeared to be about 25 years old with the rates dropping off sharply for older ages. Personal larceny showed the highest rates under 20 years old. These crimes included purse snatching, pocket picking and thefts of property without contact with the victim.

Significant differences in victimizations are evident for women by marital status, with never-married and separated and divorced women having the highest rates and widowed women having the lowest. These are considered functions of age and life style.

According to National Crime Panel data, the majority of rape and robbery victims among women reported that the assailants were strangers, while half of the victims of assault reported that the assault was by a family member, friend or acquaintance. Only about half of the female victims of violent crimes reported the crimes to police.

---

* Source: U.S. Bureau of the Census, 1976.

Table 35-22   Victimization rates for crimes against persons by sex and age: 1973
(Per 1,000 population age 12 and over)

Sex and age		Total crimes against persons	Crimes of violence						Personal larceny
					Robbery		Assault		
			Total	Rape	With injury	Without injury	Aggravated	Simple	
Women	(85,075)[1]	105.0	22.7	1.8	1.4	2.3	5.5	11.6	82.3
12 to 15 years	(8,144)	203.9	39.7	1.8	0.9	3.1	9.6	24.3	164.2
16 to 19 years	(7,872)	189.4	44.2	5.3	2.3	2.7	10.7	23.2	145.2
20 to 24 years	(9,015)	159.1	42.7	5.4	2.2	3.0	10.9	21.2	116.4
25 to 34 years	(14,432)	113.8	25.6	2.3	1.9	2.5	6.2	12.7	88.2
35 to 49 years	(17,556)	86.8	16.6	[2]0.5	0.9	1.9	4.8	8.6	70.2
50 to 64 years	(16,157)	54.4	8.4	[2]0.3	1.0	1.7	1.5	4.0	46.0
65 years and over	(11,901)	25.6	6.8	[2]0.3	1.5	2.4	1.0	1.6	18.8
Men	(77,161)	151.9	46.2	[2]0.1	3.4	7.0	15.7	20.0	105.7
12 to 15 years	(8,415)	267.0	79.9	[2]0.4	5.0	14.7	22.2	37.5	187.1
16 to 19 years	(7,712)	285.7	92.5	—	5.0	10.3	38.7	38.5	193.2
20 to 24 years	(8,330)	246.7	87.9	[2]0.1	5.8	11.8	33.1	37.1	158.8
25 to 34 years	(13,708)	161.0	47.9	[2]0.1	2.1	6.2	17.3	22.2	113.1
35 to 49 years	(16,281)	104.3	26.8	—	3.0	4.1	8.9	10.8	77.5
50 to 64 years	(14,344)	67.8	17.8	—	3.0	3.3	3.9	7.6	50.0
65 years and over	(8,371)	40.3	11.2	—	1.9	4.3	1.4	3.6	29.1

[1] Total number of persons in age group (in thousands).
[2] Estimate, based on about ten or fewer sample cases, is statistically unreliable.

Source: U.S. Department of Justice.

Women Criminals*

Female criminality has received much less attention by criminologists, law enforcement officials and community and clinical psychologists than has male criminality. One reason for the lack of interest in women prisoners is that the crimes women commit are usually ones that inconvenience society less than the crimes men commit. The overwhelming majority of women offenders have not been involved with organized crime, with crime involving high losses of property or with crimes that have endangered large numbers of people.

Generally, women account for only a small proportion of all crimes. Some theorists assert that the statistics distort rather than describe the real picture of the amount of crime that women commit. They argue that if male victims, police, prosecutors and judges would forego their chivalrous behavior, the proportion of women arrested and convicted would be vastly increased.

To summarize the picture today of how women fare at various stages in the criminal justice system: 1 in 6.5 arrests is a woman, and 1 in 9 convictions is a woman, but only about 1 in 30 of those sentenced to prison is a woman. These ratios have not changed drastically over the past two decades.

What the statistics show about the proportion of women in crime in 1972 is that there are more women involved today than at any time since the end of World War II, and probably before that. But the increase has been in certain types of offenses—forgery, fraud and embezzlement—not in crimes of violence or in the traditional female crimes, such as prostitution and child abuse.

As of 1972, 30% of all persons arrested for major larceny were women; 30% of all persons arrested for fraud and embezzlement were women; and 25% of all persons arrested for forgery were women. These proportions are much higher (by at least twice) than they are for any other offenses committed by women. If present trends continue, in 20 years women will probably be involved in white-collar crimes in a proportion commensurate with their representation in the society.

* Source: National Institute of Mental Health, 1975.

Table 35-23   Arrests by type of crime and sex: 1960 and 1974 (1,824 local jurisdictions; 1974 estimated population 69,222,000)

Type of crime	Women		Men		Percent women	
	1974	1960	1974	1960	1974	1960
All arrests	540,987	259,038	2,665,339	2,155,159	16.9	10.7
Violent crime	19,720	7,563	161,803	66,220	10.9	10.3
Murder and nonnegligent manslaughter	1,247	577	6,917	2,910	15.3	16.5
Forcible rape			10,546	5,059		
Robbery	5,059	1,247	65,214	23,933	7.2	5.0
Aggravated assault	13,414	5,739	79,126	34,318	14.5	14.3
Property crime	139,159	29,292	497,676	244,562	21.9	10.7
Burglary (breaking and entering)	10,212	2,952	175,689	85,188	5.5	3.3
Larceny (theft)	124,838	24,769	262,949	118,916	32.2	17.2
Motor vehicle theft	4,109	1,571	59,038	40,458	6.5	3.7
Other	382,108	222,183	2,005,860	1,844,377	16.0	10.8

Source: Federal Bureau of Investigation, 1974.

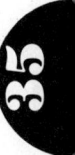

Women's Organizations and Associations

American Association of University Women
American Association of Women Ministers
American Medical Women's Association
American Newspaper Guild
American Nurses Association
American Society of Women Accountants
American Women In Radio and Television
American Woman's Society of Certified Public Accountants
Association of American Women Dentists
Citizens' Advisory Council on the Status of Women
Ecumenical Task Force on Women and Religion (Catholic Caucus)
Federally Employed Women (FEW)
Federation of Organizations for Professional Women
General Federation of Women's Clubs
Intercollegiate Association of Women Students
League of American Working Women
League of Women Voters
National Association of Colored Women's Clubs
National Association of Commissions for Women
National Association of Negro Business and Professional Women's Clubs
National Association of Railway Business Women
National Association of Women Deans and Counselors
National Association of Women Lawyers
National Black Feminist Organization
National Board of the Leadership Conference of Religious Women
National Coalition of American Nuns
National Council of Jewish Women
National Federation of Business and Professional Women's Clubs
National Federation of Republican Women's Clubs
National Organization for Women (NOW)
National Secretaries Association
National Welfare Rights Organization
National Woman's Party
National Women's Political Caucus
President's Task Force on Women's Rights and Responsibilities
Professional Women's Caucus
Unitarian Universalist Women's Federation
Women's Equity Action League
Women In Communications, Inc.
Women's International League for Peace and Freedom
Women's Joint Legislative Committee for Equal Rights
Women United
YWCA in Convention

36

THE HEALTH OF MINORITIES

Overview

- Black Americans, Spanish-surnamed Americans and American Indians are minorities with some of the worst health problems in the United States.
- Almost one of every six Americans is a member of one of these minorities. In 1970 they comprised more than 16% of the total population of 203 million. About 22.6 million (11.1%) were blacks. About 10.1 million (5%) were Americans of Spanish heritage and 800,000 (0.4%) were American Indians.
- Clustered in big city ghettos and barrios and hinterland villages and reservations, minorities have extraordinary health problems. In comparison to whites:

1. Nonwhite Americans die seven years sooner;
2. Nonwhite babies die in infancy almost twice as often;
3. Nonwhite mothers die in childbirth four times as often.

Table 36-1   Birth, death and fertility rates by race. (Rates per 1,000 population)

Item	Total	White	Negro
1975 (calendar year)			
Net growth rate	7.9	5.8	13.3
Birth rate	14.8	13.9	20.6
Death rate	9.0	9.0	9.0
General fertility rate	66.8	63.4	88.0

Source: *U.S. Statistical Abstracts, 1976.*

Measures of Health and Income*

On measures such as number of untreated conditions, number of dental caries and general level of nutrition, low-income persons are in poorer health than persons with higher income. The average number of bed-disability days, restricted-activity days and work-loss days per person is inversely related to income (National Center for Health Statistics, 1969). In fact, the differences are probably understated since low-income persons more frequently hold jobs which do not have sick leave and may therefore be forced to work when ill rather than lose a day's pay.

---

* Source: National Center for Health Statistics.

It is also becoming increasingly certain that low-income persons have less access to medical care and that the quality and range of services is much lower than those available to persons with more money.

Fewer services exist in the immediate residential area of low-income persons. The ratio of doctors (other than certain specialists) to the population is much lower in the cities than in the suburbs. Many low-income persons rely on hospital emergency rooms and public clinics for health care.

Also various sociological and psychological factors, as well as the obvious economic ones, limit the use by the poor of many of the resources that do exist.

Further, persons with incomes of less than $5,000 have more limitation of activity, more disability and more hospital episodes than the total population. They have fewer resources for obtaining medical care: fewer have hospital insurance; and, of course, they have less cash to pay expenses on their own. Within the low-income group, aid recipients have poorer health than nonrecipients. On all health measures, they have higher rates than nonrecipients—in many cases, twice as high.

Clearly the low-income persons have higher levels of activity limitation, disability and hospitalization than did the total population but had similar utilization of physicians; thus, apparently, for greater health needs, low-income persons had relatively fewer services.

An overall summary of health characteristics and the relative position of poverty groups is provided in Tables 36-2 to 36-6.

Table 36-2   Health characteristics of persons with family income under $5,000 and total population: United States, 1968

Characteristic	Family income under $5,000	Total population
	Per Cent	
Limitation of activity from chronic conditions	20.9	10.9
Hospital episodes	11.4	9.6
	Number per person	
Restricted-activity days	23.7	15.3
Bed-disability days	9.4	6.3
Short-stay hospital days per person	1.6	1.0
Short-stay hospital days per person with episodes	13.8	10.4

Source: National Center for Health Statistics.

Table 36-3 Physician visits by race and income: 1973

	Income			
	Under $5,000		$10,000 and over	
Characteristic	Black	White	Black	White
Average physician visits, per person	4.8	5.6	4.5	5.0
Place of visit: percent				
Physician's office	54	69	69	69
Hospital clinic	27	11	17	9
Other	19	19	13	21

Source: National Center for Health Statistics.

The Urban Condition

There are wide differences in the health status of the populations living in poverty and non-poverty areas of our largest cities. There are also substantial differences in the health status of the white population and that of the population of all other races.

In a select review of vital and health data from 19 major cities, the Health Resources Administration concluded that the health condition of persons of races other than white is less favorable than that of the white population, regardless of residence in poverty or non-poverty areas.

Table 36-4 Number of persons residing in poverty areas of 19 selected cities—1970

	Poverty areas		
City	Total	White	All other races
Atlanta	180,444	35,590	144,854
Baltimore	321,271	73,084	248,187
Buffalo	108,216	41,186	67,030
Chicago	833,425	188,180	645,245
Cincinnati	143,081	57,879	85,202
Cleveland	213,435	53,860	159,575
Dallas	217,069	55,907	161,162
Denver	120,241	98,051	22,190
Indianapolis	95,461	40,064	55,397
Los Angeles	583,598	233,137	350,461
Memphis	253,623	40,732	212,891
Minneapolis	73,474	60,462	13,012
New York City	2,031,586	974,462	1,057,124
Philadelphia	505,880	156,619	349,261
Pittsburgh	119,163	50,032	69,131
San Diego	97,244	60,826	36,418
San Francisco	152,435	80,022	72,413
Seattle	43,988	29,016	14,972
Washington, D.C.	246,191	19,130	227,061

Source: U.S. Bureau of the Census.

Table 36-5 Vital statistics on poverty areas in 19 selected cities: 1969–71

Vital statistics measure	United States, 1969–71	Poverty areas		
		Total	White	All other
Crude birth rate (per 1,000 population)	17.9	23.5	21.6	24.5
Fertility rate (per 1,000 women 15–44 years)	85.5	105.2	103.7	106.0
Crude death rate (per 1,000 population)	9.5	12.0	14.6	10.5
Low birth weight (2,500 grams or less) (per 100 live births)	7.9	13.1	9.3	15.1
Illegitimate births (per 100 live births)	10.7	40.8	23.7	49.5
Lack of prenatal care (live births to mothers with no care) (per 100 live births)	1.7	5.0	4.2	5.3
Education of mother (live births to mothers with less than 12 years of education) (per 100 live births)	31.1	58.5	54.8	60.4
Infant mortality rate (per 1,000 live births)	20.0	30.2	24.2	33.4

Table 36-5 (continued)

Vital statistics measure	United States, 1969–71	Poverty areas		
		Total	White	All other
Fetal death ratio (per 1,000 live births)	13.9	23.5	17.4	25.9
Death rate for tuberculosis (per 100,000 population)	2.5	9.5	8.7	10.0
Death rate for violent causes (per 100,000 population)	76.4	115.5	112.7	117.1

Source: National Center for Health Statistics.

Table 36-6 Black population, by region and residence: 1960 to 1974

Residence	1960	1970	1974
Population (millions)	18.9	22.6	23.5
Percent distribution	100	100	100
Metropolitan areas	68	74	76
Central cities	53	58	58
Outside central cities	15	16	17
Nonmetropolitan areas	32	26	24

Special Health Problems*

Blacks

Afro-Americans were cited by the 1970 census as comprising 11.1% of the population in the United States. They live in many parts of America. In the ten largest cities their popula-

*Source: "Ethnicity and Health Care," National League for Nursing, 14-625.

Death Rates

Table 36-7 Death rates for selected causes, by color and sex: 1973. (Based on age-specific death rates per 100,000 population in specified group)

Cause of death and race	1973		Cause of death and race	1973	
	Male	Female		Male	Female
Black and other races			White		
All causes	1,084.6	755.4	All causes	1,071.2	823.0
Major cardiovascular diseases	425.4	361.7	Major cardiovascular diseases	555.7	465.1
Diseases of heart	305.9	239.7	Diseases of heart	430.9	319.4
Hypertension	6.1	5.8	Hypertension	3.3	3.1
Cerebrovascular diseases	96.1	99.9	Cerebrovascular disease	91.2	113.7
Arteriosclerosis	8.5	9.2	Arteriosclerosis	13.8	19.1
Malignant neoplasms, including neoplasms of lymphatic and hemotopoietic tissues	170.1	117.9	Malignant neoplasms, including neoplasms of lymphatic and hemotopoietic tissues	189.6	153.0
Accidents	98.5	33.6	Accidents	75.9	32.7
Influenza and pneumonia	39.7	24.1	Influenza and pneumonia	32.6	26.7
Diabetes mellitus	18.2	28.2	Diabetes mellitus	14.9	19.9
Cirrhosis of liver	26.6	15.2	Cirrhosis of liver	20.5	10.1
Suicide	10.0	3.0	Suicide	18.8	7.0
Homicide	65.8	14.6	Homicide	8.3	2.8
Certain causes of mortality in early infancy	36.8	25.7	Certain causes of mortality in early infancy	14.6	9.7

Source: National Center for Health Statistics and U.S. Bureau of Census, July 1975.

36

tion ranges from 71.1% in Washington, D.C., to 17.9% in Los Angeles, California.

The following statistics highlight the extent to which some health problems are affecting Afro-Americans:

- Death rate of mothers at childbirth—eight and a half deaths per 10,000 live births for blacks and two deaths for whites.
- The tuberculosis rate for blacks is three times greater than for whites.
- Death rate from childhood diseases is six times higher among black children than whites.
- There are 33 cases of cancer *in situ* and 15 of invasive cancer per 100,000 women for whites and 63 cases of *in situ* and 33.3 invasive cancer for blacks.
- 13 million Afro-Americans have hypertension, and 50% of them are not aware of their condition. Of the 50% who are aware half are receiving no treatment.*

In addition to these "everyday major health problems," one out of every 500 Afro-Americans has sickle cell anemia, and one out of every 12 carries the trait.

The rate of patient noncompliance among black women is 75%. One can only speculate as to this amazing phenomenon until someone does significant research of black female patients to ascertain why medical orders and instructions are not followed. Some guesses might be:

- Money to purchase drugs and other medical supplies is used to buy food and other necessities for the children and other family members.
- Lack of education about her diagnosis and the reasons for certain drugs, their actions and side effects and explanations of all tests and treatments given.
- Impersonality and long waiting periods at clinics.
- Immobilized by a sense of powerlessness suffered by some disadvantaged black persons.
- Cold, superior attitude of health workers.

Binding Ties Vol. II, Special Issue on the Physical and Emotional Health Problems of Black Women. Prepared by the Black Women's Community Development Foundation, Washington, D.C.: May 1974, pp. 1–5.

Mexican Americans

There are various diseases frequently found or diagnosed among Mexican-Americans that may be considered superstitions by the dominant American culture.

Espanto (fright caused by seeing supernatural beings, spirits or events) or *susto* (fright caused by natural phenomena such as lightning, loud unexpected noises, etc.) results in a syndrome complex involving easily recognized symptoms such as insomnia, restlessness, loss of appetite and nervousness. Literally translated, *susto* means "fright." Women and children are more prone to this disorder than men.

Mal de ojo (evil-eye) is caused by someone's nonintentional admiration of a body part of the victim. Beautiful hair, pretty eyes, a clear complexion or another physical attribute may be the object of great admiration. If a person strongly admires these attributes, the victim may well lose the admired attribute or at least fall ill for a period of time. Infants, women and children are especially susceptible to this disorder. High fever, prostration, headaches, excessive fatigue or general malaise are symptomatic of the disorder.

Maintenance of health is closely tied to being in good accord with God. That is, individuals who are chronically ill or develop certain disorders, especially those which are extremely painful or disfiguring, may be suffering due to action carried out by God as punishment for evil deeds or moral indiscretions.

In order to maintain good health, certain foods must be avoided. Rice, bananas, greasy fried foods, apples, coffee and tamales are to be avoided in the evening meal.

Mexican-Americans of the same sex may be quite reticent to participate in activities such as group showers or physical examinations by a physician, in contrast with the dominant American culture. The natural functions such as urinating, defecating and bathing are considered one's private activities not to be observed by others. Nurses can allow for this factor by providing more privacy than is normally expected by the typical American patient.

Indians

While the health needs in the Indian community are great, the health resources are few. There are approximately 42 American Indian physicians, 500 American Indian nurses, five dentists, four Ph.D. social scientists and five Ph.D. physical scientists.* It is in part due to lack of American Indian scientists that diseases most prevalent within the Indian community have received little attention. There

*Cresap, McCormick and Paget, Inc. *Evaluation of the DHEW Health Manpower Training Programs Relative to Indians,* DHEW, 1972.

are data suggesting that the clinical picture for diabetes, hypertension and alcoholism is different within the American Indian population than among the majority population. For example, the Indian people may remain asymptomatic with a blood sugar level of 500 mg/ml; thus the nurse must have different information when screening Indian patients for this disease.

37

MINORITIES IN THE HEALTH CARE FIELD

Overview

Minority Employment by Occupation

Table 37-1   Employed persons by occupation and race: 1960 and 1975 (covers persons 16 years old and over)

Occupation	White		Black and other	
	1960	1975	1960	1975
Total employed (1,000)	58,850	75,713	6,927	9,070
Percent	100.0	100.0	100.0	100.0
White-collar workers	46.6	51.7	16.1	34.2
Professional, technical, and kindred	12.1	15.5	4.8	11.4
Medical and other health	2.1	2.5	0.8	2.7
Teacher, except college	2.6	3.6	1.7	3.1
Managers, administrators, exc. farm	11.7	11.2	2.6	4.4
Salaried workers	5.9	9.0	0.9	3.4
Self-employed	5.8	2.2	1.7	1.0
Salesworkers	7.0	6.9	1.5	2.7
Retail trade	4.1	3.8	1.0	2.0
Clerical workers	15.7	18.1	7.3	15.7
Stenographers, typists, and sec'ys.	3.9	5.4	1.4	3.4
Blue-collar workers	36.2	32.4	40.1	37.4
Craft and kindred workers	13.8	13.4	6.0	8.8
Carpenters	1.4	1.2	0.4	0.6
Constr. craftworkers, exc. carpenters	2.7	2.7	1.6	2.1
Mechanics and repairers	3.2	3.6	1.7	2.1
Metalcraft workers, except mechanics	1.8	1.4	0.6	0.8
Blue-collar supervisors, n.e.c.	1.9	1.7	0.4	1.0
Operatives	17.9	14.6	20.4	20.0
Operatives, except transport	(NA)	10.9	(NA)	15.0
Transport equipment operatives	(NA)	3.7	(NA)	5.0
Drivers, motor vehicles	3.5	3.1	4.4	4.0
Nonfarm laborers	4.4	4.4	13.7	8.7
Service industries	9.9	12.3	31.7	25.8
Private household workers	1.7	1.0	14.2	4.9
Service workers, exc. priv. household	8.2	11.3	17.5	20.9
Protective service workers	1.2	1.5	0.5	1.7
Farmworkers	7.4	3.6	12.1	2.6
Farmers and farm managers	4.3	2.0	3.2	0.6
Farm laborers and supervisors	3.0	1.5	9.0	2.0
Paid workers	1.7	1.1	6.6	1.8
Unpaid family workers	1.3	0.5	2.4	0.2

Source: U.S. Bureau of Labor Statistics.

Figure 37-1   Percent of population employed in selected health occupations who are Black or of Spanish heritage, by sex: United States, 1970

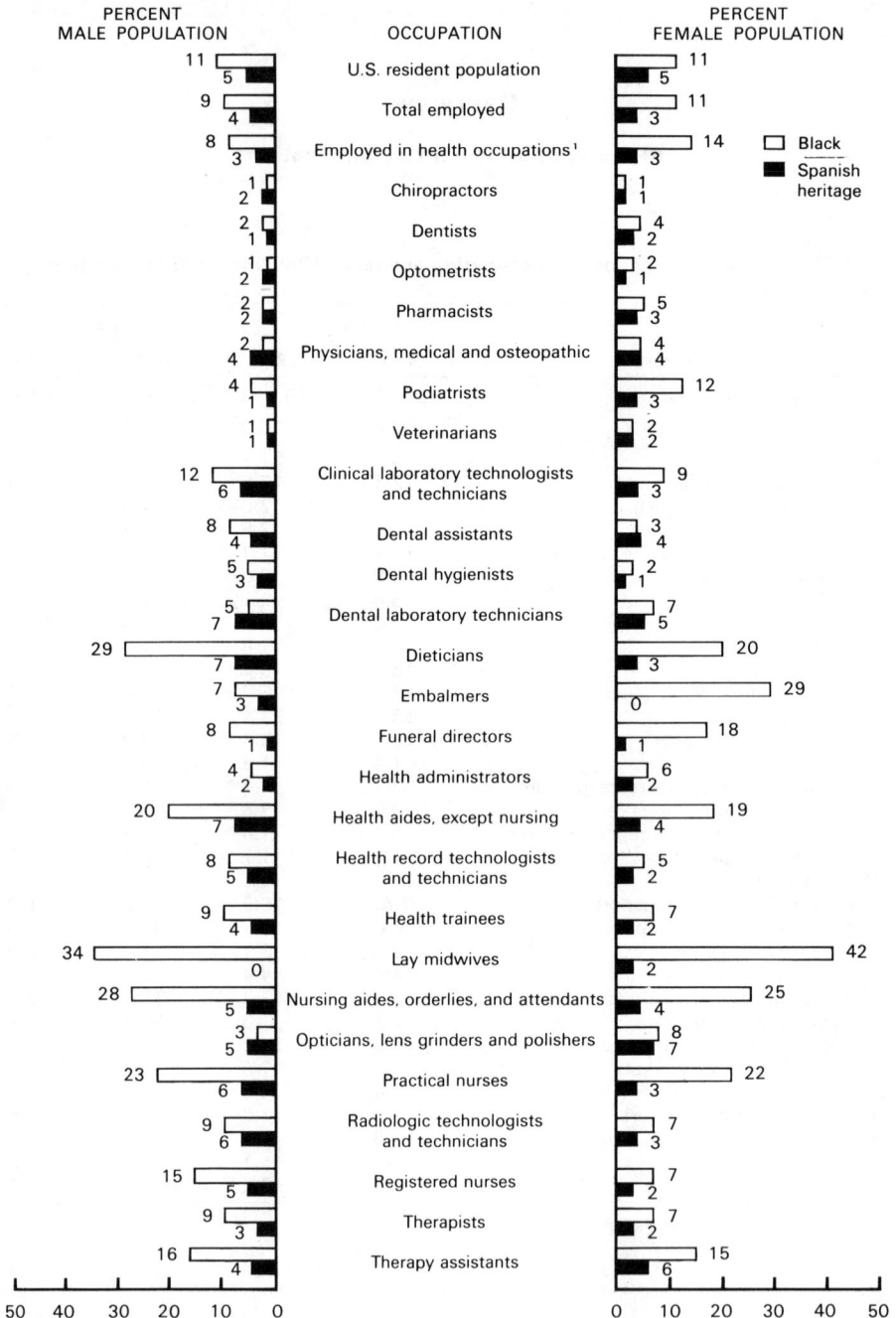

PERCENT MALE POPULATION	OCCUPATION	PERCENT FEMALE POPULATION
11 / 5	U.S. resident population	11 / 5
9 / 4	Total employed	11 / 3
8 / 3	Employed in health occupations[1]	14 / 3
1 / 2	Chiropractors	1 / 1
2 / 1	Dentists	4 / 2
1 / 2	Optometrists	2 / 1
2 / 2	Pharmacists	5 / 3
2 / 4	Physicians, medical and osteopathic	4 / 4
4 / 1	Podiatrists	12 / 3
1 / 1	Veterinarians	2 / 2
12 / 6	Clinical laboratory technologists and technicians	9 / 3
8 / 4	Dental assistants	3 / 4
5 / 3	Dental hygienists	2 / 1
5 / 7	Dental laboratory technicians	7 / 5
29 / 7	Dieticians	20 / 3
7 / 3	Embalmers	29 / 0
8 / 1	Funeral directors	18 / 1
4 / 2	Health administrators	6 / 2
20 / 7	Health aides, except nursing	19 / 4
8 / 5	Health record technologists and technicians	5 / 2
9 / 4	Health trainees	7 / 2
34 / 0	Lay midwives	42 / 2
28 / 5	Nursing aides, orderlies, and attendants	25 / 4
3 / 5	Opticians, lens grinders and polishers	8 / 7
23 / 6	Practical nurses	22 / 3
9 / 6	Radiologic technologists and technicians	7 / 3
15 / 5	Registered nurses	7 / 2
9 / 3	Therapists	7 / 2
16 / 4	Therapy assistants	15 / 6

Legend: □ Black   ■ Spanish heritage

[1] Includes health practitioners and health technologists.

Source: U.S. Bureau of the Census.

Organizations for Minorities in Nursing*

The first organization for black nurses was the National Association of Colored Graduate Nurses (NACGN), founded by Martha Franklin in 1908. This was 29 years after the first black trained nurse, Mary Eliza Mahoney, was graduated from the New England Hospital for Women and Children in Boston. While the Nurses' Associated Alumnae of the United States and Canada (forerunner of ANA) allowed black nurses to be members, it granted them few membership privileges other than paying dues.

The objectives of NACGN were in keeping with the highest professional standards and traditions: to advance the standards and best interest of trained nurses, break down discrimination in the nursing profession, and develop leadership within the ranks of black nurses.

Then in 1948, the ANA house of delegates voted to remove as rapidly as possible all barriers that prevented full participation of racial minority nurses in the association. At that time, ANA made provisions for black nurses denied membership in state nurses associations to have direct individual membership in ANA. It also called for an end to all discriminatory policies and urged the various states to follow suit. Not until 1961, did the last state (Georgia) abandon its color bar, and one district in another state held out until 1964.

Encouraged by the developments on the national level, the black nurses voted in 1949 to dissolve NACGN and formal dissolution occurred on January 31, 1951. However, in December, 1971, noting that there were issues of common concern to black nurses—among them that there had been no significant increase in the number of black nurses since 1950—the National Black Nurse's Association was formed. Among the purposes and objectives listed were the following:

● Define and determine nursing care for black consumers by acting as their advocates.

● Compile and maintain a national directory of black nurses to assist with the dissemination of information regarding black nurses and nursing on national and local levels by the use of all media.

● Recruit, counsel and assist black persons interested in nursing to insure a constant procession of blacks into the field.

Black Nurses in History

Susie King Taylor—born in slavery in Georgia, served as a volunteer battlefront nurse in the Civil War.

Namahyoke S. Curtis—instrumental in motivating the establishment of Chicago's Provident Hospital, a hospital which cared for black patients and trained black nurses and physicians. Active as a contract nurse in Spanish-American War.

Mary E. P. Mahoney—first professionally trained black nurse, graduated New England Hospital School around 1878.

Jessie C. S. Scales—first black district nurse, in New York City, 1901.

Martha Franklin—cofounder and first president of National Association for the Advancement of Colored Graduate Nurses.

Adah Thoms—cofounder of NAACGN; credited with gaining acceptance of black nurses by the army, 1917–18; winner of the first Mahoney Medal.

Estelle M. Osborne—achieved many firsts in nursing education, administration and professional organization.

Representation of Minorities in Health Fields

Among 19 health occupations, the groupings of nursing aides, orderlies and attendents have the highest proportion of minority race members (27%), according to data from the 1970 census. Over 20% of practical nurses and dietitians are members of a minority race. The proportion of Spanish-origin persons varies from .4% representation as podiatrists to 8.4% as lay midwives.

*Source: Adapted from "From Invisibility to Blackness" by Gloria Smith, *Nursing Outlook,* April 1975. © American Journal of Nursing Company.

770

Minority Representation in Health Occupations

Table 37-2   Persons employed in health occupations in the United States, by racial/ethnic category, 1970

Occupation	Total employed[1]	Racial/ethnic category							
		Total minority[1]	Negro	American Indian	Japanese	Chinese	Filipino	White	Spanish origin
Physicians (M.D. & D.O.)	100.0	6.9	2.1	0.1	0.6	0.9	2.0	93.1	3.7
Dentists	100.0	4.0	2.6	0.1	0.7	0.5	0.1	96.0	1.1
Optometrists	100.0	1.7	0.8	—	0.3	0.4	0.1	98.3	1.7
Pharmacists	100.0	4.3	2.5	0.1	0.8	0.7	0.1	95.7	1.9
Podiatrists	100.0	4.3	3.6	—	0.3	0.4	—	95.7	.4
Veterinarians	100.0	0.9	0.5	0.1	—	0.1	—	99.1	.5
Registered nurses	100.0	9.6	7.8	0.2	0.3	0.1	0.8	90.4	2.0
Dietitians	100.0	21.7	18.3	0.2	0.9	0.5	1.6	78.3	2.9
Health administrators	100.0	5.6	4.6	0.3	0.4	—	0.1	94.4	1.3
Clinical laboratory technologists, technicians	100.0	12.8	9.3	0.1	0.5	0.9	1.5	87.2	4.0
Dental hygienists	100.0	3.0	1.7	—	0.5	0.3	0.1	97.0	0.9
Health record technologists, technicians	100.0	6.6	5.0	—	0.6	—	0.8	93.4	1.7
Radiologic technologists, technicians	100.0	7.8	6.7	0.3	0.3	0.1	0.2	92.2	3.8
Dental laboratory technicians	100.0	8.6	5.4	0.1	1.9	0.5	0.5	91.4	6.8
Opticians and lens grinders and polishers	100.0	5.2	4.3	0.1	0.4	0.1	0.2	94.8	4.3
Dental assistants	100.0	4.9	3.5	0.2	0.7	0.3	0.2	95.1	3.5
Lay midwives	100.0	39.9	39.9	—	—	—	—	60.1	8.4
Practical nurses	100.0	22.9	21.7	0.5	0.2	0.1	0.3	77.1	3.7
Nursing aides, orderlies and attendants	100.0	26.6	25.3	0.6	0.2	0.1	0.2	73.4	4.1

[1] Includes other races, not shown separately.

Source: U.S. Bureau of the Census.

Minority Representation in Government Hospitals

State and local governmental hospitals account for approximately one-quarter of all employment in hospitals and convalescent institutions. Employment in these governmental hospitals has been steadily rising, increasing by 27% between 1967 and 1974. Currently, minority women alone account for 22% of all employment in public hospitals.

The rates of participation by minorities in different type governmental hospitals are described in Table 37-3.

Table 37-3   Full-time employees in state and local government hospitals and sanatoria by ethnic group, sex and type of government, 1973

Employee group	State		County		Municipality		Township		Special district	
	Number	Percent	Number	Percent	Number	Percent	Number	Percent	Number	Percent
All employees	212,276	100.0	154,364	100.0	87,472	100.0	1,167	100.0	73,986	100.0
White	159,964	75.4	110,689	71.7	43,247	49.4	1,086	93.1	53,490	72.3
Black	43,236	20.4	33,906	22.0	34,831	39.8	71	6.1	16,572	22.4
Spanish surnamed	5,891	2.8	6,455	4.2	7,252	8.3	6	.5	2,987	4.0
Asian American	947	.4	1,948	1.3	1,599	1.8	—	—	621	.8
American Indian	615	.3	580	.4	66	.1	4	.3	180	.2
Other	1,623	.8	786	.5	477	.5	—	—	186	.3
Total minority	53,312	24.7	43,675	28.4	44,225	50.5	81	6.9	20,496	27.7
Total female	135,916	64.0	118,492	76.8	60,500	69.2	962	82.4	60,113	81.2

Note: Due to rounding, percentages may not add to 100.0.

Source: Equal Employment Opportunity Commission, 1973.

Minority Representation in Private Hospitals

Table 37-4   Employees in private hospitals by minority group and sex, United States, 1973

Item, minority group and sex	Total employment	White collar occupations						Blue collar occupations				
		Total white collar employment	Officials and managers	Profes-sionals	Techni-cians	Sales workers	Office and clerical	Total blue collar employment	Skilled craft	Opera-tives	Labor-ers	Service workers
Number employees—												
5,266 units—												
All employees	2,017,666	1,213,617	107,154	494,851	303,344	4,116	304,152	119,067	30,798	53,784	34,485	684,982
Male	400,742	187,734	47,183	70,940	48,649	1,022	19,940	61,680	23,418	25,197	13,065	151,328
Female	1,616,924	1,025,883	59,971	423,911	254,695	3,094	284,212	57,387	7,380	28,587	21,420	533,654
Percentage of total employed												
All employees	100.0	100.0	100.0	100.0	100.0	100.0	100.0	100.0	100.0	100.0	100.0	100.0
Male	19.9	15.5	44.0	14.3	16.0	24.8	6.6	51.8	76.0	46.8	37.9	22.1
Female	80.1	84.5	56.0	85.7	84.0	75.2	93.4	48.2	24.0	53.2	62.1	77.9
White	78.4	86.1	91.4	89.1	79.0	81.1	86.5	74.2	82.7	71.6	70.8	65.4
Male	14.6	12.8	40.2	11.8	12.6	21.6	5.0	40.7	66.0	35.9	25.5	13.2
Female	63.8	73.3	51.2	77.4	66.4	59.5	81.5	33.6	16.7	35.8	45.3	52.2
Minority	21.6	13.9	8.6	10.9	21.0	18.9	13.5	25.8	17.3	28.4	29.2	34.6
Male	5.3	2.6	3.8	2.6	3.4	3.2	1.5	11.1	10.0	11.0	12.4	8.9
Female	16.3	11.2	4.8	8.3	17.6	15.7	11.9	14.6	7.3	17.4	16.8	25.7
Black	16.0	8.8	5.6	4.6	16.0	15.7	9.6	18.8	12.3	21.0	21.0	28.3
Male	3.4	1.2	2.3	.6	2.0	2.5	.9	7.4	6.4	7.3	8.4	6.6
Female	12.6	7.6	3.4	3.9	14.0	13.2	8.7	11.4	5.9	13.7	12.6	21.7
Spanish surnamed American	3.6	2.4	1.7	1.8	3.2	2.4	3.0	5.7	3.9	6.3	6.6	5.2
Male	1.3	.7	1.0	.6	.9	.6	.5	3.2	2.8	3.1	3.4	1.9
Female	2.3	1.8	1.0	1.2	2.3	1.8	2.6	2.6	1.0	3.1	3.1	3.2
Asian American	1.7	2.4	.4	4.3	1.5	.5	.7	.8	.7	.8	1.0	.8
Male	.5	.7	.1	1.3	.5	.1	.1	.4	.5	.4	.4	.2
Female	1.2	1.7	.2	3.0	1.0	.4	.5	.4	.1	.5	.6	.6
American Indian	.3	.2	.1	.2	.3	.2	.2	.4	.4	.2	.7	.3
Male	.1	.0	.1	.0	.1	.0	.0	.2	.2	.1	.1	.1
Female	.2	.2	.1	.2	.3	.2	.1	.3	.2	.1	.5	.3

Source: U.S. Equal Employment Opportunity Commission, 1975.

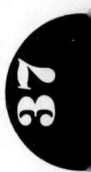

Salaries

Black nurses on the average earn more per hour than their white nurse peers. This pattern probably reflects the propensity for black nurses to work in larger cities where living costs and, hence, wages are higher. To the extent that hospital employer discrimination against black nurses exists (if it exists at all), it is not sufficiently great to offset factors (such as location) that boost relative wage rates of R.N.s.*

Table 37-5   Occupations and salaries of full-time employees in state and local government hospitals and sanatoria, 1973

| | | | Occupational distribution | | | | |
Job category	All employees	White	Total minority	Black	Spanish surnamed American	Asian American	American Indian
Total	529,265	368,476	160,789	128,616	22,591	5,115	1,395
Total percent	100.0	100.0	100.0	100.0	100.0	100.0	100.0
Officials/administrators	3.5	4.6	1.1	.9	1.4	2.9	3.4
Professionals	18.4	21.5	11.3	8.1	11.5	69.9	20.4
Technicians	15.1	15.5	14.3	15.4	10.4	5.7	11.4
Protective service	1.4	1.3	1.7	1.8	1.6	.4	.5
Paraprofessionals	24.5	21.9	30.3	32.5	23.6	7.3	33.6
Office/clerical	12.6	13.6	10.5	9.9	16.1	6.2	7.3
Skilled craft	4.4	4.9	3.1	3.2	3.2	.8	2.7
Service/maintenance	20.0	16.7	27.7	28.3	32.1	6.9	20.6
			Median annual salary				
Total	$ 6,961	$ 7,124	$ 6,711	$ 6,539	$ 6,662	$11,026	$ 6,543
Officials/administrators	12,398	12,357	12,939	12,325	13,111	18,250	12,471
Professionals	10,808	10,661	11,293	10,993	11,548	11,909	12,192
Technicians	7,142	7,112	7,217	7,197	7,216	9,023	7,226
Protective service	8,512	8,013	9,547	9,705	8,384	11,200	7,333
Paraprofessionals	5,766	5,586	6,144	6,189	5,945	6,741	5,309
Office/clerical	6,455	6,336	6,752	6,799	6,559	7,295	5,920
Skilled craft	7,509	7,874	6,310	6,097	7,402	7,833	6,286
Service/maintenance	5,817	5,908	5,437	5,593	6,186	6,843	6,037

Source: Equal Employment Opportunity Commission, 1973.

Minorities and Nurse Training

The Equal Employment Opportunity Commission claims that minorities and women are obtaining the training necessary to break into the top-paying occupations in the hospitals and sanatoria field at rates greater than ever before. For example, in the academic year 1973–74, 9.5% of all students enrolled in schools of medicine were members of minority groups (up from 3.6% in 1968–69), and 15.4% were women (up from 8.8% in 1968–69). Minorities and women represented even higher proportions of the first year enrollments for 1973–74; 11.5% and 19.7%, respectively. In addition, the proportion that blacks represented of admissions to nursing programs had risen from 3.2% in 1965–66 to 8.5% in 1971–72. The number of women in nursing programs rose during the period 1966–72, but their proportion of admissions decreased from 98.2 to 93.9%. This latter situation reflects the increased interest in nursing shown by men, as well as the opening up of other health occupations to women.**

---

* Source: DHEW, 1975 (1973 Survey).
** Source: *State and Local Government Functional Profiles; Hospitals, 1973*, EEOC.

Table 37-6   Number of minority students admitted, enrolled, and graduated from schools of nursing, 1975

Students	Associate degree	Diploma	Baccalaureate	Practical or vocational
Blacks:				
Number of admissions reported	3,495	1,014	3,650	5,795
Percent blacks enrolled	9	5	9	15
Percent blacks graduated	10	8	9	16
Spanish background:				
Number of admissions reported	1,069	204	807	1,927
Percent Spanish enrolled	5	2	3	9
Percent Spanish graduated	6	6	5	10
American Indian/Orientals:				
Number of admissions reported	532	97	454	591
Percent American Indian/ Orientals enrolled	2	1	2	4
Percent American Indians/ Orientals graduated	4	3	3	5

Source: *Nursing Outlook,* September 1976. © American Journal of Nursing Company.

Minority Recruitment

The federal government has been active in attempts to recruit minority members into the nursing profession.

Under the Health Manpower Education Initiative Awards program, Special Health Career Opportunity grants are authorized to recruit into the health professions and other health fields disadvantaged students, especially from minorities, and students likely to practice in underserved areas.

Grants are awarded to: (1) identify disadvantaged students with potential for health training, (2) enroll them in health schools and (3) assist them in completing training. For students not qualified to enroll, postsecondary or other training to prepare them for admission is authorized. This section applies to poor or otherwise disadvantaged students as well as U.S. military veterans with health training or experience.

These grants are administered by the Office of Health Manpower Opportunity within the Bureau of Health Manpower Education.*

The Division of Nursing has had a program for special project grants since 1965. These grants have been awarded for special projects focusing on the educational needs of nursing students from disadvantaged backgrounds. Among the grants to schools concerned with minority students were:

- new baccalaureate and associate degree programs, including the only R.N. program on an Indian reservation, and one other Arizona school geared particularly to the instructional needs of Mexican-Americans;
- remedial services for disadvantaged students in eleven baccalaureate, ten diploma, and three associate degree institutions.

Minority Recruitment Sources**

Following are some regional and local sources for recruitment. Organizations are listed by the seven geographic areas in which EEOC has regional offices. Employers may contact EEOC Voluntary Programs staff in the appropriate region for suggestions on additional and current local referral sources.

*Source: DHEW.

**Source: "A Directory of Resources for Affirmative Recruitment," EEOC, March 1975.

Public Agencies

U.S. Equal Employment Opportunity Commission (Regional Offices)

States

Atlanta Regional Office
Citizens Trust Building
Suite 1150
75 Piedmont Avenue N.E.
Atlanta, Ga. 30303
(404) 526-6991

Alabama, Canal Zone, Florida,
Georgia, Kentucky, N. Carolina,
Mississippi, S. Carolina,
Tennessee

Chicago Regional Office
600 S. Michigan Ave., Rm. 611
Chicago, Ill. 60605
(312) 353-1488

Illinois, Indiana, Michigan,
Minnesota, Ohio, Wisconsin

Dallas Regional Office
1100 Commerce St., Rm. 5A4
Dallas, Texas 75202
(214) 749-1841

Arkansas, Louisiana, New Mexico,
Oklahoma, Texas

Kansas City Regional Office
601 E. 12th St., Rm. 113
Kansas City, Mo. 64106
(816) 374-2781

Iowa, Kansas, Missouri,
Nebraska

New York Regional Office
Federal Office Building
26 Federal Plaza, Rm. 1615
New York, New York 10007
(212) 264-3640

Connecticut, Maine, Massachusetts,
New Hampshire, New Jersey, New
York, Puerto Rico, Rhode Island,
Vermont

Philadelphia Regional Office
127 N. 4th Street, 3rd Floor
Philadelphia, Pa. 19106
(215) 597-7784

Delaware, District of Columbia,
Maryland, Pennsylvania, Virginia,
West Virginia

San Francisco Regional Office
300 Montgomery St., Suite 740
San Francisco, Calif. 94104
(415) 556-1775

Alaska, Arizona, California,
Colorado, Guam, Hawaii, Idaho,
Montana, Nevada, N. Dakota,
Oregon, Samoa, S. Dakota, Utah,
Wake Island, Washington, Wyoming

State Employment Services (State and Local Offices)

These are primary referral sources in all regions (see under state "Employment Service" in local telephone directory) for locating professional, as well as clerical, technical, skilled and unskilled workers. Many have computerized job banks. These offices also serve as placement centers for many publicly funded, job-training programs.

Regional Offices, Manpower Administration, U.S. Dept. of Labor

Central information sources for current federally funded training programs (see regional listings).

State, County and City Human Resources Departments

These (or similarly titled) agencies, along with the Employment Service and Regional

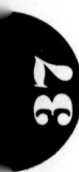

Manpower Office, are sources of information and referrals for many publicly funded training programs and organizations serving minorities and females, such as:

- Apprenticeship Training; Apprenticeship Outreach (including many skilled crafts);
- Job Corps; Neighborhood Youth Corps;
- Women in Community Service (WICS);
- Work Incentive Program (WIN);
- Concentrated Employment Program (CEP);
- JOBS Program (federally funded, on-the-job training);
- American Indian Training Programs; and
- Community Action and other special local training programs.

(Only a few of these local programs are in the following regional listings.)

State and City Human Rights Agencies

Consult local telephone directory.

Private Agencies

League of United Latin American Citizens (LULAC)

National Office
3033 N. Central Ave., Suite 402
Phoenix, Ariz. 85012

About 2000 local councils in 33 states provide informal referrals for jobs at all levels. Some local councils have job placement service (see national listing). Contact national office for referral to appropriate local councils.

National Association for the Advancement of Colored People (NAACP)

National membership organization. Does not have formal job referral service, but regularly services employers' job requests, directly or by contacting appropriate regional office and/or local branches (1,700 nationwide). Local branches have broad community contacts with many potential qualified job applicants. Contact regional offices or consult telephone directory for local NAACP branch listing.

Opportunities Industrialization Centers (OICs) of America, Inc.

Approximately 115 local OICs conduct varied skill training programs and provide referral and placement services.

SER/Jobs for Progress, Inc.

National Office
9841 Airport Boulevard
Los Angeles, Calif. 90045

Manpower agency specializing in Spanish-surnamed Americans. Varied training programs, job development and placement services provided by 50 SER offices in 43 cities. Contact national office for regional listings and local programs.

Urban Leagues

Local Urban Leagues provide referrals for jobs at all levels and participate in National Skills Bank. Local leagues also conduct varied skill training and apprenticeship programs for women and minorities. Contact regional office or consult local telephone directory for address and telephone of Urban League cities in various regions.

Boone, Young & Associates, Inc.

551 Fifth Ave., Room 2015
New York, New York 10017

Management consulting firm: specialties in executive search; health and social services; housing and real estate; economic development; management services. Works on contractual assignments to locate specific individuals for specific jobs. Also, contingency referrals of professionals. Services consumer products, package goods, advertising, broadcasting and banking industries. Specializes in professionals in banking, finance, accounting, communications, marketing, sales and personnel. Fee charged.

CAI Associates

803 W. Broad Street
Falls Church, Va. 22046

Locates, interviews and screens best qualified candidates for professional positions. Recruits for retail, insurance, manufacturing, construction and health care organizations. Arranges an initial meeting between candidates and clients; arranges appointments; follows through until point of agreement; for six months, maintains contact to be certain that an effective working relationship is established. Fee charged.

37

776

Catalyst
6 East 82nd Street
New York, New York 10028

National non-profit organization recruiting for manufacturing, sales, financial, service, health and medical, educational and governmental organizations. Issues a monthly computerized roster, listing college-educated women seeking administrative, managerial, technical or professional positions on full-time or part-time schedules. Resumés listed without charge. Employers interested in the computerized roster can request resumé from headquarters or from one of the 103 local resource centers in the Catalyst National Network. Fee charged.

Directories and Professional Rosters

Equal Employment Opportunity for Minority Group College Graduates: Locating, Recruiting, Employing (1972). Compiled by Robert Calvert, Jr. Available from: Garrett Park Press, Garrett Park, Maryland 20766. $4.95 prepaid; $5.95 if billed.

A comprehensive, useful directory. Includes: names, addresses, enrollment by degree level and field of specialization, of predominantly black colleges and universities, and of institutions with substantial number (numbers listed) of Spanish-surnamed, American Indian and Asian–American students; identified minorities at other higher educational institutions; media

(newspapers, periodicals, broadcast) serving each minority group; comprehensive listing of minority organizations and consulting firms, Human Rights Commissions and other agencies. Specific suggestions on methods and techniques of recruiting and retaining minorities.

Directory for Reaching Minority Groups. Issued by the Bureau of Apprenticeship and Training, U.S. Department of Labor, August 1973. Single copies available from Office of Information, Manpower Administration, U.S. Department of Labor, Washington, D.C. 20210.

Lists federal, state and local governmental units, community action agencies, educational institutions, fraternities, sororities, pressbroadcast media and religious and minority organizations by state and city, with addresses and telephone numbers.

A Directory of Predominantly Black Colleges and Universities in the U.S., (Revised Edition, 1973). Enrollment, types of degrees offered and numbers granted. Available from National Alliance of Businessmen, 1730 K Street N.W., Washington, D.C. 20006.

Affirmative Recruitment Package. Lists 57 national and local recruiting sources for women (including minority sources); addresses of state and local Commissions on the Status of Women; and other compilations of women's professional organizations and caucuses. Available from Women's Bureau, U.S. Department of Labor, Washington, D.C. 20210.

38

MEN IN NURSING

Profile*

A recent study of male and female student nurses at the University of Iowa indicated that the men were older than the women students, more apt to be married, had been in college longer, and had more experience in the health care field (77%). It is interesting to note, that of the married men (54.5% of the sample), four-fifths were married to nurses.

In the rank order of preference for those areas of nursing in which the students wanted to work after graduation, the men indicated a strong preference for acute care settings. In rank order, male student preferences were: emergency and outpatient departments, intensive care, medical-surgical, psychiatric and coronary care and lastly, anesthesia. Female students preferred first, pediatric nursing, then public health, medical-surgical, obstetrics/maternity and psychiatric.

As to their attitudes toward involvement in the nursing profession, men indicated greater difficulty in telling others of their occupational choice: only 66% felt easy while doing so, as compared with 83% of the women.

Table 38-1 Reasons for choosing nursing given by men and women respondents

Reasons	Men (N = 32)			Women (N = 58)		
	Rank	Number	Percentage*	Rank	Number	Percentage*
Job availability	1	18	56.3	2	20	34.5
Interest in people	2	14	43.8	1	36	62.1
Pay	3	9	28.1	—	4	6.9
Job security/mobility	4	6	18.8	5	7	12.1
Working conditions	5	6	18.8	—	6	10.3
Improve status	—	1	3.1	3	11	19.0
Interest in science	—	3	9.4	4	9	15.5
Interest in medicine	—	2	6.3	4	9	15.5

* Percentages computed on basis of number of students listing each reason.

Male Activism

In early May 1975 at the annual meeting of the Michigan Male Nurses Association, the group unanimously passed the following resolution:

Whereas, there is a national program to democratize those professions previously consisting of a majority of men; and

Whereas, these Affirmative Action Programs have had significant impact in increasing the proportion of women in previously men's professions; and

Whereas, there exist professions which are predominantly female, particularly the profession of nursing, that are not representative of the proportion of men in the general population; and

Whereas, significant barriers are encountered by men seeking careers in nursing;

Be it resolved: that each school and college of nursing in this country establish an Affirmative Action Program to recruit men students in numbers adequate to reflect the national proportion of men in the general population; and

Be it further resolved, that schools and colleges of nursing establish programs to recruit and retain men nurses on their faculties in numbers reflective of the national proportion of men; and

Be it further resolved, that the federal government, through the Department of Health, Education and Welfare, establish an enforcement program to ensure compliance on the part of the nursing profession with the word and spirit of the law of the land.

*Source: Adapted from "Men Nursing Students; How They Perceive Their Situation," by A. Shoenmaker and D. Radosevich, *Nursing Outlook,* May 1976. © American Journal of Nursing Company.

Attitudes*

Sociologists consider nursing a sex-typed feminine occupation, in part due to the preponderance of females in the field and in part, to the consistency of the nature of the nursing role with the feminine role stereotype. Several studies confirm this public attitude: children's books portray doctors as males, nurses as females; a sample of high school seniors recently ranked nursing lowest on a masculinity scale compared to other professions.

Female Nurses' Attitudes

While prospective male nurses may have to override social/cultural pressures in their choice of profession—adjust to a female peer group and a sexual minority status—their female co-workers appear to show little resentment on their "intrusion." A recent study by Myron D. Fottler at the University of Iowa on female nurse attitudes found little evidence that employment of male nurses causes role strain or role conflict among female nurses. Sex was viewed as a discretionary element of the nursing role. About 75% of the nurses surveyed indicated positive attitudes and no desire to exclude males from the practice of nursing. Among the other 25%, most negative attitudes appeared to be based upon perceptions of real or potential favoritism in favor of the male nurse. There was little evidence in this study to support the view that "many women in nursing have resisted accepting men as equals" (Silver and McAtee, 1972). Apparently the employment of males in nursing is compatible with the existing values, expectations and past experiences of female nurses. While there was an attitude among a minority of respondents that male nurses might be more effective in some clinical areas than others, the majority felt they should be utilized in all areas of nursing. This finding was further supported by the fact that there were no significant differences in attitudes of nurses employed in different employing organizations, different positions and different clinical areas.

Those female nurses expressing negative attitudes tended to be younger nurses, those

without much exposure to male nurses or those who perceived employer discrimination in favor of the male.

Table 38-2   Attitudes of female nurses toward various statements regarding the male nurse

Statement	Mean score*
The male nurse, as head of the household, should be given a larger salary than the female nurse.	1.61
Since a man can tolerate more pressure, the male nurse should be expected to assume full responsibility in an emergency situation.	1.92
Female nurses prefer males as their immediate supervisors.	2.30
Professional competition exists between male and female nurses.	3.25
The male nurse is better suited to perform some nursing functions.	3.48
On the whole, the physician seems to accept the male nurse.	3.62
Male nurses will play an increasingly important role in health care.	3.92
On the whole, the patient seems to accept the male nurse.	3.93
The nursing profession should encourage the entry of more men.	4.30
The male nurse can perform most nursing activities as well as his female counterpart.	4.43

*1 = strongly disagree, 2 = disagree, 3 = uncertain, 4 = agree, 5 = strongly agree.

A *Nursing '74* survey (October 1974) of 11,-000 nurses produced these results:

What are your feelings about male nurses?

They are a vital segment of nursing and should be given the same responsibilities as female nurses are	88%
They are useful but should never be assigned to care for female patients	10%
In general they are not as competent as female nurses	1%
Men do not belong in nursing	1%

*Source: Myron D. Fottler, "Attitude of Female Nurses Toward Male Nurses," *Journal of Health and Social Behaviour*, June 1976 (Adapted).

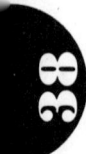

Employment Status

On the basis of the 1970 census report the following proportions of men are recorded among nursing personnel:

2.7% of registered nurses,
3.6% of practical nurses,
15.2% of aides, orderlies and attendants.

Year	R.N.s Percent male
1949	0.8
1957	0.8
1962	0.9
1966	1.1
1972	1.4

The figures on registered nurses, however, have been consistently lower than census data.

Type of Position and Field of Employment

Approximately 78.7% of male R.N.s as opposed to 64% of female R.N.s hold positions in hospitals. Within the hospital setting, less than one-third of the male nurses hold staff level positions as compared to more than one half of female R.N.s.

Table 38-3   Employed male registered nurses by field of employment and type of position, 1972

	Total	Type of position							
		Administrator or assistant	Consultant	Supervisor or assistant	Instructor	Head nurse or assistant	General duty or staff nurse	Other specified type	Not reported
Total									
Number	10,989	897	125	1,733	480	1,657	3,461	2,135	501
Percent	100.0	8.2	1.1	15.8	4.4	15.1	31.5	19.4	4.5
Hospital									
Number	8,646	568	46	1,453	194	1,452	2,893	1,697	343
Percent	100.0	6.6	0.5	16.8	2.2	16.8	33.5	19.6	4.0
Nursing home									
Number	467	166	7	123	8	63	82	—	18
Percent	100.0	35.5	1.5	26.3	1.7	13.5	17.6	—	3.9
School of nursing									
Number	361	57	2	10	261	3	6	1	21
Percent	100.0	15.8	0.5	2.8	72.3	0.8	1.7	0.3	5.8
Private duty									
Number	365	—	—	—	—	—	—	365	—
Percent	100.0	—	—	—	—	—	—	100.0	—
Public health									
Number	316	40	35	60	8	39	112	4	18
Percent	100.0	12.7	11.1	19.0	2.5	12.3	35.4	1.3	5.7
School nurse									
Number	102	7	3	12	—	11	67	2	—
Percent	100.0	6.9	2.9	11.8	—	10.8	65.7	1.9	—
Industrial									
Number	264	25	7	42	1	38	148	3	—
Percent	100.0	9.5	2.6	15.9	0.4	14.4	56.1	1.1	—
Office nurse (physician's or dentist's)									
Number	167	6	4	9	2	27	108	11	—
Percent	100.0	3.6	2.4	5.4	1.2	16.1	64.7	6.6	—
Other specified field									
Number	116	10	13	11	5	9	21	40	7
Percent	100.0	8.6	11.2	9.5	4.3	7.8	18.1	34.5	6.0
Not reported									
Number	185	18	8	13	1	15	24	12	94
Percent	100.0	9.7	4.3	7.0	0.6	8.1	13.0	6.5	50.8

Source: *The Nation's Nurses, 1972 Inventory of Nurses,* ANA, 1974.

Full or Part-Time Employment

Table 38-4   Percent of registered nurses by sex and employment status, 1972

Sex and employment status	Total	
	Number	Percent
Total	1,127,657	—
Female	1,111,206	100.0
Employed in nursing	766,416	69.0
Full-time	495,666	44.6
Regular part-time	158,807	14.3
Irregular part-time	78,025	7.0
Full or part-time not reported	33,918	3.1
Not employed in nursing	314,334	28.3
Employment status not reported	30,456	2.7
Male	14,625	100.0
Employed in nursing	10,989	75.1
Full-time	8,935	61.1
Regular part-time	628	4.3
Irregular part-time	413	2.8
Full or part-time not reported	1,013	6.9
Not employed in nursing	1,793	12.3
Employment status not reported	1,843	12.6
Sex not reported	1,826	100.0
Employed in nursing	1,065	58.3
Full-time	600	32.9
Regular part-time	174	9.5
Irregular part-time	153	8.4
Full or part-time not reported	138	7.5
Not employed in nursing	484	26.5
Employment status not reported	277	15.2

Source: *The Nation's Nurses, 1972 Inventory of Nurses*, ANA, 1974.

Male vs. Female Nurse Comparisons

Table 38-5   Employment comparisons of female and male newly licensed nurses

	Female	Male
Income		
Under $5,000	4%	6%
$5,000–5,999	7	6
$6,000–6,999	9	7
$7,000–7,999	20	19
$8,000–8,999	23	21
$9,000–9,999	12	12
$10,000–over	9	13
Other	16	16
	100%	100%
Continue education		
Definitely yes	20%	48%
Probably yes	48	30
Probably no	29	16
Definitely no	2	5
Other	1	1
	100%	100%
Distance of furthest application		
Local	72%	65%
Would require move	28	35
	100%	100%
Current/most recent employer		
Pub. Hosp.	58%	52%
Pvt. Hosp.	24	15
Nsg. Home	5	4
Govt. PH	2	5
Vol. PH	1	—
PH-MXD	—	—
Cmuty	1	3
Bd. Educ.	—	—
Sch. Nsg.	—	—
Indus.	—	1
Pvt. Duty	1	1
Office Nsg.	3	2
Military	2	11
Other	6	8
	100%	100%

Source: DHEW, May 1975.

Men in Schools of Nursing

The increase in the number of nursing students has been accompanied by a less dramatic but important change in the composition of the student body. There are more men students and students from minority groups and older age groups. More than twice as many black students were graduated in 1972 as compared with 1963.

However, less known is the fact that 1,694 men graduated in 1972, a fourfold increase over 1963, and then in 1975 the number of men graduating R.N. programs jumped to 3,807.

Table 38-6   Number and percent of men in schools of nursing—1975

Male students	Associate degree	Di-ploma	Bacca-laureate	Practical or vocational
Admissions reported	3,159	1,121	1,916	2,205
Percent of all students enrolled	7	5	6	6
Percent of all students graduated	9	6	6	5

Source: *Nursing Outlook,* September 1976.

Male Nurse Recruitment

Under The Nurse Training Act of 1971, which calls for the identification and recruitment of "individuals with a potential for education or training in the nursing profession," veterans of the Armed Forces of the United States with training or experience in the health field have been encouraged and assisted to prepare for nursing practice.

For example, a community college in Texas is the recipient of funds to prepare former medical corpsmen veterans for nursing careers.

With project grant support, a New York college has instituted a two and a half year evening program to train retiring policemen and firefighters for second careers as registered nurses. The first group of 96 men (and four women) began training in the fall of 1970. They displayed very high motivations: 87% completed the class compared with a national completion rate of 67% for all types of nursing schools. Not only was the completion

rate much above average, but the level of performance was considered exceptional by the teaching staff.

Male Figures in Nursing*

Anderson, Leslie E.—head nurse, inhalation therapy, V.A. Hospital, Albuquerque, N.M.

Bushnell, Clarence W.—administrator of 485-bed Bridgeport Hospital in Connecticut. A staff nurse and clinical instructor prior to World War II.

Craig, Leroy—pioneered in the establishment of nursing as a career for men; instrumental in obtaining legislation which authorized the commissioning of male nurses in the armed forces.

Christman, Luther—dean, College of Nursing, Rush-Presbyterian-St. Luke's Medical Center, Chicago. Background as an educator in psychiatric nursing and the area of nursing and sociology. Member of numerous panels, including the National Commission for Studying Nursing and Nursing Education (1968–70). Received award for outstanding male nurse.

Day, Philip E.—publishing director, American Journal of Nursing Company, New York. He served in many nursing positions, was an instructor, then a director of nursing, before assuming his present post.

Denny, Ernest O.—assistant professor and clinical specialist in psychiatric nursing at Ball State University. Department of Nursing, Muncie, Indiana. He recently completed work on his doctor's degree at Boston University.

Farrell, George E.—holds the office of major and received the Bronze Star for his service as a flight nurse and as assistant chief nurse of the 903rd Aeromedical Evacuation Squadron in South Vietnam.

Griffin, Gerald J.—served as director of the Department of Associate Degree Programs, National League for Nursing, New York. A former teacher, Dr. Griffin is co-author of a textbook, *Fundamentals of Patient-Centered Nursing.* With his R.N. wife, Joanne K. Griffin, he revised *Jensen's History and Trends of Nursing.*

* Source: Material in part from "Nurse: husband/father/humanitarian/specialist," National League for Nursing, NLN #41-U (Brochure).

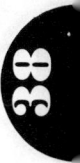

Roberts, William A.—assistant director of nursing service at renowned Menninger Clinic in Topeka, Kansas. He began his health career as a psychiatric aide, has been a pharmaceutical salesman, and pharmacist's mate in the U.S. Marine Corps.

Walker, Duane D.—assistant administrator and director of nursing services, Holy Cross Hospital, Salt Lake City. He has conducted in-service education courses for the U.S. Army Nurse Corps, been a workshop leader for the National League for Nursing.

APPENDICES

Metrics*

The establishment of a national policy to coordinate the use of metric system in the United States was put into effect with the signing of the Metric Conversion Act on December 23, 1975.

Educational materials concerning the metric system can be obtained and specific questions concerning the system will be answered by writing to the Metric Information Office, National Bureau of Standards, Washington, D.C. 20234.

Units

Compare metric and customary units

Metric	Meter	Liter	Kilogram
Customary	Inch	Teaspoon	Grain
	Foot	Tablespoon	Ounce
	Yard	Cup	Pound
	Rod	Pint	Ton
	Mile	Quart	
		Gallon	

Metric Units are in 10's
1000 millimeters = 100 centimeters = 1 meter
1000 meters = 1 kilometer

1 meter $\cong$ 1.1 yards
1 liter $\cong$ 1.1 quarts
1 kilogram $\cong$ 2.2 pounds
($\cong$ approximate)

Measure	Term	Symbol
length	meter	m
	kilometer	km
	centimeter	cm
	millimeter	mm
area	hectare	ha
weight	gram	g
	kilogram	kg
	metric ton	t
volume	liter	L
	milliliter	mL
pressure	kilopascal	kPa

Units of time and electricity will not change.

*Source: U.S. Department of Commerce, National Bureau of Standards.

Common Prefixes for Metric Units

Prefixes, added to a unit name, create larger or smaller units by factors that are powers of 10. For example, add the prefix kilo, which means a thousand, to the unit gram, to indicate 1,000 grams; thus 1,000 grams become 1 kilogram.

Factor		Prefix	Symbol
1,000,000	10^6	mega	M
1,000	10^3	kilo	k
1/100	10^{-2}	centi	c
1/1,000	10^{-3}	milli	m
1/1,000,000	10^{-6}	micro	μ

Conversions

Conversions should follow a rule of reason: do not include figures that imply more accuracy than justified by the original data. For example, 36 inches would be converted to 91 centimeters, not 91.44 centimeters (36 inches × 2.54 centimeters per inch = 91.44 centimeters), and 40.1 inches would convert to 101.9 centimeters, not 101.854.

For other exact conversions and more detailed tables, see NBS Misc. Publ. 286, Units of Weights and Measures, Price $2.25, SD Catalog No. C13.10:286.

Approximate conversions to metric measures

Symbol	When you know	Multiply by	To find	Symbol
Length				
in	inches	*2.5	centimeters	cm
ft	feet	30	centimeters	cm
yd	yards	0.9	meters	m
mi	miles	1.6	kilometers	km
Area				
in²	square inches	6.5	square centimeters	cm²
ft²	square feet	0.09	square meters	m²
yd²	square yards	0.8	square meters	m²
mi²	square miles	2.6	square kilometers	km²
	acres	0.4	hectares	ha
Mass (weight)				
oz	ounces	28	grams	g
lb	pounds	0.45	kilograms	kg
	short tons (2000 lb)	0.9	tonnes	t
Temperature (exact)				
°F	Fahrenheit temperature	5/9 (after subtracting 32)	Celsius temperature	°C

Approximate conversion from metric measures (continued)

Sym-bol	When you know	Multiply by	To find	Sym-bol
		Volume		
tsp	teaspoons	5	milliliters	ml
Tbsp	tablespoons	15	milliliters	ml
fl oz	fluid ounces	−30	milliliters	ml
c	cups	0.24	liters	l
pt	pints	0.47	liters	l
qt	quarts	0.95	liters	l
gal	gallons	3.8	liters	l
ft^3	cubic feet	0.03	cubic meters	m^3
yd^3	cubic yards	0.76	cubic meters	m^3

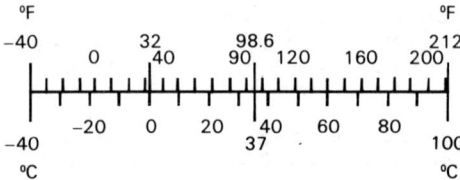

Approximate conversion from metric measures

Sym-bol	When you know	Multiply by	To find	Sym-bol
		Length		
mm	millimeters	0.04	inches	in
cm	centimeters	0.4	inches	in
m	meters	3.3	feet	ft
m	meters	1.1	yards	yd
km	kilometers	0.6	miles	mi
		Area		
cm^2	square centimeters	0.16	square inches	in^2
m^2	square meters	1.2	square yards	yd^2
km^2	square kilometers	0.4	square miles	mi^2
ha	hectares (10,000 m^2)	2.5	acres	
		Mass (weight)		
g	grams	0.035	ounces	oz
kg	kilograms	2.2	pounds	lb
t	tonnes (1000 kg)	1.1	short tons	
		Volume		
ml	milliliters	0.03	fluid ounces	fl oz
l	liters	2.1	pints	pt
l	liters	1.06	quarts	qt
l	liters	0.26	gallons	gal
m^3	cubic meters	35	cubic feet	ft^3
m^3	cubic meters	1.3	cubic yards	yd^3

Approximate conversions to metric measures (continued)

Sym-bol	When you know	Multiply by	To find	Sym-bol
		Temperature (exact)		
°C	Celsius temperature	9/5 (then add 32)	Fahrenheit temperature	°F

Temperature

°F.	to	°C.		°C.	to	°F.
0		−17.7		0		32.0
95		35.0		35.0		95.0
96		35.5		35.5		95.9
97		36.1		36.0		96.8
98		36.6		36.5		97.7
99		37.2		37.0		98.6
100		37.7		37.5		99.5
101		38.3		38.0		100.4
102		38.8		38.5		101.3
103		39.4		39.0		102.2
104		40.0		39.5		103.1
105		40.5		40.0		104.0
106		41.1		40.5		104.9
107		41.6		41.0		105.8
108		42.2		41.5		106.6
109		42.7		42.0		107.6
110		43.3		100.0		212.0

$$°C. = (°F. − 32) × 5/9$$

$$°F. = (°C. × 9/5) + 32$$

Weight

lb.	to	Kg.		Kg.	to	lb.
1		0.5		1		2.2
2		0.9		2		4.4
4		1.8		3		6.6
6		2.7		4		8.8
8		3.6		5		11.0
10		4.5		6		13.2
20		9.1		8		17.6
30		13.6		10		22
40		18.2		20		44
50		22.7		30		66
60		27.3		40		88
70		31.8		50		110
80		36.4		60		132
90		40.9		70		154
100		45.4		80		176
150		68.2		90		198
200		90.8		100		220

1 lb. = 0.454 Kg.

1 Kg. = 2.204 lb.

Approximate conversions to metric measures (continued)

Length

in.	to	cm.
1		2.5
2		5.1
4		10.2
6		15.2
8		20.3
12		30.5
18		46
24		61
30		76
36		91
42		107
48		122
54		137
60		152
66		168
72		183
78		198

1 inch = 2.54 cm.

cm.	to	in.
1		0.4
2		0.8
3		1.2
4		1.6
5		2.0
6		2.4
8		3.1
10		3.9
20		7.9
30		11.8
40		15.7
50		19.7
60		23.6
70		27.6
80		31.5
90		35.4
100		39.4

1 cm. = 0.3937 inch

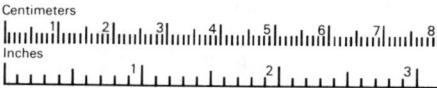

Centimeters

Inches

Useful Equivalents*

Weights

Apothecary		Apothecary		Metric
1 scruple	=	20 grains	=	1.296 grams
1 dram	=	60 grains	=	3.88 grams
1 ounce	=	480 grains (8 drams)	=	31.1 grams
1 pound	=	5.760 grains (12 ounces)	=	373.24 grams

Metric		Apothecary		Metric
1 milligram	=	1/65 grain*	=	.001 gram
1 centigram	=	1/6 grain*	=	.01 gram
1 decigram	=	1 1/2 grains*	=	.1 gram
1 gram	=	15.432 grains	=	.001 kilogram
1 kilogram	=	2.2 pounds avdp.*	=	1,000 grams

Avoirdupois		Apothecary		Metric
1 ounce	=	437.5 grains	=	28.35 grams
1 pound	=	7,000 grains	=	453.59 grams
1 ton	=	2,000 pounds avdp.	=	907.184 kilo-grams

*Approximate equivalent.

Nomogram

For converting dosage by body weight to dosage by surface area.

Nomogram
For converting dosage by body weight to dosage by surface area

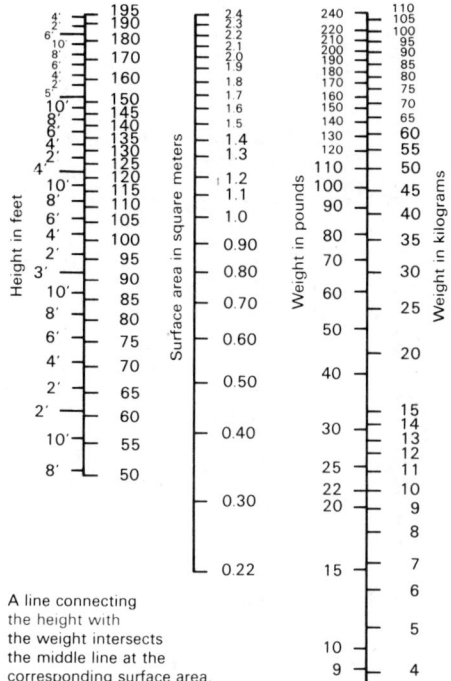

Height in feet

Surface area in square meters

Weight in pounds

Weight in kilograms

A line connecting the height with the weight intersects the middle line at the corresponding surface area.

Household Measures

1 teaspoonful	1 fl. dr.	4–5 ml.
1 dessertspoonful	2 fl. dr.	8 ml.
1 tablespoonful	1/2 fl. oz.	15 ml.
1 jigger	1 1/2 fl. oz.	45 ml.
1 wineglassful	2 fl. oz.	60 ml.
1 teacupful	4 fl. oz.	120 ml.
1 glassful	8 fl. oz.	240 ml.

786

Metric and apothecary

Metric weights milligrams		Grams		Apothecary weights grains
0.1	=	0.0001	=	1/640
0.2	=	0.0002	=	1/320
0.3	=	0.0003	=	1/210
0.324	=	0.000324	=	1/200
0.4	=	0.0004	=	1/160
0.432	=	0.000432	=	1/150
0.5	=	0.0005	=	1/128
0.54	=	0.00054	=	1/120
0.6	=	0.0006	=	1/100
0.8	=	0.0008	=	1/80
1.0	=	0.001	=	1/64
1.1	=	0.0011	=	1/60
1.3	=	0.0013	=	1/50
1.6	=	0.0016	=	1/40
1.8	=	0.0018	=	1/36
2.2	=	0.0022	=	1/30
2.6	=	0.0026	=	1/25
3.2	=	0.0032	=	1/20
4.0	=	0.004	=	1/16
6.5	=	0.0065	=	1/10
7.2	=	0.0072	=	1/9
8.1	=	0.0081	=	1/8
9.2	=	0.0092	=	1/7
11.0	=	0.011	=	1/6
13.0	=	0.013	=	1/5
16.2	=	0.0162	=	1/4
21.7	=	0.0217	=	1/3
24.3	=	0.0243	=	3/8
32.4	=	0.0324	=	1/2
43.2	=	0.0432	=	2/3
48.6	=	0.0486	=	3/4
65.0	=	0.065	=	1

Metric and apothecary

Metric weights or measures grams or ml.		Apothecary weights grains		Apothecary measures minims of water at 4° C.
0.0648	=	1	=	1.0517
0.130	=	2	=	2.11
0.194	=	3	=	3.15
0.259	=	4	=	4.20
0.324	=	5	=	5.26
0.389	=	6	=	6.31
0.454	=	7	=	7.37
0.5	=	7.72	=	8.12
0.518	=	8	=	8.41
0.583	=	9	=	9.46
0.648	=	10	=	10.52
0.713	=	11	=	11.57
0.778	=	12	=	12.63
0.842	=	13	=	13.67
0.907	=	14	=	14.72
0.972	=	15	=	15.78
1.000	=	15.4324	=	16.23
1.296	=	20	=	21.04
1.944	=	30	=	31.55

Abbreviation	Meaning
c.; c̄	with
cap.	let the patient take
caps.	capsule
celeriter	quickly
chart.	a little paper
coch. mag.	a tablespoonful
coch. med.	a dessertspoonful
coch. parv.	a teaspoonsful
cola	strain
comp.	compound
d.	day
da; det.	give; let be given
dil.	dilute
disp.	dispense
div.	divide
d.t.d. No. IV	let four such doses be given
el.	elixir
e.m.p.	after the manner prescribed
et	and
ex	from
ext.	an extract
f.; ft.	make; let be made
filt.	filter
fl.	fluid
Gm.	gram
gr.	grain
gtt.	a drop

Abbreviations Used in Prescriptions

Abbreviation	Meaning
aa; a̅a̅	of each
a.c.	before meals
ad	to; up to
add.	add
ad lib.	at pleasure
agit.	shake or stir
alb.	white
ante	before
ag.	water
ag. bull.	boiling water
ag. ferv.	warm water
ag. frig.	cold water
b.i.d.	twice daily
bis	twice

Abbreviation	Meaning	Abbreviation	Meaning
hora	hour	q.i.d.	four times a day
hor. som.	at bedtime	q.s.	a sufficient quantity
in	in; into		
liq.	a liquor	R$_x$	take; a recipe
		rept.	let it be repeated
m.	mix		
magn.	large	s.; s̄	without
mass.	a mass	s.a.	according to art
m. dict.	as directed	sat.	saturated
mixt.	a mixture	Sig.	label; let it be imprinted
m.p.	as directed or prescribed	si op. sit	If it is needed
		s.l.	according to law
no.	number	sol.	solution
non rep.	do not repeat	solv.	dissolve
		spir.	spirit
o.	a pint	ss.	one-half
o.d.	right eye	stat.	at once
o.l.	left eye	syr.	syrup
omn. hor.	every hour		
O.U.	both eyes	tab.	tablet
		tal.	of such; like this
p. ae.	equal parts	t.i.d.	three times a day
p.c.	after eating	tr.; tinct.	tincture
per	through	trit.	triturate
pil.	pills		
p.r.n.	according to circumstances	ung.	ointment
pulv.	a powder	ut dict.	as directed
q.	every		
q.d.	once a day	vin.	wine

Medical Abbreviations

Abbreviations	Meaning	Abbreviations	Meaning
Abd	abdominal	b.s.	breath sounds
ACTH	adrenocorticotrophic hormone	BUN	blood urea nitrogen
A.D.	right ear (auris dextra)	Bx	biopsy
AF	atrial fibrillation	Ca	carcinoma
A/G ratio	albumin-globulin ratio	Cath	catheter, catheterization
AH	abdominal hysterectomy	CBC	complete blood count
AI	aortic insufficiency	CC	chief complaint
Alb.	albumin	CCU	coronary care unit
alcr	alcohol rub	CM	tomorrow morning (cras mane)
Anes.	anesthesia	CN	tomorrow night (cras nocte)
Appy	appendectomy	CNS	central nervous system
AS	aortic stenosis	CPB	cardiopulmonary bypass
a.s.	left ear (auris sinistra)	CSF	cerebrospinal fluid
ATS	antitetanic serum	CV	tomorrow night (cras vespere)
AV	aortic valve replacement	CVA	cerebrovascular accident, a
AZ	Ascheim-Zondek test		stroke
Bact.	bacterium	CVI	cerebrovascular insufficiency
Ba. enem.	barium enema	D & C	dilation and curettage
Bib.	drink	D & E	dilation and evacuation
BM	bowel movement	DIFF	differential blood count
BMR	basal metabolic rate	De d. in d.	from day to day (de die in diem)
BP	blood pressure	Dieb. alt.	on alternate days (diebus
BPH	benign prostatic hypertrophy		alternis)

Abbreviations	Meaning	Abbreviations	Meaning
Dieb. tert.	every third day (diebus tertiis)	kj	knee jerk
		KO	keep open
DOA	dead on arrival	KUB	kidney, ureter, and bladder
DSD	dry sterile dressing	L_1	first lumbar vertebra
Dx	diagnosis	LA	local anesthesia
DXT	deep x-ray therapy	LFT	liver function test
		LLQ	left lower quadrant
ECG, EKG	electrocardiogram	LMP	last menstrual period
EDC	estimated date of confinement	L.O.A.	left occiput—anterior
		L.O.P.	left occiput—posterior
EDR	effective direct radiation	LRM	left radical mastectomy
EEG	electroencephalogram	LSK	liver, spleen and kidneys
EENT	eye, ear, nose and throat	L & W	living and well
EN	enema		
ESR	erythrocyte sedimentation rate	MALIG	malignant
		MCH	mean corpuscular hemoglobin
EST	electroshock therapy	MCHC	mean corpuscular hemoglobin concentration
FBS	fasting blood sugar	mEq	milliequivalent
FH	family history	MI	mitral insufficiency
FHS	fetal heart sounds	MLD	minimal lethal dose
FVL	femoral vein ligation	MS	mitral stenosis
Fx	fracture	N	normal
GB viz.	gallbladder visualization	NNR	new and nonofficial remedies
GC	gonorrhea	OBS	obstetrical service
GE	gastroenterology	O.D.	right eye (oculus dexter)
GI	gastrointestinal	OOB	out of bed
gm.	gram	OPT	outpatient treatment
GR	gastric resection	O.S.	left eye (oculus sinister)
gt., gtt.	drop; drops	OT	occupational therapy
GU	genitourinary		
Gyn	gynecology	P & A	percussion and auscultation
		PA	pernicious anemia
HED	unit of roentgen ray dosage	PAR	postanesthesia room
Hgb	hemoglobin	PAT	paroxysmal atrial tachycardia
HLR	heart-lung resuscitation	PE, Px	physical examination
HCVD	hypertensive cardiovascular disease	P.H.	past history
		pH	expression of acidity
HVD	hypertensive vascular disease	PI	present illness
		PID	pelvic inflammatory disease
IC	intensive care	PL	placebo
ICS	intercostal space	PMI	point of maximal impulse
I & D	incision and drainage	Preemy	premature infant
IMI	intramuscular injection	prog.	prognosis
I & O	intake and output	PSP	phenolsulfonphthalein test (kidney)
IOU	intensive therapy observation unit	Pt.	patient
IP	intraperitoneal	PT	physical therapy
IST	insulin shock therapy		
IUT	intrauterine transfusion	RBC	red blood cells
IV	intravenous	RCU	respiratory care unit
IVP	intravenous pyelogram (program)	R.L.Q.	right lower quadrant
		ROS	review of symptoms

Abbreviations	Meaning	Abbreviations	Meaning
RTC	return to clinic	TL	tubal ligation
Rx	prescription, therapy	TLC	tender loving care
		TPR	temperature, pulse, respiration
S	surgery	TUR	transurethal resection
s.c.	subcutaneous	TX	traction, treatment
SMR	somnolent metabolic rate		
Sp. gr.	specific gravity	UA	urinalysis
S.R.	sedimentation rate	UBI	ultraviolet blood irradiation
Stat.	at once	UTI	urinary tract infection
Stet.	let it stand		
		VD	venereal disease
TA	therapeutic abortion	VDH	valvular disease of heart
T & A	tonsillectomy and adenoi-	VDRL	serology
	dectomy	VS	venisection
TB, Tbc	tuberculosis; tubercle	WBC	white blood cells (white
	bacilli		blood count)
TDI	total-dose infusion	WBR	whole body radiation

Understanding Medical Terms

Prefixes, Suffixes and Combining Forms*

Term	Meaning	Term	Meaning
a-, an-	negative, without	cysto-, vesico-	bladder
ab-	away from	cyto-	cell
adeno-	gland	dactyl-	finger, toe
-algia	pain	diplo-	double
alve-	channel, cavity	dis-	apart
angio-	vessel	dors-	back
ankyl-	crooked, growing together	duodeno-	duodenum (1st part of small intestine)
antr-	chamber	dys-	bad, painful
apo-	detached	ect-	outside
arthro-	joint	-ectasis	dilation
blasto-	bud, embryonic form	-ectomy	excision
brachy-	short	-emia	blood
brady-	slow	endo-	inside
carcin-	cancer	entero-	small intestine
cardi-, cordi-	heart	epi-	upon, after
cata-	down	eso-	inside
-centesis	puncture	estho-	perceive, feel
cephalo-	head	en-	normal
cervico-	neck	exo-	outside
cheilo-	lips	fasci-	band
cholecyst-	gall bladder	gastro-	stomach
chondro-	cartilage	gingive-	gums
chrom-	color	gyr-	ring, circle
-clasia	breaking		
colo-	large intestine		
costo-	rib		
craneo-	skull		

---
* Source: McNeil Laboratories, Inc.

Term	Meaning	Term	Meaning
hemo-, hemato-	blood	omphal-	navel
hepato-	liver	onych-	nail
histo-	tissue	oophoro-, ovari-	ovary
hyper-	above, elevated	optic, ophth-	eye
hypo-	under, below	orchi-	testicle
		orth-	straight
-iasis	condition	-osis	condition, state resulting
iatr-	physician	oss-, ost-	bone
idio-	peculiar	osteo-	bone
ileo-	ileum (3rd part of small intestine)	-ostomy	new opening
		-otomy	incision
infra-	beneath	oto-, auri-	ear
inter-	between		
intra-	inside	pancreato-	pancreas
is-	equal	para-	beside
-itis	inflammation	-pathy	sickness, disease
		-pepsia	digestion
jejuno-	jejunum (2nd part of small intestine)	peri-	around, surrounding
		phag-	eat
kerat-	horny	pharyngo-, laryngo-, fauci-	throat
later-	side	phil-	affinity for
leuko-	white	phlebo-, vene-	vein
lipo-	fat	plasty-	shape, repair
lithio-	stone or calculus	pleuro-	membrane encasing lungs
-lysis	break down		
		pne-	breathing
macro-	long, large	pneumo-, pulmo-	lungs
mal-	abnormal	-pole-	make, produce
-malac-	soft	poly-	much, many
masto-, mammo-	breast	procto-	anus and rectum
medi-	middle	pseudo-	false
mega-	great, large	pto-	fall
melan-	black	-ptosis	prolapse
meso-	middle	pyelo-	kidney, pelvis
meta-	beyond, after	pyo-	pus
metro-, utero-, hystero-	uterus	recto-	rectum
micro-	small	retro-	backwards
morph-	shape, form	rhino-, naso-	nose
muco-	mucus	-rrhagia	break, burst
-myces	fungus	-rrhaphy	suture, sew
myco-	fungal	-rrhea	flowing
myelo-	bone marrow	-rrhexia	break, rupture
myo-	muscle		
myx-	mucus	-sect	cut
		sep-	decay
nephro-, ren-	kidney	sial-	saliva
neuro-	nerve	salpingo	fallopian tube
nod-	knot	sclero-	hardening
nos-	disease	septo	infection
		somat-	body
ocul-	eye	-some	body
-odynia	pain	spondyl-	vertebra
oligo-	few, little	sten-	narrow
-ology	study of	-sthen-	strength
-oma	tumor, swelling		

Term	Meaning
stomato-	mouth
sub-	under
super-, supra-	above, extreme
syn-	together
tax-	arrange, order
thel-	nipple
thermo-	heat
thoraco-	chest
thromb-	clot, lump
-tomy	cutting
tors-	twist
tracheo-	windpipe
tricho-	hair
trop-	turn toward
-trophy	nurture, nutrition
uria-	urine
uro-	urine

Glossary of Medical Terms*

A

abortion: Premature expulsion of fetus; miscarriage.

abruptio-placentae: Premature detachment of a normally affixed placenta.

abscess: Localized collection of pus in a cavity.

achlorhydria: Lack of hydrochloric acid in the stomach.

achondroplasia: Disorder of cartilage development resulting in imperfect bone formation.

acidosis: Reduction in alkali reserve in the body.

acne: A chronic inflammatory disease of sebaceous glands.

acrocephaly: Conical distortion of the skull.

acromegaly: An endocrine disturbance of the pituitary gland resulting in overgrowth of hands, feet and face.

adamantinoma: Epithelial tumor of the jaw.

Adams-Stokes disease, syndrome: A disorder marked by sudden loss of consciousness, caused by heart block.

Addison's disease: Disease of adrenal glands, with reduced adrenal steroid production.

adenitis: Inflammation of a gland.

adenocarcinoma: A malignant adenoma.

---

*Source: McNeil Laboratories, Inc.

adenoma: A benign tumor of glandlike structure.

adenosis: Any glandular condition.

adhesion: The stable (at times abnormal) conjoining of parts.

adrenalectomy: Excision of the adrenal glands.

adrenogenital syndrome: Appearance of secondary male sex characteristics in the female as a result of adrenal hyperfunction.

aerophagia: Swallowing of air.

afibrinogenemia: Absence of fibrinogen in the blood.

agalactia: Failure to secrete milk.

agammaglobulinemia: Absence of gamma globulin in the blood.

agranulocytosis: A disease marked by leukopenia, neutropenia, and increased susceptibility to infection.

alkalosis: A pathologic condition resulting from accumulation of alkali reserve in the body.

allergy: Hypersensitivity to a particular allergen.

alopecia: Baldness.

amblyopia: Disturbance of vision.

ameblasis: Infection with amebae, usually *Entamoeba histolytica*.

amenorrhea: Abnormal absence of menses.

anaphylaxis: Exaggerated allergic reaction to a foreign substance.

anastomosis: Surgical or pathologic formation of a communication between two normally separate parts or organs.

anemia: Deficiency of red blood cells or hemoglobin.

aneurysm: Sac formed by dilatation of wall of an artery or vein.

aneurysmectomy: Excision of an aneurysm.

angiitis: Inflammation of a blood or lymph vessel.

angina pectoris: Suppressive chest pain caused by inadequate blood supply to the heart muscle.

angioma: Tumor made up of blood or lymph vessels.

angioneurotic edema: Acute, transient edema of skin or mucous membranes, particularly the throat.

anhidrosis: Abnormal lack of sweat.

ankylosis: Immobile joint.

anorchism: Absence of one or both testes.

anorexia: Abnormal lack of appetite for food.

anovulation: Cessation of ovulation.

anoxia: Lack of oxygen.

anuria: Absence of urine production.

aphasia: Impairment of expression by speech, writing, or signs, or of recognition of these.

aplasia: Defective development of tissue.

apoplexy: Stroke, caused by acute vascular brain lesion.

appendicitis: Inflammation of the vermiform appendix.

arachnodactyly: Abnormal length and slenderness of fingers and toes.

arteriosclerosis: Thickening and hardening of the arteries.

arteriovenous fistula: Abnormal communication between an artery and a vein.

arteritis: Inflammation of an artery.

arthralgia: Joint pain.

arthritis: Inflammation of a joint.

arthropathy: Joint disease.

ascites: Collection of fluid in the peritoneal cavity.

asphyxia: Suffocation.

asthenia: Weakness.

asthma: Disease marked by paroxysms of difficult breathing, wheezing, and cough.

astigmatism: Defective curvature of one or more surfaces of the lens of the eye.

ataxia: Lack of muscle coordination.

atelectasis: Collapse of lung or part of lung.

atherosclerosis: Disease caused by fatty deposits in the inner lining of arteries.

atresia: Absence of a normal body opening.

atrophy: Wasting away; reduction in size of cell, tissue, or organ.

azotemia: Uremia.

B

bacteremia: Bacteria in the blood stream.

bacteriuria: Bacteria in the urine.

balanitis: Inflammation of the glans penis.

Basedow's disease: Exophthalmic goiter.

Bell's palsy: Facial paralysis with characteristic distortion.

beriberi: A form of polyneuritis due to deficiency of thiamine.

blepharitis: Inflammation of eyelids.

boil: Furuncle.

botulism: Food poisoning caused by *Clostridium botulinum* toxin.

bradycardia: Slowness of heartbeat.

Bright's disease: A kidney disease marked by albuminuria and edema; glomerulonephritis.

bronchiectasis: Chronic bronchial dilatation with paroxysmal coughing and purulent expectoration.

bronchitis: Inflammation of the bronchial tubes.

bronchopneumonia: Inflammation of the lungs usually originating in the bronchioles.

bubo: Inflammatory swelling of a lymphatic gland usually in groin or axilla.

bulla: A large blister filled with serous fluid.

bunion: Abnormal growth on one of the bones of the foot.

bursitis: Inflammation of a bursa.

C

cachexia: Generalized ill health characterized by weakness and emaciation.

calcinosis: Deposition of calcium salts in various tissues.

calculus: An abnormal concretion in the body, composed of mineral salts or organic matter.

callosity: Thickening of the skin, and hypertrophy of the horny layer.

callus: New bone formation deposited about the fragments of a fracture; also, callosity.

candidiasis: Infection with Candida fungi; moniliasis.

carbuncle: Necrotizing infection (usually staphylococcal) of skin and subcutaneous tissue.

carcinoma: A malignant growth of epithelial cells.

cardiopathy: Heart disease.

cardiospasm: Spasm of the stomach's cardiac sphincter.

carditis: Inflammation of the heart.

caries: Decay of teeth.

caruncle: A small fleshy eminence or nodule.

cataplexy: A state of immobility and rigidity.

cataract: Opacity of the eye's crystalline lens or its capsule.

catatonia: A form of schizophrenia marked by stupor and abnormal positioning.

celiac disease: A childhood diarrheal condition; childhood sprue.

cellulitis: Inflammation of cellular tissue.

cephalalgia: Headache.

cephalhematoma: Blood-filled tumor beneath the pericranium.

cervicitis: Inflammation of the cervix.

chalazion: A small tumor of the eyelid.

chancroid: Genital infection caused by *Hemophilus ducreyi.*

Charcot's disease: Neurogenic joint disease.

charleyhorse: Muscle spasm, soreness and stiffness.

chellosis: Fissuring and scaling of lips from B-vitamin deficiency.

Cheyne-Stokes respiration: Breathing characterized by rhythmic waxing and waning of respiratory depth.

chickenpox: An acute communicable viral disease of children.

cholangioma: A tumor of the bile ducts.

cholangitis: Inflammation of a bile duct.

cholecystectomy: Surgical removal of the gallbladder.

cholecystitis: Inflammation of the gallbladder.

cholecystojejunostomy: Surgical anastomosis of the gallbladder and the jejunum.

cholecystostomy: Surgical incision into and drainage of the gallbladder.

choledochoduodenostomy: Surgical anastomosis of common bile duct and duodenum.

choledochojejunostomy: Surgical anastomosis of common bile duct and jejunum.

choledocholithiasis: Presence of calculi in the common bile duct.

choledochostomy: Surgical opening into the common bile duct.

cholelithiasis: Gallstones.

cholestasis: Suppression of biliary flow.

chondritis: Inflammation of cartilage.

chondroma: A hyperplastic growth of cartilage tissue.

chondromalacia: Abnormal softness of cartilage.

chorea: St. Vitus' dance, a convulsive nervous disorder of muscles of extremities and face, occurring in rheumatic fever.

choriocarcinoma: A carcinoma developed from chorionic epithelium.

chylothorax: Chyle in the chest cavity.

chyluria: Chyle in the urine.

cinchonism: Tinnitus, deafness, etc., from large doses of cinchona bark or its alkaloids.

cirrhosis: A disease of the liver with progressive destruction of liver cells often occurring as a result of chronic alcoholism.

claudication: Pain in calves of legs induced by walking, as a result of decreased blood supply; usually intermittent claudication.

clavus: A corn.

climacteric: The syndrome of hormonal and psychic changes occurring in the male at the time of decreased sexual activity.

coarctation of aorta: Aortic narrowing or constriction resulting in higher than normal blood pressure in the upper extremities, and lower than normal blood pressure in the lower extremities.

coccidioidomycosis: Infection with the fungus *Coccidioides immitis.*

coccygodynia: Pain in and around caudal end of the spinal column.

colitis: Inflammation of the colon.

collagen: An albuminoid supportive protein of skin, tendon, bone, cartilage, and connective tissue.

collagen diseases: Diseases affecting collagen tissue, such as rheumatoid arthritis, systemic lupus erythematosus.

colostomy: Surgical opening of the colon onto the abdominal wall.

concretion: A calculus or other mass in a natural cavity or in tissue.

conjunctivitis: Inflammation of the conjunctiva.

contact dermatitis: Acute skin inflammation from contact with chemicals, animals, etc.

contracture: A contraction or shortening, as of a muscle.

contusion: A bruise.

cor pulmonale: Heart disease caused by obstruction of pulmonary circulation.

coronary insufficiency: Inadequacy of coronary vessels to maintain cardiac blood supply.

coronary occlusion: Obstruction of blood flow through a coronary artery.

coronary thrombosis: Formation of a clot in a coronary artery, obstructing blood flow.

coryza: Head cold.

costal chondritis: Inflammation of rib cartilage.

cretinism: A condition of arrested physical and mental development, from congenital lack of thyroid hormone.

croup: An acute respiratory illness characterized by resonant barking cough and hoarseness.

cryptorchism: A developmental defect marked by failure of testes to descend into scrotum.

curettage: Removal of material from the wall of a cavity.

Cushing's syndrome: A clinical condition caused by excess of adrenocortical hormones.

cyanosis: Bluish skin discoloration, often from cardiac malformation or poisoning, due to an excessive amount of unoxygenated blood.

cyst: A sac, especially one containing liquid or semisolid.

cystectomy: Excision of a cyst.

cystitis: Inflammation of the bladder.

cystocele: Hernial protrusion of the urinary bladder through the vaginal wall.

cystostomy: Formation of an opening into the bladder.

D

dacryoadenitis: Inflammation of a lacrimal gland.

decompensation, cardiac: Heart failure, with resultant dyspnea, venous engorgement, edema and cyanosis.

dehydration: Condition resulting from abnormal fluid loss or inadequate fluid intake.

delirium: A mental disturbance of short duration marked by illusions, hallucinations, excitement, restlessness and incoherence.

dermatitis: Inflammation of the skin.

dextrocardia: Location of the heart in the right side of the chest instead of the left.

diabetes insipidus: A metabolic disorder marked by extreme thirst and copious urination.

diathesis: A condition of the body causing tissues to react abnormally to extrinsic stimuli, with increased susceptibility to certain diseases.

dilatation: The condition of being stretched beyond normal dimensions.

diphtheria: An acute febrile, infectious disease caused by *Corynebacterium diphtheriae*, with laryngeal and pharyngeal edema, and consequent dyspnea and dysphagia.

diplegia: Bilateral paralysis of similar parts of the body.

diplopia: Visual perception of a single object as two objects.

diverticulectomy: Excision of a diverticulum.

diverticulitis: Inflammation of a diverticulum, or small pouch along the colonic border.

diverticulosis: Presence of diverticula, without inflammation.

diverticulum: Small outpouching along the border of the colon.

dropsy: Edema.

dumping syndrome: Syndrome occurring in a patient who has had part of his stomach removed, which occurs after eating and is characterized by nausea, weakness, sweating, palpitation, syncope and diarrhea.

duodenitis: Inflammation of the duodenum.

duodenotomy: Incision of the duodenum.

dysarthria: Imperfect articulation in speech.

dysentery: Inflammation of the intestines, especially the colon, with abdominal pain, tenesmus, and frequent bloody stools.

dyskinesia: Impairment of the power of voluntary movement.

dysmenorrhea: Painful menstruation.

dyspepsia: Indigestion.

dysphagia: Difficulty in swallowing.

dysphasia: Impairment of speech, caused by a central nervous system lesion.

dysplasia: Developmental abnormality.

dyspnea: Difficult breathing.

Dystonia: Disorder of muscle tension.

dystrophy: Defective nutrition, or degeneration, of a particular organ or tissue.

E

ecchymosis: Extravasation of blood beneath the skin.

eclampsia: Convulsions and coma, occurring in pregnancy and associated with proteinuria or edema, and hypertension.

eczema: An inflammatory skin disease marked by vesicles with scales and crusts, producing itching and burning.

edema: The presence of excessive fluid in intercellular tissue spaces.

elephantiasis: A chronic disease caused by nematode infestation and marked by lymphatic inflammation and obstruction, and hypertrophy, particularly of the scrotum and lower extremities.

embolectomy: Surgical removal of an embolus.

embolism: The sudden blocking of an artery or vein by a clot transported by the blood stream from one part of the body to the point of obstruction.

embryopathy: A morbid state caused by interference with normal embryonic development.

emesis: Vomiting.

emphysema: A disease characterized by overdistention of air spaces in the lung.

empyema: Accumulation of pus in a body cavity.

encephalitis: Inflammation of the brain.

encephalomalacia: Softening of the brain.

encephalomyelitis: Inflammation of the brain and spinal cord.

encephalopathy: Any disease of the brain.

endocarditis: Inflammation, infective or otherwise, of the endothelial lining of the heart.

endometriosis: A condition manifested by the occurrence, in various pelvic locations, of tissue behaving like that lining the uterus.

enteritis: Inflammation of the intestine, especially the small intestine.

enteropathy: Any intestinal disease.

enterostomy: Construction of a permanent intestinal opening through the abdominal wall.

enuresis: Involuntary discharge of urine, especially during sleep.

epididymitis: Inflammation of the epididymis (a part of the seminal duct).

epilepsy: A disease characterized by recurring excessive neuronal discharge. Symptoms may comprise recurrent loss of consciousness, involuntary excessive muscle movement and psychic, sensory and autonomic nervous system disturbances.

epistaxis: Nosebleed.

epithelioma: A malignant tumor composed of epithelial cells.

erysipelas: A contagious, infectious skin disease with erythema and edema of affected areas, and systemic symptoms.

erythema: Redness of the skin from capillary congestion, due to various causes.

erythroblastosis fetalis: Hemolytic disease of newborn caused by Rh antibodies from Rh negative mother entering circulation of Rh positive fetus.

erythrocytes: Red blood cells.

esophagitis: Inflammation of the esophagus.

esophagogastrectomy: Removal of the esophagus and stomach.

esophagogastrostomy: Surgical anastomosis between stomach and esophagus.

esophagojejunostomy: Surgical anastomosis between esophagus and jejunum.

eunuchoidism: Lack of masculine sex characteristics caused by deficiency of androgen secretion by the testes, with enunuch-like symptoms.

exacerbation: Worsening of a condition.

exanthem: An eruptive disease or fever.

exophthalmos: Abnormal protrusion of the eyeball.

exostosis: A bony growth projecting outward from a bone surface.

F

Fallot's tetralogy: A combination of congenital cardiac defects: pulmonary stenosis, interventricular septal defect, aortic dextroposition and right ventricular hypertrophy.

felon: A purulent infection or abscess involving the pulp of the distal phalanx of the finger.

fibrillation: Spontaneous local contraction of muscle fibers not under control of a motor nerve.

fibroma: A tumor composed principally of fibrous or mature connective tissue.

fibrosis: Formation of fibrous tissue.

fibrositis: Inflammatory hyperplasia of white fibrous tissue.

fissure: A cleft or groove, normal or abnormal.

fistula: An abnormal passage between two internal organs, or leading from an internal organ to body surface.

flatulence: Distention of the stomach or intestine with air or gas.

folliculitis: Inflammation of a follicle, usually a hair follicle.

fugue: A disturbance of consciousness during which purposeful acts which cannot be later remembered are performed.

furunculosis: Occurrence of a number of boils.

G

galactosemia: A congenital metabolic disorder with excess galactose in the blood.

ganglioneuroma: A tumor made up of ganglion cells.

gangrene: Local death of tissue, with putrefaction.

gargoylism: A congenital lipoid disturbance involving cartilage, bones, skin, brain, liver and spleen, and resulting in characteristic deformities.

gas gangrene: A condition often accompanying lacerated wounds and due to Clostridium bacteria.

gastrectomy: Surgical removal of the stomach.

gastritis: Inflammation of the stomach.

gastroduodenostomy: Surgical anastomosis between stomach and duodenum.

gastroenteritis: Inflammation of the stomach and intestines.

gastroesophageal: Enlarged and tortuous blood vessels of the stomach and esophagus.

gastrojejunostomy: Surgical anastomosis between stomach and jejunum.

gastrostomy: Surgical formation of an opening into the stomach.

genu valgum: Knock knee.

gigantism: Excessive size due to excessive secretion of pituitary growth hormone before puberty.

gingivitis: Inflammation involving the gums.

glaucoma: An eye disease characterized by increased intraocular pressure.

glioma: A tumor composed of connective tissue of the central nervous system.

globus hystericus: Subjective sensation of a lump in the throat.

glomangioma: A vascular tumor arising from conglomeration of small vessels.

glomerulonephritis: Inflammation of the renal glomeruli.

glossitis: Inflammation of the tongue.

glycosuria: Presence of glucose in the urine.

goiter: Enlargement of the thyroid gland, causing swelling in the front of the neck.

gonorrhea: A contagious catarrhal inflammation of genital mucous membranes caused by *Neisseria gonorrhoeae.*

gout: A disorder of purine metabolism and excess uric acid in the blood, marked by acute arthritis and formation of urate deposits in joint cartilage.

grand mal: One of the major clinical subdivisions of epilepsy.

granulocytopenia: Deficiency of granulocytes in the blood.

granuloma: A tumor or neoplasm consisting of granulation tissue.

Grave's disease: Exophthalmic goiter.

grippe: Influenza-like syndrome.

Guillain-Barré syndrome: Acute inflammatory disease of the peripheral nervous system.

gumma: A soft tumor whose constituent material resembles granulation tissue, usually occurring as a late complication of syphilis.

gynecomastia: Excessive development of the male mammary gland.

H

halitosis: Offensive breath.

hallucination: A sensory perception not resulting from objective reality.

Hansen's: Leprosy.

harelip: A congenital defect (cleft) in the upper lip.

hay fever: An acute allergic condition manifested by conjunctivitis, rhinorrhea, and occasionally asthmatic symptoms as a result of allergy to a particular pollen.

heartburn: A burning sensation in the esophagus.

heart failure, congestive: Impairment of the heart's ability to provide adequate blood flow to the tissues, with accumulations of fluid in the lung.

helminthiasis: Disease due to infestation with worms.

hemangioma: A tumor consisting of blood vessels.

hemarthrosis: Hemorrhage into a joint.

hematemesis: Vomiting blood.

hematocele: An effusion of blood into a cavity.

hematoma: A tumor containing effused blood.

hematuria: Blood in the urine.

hemiplegia: Paralysis of one side of the body.

hemoglobinuria: Presence of hemoglobin or its pigments in the urine.

hemolytic disorders: Blood disorders resulting from excessive destruction of red blood cells.

hemophilia: A hereditary disease occurring in males marked by delayed blood clotting.

hemopneumothorax: Effusion of blood accompanying accumulation of air in the chest cavity.

hemoptysis: Expectoration of blood or blood stained sputum.

hemorrhoids: A varicose dilatation of a vein of the hemorrhoidal plexus.

hemothorax: An accumulation of blood in the chest cavity.

hepatitis: Inflammation of the liver.

hepatomegaly: Enlargement of the liver.

hernia: Protrusion of part of an organ or tissue through an abnormal opening.

herpangina: An infectious viral disease with sudden onset of fever and vesicular or ulcerated lesions in the oropharynx.

herpes simplex: An acute viral disease with frequently febrile watery blisters on skin and mucous membranes (e.g., borders on the lips or the nares).

herpes zoster: Acute infection caused by varicella virus, marked by vesicular eruptions on the skin or mucous membranes and severe pain along the course of cutaneous nerves.

heterotopia: Displacement or misplacement of a part or an organ.

hiatal hernia: Upward protrusion of the stomach through the esophageal opening of the diaphragm.

hirsulism: Abnormal hairiness.

histoplasmosis: A fungal infection with *Histoplasma capsulatum,* generally of the lungs, which may also be accompanied by hepatomegaly and splenomegaly, fever, anemia, and leukopenia.

Hodgkin's disease: A generally fatal disease of the lymph glands.

hordeolum: A style of inflammation of the sebaceous glands of the eyelid.

hyaline membrane disease: Idiopathic respiratory distress of newborn.

hydrarthrosis: Accumulation of water in a joint cavity.

hydrocele: A collection of fluid, particularly in the testicle or along the spermatic cord.

hydrocephalus: A condition marked by abnormal intracranial accumulation of fluid with head enlargement, forehead prominence, brain atrophy, mental deficiency and convulsions.

hydrophobia: Rabies.

hygroma: A sac, cyst, or bursa distended by fluid.

hyperbilirubinemia: An excess of bilirubin in the blood.

hypercapnia: An excess of carbon dioxide in the blood.

hyperchloremia: An excess of chloride in the blood.

hyperchlorhydria: Excessive gastric secretion of hydrochloric acid.

hypercholesterolemia: An excess of cholesterol in the blood.

hyperemesis gravidarum: Pernicious vomiting of pregnancy.

hypergammaglobulinemia: An increased amount of gamma globulin in the blood.

hyperglobulinemia: Abnormally high globulin content of the blood.

hyperglycemia: Abnormally high glucose content of the blood.

hyperhidrosis: Excessive sweating.

hyperinsulinism: Excessive pancreatic secretion of insulin or insulin overdosage.

hyperkalemia: An excess of potassium in the blood.

hyperkeratosis: Hypertrophy of the horny layer of the skin.

hyperlipemia: An excess of fat in the blood.

hypernatremia: An excess of sodium in the blood.

hyperopia: Farsightedness.

hyperparathyroidism: Excessive parathyroid activity resulting in disturbances in calcium and phosphorus metabolism.

hyperpituitarism: A condition due to pathologically high activity of secretions of the pituitary gland.

hyperplasia: Abnormal numerical increase in normal cells in normal arrangement in tissue.

hypertension: Abnormally high blood pressure.

hyperthyroidism: Excessive functional activity of the thyroid gland.

hypertrophy: Enlargement of an organ or part resulting from enlargement of its constituent cells.

hyperuricemia: Excess of uric acid in the blood.

hyperventilation: A condition characterized by abnormally prolonged, rapid, deep breathing.

hypoadrenocorticism: Abnormally low secretion of hormones of the adrenal cortex.

hypochondriasis: Morbid anxiety about one's health, usually associated with depression.

hypoglycemia: An abnormally low glucose content of the blood.

hypogonadism: A condition of abnormally decreased functional activity of the gonads.

hypoparathyroidism: A condition produced by deficient parathyroid hormone or by removal of the parathyroids.

hypoproteinemia: A deficiency of protein in the blood.

hypoprothrombinemia: A deficiency of prothrombin in the blood.

hypotension: Lowered blood pressure; termed orthostatic if caused by change from supine to erect position.

hypothyroidism: A deficiency of thyroid activity.

hysterectomy: Excision of the uterus.

I

ichthyosis: A disease caused by hypertrophy of the horny layer of the skin and marked by dryness, scaliness and roughness.

icterus: Jaundice.

ileitis: Inflammation of the ileum.

ileocolitis: Inflammation of the ileum and colon.

ileojejunitis: Inflammation of the ileum and jejunum.

ileostomy: Opening of the ileum onto the abdominal wall.

impetigo: A bacterial, inflammatory, pustular skin disease.

incontinence: Involuntary discharge of urine or feces.

induration: Hardness.

infarct: An area of tissue necrosis resulting from circulatory obstruction.

infection: Invasion of the body by pathogenic microorganisms and the resulting tissue reaction to their presence and to their toxins.

infertility: Sterility.

influenza: An acute infectious, epidemic, viral disease with fever, nasal catarrh, neuralgic and muscular pains and gastrointestinal disturbance.

insomnia: Inability to sleep.

intertrigo: Chafing of the skin on opposed surfaces; and the resulting erythema or eczema.

iridocyclitis: Inflammation of the iris and ciliary body.

iritis: Inflammation of the iris.

ischemia: Local deficiency of blood, generally due to vascular contraction.

J

Jacksonian seizure: A form of epilepsy with involuntary clonic motion or sensation.

jaundice: A syndrome marked by hyperbilirubinemia and deposition of biliary pigment in the skin and mucous membranes.

jejunojejunostomy: Surgical anastomosis between two sections of the jejunum.

jejunostomy: Surgical opening of the jejunum onto the abdominal wall.

K

keloid: A condition caused by abnormal healing in a scar with an overgrowth of dense connective tissue.

keratitis: Inflammation of the cornea.

keratoconjunctivitis: Inflammation of the cornea and conjunctiva.

keratoconus: A noninflammatory central protrusion of the cornea.

keratomalacia: Softening of the cornea.

keratosis: A horny growth, as a wart.

kyphosis: Abnormal curvature and increased dorsal prominence of the vertebral column.

L

Laennec's cirrhosis: Atrophic cirrhosis of the liver with scarring.

laparotomy: Surgical incision into the abdominal cavity and subsequent examination.

laryngectomy: Extirpation of the larynx.

laryngitis: Inflammation of the larynx.

laryngostenosis: Narrowing or stricture of the larynx.

leiomyosarcoma: A malignant tumor derived from muscle elements.

leishmaniasis: Infection caused by Leishmania parasites transmitted by biting flies.

leukemia: A fatal disease of hematopoietic organs, with marked rise in number of blood leukocytes and enlargement and proliferation of lymphoid tissue of spleen, lymphatic glands, and bone marrow.

leukocytes: White blood cells.

leukocytosis: Increase in the number of blood leukocytes.

leukoderma: Defective pigmentation of skin in patches.

leukopenia: Reduction in the number of white cells in the blood.

leukoplakia: A disease marked by development of white, thickened patches on mucous membranes of the cheeks, gums, or tongue.

leukorrhea: A whitish, viscid vaginal discharge.

lipodystrophy: A disorder of fat metabolism with disappearance of subcutaneous fat.

lipoidosis: A condition in which lipid material is deposited in various organs.

lipoma: A tumor composed of fatty material and cells.

liposarcoma: A malignant tumor arising in fatty tissue.

lithiasis: Formation of calculi and concretions.

lithotomy: Removal of calculus by surgical incision.

lobectomy: Excision of a lobe, as in the lung.

lockjaw: Tetanus.

lordosis: Spinal curvature with forward convexity.

luxation: Dislocation.

lymphadenitis: Inflammation of lymph glands.

lymphadenopathy: Disease of lymph glands.

lymphangiectasis: Dilatation of the lymphatic vessels.

lymphangioma: A dilated or varicose condition or tumor of the lymphatics.

lymphangitis: Inflammation of a lymphatic vessel.

lymphedema: Swelling of subcutaneous tissues from excessive lymph fluid.

lymphocytosis: Excess number of lymphocytes in the blood.

lympho-epithelioma: A tumor originating in modified epithelium overlying lymphoid nasopharyngeal tissue.

M

macrocephalia: Abnormal size of the head.

malabsorption syndrome: A group of symptoms characterized by faulty absorption of various foodstuffs and vitamins.

malaria: Infectious febrile disease caused by Piasmodium protozoa and transmitted by the bite of infected Anopheles mosquitoes.

Marie-Strümpell disease: Rheumatoid spondylitis; a disease with pain, stiffness, and rigidity of the vertebral column.

mastectomy: Surgical removal of the breast.

mastitis: Inflammation of the breast or mammary gland.

mastoiditis: Inflammation of the cells and cavity of the mastoid bone.

measles: Rubeola, a contagious viral disease with cough, fever, coryza and catarrhal symptoms associated with an eruption and subsequent desquamation.

mediastinopericarditis: Inflammation of the mediastinum and the pericardium.

melanoma: A malignant tumor derived from melanophores, often highly pigmented with melanin.

menarche: Onset of menstrual function in a young female.

Meniere's syndrome: Deafness, tinnitus and dizziness, occurring in association with nonsuppurative disease of the labyrinth of the ear.

meningioma: A tumor of the meninges.

meningitis: Inflammation of the meninges, the three membranes that envelop the brain and spinal cord.

meningomyelitis: Inflammation of the spinal cord and its membranes.

menopause: The physiologic cessation of menstruation; usually in fourth or fifth decade of life.

menorrhagia: Excessive uterine bleeding occurring at regular intervals, the duration of flow being longer and/or heavier than usual.

metaplasia: Change in the type of adult cells in a tissue to an abnormal form for that tissue.

metastasis: Transfer of disease to a new focus by blood or lymph vessels, e.g., cancer.

metritis: Inflammation of the uterus.

metrorrhagia: Uterine bleeding not related to menstrual period.

microcephaly: Abnormally small size of the head.

microglossia: Abnormally small tongue.

micrognathia: An abnormally small lower jaw, with recession of the chin.

microstomia: Congenitally small mouth.

migraine: Periodic severe vascular headaches, often one sided, usually accompanied by nausea and visual disturbances.

miliaria: A skin condition with cutaneous changes associated with sweat retention and abnormal release of sweat at different levels in the skin; prickly heat.

miosis: Exaggerated contraction of the pupil.

mitral stenosis: Narrowing of the left atrioventricular orifice; usually as the result of rheumatic fever.

moniliasis: A fungal infection caused by *Monilia (Candida);* candidiasis.

mucoviscidosis: Cystic fibrosis of the pancreas; disease marked by abnormally viscous mucous secretions and frequent lung infections.

multiple sclerosis: Hardening throughout areas of the brain or spinal cord, with symptoms including weakness, incoordination, ataxia and labile emotions.

mumps: Parotitis; a contagious, febrile, viral disease with swelling of the parotid gland or sometimes the pancreas, ovaries or testicles.

murmur, cardiac: An abnormal sound originating in the heart.

muscular dystrophy: Progressive wasting of the muscles.

myalgia: Pain in a muscle or muscles.

myasthenia gravis: A syndrome of muscular fatigue and exhaustion, but without atrophy or sensory disturbance.

mydriasis: Abnormal dilation of the pupil of the eye.

myelitis: Inflammation of the spinal cord.

myleofibrosis: Replacement of marrow of the bone by fibrous tissue.

myeloma: A tumor made up of a peculiar cell called a plasma cell involving the bone marrow.

myocardial infarction: Formation of an infarct (necrotic area) in heart muscle resulting from interruption of the blood supply to the area, as in coronary thrombosis.

myocarditis: Inflammation of the muscular layer of the heart.

myocardium: Heart muscle.

myoma: A tumor derived from muscular components.

myopia: Nearsightedness. •

myositis: Inflammation of a muscle, commonly voluntary muscle.

myotonia: Tonic muscular spasm.

myxedema: A disorder caused by thyroid hormone deficiency marked by a low metabolic rate, a sallow, puffy appearance and other symptoms.

myxoma: Tumor of connective or mucous tissue.

N

nematodiasis: Infestation by nematode or roundworm parasites.

neoplasm: Any new, abnormal growth, usually referring to a tumor.

nephritis: Inflammation of the kidney.

nephrolithiasis: Presence of renal calculi (kidney stones).

nephroptosis: Prolapse or downward displacement of the kidney.

nephrosclerosis: Hardening of the blood vessels of the kidney.

nephrosis: Nephrotic syndrome.

nephrotic syndrome: Condition marked by edema, protein in the urine, blood-albumin deficiency, and infections.

neuralgia: Paroxysmal, intense pain along the course of a nerve not associated with structural changes in the nerve.

neuritis: Inflammation of a nerve with pain, hypersensitivity, numbness or burning, and loss of reflexes.

neuroblastoma: A malignant tumor of the nervous system.

neurocirculatory asthenia: Condition marked by breathlessness, giddiness, fatigue, chest pain and palpitation; called also cardiac neurosis, anxiety neurosis, neurasthenia.

neurodermatitis: Skin disorder marked by a chronic itching, lichenoid eruption associated with nervousness.

neuroma: A tumor of the nervous system made up of nerve cells and fibers.

neuromyositis: Muscle inflammation complicated by inflammation of a nerve.

neuropathy: Disease of the nervous system.

nevus: A circumscribed area of pigmentation or vascularization on the skin, as a birthmark.

nocturia: Frequent urination at night.

nodule: A small node or solid protuberance detectable by touch.

nystagmus: Involuntarily rapid movement of the eyeballs.

O

oligomenorrhea: Infrequent or scanty menstruation.

oligospermia: Deficiency of spermatozoa in semen.

oliguria: Excretion of a diminished amount of urine.

omphalitis: Inflammation of the umbilicus.

onychia: Inflammation of the nail.

onychomycosis: A fungal disease of the nails of the fingers and toes.

oophorectomy: Removal of an ovary or ovaries.

ophthalmoplegia: Paralysis of the eye muscles.

opisthotonos: Tetanic spasm of the back muscles in which the head and lower limbs are bent backward and the trunk bowed forward.

orchidectomy: Removal of one or both testicles.

orchiopexy: Surgical fixation of an undescended testicle in the scrotum.

orchitis: Inflammation of a testis with pain, swelling and a feeling of weight.

orthopnea: Inability to breathe easily other than with the head elevated.

osteitis: Inflammation of a bone.

osteoarthritis: Chronic degenerative joint disease with bony deformity.

osteochondritis: Inflammation of bone and cartilage.

osteochondroma: A tumor made of bone and cartilage.

osteodystrophy: Defective bone formation.

osteoma: A tumor containing bone tissue.

osteomalacia: Softening of the bones, leading to deformities, due to insufficient calcification.

osteomyelitis: Inflammation of bone caused by an infectious organism.

osteoporosis: Increased porosity of the bone resulting in fragility.

otitis: Inflammation of the ear.

otorrhagia: Discharge of blood from the ear.

P

palsy: Paralysis.

pancreatectomy: Removal of all or part of the pancreas.

pancreaticoduodenostomy: Surgical joining of the pancreatic duct into the duodenum.

pancreaticojejunostomy: Surgical joining of the pancreatic duct into the jejunum.

pancreatitis: Inflammation of the pancreas, with abdominal pain and tenderness, distention of abdomen and vomiting.

papilledema: Edema of the head of the optic nerve.

papillitis: Inflammation of the optic nerve.

papilloma: A benign epithelial tumor, as a wart.

paralysis agitans: Parkinson's disease.

parametritis: Inflammation of the tissue surrounding the uterus.

paraplegia: Paralysis of the lower limbs.

paresthesia: An abnormal sensation of burning, prickling, tingling or crawling of the skin.

Parkinson's disease: Paralysis agitans; characterized by progressive tremor, mask-like face, slowing of movements and stumbling gait.

paronychia: Inflammation of tissue surrounding a fingernail.

parotitis: Inflammation of the parotid glands; mumps.

pediculosis: Infestation with lice.

peptic ulcer: An ulcer of the mucous membrane of the esophagus, stomach or duodenum.

periarteritis: Inflammation of the outside layers of an artery and of surrounding tissues.

pericarditis: Inflammation of the membrane enveloping the heart.

periostitis: Inflammation of the membrane enclosing the surface of bones.

peritonitis: Inflammation of the membrane which lines the interior of the abdominal cavity and surrounds the contained viscera.

pertussis: Whooping cough.

petechiae: Small, nonraised, purplish-red spots caused by intradermal hemorrhage.

phenylketonuria: Congenital defective metabolism of the amino acid, phenylalanine, often associated with mental defects.

pheochromocytoma: Tumor of the adrenal gland and other tissues producing adrenalin, associated with paroxysmal hypertension.

phimosis: Tightness of the foreskin of the penis.

phlebitis: (Thrombophlebitis) Inflammation of a vein marked by formation of a clot of coagulated blood, edema, and pain.

phlebosclerosis: Hardening of a vein, especially the inner coats.

phlebothrombosis: Formation of a clot in a vein; venous thrombosis.

phocomelia: A developmental defect in which the hands or feet are attached to the trunk by a small, irregular bone; seal limbs.

photophobia: Exaggerated intolerance to light.

pityriasis rosea: Noninfectious skin condition characterized by a maculopapular rash.

pleurisy: Inflammation of the membrane enveloping the lung.

plumbism: Lead poisoning.

pneumoconiosis: Chronic inflammation of the lungs from inhaling dust.

pneumonectomy: Surgical removal of a lung.

pneumonia: Inflammation of the lungs.

pneumonitis: Localized inflammation of the lungs.

pneumopericardium: The presence of air in the sac encasing the heart.

pneumothorax: Accumulation of air in the cavity between the lung and the chest wall.

pollenosis: Hay fever.

polyarteritis: Simultaneous inflammation of several arteries.

polycythemia: Condition marked by increased numbers of red corpuscles in the blood.

polydactyly: Having more than the normal number of fingers or toes.

polydipsia: Excessive thirst.

polymyositis: Inflammation of many muscles at the same time.

polyneuritis: Simultaneous inflammation of many nerves; multiple peripheral neuritis.

polyp: Nodular growth of neoplastic or other tissue found usually on mucous membranes.

polyphagia: Excessive, voracious eating.

polyuria: Voiding of excessive quantities of urine.

priapism: Persistent erection of the penis, usually without sexual desire.

proctitis: Inflammation of the rectum.

progeria: Premature senility or old age.

prognathism: Projecting jaw.

prostatectomy: Surgical removal of all or part of the prostate gland.

pruritus: Itching.

psoriasis: A chronic skin disease marked by the formation of scaly red patches.

ptosis: Prolapse or falling down of an organ, especially paralytic drooping of the upper eyelid.

purpura: A condition in which hemorrhages occur in the skin.

pyarthrosis: Suppuration within a joint cavity.

pyelitis: Inflammation of the pelvis of the kidney.

pyelonephritis: Inflammation of the kidney and its pelvis.

pyloric stenosis: Obstruction of the opening between the stomach and the duodenum.

pyloroplasty: An operation to repair and enlarge the opening between stomach and duodenum.

pyoderma: Any pus-producing skin disease.

pyonephrosis: Accumulation of pus in the kidney.

pyrexia: Fever.

pyrosis: Heartburn; burning sensation in the stomach.

pyuria: Presence of pus in the urine.

R

rabies: Hydrophobia. A viral disease of animals communicated to man by the bite of an infected animal.

rales: Abnormal respiratory sound.

Raynaud's disease: A vascular disorder of the extremities, especially fingers and toes with attacks of pallor and cyanosis, due to cold or emotion.

rectocele: Protrusion of the rectum into the vagina.

retinitis: Inflammation of the retina with impaired vision, edema and exudation into the retina.

rheumatic fever: A febrile disease associated with previous hemolytic streptococcal infection, marked by joint pain and a predilection to heart damage.

rheumatic heart disease: A manifestation of rheumatic fever consisting of inflammatory changes and damaged heart valves.

rhinitis: Inflammation of the mucous membrane of the nose.

rhinorrhea: Free drainage of a thin mucous from the nose.

rickets: A bone disease of children caused by vitamin-D deficiency.

rubella: German measles.

rubeola: Measles.

S

St. Vitus' dance Chorea: A disorder of the nervous system marked by involuntary action of the muscles of the face and extremities.

salmonellosis: Infection with Salmonellae, marked by violent diarrhea.

salpingitis: Inflammation of the fallopian tube or eustachian tube.

scabies: A contagious skin disease marked by intense itching, due to the itch mite.

scarlet fever: An acute contagious streptococcal infection marked by high fever and rash.

sciatica: Pain along the course of the sciatic nerve, marked by paresthesia, tenderness, and wasting of affected muscles.

scleroderma: A systemic disease marked by hardening of connective tissue.

sclerosis: Induration or hardening.

scoliosis: Lateral curvature of the spine.

scurvy: Vitamin-C deficiency marked by weakness, anemia, spongy gums and hemorrhage, and rash.

seborrhea: Sebaceous gland disorder marked by excessive discharge of sebum.

septicemia: Blood poisoning; presence in the blood of bacterial toxins.

serum sickness: An anaphylactic reaction following serum therapy.

shigellosis: Bacillary dysentery caused by Shigella organisms.

shingles: Herpes zoster.

silicosis: Pneumoconiosis due to the inhalation of silica particles.

singuitus: A hiccup.

sinusitis: Inflammation of a sinus.

spasm: A sudden, violent, involuntary contraction of a muscle or a group of muscles with pain and disturbance of function.

sphincterotomy: The cutting of a sphincter.

splanchnicectomy: Excision of the greater splanchnic nerve; frequently combined with sympathectomy to relieve essential hypertension.

splenectomy: Removal of the spleen.

splenomegaly: Enlargement of the spleen.

spondylitis: Inflammation of the vertebrae.

status asthmaticus: Asthmatic shock; a prolonged intense episode of asthma.

stenosis: Narrowing of a duct or canal.

stomatitis: Inflammation of the oral mucosa.

stricture: The abnormal narrowing of a canal, duct, or passage.

stridor: A harsh, high-pitched respiratory sound.

stye: Hordeolum; inflammation of the sebaceous glands of the eyelids.

subluxation: Incomplete dislocation.

suppuration: Formation and discharge of pus.

sympathectomy: Surgical interruption of some portion of the sympathetic nervous pathways.

syncope: Fainting.

syndactyly: Webbing of fingers or toes.

syndrome: A group of symptoms.

syphilis: A contagious veneral disease caused by *Treponema pallidum.*

T

tachycardia: Excessively rapid heart action.

tachypnea: Excessively rapid, shallow breathing.

talanglectasia: Dilatation of capillaries in the skin.

tenesmus: Extreme lower abdominal cramping with urgency to defecate.

tenosynovitis: Inflammation of a tendon sheath.

tetanus: Lockjaw, a disease caused by a toxin elaborated by *Clostridium tetani,* marked by tonic spasm of the masseter muscles, causing trismus ("lockjaw"), and spasms of the back muscles producing opisthotonos.

tetany: A condition marked by intermittent, painful tonic spasm of the muscles.

thoracotomy: Surgical incision into the chest cavity.

thromboanglitis obliterans: Disease of the blood vessels of the extremities marked by tissue ischemia and gangrene; Buerger's disease.

thrombocytopenia: Decrease in the number of blood platelets.

thromboendarterectomy: Removal of an obstructing blood clot together with the inner lining of an obstructed artery.

thrombophlebitis: Inflammation of a vein with formation of a blood clot.

thrombosis: The formation, development or presence of a blood clot in the heart or a blood vessel.

thrush: A fungal disease caused by *Candida albicans* marked by whitish spots in the mouth, fever, and gastrointestinal irritation.

thymectomy: Removal of the thymus.

thyroidectomy: Surgical removal of the thyroid.

thyroiditis: Inflammation of the thyroid gland.

tic: A twitching, especially of the face.

tic douloureux: Trigeminal neuralgia.

tinea capitis: Fungal infection of the scalp.

tinnitus: A ringing, roaring or hissing noise in the ears.

torticollis: Wryneck; twisting of the neck and unnatural position of the head.

toxemia: A poisonous intoxication due to bacterial or cellular toxins.

tracheostomy: Surgical opening into the trachea through the neck for insertion of a tube to facilitate breathing.

trachoma: A viral infection of the eyelids affecting the conjunctiva and cornea.

trichinosis: A disease from eating undercooked pork containing *Trichinella spiralis.*

trigeminal neuralgia: Severe facial pain in the area of the trigeminal nerve.

trismus: Lockjaw; spasm of the masticatory muscles.

tuberculosis: An infectious disease caused by *Mycobacterium tuberculosis* which may affect any organ or tissue of the body.

tularemia: A disease of rodents, resembling plague, which is transmitted to man by insect bites or handling infected animals.

tumor: A swelling or abnormal enlargement; a new tissue growth which develops independently and has no physiologic use.

tympanites: Distention of the abdomen from an accumulation of gas in the intestine or peritoneal cavity.

typhoid fever: An infection due to *Salmonella typhosa.*

typhus: A rickettsial infection transmitted to man by lice and rat fleas, marked by malaise, headache, fever, and spotty eruptions.

U

ulcer: Surface disintegration of cutaneous or mucous tissue.

ulcerative colitis: Chronic ulceration in the colon.

uremia: The retention of urinary constituents in the blood and the resulting toxic condition resulting from their deficient excretion.

ureterostomy: Surgical formation of a permanent canal through which a ureter can discharge, generally via the abdominal wall.

urethritis: Inflammation of the urethra.

urethrotomy: Surgical repair of urethral stricture.

urolithiasis: The formation of urinary calculi and the resulting disease condition.

urticaria: An allergic vascular skin reaction marked by edema and severe itching.

V

vaginitis: Inflammation of the vagina marked by pain and discharge.

valvulitis: Inflammation of a valve, especially of the heart.

varicella: Chickenpox.

varices: Enlarged and tortuous veins, arteries or lymph vessels.

varicose veins: Distended, knotted and tortuous veins, especially in the lower extremities.

variola: Smallpox.

vasospasm: Spasm of the blood vessels.

venesection: Phlebotomy, or opening of a vein for blood-letting.

verruca: Wart.

vertigo: Spinning sensation.

Vincent's angina: Ulceration of mucous membranes of gums, mouth and throat.

viremia: Presence of virus in the blood.

virilism: Masculinity; the development of masculine traits in the female.

vitiligo: Leukoderma; skin disease marked by smooth, nonpigmented patches.

volvulus: Intestinal obstruction from twisting of the bowel upon itself.

vulvovaginitis: Simultaneous inflammation of the vulva and vagina.

W

wart: Localized, benign hypertrophy of the skin.

wen: Sebaceous cyst.

X

xanthochromia: Yellowish discoloration of the skin or spinal fluid.

xanthoma: A flat or slightly raised patch or nodule of new skin growth of a yellowish color.

xeroderma: Abnormal dryness of the skin.

xerophthalmia: Dry and lusterless condition of the eyeball due to vitamin-A deficiency.

xerostomia: Dryness of the mouth.

Y

yaws: A nonvenereal treponemal infection with raspberry-like lesions of the skin.

yellow fever: An acute viral disease transmitted by mosquitoes and marked by fever, jaundice and albuminuria.

Z

zona: Herpes zoster.

English-Spanish Language Guide for Nurses (phonetic pronunciation)*

Good morning.
Buenos dias (*bway*-nos *dee*-us).

Good afternoon.
Buenas tardes (*bway*-nus *tar*-days).

Good evening.
Buenas noches (*bway*-nus *no*-chess).

Please.
Por favor (pore fah-*vor*).

Write your name.
Escriba su nombre (ess-*skree*-bah soo *nohm*-bray).

Are you feeling better?
¿Se siente mejor? (say see-*yen*-tay may-*hor*).

Do you have pain?
¿Tiene usted dolor? (tea-*yeh*-nay oo-*stead* doe-*lore*).

Much pain?
¿Mucho dolor? (*moo*-choe doe-lore).

Tell me where it hurts.
Digame donde le duele (*dee* gah-may don-day lay *dwel*-ay).

Sit up.
Incorporese (een-core-*poe*-ray-say).
Lie down.
Acuestese (ah-*kwess*-teh-say).

Roll over.
Virese (*vee*-ray-seh).

Try to lie quietly.
Trate de descansar acostado (*trah*-tay day *dess*-can-sar ah-cos-*tah*-doe).

Try to sleep.
Trate de dormir (*trah*-tay day dor-*meer*).

You must not sit up.
Usted no debe sentarse (oo-*stead* no *day*-bay sen-tar-say).

Take your medicine.
Tome la medicina (*toe*-may lah may-dee-*see*-nah).

Try to drink.
Trate de beber (*trah*-tay day bay-*bair*).

You must not drink.
Usted no debe beber (oo-*stead* no *day*-bay bay-*bair*).

Try to eat.
Trate de comer (*trah*-tay day coh-*mair*).

You must not eat.
Usted no debe comer (oo-*stead* no *day*-bay coh-*mair*).

I am going to give you a bath.
Voy a darle un bano (voy ah *dahr*-lay un *bah*-noh).

I am going to make your bed.
Voy a hacerle la cama (voy ah ah-*sair*-lay lah *cah*-mah).

Have you urinated?
¿Ha orinado? (ah oh-ree-*nah*-doe).

You must collect your urine in here.
Tiene usted que recoger su orina aqui (tea-yeh-*nay* oo-*stead* kay ray-coe-*gair* soo oh-*ree*-neh ah-*key*).

Have you had a bowel movement?
¿Ha evacuado? (ah eh-vah-*kwah*-doe).

Are you constipated?
¿Tiene estrenimiento? (tea-*yeh*-nay ess-tray-nee-*meeyen*-toe).

Do you have diarrhea?
¿Tiene diarrea? (tea-*yeh*-nay dee-ah-*rhee*-ah).

You must collect your stools in here.
Tiene usted que recoger sus heces aqui (tea-*yeh*-nay oo-*stead* kay ray-coe-*gair* soos *eh*-sis ah-*key*).

I am going to take your blood pressure.
Voy a tomarle la presion arterial (voy ah toh-*mar*-lay lah pray-*seeohn* ar-tay-rhee-ahl).

I am going to give you an injection.
Voy a ponerle una inyeccion (voy ah poh-*nair*-lay *oo*-nah een-yeck-see-*ohn*).

It won't hurt.
No le dolera (noh lay doh-lay-*rah*).

I am going to change your dressing.
Voy a cambiarle el vendaje (voy ah cam-bee-*ar*-lay el ven-*dah*-hey).

*Source: *Breaking the Language Barrier,* Warner-Chilcott, Morris Plains, N.J.

Breathe deeply.
Respire profundamente (reh-*spee*-ray pro-foon-deh-*men*-tay).

Cough.
Tosa (*toe*-sah).

You must not smoke.
Usted no debe fumar (oo-*stead* no *day*-bay foo-*mar*).

I am going to take some blood from your arm.
Voy a sacarle sangre del brazo (voy ah sah-*car*-lay *sahn*-gray del *brah*-zoh).

You are going to x-ray.
Van a llevarlo a la sala de radiografia (vahn ah yea-*vahr*-loh ah lah *sah*-lah day rah-deeoh-grah-*feeah*).

You are going to the operating room.
Van a llevarlo a la sala de operaciones (vahn ah yea-*vahr*-loh ah lah *sah*-lah day oh-pay-rah-*seeoh*-nais).

Please sign this permit for an operation.
Por favor firme este permiso para una operacion (pore fah-*vor* *fear*-may *ess*-tay peir-*mee*-soh *pah*-rah oo-nah oh-pay-rah-see-*ohn*).

Health and Medical Museums*

Academy of Medicine of New Jersey Historical Museum, Bloomfield, N.J. 07003

Alexander Graham Bell National Historic Park, Baddeck, N.S. CAN.

American Institute of Radiology, Chicago, IL. 60606

American Psychiatric Museum Association, Washington, D.C. 20009

Archives and Company Museum-Eli Lilly And Company, Indianapolis, IN. 46206

Armed Forces Medical Museum, Washington, D.C. 20306

Cherokee Mental Health Institute, Cherokee, IA. 51012

Cleveland Health Education Museum, Cleveland, OH. 44106

The Country Doctor Museum, Bailey, N.C. 28707

Crawford W. E. Bong Medical Museum, Jefferson, GA. 30549

Cyclorama of Life, Department of Health Education, Philadelphia, PA. 19151

Dallas Health And Science Museum, Dallas, TX 75226

The Discovery Center, Amarillo Foundation For Health & Science Education, Inc., Amarillo, TX. 79106

Dr. John Harris Dental Museum, Columbus, OH 43215

Fort Winnebago Surgeons Quarters, Portage, WI. 53901

Heritage House Museum, Weeping Water, NV. 68463

Historic Sites Section, Parks And Historic Sites Department of Natural Resources, Atlanta, GA. 30334

Historical Dental Museum, Temple University School of Dentistry, Philadelphia, PA. 19140

Howard Dittrick Museum of Historical Medicine, Cleveland, OH. 44106

Hugh Mercer Apothecary Shop, Fredericksburg, VA. 22401

Kansas Health Museum, Halstead, KS. 67056

Kilmer Museum of Surgical Products, New Brunswick, N.J. 08901

Library of Los Angeles County Medical Assn., Los Angeles, CA. 90057

Mayo Medical Museum, Rochester, MN. 55901

Museum & Archives, The Menninger Foundation, Topeka, KS. 66601

Museum of Dentistry, Orange, CA. 92668

Museum of Electricity In Life At Medtronic, Minneapolis, MN. 55430

Museum of Medical Progress-Stovall Hall of Health, Prairie du Chien, WI. 53821

Museum of Medical Science, Houston, TX. 77004

Museum of Pharmacy At Brooklyn College of Pharmacy, Brooklyn, N.Y. 11216

Mutter Museum, College of Physicians of Philadelphia, Philadelphia, PA. 19103

Old Fort Howard Hospital, Green Bay, WI. 54303

Pathology Museum of The University of Maryland Medical School, Baltimore, MD. 21201

Rank Drug Store Museum, Virginia City, MT. 59755

Robert Crown Center For Health Education, Hinsdale, IL. 60521

Rutgers University, Serological Museum, New Brunswick, N.J. 08903

St. Joseph State Hospital Psychiatric Museum, St. Joseph, MO. 64502

St. Louis Medical Museum And National Museum of Medical Quackery, St. Louis, MO. 63108

Stabler-Leadbeater Apothecary, Alexandria, VA. 22314

Toledo Museum of Health And Natural History, Toledo, OH, 43609

Trent Collection In The History of Medicine, Durham, N.C. 27710

University of Washington School of Medicine, Seattle, WA. 98195

Washington State Board of Pharmacy, Olympia, WA. 98504

Wood Library-Museum of Anesthesiology, Park Ridge, IL. 60068

Yale Medical Library, New Haven, CT. 06510

---

*Source: *Official Museum Directory, 1977*, ed. American Association of Museums (National Register Publishing Co., Inc.).

INDEX